KU-489-463

Pathology of Domestic Animals

FOURTH EDITION Volume 2

Pathology of Domestic Animals

FOURTH EDITION Volume 2

EDITED BY

K. V. F. JUBB
School of Veterinary Science
University of Melbourne
Victoria, Australia

PETER C. KENNEDY
Department of Pathology
School of Veterinary Medicine
University of California, Davis
Davis, California, USA

NIGEL PALMER
Veterinary Laboratory Services
Ontario Ministry of Agriculture and Food
Guelph, Ontario, Canada

ACADEMIC PRESS, INC.
Harcourt Brace Jovanovich, Publishers
San Diego New York Boston
London Sydney Tokyo Toronto

This book is printed on acid-free paper. ♾

Academic Press, Inc.
1250 Sixth Avenue, San Diego, California 92101-4311

United Kingdom Edition published by
Academic Press Limited
24–28 Oval Road, London NW1 7DX

Library of Congress Cataloging-in-Publication Data

Jubb, K. V. F.
Pathology of domestic animals / K.V.F. Jubb, P.C. Kennedy, N.C. Palmer. – 4th ed.
p. cm.
Includes bibliographical references and index.
ISBN 0-12-391606-2 vol. 2
1. Veterinary pathology. I. Kennedy, Peter C. (Peter Carleton), date. II. Palmer, Nigel. III. Title.
SF769.J82 1992
636.089'607–dc20 92-12261
CIP

PRINTED IN THE UNITED STATES OF AMERICA
92 93 94 95 96 97 EB 9 8 7 6 5 4 3 2 1

Contents

CHAPTER 2

The Liver and Biliary System

W. ROGER KELLY

CHAPTER 3

The Pancreas

K. V. F. JUBB

CHAPTER 4

The Peritoneum and Retroperitoneum

IAN K. BARKER

CHAPTER 5

The Urinary System

M. GRANT MAXIE AND WITH A CONTRIBUTION BY JOHN F. PRESCOTT

Chapter 6

The Respiratory System

D. L. DUNGWORTH

Contents of Other Volumes

Volume 1

Volume 3

Contributors

Volume 1

Thomas J. Hulland, Department of Pathology, Ontario Veterinary College, University of Guelph, Guelph, Ontario, Canada N1G 2W1.

C. R. Huxtable, School of Veterinary Studies, Murdoch University, Murdoch, Western Australia, Australia 6150.

K. V. F. Jubb, School of Veterinary Science, University of Melbourne, Werribee, Victoria, Australia 3030.

Nigel Palmer, Veterinary Laboratory Services, Ontario Ministry of Agriculture and Food, Guelph, Ontario, Canada N1H 6R8.

Danny W. Scott, Department of Clinical Sciences, New York State College of Veterinary Medicine, Cornell University, Ithaca, New York, USA 14853-6401.

Brian P. Wilcock, Department of Pathology, Ontario Veterinary College, University of Guelph, Guelph, Ontario, Canada N1G 2W1.

Julie A. Yager, Department of Pathology, Ontario Veterinary College, University of Guelph, Guelph, Ontario, Canada N1G 2W1.

Volume 2

Ian K. Barker, Department of Pathology, Ontario Veterinary College, University of Guelph, Guelph, Ontario, Canada N1G 2W1.

D. L. Dungworth, Department of Pathology, School of Veterinary Medicine, University of California, Davis, California, USA 95616.

K. V. F. Jubb, School of Veterinary Science, University of Melbourne, Werribee, Victoria, Australia 3030.

W. Roger Kelly, Department of Veterinary Pathology, University of Queensland, St. Lucia, Brisbane, Queensland, Australia 4072.

M. Grant Maxie, Veterinary Laboratory Services, Ontario Ministry of Agriculture and Food, Guelph, Ontario, Canada N1H 6R8.

Nigel Palmer, Veterinary Laboratory Services, Ontario Ministry of Agriculture and Food, Guelph, Ontario, Canada N1H 6R8.

John F. Prescott, Department of Veterinary Microbiology and Immunology, Ontario Veterinary College, University of Guelph, Guelph, Ontario, Canada N1G 2W1.

A. A. van Dreumel, Veterinary Laboratory Services, Ontario Ministry of Agriculture and Food, Guelph, Ontario, Canada N1H 6R8.

Volume 3

Charles C. Capen, Department of Veterinary Pathology, The Ohio State University, Columbus, Ohio, USA 43210-1093.

Peter C. Kennedy, Department of Pathology, School of Veterinary Medicine, University of California, Davis, California, USA 95616.

P. W. Ladds, Graduate School of Tropical Veterinary Science and Agriculture, James Cook University, Townsville, Queensland, Australia 4811.

M. Grant Maxie, Veterinary Laboratory Services, Ontario Ministry of Agriculture and Food, Guelph, Ontario, Canada N1H 6R8.

Richard B. Miller, Department of Pathology, Ontario Veterinary College, University of Guelph, Guelph, Ontario, Canada N1G 2W1.

B. W. Parry, School of Veterinary Science, University of Melbourne, Werribee, Victoria, Australia 3030.

Wayne F. Robinson, School of Veterinary Studies, Murdoch University, Murdoch, Western Australia, Australia 6150.

V. E. O. Valli, College of Veterinary Medicine, University of Illinois, Urbana, Illinois, USA 61801.

Preface to the Fourth Edition

Thirty years will have elapsed since the publication of the first edition of "Pathology of Domestic Animals." In that time it has become like a living thing, changing and adapting as veterinary pathology has changed, yet retaining the generic character of the first edition. The fourth edition will be immediately recognizable to the many users of earlier editions, but it is changed in significant ways.

Yesterday's interesting new case becomes tomorrow's new syndrome. Accordingly, we have attempted to provide a more comprehensive textual inclusion of individual disease entities rather than relegate many diseases to the bibliographies as in earlier editions. This change respects and reflects current veterinary pathology practice. Our concern for the economically significant diseases remains and they are discussed in detail. However, recent rapid growth in knowledge has come from applying modern investigative techniques to comparative pathology and the diseases of companion animals.

Library resources are more readily available than when this work was first produced. The bibliographic listings have been reduced and placed closer to their subjects. These sources have been selected not only for intrinsic merit but for the comprehensive bibliographies they provide.

An essential part of the work has been the illustrations, the number and quality of which have been maintained. We are particularly grateful to our many colleagues who have provided photographs of high quality; they are acknowledged in the figure legends. We have to a large extent departed from the plate format for illustrations; this has allowed us to replace some illustrations and to locate others more appropriately in relation to the text.

The bringing together of this fourth edition has involved many people, far too many to name. Acknowledgments are made at the end of several chapters but we, as editors, are grateful to our contributing authors for their splendid and timely contributions, to Dr. Jennifer Anne Charles for meticulous editorial assistance, and to our word-processor operators Yvonne Pritchard and Kay Vincent who never allowed the way to seem too long or too weary. Edward W. Eaton of the University of Guelph prepared most of the new illustrations for this edition, and we thank him for his assistance. It remains a pleasure to work with Academic Press.

Melbourne, Australia
1993

K. V. F. Jubb
Peter C. Kennedy
Nigel Palmer

Preface to the Third Edition

Much has been happening in veterinary pathology between editions of this work. We had, from the time of the first edition, an expectation and a hope that as the number of scientists dedicated to this field of study grew, so also would the variety of publications to serve the diversity of interests. This anticipation has only partly been realized. We still have few books that address themselves to diseases of a single domestic species or to a single organ system of domestic animals. The need for a comprehensive treatment of diseases of domestic species, from the viewpoint of the pathologist, remains. The reception of earlier editions and the interest of our colleagues around the world have influenced us to try for the third time to produce a work of some universal usefulness.

The amount of information available on the pathology of animal disease has grown enormously, and the task of integrating so much new information into a coherent statement has grown on an equal or larger scale. Changes have become necessary in this book. This edition introduces the new generation of veterinary pathologists to a literary task that has grown much beyond what the original authors could handle. We take great satisfaction in this growth and in our colleagues' willingness to join us in the project. The contributors are identified with those chapters or parts of chapters for which they have been individually responsible, although this method does understate the contribution and the dedicated commitment of our coauthors to what has been very much a cooperative effort.

We have retained the original style and format. It was established as the medium for what were personal statements by the authors. We hope that we have been able to maintain some of that flavor. Some features of the style and the format have proven to be awkward in use by the busy working pathologist, and in recognition of this we have given attention to subdivisions in the text, to an expansion of tables of content, to details in indexation (including addition of a cumulative index, in Volume 3), and to an expanded selection of illustrations. The wish to preserve the original style has presented to us and to our contributing authors challenges on content and balance. We hope that these have reasonably been met. Inevitably, we have had to make choices in blending the contributions of our contributing authors into a whole. We have had to reduce excellent sections to keep these volumes within reasonable size, and we have expanded other sections for the sake of completeness. Inevitably too, some of our editorial judgments will be imperfect, and responsibility remains with us for deficiencies in the final compilation.

It is not possible adequately to acknowledge the many people who have contributed to this work; most of them will in this prefatory statement remain unnamed.

The contributors, all of whom volunteered effort without which this work could not have been completed, will find that the uses to which these volumes are put in the next few years will be a fuller tribute to their work than can be written here. The support of our many other colleagues in veterinary pathology is perhaps best indicated by their generosity in providing illustrative material. We have brought forward many of the plates or figures from the earlier editions and have added many new ones. Those brought forward or added are acknowledged in the legends, but many more excellent photographs were received than could be used. We are deeply grateful to those colleagues who offered them.

The institutions with which we are individually affiliated have made time and other resources available to us. The several chapters contain acknowledgments for assistance received, but we must here acknowledge Sandra Brown, Jean Middlemiss, and Edward W. Eaton of the University of Guelph for preparing most of the draft manuscript and many illustrations, Denise Heffernan, Lynette Magill, and Frank Oddi of the University of Melbourne for the preparation of final copy and illustrations, and Tammie Goates of that university for editing the bibliographies. We gratefully acknowledge a generous donation from Syntex Agribusiness toward the costs of preparation of the manuscript. We are grateful again to receive the courtesy and cooperation of Academic Press in this shared contribution to the study of animal disease.

Melbourne, Australia
1984

K. V. F. Jubb
Peter C. Kennedy
Nigel Palmer

Preface to the Second Edition

The first edition of "Pathology of Domestic Animals" went to press, not without some sense of satisfaction, with a philosophic acceptance of the many imperfections and a tentative hope that any future edition would provide an opportunity to refine our knowledge, understanding, and technique of communication. Alas, imperfections remain, different ones perhaps, inevitable products of the interaction of limited time, limited intellect, and unlimited supplies of scientific data.

We are impressed by the masses of data that weekly flood our libraries and by the short half-life of much of it, by the exponential increase in knowledge and the splintering of disciplines that proliferate therefrom, and by the inability of many disciplines relevant to medical science to be completely self-sustaining. More and more it is evident that the theme of pathology provides the central and connecting link in medical education and practice and the basis on which a multidisciplined structure can be supported. This is a difficult role for pathologists, but one which they will fill, not by virtue of superior intellects and capacious memories, desirable though these attributes may be, but rather by the proper application of the logic of the scientific method.

Therefore, in preparing this second edition we have attempted to incorporate new knowledge on the specific diseases of animals and, more earnestly, to find a theme of organ susceptibility and responsiveness. We do not doubt the validity of the approach even if we are unable as yet to apply it feasibly to all organs and systems. The format of this edition remains the same as for the first and for the same reasons; the logistics of suitable alternatives are too formidable.

Once again we must express our gratitude to the many people who have contributed in some way to the preparation of this edition. Especially, we are indebted to Professor T. J. Hulland of the University of Guelph for revising the chapter on muscle, to Dr. Anne Jabara, University of Melbourne for the section on mammary tumours, and to Dr. N. C. Palmer and Dr. J. S. Wilkinson of the University of Melbourne for material assistance and many fruitful conversations. As always, a heavy burden falls on those who convert our notes to manuscript and arrange the bibliography, a task shared and cheerfully and devotedly performed by Mrs. Sylvia Lewis and Miss Frances Douglas. We hope that we have done justice to those who have contributed illustrative material: Dr. A. Seawright, University of Queensland; Dr. D. Kradel, Pennsylvania State University; Dr. E. Karbe, University of

Zurich; Dr. B. C. Easterday, National Animal Disease Laboratory at Ames; Mr. J. D. J. Harding, Central Veterinary Laboratory, Weybridge; Dr. J. Morgan, University of California; Miss Virginia Osborne, University of Sydney.

Melbourne, Australia
October, 1969

K. V. F. JUBB
PETER C. KENNEDY

Preface to the First Edition

The preface offers the opportunity to an author to present his excuses for having written the book and his justification of the content and mode of presentation. Our reasons for writing "Pathology of Domestic Animals" are as insubstantial but as compelling as those which committed Captain Ahab to the pursuit of Moby Dick, and we offer no excuses. Neither shall we attempt justification because a bad book cannot be justified and a good book is its own justification.

These volumes are based on our experience and on as much of the relevant literature of the world as we have been able to find and evaluate and we offer them to our colleagues and to all students of pathology in the hope that they will contribute to an understanding of animal disease. We anticipate some criticism in offering these as student texts but in doing so we indicate our confidence in teachers of pathology to guide students in the use of such volumes and in the ability of the student to profit from the exposure. Moreover, these volumes represent, it seems to us, a fair assessment of the needs of veterinary students in these times, since we realize as we should, that the knowledge of pathology possessed by most graduating students must serve them for the rest of their lives.

We should have preferred to write at greater length and in more detail of our chosen field, but practicality and economics have dictated that we can present here no more than a précis of the wealth of information that is the gift of our predecessors and contemporaries to the veterinary profession. In compensation, we have appended to each chapter an extensive but selected bibliography by the proper use of which the earnest seeker after further knowledge will be richly rewarded. Many valuable contributions from the old and foreign literature will not be listed in our bibliolgraphies, perhaps because we have failed to appreciate their significance but largely because we have not obtained access to them.

We wish to emphasize to our younger colleagues that there exist vast gaps in our present knowledge, and we hope future work will do much to fill these gaps. For any errors of established fact that appear and for errors of interpretation of published information we tender, with our apologies, a request that they be drawn to our attention. We have not always attempted to distinguish between what we know and what we think we know, and in stating our position on many matters of controversy it is inevitable that we are sometimes in error; but we do prefer to state our positions while reserving our right to change our opinions when necessary.

The aim of the scientific method is to provide understanding, and the ultimate aim in all study of disease is to understand well enough to preserve the organism and prevent the disease. But disease and the temper of the community do not wait upon the languid spirit of most scientific enquiry; in the annals of veterinary science there are many endemic and epidemic diseases concerning which a broad search for understanding is necessarily postponed in the interest of quickly finding a way to avoid the disease or to face and exert some measure of control over it. Such hastily constructed controls are often satisfactory, but seldom enough, and usually they merely stem the tide while further enquiry can be made and understanding sought. It is from pathology, viewed broadly, that understanding comes and the need is great because there are old diseases still to be contended with, others now in existence but still to be recognized, and new ones to be anticipated. The pathologist is necessarily concerned with all matters pertaining to disease and we would enjoin him to remember this and meet his responsibilities in an age when urgency disturbs the spirit of the Groves of the Academy.

We have departed somewhat from tradition in the arrangement of these volumes. General pathology is well covered in many existing textbooks and we have not taken space for it, but have restricted our discussions to systemic or special pathology. Almost all we have to say on a particular subject or specific disease is said in one place under the organ system in which it appears most appropriate, although we have waived this general rule in an attempt to make the sections devoted to genitalia and special senses self-sufficient. A few diseases which resisted our systemic classification are relegated to an appendix in Volume 2. Detailed tables of contents are included for each volume to indicate the organization of the text and our classification of the diseases of the systems.

Guelph, Ontario
January, 1963

K. V. F. JUBB
PETER C. KENNEDY

CHAPTER 1 The Alimentary System

IAN K. BARKER
University of Guelph, Canada

A. A. VAN DREUMEL
Ontario Ministry of Agriculture and Food, Canada

NIGEL PALMER
Ontario Ministry of Agriculture and Food, Canada

I. The Oral Cavity

Examination of the oral cavity should be standard procedure during any postmortem examination. To obtain a clear view of the mucous membranes of the buccal and oral cavities, teeth, tongue, gums, and tonsils, it is essential to split the mandibular symphysis and separate the mandibles as far as possible. A thorough examination of all structures will reveal not only local lesions but often those which may be due to systemic disease. Lesions may be associated with congenital anomalies; trauma (physical and chemical); bacterial, mycotic, viral, and parasitic infections; metabolic and toxic diseases; and immune-mediated, dysplastic, or neoplastic disease. The poor physical condition of an animal may be directly related to oral lesions which result in difficulties of prehension, mastication, or swallowing of food.

A. Congenital Anomalies

The development of normal facies and the oral cavity requires the integration of many embryonic processes. The complexity and duration of this development may lead to a great variety of aberrations. These are usually expressed in the newborn in the form of clefts resulting from failures of integrated growth and fusion. A common failure of fusion is that of the maxillary processes to the frontonasal process. This may leave facial fissures, cleft lip (harelip, cheiloschisis) and uni- or bilateral primary cleft palate involving the area rostral to the incisive papilla.

Facial clefts may involve the skin only, or the deeper tissues as well. They are variously located, and not all are obviously related to normal lines of fusion. All are rare. The least uncommon is a complete cleft from one angle of the mouth to the ear of that side. This results from failure of fusion of the lateral portions of the maxillary and mandibular processes. A defect extending from a harelip to the eye results from failure of fusion of the maxillary and frontonasal processes; its least expression is superficial and a failure of closure of the nasolacrimal duct.

Cheiloschisis and primary cleft palate include developmental anomalies of the lips anterior to the nasal septum, columella, and premaxilla. They may be uni- or bilateral and superficial or extend into the nostril. The defect arises from incomplete fusion of the frontonasal process with the maxillary processes.

Secondary cleft palate (cleft palate, palatoschisis) (Fig. 1.1) is often associated with cheiloschisis and primary cleft palate. The hard palate is formed, except for a small anterior contribution from the frontonasal process, by the bilateral ingrowth of the lateral palatine shelves from the maxillary processes. At the midline, they fuse with each other and with the nasal septum, and undergo intramembranous ossification, except in their posterior part, which becomes the soft palate. Inadequate growth of the palatine shelves leaves a central defect, in either or both of the hard and soft palates, which communicates between the oral and nasal cavities. Other manifestations of disordered palatogenesis include unilateral defects in the soft palate;

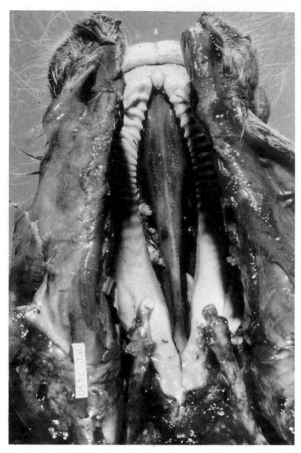

Fig. 1.1 Secondary cleft palate exposing the nasal cavity. Calf.

bilateral hypoplasia of the soft palate; or dorsal displacement of the soft palate, with excess soft tissue on the caudal portion. Affected animals have difficulty sucking, may have nasal regurgitation, and usually die within the first few days of life from aspiration pneumonia.

Cleft palates have been reported in most species of domestic animals. The etiology is usually unknown, but at least in some species, it is hereditary or due to ingestion of teratogenic agents during pregnancy. In one extensive survey of Thoroughbred foals, 4% of congenital defects were secondary cleft palates. Most of these foals had a complete cleft of the hard palate; a few had clefts or hypoplasia of the soft palate only. The cause of palatoschisis in foals is unknown.

In calves, cleft palate is one of the most common anomalies. Secondary cleft palate and arthrogryposis frequently occur together in Charolais calves, and appear to be hereditary (probably simple autosomal recessive), as in Hereford cattle. These two anomalies have also been associated with the ingestion of certain lupines by cows during gestational days 40–70. Cleft palate is uncommon in lambs, in which it may be genetic in origin (possibly simple recessive), or associated with the ingestion of *Veratrum californicum*.

In swine, primary cleft palate is less common than secondary cleft palate, although the two anomalies often occur together. The defects are probably polygenic or multifactorial developmental anomalies. Secondary cleft palates have been induced experimentally in newborn pigs by feeding gilts seeds or plants of poison hemlock (*Conium maculatum*) during gestational days 30–45. The teratogenic substance responsible for the defect is an alkaloid, γ-coniceine. Tree tobacco (*Nicotiana glauca*), a close relative of *N. tabacum*, also induces a high incidence of cleft palate in newborn pigs when fed to gilts early in pregnancy. Affected pigs also have arthrogryposis (see Bones and Joints, Volume 1, Chapter 1). Palatoschisis in piglets has also been associated with consumption of feed contaminated with *Crotalaria retusa* seed by sows during gestation.

Primary and secondary cleft palate in the German boxer dog appear to be hereditary, probably due to a single autosomal recessive gene. Secondary cleft palate occurs in Siamese and Abyssinian cats and is thought to be hereditary, although the mode of inheritance has not been determined. Griseofulvin treatment of the pregnant queen will result in palatoschisis in the offspring. The defect has also been reported in both parts of the doubled face in diprosopus cats.

Anomalies in the growth of jaws are quite common. **Brachygnathia superior,** shortness of the maxillae, is an inherited breed characteristic among dogs and swine. It has been reported in the Large White or Yorkshire breed. The condition is progressive with age, resulting in malapposition of the incisor and cheek teeth, which interferes with prehension and mastication. In swine, brachygnathia superior may be confused with atrophic rhinitis. In Jersey cattle, brachygnathia superior occurs as a single autosomal recessive trait. It may, in any species, be associated with chondrodysplasia.

Brachygnathia inferior or micrognathia, shortness of the mandibles, may be a mild to lethal defect in cattle and sheep and is a breed characteristic of long-nosed dogs. Micrognathia is a common defect in calves. It is inherited, probably as a simple autosomal recessive trait. There is a higher incidence in males. In Aberdeen Angus cattle the defect may occur concurrently with cerebellar hypoplasia, and with osteopetrosis in this and other breeds (see Bones and Joints, Volume 1, Chapter 1). Mild brachygnathia inferior, termed parrot mouth, is a common conformational defect in horses.

Prognathism refers to an abnormal prolongation of the mandibles. It too is rather common, especially in sheep. It may develop with recovery from calcium deficiency in this species (see Bones and Joints, Volume 1, Chapter 1). The malformation is relative, and it is not always easy to determine whether the jaw is absolutely long or merely apparently so, relative to a mild brachygnathia superior.

Agnathia is a mandibulofacial malformation characterized by absence of the lower jaw, due to failure of development of the first branchial arch and associated structures. The defect is one of the most common anomalies in lambs but is rare in cattle. Associated malformations in lambs may include ateloprosopia (incomplete development of the face), microglossia or aglossia, and atresia of the oropharynx. Concurrent anomalies affecting other body systems may also be evident.

A lethal glossopharyngeal hereditary defect, termed **bird tongue** and caused by a simple, recessive, autosomal gene, has been reported in dogs; the breed involved was not revealed. The affected pups have a narrow tongue, especially the anterior half where the margins are folded medially onto the dorsal surface. The pups are unable to swallow. The muscle fibers of the affected tongues are normal histologically. Hypertrophy of the tongue occurs as a congential anomaly in pigs.

Epitheliogenesis imperfecta is an anomaly causing widespread defects in cutaneous epithelium, and also affects the epithelial lining of the oral cavity, especially the tongue (Fig. 1.2) (see The Skin and Appendages, Volume 1, Chapter 5). The condition is characterized by irregular, well-demarcated, red areas from which the epithelium of the oral mucosa is absent. Histologically, these consist of abruptly defective areas in the squamous mucosa with inflammation of the submucosal connective tissues. The anomaly occurs in most species and is inherited as a simple autosomal recessive character in cattle, horses, and pigs; the mode of inheritance is unknown in the other species.

There are several hereditary skin conditions in animals, such as epidermolysis bullosa simplex in collie dogs, ovine epidermolysis bullosa in Suffolk and South Dorset Down sheep, and familial acantholysis of Aberdeen Angus calves, which have minor involvement of the lips and oral mucosa. (see The Skin and Appendages, Volume 1, Chapter 5).

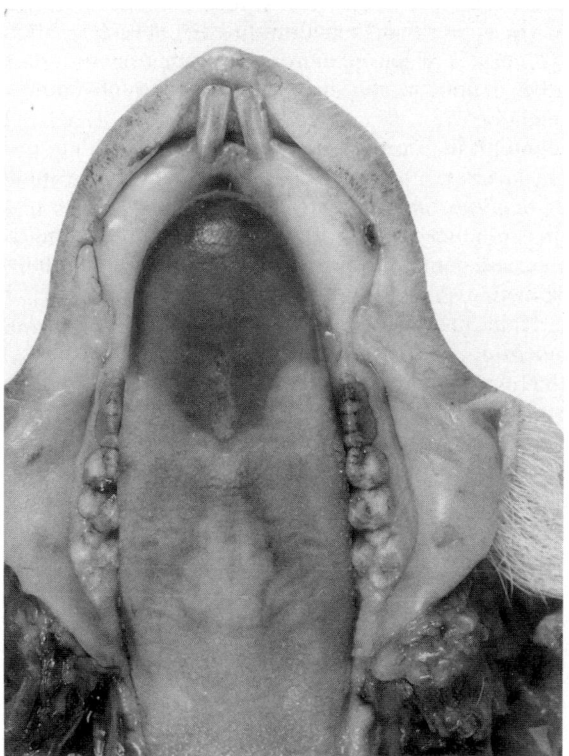

Fig. 1.2 Epitheliogenesis imperfecta. Tongue. Pig.

Bibliography

Crowe, M. W., and Swerczek, T. W. Equine congenital defects. *Am J Vet Res* **46:** 353–358, 1985.

Dennis, S. M. Perinatal lamb mortality in Western Australia. 7. Congenital defects. *Aust Vet J* **51:** 80–82, 1975.

Dennis, S. M., and Leipold, H. W. Agnathia in sheep: External observations. *Am J Vet Res* **33:** 339–347, 1972.

Donald, H. P., and Wierer, G. Observations on mandibular prognathism. *Vet Rec* **66:** 479–483, 1954.

Done, J. T. Facial deformity in pigs. *Vet Ann* **17:** 96–102, 1977.

Edmonds, L., Crenshaw, D., and Selby, L. A. Micrognathia and cerebellar hypoplasia in an Aberdeen Angus herd. *J Hered* **64:** 62–64, 1973.

Evans, H. E., and Sack, W. O. Prenatal development of domestic and laboratory mammals: Growth curves, external features, and selected references. *Anat Histol Embryol* **2:** 11–45, 1973.

Haynes, P. F., and Qualls, C. W., Jr. Cleft soft palate, nasal septal deviation, and epiglottic entrapment in a thoroughbred filly. *J Am Vet Med Assoc* **179:** 910–913, 1981.

Heidari, M., Vogt, D. W., and Nelson, S. L. Brachygnathia in a herd of Angus cattle. *Am J Vet Res* **46:** 708–710, 1985.

Hooper, P. T., and Scanlan, W. A. *Crotalaria retusa* poisoning of pigs and poultry. *Aust Vet J* **53:** 109–114, 1977.

Hutt, F. B., and de Lahunta, A. A lethal glossopharyngeal defect in the dog. *J Hered* **62:** 291–293, 1971.

Johnson, J. H., Hull, B. L., and Dorn, A. S. The mouth. *In* "Veterinary Gastroenterology," N. V. Anderson (ed.), pp. 337–372. Philadelphia, Pennsylvania, Lea & Febiger, 1980.

Keeler, R. F., and Crowe, M. W. Congenital deformities in swine induced by wild tree tobacco (*Nicotiana glauca*). *Clin Toxicol* **20:** 49–58, 1983.

Leipold, H. W., and Schalles, R. Genetic defects in cattle: Transmission and control. *Vet Med Small Anim Clin* **72:** 80–85, 1977.

Logue, D. N., Breeze, R. G., and Harvey, M. J. A. Arthrogryposis–palatoschisis and a 1/29 translocation in a Charolais herd. *Vet Rec* **100:** 509–510, 1977.

Mulley, R. C., and Edwards, J. J. Prevalence of congenital abnormalities in pigs. *Aust Vet J* **61:** 116–120, 1984.

Mulvihill, J. J. Congenital and genetic disease in domestic animals. *Science* **176:** 132–137, 1972.

Noden, D. M., and de Lahunta, A. "The Embryology of Domestic Animals. Developmental Mechanisms and Malformations." Baltimore, Maryland, Williams & Wilkins, 1985.

Panter, K. E., Keeler, R. F., and Buck, W. B. Induction of cleft palate in newborn pigs by maternal ingestion of poison hemlock (*Conium maculatum*). *Am J Vet Res* **46:** 1368–1371, 1985.

Riley, C. C, Yovich, J. V., and J. R. Bolton. Bilateral hypoplasia of the soft palate in a foal. *Aust Vet J* **68:** 178–179, 1991.

Sekeles, E., Aharon, D. C., and Fass, U. Craniofacial duplication (diprosopus) in the cat—case report and review of the literature. *Zbl Vet Med A* **32:** 226–233, 1985.

Selby, L. A., Hopps, H. C., and Edmonds, L. D. Comparative aspects of congenital malformations in man and swine. *J Am Vet Med Assoc* **159:** 1485–1490, 1971.

Swartz, H. A., Vogt, D. W., and Kintner, L. D. Chromosome evaluation of Angus calves with unilateral congenital cleft lip and jaw (cheilognathoschisis). *Am J Vet Res* **43:** 729–731, 1982.

Turba, E., and Willer, S. Untersuchungen zur Vererbung von Hasenscharten und Wolfsrachen beim Deutschen Boxer. *Mh Vet Med* **42:** 897–901, 1987.

B. Diseases of Teeth and Dental Tissues

Dental examinations in animals are usually cursory, except to assess age, but dental disease is common and often is the factor which limits the useful life span, especially of sheep. The comments on dental development and anatomy are intended to assist the understanding of dental disease.

Teeth develop from horseshoe-shaped thickenings in the oral ectoderm called dental laminae. Neural crest cells beneath the laminae induce formation of tooth buds, which generate the enamel organs. These epithelial structures grow into the underlying ectomesenchyme and organize it to form dental papillae, which they enclose like a cap. Surrounding both is another mesenchymal condensation, the dental sac, which has a collagenous inner layer, the dental follicle, and an outer fibrovascular layer. In dogs the dental follicle is thought to coordinate resorption of alveolar bone that is necessary for tooth eruption.

The inner enamel epithelium of the enamel organ induces differentiation of odontoblasts from the mesenchyme of the papilla. Odontoblasts produce dentin, which in turn induces enamel formation by the inner enamel epithelium. Formation of dentin is essential for formation of enamel. These inductive interactions of epithelium and mesenchyme are considered important in the histodifferentiation of some tumors of dental tissues.

The free edge of the enamel organ extends beyond the enamel–dentin junction, and this extension is called Hertwig's epithelial root sheath. It molds the dental papilla to form the root or apex of the tooth. Subsequently it fragments, allowing mesenchymal cells from the dental sac to contact the root dentin, differentiate into cementoblasts, and deposit cementum on the dentin. Remnants of the root sheath are called epithelial rests of Malassez. They persist in the periodontal ligament, and may give rise to tumors or cysts. They may be important in the induction or repair of cementum, and in periodontal reattachment following injury. In pigs and sheep, the rests may be incorporated into the junctional epithelium as it migrates apically in chronic periodontal disease. Cells of the root sheath that adhere to the dentin can produce enamel pearls.

Once the dental lamina has produced the buds of the permanent teeth, it degenerates. Epithelial remnants persist as epithelial pearls or islands in the gingiva and jaws. These remnants also may give rise to tumors and cysts.

There are important differences between the brachydont teeth of humans, carnivores, and swine, in which the enamel is restricted to the tooth crown, and the hypsodont teeth of herbivores. In hypsodont teeth, enamel extends far down on the roots, and is invaginated into the dentin to form infundibula. Also, the hypsodont teeth of herbivores, except the mandibular premolars of ruminants, are covered by cementum, which more or less fills the infundibula. Exceptions to these rules are provided by the tusks of boars, which are hypsodont, but not covered by cementum, and by ruminant incisors, which are brachydont but do have enamel covering part of the root dentin and cementum covering the root enamel.

The three hard tissues of teeth are dentin, enamel, and cementum. **Dentin** is light yellow and constitutes most of the tooth. It consists of ~35% organic matter and 65% mineral. Thus its composition is similar to that of bone, and like bone, it contains type I collagen. Dentin is produced by columnar cells with basal nuclei called odontoblasts, which differentiate from mesenchyme of the dental papilla. It is formed as unmineralized predentin. The odontoblasts move away from the dentin–enamel junction, gradually encroaching on the pulp cavity as they produce dentin. Each odontoblast has a process extending into the dentin, encased in a dentinal tubule, which arborizes at the dentin–enamel junction. The process also anastomoses with the processes of other odontoblasts. Dentinal tubules are visible in histologic sections, but the anastomoses are not. Except for the processes, and nerve endings in the dentinal tubules near the pulp, dentin is acellular.

Normal dentin contains incremental or imbrication lines of von Ebner, which are fine basophilic lines running at right angles to the dentinal tubules. They represent normal variations in the structure and mineralization of dentin. Sublethal injury caused by certain infections, metabolic stresses, or toxic states may injure the odontoblasts, which then produce accentuated incremental lines known as the contour lines of Owen. Sometimes irregular zones of unmineralized or poorly mineralized dentin form between foci of normal mineralization. These are zones of interglobular dentin, which may be caused by hypophosphatemia.

Odontoblasts normally are active throughout life, producing layers of secondary dentin, which often contain fewer dentinal tubules than primary dentin. Reparative dentin is produced locally in response to injury to dentinal tubules, and contains a limited number of twisted tubules and sometimes a few odontoblasts, which soon die. Reparative dentin may resemble bone and is sometimes called osteodentin. Sclerotic (transparent) dentin is formed when dentinal tubules are occluded by calcium salts. The junctions between primary, secondary, and reparative dentin are usually demarcated by basophilic lines.

Enamel has ~5% organic matter and 95% mineral. It is produced by the tall columnar ameloblasts of the inner enamel epithelium. Enamel is produced in the form of prisms or rods, cemented together by a matrix. Mineralization begins as soon as it is formed and is a two-stage process, somewhat similar to that in bone, but much more rapid. The cells of the inner enamel epithelium also move away from the dentin–enamel junction as the tooth is formed, but unlike odontoblasts, they do not have processes. Enamel is hard, dense, brittle, and permeable, and is translucent and white. Mature enamel is not present in demineralized sections, but some of the matrix of immature enamel may be visible near ameloblasts of developing teeth.

Ameloblasts are very sensitive to environmental changes. Normal enamel contains incremental lines of Retzius, which are analogous to the incremental lines of von Ebner in dentin, and also reflect variations in structure and mineralization. The incremental lines are accentuated during periods of metabolic stress. More severe injury in fluorosis, or infections by some viruses (Fig. 1.3A,B), can produce focal **hypoplasia or aplasia of enamel.**

Formation of enamel ends before tooth eruption. The inner enamel epithelium then merges with the cells of the underlying stratum intermedium and the outer enamel epithelium to form the reduced enamel epithelium. It protects the enamel of the formed tooth prior to eruption. Degeneration of this protective layer permits connective tissue to contact the enamel, and there may be resorption of enamel or deposition of a layer of cementum on it. This normally occurs during odontogenesis in horses.

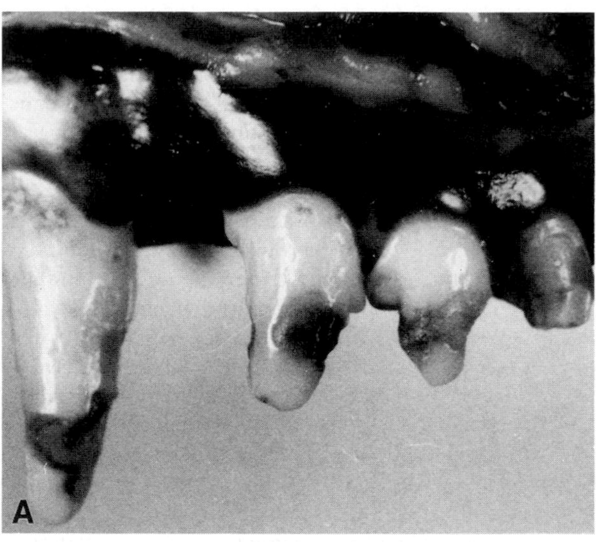

Fig. 1.3A Focal enamel hypoplasia, sequel to canine distemper. Dog.

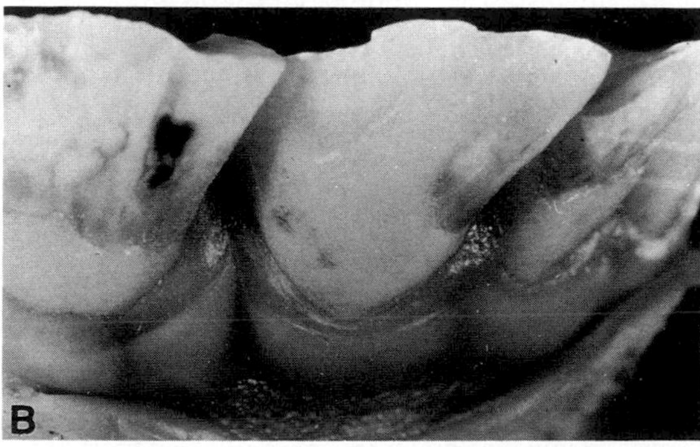

Fig. 1.3B Enamel hypoplasia. Calf. Sequel to intrauterine infection by bovine virus diarrhea virus. (Courtesy of R. B. Miller.)

Cementum is an avascular, bonelike substance, produced by cementoblasts; it contains ~55% organic and 45% inorganic matter. In general, the dentin of brachydont teeth is covered by cementum wherever it is not covered by enamel. When dentin formation has begun in the root, degeneration of Hertwig's epithelial root sheath begins and permits mesenchymal cells from the dental sac to contact dentin. They differentiate into cementoblasts, which produce cementoid, and later mineralize it. Some layers of cementum do not contain cells (acellular cementum), but in other layers, cementocytes are enclosed in lacunae. Sharpey's fibers from alveolar bone are embedded in the cementum. Cementum is more resistant to resorption than is bone, and unlike bone, normally is not resorbed and replaced as it ages; instead a new layer of cementum is deposited on top of the old layer. In some pathologic conditions cementum is resorbed; subsequently, cellular or acellular cementum is deposited, and more or less repairs the defect.

Hypercementosis is abnormal thickening of cementum and may involve part or all of one or many teeth. When extra cementum improves the functional properties of teeth, it is called cementum hypertrophy; if not, it is called cementum hyperplasia. Extensive hyperplasia often is associated with chronic inflammation of the dental root.

The **periodontal ligament** is a very cellular, well-vascularized connective tissue that develops from the dental sac. The periodontium comprises the periodontal ligament, gingival lamina propria, cementum, and alveolar bone. The ligament supports the tooth and adjusts to its movement during growth. It is well supplied with nerves and lymphatics, which drain into alveolar bone. The periodontal ligament also is a source of the cells that remodel alveolar bone and, in disease, cementum.

Epithelial rests of Malassez are present in the periodontal ligament and are particularly numerous in the incisor region of sheep. In all species, they may proliferate and become cystic when there is inflammation of the periodontium. The periodontium is also a site of origin of tumors. The periodontal ligament normally is visible in radiographs as a radiolucent line between tooth and alveolar bone. In prolonged hyperparathyroidism, alveolar bone is resorbed, and the ligament is no longer outlined radiographically, a change referred to as loss of the lamina dura.

1. Developmental Anomalies of Teeth

Anodontia, absence of teeth, is inherited in calves, probably as a sex-linked recessive trait in males, and is associated with skin defects. **Oligodontia,** fewer teeth than normal, occurs sporadically in horses, cats, and dogs, and also as an inherited trait in dogs. In brachycephalic breeds, the cheek teeth are deficient; in toy breeds, the incisors are deficient. Pseudo-oligodontia and pseudoanodontia result from failed eruption. These defects may be associated with bone-modeling defects in gray lethal mice with osteopetrosis. Delayed eruption of permanent teeth occurs in Lhasa apso and Shih Tsu dogs. **Polyodontia,** excessive teeth, occurs in brachycephalic dogs; the incisors are involved, and the defect is probably related to breeding for broad muzzles. A high incidence of canine polyodontia, involving particularly an extra maxillary premolar, is reported from the Netherlands. Polyodontia also occurs in horses and cats, involving either incisors or cheek teeth. Pseudopolyodontia is retention of deciduous teeth after eruption of the permanent dentition. It occurs in horses, cats, and dogs, especially in the miniature breeds.

Heterotopic polyodontia is an extra tooth, or teeth, outside the dental arcades. The best-known example is the ear tooth of horses, which develops in a branchiogenic cyst. The cysts originate from failure of closure of the first branchial cleft, or from the inclusion of cellular rests in this area. They are lined by a stratified mucous- or cutaneous-type epithelium, and may contain one or more teeth, either loosely attached in the cyst wall or deeply embedded in the petrous temporal bone. The tooth is derived from misplaced tooth germ of the first branchial arch, which is displaced toward the ear with the first branchial cleft. The cysts form in the parotid region and may fistulate to the exterior. They are occasionally bilateral, and rarely the tooth may form a pedunculated mass enclosed by skin, and attached by a pedicle to the skin of the head. Heterotopic polyodontia also occurs in cattle, dogs, pigs, and sheep.

Developmentally **misshapen teeth** are classified as geminous (dichotomous) when there is a single root and partially or completely separate crowns; fused, when the dentin of two teeth is confluent; and concrescent when the dentin is separate but the roots are joined by cementum. Gemination represents the embryologic partial division of a tooth primordium. It occurs in dogs, usually involving the incisors, and the affected tooth usually has a groove dividing the crowns. Fusion and concrescence represent the joining of two adjacent tooth primordia, one of which may be supernumerary. Malformation and malpositioning of teeth accompany abnormalities of the jaw bones. Aberdeen Angus and Hereford calves with congenital osteopetrosis have brachygnathia inferior, malformed mandibles and impacted cheek teeth, (see Bones and Joints, Volume 1, Chapter 1). Impacted molars occur as an inherited lethal in shorthorns; an association with osteopetrosis apparently has not been investigated in this breed.

Odontogenic cysts are epithelium-lined cysts derived from cell rests of Malassez, cell rests of dental laminae, reduced enamel epithelium, or malformed enamel organs. **Dentigerous cysts** are, by definition, cysts which contain part or all of a tooth, which often is malformed. Of the odontogenic cysts listed, all except those derived from cell rests of Malassez are potentially dentigerous. (The rests of Malassez are the probable source of periodontal cysts.) Dentigerous cysts originating in malformed enamel organs should include malformed teeth, since development of enamel is incomplete until the organ degenerates. Those teeth in cysts of reduced enamel epithelium or rests of dental laminae are not necessarily abnormal. The affected teeth probably erupt into the preformed cysts. Dentigerous cysts enclose at least the crown of the tooth, but may include it all. The most common forms of odontogenic dentigerous cysts in animals are those involving the vestigial wolf teeth of horses and the vestigial canines, especially of mares. The smaller cysts appear as tumors of the gums, whereas some of the larger ones may cause swelling of the jaw or adjacent maxillary sinus. Dentigerous cysts of animals are not so destructive as those in humans, in which species they are regarded as the most common benign destructive lesion of the skeleton.

The ear tooth of horses is probably the most common nonodontogenic dentigerous cyst (see heterotopic polyodontia earlier in this section). Occasionally true dentigerous cysts form when a tumor prevents normal eruption or when there is maleruption due to odontodystrophy.

Cystic dental inclusions about vestigial supernumerary teeth also occur in the juxtamolar positions in cattle but are insignificant. These too may be dentigerous, or they may be primordial cysts developed before the stage of enamel formation, and hence containing no mineralized tooth structures. Either type of cyst may give rise to ameloblastomas.

A high incidence of dentigerous cysts involving incisors occurs in some sheep flocks in Scotland and New Zealand. A congenital disease involving the jaws and teeth of calves in Germany (odontodysplasia cystica congenita) is characterized by massive fibro-osseous enlargement of the maxillae and horizontal rami of the mandibles. Some teeth are malformed, misshapen, or absent. Cystic spaces in the jaws are lined by fibrous tissue or epithelium, the latter probably derived from enamel organs. The dental changes are thought to be secondary to those in bone. Most affected calves are aborted or stillborn, and many have ascites and hydrocephalus. The disease may be caused by environmental influences.

The permanent teeth are unique in that their development continues for a long time after birth. Thus, inflammatory and metabolic disease of postnatal life can produce hypoplasia of dentin and enamel. Hypoplasia of enamel of deciduous teeth occurs in some calves with intrauterine bovine virus diarrhea infection (Fig. 1.3B). It has also been described in calves and pigs following irradiation of the dam during gestation. Dysplastic proliferation of dentin and enamel involving mandibular PM_1 and M_1 has been seen in young uremic dogs. Extreme fragility of deciduous teeth is a feature of bovine osteogenesis imperfecta (see Bones and Joints, Volume 1, Chapter 1). Dental dysplasia characterized by normal dentin, absence of enamel matrix, and excess, irregular cementum is described in a foal with epitheliogenesis imperfecta involving the oral mucosa.

2. Degenerative Conditions of Teeth and Dental Tissue

a. Pigmentation of the Teeth Normal enamel is white and shiny, but normal cementum is off-white to light yellow, and normal dentin is slightly darker yellow. Depending on the tooth, or the part of the tooth being examined, the normal color may be any one of these. Normal enamel is never discolored. Hypoplastic enamel of chronic fluorosis is discolored yellow through brown to almost black. Discoloration of brachydont teeth results from pigmentation of dentin, which is then visible through the semitransparent enamel, or pigmentation of the cementum of the root. Dentin may be colored red-brown by pulpal hemorrhages or inflammation, gray-green in putrid pulpitis, and yellow in icterus. Congenital erythropoietic porphyrias of calves, cats, and swine discolor the dentin red in young animals (pink tooth) and darker brown in adults, although in swine, the discoloration may disappear with aging. Transient porphyria with pink discoloration of teeth is reported in a dog.

Yellow to brown discoloration of teeth, and bright yellow fluorescence in ultraviolet light, due to deposition of tetracycline antibiotics in mineralizing dentin, enamel, and probably cementum, occurs in all species. Treatment of the pregnant dam may cause staining of deciduous teeth in the offspring. Tetracyclines are toxic to ameloblasts in the late differentiation and early secretion stages and, at high dose rate, may produce enamel hypoplasia.

Black discoloration of ruminant cheek teeth is extremely common, and is caused by impregnation of mineral salts with chlorophyll and porphyrin pigments from herbage.

b. DENTAL ATTRITION Attrition is loss of tooth structure caused by mastication. The mature conformation of teeth is largely the outcome of opposed growth and wear, and the degree of wear depends on the type of tooth, the species of animal, and the matter chewed. Wear is most evident in herbivores, and irregularities of wear are perhaps the most common dental abnormalities. In general, with normal occlusion and use, the extra-alveolar portion of the tooth does not shorten. Its length is maintained initially by growth—the period of growth depending on the species—then by hypertrophy of the root cementum and/or dentin and by proliferation of alveolar bone, which serves to push the tooth out. Finally, senile atrophy of the alveolar processes and gingival recession may maintain or increase the length of the clinical crown. Cementum hypertrophy and alveolar atrophy may also result in loss of teeth in senility, or, if combined with subnormal wear, produce teeth which in old age are excessively long. Normal wear of the complicated cheek teeth of horses and cattle causes smoothing of the occlusal surfaces. As soon as wear of enamel exposes the dentin, which being softer wears more rapidly, secondary or irregular dentin is deposited to protect the pulp. In time, this may fill the pulp cavity and cause death of the tooth.

Abnormalities of wearing are most common in herbivores (Fig. 1.4). Excessive wear of the deciduous and permanent central incisors occurs in certain sheep flocks in New Zealand. The wear is intermittent and may be severe enough to expose the pulp cavity. The cause is unknown but may be related to delayed eruption of adjacent teeth, leading to increased use of the affected pairs.

Subnormal wear, due to loss of the opposing tooth, occurs in oligodontia, abnormal spacing of adjacent teeth, and acquired loss of teeth; it results in abnormal lengthening. Such elongated teeth may grow against the opposing gum or, if deviated, into an adjacent soft structure such as cheek or lip. These teeth usually wear in abnormal places because complete loss of antagonism is unusual, since the upper and lower arcades do not coincide exactly, and the coincidence is further reduced by the displacement of chewing. Incomplete longitudinal coincidence of the molar arcades allows irregular wear and hook formation on the first and last cheek teeth. Abnormal wear due to abnormal chewing is caused by voluntary, as in painful conditions, or mechanical impairment of jaw movement. Lateral movements of the jaws without the normal rotary grinding movements allow the ridges of the teeth of herbivores to become accentuated. Steep angulation of the occlusal surfaces results from inadequate lateral movement of the jaws, and sharp edges form on the buccal aspect of the maxillary teeth and the lingual aspect of the mandibular teeth. This may be unilateral when the animal chews with only one side of its mouth, the other side then being affected. The teeth wear progressively sharper, and pass each other like shear blades; hence, the term shear mouth. Subnormal resistance to wear on the part of the molar teeth is common, and results in weave mouth or step mouth, in which successive teeth in an arcade wear at different rates. The weave or step form of the antagonistic arcade is reversed, so that the teeth of the two arcades interdigitate. This pattern of attrition is caused by variation in the hardness of opposing teeth, and usually is caused by intermittent odontodystrophy. Opposing teeth of the upper and lower jaws do not develop at the same time; thus, discontinuous nutritional deficiencies often result in unequal wear. Certain vices, such as crib biting, also produce abnormal wear. In severely worn ruminant incisors, a central black core may be visible, which is secondary dentin deposited in the pulp cavity. It is not

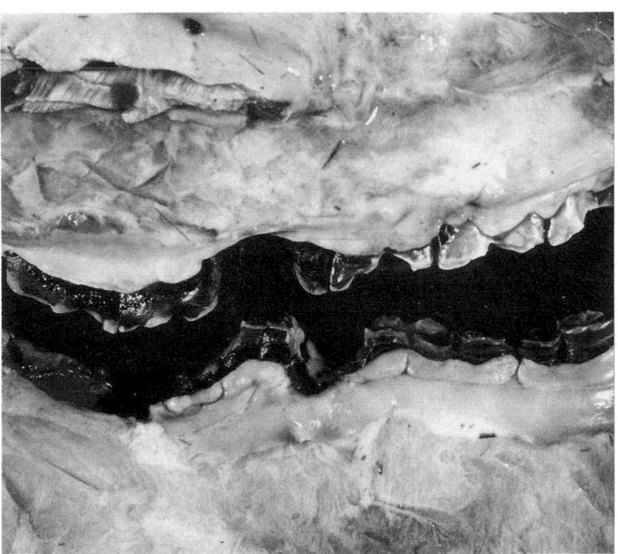

Fig. 1.4 Irregular wear of teeth. Horse.

carious, but stains darker than the surrounding primary dentin.

c. ODONTODYSTROPHIES Odontodystrophies are diseases of teeth caused by nutritional, metabolic, and toxic insults. They are manifest by changes in the hard tissues of the teeth and their supporting structures. Lesions of enamel and dentin are emphasized here. The most prominent effects of odontodystrophies appear in enamel, and lesions of enamel are most significant because they are irreparable.

Formation of enamel occurs in a set pattern. It begins at the occlusal surface and progresses toward the root. Mineral maturation occurs in the same sequence, but for each level, it begins at the dentin–enamel junction and moves toward the ameloblast. Deleterious influences have their most severe affects on those ameloblasts which are forming and mineralizing enamel. Depending on the severity on the insult, ameloblasts may produce no enamel, a little enamel, or poorly mineralized enamel. Removal of the insult permits those ameloblasts which were not yet active to begin making normal enamel. Thus, enamel defects vary in severity from isolated opaque spots or pits on the surface to deep and irregular horizontal indentations. These defects are most clearly seen on the incisor teeth and canine teeth and are usually bilaterally symmetrical. Similar lesions are also produced by infectious agents which injure ameloblasts, such as the viruses of canine distemper and bovine virus diarrhea (Fig. 1.3A,B).

Odontoblasts are susceptible to many of the same influences as ameloblasts, but they can be replenished from the undifferentiated cells of the dental pulp. Thus, lesions in actively forming dentin may be repaired, whereas those in enamel are permanent.

Because of their close anatomical association with the jaws, teeth are very susceptible to disruption in the harmony of growth. This harmonious arrangement often is upset in the odontodystrophies and osteodystrophies, and leads to malocclusion and anomalous development of teeth.

Several nutritional and toxic conditions produce odontodystrophy. Fluorine poisoning is exemplary (see Metabolic Diseases of Bone, Volume 1, Chapter 1). In vitamin A deficiency, ameloblasts do not differentiate normally, and their organizing ability is disturbed. As a result, odontoblastic differentiation is abnormal. Several lesions develop including enamel hypoplasia and hypomineralization, cellular, vascularized dentin (osteodentin), and retarded or obviated eruption.

Calcium deficiency retards eruption, and causes enamel hypoplasia and mild dentin hypoplasia. Teeth formed during the period of deficiency are very susceptible to wear. In sheep, recovery from prolonged calcium deficiency results in malocclusion due to inferior prognathia. This reflects inadequate maxillary, but normal mandibular repair during the recovery phase.

Phosphorus deficiency, combined with vitamin D deficiency, depresses dentin formation slightly, but has virtually no effect on enamel, at least not in sheep. Hypophosphatemia is associated with formation of interglobular dentin in humans. Malocclusion and abnormalities of bite in rachitic sheep are secondary to mandibular deformity.

Severe, experimental **malnutrition** also produces malocclusion. Recovery from malnutrition does not correct the lesion, and in addition, is associated with misshapen, malformed teeth, oligodontia, and polyodontia.

The major effects of odontodystrophies in herbivores, are **malocclusion,** and/or accelerated **attrition.** Sometimes a high incidence of these abnormalities is attributable to one of the causes previously discussed, but often they are idiopathic. Most of the lesions described in experimental odontodystrophies also occur in natural diseases. A syndrome of dental abnormalities of sheep in the North Island of New Zealand is characterized by excessive wear of deciduous teeth, maleruption and excessive wear of permanent teeth, periodontal disease involving permanent teeth, and development of dentigerous cysts involving permanent incisors. Mandibular osteopathy is also present. All animals older than 5 years are culled for dental problems. The odontodystrophy (and osteodystrophy) possibly is caused by deficiencies of calcium and copper, and perhaps other nutrients, such as protein, and energy. Sheep from an affected flock, pastured elsewhere, have minimal lesions.

This syndrome exemplifies the naturally occurring odontodystrophies in that it probably has a complex pathogenesis, and is associated with an osteodystrophy. The latter association is to be expected, since bones and teeth usually are susceptible to the same insults.

3. Infectious and Inflammatory Diseases of Teeth and Periodontium

The role of viruses in enamel hypoplasia is mentioned in Section I,B,2,c of this chapter. Bacterial plaque is discussed in succeeding sections along with other tooth-accumulated materials.

Bacterial diseases involving tooth surfaces are caused by the development of supragingival and subgingival **plaque.** Supragingival plaque is located on the exposed crown of the tooth and causes dental caries. Subgingival plaque is found in the crevicular groove and causes periodontal disease. Tooth enamel is covered by a translucent pellicle, the acquired enamel pellicle, which is formed by selective adsorption of complex salivary proteins, and which is essential to the development of supragingival plaque. It is a dense, nonmineralized, bacterial mass, firmly adherent to tooth surfaces, which resists removal by salivary flow and prevents the buffering capacity of saliva from influencing plaque metabolites. Formation of this plaque involves adhesion of bacteria to the pellicle, and adhesion of bacteria to each other. Only organisms with the ability to adhere to the pellicle can initiate the formation of supragingival plaque; those that cannot are removed by oral secretions and mechanical action. Pathologic reduction of salivary flow increases the prevalence of caries in some species.

The bacteria in supragingival plaque are members of the indigenous oral flora and are usually Gram-positive. Most are streptococci and *Actinomyces* spp., which form an organized array on the tooth surface. Some plaque-forming bacteria synthesize extracellular polymers, which constitute the matrix of the plaque and permit adhesion between organisms of the same species. Some utilize polymers derived from host secretions to adhere to the pellicle, whereas others attach to bacteria of a different species which are already fixed to the tooth. Plaque increases in mass with time, and its composition becomes more complex as Gram-negative bacteria join the streptococci and actinomycetes which initiated plaque formation.

Supragingival plaque is metabolically active. It utilizes dietary carbohydrates to produce the adhesive polymers and the acids needed to demineralize enamel, and as energy sources for maintenance and the production of various enzymes and mediators of inflammation. Enamel may harbor extensive deposits of supragingival plaque that are virtually invisible unless treated with a disclosing solution.

Subgingival plaque is less organized than the supragingival variety, and many of the organisms that compose it are Gram-negative anaerobes that are asaccharolytic, weakly adherent, and motile. They derive their nutrients from the crevicular fluid. The flora of subgingival plaque is less well characterized than that in the supragingival location. Culture results vary with sample collection technic, site of collection, and selectivity of media. Further, the taxonomy of many of the periodontal residents is unresolved. *Haemophilus* spp., *Bacteroides* spp., and spirochetes are likely periodontal pathogens.

Dental calculus (tartar) is mineralized plaque. It is formed by the deposition of mineral, mainly from saliva, in the dead bacteria. In horses and dogs, calculus is predominantly calcium carbonate. Calculus is often found in old dogs and cats, occasionally in horses and sheep, and rarely in other species. The distribution is often uneven, but it is usually most abundant next to the orifices of salivary ducts. Calculus on horses' teeth is chalky and easily removed. In dogs, it is hard, firmly attached, and often discolored. Red-brown to black calculus with a metallic sheen develops in pastured sheep and goats. It usually involves all the incisors, principally on the neck of the buccal surface. Minor amounts are common along the gum–tooth junction of the molar teeth, but occasionally larger (to 2 cm) hard, black, rounded concretions may protrude from between opposed surfaces of the premolars. A high prevalence of calculus in sheep on the Scottish island of North Ronaldsay was related to their predominantly seaweed diet. Calculus was most severe around the cranial cheek teeth, increased in severity with age, was associated with periodontal disease, and contained large amounts of calcium, magnesium, and phosphorus.

Materia alba which adheres to teeth, is a mixture of salivary proteins, desquamated epithelial cells, disintegrating leukocytes, and bacteria. The bacteria are not organized, and materia alba is easily removed. It is distinct from dental plaque, and from food debris, which also accumulates between uncleaned teeth.

a. Dental Caries Dental caries is a disease of the hard tissues of teeth, characterized by demineralization of the inorganic part and enzymatic degradation of the organic matrix. Erosions of teeth are characterized by removal of hard tissues layer by layer. These definitions permit the inclusion of equine infundibular necrosis as a form of caries (see following sections).

Dental caries is the principal disease of teeth in humans to about the age of 30 years. It is then superseded by periodontal disease. Caries is common in horses and sheep but rare in dogs and cats.

There are two types of caries, pit or fissure caries, and smooth-surface caries. The first type develops in irregularities or indentations, which trap food and bacteria, usually on the occlusal surface of the tooth. Plaque is not essential for initiation of this form of caries, of which equine infundibular necrosis is an example. Smooth-surface caries usually occurs on proximal (adjacent) surfaces of teeth, typically just below contact points, or around the neck, and requires dental plaque for its initiation.

The organic acids, principally lactic, which initiate demineralization, are produced by bacterial fermentation of dietary carbohydrates. In smooth-surface caries, plaque produces the acid and maintains a low pH on the surface of the tooth. Progression of lesions depends on various factors such as salivary pH, hardness and resistance to demineralization of enamel, and frequency of access to carbohydrate. Demineralization of enamel occurs often in the subsurface enamel but progresses to caries only with prolonged exposure to acid. Infrequent exposure allows remineralization of enamel between meals. The enzymes which lyse the organic matrix probably are produced by plaque, but may be derived from leukocytes, for which plaque is chemotactic. Carious enamel loses its sheen and becomes dull, white, and pocked. When dentin is exposed, it becomes brown or black. Dentin is softer and more readily demineralized than enamel, and a pinpoint lesion in enamel may lead to a large defect when the carious process reaches the dentin. Nerve endings have not been identified at the enamel–dentin junction, and the pain of caries is thought to be caused by chemical or pressure changes in the dentinal tubules. Spread of infection along the tubules to the pulp cavity may result in formation of secondary or reparative dentin, pulpitis, or tooth loss.

In horses and dogs, caries develops most often on the occlusal surface of the maxillary first molar. In sheep the proximal surfaces of mandibular teeth are usually affected, and caries is commonly accompanied by periodontitis. Cats, whose teeth do not have retaining centers where food can collect, sometimes develop carieslike lesions of the neck region of cheek teeth. Some workers regard these lesions as a form of periodontal disease since the resorptive lesions at the cemento–enamel junction are associated with gingivitis and periodontal destruction including loss of alveolar bone. Attempted repair of the lesions is by deposition of cementum. Carieslike lesions associated with hypervitaminosis A in cats seem to be distinct from conventional caries, but their pathogenesis is not known. Erosions of the neck region of the deciduous teeth occurred in sheep in New Zealand. The lesions were mainly located apical to the enamel–dentin junction on the labial or lingual surface. They did not seem to be related to the usual causes of localized tooth destruction.

The enamel invaginations (infundibula) in the cheek teeth of horses normally are filled with cementum before the teeth erupt. Filling proceeds from the occlusal surface toward the apex, but often is not completed before eruption. At this time the blood supply is cut off, and ischemic necrosis of any residual cementogenic tissue in the infundibula occurs. The deficiency of cementum is called hypoplasia. Anterior infundibula are affected more frequently than are posterior, and the first molar, more often than other teeth (Fig. 1.5A).

Teeth with incompletely filled infundibula may accumulate food material and bacteria (Fig. 1.5B), and in some animals, the necrotic area expands to involve all the cementum and the adjacent enamel and dentin. Decay of the mineralized tissues sometimes progresses to coalescence of the cement lakes, fracture of the tooth, root abscess, and empyema of the paranasal sinuses. The incidence of infundibular necrosis increases with age, and 80–100% of horses older than 12 years may have the lesion. Most are without signs, and in most, the lesion does not progress. Inflammation of the dental pulp, in horses and in other species, may result from direct expansion of caries, or

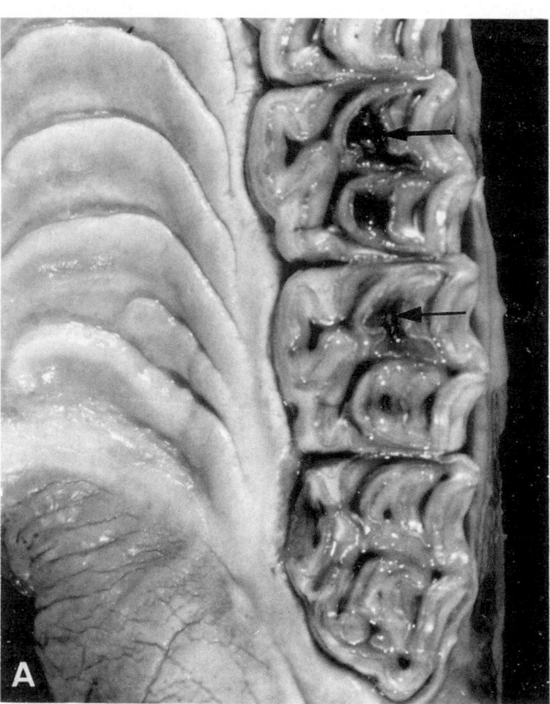

Fig. 1.5A Infundibular necrosis of first and second maxillary molars (arrows). Horse. Necrosis confined to cement lakes.

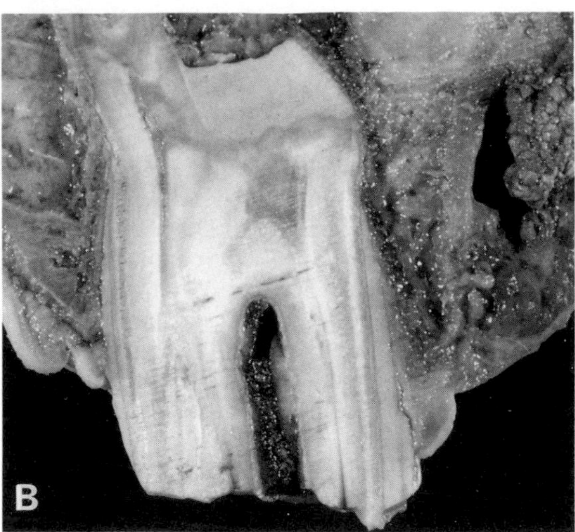

Fig. 1.5B Section through (A) showing black discoloration of infundibulum.

from penetration of bacteria and bacterial degradation products along the dentinal tubules. Production of reparative dentin in the pulp cavity is expected.

b. PULPITIS The dental pulp is derived from the dental papilla. It is surrounded by odontoblasts and dentin, except at the apical foramen, through which vessels and nerves pass. Pulp is a loose syncytium of stellate fibrocytes, and contains histiocytes and undifferentiated mesenchymal cells. The latter are odontoblastic precursors.

The apical foramen is narrow, and this predisposes to vascular occlusion, ischemic necrosis of the pulp, and death of the tooth. Production of abundant secondary dentin and reparative dentin can cause occlusion, but the usual cause is inflammation. Normally pulp is the only vascular tissue of the tooth, and, along with the periodontium, the only site of conventional inflammation. Pulpitis is always related to infection, the effector bacteria or their products entering through fractures, carious perforations (especially in teeth with enamel defects), perforations resulting from abnormal wear or trimming, from periodontitis, and possibly hematogenously. In herbivora, in which the pulp is divided by enamel foldings, inflammation usually is limited to one division, and is usually purulent. Very mild pulpitis may heal, but usually it terminates in necrosis, suppuration, or gangrene.

Inflammation of the pulp may extend to the periodontium and the jaws. Periapical abscess and osteomyelitis of the jaws are complications of pulpitis that may follow clipping the tusks (needle teeth) of piglets. Trimming of the incisor teeth of sheep to avoid the effects of brokenmouth often exposes the pulp cavity, but the pulpitis that ensues is rarely chronic. The exposed pulp canal is healed in 30–50 days by deposition of reparative dentin and secondary dentin. Similar healing presumably occurs in most piglets. Maxillary (malar) abscess of dogs involves the periapical tissues usually of the carnassial tooth, and may cause a discharging sinus beneath the eye. The pathogenesis of the abscess is obscure, but it may be a sequel to crown fractures or to pressure necrosis of periapical tissues. Some chronic inflammations of the pulp are confined to the periodontium and become slowly expansive spherical granulomas about the root apex (root granulomas). Occasionally these granulomas are enclosed by an epithelial cyst (periodontal cyst) derived from cell rests of Malassez. The epithelium contains plasma cells, and the combination may have a protective role in periapical sepsis.

c. Periodontal Disease Periodontal disease is the most common chronic disease of humans, the most common dental disease of sheep and dogs, and an important problem in horses, other ruminants, and cats. Although there are minor differences between species, in general, periodontal disease begins as gingivitis associated with subgingival plaque, and may progress through gingival recession and loss of alveolar bone to chronic periodontitis and exfoliation of teeth.

The gingival sulcus or crevice is an invagination formed by the gingiva as it joins with the tooth surface at the time of eruption. Clinically normal animals have a few lymphocytes, plasma cells, and macrophages under the crevicular epithelium of the gingiva, which forms the outer wall of the crevice, and under the junctional epithelium, which is apposed to the enamel of the tooth.

Clinical **gingivitis** usually is initiated by accumulation of plaque in the crevice, but may be associated with impaction of feed, especially seeds, between teeth. The gingivitis initially is characterized by increased leukocytes and fluid in the gingival crevice, and then by acute exudative inflammation and accumulation of plasma cells, lymphocytes, macrophages, and neutrophils in the marginal gingiva. If the disease progresses, marked loss of gingival collagen occurs in a few days due to the activity of enzymes from neutrophil lysosomes, or possibly from plaque bacteria such as *Bacteroides gingivalis,* which produce a trypsinlike enzyme. Grossly the gingiva is red. Acute gingivitis may become quiescent, with lymphocyte aggregations beneath the junctional epithelium.

Continuation and exacerbations of the inflammation cause apical recession of the tooth–gingiva attachment, and resorption of alveolar bone (Fig. 1.6). Shifts in the periodontal flora may be responsible for these exacerbations. If gingival recession precedes bone loss, the sulcus is deepened to form a periodontal pocket, which is the site of chronic active inflammation. When gingival recession is accompanied by concomitant loss of alveolar bone and gingival collagen, pockets do not form. In either case, destruction of the periodontium, and resorption of alveolar bone, cementum, and root dentin, leads to exfoliation of teeth. In dogs, pocket formation is quite unpredictable and may be present on one root of a tooth and absent on the other. Gingivitis in dogs is unusually proliferative, the gingiva being replaced by collagen-poor, highly vascular granulation tissue, which appears as a red, rolled edge next to the tooth. Bone loss in dogs is often more severe at the bifurcation of two-rooted teeth than in interproximal areas. Resorption of bone is associated with osteitis as the inflammation extends from the periodontium into alveolar bone. In dogs, the premolars and, to a lesser extent the first molars and central incisors, are most severely affected, whereas the second molars and mandibular canines are quite resistant.

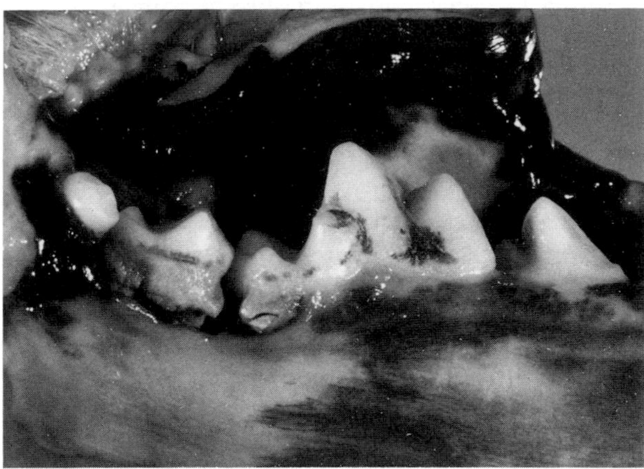

Fig. 1.6 Periodontal disease. Dog. Marked gingival recession with exposure of roots of the molar teeth.

In sheep, periodontal disease may involve all teeth, but the effects are most severe on the incisors, and periodontal disease is a major cause of premature exfoliation. Sheep develop acute gingivitis during tooth eruption, in association with accumulation of subgingival plaque around the tooth. In some sheep chronic gingivitis involving the lingual aspect of the incisors ensues, and on farms with a high incidence of broken-mouth (lengthening of the incisor crown, forward protrusion and loosening of the teeth), this progresses to chronic active periodontal disease.

Cara inchada (swollen face) is a periodontal disease of cattle in the west central part of Brazil. Animals of 2–14 months are mostly affected, and herd prevalences of more than 50% are recorded. When progressive, cara inchada causes loss of teeth leading to malnutrition. It is associated with a variety of Gram-negative bacteria including *Bacteroides melaninogenicus.*

A major part of chronic periodontal disease is resorption of alveolar bone, which modifies the attachment site of the periodontal ligament. Lipopolysaccharides that stimulate bone resorption and inhibit bone collagen production are produced by *Bacteroides gingivalis,* and these could be involved. Evidence that periodontal disease in humans and other animals is primarily a nutritional disease, and that the bone resorption is caused by hyperparathyroidism, has been presented, but is not generally accepted. It seems reasonable, however, that the less bone that is present when the disease is initiated, the more rapid will be the progression of this aspect of the disease.

The sequelae of suppurative periodontitis are many, being variations on a theme of osteomyelitis. The osteomyelitis of actinomycosis is discussed with Bones and Joints (Volume 1, Chapter 1). If the mandible is involved, the fistula usually develops on the ventral margin. If the maxillary molars are involved, fistulation may occur into the maxillary sinus. If the premolars are involved, fistulation may develop into the nasal cavity or externally. In dogs, involvement of the canine teeth may produce internal or external fistulae, and involvement of the maxillary carnassials usually produces a fistula beneath the eye, and orbital inflammation. Fistulation may be prevented for some time or permanently by ossifying periostitis over the involved bone. Fistulae in the upper jaw tend to be persistent. In the lower jaw, they may heal, usually with extensive deposition of new bone. Occasionally, especially in horses, chronic mild periodontitis may be confined by the periodontium, which is, however, expanded by granulation tissue to form a root granuloma. Under the same circumstances there may be hyperplastic exostosis of the cementum.

Bibliography

Baker, J. R., and Britt, D. P. Dental calculus and periodontal disease in sheep. *Vet Rec* **115:** 411–412, 1984.

Bell, A. F. Dental disease in the dog. *J Small Anim Pract* **6:** 421–428, 1965.

Blobel, H. *et al.* Bakteriologische Untersuchungen an der "Cara inchada," einer periodontalen Erkrangung bei Rindern in Brasilien. *Tierarz Umschau* **42:** 152–157, 1987.

Dubielzig, R. R., Higgins, R. J., and Krakowka, S. Lesions of the enamel organ of developing dog teeth following experimental inoculation of gnotobiotic puppies with canine distemper virus. *Vet Pathol* **18:** 684–689, 1981.

Dubielzig, R. R. *et al.* Dental dysplasia and epitheliogenesis imperfecta in a foal. *Vet Pathol* **23:** 325–327, 1986.

Dubielzig, R. R. *et al.* Dental dysplasia in two young uremic dogs. *Vet Pathol* **23:** 333–335, 1986.

Frisken, K. W. *et al.* Black-pigmented *Bacteroides* associated with broken-mouth periodontitis in sheep. *J Periodont Res* **22:** 156–159, 1987.

Harris, M., and Toller, P. The pathogenesis of dental cysts. *Br Med Bull* **31:** 159–163, 1975.

Miles, A. E. W., and Grigson, C. "Colyer's Variations and Diseases of the Teeth of Animals." Cambridge, England, Cambridge University Press, 1990.

Page, R. C., and Schroeder, H. E. Spontaneous chronic periodontitis in adult dogs. A clinical and histopathological survey. *J Periodontol* **52:** 60–73, 1981.

Page, R. C., and Schroeder, H. E. "Peridontitis in Man and Other Animals. A Comparative Review." Basel, Switzerland, S. Karger AG, 1982.

Ranney, R. R. Immunologic mechanisms of pathogenesis in periodontal diseases: An assessment. *J Periodont Res* **26:** 243–254, 1991.

Rieck, G. W. Multiple adamantinogene Zysten der Alveolarfortsatze beim Rind, die *Odontodysplasia cystica congenita,* eine angeborene Erkrankung de Kiefer und des Zahnapparates. *J Vet Med A* **33:** 588–599, 1986.

Schneck, G. W. A case of enamel pearls in a dog. *Vet Rec* **92:** 115–117, 1973.

Socransky, S. S., and Haffajee, A. D. Microbial mechanisms in the pathogenesis of destructive periodontal diseases: A critical assessment. *J Periodont Res* **26:** 195–212, 1991.

Thesleff, I., and Hurmerinta, K. Tissue interactions in tooth development. *Differentiation* **18:** 75–88, 1981.

Thurley, D. C. The pathogenesis of excessive wear in the permanent teeth of sheep. *N Z Vet J* **33:** 24–26, 1985.

Thurley, D. C. Erosion of the nonocclusal surfaces of sheeps' deciduous teeth. *N Z Vet J* **33:** 157–158, 1985.

Verstraete, F. J. M. Anomalous development of the upper third premolar in a dog and a cat. *J S Afr Vet Assoc* **56:** 131–134, 1985.

West, J. L. Enamel hypoplasia of the deciduous incisor teeth of a calf. *Am J Vet Res* **34:** 839–840, 1973.

C. Diseases of the Buccal Cavity and Mucosa

1. Pigmentations

Melanotic pigmentation is normal and common in most breeds of animals and increases with age. It may be irregular, or the mucosa may be entirely pigmented. Diffuse yellow discoloration may be seen in icterus.

2. Circulatory Disturbances

Examination of the mucous membranes is an essential detail in any clinical or autopsy examination. Pallor may indicate anemia but is misleading in a cadaver. In cyanosis, the mucosa is dark reddish blue. The mucosae are muddy in methemoglobinemia. Congestion and edematous swelling of the tongue and buccal mucosa are specific lesions of bluetongue of sheep. An acute congestion and cyanosis associated with ulceration is common in dogs and sometimes in cats in chronic uremia. Hemorrhages are indicative of septicemia, and larger ones may accompany local inflammation, trauma, and the hemorrhagic diatheses. Petechiae on the ventral surface of the tongue and frenulum in horses are consistent with equine infectious anemia, or other thrombocytopenic or purpuric conditions. The active hyperemia which gives the diffuse pink coloration to the mucosa in diffuse stomatitis disappears immediately at death, so that at autopsy the inflamed mucosa is disappointingly blanched.

3. Foreign Bodies in the Oral Cavity

The presence of feed in the mouth of a cadaver is abnormal. In most cases it is attributable to disease, which results in paralysis of deglutition or semiconsciousness. It is common in horses with encephalitis, leukoencephalomalacia, and hepatic encephalopathy. The food in such cases is usually poorly masticated and readily differentiated from that refluxed postmortem. Bones or other large foreign bodies lodged in the pharynx of cattle suggest pica of phosphorus deficiency. They may cause asphyxiation or pressure necrosis in the wall of the pharynx. Large portions of root crops may also lodge in the pharynx. In dogs, bones, sticks, and balls may be found. The bones and sticks tend to be wedged across the palate behind the carnassial teeth.

In dogs a foreign-body stomatitis occurs, caused by

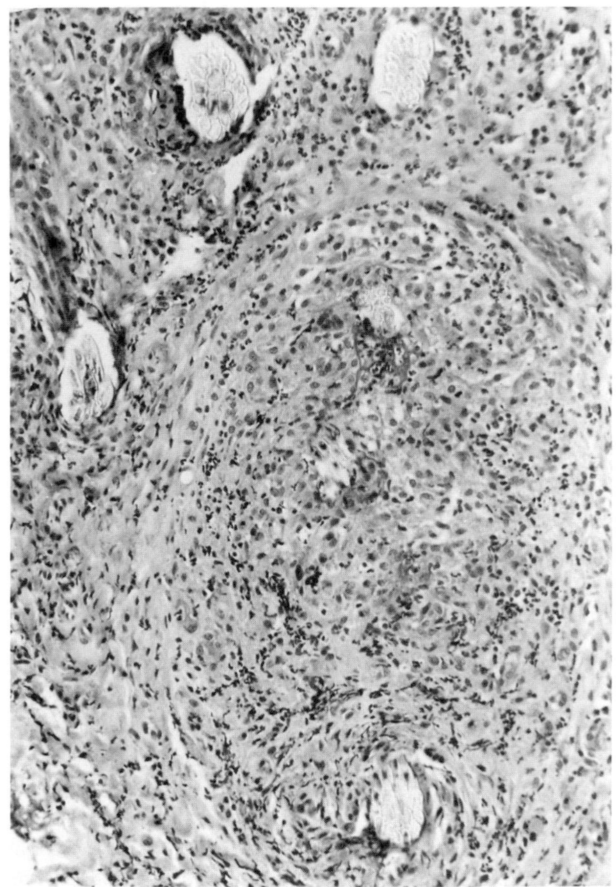

Fig. 1.7 Granulomatous reaction to plant material. Tongue. Dog. Foreign-body glossitis or burr tongue.

plant fibers, burrs, or quills (Fig. 1.7). In mild cases there is a gingivitis surrounding the incisors and canine teeth. Small papules or vesicles and shallow ulcers may be evident on the tongue. Plant fibers may protrude from the lesions. Chronic cases are characterized by exuberant granulomas and gingival hyperplasia with plant fibers deeply embedded in these lesions. Long-haired dogs are especially prone to develop this type of lesion when they attempt to remove plant material that is trapped in their hair coat. The granulomas must be differentiated from neoplasms.

Sharp foreign bodies which cause laceration of the mucosa predispose to necrotic and deep stomatitis. Grass seeds and awns frequently impact between the retracted gingival margin and teeth in periodontitis of ruminants and exacerbate the local initial lesion, perhaps predisposing to the development of osteomyelitis. Horses fed dry triticale hay, a hybrid between wheat and rye grass, may develop severe oral ulceration with masses of awns embedded in the ulcers. The ulcers vary in size from 1 mm to 5 cm in diameter and are mainly located at the junction of the labial and gingival mucosa adjacent to the upper corner incisors, the lingual frenulum, the sublingual folds, the base of the dorsum of the tongue, and the soft palate. Triticale is grown primarily as a grain crop in irrigated areas of Queensland, Australia; it appears to be harmless when grazed by cattle as a forage crop at an early stage of growth.

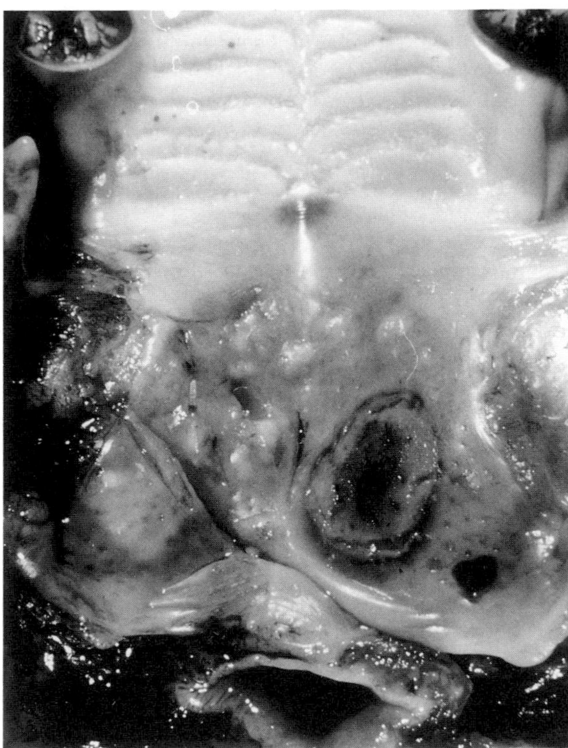

Fig. 1.8 Necrotic palatine tonsillitis. Pig.

Swine have a diverticulum of the pharynx in the posterior wall immediately above the esophagus, and barley awns and other rough plant fibers occasionally lodge here and penetrate the pharynx. This occurs mainly in young pigs, and death follows pharyngeal cellulitis. Similar problems occur in sheep, following improper use of drenching guns, and in cattle injured by balling guns.

4. *Inflammation of the Oral Cavity*

Inflammatory processes of the oral cavity may be diffuse (stomatitis) or localized predominantly in certain regions to produce if (1) the pharynx is involved, pharyngitis; (2) the tongue, glossitis; (3) the gums, gingivitis; (4) the tonsils, tonsillitis (Fig. 1.8); and (5) the soft palate, angina. Lesions limited to the mucosa of the oral cavity are termed superficial stomatitides. Processes seated in connective tissues of the mouth, the deep stomatitides, are usually sequelae to transient superficial lesions.

a. Superficial Stomatitis Inflammatory changes may be associated with ingestion of irritating chemicals such as caustic or toxic compounds. An example is paraquat, a herbicide, which may cause a severe erosive stomatitis in dogs. Dogs that chew on the plant *Dieffenbachia* may develop oral erosions and ulcers. Electrical burns are occasionally seen in puppies or kittens that chew through electrical wires. It is often not possible to differentiate the cause of diffuse stomatitides, but an attempt to do so is important because it may indicate a systemic disease state. Viral diseases causing stomatitis will be considered in detail in the section on Infectious and Parasitic Diseases of the Gastrointestinal Tract (Section VII of this chapter).

Inflammatory disease, localized to the buccal cavity, and not part of systemic viral disease, is also common and important. It is generally due to the indigenous bacterial flora. The oral microbiota ordinarily contains many microbial species, mainly anaerobes such as *Actinomyces, Fusobacterium,* and spirochetes, which exist in balance with each other and in harmony with the host. Disruption of this microfloral balance may lead to stomatitis. The oral mucosa is quite resistant to microbial invasion for several reasons. These include the squamous mucosal lining, antibacterial constituents of saliva such as lysozyme, immunoglobulins, especially immunoglobulin A (IgA), in oral secretions, and the presence of a rich submucosal vascular network and inflammatory cells. Factors altering the balance of indigenous organisms are not well delineated. Systemic illness, stress, and nutritional and hormonal imbalances may alter the microbial population by altering the amount, composition, and pH of saliva. The integrity of the oral epithelium depends on a high rate of epithelial regeneration to balance loss due to a high rate of abrasion and desquamation. Rapid epithelial replication promotes quick healing of superficial lesions.

The lamina propria of the oral epithelium is well vascularized, but generally dense and relatively inelastic. For this reason, there is little distension of lymphatics and tissue spaces with fluid exudate, and therefore, swelling due to edema is not a significant part of stomatitis involving gums and hard palate.

b. Catarrhal Stomatitis Catarrhal stomatitis is a superficial inflammation of the oral mucosa, which usually involves the posterior fauces and may be associated with mild gingivitis. It is a common nonspecific lesion, which often develops in the course of debilitating diseases. The mucosae are hyperemic, and the loose texture of the submucosa in the fauces permits development of edema. The swelling is aggravated by edema and hyperplasia of the abundant lymphoid tissues of the soft palate, tonsil, and pharyngeal mucosa. The epithelium accumulates, producing a dull gray mucosal surface. There is excessive mucus production by palatine glands. Catarrhal stomatitis resolves with the return of normal oral function.

Thrush, or oral candidiasis, occurs most commonly in foals, pigs, and dogs. It involves the proliferation of yeasts and hyphae in the parakeratotic superficial layers of the oral epithelium. It appears grossly as patchy pale pseudomembranous material on the oral mucosa and back of the tongue, and probably reflects alterations in epithelial turnover and oral flora (see Infectious and Parasitic Diseases of the Gastrointestinal Tract, Section VII of this chapter). Gingivitis and ulceration of the oral mucosa may, in dogs, be associated with infection due to *Nocardia* spp.

c. Vesicular Stomatitides Stomatitis, characterized by the formation of vesicles, occurs in most species of domestic animals. The vesicles develop as accumulations of serous fluid within the epithelium or between the epithelium and the lamina propria. These may coalesce to form bullae, and the elevated epithelium is easily rubbed off during chewing to leave raw eroded patches with bits of epithelium still adherent. The transition from vesicle to erosion occurs rapidly so that, in individual animals, vesicles may not be seen. This is especially so in dogs and cats because the oral mucosa is very thin. Because the basal epithelium or basement membrane remains intact, regeneration and healing are complete in a few days unless the local lesions are complicated by bacterial or mycotic infections. However, foci of previous erosion may be identifiable for some months by their slight depression and lack of pigmentation.

Traditionally vesicular stomatitides in animals were mainly associated with viral infections, and these are still the most important causes. In horses, ruminants, and swine, oral vesicles should be regarded, in the appropriate species, as indicating one of the vesicular diseases that the species is susceptible to until proven otherwise (see Infectious and Parasitic Diseases of the Gastrointestinal Tract, Section VII of this chapter). In swine, sunburn and lesions associated with porcine parvovirus infection may cause lesions of the snout resembling vesicular diseases. Bullous immune skin diseases are recognized with increased frequency, especially in dogs, and some of these have severe oral lesions, which will be described here; (see also The Skin and Appendages, Volume 1, Chapter 5).

Pemphigus vulgaris is a severe, acute or chronic, vesicular, bullous autoimmune disease. It is characterized by acantholysis of the epidermis, which results in formation of flaccid bullae and erosions involving mainly mucocutaneous junctions, oral mucosa and, to a lesser extent, skin. The disease is similar, if not identical, to pemphigus vulgaris in humans. Clinically affected dogs and cats show excessive salivation, halitosis, and erosions and ulcerations of the oral mucosa. The oral lesions are generally more prominent than, and precede, the skin lesions. They are most obvious on the dorsal surface of the tongue, which is bright red with a few scattered pink raised areas representing islands of normal mucosa. The lesions vary greatly in severity and distribution, although the hard palate is often severely ulcerated. Bullae are rarely seen in the oral cavity because they ulcerate rapidly.

Microscopically, the earliest lesion consists of suprabasilar acantholysis, which is followed by the formation of clefts. These lead to ulceration of the mucosa. The basal cells of the epidermis remain attached to the basement membrane and form a so-called row of tombstones. A few neutrophils and eosinophils may infiltrate the epithelium.

There is a variable lymphocytic and plasmacytic lichenoid reaction in the propria.

The presence of suprabasilar clefts and bullae due to acantholysis is considered to be diagnostic of pemphigus vulgaris. However, extensive erosion and ulceration of the mucosa and secondary bacterial infections frequently obscure these clefts and bullae. Several biopsies from different areas of the oral mucosa may be required to demonstrate the characteristic lesions. A presumptive histologic diagnosis should be supported by direct immunofluorescence tests which show autoantibodies (usually IgG) and complement in the intercellular spaces of stratified squamous epithelium.

Bullous pemphigoid is characterized by mucocutaneous, superficial vesicobullous or ulcerative disease of mucous membranes (including the oral mucosa) and skin. Clinically the disease is often impossible to distinguish from pemphigus vulgaris. Bullous pemphigoid has been reported in humans, horses, dogs, and possibly cats. The characteristic microscopic lesions are transient subepidermal blisters, which may contain fibrinocellular exudate. Acantholysis is not a feature of the lesion. Direct immunofluorescence of lesions shows autoantibody (IgG) and complement deposits along the basement membrane.

The oral lesions of pemphigus vulgaris and bullous pemphigoid must be differentiated from lesions due to trauma, toxic epidermal necrolysis, drug eruptions, chronic uremia, mucocutaneous candidiasis, and lymphoreticular malignancies.

Feline calicivirus belongs to the Picornaviridae and causes mainly a respiratory infection in cats. The disease is complicated by lingual and oropharyngeal ulcers, which start out as vesicles. They are 5–10 mm in diameter, smooth, and well demarcated from the surrounding normal mucosa. They occur mainly on the anterodorsal and lateral surfaces of the tongue and each side of the midline of the hard palate. The palatine lesions are apparently more severe in cats fed dry food. Microscopically, the earliest lesions consist of foci of pyknotic cells in the stratum corneum and superficial stratum spinosum. They progress to foci of necrosis with vesicle formation and subsequent erosion and ulceration of the mucosa. Regeneration of the oral mucosa in the ulcerated areas generally occurs within 10–12 days. A single layer of squamous epithelial cells extends from the margins of the ulcer beneath a layer of exudate. Active viral replication also takes place in the tonsillar crypt epithelial cells, and virus may be recovered from these areas for weeks postinfection. Inclusions have not been observed in oral epithelial cells. The virus is isolated from a high percentage of cats with chronic stomatitis, as discussed in the following section.

d. Erosive and Ulcerative Stomatitides This form of stomatitis is characterized by local epithelial defects of the oral mucosa and nasolabium and is usually associated with acute diffuse stomatitis and pharyngitis. Erosions are circumscribed areas of loss of epithelium which leave the stratum germinativum and basement membrane more or less intact. They are usually associated with acute inflammation in the underlying propria. The erosions vary in size and shape, and although they are often a nonspecific development in a wide variety of conditions, they are also an essential part of a number of important diseases. They heal cleanly and quickly, but if secondarily infected or complicated, may develop into ulcers.

Ulcers, in contrast to erosions, are deeper deficiencies which extend into the substantia propria. They too vary greatly in size and shape; the edges tend to be elevated and ragged, and when they heal, it is with scar formation.

The causes of ulcerative stomatitis are in general those of erosive stomatitis. There are, however, a number of recognized syndromes and specific diseases in which the predominant change is ulcerative. Phenylbutazone intoxication in horses may cause oral ulcers in concert with ulcers of the stomach, intestine, and colon; the syndrome is discussed fully with ischemic diseases of the gut. Erosive/ulcerative conditions are discussed in succeeding paragraphs.

Feline ulcerative stomatitis and glossitis is an ulcerative and chronic inflammation of the mucosa of the fauces, the angle of the jaws and, less commonly, the hard palate, gingiva, and tongue. It is more common in older cats. These lesions may form the largest group of feline oral clinical conditions. The cause is unknown, but is probably multifactorial, involving imbalance in the oral microbial flora, with predominance of spirochetes.

Some workers have reported the isolation of feline calicivirus from a significant number of cats with lesions of chronic stomatitis compared to those of controls. The role of this virus in the etiology of this disease remains to be resolved. Feline leukemia and feline immunodeficiency viruses may predispose some cats to chronic stomatitis because of their immunosuppressive effects. Microscopically, there is chronic active inflammation of the oral mucosa and submucosal connective tissues.

Feline plasma cell gingivitis–pharyngitis is characterized by raised erythematous, proliferative lesions, mainly in the glossopalatine arches, extending caudally to the palatopharyngeal arch and cranially to the gingiva. Microscopically the lesions are characterized by a hyperplastic and frequently ulcerated mucosa, with a marked submucosal inflammatory cell reaction, mainly plasmacytes, including binucleate cells and cells containing Russell bodies. Neutrophils, lymphocytes, and histiocytes are scattered among the plasma cells. Affected cats have elevated serum gamma globulin levels. The polyclonal gammopathy and the plasmacytic, lymphocytic reaction are suggestive of an immune-mediated lesion.

Eosinophilic ulcer (eosinophilic granuloma, lick granuloma, labial ulcer, rodent ulcer) is a chronic, superficial ulcerative lesion of the mucocutaneous junctions of the lips, and to a lesser extent, the oral mucosa and skin, in cats of all ages. The cause is unknown but the lesions may respond to corticosteroid, oral progestagens, cryosurgery, or radiation therapy, although recurrences are common.

Typically, well-demarcated, red-brown, shallow ulcers,

often with elevated margins, occur on the upper lip on either side of the midline. They are usually a few millimeters wide and several centimeters long. Occasionally, ulcers are present elsewhere in the mouth, such as on the gums, palate, pharynx, and tongue. Skin lesions are located in those areas which are frequently licked, such as the neck, lumbar area, and abdomen. Microscopically, eosinophilic ulcer is characterized by ulceration of the squamous mucosa, with large areas of necrosis of the underlying connective tissues, accompanied by a marked inflammatory cell reaction. The cellular reaction consists predominantly of neutrophils at the periphery of the ulcers, with a mainly mononuclear cell reaction (plasma cells and mast cells) in the propria, eosinophils and histiocytes being only occasionally seen. In some cases, the eosinophils and mast cells may predominate, but this difference may be a reflection only of the evolution of the lesion.

Eosinophilic ulcer is considered to be one of the three different types of lesions that have been associated with the so-called eosinophilic granuloma complex. The other two conditions, eosinophilic plaque and linear granuloma, cause mainly skin lesions, which are different clinically and morphologically from eosinophilic ulcer. The differences are discussed in The Skin and Appendages (Volume 1, Chapter 5).

Oral eosinophilic granuloma (linear granuloma) in dogs occurs as a familial disease in young Siberian huskies. Sporadic cases have been reported in other breeds. Affected dogs have single or multiple firm, often ulcerated, raised plaques, which are covered by a yellow-brown exudate, on the lateral or ventral surfaces of the tongue. Lesions on the soft palate are less common, and here they tend to be oval to circular ulcers with slightly elevated borders. Cytologic preparations made from scrapings of the oral lesions show many eosinophils, a few neutrophils, occasional macrophages, and epithelial cells.

Microscopically, the lesions are characterized by foci of collagenolysis (necrobiosis), in the mid and deep zones of the lingual submucosa, which are surrounded by a mainly histiocytic granulomatous inflammatory reaction, with giant cells, lymphocytes, plasma cells, and mast cells. Eosinophils are a constant feature, but their numbers vary from few to many. The lesions are identical to those seen in linear granuloma of cats.

The cause is unknown, although the morphology of the lesion and the response to corticosteroid therapy are suggestive of hypersensitivity. The familial tendency in Siberian huskies indicates that hereditary factors are involved. Eosinophilic granuloma must be differentiated from oral mast cell tumors, which also affect the tongue in dogs. Necrobiosis of collagen fibers is often a feature of mast cell tumors; however, in mastocytoma, the characteristic mixture of mast cells and eosinophils infiltrates the tongue and connective tissues more diffusely. The mast cells may be in various stages of degranulation, and inflammation is minimal or absent in mast cell tumors.

Horses with eosinophilic epitheliotropic disease (see The Skin and Appendages, Volume 1, Chapter 5 and Eosinophilic gastroenteritis, this chapter) may also have eosinophilic stomatitis and lingual ulceration.

Cyclic hematopoiesis (gray collie syndrome), discussed with The Hematopoietic System (Volume 3, Chapter 2), may cause recurring oral ulcers in silver-gray collies.

Feline viral rhinotracheitis is a common upper respiratory tract infection of cats caused by feline herpesvirus-1 (see The Respiratory System, Chapter 6 of this volume). This virus may cause ulcerative lesions in the mouth, especially on the tongue. Rarely, oral and skin ulcers may occur, without evidence of concurrent respiratory tract infection. Microscopic lesions are characterized by foci of cytoplasmic vacuolation in squamous epithelium, which evolve into areas of necrosis and ulceration. The ulcers are often covered by a layer of fibrinocellular exudate. Herpetic inclusions may be present in epithelial cells at the periphery of the ulcers.

Uremia associated with chronic renal disease often causes fetid ulcerative stomatitis in dogs, and less commonly in cats. The buccal mucosa, and especially the tongue, are deeply cyanotic. Dirty grayish-brown ulcers occur on the gums, lateral surface and margin of the tongue, and on the inner surface of the lips and cheeks. The margins of the ulcers are swollen and hyperemic.

The pathogenesis of the oral lesions in uremia is still poorly understood. Elevations in blood and salivary urea levels may predispose to bacterial infection, and urease-producing bacteria, normally present in the oral microflora, generate ammonia from salivary urea. Ammonia has a caustic effect on the oral mucous membranes. This may explain why the lesions are located mainly where salivary ducts enter the oral cavity, or in proximity to teeth, on which bacterial plaque or calculus is present. There is apparently a poor correlation between the levels of blood urea nitrogen and the development of uremic stomatitis, suggesting that other factors, such as a decreased local and systemic immune response, are involved in its pathogenesis.

Salivary glucose levels may be elevated in dogs and cats with diabetes mellitus, resulting in an imbalance of the oral microflora and explaining chronic gingivitis in diabetic animals.

Ulcerative glossitis and stomatitis in swine is commonly part of **exudative epidermitis** (greasy pig disease) of preweaning pigs (see The Skin and Appendages, Volume 1, Chapter 5). In addition to the characteristic skin lesions, about a third of the piglets may develop ulcers on the dorsum of tongue. Erosions and ulcers of the hard palate occur in a small number of piglets. Microscopically, there is ulceration of the squamous mucosa with coagulation necrosis, and vesicle and pustule formation in the superficial epithelium over the rete pegs. A pleocellular inflammatory reaction is evident in the connective tissue below the ulcers.

Oral erosions and ulcers have been reported in pigs with congenital swinepox. Microscopically, there is swelling and degeneration of squamous epithelial cells with numerous eosinophilic intracytoplasmic inclusions. The central areas of the lesions are necrotic. There is a mixture of lymphocytes, neutrophils, eosinophils, and histiocytes in the submucosa. Poxvirus may be demonstrated by electron-microscopic examination of the lesions.

Bibliography

Ackerman, L. J. Canine and feline pemphigus and pemphigoid. Part I. Pemphigus. Part II. Pemphigoid. *Compend Cont Ed Pract Vet* **7:** 89–98, and 281–286, 1985.

Andrews, J. J. Ulcerative glossitis and stomatitis associated with exudative epidermitis in suckling swine. *Vet Pathol* **16:** 432–437, 1979.

Arnbjerg, A. *Pasteurella multocida* from canine and feline teeth, with a case report of glossitis calcinosa in a dog caused by *P. multocida*. *Nord Vet Med* **30:** 324–332, 1978.

Baker, G. J. *et al.* Oral dermatophilosis in a cat: A case report. *J Small Anim Pract* **13:** 649–653, 1972.

Borst, G. H. A. *et al.* Four sporadic cases of congenital swinepox. *Vet Rec* **127:** 61–63, 1990.

Crandell, R. A. Feline viral rhinotracheitis (FVR). *Adv Vet Sci Comp Med* **17:** 201–224, 1973.

Evermann, J. F. *et al.* Isolation of a calicivirus from a case of canine glossitis. *Canine Pract* **8:** 36–39, 1981.

Gaskell, R. M., and Gruffydd-Jones, T. J. Intractible feline stomatitis. *Vet Annu* **17:** 195–199, 1977.

Gaskell, C. J., and Gruffydd-Jones, T. J. The alimentary system. *In* "Feline Medical Therapy," E. A. Chandler, C. J. Gaskell, and A. D. R. Gilberg (eds.), pp. 158–175. Oxford, England, Blackwell Scientific Publications. 1985.

Gaskell, C. J. *et al.* Chronic stomatitis in the cat. *Vet Annu* **28:** 246–250, 1988.

Gillespie, J. H., and Scott, F. W. Feline viral infections. *Adv Vet Sci Comp Med* **17:** 163–200, 1973.

Gupta, P. P., and Tisha, B. P. Oral dermatophilosis associated with actinomycosis in cattle. *Zentralbl Veterinaermed [B]* **25:** 211–215, 1978.

Hoover, E. A., and Kahn, D. E. Lesions produced by feline picornaviruses of different virulence in pathogen-free cats. *Vet Pathol* **10:** 307–322, 1973.

Hoskins, W. J., and Potten, C. S. Advances in epithelial kinetics—An oral view. *J Oral Pathol* **8:** 3–22, 1979.

Johnessee, J. S., and Hurvitz, A. I. Feline plasma cell gingivitis–pharyngitis. *J Am Anim Hosp Assoc* **19:** 179–181, 1983.

Johnson, R. P., and Povey, R. C. Effect of diet on oral lesions of feline calicivirus infection. *Vet Rec* **110:** 106–107, 1982.

Kaplan, M. L., and Jeffcoat, M. K. Acute necrotizing ulcerative gingivitis. *Canine Pract* **5:** 35–38, 1978.

Kharole, M. U. *et al.* Oral streptothricosis in cow calves and a buffalo calf. *Indian J Anim Sci* **45:** 119–122, 1975.

Knowles, J. O. *et al.* Prevalence of feline calicivirus, feline leukaemia virus, and antibodies to FIV in cats with chronic stomatitis. *Vet Rec* **124:** 336–338, 1989.

MacDonald, J. M. Stomatitis. *Vet Clin North Am: Small Anim Pract* **13:** 415–436, 1983.

McCosker, J. E., and Keenan, D. M. Ulcerative stomatitis in horses and cattle caused by triticale hay. *Aust Vet J* **60:** 259, 1983.

McKeever, P. J., and Klausner, J. S. Plant awn, candidal, nocardial, and necrotizing ulcerative stomatitis in the dog. *J Am Anim Hosp Assoc* **22:** 17–24, 1986.

Mebus, C. A. *et al.* Exudative epidermitis. *Pathol Vet* **5:** 146–163, 1968.

Nesbitt, G. H., and Schmitz, J. A. Contact dermatitis in the dog: A review of 35 cases. *J Am Anim Hosp Assoc* **13:** 155–163, 1977.

Neufeld, J. L. *et al.* Eosinophilic granuloma in a cat. Recovery of virus particles. *Vet Pathol* **17:** 97–99, 1980.

Parker, W. M. Autoimmune skin diseases in the dog. *Can Vet J* **22:** 302–304, 1982.

Potter, A. Eosinophilic granuloma of Siberian huskies. *J Am Anim Hosp Assoc* **16:** 595–600, 1980.

Povey, R. C. A review of feline viral rhinotracheitis (feline herpesvirus 1 infection). *Comp Immunol Microbiol Infect Dis* **2:** 373–387, 1979.

Povey, R. C., and Hale, C. J. Experimental infections with feline caliciviruses (picornaviruses) in specific pathogen-free kittens. *J Comp Pathol* **84:** 245–256, 1974.

Scott, D. W. *et al.* The comparative pathology of nonviral bullous skin diseases in domestic animals. *Vet Pathol* **17:** 257–281, 1980.

Thompson, R. R. *et al.* Association of calicivirus infection with chronic gingivitis and pharyngitis in cats. *J Small Anim Pract* **25:** 207–210, 1984.

Walsh, K. M. Oral eosinophilic granuloma in two dogs. *J Am Vet Med Assoc* **183:** 323–324, 1983.

e. DEEP STOMATITIDES Lesions of the oral mucosa may permit the entry of pyogenic bacteria, often normal oral flora, into the connective tissues of the submucosa and muscle. Purulent inflammation or cellulitis may develop in the lips, tongue, cheek, soft palate, and pharynx. Abscesses may form and may fistulate through the mucosa or skin. Abscesses in the wall of the pharynx may result from necrosis of retropharyngeal lymph nodes. Necrotic stomatitis with simple necrosis of the epithelium and lamina propria may be produced by thermal or chemical agencies, but, in animals, it is usually caused by *Fusobacterium necrophorum* and other anaerobes.

i. *Oral Necrobacillosis* *Fusobacterium necrophorum* is the principal cause of **oral necrobacillosis** or **necrotic stomatitis** in animals. It is also associated with necrotizing lesions elsewhere in the upper and lower alimentary tract, and liver. Wherever it occurs, it is usually a secondary invader following previous mucosal damage. The organism produces a variety of exo- and endotoxins, whose exact role in the pathogenesis of the lesions has yet to be determined. The exotoxins include leukocidins, hemolysins, and a cytoplasmic toxin, all of which probably enhance the necrotizing ability of the organism. Once established in a suitable focus, *F. necrophorum* proliferates, causing extensive coagulation necrosis.

The best-known form of necrobacillary stomatitis is calf diphtheria, an acute necrotizing ulcerative inflammation of the buccal and pharyngeal mucosa. The predisposing lesions may include trauma, infectious bovine rhinotracheitis, and papular stomatitis. Necrosis of palatine and pharyngeal tonsils may be seen. The incidence of diphtheria in slaughtered beef cattle may be as high as 1.4%. The same syndrome is rather common in housed lambs as a complication of contagious ecthyma. The infection also may be initiated in the gums about erupting teeth in any species, and by the trauma produced in baby pigs by removing the needle teeth (Fig. 1.9A). It is frequently fatal in young animals, in which extension often occurs to other organs. In adults, oral necrobacillosis tends to remain localized to the oral cavity, where it may complicate vesicular and ulcerative stomatitides. It is not unusual, however, for the infection to spread down the alimentary tract. In the lower alimentary tract, the Peyer's patches especially are involved, perhaps as a complication of bovine virus diarrhea.

The early lesions are large, well-demarcated, yellowish-gray, dry areas of necrosis, surrounded by a zone of hyperemia (Fig. 1.9B). They are found on the sides or dorsal groove of the tongue, on the cheeks, gums, palate, and pharynx, especially the recesses beside the larynx. Primary foci may occur in the laryngeal ventricles. Death may be associated with asphyxia. The necrotic tissue projects slightly above the normal surface and is friable but adherent and is not easily detached. In time it may slough and leave deep ulcers, which may heal by granulation. The necrotic tissues are histologically structureless and are surrounded at first by a zone of vascular reaction, later by a dense but narrow rim of leukocytes, and later still by thick encapsulating granulation tissue. The bacteria are arranged in long filaments, particularly at the advancing edge of the lesions. The submucosal extension of the lesions may take them deeply into the underlying soft tissues and bone.

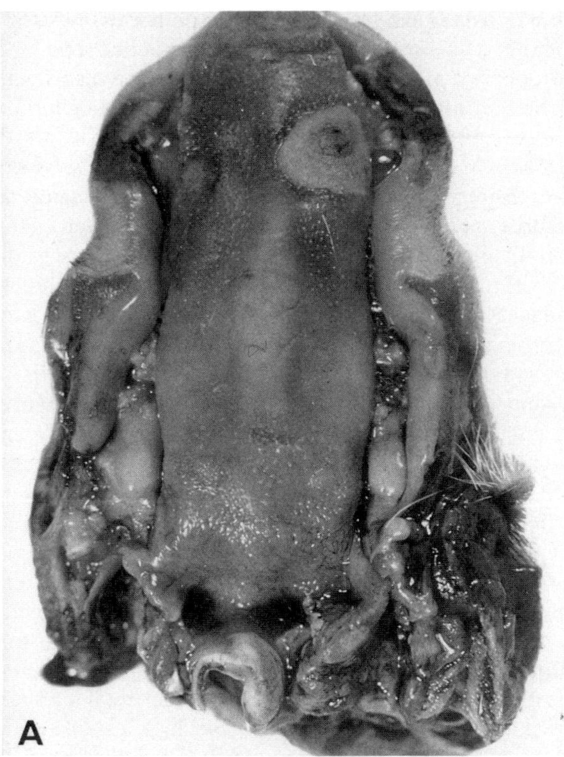

Fig. 1.9A Necrotic glossitis and stomatitis. Pig. *Fusobacterium necrophorum* infection associated with trauma by needle teeth.

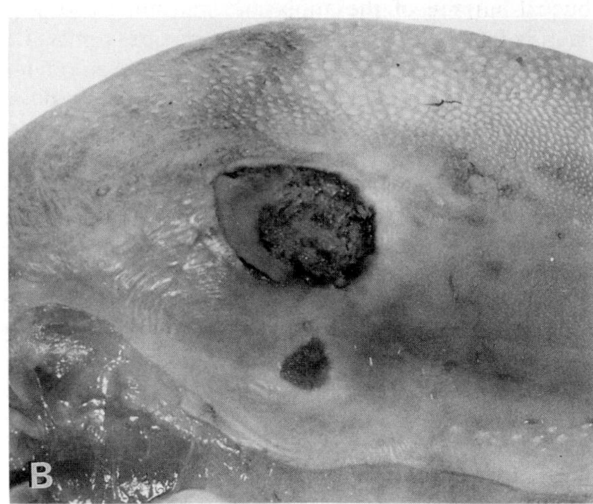

Fig. 1.9B Lingual necrobacillosis. Calf.

Spread from the oral foci occurs down the trachea (causing aspiration pneumonia), down the esophagus, and via blood vessels. Death may occur acutely in septicemia with only multiple small serosal hemorrhages as evidence, or metastases may occur in other tissue. Venous drainage from the face to the vascular sinuses of the meninges may lead to pituitary and cerebral abscessation.

Fusobacterium necrophorum has also been associated with a syndrome of necrotic stomatitis, enteritis, and granulocytopenia in calves. Affected calves have a nonregenerative anemia, leukopenia, absolute neutropenia, hypoproteinemia, and increased fibrinogen levels. In addition to the characteristic oral lesions, there is marked depletion of lymphoid tissues and necrotic enteritis. *Fusobacterium*-like organisms are present in large numbers in a variety of organs including the bone marrow. Possibly very virulent strains of *F. necrophorum* produce enough leukotoxins, especially in immunodeficient calves, to suppress bone marrow activity.

A gross diagnosis of oral necrobacillosis is ordinarily possible, but may be confirmed by a smear from the margin of the lesion. The organism is difficult to cultivate because of its strict anaerobiasis.

ii. *Noma* This is a rapidly spreading pseudomembranous or gangrenous stomatitis; it is not caused by a specific pathogen but is associated with tissue invasion by the normal oral flora, particularly spirochetes and fusiforms. The predisposing factors are unknown, but they are probably nonspecific and associated with mucosal trauma and debility. The disease, which is observed occasionally in horses, dogs, and monkeys, is in many respects similar to oral necrobacillosis. In the lesions, the spirochetes can be found in large numbers at the advancing margins as well as in peripheral viable tissue. In the deep layers of necrosis, fusiforms predominate, and toward the surface, there is a variety of other organisms, chiefly cocci.

The initial lesion is a small tattered ulcer of the cheek or gum, which spreads rapidly and may involve much of the buccal surface of the gums and the mucosa of the cheek. It is intensely fetid and consists of a dirty necrotic pseudomembrane surrounded by a zone of acute inflammation. The necrotic tissue may slough to leave deep ulcers; the cheek may be perforated to leave a gaping defect, or gangrene may supervene.

iii. *Actinobacillosis* This is a deep stomatitis caused in cattle by *Actinobacillus lignieresii,* a member of the normal oral flora. When introduced into the submucosa, it causes pyogranulomatous inflammatory foci centered on club colonies containing Gram-negative coccobacilli. Morphologically similar lesions may be caused by a variety of organisms (Fig. 1.10). *Actinomyces* (*Corynebacterium*) *pyogenes* may be isolated from lingual ulcers and granulomas in lambs. Microscopic examination of these lesions reveals well-demarcated submucosal granulomas with plant fibers in the center, surrounded by a marked neutrophilic reaction. The organisms most likely gain entry after the mucosa is damaged by hard fibrous plant fibers from the weed lambsleeve sage (*Salvia reflexa*), present in the bedding. *Actinomyces bovis,* a Gram-positive filamentous organism, causes pyogranulomatous mandibular and maxillary osteomyelitis in cattle, and mastitis in sows. Staphylococci may cause pyogranulomatous lesions (botryomycosis) in any species, especially mastitis in sows. Less-common causes of similar microscopic lesions include *Nocardia* and the various agents associated with mycetomas (see The Skin and Appendages, Volume 1, Chapter 5).

Actinobacillosis is typically a disease of soft tissue, spreading as a lymphangitis and usually involving the regional lymph nodes. This distinguishes it from actinomycosis, which causes bone lesions. The tongue is often involved in actinobacillosis, and the chronic condition produces clinical wooden tongue.

Entry of actinobacilli to the tongue may be gained through traumatic erosions along its sides, but often the primary lesion is in the lingual groove. Here, trapped grass seeds and awns may provoke the initial trauma. Lesions elsewhere in the soft tissue of the mouth may be attributed to disruption of the mucosa by similar types of insults, and eruption of, or abrasion by, teeth.

Microscopically, the lesion is a pyogranuloma, centered on a mass of coccobacilli, surrounded by radiating eosinophilic clubs, probably made up of immune complexes (Fig. 1.11). The club colonies, in turn, are surrounded by variable numbers of neutrophils, and are invested by macrophages or giant cells. Lymphocytic and plasmacytic infiltrates are present in the surrounding reactive fibrous stroma or granulation tissue. An individual inflammatory focus appears grossly as a nodular, firm, pale, fibrous mass a few millimeters to one centimeter in diameter containing in the center minute yellow "sulfur" granules, which are the club colonies.

Actinobacillosis causes a lymphangitis, and lymphogenous spread is common. Affected lymphatics are thickened, and nodules are distributed along their course. This distribution is best seen beneath the mucosa of the dorsum and the lateral surface of the tongue and can often be traced through to the pharyngeal lymphoid tissue (Fig. 1.12A,B). Some of these more superficial nodules erode the overlying epithelium, and coalescence may produce quite large ulcers. The most common form of lingual actinobacillosis consists of granulation tissue in which are embedded many small abscesses surrounded by a dense connective tissue capsule. The epithelium overlying these large granulomas may be intact or ulcerated. Diffuse sclerosing actinobacillosis of the tongue (wooden tongue) is firm, because of extensive proliferation of connective tissue, which replaces the muscle fibers. Granulomatous nodules are sparsely scattered in the fibrous stroma.

Although actinobacillosis in cattle is best known as a disease of the tongue, the infection may occur in any of the exposed soft tissues, especially those of mouth and neck; occasionally it involves the wall of the forestomachs, any portion of skin, and the lungs. Lesions in these sites resemble those described in the tongue.

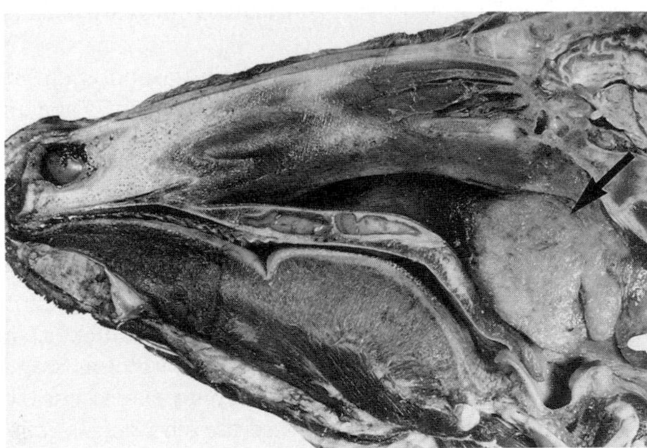

Fig. 1.10 Pharyngeal actinomycosis. Cow. Fleshy mass in pharynx (arrow), which resembles actinobacillosis.

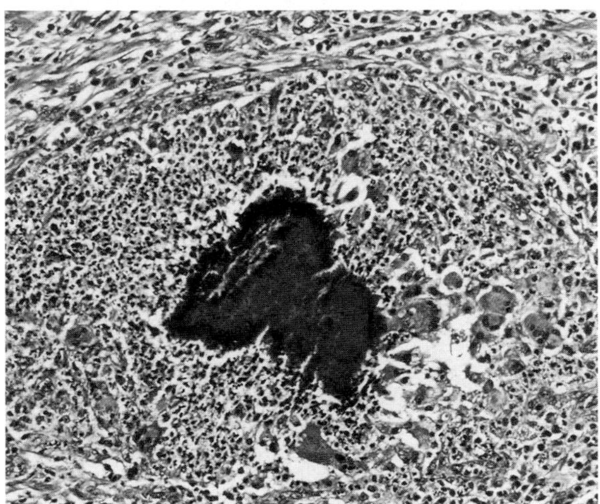

Fig. 1.11 Actinobacillosis. Cow. Pyogranulomatous focus containing club colony of *Actinobacillus lignieresii*.

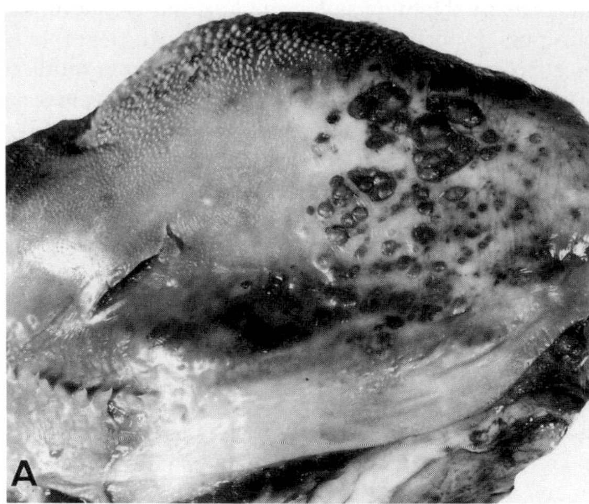

Fig. 1.12A Actinobacillosis. Cow. Granulomas bulging on lateral surface of tongue.

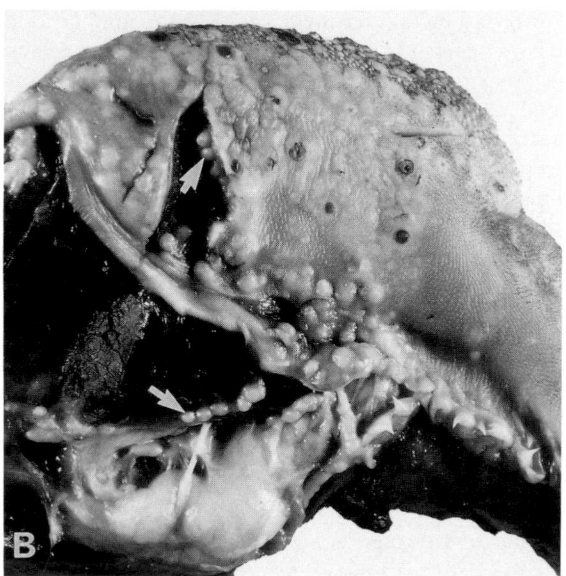

Fig. 1.12B Actinobacillosis. Cow. Granulomatous nodules (arrows) along course of lymphatics.

Actinobacillosis causes regional lymphadenitis. The cut surface of the node reveals small, soft yellow or orange granulomatous masses, which project somewhat above the capsular contour and which contain "sulfur" granules. There is also sclerosing inflammation of the surrounding tissues, which may cause adhesion to overlying skin or mucous membranes. The retropharyngeal and submaxillary nodes are most often affected, as well as the lymphoid tissues of the submucosa of the soft palate and pharynx. Involvement of the pharynx and the retropharyngeal lymph nodes may cause dyspnea and dysphagia.

Oral actinobacillosis in swine causes lesions similar to those in cattle, including glossitis. Actinobacillosis may also occur sporadically or as outbreaks in sheep, but in this species the tongue seems to be exempt. The characteristic lesions in sheep occur in the subcutaneous tissue of the head, especially of the cheeks, nose, lips, and submaxillary and throat regions, and on the nasal turbinates. They may also occur on the soft palate and pharynx as complications of wounds received at drenching. The organism has been isolated from a horse with a greatly enlarged tongue.

iv. *Oral Dermatophilosis of Cats* This is caused by *Dermatophilus congolensis*, a bacterium which commonly causes an exudative dermatitis in a wide variety of species (see The Skin and Appendages, Volume 1, Chapter 5). In cats, the organism is uncommonly associated with oral granulomas, especially affecting the tongue and tonsillar crypt. Large numbers of Gram-positive, filamentous, branching organisms, with longitudinal and transverse divisions, may be demonstrated in the necrotic centers of submucosal granulomas. The organisms are most likely to enter through damaged mucosa. The lesion must be differentiated from the more common squamous cell carcinomas of the tongue. In cattle, cutaneous streptothricosis involving the muzzle may extend into the oral cavity.

Bibliography

Baum, K. H. *et al.* Isolation of *Actinobacillus lignieresii* from enlarged tongue of a horse. *J Am Vet Med Assoc* **185:** 792–793, 1984.

Davis, C. L., and Stiles, G. W. Actinobacillosis in rams. *J Am Vet Med Assoc* **95:** 754–756, 1939.

Emery, D. L. *et al.* Biochemical and functional properties of a leucocidin produced by several strains of *Fusobacterium necrophorum*. *Aust Vet J* **61:** 382–387, 1984.

Hayston, J. T. Actinobacillosis in sheep. *Aust Vet J* **24:** 64–66, 1948.

Jensen, R. *et al.* Laryngeal diphtheria and papillomatosis in feedlot cattle. *Vet Pathol* **18:** 143–150, 1981.

Johnston, K. G. Nasal actinobacillosis in a sheep. *Aust Vet J* **30:** 105–106, 1954.

Langworth, B. F. *Fusobacterium necrophorum:* Its characteristics and role as an animal pathogen. *Bacteriol Rev* **41:** 373–390, 1977.

M'Fadyean, J. Actinomycosis and actinobacillosis. *J Comp Pathol* **45:** 93–105, 1932.

Newsom, I. E., and Cross, F. Some complications of sore mouth in lambs. *J Am Vet Med Assoc* **78:** 539–544, 1931.

Nimmo-Wilkie, J. S., and Radostits, O. Fusobacteremia in a calf with necrotic stomatitis, enteritis, and granulocytopenia. *Can Vet J* **22:** 166–170, 1981.

Rossiter, D. L. *et al.* Lingual abscesses in suckling and weaned lambs. *J Am Vet Med Assoc* **185:** 1552, 1984.

Till, D. H., and Palmer, F. P. A review of actinobacillosis with a study of the causal organism. *Vet Rec* **72:** 527–533, 1960.

5. *Parasitic Diseases of the Oral Cavity*

These are of minor significance. Sarcosporidiosis and cysticercosis occur in the striated muscles of the tongue and produce the same lesions as they do elsewhere (see Muscle and Tendons, Volume 1, Chapter 2). *Trichinella spiralis* may be found in muscles of the tongue and mastication. *Gongylonema* spp. are found in the mucosal lining of the tongue, especially in swine allowed to graze, and less commonly in cattle and sheep. They evoke little or no inflammation of the mucosa, but a mild to moderate lymphocytic and eosinophilic reaction may be evident in the underlying lamina propria. The larvae of *Gasterophilus* spp. in the horse and of *Oestrus ovis* in sheep are found attached to the pharyngeal mucosa, where they may cause focal ulceration and excite mild inflammation. The larvae of *G. nasalis* migrate from the lips and invade the gums around and between the teeth and behind the alveolar processes to cause small suppurating pockets. *Micronema* spp. have been observed in proliferative granulomas of the mandibular gingiva in a horse.

Bibliography

Cho, D. Y. *et al.* *Micronema* granuloma in the gingiva of a horse. *J Am Vet Med Assoc* **187:** 505–507, 1985.

Zinter, D. E., and Migaki, G. *Gongylonema pulchrum* in tongues of slaughtered pigs. *J Am Vet Med Assoc* **157:** 301–303, 1970.

D. Diseases of the Tonsils

The tonsils are normally prominent and protrude slightly from the tonsillar fossa in the dog and cat. In swine, tonsillar lymphoid tissue is concentrated in the posterior soft palate. In other species, the tonsils are diffuse. They are subject to the usual conditions involving lymphoid tissue, and undergo progressive atrophy with age.

Tonsils are constantly exposed to antigenic stimuli, by virtue of their function in immune surveillance in the oropharynx. As a result, they are a site of functional lymphoid hyperplasia and physiologic inflammation. Many bacteria native to the oropharyngeal mucosa probably inhabit the tonsillar crypts. They consequently may serve as portal of entry for a variety of bacterial agents, including *Streptococcus suis* and intracellular organisms, and for lymphotropic viruses. A significant percentage of swine may carry *Erysipelothrix rhusiopathiae* and *Salmonella* spp. in the tonsils.

Desquamated epithelium, bacteria, necrotic debris, and neutrophils may normally be present to moderate degree in tonsillar crypts. This reaction is exaggerated, and may be associated with ulceration of the crypt and suppuration of involuted tonsillar lymphoid tissue, in certain bacterial infections, causing the formation of visible yellowish nodules. Conditions in which such bacterial tonsillitis may occur include pasteurellosis in sheep and pigs, and necrobacillosis in all species (Fig. 1.8). In porcine anthrax, hemorrhagic necrotizing tonsillitis is reported.

The tonsil is the site of primary virus multiplication in pseudorabies (Aujeszky's disease) in swine. The virus causes a necrotizing tonsillitis, and intranuclear inclusions may be seen in cryptal epithelial cells.

Involution of B-dependent tonsillar lymphoid follicles due to viral lymphocytolysis may occur during the early phase of a number of lymphotropic diseases such as feline panleukopenia, canine parvovirus infection, canine distemper, bovine virus diarrhea, rinderpest, and swine vesicular disease. Numerous karyorrhexic nuclei, lymphocyte depletion, and prominent histiocytes signal such damage. In distemper, involuted tonsils are susceptible to secondary bacterial invasion and suppuration. Compensatory lymphoid hyperplasia may occur during the postviremic phase of parvoviral infections and distemper. The tonsil often appears to be the preferred organ of viral persistence in a symptomatic carrier infected with, for example, feline picorna- and caliciviruses. Rabies virus may persist for several months in tonsils of dogs after experimental infection.

Inflammatory polyps of the tonsils occur infrequently in old dogs. They are flat to pedunculated rubbery masses (1–3 cm in length), attached to the tonsillar sinus, with a smooth to verrucose surface. Histologically, the lesions are composed of mature, sometimes edematous, highly vascularized connective tissue that is covered by squamous epithelial cells. Aggregates of lymphocytes and plasma cells are scattered throughout the connective tissue. The lesions are probably the result of chronic recurrent episodes of subclinical tonsillitis. They are usually asymptomatic but may cause gagging and retching.

Bibliography

Fekadu, M. *et al.* Rabies virus in the tonsils of a carrier dog. *Arch Virol* **78:** 37–47, 1983.

Lucke, V. M. *et al.* Tonsillar polyps in the dog. *J Small Anim Pract* **29:** 373–379, 1988.

Narita, M., Inui, S., and Shimizu, Y. Tonsillar changes in pigs given pseudorabies (Aujeszky's disease) virus. *Am J Vet Res* **45:** 247–251, 1984.

E. Neoplastic and Similar Lesions of the Oral Cavity

Many of the lumps, bumps, and cysts which develop in and around the oral cavity are malformations, hyperplasias, and neoplasias originating in tooth germ or teeth. The classification of these masses, especially those containing more than one tissue, is not established, and must be arbitrary. Malformations of dental origin have been considered previously under developmental anomalies of teeth. Gingival masses of all types, many of which are of tooth germ origin, are common in dogs, and rarely occur in other species. The oral and pharyngeal mucosa is the fourth most common site of malignant tumors in the dog. It is also a common site of malignant tumors in cats. Malignant oral tumors account for ~6% of all canine and ~7% of all feline neoplasms. Large domestic animals have a low prevalence of such tumors. When they do occur in ungulates, they are usually nonaggressive.

Regional geographic differences exist in the prevalence of certain oral tumors, especially in dogs and cattle. These differences may be related to types and levels of carcinogens in the environment and warrant further investigation from the point of view of comparative oncology. An example may be the reported higher prevalence of tonsillar squamous cell carcinomas in dogs in certain urban areas with high levels of atmospheric pollution, compared to that in more rural areas.

The most common types of malignant oral tumors in dogs and cats are squamous cell carcinomas, fibrosarcomas and, in dogs only, malignant melanomas. They vary considerably in their behavior depending on the species in which they occur, and the type and location of the tumor. Dogs and cats, 7 years of age or older, are mainly affected. Typical clinical signs associated with these tumors are excessive salivation, halitosis, pain, dysphagia, loose teeth, oral bleeding, noisy respiration, coughing, and a change in voice. All of these signs are determined by the location of the tumor.

Both breed and sex predilection have been reported for malignant oral tumors in dogs. Boxers, cocker spaniels, German shorthaired pointers, Weimaraners, and golden retrievers apparently have a higher prevalence of these tumors than do other breeds. Dachshunds and beagles apparently have a very low prevalence. The male-to-female ratio for these tumors has been reported to be as high as 6 : 1 for melanomas, 3 : 1 for tonsillar carcinomas, and 2 : 1 for fibrosarcomas. The ratios have to be interpreted with some caution since they may be partly related to differences in the ratio of males to females in the general population.

All malignant oral tumors in dogs and cats tend to follow a rapid course, and regardless of the type of malignancy, the prognosis is poor.

1. Oral Papillomatosis

These benign epithelial tumors (warts) in dogs and cattle are caused by papovaviruses. In dogs, they occur mainly in young animals, but older dogs in close contact may become infected. The virus is host specific and fairly site specific. It can be readily transmitted to the scarified oral mucosa but less easily to the conjunctiva and skin. Infection with canine oral papilloma virus apparently elicits two different responses in the squamous mucosa of benign papillomas. In some basal cells the virus stimulates increased mitosis, whereas in the more differentiated cells of the stratum spinosum, it results in the expression of virions and degeneration of the cells. The incubation period is generally 1 month. Spontaneous recovery, followed by solid immunity, usually occurs within 2–3 months. The warts first develop on the lips as single, smooth papular elevations, which are pale or the color of the mucosa. These lesions progress to multiple, proliferative cauliflower-like, firm, white-to-gray growths (Fig. 1.13). Similar lesions develop on the inside of the cheeks, the tongue, the palate, and the walls of the pharynx. The gingiva are usually not affected. The esophagus may be involved.

The microscopic structure is typically papillomatous with a very thick squamous epithelium covering thin, branching, often pedunculated, cores of proprial papillae. Individual or small groups of epithelial cells in the upper areas of the stratum spinosum undergo hydropic or acidophilic degeneration with loss of intercellular bridges.

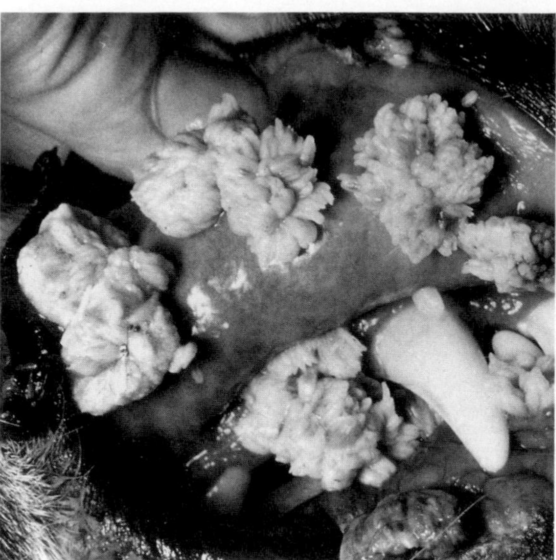

Fig. 1.13 Oral papillomatosis. Dog. (Courtesy of W. R. Kelly.)

There is also marked acanthosis. Intranuclear basophilic inclusions may be found in the cells in the outer spinose layers. Transformation of spontaneous oral papillomas to squamous cell carcinomas is apparently rare. Experimental injections of live canine oral papillomavirus vaccine into the skin of dogs may result in a spectrum of lesions including epidermal hyperplasia, papillomas, epidermal cysts, basal cell tumors, and squamous cell carcinomas. This virus may be involved in the development of spontaneous dermal squamous cell carcinomas in dogs.

Oral papillomas, due to bovine papillomavirus type 4, occur commonly in cattle. Their morphology and distribution are similar to those of the papillomas of dogs, and they are considered more fully under tumors of the esophagus and reticulorumen.

Oral papillomas, due to a papovavirus, also occur in domestic rabbits. The prevalence of this tumor may be greater than reports indicate, since they are usually incidental findings due to their small size and their location on the ventral surface of the tongue.

2. Epulides

Epulis is the generic and clinical term for tumorlike masses on the gingiva. This includes developmental, inflammatory, and hyperplastic lesions as well as the neoplastic epulides, which are numerous in dogs, and develop occasionally in cats. A feature of hyperplastic and neoplastic epulides that is potentially confusing is the nature of the epithelium and of the hard tissues that often are found in the stroma. Epithelial remnants from tooth embryogenesis commonly occur in the gingiva and the periodontium, and it is not unusual to find nests of dental epithelium in any proliferative lesion in this region. Characteristically dental epithelial cells show reverse polarity, their nuclei being located at the apex of the cell distal to the basement membrane. Often the cell nests are surrounded by a relatively clear halo that contains a few strands of collagenous tissue. Also, gingival epithelium commonly proliferates extravagantly in response to irritation, and may form complex plexiform patterns. Unless there is neoplastic change, the epithelial component is not of primary significance. Similarly, many stromal proliferations in the regions of the jaws include mineralized tissues or amorphous, apparently mineralizable tissues, which may develop by metaplasia of fibrous tissue or by *de novo* cellular differentiation. Whether this is bone, cementum, or dentin, or their precursors, is often difficult to determine, and is prognostically irrelevant, as is the abundance of the tissues themselves.

Pyogenic granuloma is a bright red or blue mass on the gums of dogs. It is composed of extremely vascular, chronic granulation tissue covered by gingival epithelium. It ulcerates and bleeds easily. Pyogenic granuloma is probably an exaggerated response to local irritation and infection. In horses exuberant granulation tissue of periodontal origin sometimes develops at the site of extracted teeth to produce a tumorlike mass in the dental arcade. Epithelial remnants and proliferative bone may be associated with the granulation tissue.

Giant-cell epulis (peripheral giant cell granuloma) occurs in dogs and cats as gingival masses, often red, that may be smooth and sessile, or pedunculated. The gingival epithelium is hyperplastic or ulcerated and extends deeply into the underlying mass, which is well vascularized and often contains hemosiderin. Characteristic of the tumor are numerous giant cells, with multiple central nuclei and abundant eosinophilic cytoplasm, which are located in a densely cellular stroma. Foci of hard tissue may be present. The giant-cell epulis is regarded as a hyperplastic or granulomatous lesion and has occurred at the site of tooth extraction.

Hamartomas are focal disorganized overgrowths of mature tissue endogenous to the organ involved. **Gingival vascular hamartomas** are rare congenital anomalies that occur on the gums of young calves. Because of their location, they usually have an inflamed surface, and may resemble, superficially, granulation tissue. They are pink to red lobulated masses, as much as several centimeters in diameter, often pedunculated, on the rostral mandibular gingiva adjacent to the incisors, which may be displaced. They may also be located in the tongue. Microscopically the tumors consist of irregular, thin-walled vascular channels containing erythrocytes or proteinaceous material, and lined by well-differentiated endothelial cells. The vascular spaces are separated by loose fibrous stroma. Vascular hamartomas are completely benign. Those in the oral cavity must be differentiated from oral papillomatosis and granulomas.

Fibrous hyperplasia (fibrous epulis) is common in dogs, and is either generalized, or localized to one or more teeth. When localized, it is a discrete tumorlike mass and, whether local or general, may cover part of the crown

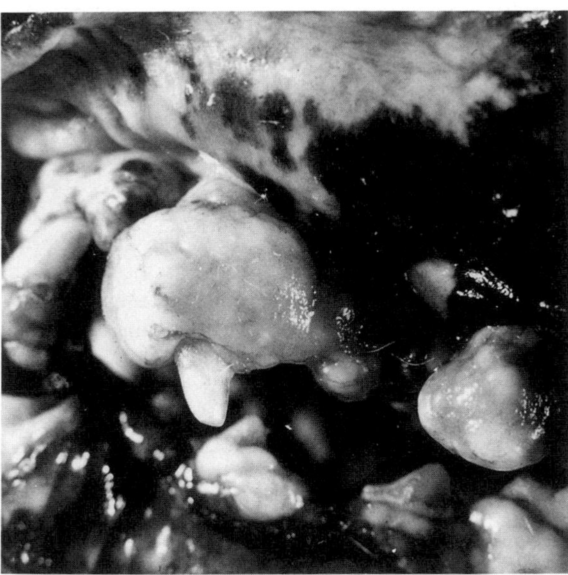

Fig. 1.14 Fibrous hyperplasia (fibrous epulis.) Boxer dog.

(Fig. 1.14). The stromal component of the mass consists of mature fibrous tissue with low cellular density. Foci of hard tissue and epithelial nests may be present. Local enlargement is caused by chronic, probably painless, inflammation. It may be associated with periodontal disease, in which case it is often accompanied by a more or less extensive chronic or chronic-active inflammatory reaction. Characteristically there is a band of mononuclear cells, predominantly plasma cells, in the gingival stroma adjacent to the epithelium, which is often hyperplastic, sometimes markedly so. When the epithelium is ulcerated, neutrophils may be prominent, marginating in vessels, in the stroma, and migrating through the epithelium.

Diffuse gingival hypertrophy is familial in boxer dogs, and a more severe overgrowth, termed hyperplastic gingivitis, occurs as a recessive inherited disease in Swedish silver foxes. In the foxes, both jaws are affected, and the hypertrophy causes displacement and malalignment of teeth, eventually reaching such proportions that the mouth cannot be closed. Diffuse gingival hypertrophy sometimes is associated with prolonged anticonvulsant therapy in humans.

Fibromatous epulis, which is a peripheral odontogenic neoplasm, peripheral here indicating an origin outside the jaws, is indistinguishable clinically from fibrous hyperplasia. The distinction is academic since prognosis following surgical removal is good for both lesions. Fibromatous epulis of dogs is a neoplasm, however, comparable to the rare human tumor called peripheral odontogenic fibroma. Similar tumors occur rarely in cats. Fibromatous epulides are firm to hard, gray-pink neoplasms, often projecting from between the teeth or from the hard palate near the teeth. Often they are mushroom shaped and have a smooth, lobulated surface. They are attached to the periosteum, and may displace teeth mechanically, but do not invade bone. Fibromatous epulides are most common around the carnassial and canine teeth of brachycephalic breeds.

Fibromatous epulides are stromal tumors, and the stroma consists of interwoven bundles of cellular fibroblastic tissue that is often well vascularized (Fig. 1.15). They are distinguished from fibrous hyperplasia by the immaturity of this stroma, and their tendency to contain less inflammatory tissue and more hard tissue. About 60% contain branching cords or islands of epithelium, which usually are continuous with the gingiva. The epithelium is bordered by a row of cuboidal cells somewhat resembling odontogenic epithelium (Fig. 1.16). Epulides sometimes are divided into fibromatous and ossifying types, depending on the abundance of the hard tissue that is present, in about 60% of affected dogs. There is no prognostic value in this distinction since these are all benign tumors, which are cured by excision.

Acanthomatous epulis, an epithelial tumor variously called oral adamantinoma and basal cell carcinoma probably arising from the gingival epithelium, is easily confused with the benign canine epulides. It arises from the gingiva and from epithelial rests. Clinically these tumors initially may resemble stromal epulides, but in many dogs, recurrence and local invasion of alveolar bone (Fig. 1.17) with loss of teeth follows conservative treatment. Grossly they

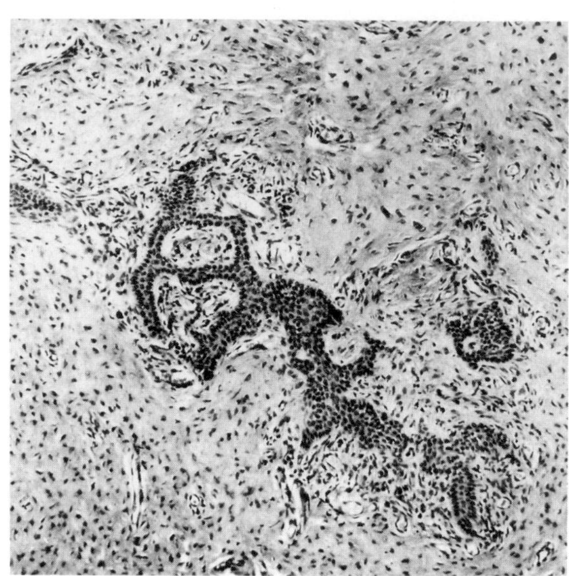

Fig. 1.16 Branching cords of epithelium in mesenchymal stroma. Epulis. Dog.

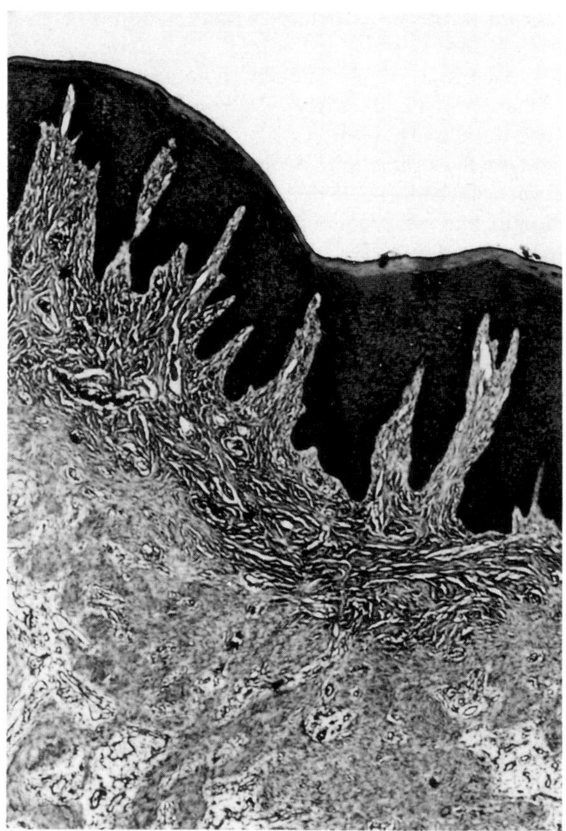

Fig. 1.15 Fibromatous epulis. Dog. Note demarcation between tumor (below) and gingival stroma.

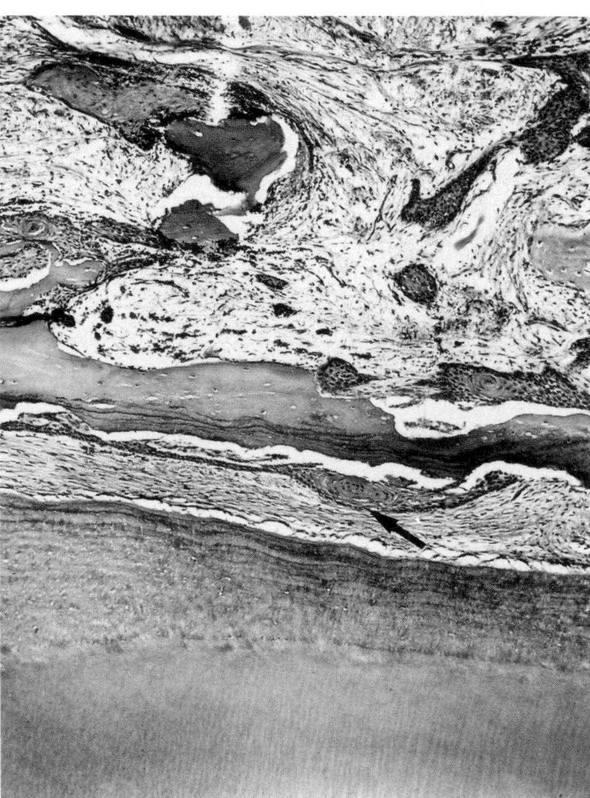

Fig. 1.17 Acanthomatous epulis invading periodontal ligament (arrow) and resorbing alveolar bone (center). Cementum and dentin (below).

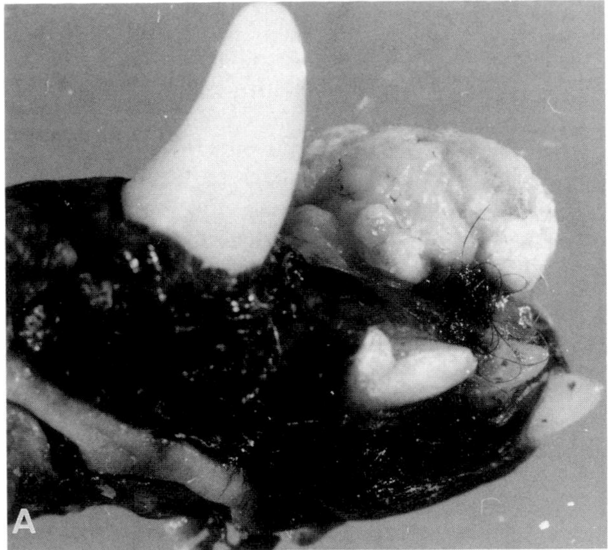

Fig. 1.18A Acanthomatous epulis. Dog. Tumor is destroying mandibular symphysis and displacing teeth.

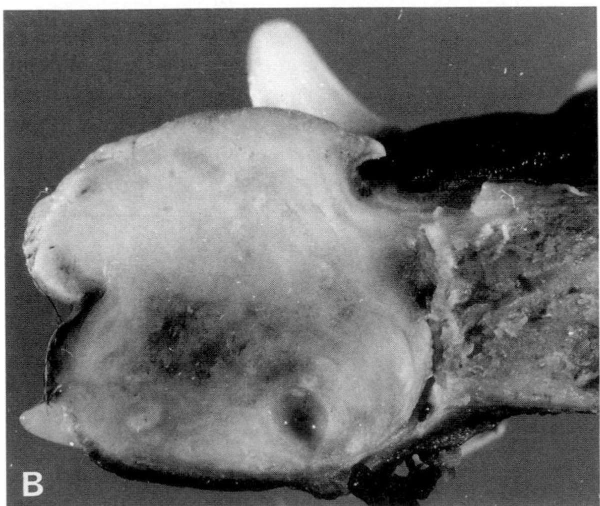

Fig. 1.18B Medial view of A. symphysis split.

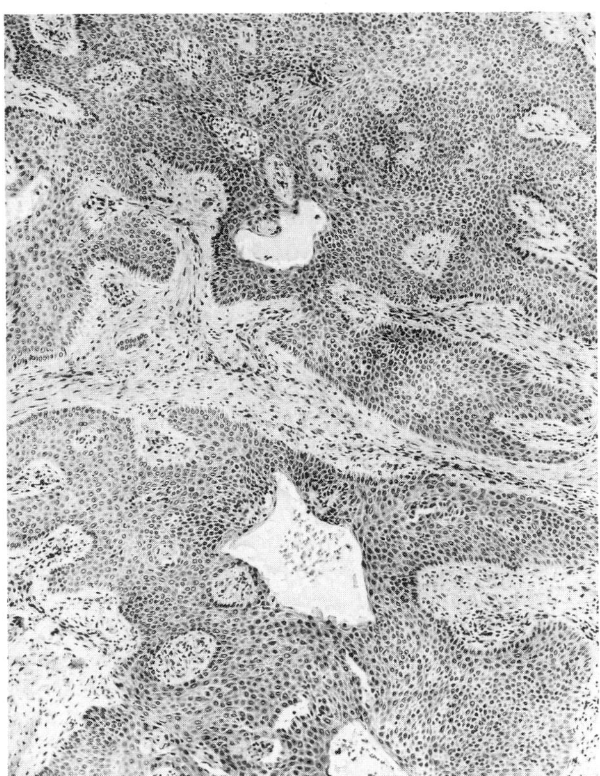

Fig. 1.19 Acanthomatous epulis. Dog.

may be papillary to sessile, and gray-pink (Fig. 1.18A,B). Histologically the tumor is composed of sheets, nodules, and anastomosing cords of epithelium bordered by a row of cuboidal to columnar cells with round to oval nuclei and moderate amounts of cytoplasm. Prominent intercellular bridges are present between many of the central polyhedral cells. In some tumors there are intraepithelial cysts containing vacuolated, otherwise structureless, eosinophilic material and cellular debris (Fig. 1.19). These cysts probably form from degenerate epithelium. Small masses of hard tissues may develop in the stroma between the epithelium.

It is sometimes difficult to distinguish an acanthomatous epulis developing from the gingiva and the epithelial proliferation accompanying gingivitis. Besides the usual prudence required when identifying neoplastic cells in areas of inflammation, other criteria for differentiation include the predominance of broad sheets of epithelium and the mitotic figures sometimes present in the acanthomatous epulis. Evidence of invasion of bone is clearly relevant to the diagnosis, care being taken to differentiate alveolar bone from stromal hard tissues.

The origin and naming of these tumors are debated. Acanthomatous epulis of periodontal origin and basal cell carcinoma probably arising from gingival epithelium are current. Adamantinoma is now rarely used. The tumors arise in both gingival epithelium and periodontal ligament and have varied gross and microscopic appearances. Acanthomatous epulis does carry the implication of a benign tumor, but until a more suitable alternative is established, we find it least confusing.

Some acanthomatous epulides show characteristics of squamous cell carcinoma when they escape the influence of the subgingival stroma and invade bone, but metastases are not recorded. Squamous cell carcinoma, fibrosarcoma, and osteosarcoma have been reported from the site of irradiated acanthomatous epulides. These tumors developed several months to several years after irradiation.

3. Tumors of Dental Tissues

Tumors of dental tissues are classified as either epithelial or stromal neoplasms, and malformations. Other than the canine fibromatous epulis (see the preceding), stromal neoplasms are very rare in animals. Tooth development provides the classic example of epithelial–mesenchymal interactions, and it is generally accepted that inductive influences are active in some tumors. Familiarity with dental embryology assists an understanding of the origin, appearance, and classification, of these tumors.

Most tumors of dental tissues are rare, nonmalignant, and infiltrative or expansive. However, their location predetermines destruction of bone and displacement of teeth, and they are difficult to remove.

Ameloblastoma is an invasive tumor consisting of proliferating odontogenic epithelium in a fibrous stroma. The proportions of epithelium and stroma vary widely. Ameloblastoma is preferable to the synonyms adamantinoma and enameloblastoma. These tumors are more common in dogs and cattle than in cats and horses, and seem to occur more often in the mandible than in the maxilla.

Ameloblastomas occur at any age, and originate from the dental lamina, the outer enamel epithelium, the dental follicle around retained unerupted teeth, the oral epithelium, or odontogenic epithelium in extraoral locations. They are predominantly intraosseous and because of their location, they may destroy large amounts of bone, and extend into the oral cavity or sinuses. Large tumors undergo central degeneration and become cystic.

The odontogenic epithelium, which is the criterion for diagnosis of ameloblastoma, may form any one of several patterns (Fig. 1.20). Follicular and plexiform patterns are

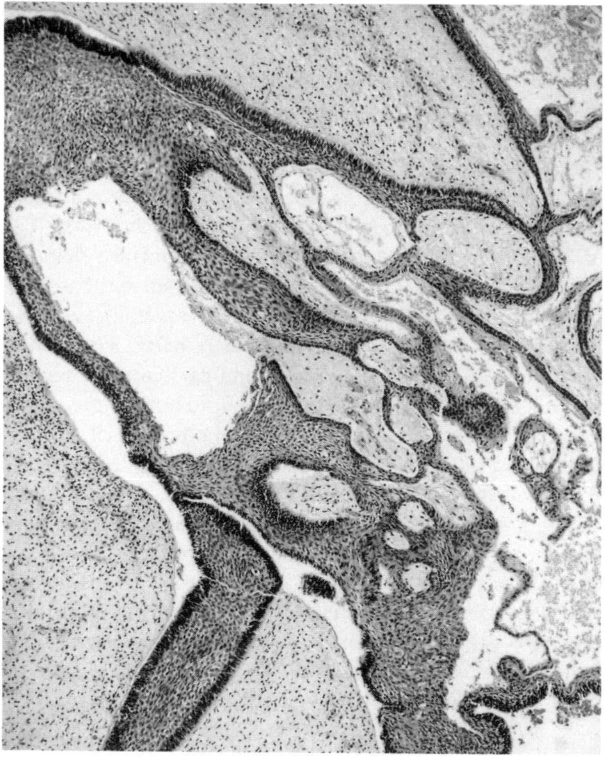

Fig. 1.20 Ameloblastoma. Cow. Tall enamel-type epithelium and cyst formation.

most common, consisting of discrete islands, or irregular masses and strands of epithelium, respectively. Many tumors contain both patterns. In both, central masses of cells, often resembling the stellate reticulum of the enamel organ, but sometimes with an acanthomatous appearance, are surrounded by a single layer of cuboidal or columnar cells, which resemble inner enamel epithelium. Cysts originate from degeneration of the centers of epithelial islands, or from stromal degeneration. Small cysts may coalesce to form gross cavities. Ameloblastomas occasionally undergo keratinization. In some, stromal osteoid and bone develop, which may be an epithelial inductive effect. Acanthomatous epulis, a more common tumor of dental epithelium, is discussed with epulides.

Calcifying epithelial odontogenic tumors, (Pindborg tumor) are rare tumors that occur as unencapsulated gingival masses in dogs and cats. Intra-osseous occurrence has not been described in animals. These tumors are characterized by epithelium, often of dental type, mineralization in epithelium and stroma, and also deposits of amyloid or amyloidlike material in epithelium and stroma. The epithelium may be arranged in strands, nests, or masses and may contain areas of stellate reticulum. The mineral may be in the form of small nodules often with Liesegang rings, or amorphous masses. The amyloid may also be nodular or amorphous and may be intermingled with the mineral. It shows apple-green birefringence when stained with congo red. Trabeculae of osteoid/dentinoid may be present in these tumors and are often a dominant feature. All reported tumors have been cured by surgical excision.

Ameloblastic fibroma (fibroameloblastoma, inductive fibroameloblastoma) is a rare tumor in calves but occurs more often in the bone or soft tissues of the maxilla of young cats. It consists of cords of epithelium resembling dental lamina, intimately associated with spindle cells resembling dental pulp. It behaves like an ameloblastoma.

Ameloblastic fibroma corresponds to that stage of odontogenesis at which dental epithelium invests the dental papilla, but odontoblasts have not yet differentiated.

Ameloblastic odontoma (ameloblastic fibro-odontoma) resembles ameloblastic fibroma, but contains dentin and enamel, and the epithelium is more typical of the enamel organ. It occurs in horses, cows, and dogs, often in immature animals.

Complex and compound odontomas are malformations in which all of the dental tissues are represented. In complex odontomas the tissues are disorganized, whereas in compound odontomas, toothlike structures (denticles) are present, each one containing enamel, dentin, cementum, and pulp, arranged as in a normal tooth. Distinction of the two may be arbitrary. Separate areas of ameloblastic epithelium are not present in complex and compound odontomas. A tumor which contains ameloblastic epithelium and separate areas of complex or compound odontoma is an **odontoameloblastoma.**

Odontomas are usually located in the mandibular or maxillary arch, and are less rare in cattle and horses than in other species. They are connected with existing dental alveoli and are detected when they bulge the contour of the host bone or interfere with other teeth. They may originate from normally or abnormally placed dental anlage as well as from supernumerary dental anlage.

4. Squamous Cell Carcinoma

This tumor is the most common oral malignancy of cats, in which it is most frequently located on the ventral surface near the frenulum of the tongue. The tonsils and gingiva are less common sites. Grossly, these tumors are irregular, slightly nodular, red-gray, friable masses, often with an ulcerated surface that bleeds easily. In the early stages gingival squamous cell carcinomas are often mistaken for gingivitis. Microscopically the tumor is conventional in appearance. It is locally invasive, especially into bone, and metastatic to regional lymph nodes, and rarely to the lungs.

In the dog, this tumor is second to melanoma in prevalence in the oral cavity. It usually involves the tonsils, although the gingivae are also common sites.

Grossly, tonsillar carcinoma usually appears unilateral. The earliest lesion appears as a small, slightly elevated, granular plaque on the mucosal surface. In the advanced stages, the affected tonsil is two to three times normal size, nodular, firm, and white, and the surface is often ulcerated. There is usually extensive infiltration of the surrounding tissues. Histologic examination of the grossly unaffected tonsil frequently also shows early carcinoma. Squamous cell carcinomas originating in the tongue and tonsils often metastasize to the regional nodes, with distant metastases to visceral organs, especially the lungs, in dogs. Tonsillar carcinoma must be differentiated from involvement of the tonsil in lymphosarcoma.

Gingival squamous cell carcinomas may be associated with chronic periodontitis in dogs. It is not always clear whether they have predisposed to periodontitis, or resulted from chronic irritation of the gingiva. Their appearance is conventional, though often obscured by chronic active inflammation. They are most common about the incisor and canine teeth and are locally invasive, and may invade bone (Fig. 1.21). However, they are less likely to metastasize than is squamous cell carcinoma of the tonsil. It is assumed that some originate in the gingiva and others, in subgingival or periodontal epithelium (see also acanthomatous epulis, Section I,E,2 of this chapter). This tumor may also be found elsewhere in the oropharynx, e.g., in the labial mucosa, palate, and pharynx.

In horses squamous cell carcinomas are found rarely on the gums and hard palate, possibly arising in chronically irritated hyperplastic alveolar epithelium in cases of chronic periodontitis. They are slow growing, exceedingly destructive, and metastatic mainly to the regional lymph nodes. Such tumors are large when first observed and may project from the palate or gums as grayish extensively ulcerated masses, or appear as craterous ulcers. The large ones are extensively necrotic and putrid, and the teeth are lost or loosely embedded in the tumor. These tumors of the maxilla rapidly fill the adjacent sinuses and cause bulging of the face and may extend further into the nasal, orbital, and cranial cavities. The microscopic appearance of the tumors varies considerably, from well differentiated with keratinization of individual epithelial cells and formation of keratin pearls, to poorly differentiated with little evidence of keratinization.

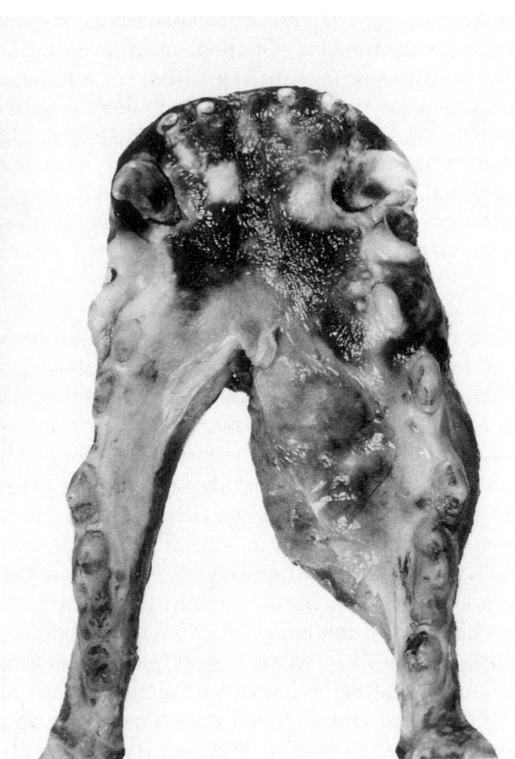

Fig. 1.21 Squamous carcinoma arising from alveolus of right canine tooth and invading mandible. Dog.

In cattle, oral squamous cell carcinomas are very rare, with the exception of a few geographic foci, where they are associated with oral papillomatosis and ingestion of bracken fern. A similar association is made in the etiology of squamous carcinomas of the esophagus and forestomachs in cattle, and is considered more fully in that section. There are sporadic reports of this tumor in the lower lip of sheep.

5. Melanoma

Melanomas are the most common oral tumor in dogs. In contrast to cutaneous melanomas in the dog, which are usually benign, melanomas of the oral mucosa are almost always malignant. Most are considered to have metastasized by the time they are diagnosed. They arise from the melanocytes in the mucosa or superficial stroma, and are usually located on the gingiva, gums, buccal mucosa, lips, and palate, and less often on the tongue. The prevalence is higher in males than females. They tend to be more common in breeds that have a dark hair coat and pigmented mucous membranes, such as Scottish and Boston terriers, black cocker spaniels, German shepherds, and possibly Airedales. The degree of pigmentation of these tumors varies considerably, but there appears to be no relationship between the amount of pigment and biological behavior. They grow rapidly; necrosis and ulceration are common (Fig. 1.22A), and 70–90% metastasize to the regional lymph nodes, mainly the submandibular nodes. They may spread via hematogenous and lymphatic routes to more distant sites, especially the lungs. The median survival time for untreated dogs has been reported as 65 days.

The histologic appearance of melanomas varies greatly, from a fairly well differentiated, heavily pigmented type, to a highly anaplastic amelanotic type. The diagnosis of the latter is often difficult. However, certain features are evident in most of these tumors. Anaplastic melanocytes, which have large, oval or elongated nuclei with distinct nucleoli and abundant cytoplasm, show junctional activity, infiltrating the junction between the basilar epithelial cells and the submucosa (Fig. 1.22B). Frequently there is a characteristic mixture of epithelial-like and spindle-shaped cells, which have a marked tendency to form nests extending deep into the submucosa. Multinucleated giant cells may also be present. About 75% of melanomas have melanin pigment, but detection of this pigment often requires careful examination of individual tumor cells. Metastases are usually pigmented, but in a few cases the primary tumor is pigmented, and the metastases are not, and vice versa.

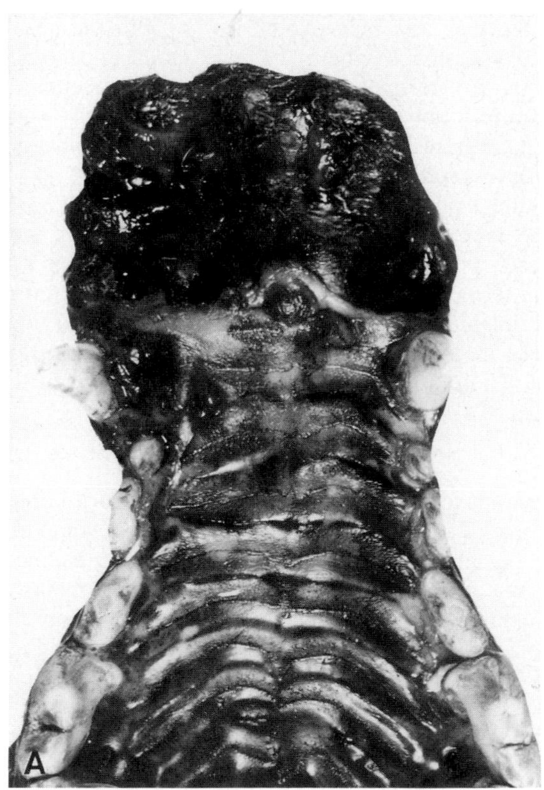

Fig. 1.22A Malignant melanoma of palate. Dog.

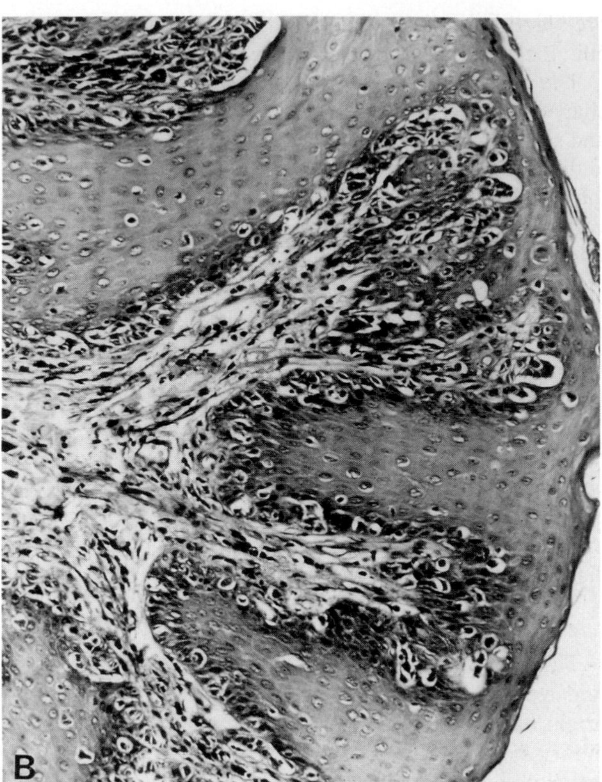

Fig. 1.22B Junctional activity in oral mucosa adjacent to melanoma.

Pigmented basilar epithelial cells are frequently present in superficial areas of the submucosa in a variety of non-neoplastic lesions resulting from irritation to the mucosa. This so-called pigmentary incontinence must be differentiated from malignant melanoma.

Although cutaneous melanomas are common tumors in horses and certain breeds of swine, these species have no tendency to develop oral melanomas. These tumors are also rare in cats.

6. *Fibrosarcoma*

Fibrosarcoma is the third most common oral malignant tumor in dogs, but the most common sarcoma of the oral cavity. This tumor is frequently seen in younger dogs; e.g., one report indicated 25% occurred in dogs younger than 5 years. It occurs mainly on the gums of the upper molars and adjacent soft palate, and the anterior half of the lower mandible, and less often in the buccal mucosa, lips, tongue, and palate. Infiltration of maxillary and mandibular bone is common. It grows rapidly, and frequently recurs after surgical removal. About 35% metastasize to regional nodes, and pulmonary metastases occur early in its course.

In cats, this tumor is the second most common oropharyngeal malignant neoplasm. The gingiva, ventral surface of the tongue, and palate have been reported as sites of predilection by some, but others did not observe any specific location. As in dogs, invasion of bone is common.

The tumors are gray to red, large, firm, irregularly shaped to nodular fleshy masses that are often ulcerated and secondarily infected. Microscopically the submucosa is diffusely infiltrated by densely cellular sheets of pleomorphic fibroblasts arranged in interwoven bundles with variable amounts of collagen. The mitotic index is high. There may be multinucleated giant cells scattered throughout the tumor.

7. Mast Cell Tumor

This tumor occurs occasionally in the oral cavity of the dog and cat. It may be an extension of cutaneous tumors on the lip, or it may arise in submucosal areas, especially on the tongue of dogs. The tumor should be considered potentially malignant, with metastasis to regional lymph nodes a possibility. Mast cell tumor should be considered in the differential diagnosis of oral lesions resembling granulation tissue or eosinophilic granuloma in dogs and cats.

8. Granular Cell Tumor (Myoblastoma)

This rare tumor or tumorlike lesion occurs in older dogs (mean age 9 years), mainly in the base of the tongue. The origin of granular cell tumors is still uncertain. Current theory suggests that it originates from a fibroblastlike interstitial cell believed to be the multipotential precursor of both Schwann cells and granular cells. It is elevated, red, and granular or smooth on the mucosal surface. The cut surface is white and firm. Microscopically, the mass consists of large, polyhedral to round epithelioid cells which have abundant acidophilic granular cytoplasm. The cytoplasmic granules are strongly periodic acid–Schiff (PAS) positive. The nuclei are round to oval, centrally or eccentrically located, and have one to two nucleoli. Mitotic figures are rare. The tumor cells have a marked tendency to form nests or cords, which are separated by a delicate network of reticulin fibers. None of these tumors in dogs has recurred after excision, nor have they metastasized. Similar tumors occur in humans, where they are also most common in the tongue, but they may occur in a variety of organs. There is a single report of this tumor in the tonsil of a cat. In horses, granular cell tumors are located in the lungs (see The Respiratory System, Chapter 6 of this volume).

9. Neuroendocrine (Merkel) Cell Tumors

Merkel cells occur in the epidermis of many animals and in the oral mucosa of several mammalian species, where they are closely associated with nerve endings. These cells are part of the neuroendocrine system, and they are thought to function as pressure receptors.

Rarely, they form tumors of the skin and the oral mucosa in the dog. In the latter site they tend to be pedunculated, and are located on the gums and lips. Histologically, they consist of well-circumscribed, densely packed nests and sheets of polygonal to round cells in the submucosa, resulting in an organoid appearance. The cells have a moderate amount of pale basophilic cytoplasm. The nuclei are pleomorphic, the nuclear membrane is indented, and there are one to two centrally located nucleoli. The mitotic index varies from few to two to three mitotic figures per high-power field. Multinucleate giant cells are often present. The cells stain negatively with the PAS stain but have a positive argyrophilic reaction. These are useful features to differentiate this tumor from granular cell tumors. The tumor must also be differentiated from malignant melanoma.

10. Plasmacytoma

Extramedullary plasmacytomas are an uncommon tumor of the oral mucosa and skin of mainly older dogs (mean age 9–10 years). They arise as primary tumors from plasma cells in the soft tissue, or rarely as metastases from primary osseous myeloma.

This tumor has probably been underdiagnosed in the past, being mistaken for undifferentiated round cell tumor, reticulum cell sarcoma, or a variant of dermal lymphoma. In the oral cavity it has been misdiagnosed as malignant melanoma. Grossly the tumor is a red, lobulated, raised mass usually located on the gingiva. It rarely invades bone. Plasmacytoma also occurs sporadically in the stomach, colon, and rectum.

Histologically the tumor is well circumscribed, nonencapsulated, and the overlying mucosa is usually intact, unless it has been traumatized in large tumors. The tumor cells are pleomorphic with variable amounts of amphophilic to basophilic cytoplasm. The nuclei are round to oval, and the nuclear membrane is indented. The cells are densely packed into nests and sheets that are divided by scant fibrovascular stroma. Bi- and multinucleated cells are frequently present in the center of the tumor. The most-differentiated plasma cells are usually evident at the periphery of the tumor. The mitotic index varies widely from one tumor to another. Immunoglobulins, especially IgG, can frequently be demonstrated in the neoplastic cells. Electron-microscopic examination reveals typical features of plasma cells, notably prominent rough endoplasmic reticulum and intracytoplasmic filaments, which are likely to represent immunoglobulins. Amyloid is rarely present among the tumor cells.

In spite of the anaplastic appearance and the presence of mitotic figures, the biological behavior of these tumors is benign.

Similar tumors also occur in humans, usually in the head and neck, in the submucosa of the air passages and paranasal sinuses.

11. Undifferentiated Malignant Tumors

There are uncommon, highly malignant oral tumors that lack specific features of either carcinomas or sarcomas. They occur mainly in dogs younger than 2 years, and are usually located in the upper molar and premolar areas. The tumors are soft, gray-tan to dark red, and poorly demarcated. They frequently extend into maxillary and nasal sinuses, orbital areas, and occasionally into the cranial cavity. Histologically the tumors are composed of nests and sheets of undifferentiated small to medium-sized, round to spindle-shaped cells that have a finely granular cytoplasm. The nuclei are round to oval. Large areas of necrosis are usually present within the tumor. The mitotic index is high. These tumors are highly malignant, resulting in widespread metastases.

12. Miscellaneous Tumors

A variety of benign and malignant neoplastic and similar lesions in the oropharynx have been reported sporadically. In the dog benign tumors include histiocytoma, lipoma, lymphangioma, hemangioma, and calcinosis circumscripta (of the tongue). Malignant tumors that have been reported, mainly in the tongue, are hemangiosarcoma, leiomyosarcoma, ectopic thyroid carcinoma, hemangiopericytoma, and rhabdomyosarcoma.

In cats, benign tumors include hemangioma and fibroxanthoma, and malignant examples are oral and tonsillar lymphosarcoma. Pharyngeal lymphomas have been described in horses.

Salivary tumors are described with the salivary glands.

Bibliography

Adams, R., Calderwood-Mays, M. B., and Peyton, L. C. Malignant lymphoma in three horses with ulcerative pharyngitis. *J Am Vet Med Assoc* **193:** 674–676, 1988.

Beck, E. R. *et al.* Canine tongue tumors: A retrospective review of 57 cases. *J Am Anim Hosp Assoc* **22:** 525–532, 1986.

Borthwick, R., Else, R. W., and Head, K. W. Neoplasia and allied conditions of the canine oropharynx. *Vet Ann* **22:** 248–269, 1982.

Bostock, D. E., and Curtis, R. Comparison of canine oropharyngeal malignancy in various geographical locations. *Vet Rec* **114:** 341–342, 1984.

Bostock, D. E., and White, R. A. S. Classification and behaviour after surgery of canine "epulides." *J Comp Pathol* **97:** 197–206, 1987.

Bradley, R. L. Selected oral, pharyngeal, and upper respiratory conditions in the cat. *Vet Clin North Am: Small Anim Pract* **14:** 1173–1184, 1984.

Bradley, R. L., Sponenberg, D. P., and Martin, R. A. Oral neoplasia in 15 dogs and four cats. *Sem Vet Med Surg (Small Anim)* **1:** 33–42, 1986.

Bregman, C. L. *et al.* Cutaneous neoplasms in dogs associated with canine oral papillomavirus vaccine. *Vet Pathol* **24:** 477–487, 1987.

Brodey, R. S. Alimentary tract neoplasms in the cat: A clinicopathologic survey of 46 cases. *Am J Vet Res* **27:** 74–80, 1966.

Brodey, R. S. The biological behaviour of canine oral and pharyngeal neoplasms. *J Small Anim Pract* **11:** 45–53, 1970.

Dorn, C. R., and Priester, W. A. Epidemiologic analysis of oral and pharyngeal cancer in dogs, cats, horses, and cattle. *J Am Vet Med Assoc* **169:** 1202–1206, 1976.

Dubielzig, R. R. Proliferative dental and gingival diseases of dogs and cats. *J Am Anim Hosp Assoc* **18:** 577–584, 1982.

Dubielzig, R. R., and Thrall, D. E. Ameloblastoma and keratinizing ameloblastoma in dogs. *Vet Pathol* **19:** 596–607, 1982.

Dubielzig, R. R., Adams, W. M., and Brodey, R. S. Inductive fibroameloblastoma, an unusual dental tumor of young cats. *J Am Vet Med Assoc* **174:** 720–722, 1979.

Dubielzig, R. R., Goldschmidt, M. H., and Brodey, R. S. The nomenclature of periodontal epulides in dogs. *Vet Pathol* **16:** 209–214, 1979.

Dyrendahl, S., and Henricson, B. Hereditary hyperplastic gingivitis in silver foxes. *Acta Vet Scand* **1:** 121–139, 1960.

Gardner, D. G., and Baker, D. C. Fibromatous epulis in dogs and peripheral odontogenic fibroma in human beings: Two equivalent lesions. *Oral Surg Oral Med Oral Pathol* **71:** 317–321, 1991.

Harvey, H. J. *et al.* Prognostic criteria for dogs with oral melanoma. *J Am Vet Med Assoc* **178:** 580–582, 1981.

Head, K. W. Tumors of the upper alimentary tract. *Bull WHO* **53:** 145–166, 1976.

Henson, W. R. Carcinoma of the tongue in a horse. *J Am Vet Med Assoc* **94:** 124, 1939.

Hoyt, R. F., Jr., and Withrow, S. J. Oral malignancy in the dog. *J Am Anim Hosp Assoc* **20:** 83–92, 1984.

Ladds, P. W., and Webster, D. R. Pharyngeal rhabdomyosarcoma in a dog. *Vet Pathol* **8:** 256–259, 1971.

Lantz, G. C., and Salisbury, S. K. Surgical excision of ectopic thyroid carcinoma involving the base of the tongue in dogs: Three cases (1980–1987). *J Am Vet Med Assoc* **195:** 1606–1608, 1989.

Morton, L. D. *et al.* Oral extramedullary plasmacytomas in two dogs. *Vet Pathol* **23:** 637–639, 1986.

Patnaik, A. K., and Mooney, S. Feline melanoma: A comparative study of ocular, oral, and dermal neoplasms. *Vet Pathol* **25:** 105–112, 1988.

Patnaik, A. K., Hurvitz, A. I., and Johnson, G. F. Canine gastrointestinal neoplasms. *Vet Pathol* **14:** 547–555, 1977.

Patnaik, A. K. *et al.* Extracutaneous mast-cell tumor in the dog. *Vet Pathol* **19:** 608–615, 1982.

Patnaik, A. K. *et al.* A clinicopathologic and ultrastructural study of undifferentiated malignant tumors of the oral cavity in dogs. *Vet Pathol* **23:** 170–175, 1986.

Pirie, H. M. Unusual occurrence of squamous carcinoma of the upper alimentary tract in cattle in Britain. *Res Vet Sci* **15:** 135–138, 1973.

Rakich, P. M. *et al.* Mucocutaneous plasmacytomas in dogs: 75 cases (1980–1987). *J Am Vet Med Assoc* **194:** 803–810, 1989.

Roberts, M. C., Groenendyk, S., and Kelly, W. R. Ameloblastic odontoma in a foal. *Equine Vet J* **10:** 91–93, 1978.

Samuel, J. L. *et al.* Oral papillomas in cattle. *Zbl Vet Med B* **32:** 706–714, 1985.

Schuh, J. C. L. Squamous cell carcinoma of the oral, pharyngeal, and nasal mucosa in the horse. *Vet Pathol* **23:** 205–207, 1986.

Stebbins, K. E., Morse, C. C., and Goldschmidt, M. H. Feline oral neoplasia: A ten-year survey. *Vet Pathol* **26:** 121–128, 1989.

Sundberg, J. P., Junge, R. E., and El Shazly, M. O. Oral papillomatosis in New Zealand white rabbits. *Am J Vet Res* **46:** 664–668, 1985.

Sundberg, J. P. *et al.* Cloning and characterization of a canine oral papillomavirus. *Am J Vet Res* **47:** 1142–1144, 1986.

Todoroff, R. J., and Brodey, R. S. Oral and pharyngeal neoplasia in the dog: A retrospective survey of 361 cases. *J Am Vet Med Assoc* **175:** 567–571, 1979.

Turk, M. A. M. *et al.* Canine granular cell tumour (myoblastoma): A report of four cases and review of the literature. *J Small Anim Pract* **24:** 637–645, 1983.

Valentine, B. A., and Eckhaus, M. A. Peripheral giant-cell granuloma (giant-cell epulis) in two dogs. *Vet Pathol* **23:** 340–341, 1986.

Vos, J. H., and van der Gaag, I. Canine and feline oral–pharyngeal tumours. *J Vet Med A* **34:** 420–427, 1987.
Walsh, K. M., Denholm, L. J., and Cooper, B. J. Epithelial odontogenic tumours in domestic animals. *J Comp Pathol* **97:** 503–521, 1987.
White, R. A. S., Jefferies, A. R., and Gorman, N. T. Sarcoma development following irradiation of acanthomatous epulis in two dogs. *Vet Rec* **118:** 668, 1986.
Whiteley, L. O., and Leininger, J. R. Neuroendocrine (Merkel) cell tumors of the canine oral cavity. *Vet Pathol* **24:** 570–572, 1987.
Wilson, R. B. Gingival vascular hamartoma in three calves. *J Vet Diagn Invest* **2:** 338–339, 1990.
Wilson, R. B. *et al.* Tonsillar granular cell tumour in a cat. *J Comp Pathol* **101:** 109–112, 1989.

II. The Salivary Glands

The most common conditions of the salivary glands are functional, ptyalism being an increased secretion of saliva and aptyalism being a reduced or ceased secretion. Ptyalism (to be differentiated from failure to swallow) is seen as abnormal accumulation of saliva in the mouth. It occurs in a variety of conditions including heavy-metal poisoning, poisoning with organophosphates, encephalitis, and most often, stomatitis. Decreased secretion of saliva is less common but accompanies fever, dehydration, and salivary gland disease.

Ptyalism in cattle and horses may be an expression of a mycotoxicosis. *Rhizoctonia leguminicola,* which causes blackpatch disease of several legumes, is the fungus. On well-cured legume hay, the mycelial growth is not visible grossly. The fungus has a wide geographic distribution. The toxic principle is a parasympathomimetic alkaloid called slaframine, which literally means "an amine that causes an animal to salivate." In addition to excessive salivation, other signs include anorexia, excessive lacrimation, diarrhea, frequent urination, and bloat. Milk production is reduced, and there is loss of body weight. No specific lesions have been associated with slaframine toxicosis. Guinea pigs are extremely sensitive to the toxin. Presumptive diagnosis may be based on feeding trials in that species, if chromatographic analysis for slaframine is not readily accessible.

Foreign bodies occasionally are present in the ducts, usually the parotid duct, but sometimes the submaxillary. They are usually plant awns or fiber. They invariably cause some degree of inflammation with secondary infection; if the duct epithelium is destroyed, a local cellulitis occurs. **Salivary calculi** (sialoliths) may also cause obstruction and inflammation. They are more common in horses than in other species. Calculi are composed largely of calcium carbonate, possibly centered on a small foreign body, and are whitish, hard, and laminated. Calculi are usually single and cylindrical, and they may be quite large. Most of them lodge at the orifice and cause some degree of salivary retention, glandular atrophy, and a predisposition to infection and further inflammation.

Dilations of the duct are due to stagnation of flow, and this in turn is a result of obstruction due to congenital atresia or by foreign bodies, calculi, and inflammatory strictures. The dilated ducts appear as fluctuating cords, sometimes with local diverticula. **Ranula** is the term applied to a cystic distension of the duct in the floor of the mouth. These present a smooth, rounded prominence with a bluish tinge and fluctuations. The contents may be serous or of thick, tenacious mucus. Rupture of a duct or a gland to an epithelial surface results in a permanent fistula as the continued flow of saliva prevents normal restoration, the duct epithelium fusing with that of the surface.

Ranula by definition is a dilation of a duct with its lining epithelium more or less intact. Accumulation of salivary secretions in single or multiloculated cavities adjacent to ducts is now referred to as **salivary mucocele** or **sialocele.** These cystic formations do not have an epithelial lining. Small mucoceles, seldom exceeding 0.5 cm in size, are occasionally observed on the side of the bovine tongue. Their origin is presumably from rupture of the fine tortuous ducts of the dorsal part of the sublingual gland.

Mucoceles in dogs are well known because they are large enough to be a surgical problem. They occur in dogs of any breed. There may be a history of an antecedent ranulalike swelling in the mouth. Many mucoceles are probably the result of trauma to the duct. They may be located anywhere from the mandibular symphysis to the middle of the neck, the latter due to gravitational displacement. Most are ventrolateral, sometimes bilateral or midline, at the angle of the mandible. It appears that they arise most commonly from the sublingual salivary gland, either from individual units of the polystomatic portion or from the duct of the monostomatic portion. Zygomatic salivary mucoceles also occur, associated with local swelling and exophthalmos. Most mucoceles are subcutaneous and are as large as 10 cm in diameter, the larger ones being pendulous. The wall is of soft, pliable connective tissue, well vascularized, with a glistening lining. The contents are brown and mucinous, becoming progressively inspissated and tenacious with time.

The histologic appearance of mucoceles varies greatly, apparently depending on the stage of development. Initially, the wall consists of an outer, highly vascularized layer of immature connective tissue and an inner zone of loosely arranged fibroblasts. A pleocellular inflammatory reaction is evident in the central area, which also contains much amorphous acidophilic or amphophilic debris. Collagenous connective tissue forms the wall in later stages. The inflammatory cells are mainly mononuclear, and plasma cells often predominate. The debris in the center becomes progressively more basophilic.

Cysts of other origins do occur in this region. Cysts of the thyroglossal duct are midline and are distinguishable readily when they contain thyroid follicles. Cystic salivary adenomas are rare. Branchial cleft cysts may be located ventrolaterally, as are the salivary cysts, or dorsolateral on the neck. Their distinction is probably valid when no demonstrable connection occurs with a salivary duct, and a pseudostratified or stratified squamous or columnar lining epithelium is present.

Sialoadenitis, inflammation of the salivary glands, is uncommon in animals. It is, after mucoceles and malignant neoplasms, the most commonly diagnosed lesion involving salivary glands of dogs and cats. The submandibular gland is most frequently affected. Inflammation of the zygomatic gland in dogs is a cause of retrobulbar abscess. The infection usually gains entrance via the excretory duct, although it may be hematogenous or locally traumatic. Inflammation of the duct results in its obstruction by exudate, desquamated epithelial cells, and mucus. Some of this may be expressed from the ductal orifice as pus; the orifice is usually acutely inflamed. Obstruction of the duct, whether partial or complete, produces secondary atrophic changes in the glands, although there is initial enlargement due to the combined effects of retained secretion and inflammation. The ducts throughout the gland dilate, and leukocytes infiltrate the lumen and stroma. The acini undergo compression atrophy or swell and rupture from retained secretion. In acute infections this often leads to suppuration, and in chronic ones, only remnants of atrophic epithelium remain in a mass of inflamed scar tissue.

Specific inflammations of the salivary glands in domestic animals are unusual, although sialoadenitis does occur in rabies and malignant catarrhal fever. In rabies there is often focal lysis of acinar cells, and a mononuclear infiltration and, uncommonly, Negri bodies in the ganglionic neurons. The lesions of malignant catarrhal fever will be described in the section on Infectious and Parasitic Diseases (Section VII of this chapter). Eosinophilic sialoadenitis is found in an eosinophilic epitheliotropic syndrome in horses discussed with eosinophilic enteritis and dermatitis. Probably the most common associations with sialoadenitis in animals are strangles in horses and distemper in dogs. Mumps virus may infect dogs. Sialoadenitis also occurs in vitamin A deficiency in calves and pigs and in cattle poisoned with highly chlorinated naphthalenes. In these conditions, the inflammations, often purulent, are secondary to squamous metaplasia of the ducts with stasis of flow and secondary infection; squamous metaplasia of interlobular ducts is an early and rather specific lesion of vitamin A deficiency.

Infarction of the salivary gland is uncommon; it affects cats more often than dogs, perhaps due to fighting by the former. There may be a history of trauma to the head or neck regions, and it is uncertain whether the lesion is genuinely infarction or acute necrotizing sialoadenitis. The submandibular gland is most frequently affected. Clinically, there is firm local swelling, fever, leukocytosis, and anorexia. Histologically, the lesion is characterized by well-demarcated areas of necrosis with a mixture of inflammatory cells and hemorrhage at the periphery. Thrombi may be present in vessels within the infarcted areas. Marked regenerative hyperplasia, and in some cases squamous metaplasia, is often seen in the gland surrounding the infarcts. The latter changes must be differentiated from neoplasia. Infarcts in salivary glands usually resolve in 7–10 days.

Neoplasms of the salivary glands are rare in all species; they have been reported in cattle, sheep, goats, horses, dogs, and cats, but apparently not in swine. Only in dogs and cats do salivary tumors occur often enough to permit a general statement. They may arise from either the major or the minor salivary glands, involvement of the major glands being three times as frequent; of these, the most susceptible is the parotid. The tumors develop almost exclusively in aged animals; the majority are malignant, grow rapidly, become fixed to the overlying skin, and are painful. Metastasis to regional nodes and distant sites, especially the lungs, is common.

Salivary tumors have two main sites of origin within the gland: the ducts and the glandular tissue. In most cases, the histogenesis can be recognized, the duct neoplasms being papillomatous if benign, and squamous or mucoepidermoid carcinomas if malignant. Tumors arising in the glandular tissue are usually adenomatous (Fig. 1.23). Their malignant potential may be manifest only by carcinomatous areas at the periphery of the neoplasm.

The histologic structure of salivary tumors in animals is as diverse as that in humans, and the accepted classifications apply. The most frequent variety in dogs is of acinar cell origin and, although there are various structural

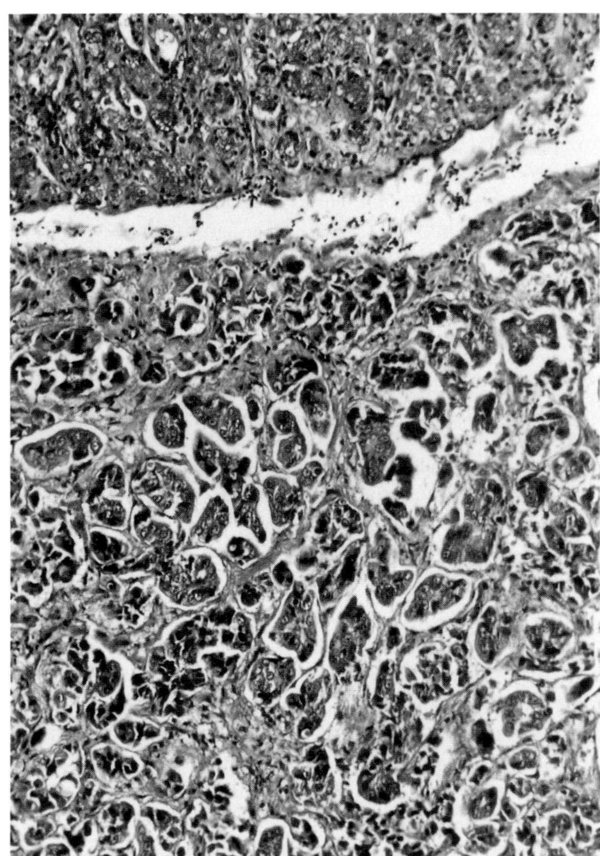

Fig. 1.23 Salivary adenocarcinoma of glandular origin. Cat.

patterns, an acinar arrangement is usually evident. This arrangement is emphasized by the common occurrence of pseudocystic dissolution, in which tumor cells with clear vesicular cytoplasm rupture, the secretion forming cyst-like spaces.

Acinic cell carcinomas have been rarely recognized in domestic animals. They occur mainly in dogs and sporadically in the horse and cow. They are composed of glandular epithelial cells that form a pronounced acinar pattern. The cells are round to polyhedral with basophilic cytoplasm and have small oval nuclei. A clear cell variant of this tumor has been reported in the minor salivary glands of the tongue in a dog. These tumors are locally invasive; metastases to the regional nodes are rare.

Mixed tumors, comparable to those of the mammary gland, occur. The mesenchymal component probably originates from myoepithelial cells. It is similar to that in mammary tumors, with areas of myoepithelial cells embedded in a mucinous matrix, which also contains neoplastic epithelial cells. Bone and cartilage form in these areas.

Bibliography

Booth, A., Reid, M., and Clark, T. Hypovitaminosis A in feedlot cattle. *J Am Vet Med Assoc* **190:** 1305–1308, 1987.

Brunnert, S. R., and Altman, N. H. Canine lingual acinic cell carcinoma (clear cell variant) of minor salivary gland. *Vet Pathol* **27:** 203–205, 1990.

Bundza, A. Primary salivary gland neoplasia in three cows. *J Comp Pathol* **93:** 629–632, 1983.

Carberry, C. A. *et al.* Salivary gland tumors in dogs and cats: A literature and case review. *J Am Anim Hosp Assoc* **24:** 561–567, 1988.

Crump, M. H. Slaframine (slobber factor) toxicosis. *J Am Vet Med Assoc* **163:** 1300–1302, 1973.

Eversole, L. R. Histogenic classification of salivary tumors. *Arch Pathol* **92:** 433–443, 1971.

Field, J. R., Trout, D., and Physick-Sheard, P. W. Ablation of a congenital neck mass in a foal. *Can Vet J* **31:** 643–644, 1990.

Glen, J. B. Canine salivary mucoceles: Results of sialographic examination and surgical treatment of 50 cases. *J Small Anim Pract* **13:** 515, 1972.

Hagler, W. M., and Behlow, R. F. Salivary syndrome in horses: Identification of slaframine in red clover hay. *Appl Environ Microbiol* **42:** 1067–1073, 1981.

Harrison, J. D., and Garrett, J. R. An ultrastructural and histochemical study of a naturally occurring salivary mucocele in a cat. *J Comp Pathol* **85:** 411–416, 1975.

Harvey, C. E. Parotid salivary duct rupture and fistula in the dog and cat. *J Small Anim Pract* **18:** 163–168, 1977.

Harvey, H. J. Pharyngeal mucoceles in dogs. *J Am Vet Med Assoc* **178:** 1282–1283, 1981.

Head, K. W. Tumors of the alimentary tract. *In* "Tumors in Domestic Animals," J. E. Moulton (ed.), 3rd Ed., pp. 340–373. Berkeley, CA. Univ. of California Press, 1990.

Karbe, E., and Nielsen, S. W. Canine ranulas, salivary mucoceles, and branchial cysts. *J Small Anim Pract* **7:** 625–630, 1966.

Karbe, E., and Schiefer, B. Primary salivary gland tumours in carnivores. *Can Vet J* **8:** 212–214, 1967.

Kelly, D. F. *et al.* Histology of salivary gland infarction in the dog. *Vet Pathol* **16:** 438–443, 1979.

Koestner, A., and Buerger, L. Primary neoplasms of the salivary glands in animals compared to similar tumors in man. *Pathol Vet* **2:** 201–226, 1965.

Lane, V. M., and Anderson, B. C. Adenocarcinoma of the mouth of a goat. *J Am Vet Med Assoc* **183:** 1099–1100, 1983.

Mitten, R. W., Fleming, C., and Gooey, P. D. Concurrent parotiditis (mumps) in a child and a dog. *Aust Vet J* **58:** 39, 1982.

Schmidt, G. M., and Betts, C. W. Zygomatic salivary mucoceles in the dog. *J Am Vet Med Assoc* **172:** 940–942, 1978.

Spangler, W. L., and Culbertson, M. R. Salivary gland disease in dogs and cats: 245 cases (1985–1988). *J Am Vet Med Assoc* **198:** 465–469, 1991.

Spreull, J. S. A., and Head, K. W. Cervical salivary cysts in the dog. *J Small Anim Pract* **8:** 17–35, 1967.

Stackhouse, L. L., Moore, J. J., and Hylton, W. E. Salivary gland adenocarcinoma in a mare. *J Am Vet Med Assoc* **172:** 271–273, 1978.

Talley, M. R. *et al.* Congenital atresia of the parotid salivary duct in a 7-month-old quarter horse colt. *J Am Vet Med Assoc* **197:** 1633–1634, 1990.

Wells, G. A. H., and Robinson, M. Mixed tumour of salivary gland showing histological evidence of malignancy in a cat. *J Comp Pathol* **85:** 77–85, 1975.

Youssef, H. *et al.* Effect of duct ligation on the parotid salivary gland of the dog. *Assiut Vet Med J* **19:** 144–151, 1988.

III. The Esophagus

The esophagus merits particular attention during the examination of animals with inadequate growth rate, cachexia, ptyalism, dysphagia, regurgitation, vomition, and aspiration pneumonia. In the ruminant, tympany may be a sequel to esophageal disease. The presence of a bloat line in the esophagus at the thoracic inlet may indicate a condition causing increased intra-abdominal pressure, such as gastric dilation or ruminal tympany. The squamous mucosa is frequently eroded or ulcerated in viral diseases which cause similar lesions elsewhere in the upper alimentary tract. Conditions of striated muscle, such as nutritional myodegeneration and eosinophilic myositis in the ruminant, or polymyositis, systemic lupus erythematosus, and trypanosomiasis in the dog, will involve the esophageal muscle. Diseases of the neuromuscular junction, as in myasthenia gravis, and peripheral neuropathies, such as giant axonal neuropathy and polyneuritis, will result in esophageal disease.

Bibliography

Henk, W. G., Hoskins, J. D., and Abdelbaki, Y. Z. Comparative morphology of esophageal mucosa and submucosa in dogs from 1 to 337 days of age. *Am J Vet Res* **47:** 2658–2665, 1986.

Jones, B. D., Jergens, A. E., and Guilford, W. G. Diseases of the esophagus. *In* "Textbook of Veterinary Internal Medicine," S. J. Ettinger (ed.), 3rd Ed., pp. 1255–1277. Philadelphia, Pennsylvania, W. B. Saunders, 1989.

Slocombe, R. F., Todhunter, R. J., and Stick, J. A. Quantitative ultrastructural anatomy of esophagus in different regions in the horse: Effects of alternate methods of tissue processing. *Am J Vet Res* **43:** 1137–1142, 1982.

Strombeck, D. R., and Guilford, W. G. Pharynx and esophagus—Normal structure and function. *In* "Small Animal

Gastroenterology," 2nd Ed., pp. 129–139. Davis, California, Stonegate Publishing, 1990.

A. Anomalies, Epithelial Metaplasia, and Similar Lesions

Congenital anomalies of the esophagus are very rarely recorded in domestic animals, and their interpretation as such can be difficult, since some similar defects may develop as sequelae of esophageal trauma or inflammation.

Congenital duplication of the esophagus is rare in domestic animals. It may result in a cystic mass, usually in the vicinity of the esophagus, lined by variably columnar to squamous epithelium, and with a double muscle layer in the wall; such cysts may become manifest as space-occupying lesions as they fill with cellular debris and secretion. Tubular duplications of the esophagus are usually clinically silent; they are contiguous with the wall of the true esophagus, with which they communicate.

Rare segmental aplasia of the proximal esophagus may be apparent in the neonate. A short blind pouch communicates with the pharynx, and a thin fibrous band connects it to the distal patent esophagus, which follows a normal course to the stomach. Esophageal atresia and congenital esophagorespiratory communications result from anomalies occurring when the respiratory primordium buds from the embryonic foregut. The epithelium of the anterior esophagus may be absent in epitheliogenesis imperfecta in foals.

Esophagorespiratory fistulae without esophageal atresia are more commonly recognized in animals; in calves and dogs, strong circumstantial evidence suggests that some of these are congenital. Short fibrous bands with a narrow mucosa-lined lumen, connecting an esophagus of normal diameter with the trachea or bronchus, are reported, as are small apertures connecting the lining of esophageal diverticula with the respiratory tree. The lining of such defects changes from stratified squamous to columnar respiratory epithelium in the fistula or wall of the diverticulum. Gastric distension by air in calves, and pneumonia due to aspiration, have been associated with esophagorespiratory fistulae.

The diagnosis of esophagorespiratory fistulae and diverticula as congenital anomalies is best based on recognition early in life, since both may be acquired following esophageal obstruction. Acquired fistulae result from gradual pressure necrosis caused by an intraluminal mass, and adhesion of esophagus to underlying trachea, or lung, with development of a fistula into the adjacent airway. This may be lined eventually by epithelium of esophageal or respiratory origin. In dogs, acquired esophagobronchial fistulae most commonly communicate with the bronchus of the intermediate or right caudal lung lobe.

Esophageal diverticula are irregular outpouchings or herniations of the esophageal mucosa through the muscularis. They communicate with the esophagus by various sized, often slitlike, apertures. Most are probably acquired, and they are commonest in the lower cervical esophagus, or in the distal thoracic esophagus, just cranial to the diaphragm. Increased intraluminal pressure, associated with foreign bodies, obstruction, or stenosis, is considered the cause of pulsion diverticula, in which the mucosa is forced out through the distended or ruptured muscularis. Such diverticula may be large spherical structures, with a narrow neck. They are most common in the horse and dog. The rare traction diverticulum is the result of contraction of a paraesophageal fibrous adhesion, following perforation and inflammation, drawing with it a pouch of esophageal mucosa, which is usually small and inconsequential. In contrast to pulsion diverticula, which have a layer of epithelium lining the inner aspect of a wall of fibrous connective tissue, traction diverticula have a wall comprising all layers of the esophagus. Ingesta and foreign bodies may accumulate in diverticula, causing gradual enlargement, with the potential for local esophagitis, ulceration and perforation, or formation of a fistula.

Rare anomalies of the mucosa include epithelial inclusion cysts, the presence of papillae resembling those of the rumen in the distal esophagus of cattle, and gastric heterotopia. The presence of gastric glands of the cardiac mucous type in the distal esophagus of dogs and cats is uncommon, and whether it is a developmental anomaly or a metaplastic response to mucosal injury, perhaps gastric reflux, is unclear.

Hyperkeratosis and thickening of the epithelium may be signs of vitamin A deficiency, or chlorinated naphthalene toxicity. Squamous metaplasia in the ducts of submucosal esophageal mucous glands, and in ducts and glands elsewhere, should be sought. Mild hyperkeratosis may be difficult to assess since in herbivores some degree of keratinization may be normal, and anorexia or failure to swallow results in loss of the abrasive effect of food passage, with accumulation of keratinized squames. Parakeratotic thickening and basal hyperplasia of the epithelium should be considered indicative of response to epithelial injury, and in the distal esophagus of pigs, is a concomitant of ulceration of the pars esophagea of the stomach. Parakeratosis of the esophagus occurs in pigs with cutaneous parakeratosis of zinc deficiency.

Bibliography

Bishop, L. M. *et al.* Megaloesophagus and associated gastric heterotopia in the cat. *Vet Pathol* **16:** 444–449, 1979.

Caywood, D. D., and Feeney, D. A. Acquired esophagobronchial fistula in a dog. *J Am Anim Hosp Assoc* **18:** 590–594, 1982.

Dodman, N. H., and Baker, G. J. Tracheo-oesophageal fistula as a complication of an oesophageal foreign body in the dog—a case report. *J Small Anim Pract* **19:** 291–296, 1978.

Keane, D. P., Horney, F. D., and Ogilvie, T. H. Congenital esophagotracheal fistula as the cause of bloat in a calf. *Can Vet J* **24:** 57–59, 1983.

MacDonald, M. H. *et al.* Esophageal phytobezoar in a horse. *J Am Vet Med Assoc* **191:** 1455–1456, 1987.

Orsini, J. A. *et al.* Esophageal duplication cyst as a cause of choke in the horse. *J Am Vet Med Assoc* **193:** 474–476, 1988.

Park, R. D. Bronchoesophageal fistula in the dog: Literature

survey, case presentations, and radiographic manifestations. *Compend Cont Ed Pract Vet* **6:** 669–678, 1984.
Pearson, H., Gibbs, C., and Kelly, D. F. Oesophageal diverticulum formation in the dog. *J Small Anim Pract* **19:** 341–355, 1978.
Scott, E. A. *et al.* Intramural esophageal cyst in a horse. *J Am Vet Med Assoc* **171:** 652–654, 1977.
van Ee, R. T. *et al.* Bronchoesophageal fistula and transient megaesophagus in a dog. *J Am Vet Med Assoc* **188:** 874–876, 1986.

B. Esophagitis

Erosive and ulcerative esophagitis is a common finding associated with viral diseases, causing similar lesions in the oropharynx or reticulorumen. Mucosal disease, rinderpest, and malignant catarrhal fever tend to produce longitudinal epithelial defects in cattle. Bovine papular stomatitis, infectious bovine rhinotracheitis, the herpesviruses of small ruminants, and calicivirus in cats may produce focal necrotizing esophageal lesions, which tend to be punctate or approximately round, perhaps with a raised periphery. Healing focal esophageal ulcers repair by granulation. Local epithelial proliferation and thickening produce an opaque pearly appearance of the margin of the lesion or surface of the scar.

Caustic or irritant chemicals, ionizing radiation, electrochemical reactions, and hot ingesta may cause mucosal injury, the severity of which depends on the nature of the insult and duration of exposure. Mild acute insult may result in diffuse or local reddening of the mucosa. Deep sloughing of the mucosa, liquefactive necrosis associated with alkalis, and coagulation necrosis following acid and toxins (paraquat, oak toxicosis), reflect more severe insult and may result in ulceration extending to deeper layers of the esophagus.

Superficial epithelial damage heals uneventfully, though repeated insult may cause thickening of the epithelium with the development of prominent rete pegs. Ulcerated mucosa will granulate, and raised islands of surviving pearly proliferative epithelium may be present over the surface. The inflammatory reaction in ulceration frequently involves muscularis and adventitia. The ultimate development of a contracted fibrous scar causes stricture or stenosis, if the original mucosal defect involved a significant portion of the esophageal circumference.

Reflux esophagitis results from the action on the esophageal mucosa of gastric acid, pepsin, probably regurgitated bile salts, and possibly pancreatic enzymes (Fig. 1.24A). Stratified squamous epithelium appears more susceptible to the corrosive effects of gastric secretion than other types of mucosa in the lower gastrointestinal tract. Relatively short duration of exposure to refluxed gastric content is required to induce epithelial damage, which is signaled by hyperemia or linear erosions and ulcers, perhaps with superficial fibrinonecrotic debris, and erythematous margins. Such damage is most common in the distal esophagus, but may extend well forward, in some instances nearly to the pharynx. The expected microscopic basal epithelial activation, rete peg elongation, and epithelial transmigration by neutrophils occur in response to mild superficial epithelial necrosis. A thinned epithelium following recent moderate insult, or granulation of an ulcerated surface may be evident. Re-epithelialization with a columnar mucous cell type may occur in distal esophagus adjacent to the cardia. Papillomatous esophagitis of unknown etiology has been reported in the distal esophagus of the cat, which normally has a somewhat corrugated or herringbone pattern to the mucosa.

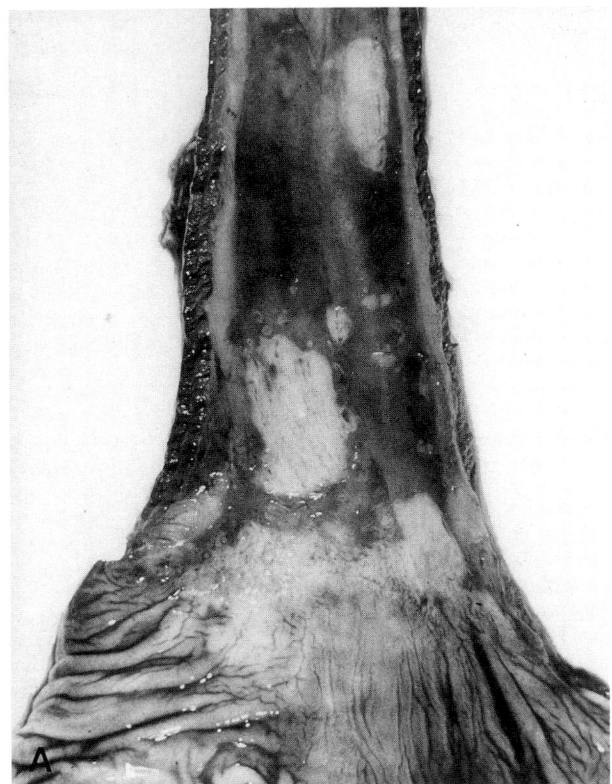

Fig. 1.24A Reflux esophagitis following chronic vomition. Dog. Islands of squamous epithelium remain surrounded by ulcerated mucosa.

Functional integrity of the lower esophageal sphincter may be compromised or overwhelmed by airway occlusion and increased intra-abdominal pressure, the pharmacologic effects of preanesthetic agents, or abnormality of the hiatus. Reflux esophagitis is thus most common in dogs and cats as a sequel to surgery involving general anesthesia, though it may follow chronic gastric regurgitation or vomition for any cause. In swine and horses, it may be associated with ulceration of the squamous esophageal portion of the stomach (Fig. 1.24B). In dogs, it is associated with rare hiatus herniation.

Hiatus hernia usually involves sliding herniation of all or part of the abdominal esophagus, cardia, and stomach into the thoracic esophagus, rather than periesophageal herniation. It is generally self-reducing, and its effect is

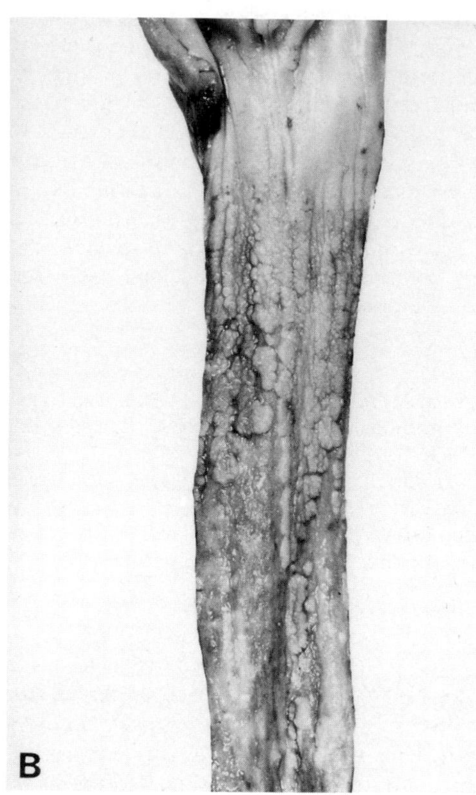

Fig. 1.24B Reflux esophagitis. Pig. Associated with esophagogastric ulceration.

usually lower esophageal sphincter failure and reflux, rather than gastric herniation and obstruction. Gastroesophageal intussusception is a very rare event, most reported in puppies of large breeds of dogs, and may be associated with congenital megaesophagus. The entire stomach everts into the esophagus, and occasionally the spleen and pancreas may be involved.

Thrush, or mycotic esophagitis caused by *Candida albicans,* is seen in piglets and weaner swine, in which the lesions may involve squamous mucosa of the entire upper alimentary canal. The condition is probably secondary to other intercurrent problems, including antibiotic therapy, inanition, and esophageal gastric reflux, and is considered more fully in the section on mycotic lesions of the gastrointestinal tract (Section VII,C of this chapter). Similarly, secondary phycomycotic granulomatous involvement of the esophagus is a rarely recorded complication of debilitating systemic disease states and heavy use of glucocorticoids and antibiotics.

Bibliography

Alexander J. W. *et al.* Hiatal hernia in the dog: A case report and review of the literature. *J Am Anim Hosp Assoc* **11:** 793–797, 1975.

Gaskell, C. J., Gibbs, C., and Pearson, H. Sliding hiatus hernia with reflux esophagitis in two dogs. *J Small Anim Pract* **15:** 503–509, 1974.

Hamilton, S. R. Reflux esophagitis and Barrett esophagus. *In* "Gastrointestinal Pathology," H. Goldman *et al.* (eds.), pp. 11–68. Baltimore, Maryland, Williams & Wilkins, 1990.

Leib, M. S., and Balss, C. E. Gastroesophageal intussusception in the dog: A review of the literature and a case report. *J Am Anim Hosp Assoc* **20:** 783–790, 1984.

Pearson, H. *et al.* Reflux esophagitis and stricture formation after anaesthesia: A review of seven cases in dogs and cats. *J Small Anim Pract* **19:** 507–519, 1978.

Peterson, S. L. Esophageal hiatal hernia in a cat. *J Am Vet Med Assoc* **183:** 325–326, 1983.

Strombeck, D. R., and Guilford, W. G. Diseases of swallowing. *In* "Small Animal Gastroenterology," 2nd Ed., pp. 140–166. Davis, California, Stonegate Publishing, 1990.

Wilkinson, T. Chronic papillomatous oesophagitis in a young cat. *Vet Rec* **87:** 355–356, 1970.

Yamashita, M. *et al.* Esophageal electrochemical burn by button-type alkaline batteries in dogs. *Vet Hum Toxicol* **29:** 226–230, 1987.

C. Esophageal Obstruction, Stenosis, and Perforation

"Choke," obstruction, or impaction of the esophagus occurs when large or inadequately chewed and lubricated foods, such as beets, potatoes, corn cobs, apples, bones, masses of grain or fibrous ingesta, lodge in the lumen of the esophagus (Fig. 1.25). This often occurs where the esophagus deviates or is slightly restricted normally, at the area over the larynx, the thoracic inlet, the base of

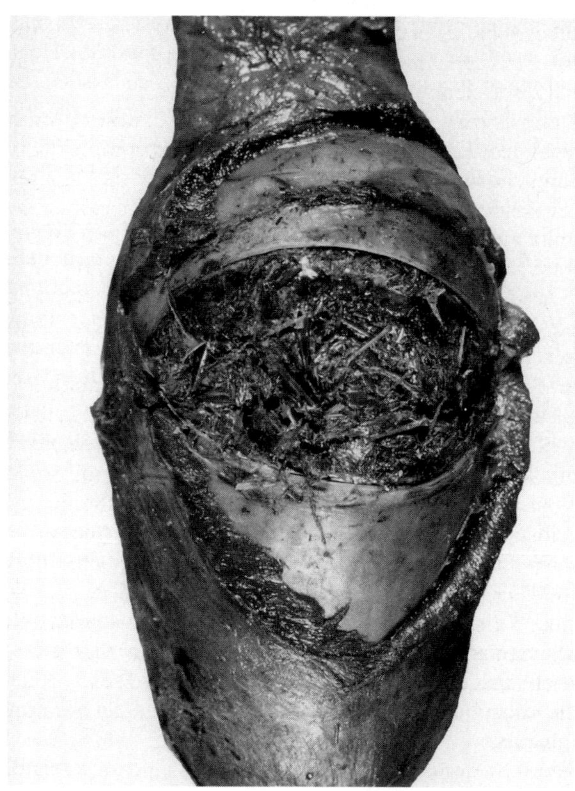

Fig. 1.25 Impaction of esophagus with rupture of muscularis. Horse.

the heart, and immediately anterior to the diaphragmatic hiatus.

Complications of obstruction include pressure necrosis and ulceration of the mucosa, which may progress to perforation. Sharp objects, such as bones, are most likely to cause perforation. Usually fatal cellulitis of the periesophageal tissue ensues, which may involve the mediastinum directly, or by extension along fascial planes from the cervical region, depending on the site of perforation. Alternatively, perforation of the thoracic esophagus may lead to sepsis of the pleural space, and pleuritis. Perforations of the pharyngoesophageal diverticulum above the cricoid cartilage, due to injuries caused by administration of medication by balling or drenching guns, or by passage of a stomach tube, probang, or endoscope, may have similar consequences.

Sharp objects such as needles, quills, grass seeds, or awns may penetrate and track from the esophagus. Diverticulum, and esophagorespiratory or esophagoaortic fistulae may also ensue following obstruction by foreign bodies. The cervical esophagus may be perforated by sharp objects such as wire or needles penetrating from the external surface of the skin.

Removal or dissolution of an obstructing object may be followed by scarring of the segmentally ulcerated esophagus, resulting in a narrowing of the lumen, stricture, or stenosis. Esophagitis, especially due to gastric reflux, may have a similar sequel. Although hypertrophy of internal and external muscle layers is seen occasionally in the distal esophagus of cattle and horses (in which species the distal esophageal muscle is normally relatively thick), it is usually not clearly the result of obstruction.

Stenosis may also result from rare intramural or intraluminal neoplasia, or commonly by external compression. Among causes of external compression may be enlarged hyperplastic or neoplastic thyroids, and neoplasia of the thymus and of cervical and mediastinal lymph nodes.

Vascular ring anomalies, seen in dogs, occasionally in cats, and rarely in other species, are the most common causes of external constriction of the esophagus. Dextroaorta, the development of the aortic arch from the right, instead of the left, fourth arch, is the most common of these anomalies. This results in entrapment and constriction of the esophagus between the heart and pulmonary artery ventrally, the anomalous aortic arch on the right, and the ligamentum arteriosum or remnant of the ductus arteriosus dorsally on the left. Other vascular anomalies that may constrict the esophagus, and are reported only in the dog, are persistence of both right and left aortic arches; persistent right ductus arteriosus; aberrant left subclavian artery, in association with persistent right aortic arch; and aberrant right subclavian artery arising distal to the left subclavian artery, and passing dorsally over the esophagus.

The Irish setter, German shepherd, and Boston terrier are the breeds most commonly afflicted with vascular ring anomalies. Esophageal deviation and stenosis have been associated in English bulldogs with thoracic shortening due to hemivertebra and esophageal compression between the left subclavian artery and the brachiocephalic artery.

The site of stricture, with its narrowed esophageal lumen, is readily identified at necropsy. Constricting mural fibrosis or other causative internal or external obstructive lesions will be obvious. The mucosa at the site of stricture may be ulcerated, as the result of impaction of ingesta, or as a sequel to antecedent esophagitis, pressure necrosis, or neoplasia. The esophagus anterior to the stenotic area is dilated, may contain retained ingesta, and itself may have evidence of esophagitis.

Bibliography

Murray, M. J., Ball, M. M., and Parker, G. A. Megaesophagus and aspiration pneumonia secondary to gastric ulceration in a foal. *J Am Vet Med Assoc* **192:** 381–383, 1988.

VanGundy, T. Vascular ring anomalies. *Compend Cont Ed Pract Vet* **11:** 36–48, 1989.

Woods, C. B. *et al.* Esophageal deviation in four English bulldogs. *J Am Vet Med Assoc* **172:** 934–940, 1978.

D. Dysphagia

Dysphagia, or disorder of swallowing, is a major sign of esophageal disease. It must be differentiated from vomition or emesis, which is the violent or active regurgitation of the contents of the stomach, a sequel to the ingestion of emetic agents, toxins such as vomitoxin or other trichothecenes, gastric irritation, and upper intestinal obstruction.

Swallowing is a complex and highly coordinated physical act, which may be conveniently divided into three phases. **Oral-phase dysphagias** are the product of painful physical lesions of the oral cavity and tongue, such as stomatitis, glossitis, gingivitis, or lesions such as hyoid damage, which limit movement of the tongue or delivery of the bolus to the pharynx. Loss of hypoglossal nerve function associated with hydrocephalus, trauma, or myasthenia gravis impairs lingual function. Cleft palate results in nasal regurgitation at this phase.

Pharyngeal dysphagia may be associated with painful pharyngitis, tonsillitis, retropharyngeal abscesses, and granulomas. Abscesses, granulomas, and neoplastic processes involving the tonsils and regional lymph nodes may physically intrude on the pharyngeal space. Encephalitis involving the medulla oblongata and the nuclei or tracts of the major cranial nerves involved in pharyngeal contraction and lingual function (V, IX, X, XII) should be sought in pharyngeal dysphagia, unexplained on physical grounds. Rabies and brain abscess in all species, and infectious bovine rhinotracheitis and listeriosis in ruminants are candidate central causes of pharyngeal paralysis. Retropharyngeal abscesses and lesions of the equine guttural pouch may cause peripheral nerve damage and paralysis. Idiopathic myodegeneration and myasthenia gravis have been reported as causes of impaired pharyngeal muscle function. Bluetongue and Ibaraki disease cause necrosis of lingual, pharyngeal, and esophageal muscle, resulting in dysphagia and aspiration of ingesta.

Cricoesophageal incoordination or **achalasia** may impede the first stage of the esophageal phase of swallowing—the opening of the upper esophageal sphincter to accept the approaching bolus. This condition is recognized in the dog, but not the cat. It is probably a result of a neurologic, rather than local physical or muscular deficit. Microscopic examination of the cricopharyngeal muscle has produced inconsistent observations, though either hypertrophy or degeneration might impede relaxation of the muscle and opening of the esophagus.

Megaesophagus or **esophageal ectasia** is the result of atony of the esophageal muscle, flaccidity, and luminal dilatation (Fig. 1.26). This is the product of segmental or diffuse motor dysfunction of the body of the esophagus. This results in failure of peristaltic propulsion of the food bolus to, and through, the lower esophageal sphincter to the stomach. Ingesta accumulates in the esophageal lumen, with eventual regurgitation of undigested food. Retention of some ingesta in the esophagus may lead to putrefaction and esophagitis in dilated or dependent areas. The volume of the dilated thoracic and cervical esophagus may greatly exceed that of the stomach, and the intrathoracic trachea and heart may be displaced ventrally. Animals presenting with esophageal hypomotility or megaesophagus may have signs of marked malnutrition including emaciation, dehydration, and osteopenia, often in association with rhinitis and aspiration pneumonia resulting from regurgitation.

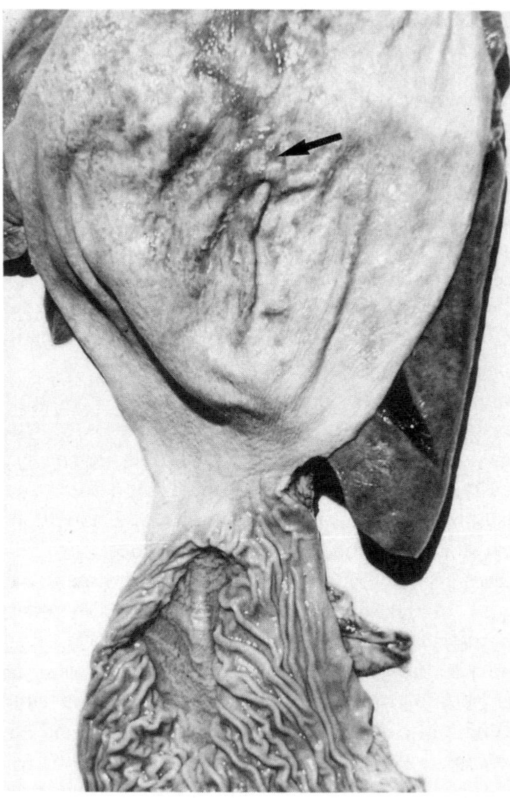

Fig. 1.26 Congenital esophageal dilation. Dog. Mucosal erosions (arrow). Capacity of distal esophagus exceeds that of stomach.

Idiopathic megaesophagus is a relatively common congenital disease in dogs. It is considered to be a neuromuscular developmental disorder or immaturity, which may improve functionally to some extent with time. Megaesophagus in this manifestation is not secondary to physical obstruction or failure of the lower esophageal sphincter to open. Hence, it is not comparable to esophageal achalasia in humans. No consistent reduction in number of ganglia in the esophageal myenteric plexus has been recognized. The functional defect in the dog has no basis in the vagal dorsal motor nucleus, since the external muscle layers of the entire esophagus are striated, and are innervated directly by fibers arising from lower motor neurons in the nucleus ambiguus. These fibers are not parasympathetic, despite being carried in the vagus nerve. The striated esophageal muscle does not show consistent signs of denervation atrophy in idiopathic megaesophagus, and vagal stimulation causes contraction. Hence it is inferred that the lower motor unit is intact. The functional lesion may reside in the upper motor neurons of the central swallowing center, or in the afferent sensory arm of the reflex controlling peristalsis, which arises in the esophagus.

Congenital idiopathic megaesophagus in dogs has its highest prevalence in Great Danes, followed by German shepherds and Irish setters. The condition appears to be heritable, with a pattern in miniature schnauzers compatible with a simple autosomal dominant, or a 60% penetrance autosomal recessive mode of inheritance.

Analogous idiopathic functional and morphologic defects may also develop in mature dogs, in which, in some studies, the majority of cases of megaesophagus are reported to occur. In addition, megaesophagus may be acquired secondary to glycogen storage disease in Lapland dogs, myasthenia gravis, administration of cholinesterase inhibitors, hypoadrenocorticism, canine giant axonal neuropathy, immune-mediated polymyositis, polyradiculoneuritis, canine distemper, systemic lupus erythematosus, lead poisoning, and Chagas' disease.

Megaesophagus in the cat may be congenital, with signs appearing about weaning, and it seems most common in the Siamese breed. The pathogenesis is unclear. Since the esophageal muscle of the cat is smooth in the distal half, dependent on the myenteric plexus for motor control and the vagus for coordination of peristalsis, the pathogenesis probably differs from that in the dog. Neuronal degeneration or neurogenic atrophy of muscle are not recognized in the esophageal wall. Megaesophagus in cats also has been associated with functional pyloric stenosis, hiatus hernia, and lead poisoning.

Several foals have been reported with esophageal dilation or ectasia, apparently congenital. Dilation of the anterior portion, with a normal or thickened caudal thoracic esophagus, was found in two cases. Examination of the wall, which is smooth muscle in the caudal half, revealed equivocal muscle abnormalities, and no anomalies of the autonomic ganglia in those animals. However, aganglionosis has been implicated in megaesophagus in a third case. Megaesophagus may also be acquired in foals with ulceration and fibrosis of the cardia and lower esophagus, associated with ulceration of the pars esophagea of the stomach.

Acquired megaesophagus in cattle has been associated with hiatus hernia, and with pharyngeal trauma presumably causing vagus nerve damage. Segmental megaesophagus is reported in the cervical region, in one case associated with marked fatty replacement of esophageal myofibers. Megaesophagus is rarely reported in small ruminants.

Bibliography

Anderson, N. V. *et al.* Hiatal hernia and segmental megaesophagus in a cow. *J Am Vet Med Assoc* **2:** 193–195, 1984.

Barber, S. M., McLaughlin, B. G., and Fretz, P. B. Esophageal ectasia in a quarterhorse colt. *Can Vet J* **24:** 46–49, 1983.

Boudrieau, R. J., and Rogers, W. A. Megaesophagus in the dog: A review of 50 cases. *J Am Anim Hosp Assoc* **21:** 33–40, 1985.

Braun, U., *et al.* Regurgitation due to megaesophagus in a ram. *Can Vet J* **31:** 391–392, 1990.

Coppock, R. W. *et al.* Preliminary study of the pharmacokinetics and toxicopathy of deoxynivalenol (vomitoxin) in swine. *Am J Vet Res* **46:** 169–174, 1985.

Cox, V. S. *et al.* Hereditary esophageal dysfunction in the miniature schnauzer dog. *Am J Vet Res* **41:** 326–330, 1980.

Guilford, W. G. Megaesophagus in the dog and cat. *Sem Vet Med Surg (Small Anim)* **5:** 37–45, 1990.

Hoenig, M. *et al.* Megaesophagus in two cats. *J Am Vet Med Assoc* **196:** 763–765, 1990.

Klein, H.-J. *et al.* Megaösophagus bei einem Fohlen infolge einer lokalen Aganglionose. *Pferdeheilkunde* **5:** 31–39, 1989.

Leib, M. S. Megaesophagus in the dog. Part I. Anatomy, physiology, and pathophysiology. *Compend Cont Ed Pract Vet* **5:** 825–833, 1983.

Levitt, L. *et al.* Unilateral stylohyoid disarticulation as a cause of dysphagia in a dog. *Can Vet J* **31:** 647–649, 1990.

Maddison, J. E., and Allan, G. S. Megaesophagus attributable to lead toxicosis in a cat. *J Am Vet Med Assoc* **197:** 1357–1358, 1990.

Pearson, H. *et al.* Pyloric and oesophageal dysfunction in the cat. *J Small Anim Pract* **15:** 487–501, 1974.

Strombeck, D. R., and Guilford, W. G. Diseases of swallowing. *In* "Small Animal Gastroenterology," 2nd Ed., pp. 140–166. Davis, California, Stonegate Publishing, 1990.

Vestweber, J. G., Leipold, H. W., and Knighton, R. G. Idiopathic megaesophagus in a calf: Clinical and pathologic features. *J Am Vet Med Assoc* **187:** 1369–1370, 1985.

Walvoort, H. C. Glycogen storage disease type II in the Lapland dog. *Vet Q* **7:** 187–190, 1985.

Willard, M. D. *et al.* Progressive oropharyngeal dysfunction in a dog. *J Am Vet Med Assoc* **183:** 1009–1011, 1983.

E. Parasitic Diseases of the Esophagus

Sarcosporidiosis occurs in the striated esophageal muscle of sheep. Esophageal sarcocysts appear as ovoid white thin-walled nodules ~1 cm long, projecting from the esophageal muscle. *Sarcocystis gigantea,* the species producing large esophageal cysts and similar large cysts in skeletal muscle, is spread by cats. Microscopic sarcocysts of other species also may be encountered in esophageal striated muscle of a variety of hosts [see Protozoal Gastroenteritis (Section VII,F of this chapter), and Muscles and Tendons (Volume 1, Chapter 2)]. Sarcocysts in esophageal muscle normally incite little or no local inflammatory reaction and are of significance only in meat inspection. However, lesions of eosinophilic myositis, possibly associated with rupture of cysts, are found in the esophageal muscle, and megaesophagus has been reported in a sheep with esophageal myositis associated with sarcocysts.

Larvae of *Gasterophilus* spp. may be temporarily attached to the caudal pharyngeal and cranial esophageal mucosa, and to the mucosa cranial to the cardia, in horses. Insignificant focal ulceration may occur at the sites of attachment.

The larvae of the warble fly *Hypoderma lineatum* migrate to the dermis of the back following a period of residence in the submucosa or adventitia of the bovine esophagus. The easily overlooked translucent larvae may be only 2–4 mm in length, but instigate local hemorrhage and neutrophil infiltration. *Hypoderma* assume significance in a small proportion of animals treated with systemic organophosphate insecticides while larvae reside in the esophageal wall. An acute inflammatory reaction, probably an allergic response to products of dead larvae, develops in the esophageal submucosa. This leads to swelling, hemorrhage, and necrosis, causing fatal esophageal obstruction, tympany, and esophageal perforation.

Spirurid nematodes of the genus *Gongylonema* may be encountered in the stratified squamous mucosa of the upper alimentary tract including the esophagus, in ruminants and swine. White threadlike worms 10–15 cm long, they burrow in the epithelium, and occasionally the propria, of the esophageal wall. They usually produce white or red blood-filled zigzag tracks in the mucosa (Fig. 1.27). Their presence is inconsequential to the host.

Spirocerca lupi is a spirurid nematode which parasitizes the esophageal wall of Canidae and some other carnivores. It is most common in warm climates where appropriate species of dung beetles act as intermediate hosts, and where the opportunity for dogs to obtain access to larvae in vertebrate transport hosts is high. The normal site for the adult nematode is in large, thick-walled cystic granulomas in the submucosa of the caudal portion of the esophagus or gastric cardia, where one or more pink worms, surrounded by purulent exudate, are found. A fistulous tract to the esophageal lumen is usually present, through which the tail of the female worm may protrude, and which provides the outlet for ova to the gastrointestinal tract (Fig. 1.28A,B).

Third-stage larvae of *Spirocerca,* ingested with dung beetles or encysted in the insectivorous transport hosts, penetrate the gastric mucosa and move along arteries to the aorta. Here they migrate, often subintimally, forward

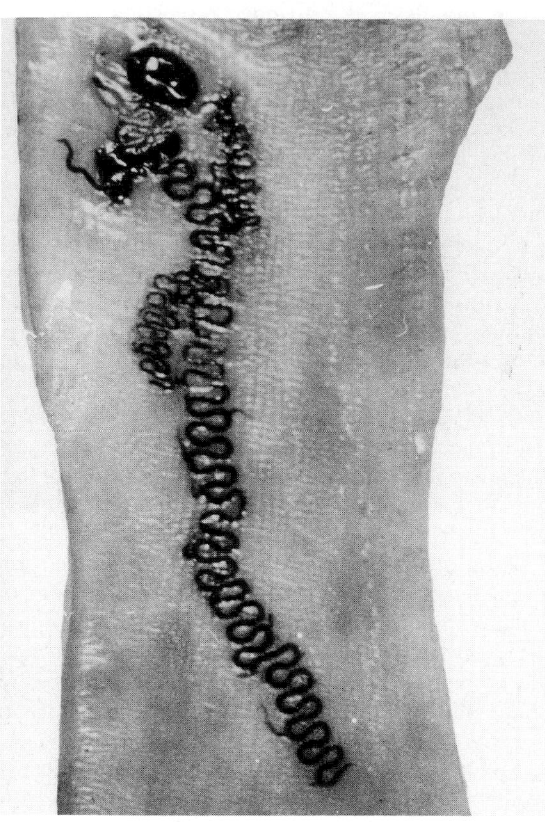

Fig. 1.27 Blood-filled tracks and small hematoma in esophageal mucosa. *Gongylonema pulchrum*. Cow.

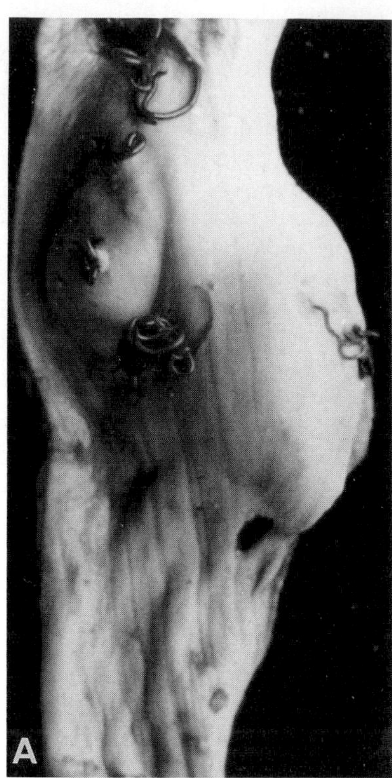

Fig. 1.28A *Spirocerca lupi* nodules in distal esophagus. Dog. Worms protrude through fistulae into esophageal lumen. (Courtesy of R. G. Thomson.)

to the caudal thoracic area, which they attain within several weeks of infection. Following 2–4 months in an inflammatory granuloma in the aortic adventitia, worms migrate to the subjacent esophagus where they develop to adulthood in the submucosa and perforate the epithelium. Larvae which adopt aberrant migratory pathways may be found in granulomas in sites such as the subcutis, bladder, kidney, spinal cord, as well as stomach and intrathoracic locations.

Aortic lesions associated with *Spirocerca* are described with The Cardiovascular System (Volume 3, Chapter 1), but include subintimal and medial hemorrhage and necrosis, with eosinophilic inflammation, intimal roughening with thrombosis, aneurysm with rare aortic rupture, subendothelial and medial mineralization, and heterotopic bone deposition. The presence of persistent aortic lesions in the dog, even in the absence of esophageal granuloma, is evidence for prior infection with *S. lupi*. Spondylosis of the ventral aspects of thoracic vertebral bodies 5–10 occurs in some cases. Exostoses or bony spurs arise from one or both ends of the vertebral bodies, and presumably are instigated by the local irritant effects of migrating worms.

In some animals with *S. lupi,* mesenchymal neoplasms develop in the wall of the esophageal granuloma, and pulmonary fibrosarcoma has been associated with an

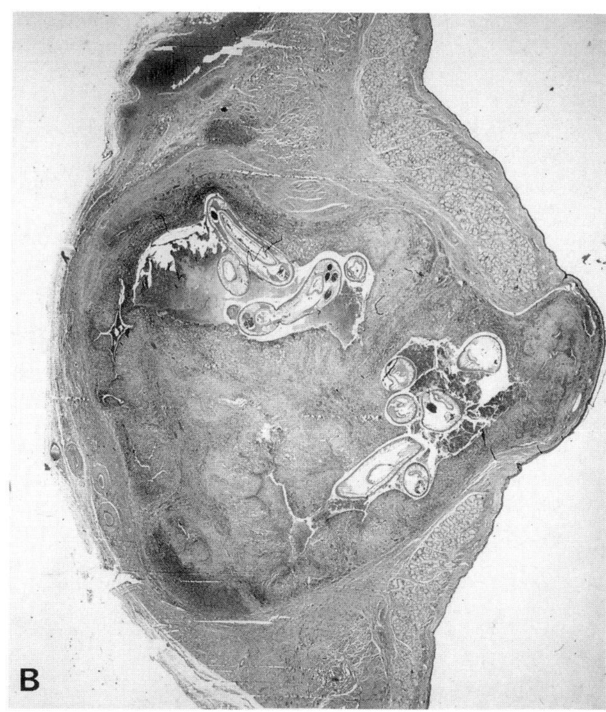

Fig. 1.28B Section through esophageal nodule containing *Spirocerca lupi*. Dog.

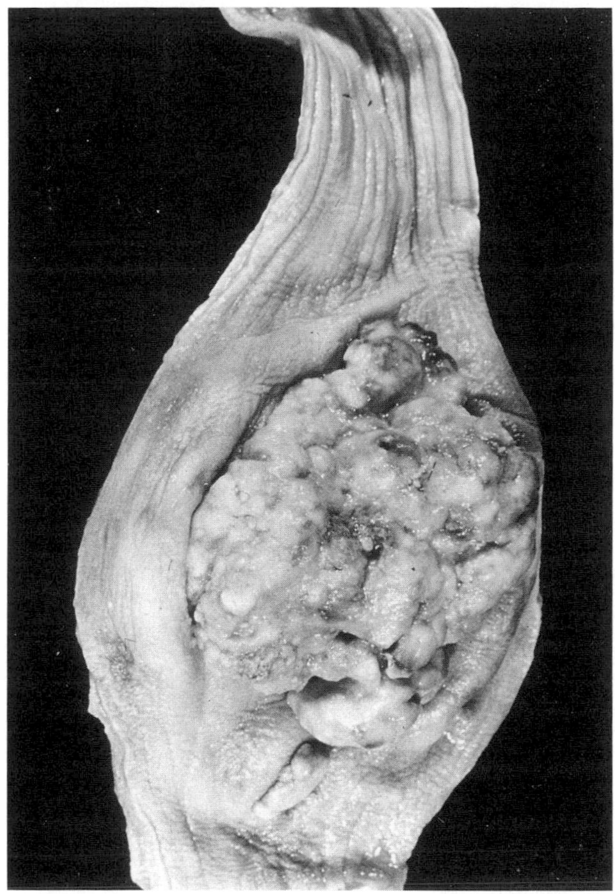

Fig. 1.29 Ulcerating fibrosarcoma associated with *Spirocerca* granuloma. Distal esophagus. Dog. (Courtesy of R. G. Thomson.)

ectopic worm (Fig. 1.29). The granulomas around *Spirocerca* contain highly reactive pleomorphic fibroblasts with large open nuclei and numerous mitotic figures. Neoplasms arising from such lesions have cytologic characteristics typical of fibrosarcoma and osteosarcoma, with local tissue invasion, and in many cases, pulmonary metastasis. The carcinogenic stimuli associated with the development of these tumors are unknown. Hypertrophic osteopathy is occasionally found in animals with *Spirocerca*-associated sarcoma and rarely, granuloma. Clinical disease, exclusive of that associated with neoplasia, is uncommon in animals with *S. lupi,* and is restricted to aortic thrombosis or aneurysmal rupture, occasional partial esophageal obstruction, and rare perforation.

Bibliography

Collins, G. H., Atkinson, E., and Charleston, W. A. G. Studies on *Sarcocystis* species III: The macrocystic species of sheep. *N Z Vet J* **27:** 204–206, 1979.

Fox, S. M., Burns, J., and Hawkins, J. Spirocercosis in dogs. *Compend Cont Ed Pract Vet* **10:** 807–822, 1988.

Munday, B. L., and Obendorf, D. L. Growth and development of *Sarcocystis gigantea* in experimentally infected sheep. *Vet Parasitol* **15:** 203–211, 1984.

Stephens, L. C., Gleiser, C. A., and Jordine, J. H. Primary pulmonary fibrosarcoma associated with *Spirocerca lupi* infection in a dog with hypertrophic pulmonary osteoarthropathy. *J Am Vet Med Assoc* **182:** 496–498, 1983.

IV. The Forestomachs

The importance of closely examining the rumen contents is often overlooked during routine autopsy. The first, and sometimes only, indication of the presence of certain toxic substances may be provided by the odor and appearance of the rumen content. Urea toxicity may be indicated by an ammoniacal odor and alkaline pH. Organophosphates have a characteristic pungent insecticidal smell reminiscent of cooked turnip. *Taxus* spp. toxicity is signified by an aromatic odor like cedar oil, and the presence of needles in the ingesta. In other suspected plant poisonings, characteristic foliage should be sought in rumen contents. The presence of paint flakes, pieces of metallic lead, and oily content and odor (from used crankcase oil) point to lead poisoning. Frothy voluminous rumen content will support a diagnosis of primary tympany. Porridgelike content with a fermentative odor and perhaps acid pH (<5.0) suggests grain overload.

A. Dystrophic and Hyperplastic Changes in the Ruminal Mucosa

The ruminal papillae in the newborn are rudimentary, which gives the mucosa a relatively smooth and pale appearance. Subsequent development of the ruminal papillae depends mainly on the type of diet fed. Little or no growth of papillae occurs in animals as long as they are fed milk. Animals on rations containing adequate levels of roughage develop long, slender, regular, white to gray ruminal papillae. The ruminal pillars normally lack papillae. Microscopically, the normal papillae are covered by a thin layer of keratinized squamous epithelial cells.

Rations high in concentrate give rise to black, club- and tongue-shaped papillae, which have a tendency to form clumps, nodules, and rosettes. They are distributed over the entire mucosa, except for a small area in the dorsal sac where the gas cap would be located. The most prominent changes are mainly in the atrium ruminis and ventral caudal sac, depending somewhat on the age of the animal and the type of concentrate. Microscopically, there is marked acanthosis, hyper- and parakeratosis, and hyperpigmentation of the papillary epithelial cells. Hyperplasia of secondary papillae is also prominent, which may explain the formation of clumps and rosettes seen grossly. The wall is thickened due to fibroplasia of the lamina propria and submucosa. Rumens in animals fed barley rations have similar changes. In addition, animal and vegetable hairs, from the rachilla of the barley, adhere to the mucosa, especially in the interpapillary areas, giving it a distinct matted appear-

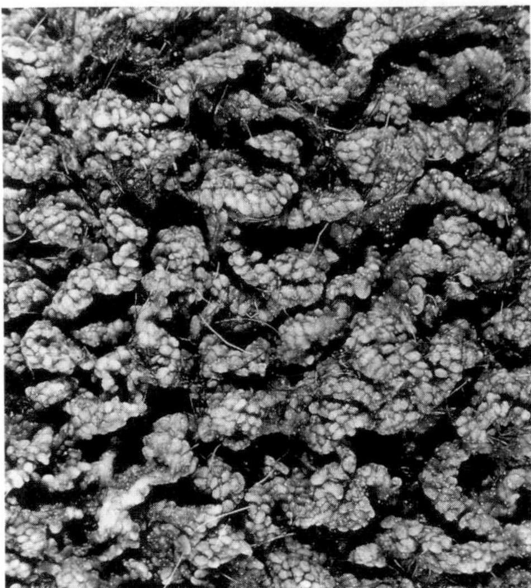

Fig. 1.30 Clubbing and adhesion of rumen papillae with parakeratotic epithelium, associated with feeding a ration high in barley. Plant fibers and hairs are among the matted papillae.

ance (Fig. 1.30). Large numbers of hairs are seen in sections of the mucosa. They penetrate the mucosa and lamina propria, where they evoke a leukocytic inflammatory reaction, often causing microabscesses. A diffuse pleocellular reaction is evident in the thickened fibrotic wall.

The pathogenesis of morphologic variations in the ruminal papillae depends on several factors. These include the level, type, and proportion of volatile fatty acids evolved in the ruminal contents, the pH, and the proportion and coarseness of the roughage fed. Other factors are probably involved. High-concentrate rations result in increased levels of propionic and butyric acids and lower concentrations of acetic acid. The mucosal adaptation is of major importance for the stabilization of the pH of the rumen contents in ruminants fed high-energy rations. The pH is also lowered, but not enough to cause chemical rumenitis. Hyper- and parakeratosis do not occur when ruminants are fed rations containing adequate levels (approximately 15%) of coarse roughage. The dystrophic changes in the mucosa are reversible when high concentrates are replaced by such levels of roughage. Such a change in the ratio of roughage to concentrate in the diet results in a rise in pH and a shift in the proportions of fatty acids: acetic acid levels increase; propionic and butyric acids decrease. Roughage is also thought to remove keratinaceous debris and food particles from the mucosal surface. The animal and vegetable hairs in barley rations may provide the portal of entry for bacteria, which cause the mild rumenitis and microabscesses in the ruminal wall.

Hyperkeratosis of the ruminal epithelium also occurs in calves deficient in vitamin A.

Bibliography

Landsverk, T. Indigestion in young calves. IV. Lesions of ruminal papillae in young calves fed barley and barley plus hay. *Acta Vet Scand* **19:** 377–391, 1978.

Leek, B. F. Reticuloruminal function and dysfunction. *Vet Rec* **84:** 238–243, 1969.

Liebich, H. G., and Scharrer, E. Entwicklungsbedingte Veränderungen von Struktur und Funktion des Pansenepithels. *Zbl Vet Med C* **13:** 25–41, 1984.

Mayer, E. Changements de régimes alimentaires et variations morphologiques des papilles du rumen chez la vache laitière à haute production. *Bull Acad Vét France* **59:** 159–174, 1986.

McGavin, M. D., and Morill, J. L. Scanning electron microsopy of ruminal papillae in calves fed various amounts and forms of roughage. *Am J Vet Res* **37:** 497–508, 1976.

Scheurmann, E., and Weyrauch, K. D. Einfluss der Ernährung auf den Papillarkörper der Pansenschleimhaut bei Kälbern. *Zbl Vet Med C* **12:** 126–138, 1983.

Warner, E. D. The organogenesis and early histogenesis of the bovine stomach. *Am J Anat* **102:** 33–63, 1958.

B. Postmortem Change

The ruminal mucosa usually sloughs within a few hours after death. It separates from the lamina propria in large gray patches, which cover the ingesta when the rumen is opened.

Persistent firm attachment of epithelium is abnormal. This undue adhesion occurs in dystrophic changes, described earlier, in acute rumenitis, especially if caused by fungi, and about healed lesions of necrobacillary rumenitis. Adhesion may not occur in the early stages of ruminal acidosis.

C. Dilation of the Rumen

Tympanitic distension of the forestomachs (tympany, hoven, bloat) may be acute, or chronic and recurrent, and there is a basic distinction between the two. The acute tympany of cattle fed legumes is characterized by foaming of the rumen contents, whereas in chronic or recurrent tympany, the gas is free but retained because of some physical or functional defect of eructation.

Primary tympany is also called frothy bloat. Foam production in ruminal contents occurs normally. However, the amount of foam produced is small and unstable. There is apparently a delicate balance between pro- and antifoaming factors. These factors are multiple, and there is considerable controversy as to the extent that each one influences the production of the foamy, viscous ruminal content so characteristic of frothy bloat, the most common cause of rumen distension.

The formation of foam is dependent on soluble proteins, especially fraction I proteins, which are present in high levels (to 4.5%) in bloat-inducing legumes. These soluble proteins are released from chloroplasts. When they are degraded by the rumen microflora, they rise to the surface where they are denatured, become insoluble, and stabilize the foam. The optimal pH (isoelectric point) for foam production by soluble proteins ranges from 5.4 to 6.0. Pectins are considered to increase viscosity of ruminal fluid and may act as foam-stabilizing agents. Plant lipids may act as antifoaming agents by competing for metal ions with the soluble proteins, thus inhibiting the denaturation of these proteins and resulting in decreased foam production.

Chloroplasts and particulate matter may play a more important role than the soluble proteins in the pathogenesis of frothy bloat by providing a matrix for colonization by rumen microorganisms, stimulating rapid fermentations of ingesta, resulting in increased gas production. The fermentation gases are trapped by buoyant frothy ingesta. Excessive foam production causes distension of the rumen because the animals are unable to eructate foam. Frothy ruminal contents prevent the clearing of the cardia, which is essential for normal eructation to take place. When foam enters the esophagus, it stimulates the swallowing reflex, which also interferes with normal eructation.

Animal factors which may contribute to bloat are less accessible to study, and little is known of them. Certain sires are known to produce cows which have a high susceptibility to bloating. These differences in susceptibility to bloat do not appear to be due to differences in anatomical structure and function of the ruminoreticulum. Monozygotic twins may have similar bloating tendencies.

The variation among animals in their susceptibility to bloat may be determined in part by variations in the amount and composition of saliva secreted. Saliva apparently has properties which may promote or prevent foaming in the rumen. When secretion of saliva decreases, the viscosity of ruminal contents increases, which in turn promotes foaming. Cows that have a high susceptibility to bloating produce less saliva than cows which have a low susceptibility. Succulent and high-concentrate feeds reduce salivary secretion, thus increasing viscosity of rumen contents. The composition of saliva affects foam production in several ways. Combination of salivary bicarbonate with organic acids such as citric, malonic, and succinic acids, which are present in high levels in legumes, results in the production of large amounts of carbon dioxide, enhancing bubble formation. Carbon dioxide accounts for 40–70% of the total gas produced in the rumen.

Salivary mucoproteins increase viscosity, whereas mucins reduce viscosity. The levels of the various pro- and antifoaming compounds in saliva are dependent on the gland of origin. The parotid and submaxillary glands produce saliva with a high concentration of mucins. These glands actively secrete saliva when the animal is eating and when ruminal pressure is high. The buffering action of saliva may raise the pH of the ruminal contents above the range at which soluble proteins are most likely to produce stable foam. Cattle that have a high susceptibility to bloating have higher levels of chlorophyll that originates from chloroplasts, more buoyant particulate matter, and higher rates of gas production in the ruminal contents compared to cattle that do not bloat. High and low susceptibility to bloat can be temporarily transferred between animals by exchange of total reticulorumen contents. The understanding of the full role played by these various factors in bloat is still incomplete, and other factors may be involved.

Rations high in concentrate and low in roughage not only reduce saliva secretion, but they also change the ruminal microflora. They promote the growth of large numbers of encapsulated bacteria, which increase the concentration of polysaccharides, and these, in turn, increase the viscosity. These bacteria are also often mucinolytic and may destroy the salivary mucins. Perhaps this explains the more gradual onset of **feedlot bloat,** since it takes time for the ruminal flora to change.

The cause of death in bloat is probably the combined effects of increased intra-abdominal pressure on the diaphragm inhibiting respiration, and the shunting of a large volume of blood away from the abdominal viscera. Anoxia may be caused by respiratory embarrassment. Increased intra-abdominal pressure also has a marked effect on the hemodynamics of the abdominal viscera. There is compression of the posterior vena cava, which results in a redirection of blood flow from the caudal areas of the animal. The blood is shunted through the lumbar veins, into the longitudinal vertebral sinuses, from there to the intercostal veins and into the hemiazygos or costocervical vein.

The bloated animal is often found dead and distended with gas; blood exudes from the orifices, and because of the gaseous distension, the carcass often rolls on its back and assumes a sawhorse posture. The blood is dark and clots poorly; both features are indicative of death due to anoxia. Subcutaneous hemorrhages are prominent in the neck and the trunk. There is marked edema, congestion, and hemorrhage of the cervical muscles and of the lymph nodes of the head and neck. An inconsistent, but significant finding, is the so-called bloat line in the esophageal mucosa (Fig. 1.31A). This lesion is formed due to congestion with petechial and ecchymotic hemorrhages in the mucosa of the cervical esophagus, which changes abruptly

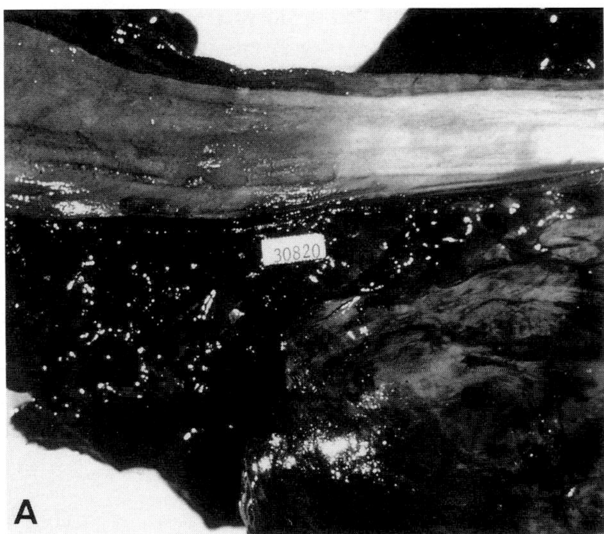

Fig. 1.31A Bloat line. Cow. Ruminal tympany. Congestion of esophagus and connective tissue cranial to thoracic inlet and blanching of esophagus caudal to thoracic inlet.

or gradually to a pale mucosa at the level of the thoracic inlet. The tracheal mucosa is hemorrhagic, especially anterior to the thoracic inlet. Blood clots are frequently seen in the bronchi, and paranasal and frontal sinuses. The lungs are compressed into the anterior thorax by the bulging diaphragm. There is pressure ischemia of the abdominal viscera, especially the liver. The extreme margins of the hepatic lobes may be congested. Lymph nodes and the muscles of the hind legs are pale. There may be marked subcutaneous edema, particularly of the vulva and perineum. If the autopsy is done soon after death, the ruminal contents are bulky and foamy (Fig. 1.31B). The foam gradually disappears after death and is usually absent if the autopsy is delayed for 10–12 hr. Inguinal hernia and diaphragmatic rupture may occur after death.

Secondary tympany (free gas or secondary bloat) may be acute, but is usually chronic, with periods of acute exacerbation. It is usually the result of a physical or functional defect in eructation of gas produced by normal rumen fermentation. The more common physical problems include internal or external obstructions of esophagus or esophageal groove by tumor, papilloma, or foreign body, and esophageal stenosis of any cause. Reticular adhesions, abscesses, peritonitis, or tumor masses that interfere with contractions of the forestomach can result in bloat. Functional causes of secondary tympany include organophosphate intoxication, and vagal damage due to adhesion or lymphosarcomatous infiltrates. It is a component of the syndromes collectively termed vagus indigestion.

Secondary tympany, sometimes fatal, occurs in bucket-fed calves. They ingest large amounts of milk, which escape the esophageal groove and flow into the rumen, where it putrefies because of digestion by proteolytic bacteria. Failure of the esophageal reflex may be a persistent problem in some veal calves, which are known as ruminal drinkers. The clinical signs are characterized by inappetence, unthriftiness, recurrent tympany, abdominal distention, and claylike feces. The presence of partly digested milk in the rumen results in hyper- and parakeratosis of the mucosa and perhaps a mild rumenitis. Casein clot formation in the abomasum is inhibited. The affected calves have villus atrophy in the small intestine resulting in malabsorption. The pathogenesis of the latter remains to be resolved.

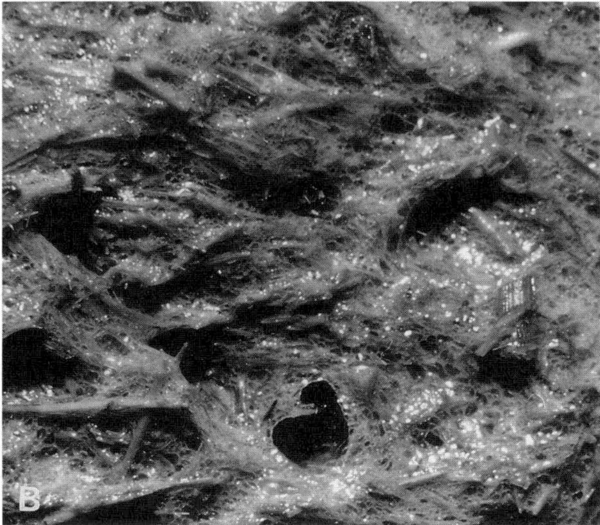

Fig. 1.31B Frothy bloat. Cow. Fine bubbles are evident in the rumen content.

Animals fed rations that have too much roughage may have recurrent episodes of bloat. Feed must contain adequate proportions of protein, starch and/or sugars, and cellulose to stimulate growth of the cellulytic microflora. Undigestible roughage accumulates in the rumen and reticulum when the intake of digestible nutrients (starches and sugars) is inadequate. As a result the forestomachs become dilated, which in turn inhibits rumenoreticular contractions that are required for clearance of the cardia and subsequent eructation.

A diagnosis of secondary bloat at autopsy is based on physical findings like those described in primary bloat, but without frothy rumen content, and with the addition of any physical causes of impaired eructation. Postmortem distension of the rumen must not be mistaken for antemortem tympany. Extraruminal lesions must be present to establish a diagnosis of bloat.

Bibliography

Breukink, H. J. *et al.* Consequences of failure of the reticular groove reflex in veal calves fed milk replacer. *Vet Q* **10:** 126–135, 1988.

Clarke, R. T. J., and Reid, C. S. W. Foamy bloat of cattle: A review. *J Dairy Sci* **57:** 753–785, 1974.

Constable, P. D. *et al.* The reticulorumen: Normal and abnormal motor function. Part II. Secondary contraction cycles, rumination, and esophageal groove closure. *Compend Cont Ed Pract Vet* **12:** 1169–1174, 1990.

Dirksen, G. U., and Gary, F. B. Diseases of the forestomachs in calves. Parts I, II. *Compend Cont Ed Pract Vet* **9:** F140–F147, F173–F179, 1987.

Howarth, R. E. A review of bloat in cattle. *Can Vet J* **16:** 281–294, 1975.

Keane, D. P. *et al.* Congenital esophagotracheal fistula as the cause of bloat in a calf. *Can Vet J* **24:** 57–59, 1983.

Majak, W. *et al.* The distribution of chlorophyll in rumen contents and the onset of bloat in cattle. *Can J Anim Sci* **66:** 97–102, 1986.

Mills, J. H. L., and Christian, R. G. Lesions of bovine ruminal tympany. *J Am Vet Med Assoc* **157:** 947–952, 1970.

Waghorn, G. C., and Reid, C. S. W. Bloat in cattle. 43. Resting level and vertical displacement of the cranial pillar and other structures in the ruminoreticulum of cattle of known bloat susceptibility. *N Z J Agric Res* **27:** 481–490, 1984.

D. Foreign Bodies in the Forestomachs

Cattle are notoriously lacking in alimentary finesse, a deficiency that allows an amazing variety of foreign bodies, prehended with the food, to be deposited in the forestomachs. Sheep are largely immune because of their more selective eating habits. Foreign bodies are rarely found in the rumen of goats, despite their reputation for indiscriminate feeding habits. In consequence, a large proportion of adult cattle, and very few goats or sheep, have foreign bodies in the rumen and reticulum, but rarely in the omasum. It is possible that many of the lighter and smaller foreign bodies are regurgitated.

Foreign bodies consisting largely of hair or wool (trichobezoars), or plant fibers (phytobezoars) may also form in these compartments. Hairballs are most common in younger ruminants, the hair being swallowed after licking, particularly by animals deprived of dietary fiber. They may have some other foreign body as a nucleus and contain a proportion of plant fibers, the whole mass concreted by organic substances and inorganic salts. The same general comments apply to phytobezoars. Being smooth, neither are important unless regurgitated to lodge in the esophagus or passed on to obstruct the reticulo-omasal orifice, the pylorus, or the intestine, which is infrequent.

The important foreign bodies are those (such as lead) which cause intoxication when dissolved, and those which (being abrasive or sharp) penetrate the mucosa. In calves on diets low in roughage, ingestion of wood shavings or straw may lead to diffuse cellulitis of the forestomachs and sometimes the abomasum. A mixed bacterial flora containing clostridia is responsible, presumably following mucosal trauma. The sequel to penetration by sharp objects in adult cattle is traumatic reticuloperitonitis.

Bibliography

Osborne, A. D. Hairballs in veal calves. *Vet Rec* **99:** 239, 1976.

E. Traumatic Reticuloperitonitis and Its Complications

Perforation of the forestomachs by foreign bodies virtually always is a penetration of the reticular wall by a sharp foreign body, usually a piece of wire or a nail 4 cm or more in length. Incomplete perforation of the wall is usually without significant effect, although in some cases a suppurative or granulomatous inflammation develops in the wall of the reticulum, with minor overlying peritonitis. There are no adequate answers as to why perforation occurs or why it is so frequently in the anteroventral direction. It is probably caused by forceful contraction of the reticulum, and many cases seem to be precipitated by the increased intra-abdominal pressure of late pregnancy and parturition.

There is a rather uniform train of events when complete perforation occurs, but variations of the pattern are common. The perforation is usually in the anteroventral direction and is followed immediately by an acute local peritonitis. If the foreign body is short or bent, it may progress no further, and some foreign bodies are apparently withdrawn with the next reticular movement; in such instances, a chronic local peritonitis with adhesions develops. The foreign body may advance to perforate the diaphragm and pericardium, resulting in traumatic pericarditis, but this advancement may be delayed.

A ventral penetration may result in subperitoneal and subcutaneous abscess near the xiphoid. Rare perforation of one of the larger regional arteries may result in sudden death from hemorrhage, and sudden death may also occur if there is penetration of the myocardium or rupture of a coronary artery. Penetration of the thoracic cavity may occur without perforation of the pericardium and causes pneumonia and pleuritis. Right lateral deviation of the penetrating agent causes involvement of the wall of the abomasum. It is unusual for the liver or spleen to be penetrated, but metastatic abscesses in the liver are common.

As soon as the foreign body penetrates the serosa, a local fibrinous peritonitis develops, which later leads to dense adhesion of variable extent between the reticulum and adjacent structures. Further progression of the foreign body is ordinarily slow and produces a canal surrounded by chronic granulation tissue and containing, besides the foreign body, ingesta, purulent exudate, and detritus. The bacteria commonly active in the tract are *Actinomyces pyogenes, Fusobacterium necrophorum,* and a variety of putrefactive types. In many cases, a foreign body cannot be found, perhaps because it has rusted away or been withdrawn into the reticulum.

Traumatic pericarditis is a less common sequel now, perhaps because so many of the initial penetrations are diagnosed and the foreign body removed surgically. The pericardial reaction is copious, fibrinopurulent, and putrid. There are usually additional lesions of traumatic pneumonia and pleurisy.

The prophylactic use of magnets has become common in many herds, and this probably contributes to the marked decrease in fatal cases. Frequently, these magnets are found incidentally in the reticulum, completely covered with metal foreign bodies, including nails and wires, which might otherwise have penetrated the reticular wall. The replacement of baling wire with binder twine is another reason for the apparent decline in the prevalence of this disease.

One of the variants in the usual pattern of migration of the foreign body is penetration of the side of the reticulum, leading to a suppurative inflammation in the grooves between the reticulum, omasum, and abomasum. Although the acute local peritonitis causes immediate cessation of ruminal movements, a persistent ruminal atony or irregular motility and gradual onset of bilateral abdominal distension, inappetence, and decreased milk production may ensue. Clinically, this is referred to as **vagus indigestion,** and at autopsy there are very characteristic changes in the stomachs.

In vagus indigestion, the abomasum may be distended and impacted with dry ingesta, presumably because of functional pyloric stenosis or abomasal stasis. The omasum in this condition can be very large and impacted with dehydrated ingesta. The rumen is distended with enough fluid to cause sloshing if the carcass is jolted. There is no ruminal fermentation or odor, and bits of unmacerated straw and food particles float on the watery fluid. The more-normal ingesta has sedimented.

The question of the importance of vagal nerve damage in the pathogenesis of so-called vagus indigestion remains unresolved. The consensus is that this syndrome is associated with mechanical or functional impairment of outflow of ingesta from the forestomachs or abomasum, but in some cases the primary defect appears to reside in flaccidity of the esophageal groove and in degeneration of its muscle and intramuscular nerve plexus. The rumen and reticulum are dependent on intact vagi for normal movement, and a minority of cases of vagus indigestion appear to be associated with damaged nerves. Vagal lesions may be in the pharyngeal and cervical areas, or intrathoracic, such as lymphosarcomatous infiltration, or abdominal. The latter are usually investment of the nerve in adhesions following reticular perforation, or trauma following abomasal volvulus.

In other cases, degeneration of the vagus is not evident. In these, the dysfunction and lesions are more likely to be due to peritonitis and the subsequent abscessation, or adhesions which disrupt the normal tension-receptor activity, or cause a pain response that interferes with normal motility of the forestomachs and abomasum. In **failure of omasal transport,** (type II vagus indigestion), there is impairment of movement of ingesta from the rumenoreticulum to the omasum, associated with abscesses adjacent to the reticulo-omasal orifice. There, lesions probably result in mechanical or neural interference to emptying of the ruminoreticulum. A diagnosis of vagal indigestion at autopsy is ordinarily dependent on evidence of abnormal abomasal, omasal, or reticuloruminal motility, in association with morphologic lesions of the vagus nerves, or adhesions, or neoplasms involving the forestomachs and abomasum.

Bibliography

Fubini, S. S. *et al.* Failure of omasal transport attributable to perireticular abscess formation in cattle: 29 cases (1980–1986). *J Am Vet Med Assoc* **194:** 811–814, 1989.

Misra, S. S., and Angelo, S. J. Traumatic reticulopericarditis in bovines. *Vet Res J* **4:** 89–113, 1981.

Rebhun, W. C. *et al.* Vagus indigestion in cattle: Clinical features, causes, treatments, and long-term follow-up of 112 cases. *Compend Cont Ed Pract Vet* **10:** 387–392, 1988.

F. Rumenitis

Inflammatory lesions in the forestomachs occur in a number of viral diseases of the alimentary tract in ruminants. In neonatal calves, necrosis of ruminal mucosa is an important sequel to infectious bovine rhinotracheitis infection. Bovine papular stomatitis and contagious ecthyma will rarely cause rumen lesions. Ruminal erosions and ulcers are present in some cattle with mucosal disease; they are reported to be less common in rinderpest. Extensive hemorrhage and ulceration of the reticuloruminal mucosa may be seen in bluetongue in sheep. Adenovirus infection occasionally causes a multifocal fibrinohemorrhagic rumenitis. Focal or diffuse rumenitis may be present in cattle with malignant catarrhal fever. These conditions are described fully with Infectious and Parasitic Diseases of the Gastrointestinal Tract (Section VII of this chapter).

A mild inflammation of the forestomachs occurs in some young calves fed milk from a pail, when, because of laxity of the esophageal-groove reflex, the milk spills into the rumen and reticulum in large quantity. A similar problem occurs with feeding by stomach tube. Putrefaction in these compartments leads to mild rumenitis, with edema and mild neutrophil infiltration of the mucosa.

Accidental consumption of excessive quantities of urea, in the form of nonprotein nitrogen supplement, or fertilizer, in liquid or powder form, results in the production of ammonia in the rumen. The toxic effect is accelerated by urease in soy-based rations, and is based on the production of high blood levels of ammonia. Rumen contents smell ammoniacal when the organ is opened; the content is alkaline; and there may be congestion or coagulation necrosis of the anteroventral wall of the rumen. Elevated ruminal and abomasal pH values ($\geq$7.0), without specific lesions, have been associated with ingestion of boron fertilizer by cattle and goats.

Ingestion of toxic levels of sulfur results in chemical rumenitis due to the conversion of sulfur to H_2S, and possibly sulfurous acid, in the rumen. Large amounts of yellow sulfur granules are usually found in the rumen and abomasum. Eructation and subsequent inhalation of H_2S results in acute alveolitis. Absorption of the sulfides from the lungs leads to marked depression of the respiratory and cardiovascular centers in the central nervous system. Affected animals also develop acidosis, probably due to the absorption of acids, and impaired renal function associated with the direct toxic effects of sulfur metabolites on tubular epithelial cells.

Inflammation of the forestomachs may be associated with certain plant toxicoses, mainly in Australia and southern Africa. Examples are Kikuyu grass (*Pennisetum clandestinum*) and prickly paddy melon (*Cucumis myriocarpus*).

A more common form of acute chemical rumenitis develops after overeating on rapidly fermentable carbohydrate, usually grain.

Bibliography

Bartley, E. E. *et al.* Ammonia toxicity in cattle. I. Rumen and blood changes associated with toxicity and treatment methods. *J Anim Sci* **43:** 835–841, 1976.

Davidovich, A. *et al.* Ammonia toxicity in cattle. III. Absorption of ammonia gas from the rumen and passage of urea and ammonia from the rumen to the duodenum. *J Anim Sci* **46:** 551–558, 1977.

Fell, B. F. *et al.* The role of ingested animal hairs and plant spicules in the pathogenesis of rumenitis. *Res Vet Sci* **13:** 30–36, 1972.

Gunn, M. F. *et al.* Accidental sulfur poisoning in a group of Holstein heifers. *Can Vet J* **28:** 188–192, 1987.

Kennedy, P. M., and Milligan, L. P. The degradation and utiliza-

tion of endogenous urea in the gastrointestinal tract of ruminants: A review. *Can J Anim Sci* **60:** 205–221, 1980.
McKenzie, R. A. *et al.* Prickly paddy melon (*Cucumis myriocarpus*) poisoning of cattle. *Aust Vet J* **65:** 167–170, 1988.
Peet, R. L. *et al.* Kikuyu poisoning in goats and sheep. *Aust Vet J* **67:** 229–230, 1990.
Sisk, D. B. *et al.* Acute, fatal illness in cattle exposed to boron fertilizer. *J Am Vet Med Assoc* **193:** 943–945, 1988.

G. Rumenitis and Acidosis Caused by Carbohydrate Overload

Ruminal acidosis and rumenitis associated with ingestion of excess carbohydrate is a problem mainly of intensive beef and dairy production. Sheep, and especially goats, are also susceptible to this problem. Its importance lies partly in loss of production and partly in mortality due to the acute disease, in which the rumenitis is of minor significance, and the lactic acidosis is the major cause of morbidity and mortality. Rumenitis assumes significance in subclinical disease or in survivors of acute episodes by providing a portal for the entry for fungi and *F. necrophorum*. These complications are discussed subsequently. There are other complications. Primary tympany (frothy bloat) may coexist and be the fatal partner of grain overload in feedlot cattle.

Ruminal acidosis usually follows the ingestion of excess carbohydrate in the form of grain, or other fermentable feedstuffs occasionally used, such as root crops, bread, brewers' waste, and apples. There is a wide variation in the amount of carbohydrate necessary to kill an animal, because tolerance to rations high in starch does develop. Sudden increments in the amount of carbohydrate ingested are of more importance than the actual amount, provided this increases slowly. In sheep, for which some information is available, about 60 gm of wheat per kg of body weight must be ingested to cause death; probably this figure is generally applicable to cattle also. Lesser amounts than this may cause illness but permit eventual recovery. Even after cattle are accustomed to high-concentrate rations, they may still develop ruminal acidosis. Sudden changes from concentrates with lower energy values to those with higher values may predispose to acidosis. Extreme environmental temperature changes, either hotter or cooler, may result in temporary reductions in feed consumption, and acidosis may develop once such animals return to full feed.

Shortly after the ingestion of a toxic amount of carbohydrate, the ruminal pH begins to fall. The decrease in pH during the first 8 hr is mainly due to an increase in dissociated volatile fatty acids, not lactic acid. The production of the latter increases after there has been a marked change in the ruminal flora, which is very responsive to the substrate available for fermentation. The normal pH of ruminal fluid in cattle and sheep varies between 5.5 and 7.5, depending on the diet fed.

The Gram-negative bacteria which predominate in the normal flora and the protozoa are very sensitive to changes in the pH. Most of these organisms die at a pH of 5.0 or less. Once the pH of the ruminal contents starts to decrease, there is a rapid proliferation of streptococci, mainly *Streptococcus bovis,* and these bacteria are the main source of lactic acid. When the pH reaches 5.0–4.5, the numbers of streptococci decrease, with a concomitant increase in lactobacilli. The pH of rumen content may be as low as 4.0–4.5 in fatal cases.

As the ruminal pH drops, ruminal atony develops, mainly as the result of an increase in the concentration of nondissociated fatty acids, rather than of lactic acid, as was once thought. There are many epithelial receptors in the forestomachs that are excited by one or more of the three volatile fatty acids: lactic, propionic, and butyric acid. Loss of ruminal motility may result from activation of these receptors by elevated levels of these acids. The receptors mediate inhibition of reticuloruminal motility via a vagovagal reflex. Lactic acid is apparently not responsible for receptor activation despite being present in high levels, although it may facilitate the excitation of the other receptors because of its erosive action on the mucosa. Loss of forestomach motility in ruminal acidosis is apparently not dependent on the development of systemic acidosis. There is also a cessation of salivary secretion so that the buffering effect of saliva is absent.

The increase in ruminal organic acids, mainly lactate, causes an increase in ruminal osmotic pressure. This results in movement of fluid from the blood into the rumen, producing bulky and liquid ruminal contents and severe dehydration. There is a reduction in plasma volume; hemoconcentration, anuria, and circulatory collapse follow. Serum protein levels, urea, inorganic phosphorus, lactate, pyruvate, and liver enzymes are all elevated. The osmotic pressure of the intestinal contents also increases when the ingesta with the high lactate concentrations arrives there. Loss of fluid at this level probably contributes further to the dehydration, and it may also play a significant role in the development of the diarrhea, which is commonly seen clinically.

In those animals which survive the acute phase of ruminal acidosis, complete recovery is delayed until a normal ruminal flora is reestablished through contact with other animals. A temporary recovery may be followed by what appears clinically to be a relapse in acidosis, but which is a developing mycotic rumenitis. If treatment of the initial fluid imbalance is delayed, death may occur in a week or so from ischemic renal cortical necrosis.

In addition to the osmotic effects, there is acidosis due to the absorption of lactate from the rumen, and possibly from the intestine. Almost equal concentrations of D- and L-isomers of lactic acid are produced in the rumen. However, the D-isomer of lactic acid is poorly metabolized by the host and hence accumulates eventually to a much higher concentration in plasma than does the L-isomer. This is probably reinforced by endogenous lactate produced in the state of relative anaerobiosis of peripheral circulatory failure. The blood pH may be as low as 7.0, which causes a marked depletion of alkali reserves. Absorption of D-lactate exceeds the rate of metabolic breakdown, and further aggravation of the acidosis may occur when the excretion of this isomer is impaired due to reduced renal function. Such a reduction in the plasma clearance of lactic acid occurs only after the blood pH decreases to 7.14 or less, and lactic acid levels have increased to approximately 25 ml/liter or higher. There are other toxic factors, including histamine, produced in this disease, but the amounts absorbed from an acid rumen are probably too low to have any effect.

The low ruminal pH which develops is lethal to much of the normal flora and fauna. The protozoa appear to be particularly sensitive, but many types of bacteria are also lost. Therefore, in animals which show signs of immediate recovery, with or without therapeutic aid, the reestablishment of normal fermentation reactions may be delayed.

The morbid anatomy of this metabolic disease is not specific, and a practical diagnosis requires knowledge of access to fermentable carbohydrate and a clinically observed circulatory failure. At autopsy, the eyes are sunken, the blood may be thick and dark due to dehydration and hypoxia, and there is general venous congestion. The appearance of the ruminal contents varies with the time interval between ingestion of the carbohydrate and the autopsy. In the early stages, there is a copious amount of porridgelike rumen contents, which has a distinct fermentative odor. The amount of grain or corn varies considerably and is an unreliable indication of acidosis, and the presence of finely ground concentrate may be overlooked. Ruminal pH is helpful only when it is low (<5.0), since it may increase in later stages of the disease. Although the ruminal contents may appear relatively normal in more advanced cases of acidosis, the intestinal contents tend to remain very watery. Absence of protozoa is consistent with chemical rumenitis, but is also influenced by the interval between death and the postmortem examination.

The diagnosis of ruminal acidosis at autopsy can be difficult. The most suggestive abnormality is the rumenitis. It is probably chemical and dependent on the low pH, and is not readily discerned grossly. There may be a slight poorly defined bluish coloration in the ventral sac of the rumen and reticulum and in the omasum, visible through the serosa. When the epithelium is detached, the lamina propria is seen to be hyperemic in patches.

Microscopic examination of the ruminal mucosa is the most reliable way to confirm a diagnosis of chemical rumenitis. The ruminal papillae appear enlarged. There is marked cytoplasmic vacuolation of the epithelial cells, often leading to vesiculation. A mild to marked neutrophilic reaction is evident in the mucosa and submucosa (Fig. 1.32). Focal areas of erosion and ulceration may or may not be present.

Fusobacterium necrophorum is a normal inhabitant of the anaerobic ruminal environment. This bacterium is usually responsible for the infective complications of ruminal acidosis, and it produces characteristic lesions in the forestomachs (Fig. 1.33A,B) and in the liver. Invasion of the wall of the rumen probably does not occur with significant

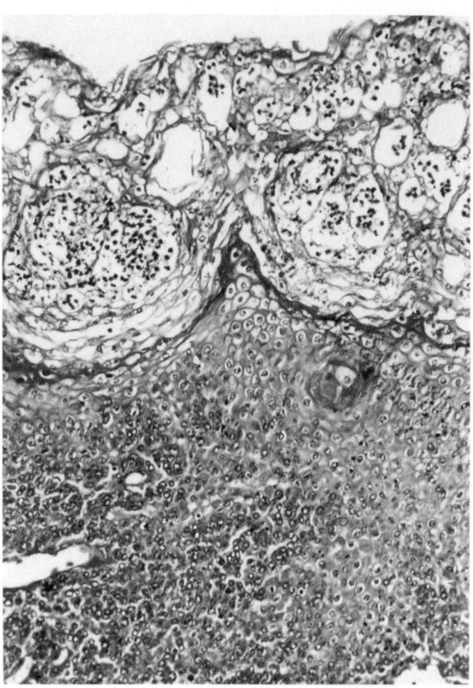

Fig. 1.32 Vacuolation and neutrophil infiltration into superficial epithelium of rumen papilla. Chemical rumenitis (ruminal acidosis) due to excess carbohydrate intake.

frequency unless a foothold is provided by the superficial necrosis and inflammation of acidosis. Necrobacillary rumenitis is common in feedlot cattle, probably a product of mild acidosis following a too-rapid introduction to a high-concentrate ration. It is also a problem in other cattle, especially dairy cows which gain access to unusual amounts of grain, and in sheep under the same circumstances.

Necrobacillary rumenitis affects the papillated areas of the ventral sac and occasionally the pillars. On the inner surface, the early lesions are visible as multiple irregular patches from 2 to 15 cm across, in which the papillae are swollen, dark, slightly mushy, and are matted together by fibrinocellular inflammatory exudate. The affected papillae are necrotic, but ulceration may be delayed if there is ruminal atony and stasis. If the animal recovers from the immediate effects of overeating, the necrotic epithelium sloughs, the ulcer contracts, and epithelial regeneration begins from the margins. The regenerated epithelium is flat and white, and the papillae do not completely return. A stellate scar often remains, but many of the smaller lesions may disappear completely (Fig. 1.33C). Hepatic lesions are initially typical of necrobacillosis, being of coagulative necrosis, but in time they liquefy to form typical abscesses, and these often persist long after the initial ruminal lesions have healed, cicatrized, and disappeared.

It is unusual for ruminal necrobacillosis in cattle to be more than a superficial infection, and although the muscle layers are involved in the inflammation, they are not ordinarily invaded by the organism. However, perforation of

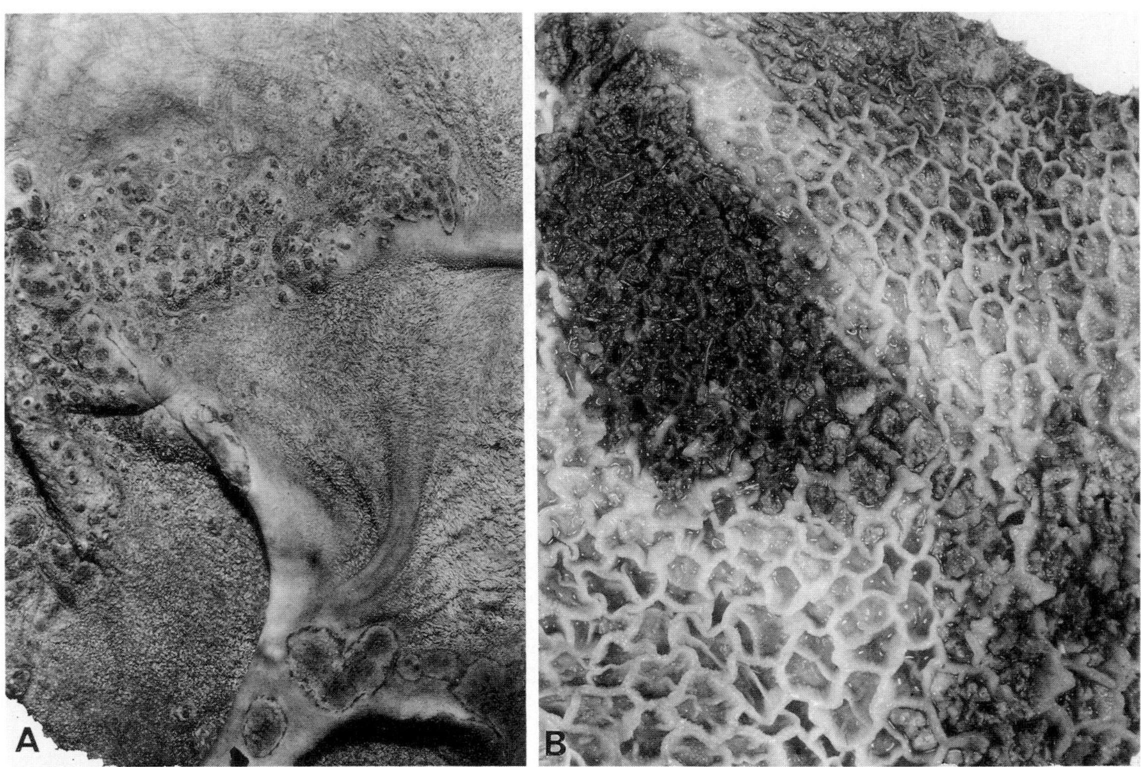

Fig. 1.33A,B Acute necrobacillosis in rumen and reticulum. Cow.

the omasal leaves is common. In sheep, the infection is more progressive than it is in cattle.

Mycotic infection should be suspected when inflammation in the wall of the forestomachs extends to the serosa and is hemorrhagic. The fungi, which are opportunists like *F. necrophorum,* are usually zygomycetes of the genera *Mucor, Rhizopus,* and *Absidia,* and these cannot be differentiated from each other in histologic sections. In the few cases cultured, the incriminated organism was *Rhizopus.*

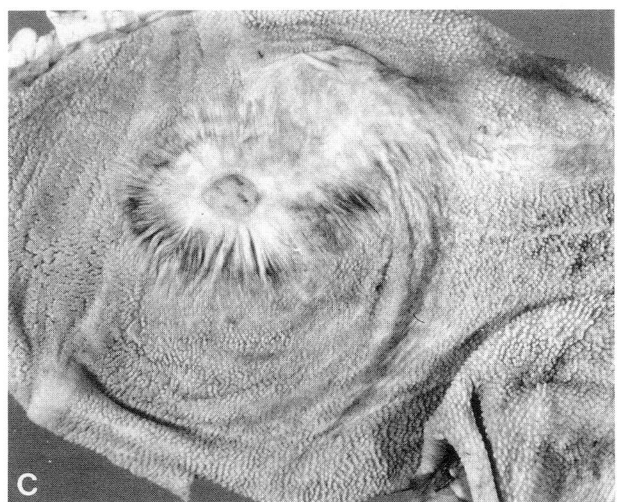

Fig. 1.33C Stellate scarring of incompletely healed ulcer in rumen mucosa in fusobacterial rumenitis.

Mycotic rumenitis is much more severe and extensive than necrobacillary rumenitis, and is often fatal. The inflammation extends to the peritoneum, causing a hemorrhagic and fibrinous peritonitis which mats the omentum to the rumen. In fatal cases, most of the ventral sac and parts of the reticulum and/or omasum are involved. The lesions are very striking and suggest on initial inspection that the walls have been massively infarcted, which in part they have (Fig. 1.34A). The margins are well demarcated, usually by a narrow zone of congestive swelling. The affected areas are red to black, thickened to 1 cm or more, and firm and leathery. There is acute fibrinohemorrhagic inflammation of the overlying peritoneum, and beneath it in the grooves there is a bloodstained, inflammatory edema. Thrombosis, as the result of vasculitis due to the invasion of the vessels by the fungus, is the basis for this lesion.

On the inner surface of the rumen, the lesions are more hemorrhagic than those of necrobacillosis, and more irregular in outline (Fig. 1.34B), and the necrotic epithelium is difficult to detach. Histologically, the rumenitis is characterized by hemorrhagic necrosis of all structures in the wall; by copious fibrinous exudate, and by rather scant leukocytic reaction. A severely necrotizing vasculitis is characteristic, and the fungus is readily visible in the necrotic tissues and the lumina of the blood vessels. More

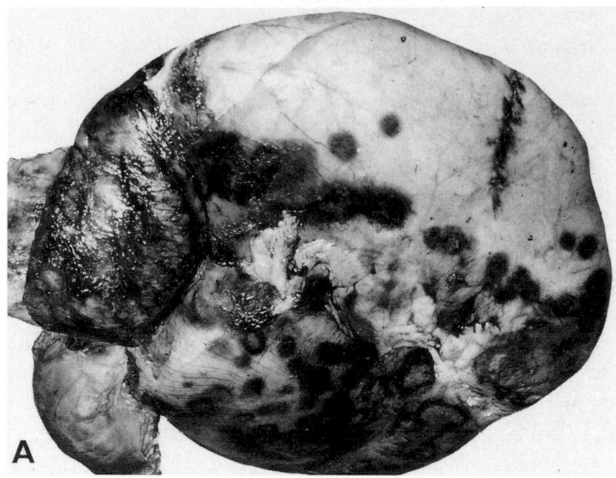

Fig. 1.34A Mycotic rumenitis following acidosis. Cow. Dark areas of infarction involving rumen and reticulum. *Aspergillus* and *Rhizopus*.

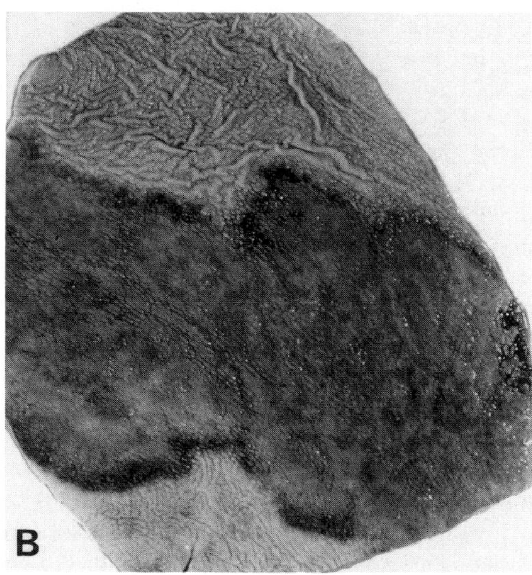

Fig. 1.34B Mycotic rumenitis following acidosis. Cow. Appearance of mucosal surface of rumen.

chronic cases are characterized by granulomatous inflammation in the deeper parts of the mucosal lesion.

Mycotic rumenitis and omasitis may occur in cows that do not have a history of acidosis. It has been suggested that these cases may be a sequel of sepsis, with reflux of abomasal fluid into the forestomachs, and therapy with broad-spectrum antibiotics acting as predisposing factors for mycotic infections.

Metastases sometimes occur in the liver and cause a necrotizing thrombophlebitis of the portal radicles visible as small irregular tan areas of infarction surrounded by a deep red margin (Fig. 1.35).

Other conditions which have been associated with ruminal acidosis are laminitis and an encephalopathy which morphologically resembles the lesions of early poli-

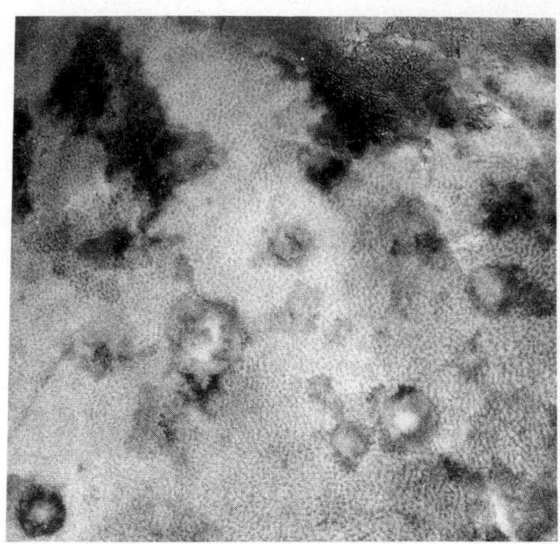

Fig. 1.35 Necrosis in liver. Cow. Due to metastasis of fungi via portal circulation from primary foci of zygomycotic rumenitis.

oencephalomalacia (see The Skin and Appendages, Volume 1, Chapter 5, and The Nervous System, Volume 1, Chapter 3).

Bibliography

Allison, M. J. *et al.* Grain overload in cattle and sheep: Changes in microbial populations in the cecum and rumen. *Am J Vet Res* **36:** 181–185, 1975.

Chihaya, Y. *et al.* Ruminant forestomach and abomasal mucormycosis under rumen acidosis. *Vet Pathol* **25:** 119–123, 1988.

Crichlow, E. C. Ruminal lactic acidosis: Forestomach epithelial receptor activation by undissociated volatile fatty acids and rumen fluids collected during loss of reticuloruminal motility. *Res Vet Sci* **45:** 364–368, 1988.

Crichlow, E. C. Loss of forestomach motility in sheep experiencing ruminal lactic acidosis is not dependent on duodenal acidification by lactic acid. *J Vet Med A* **36:** 39–45, 1989.

Huber, T. L. Physiological effects of acidosis on feedlot cattle. *J Anim Sci* **43:** 902–909, 1976.

Jensen, R. *et al.* Rumenitis and its relation to rate of change of ration and the proportion of concentrate in the ration of cattle. *Am J Vet Res* **15:** 425–428, 1954.

Kay, M. *et al.* The relationship between the acidity of the rumen contents and rumenitis, in calves fed on barley. *Res Vet Sci* **10:** 181–187, 1969.

Russell, J. B., and Hino, T. Regulation of lactate production in *Streptococcus bovis:* A spiraling effect that contributes to rumen acidosis. *J Dairy Sci* **68:** 1712–1721, 1985.

Slyter, L. L. Influence of acidosis on rumen function. *J Anim Sci* **43:** 910–929, 1976.

Suber, R. L. *et al.* Blood and ruminal fluid profiles in carbohydrate-foundered cattle. *Am J Vet Res* **40:** 1005–1008, 1979.

Sweeney, R. W. *et al.* Mycotic omasitis and rumenitis as sequelae to sepsis in dairy cattle: Six cases (1979–1986). *J Am Vet Med Assoc* **194:** 552–553, 1989.

Telle, P. O., and Preston, R. L. Ovine lactic acidosis: Intraruminal and systemic. *J Anim Sci* **33:** 698–705, 1971.

Vestweber, J. G. E., and Leipold, H. W. Experimentally induced ovine ruminal acidosis: Pathologic changes. *Am J Vet Res* **35:** 1537–1540, 1974.

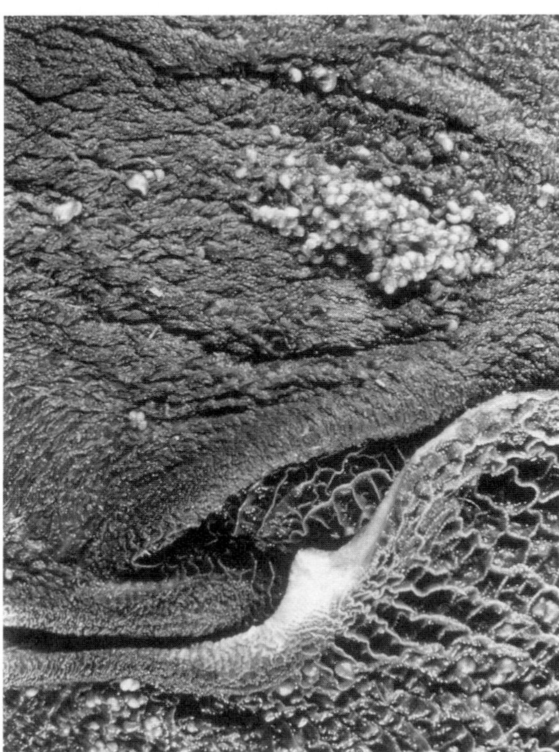

Fig. 1.36 *Paramphistomum* sp. flukes on the mucosa of the reticulorumen.

H. Parasitic Diseases of the Forestomachs

Gongylonema spp. occur in the epithelium of the rumen. They appear as described in the esophagus, and are not pathogens.

More important parasites are the conical flukes belonging to the family Paramphistomatidae. They are found in cattle and sheep in warm temperate, subtropical, and tropical regions. These reddish, plump, droplet-shaped flukes are about the size of the papillae between which they reside in the rumen, where they are nonpathogenic (Fig. 1.36). Their importance lies in the potential for larval paramphistomes in the duodenum to cause disease. The biology and pathogenicity of paramphistomes is discussed with Infectious and Parasitic Diseases of the Gastrointestinal Tract (Section VII of this chapter).

Myiasis of the rumen caused by larvae of the "screwworm" fly *Callitroga hominovorax* is occasionally a cause of mortality in young calves in South America. The larvae are presumed to be licked from cutaneous wounds and swallowed. They lodge in the rumen and perforate it.

Bibliography

Boray, J. C. The pathogenesis of ovine intestinal paramphistomosis due to *Paramphistomum ichikawai*. *In* "The Pathology of Parasitic Diseases," S. M. Gaafar (ed.), pp. 209–216. Lafayette, Indiana, Purdue University Press, 1971.

Bouvry, M., and Rau, M. E. *Paramphistomum* spp. in dairy cattle in Quebec. *Can Vet J* **25:** 353–356, 1984.

I. Neoplasia of the Esophagus and Forestomachs

Neoplasia of the esophagus and reticulorumen is, with the exception of papilloma, rare in domestic animals.

Papillomas of the esophagus in dogs are uncommon and may be associated with oral papilloma. In cattle, papillomata of the esophagus and reticulorumen are common in some areas. They are caused by bovine papillomavirus type 4 (BPV-4), which infects only squamous mucosa of the mouth, pharynx, and upper alimentary tract. Bovine alimentary papillomata are usually solitary, though a minority of infected animals may have multiple lesions. Most are small (<1 cm), broadly pedunculate, tapering, acuminate masses. They are composed of a number of closely packed fronds of squamous epithelium, each supported by a light core of fibrous stroma, and arising from a common fibrous base.

Fibropapillomas, limited to the esophagus, esophageal groove, and rumen, are caused by bovine papillomavirus-2 (BPV-2), normally associated with cutaneous papillomas and fibropapillomas. Alimentary fibropapillomas are smooth, nodular, pearly white masses, usually about 0.5 to 1.0 cm in diameter, but occasionally up to 3.0 cm and plaquelike. They are composed of fibromatous stroma covered by acanthotic epithelium, which may occasionally be ulcerated. In a low proportion of typical alimentary papillomata in cattle, eosinophilic intranuclear inclusion bodies may be present in keratinizing cells. In these, and in vacuolate nuclei containing amphophilic material, papovaviruses may be found by electron microscopy. No evidence of expression of BPV-2 is found in alimentary fibropapillomas, the viral genome being identified by nucleic acid hybridization.

Papillomas and fibropapillomas are normally asymptomatic, though large lesions of the reticular groove and esophagus may interfere with eructation and deglutition.

Malignant neoplasms of the esophagus and forestomachs in ruminants are ordinarily extremely rare. However, in several localities, squamous cell carcinoma is relatively commonly found, in association with BPV-4–induced papilloma (but not with fibropapilloma due to BPV-2). However, BPV-4 viral antigens or genome are not detected in these carcinomas. It has been suggested that an interaction between papilloma virus and ingestion of carcinogens in bracken fern predisposes to the development of squamous cell carcinomas of the esophagus and forestomachs in the hill country of Scotland and northern England. In Brazil a similar association is made with carcinomas of the oropharynx and esophagus. A high prevalence of carcinoma of the esophagus and forestomachs also has been reported from a single valley in Kenya, in association with papillomata, not confirmed as viral, and with a carcinogen apparently ingested with or derived from native forest plants.

Esophageal and ruminal carcinomas are associated with dysphagia or difficult deglutition, rumen tympany, and apparent abdominal pain with progressive cachexia. Concurrent papillomas, carcinomas, and hemangiomas of the bladder like those causing enzootic hematuria are often found in cattle with esophageal or ruminal cancer. In Scotland intestinal adenomas or adenocarcinoma were also found in many cases.

Esophageal and ruminal carcinoma may be seen developing from recognizable papillomas, as brownish, irregular, roughened hyperplastic epithelium, or as ulcerated or irregular proliferative fungating lesions. Distal esophagus, reticular groove, and the adjacent ruminal wall are the sites most commonly affected with carcinoma. Microscopically, they are typical squamous cell carcinomas, and invade locally, causing induration of the wall of the organ. They may metastasize to local lymph nodes, and to distant sites such as liver and lung.

Squamous cell carcinomas may also be encountered rarely in the esophagus of cats, where they develop in the midthoracic portion, forming proliferative plaques of neoplastic cells, which eventually ulcerate and invade the wall of the esophagus and adjacent mediastinum. In horses, squamous cell carcinomas of the stomach may also involve the adjacent terminal esophagus.

Rare squamous carcinomas, and adenocarcinomas arising from the esophageal glands, are reported in dogs.

Mesenchymal tumors of the esophagus, with the exception of the *Spirocerca*-associated fibrosarcomas and osteosarcomas in dogs, referred to previously, are very rare. Connective tissue tumors of the rumen are similarly rare, though fibromas of the reticular groove have been reported. Occasional involvement of the rumen, omasum, and reticulum may occur in cattle with lymphosarcoma, usually also involving the abomasum and more distant sites. Invasion of, or metastasis to, the canine esophagus by thyroid, respiratory, and gastric carcinomas is also reported.

Bibliography

Bailey, W. S. *Spirocerca* associated esophageal sarcomas. *J Am Vet Med Assoc* **175:** 148–150, 1979.

Campo, M. S. Papillomas and cancer in cattle. *Cancer Surv* **6:** 39–54, 1987.

Carb, A. V., and Goodman, D. G. Oesophageal carcinoma in the dog. *J Small Anim Pract* **14:** 91–99, 1973.

Doige, C. E. Omasal squamous cell carcinoma in a ewe. *Can J Comp Med* **47:** 382–384, 1983.

Georgsson, G. Carcinoma of the reticulum of a sheep. *Vet Pathol* **10:** 530–533, 1973.

Jarrett, W. F. H. *et al.* Alimentary fibropapilloma in cattle: A spontaneous tumor, nonpermissive for papillomavirus replication. *J Nat Cancer Inst* **73:** 499–504, 1984.

Plowright, W., Linsell, C. A., and Peers, F. G. A focus of rumenal cancer in Kenyan cattle. *Br J Cancer* **25:** 72–80, 1971.

Randolph, J. F. *et al.* Hypertrophic osteopathy associated with adenocarcinoma of the esophageal glands in a dog. *J Am Vet Med Assoc* **184:** 98–99, 1984.

Sundberg, J. P., and O'Banion, M. K. Animal papillomaviruses associated with malignant tumors. *Adv Viral Oncol* **8:** 55–71, 1989.

V. The Stomach and Abomasum

A. Normal Form and Function

The stomach should be examined carefully in animals of any species with a history of inappetence or anorexia, cachexia, hypoproteinemia, diarrhea, regurgitation, or vomition. Abdominal distension may be associated with gastric dilation or displacement. Hematemesis, melena, or anemia may signify gastric bleeding. Many infectious diseases, with major systemic or alimentary tract signs elsewhere, produce gastric lesions. Systemic states such as uremia and endotoxemia cause characteristic gastric lesions in some species.

In the horse and pig, an obvious smooth white or yellowish esophageal region is present. It is covered by stratified squamous epithelium, with susceptibility to insult and reparative capacity similar to that of the esophageal lining. Chronic inflammatory infiltrates and lymphoid follicles are normally present in the lamina propria and submucosa of the cardiac gland mucosa abutting the esophageal region, especially in the pig. The cardiac gland zone has a grayish color and is particularly well developed in this species, lining the gastric diverticulum, fundus, and about half the body of the stomach. In the dog, cat, and ruminant, cardiac glands are limited to a narrow zone at the cardia or omasal opening. Cardiac glands are branched tubular structures, lined almost exclusively by columnar mucous cells. The anterior portions of the equine and porcine stomach are so modified to permit bacterial fermentation and evolution of organic acids in an environment of relatively high pH (>pH 5), buffered by saliva and cardiac gland secretions.

The fundic or oxyntic gland acid-secretory mucosa in the horse and pig is reddish brown and slightly irregular but not highly folded. More prominent longitudinally oriented rugae or plicae are present in the dog and cat, and in the abomasum. Gastric secretion undiluted by ingesta in the dog or cat normally should be <pH 3. Abomasal content should be <pH 3.5–4.0. Tall columnar mucous cells cover the gastric surface, and line pits or foveolae. The junction of the base of the foveola and the upper portion of the neck of the fundic gland proper is termed the isthmus. Cuboidal or low columnar mucous neck cells in a narrow zone in this area undergo mitosis. Some daughter cells differentiate into foveolar mucous cells, migrating up onto the gastric surface, where they are lost, probably in about 4–6 days. The neck of the oxyntic gland below the isthmus is lined by pyramidal, peripherally located acid- and intrinsic factor-producing parietal cells. Interspersed are inconspicuous mucous neck cells, mainly in the upper neck, and scattered endocrine cells. In the base of the gland, pepsinogen-producing zymogen or chief cells are concentrated.

Mucous neck cells, like foveolar and surface mucous cells, stain PAS positive. The cytoplasm of these cells contains, in addition to mucous granules, many polyribosomes and rough endoplasmic reticulum, suggesting poor specialization. Parietal cells differentiate from mucous neck cells proliferating at the isthmus, and appear to be relatively long lived, that is, of the order of weeks to months. They contain many mitochondria, and hence stain well with eosin. A complex tubulovesicular/canalicular structure opens at the luminal apex of the cell in the secretory state. A number of long-lived endocrine cells, derived from proliferative cells at the isthmus, are recognized in the oxyntic gland, secreting histamine, serotonin, and somatostatin, among other endocrine/paracrine agents. Endocrine cells usually abut the basement membrane of the gland, lack exposure to the gland lumen, and have characteristic basal granules. The chief cells are apparently long-lived cells, probably derived from stem cells at the isthmus, but possibly autonomously replicative at a slow rate. Ultrastructurally they have extensive rough endoplasmic reticulum, a prominent Golgi zone, and numerous zymogen granules.

Normally, mitotic figures are not common in cells at the isthmus of fundic glands, and virtually never are seen at any distance from the isthmus. The fundic mucosa of newborn ruminants and especially piglets may be relatively poorly differentiated and proliferative. The proliferative compartment is sensitive to radiomimetic insults. This is reflected in attenuation of the lining epithelium and narrowing of the isthmus and upper neck of oxyntic glands in dogs with parvovirus infection (Fig. 1.114A), and in animals treated with cytotoxic agents such as cyclophosphamide.

The pyloric mucosa forms a slightly pitted or irregular surface in the distal portion of the stomach; it extends further cranially along the lesser than the greater curvature. The knoblike torus pyloricus at the pylorus of the pig is a normal structure. The tubular glands of the pyloric mucosa open into deep gastric pits, which may extend half the thickness of the mucosa. The glands are lined by pale mucous cells, with interspersed endocrine elements, mainly G (gastrin) and D (somatostatin) cells. Scattered parietal cells may be present, especially in glands in the zone intergrading with fundic mucosa.

The stromal elements of the gastric lamina propria are relatively inconspicuous, in fundic mucosa in particular. Normally, few lymphocytes and plasma cells and scattered mast cells are present, mainly deep between glands. Occasional lymphocytic nodules or follicles may be present, usually near the muscularis mucosae. Lymphoid infiltrates are more common in antral mucosa.

Rapid fixation of the gastric mucosa is desirable to avoid postmortem artefacts.

Hydrolysis of protein in preparation for subsequent intestinal digestion and absorption is accomplished in the stomach by acid and by pepsin, activated by autocatalysis from pepsinogen at low pH. Secretion of acid is the function of the oxyntic or parietal cells, about 1 billion of which are present in the stomach of a 20-kg dog. Regulation of the volume and acidity of gastric secretion is physiologically complex and highly integrated, involving neurocrine, endocrine, and paracrine mechanisms.

The parietal cell secretes hydrochloric acid in response to stimulation by histamine, acetylcholine, and gastrin. All three agonists are probably continuously present and involved in basal acid secretion. However, the effects of acetylcholine and gastrin are largely dependent on concurrent stimulation by the permissive agonist, histamine.

Histamine is a paracrine stimulant, continuously present in the environment of the oxyntic cells. Occupation of the H_2 histamine receptor on the oxyntic cell causes enhanced generation of cyclic adenosine monophosphate (AMP). This in turn stimulates intracellular metabolic events culminating in acid secretion.

Acetylcholine, the neurocrine agonist, is released near the oxyntic cell from processes of parasympathetic postganglionic neurons. Its release is enhanced by vagal activity during the central stimulation of the cephalic phase—the Pavlovian response. Gastric distension also stimulates the parietal cell via vagovagal and short intramural reflex pathways. The effect of acetylcholine is associated with calcium ion influx as second messenger.

Gastrin is released into the bloodstream by G cells, located mainly in the pyloric antrum. Calcium, amino acids, and peptides in ingesta, impinging on G cells, stimulate gastrin release. Vagal stimulation during the cephalic phase, and fundic–pyloric vagovagal reflexes, in concert with local pyloric reflexes, initiated by distension, also cause G cells to release gastrin. Gastrin alone is a weak calcium-ion-dependent stimulator of acid production, but it contributes to the synergistic effects on secretion by oxyntic cells exposed to histamine and acetylcholine. In addition, gastrin has an important trophic effect, increasing the number of parietal and endocrine cells in fundic mucosa.

Acid production during the gastric phase of secretion is depressed by the negative-feedback effect of acid in the antrum, possibly through the inhibitory effect of somatostatin on the G cell below pH 3. Acid, fat, and hyperosmolal solutions in the proximal small intestine also inhibit acid secretion, perhaps by the mediation of neural reflexes, and secretin, gastric inhibitory polypeptide, epidermal growth factor, or other enterogastrones. Prostaglandin E_2 (PGE_2) also inhibits acid production by parietal cells. The chief cell is probably susceptible to the same general stimuli for secretion as is the parietal cell.

B. Gastric Mucosal Barrier

The gastric mucosal barrier to acid back-diffusion and autodigestion resides largely in the single layer of foveolar and surface mucous cells. Integrity of the gastric mucosal barrier implies continuity of the mucosal surface epithelium. The capacity of these cells to maintain tight junctions, to migrate rapidly to fill defects, and possibly to secrete mucus and bicarbonate, is central to protecting the gastric mucosa against progressive injury by insults arising in the lumen.

Gastric mucus is freely permeable to hydrogen ions and has little innate buffering capacity. Cardiac gland mucosa in the pig, and pyloric mucosa secrete bicarbonate in considerable quantities, and normally resist acid attack. Fundic surface mucous cells also actively secrete bicarbonate, into a thin, unstirred layer of surface mucus. Bicarbonate and mucus secretion by mucous cells is stimulated by PGE_2. Though it has been suggested that acid is buffered by bicarbonate in mucus on the gastric surface, the significance of this mechanism in protecting the mucosa against ulceration is questioned.

Prostaglandins, ubiquitous in gastric mucosal lamina propria, may have protective effects other than by stimulation of bicarbonate and mucus secretion by mucous cells, and by inhibition of histamine-stimulated acid secretion by parietal cells. They cause proliferation, resulting in an increased mass of foveolar mucous epithelium. They may promote incorporation of surfactant molecules into the apical cell membrane of surface mucous cells, increasing its hydrophobicity and imparting greater resistance to water-soluble insults. They also may be involved in gastric mucosal cytoprotection by sulfhydryl compounds, which may neutralize free radicals and other toxic metabolites.

Prostaglandins cause vasodilation and increased blood flow, in addition to inhibiting acid secretion. The high metabolic rate of the gastric mucosa requires a high blood flow to maintain an intact, functional surface epithelium. Bicarbonate in the local circulation, resulting from the alkaline tide generated by acid secretion in glands deeper in the mucosa, is probably important in buffering the superficial lamina propria against back-diffusion of acid, and adequate blood flow flushes injurious free radicals from the vicinity of surface cells. Experimentally, high blood flow is protective against many mucosal insults, whereas ischemia is ulcerogenic.

The peptides, epidermal growth factor, originating in salivary glands, and transforming growth factor-α (TGFα), produced locally in the gastric mucosa, also appear protective, in that they may promote cell proliferation and migration to fill defects, and suppress acid production.

Bibliography

Al-Tikriti, M. *et al.* The normal structure of regional feline gastric mucosae: Scanning electron microscopic study. *Scanning Microsc* **1:** 1871–1880, 1987.

Anderson, W. D., and Anderson, B. G. Comparative anatomy. *In* "Veterinary Gastroenterology," N. V. Anderson (ed.), pp. 127–171. Philadelphia, Pennsylvania, Lea & Febiger, 1980.

Argenzio, R. A, Southworth, M., and Stevens. C. E. Sites of organic acid production in the equine gastrointestinal tract. *Am J Physiol* **226:** 1043–1050, 1974.

Asari, M. *et al.* Histological development of bovine abomasum. *Anat Anz Jena* **159:** 1–11, 1985.

Beauchamp, R. D. *et al.* Localization of transforming growth factor α and its receptor in gastric mucosal cells. *J Clin Invest* **84:** 1017–1023, 1989.

Goodlad, R. A. *et al.* Prostaglandins and the gastric epithelium: Effects of misoprostol on gastric epithelial cell proliferation in the dog. *Gut* **30:** 316–321, 1989.

Hall, J. A., Burrows, C. F., and Twedt, D. C. Gastric motility in dogs. Part I. Normal gastric function. *Compend Cont Ed Pract Vet* **10:** 1282–1293, 1988.

Henagan, J. M., Schmidt, K. M., and Miller, T. A. Prostaglandin prevents aspirin injury in the canine stomach under *in vivo* but not *in vitro* conditions. *Gastroenterology* **97:** 649–659, 1989.

Johnson, L. R. (ed.). "Physiology of the Gastrointestinal Tract," New York, Raven Press, 1987. (Includes chapters on functional gastric morphology, proliferation and differentiation of normal and diseased cells, gastric mucosal defence and repair, gastrointestinal hormones, prostanoids as regulators of gastrointestinal function.)

Johnson, L. R. Regulation of gastrointestinal mucosal growth. *Physiol Rev* **68:** 456–502, 1988.

Langer, P. Comparative anatomy of the stomach in mammalian herbivores. *Q J Exp Physiol* **69:** 615–625, 1984.

McLeay, L. M., and Titchen, D. A. Gastric, antral, and fundic pouch secretion in sheep. *J Physiol* **248:** 595–612, 1975.

Miller, T. A. Gastroduodenal mucosal defense: Factors responsible for the ability of the stomach and duodenum to resist injury. *Surgery* **103:** 389–397, 1988.

Murray, M. The fine structure of bovine gastric epithelia. *Res Vet Sci* **11:** 411–416, 1970.

Nicholls, C. D., and Lee, D. L. Post-mortem changes in the abomasal mucosae of sheep infected with *Haemonchus contortus* compared with those in uninfected sheep. *J Comp Pathol* **100:** 19–25, 1989.

Prokopiw, I. *et al.* The microvascular anatomy of the canine stomach. *Gastroenterology* **100:** 638–647, 1991.

Samloff, I. M. Peptic ulcer: The many proteinases of aggression. *Gastroenterology* **96:** 586–595, 1989.

Shorrock, C. J., and Rees, W. D. W. Overview of gastroduodenal mucosal protection. *Am J Med* **84** (Suppl. 2A): 25–34, 1988.

Strombeck, D. R., and Guilford, W. G. Gastric structure and function. *In* "Small Animal Gastroenterology," 2nd Ed., pp. 167–186. Davis, California, Stonegate Publishing, 1990.

Twedt, D. C., and Magne, M. L. Diseases of the stomach. *In* "Textbook of Veterinary Internal Medicine," S. J. Ettinger (ed.), pp. 1289–1322, Philadelphia, Pennsylvania, W. B. Saunders, 1989.

Wallace, J. L. Gastric resistance to acid: Is the "mucus–bicarbonate barrier" functionally redundant? *Am J Physiol* **256:** G31–G38, 1989.

Youngberg, C. A. *et al.* Radiotelemetric determination of gastrointestinal pH in four healthy beagles. *Am J Vet Res* **46:** 1516–1521, 1985.

C. Response of the Gastric Mucosa to Injury

Repair of acute erosive physical or chemical trauma to the mucosal surface, such as that caused by aspirin, and presumably abrasion, is by rapid (minutes to hours) immigration of surviving attenuated surface and foveolar cells. Within a day or two, proliferation of cells in the isthmus follows, if the erosive lesion is superficial, and spares the progenitor cells. A cap of mucus, exfoliated epithelium, and fibrin over a mucosal defect may form a protective barrier conducive to effective restitution of the mucosal epithelium. An acute inflammatory reaction demarcates severely eroded or superficially necrotic mucosa, and hemorrhage may be evident on the surface and in adjacent mucosa. Mitoses become common in the upper gland.

During the early phase of repair, cells lining shallow foveolae and covering the surface are basophilic, poorly differentiated and flattened, cuboidal, or low columnar. Sites of epithelial exfoliation and neutrophil transmigration or effusion into the lumen may be evident. Congestion, edema, mild neutrophilia, and fibroplasia are seen in the superficial lamina propria. The evolution and repair of gastric ulceration, to which erosion may be antecedent, are discussed later. The progenitor cells of the fundic mucosa have the potential to produce tall columnar mucous cells of the foveolar or surface type, to produce mucous neck cells, and, by further differentiation, to evolve parietal cells.

Atrophy of parietal cell mass without extensive mucous cell hyperplasia occurs in animals, particularly ruminants, which have signs of gastrointestinal disease, including inappetence. The change is not evident grossly. Microscopically, fewer parietal cells are seen in the upper neck of fundic glands, and often in the depth of the gland. This is accompanied by epithelial proliferation, indicated by moderate numbers of mitotic figures at the isthmus and in the neck of the gland. Mucous neck cells become the predominant cell in the upper gland. The PAS stain demonstrates the encroachment of increased numbers of such cells into the deeper portion of fundic glands. In extreme cases, mucous neck cells are present to the base of glands, and achlorhydria occurs.

The cause of this change is unclear. It has been demonstrated in sheep infected with intestinal nematodes, but similar findings occur in animals with a wide variety of syndromes involving loss of appetite. Starvation of moderate duration does not produce comparable lesions. Reduction in, or interference with, factors trophic for parietal cell mass, might be the mechanism in parietal cell atrophy of this type.

Mucous metaplasia and hyperplasia of glands in the fundic stomach in all species is associated with chronic inflammation of the mucosa. As the lesion evolves, parietal cells are present only in the basal portion of the glands, and they appear to be progressively displaced from above by hyperplastic mucous cells. Mitotic figures may be numerous throughout the neck of the gland, which elongates. The metaplastic epithelium in early lesions tends to resemble mucous neck cells. In established lesions, columnar mucous cells with regular nuclear polarity, similar to foveolar mucous cells, may be present. When inflammatory infiltrates are local, the mucous change is limited to a few surrounding glands. More diffuse inflammation is associated with the development of widespread epithelial mucous metaplasia. Focal or diffuse, superficial or mucosal, proprial infiltrates of plasma cells and lymphocytes are typical. Often, neutrophils, eosinophils, and Russell-body cells will be present in the lamina propria, and lymphocytes may be between epithelial cells in glands. Globule leukocytes may be present in the epithelium of glands, especially in the parasitized abomasum.

Mucous metaplasia and hyperplasia of fundic mucosa may be caused by local immune events or inflammation in the lamina propria. Interactions between immune processes in the stomach and epithelial differentiation are poorly explored. Secretion of lysozyme, and of secretory piece and IgA, are properties of mucous neck cells in gastritis in humans. Cell-mediated immune events in the lamina propria of the small intestine are increasingly implicated in altered proliferation and differentiation of enteric epithelium by as yet undefined mechanisms. It may be that similar phenomena in the stomach await recognition and investigation.

Such atrophy of the parietal cells and mucous metaplasia and hyperplasia apparently do not result from withdrawal of the trophic stimulus of gastrin. At least in *Ostertagia*-induced gastritis, it occurs in the face of gastrin concentrations many times above normal levels, which are not simply the result of achlorhydria and failure of suppression of gastrin-releasing G cell secretion by antral acidification.

This mucous metaplasia, hyperplasia, and chronic inflammation is associated with a variety of causes, including chronic traumatic insults, such as those due to implanted foreign bodies. Chronic abomasal involvement in mucosal disease or herpes rhinotracheitis, and in the retrovirus infections caprine arthritis/encephalitis and ovine progressive pneumonia, may be associated with mucosal lesions of this type. The specific agency most commonly recognized is gastric parasitism by nematodes such as *Ostertagia* spp., *Trichostrongylus axei*, *Hyostrongylus* spp., and *Ollulanus tricuspis*, in which the distribution of the lesion often is closely related to the physical presence of nematodes and to the interstitial inflammatory reaction they incite. Hypertrophic gastritis in dogs may in part reflect chronic inflammation as well. Mucous metaplasia and hyperplasia are also typically present around the healing margins of chronic ulcers, perhaps in response to local inflammation.

The mucosa affected in these circumstances is grossly thickened, as on the overhanging margin of an ulcer, or in an *Ostertagia* nodule, with a pebbled or convoluted surface if the lesion is widespread. Gastric rugae or plicae are thickened, partially as a result of mucosal hypertrophy, perhaps with submucosal edema. The surface of the stomach is usually paler than normal in affected areas; however, local congestion or hyperemia may be evident. Though the surface may be glistening, profuse mucus secretion is not usually obvious. Achlorhydria is the consequence of widespread change of this type. Mucous metaplasia and hyperplasia are differentiated on the basis of the degree of mucous cell hyperplasia and differentiation, and the presence of inflammatory cells, from fundic atrophy associated with loss of appetite.

Antral mucosa also undergoes hyperplasia and thickening in antritis. Some chronic inflammatory infiltrate between antral glands and at the base of the mucosa is usual, and lymphoid follicles may be present in the lamina propria. Expansion of the proliferative compartment in the antral glands is recognized as mitotic figures scattered in the neck of the gland. Foveolar and glandular mucous cells increase in number, and the antral mucosa is thickened and superficially rugose, perhaps with local congestion or erythema. The stimulus for antritis if often unclear. Gastric reflux of duodenal contents containing bile may be of some significance in the dog. In ruminants, the pyloric mucosa may be colonized by abomasal nematodes, and by a few worms of species normally found in the small intestine, if enteric populations are high.

The functional significance of gastric mucous metaplasia is unclear. Presumably hyperplasia of cells is partly a response to soluble local immune-mediated stimuli or products of inflammation. Replacement of parietal cells by mucous neck cells, or an apparently more fully differentiated mucous cell in chronic gastritis, may be a protective response. It may eliminate the threat of local acid corrosion, and promote the transfer into the lumen of protective soluble factors such as lysozyme and IgA or its analogs.

Achlorhydria ensues in severe chronic gastritis and mucous metaplasia. The pH of gastric secretion approaches or exceeds neutrality under some circumstances, as sodium ion replaces hydrogen ion in gastric content and bicarbonate is secreted. With diminished gastric acid concentration, progressive microbial colonization of the stomach and upper intestine ensues. Parietal cell atrophy and replacement by mucous neck cells in ruminants with anorexia due to enteric disease may predispose to mycotic invasion of the mucosa, if it is physically disrupted. Mucous metaplasia and hyperplasia, as seen in chronic gastritis or conditions like ostertagiosis, does not seem to render the mucosa prone to mycosis. Loss of the hydrolytic effects of acid and pepsin, in achlorhydria, seems to have little effect on digestion of protein and uptake of nitrogen at least in animals with ostertagiosis, and the effect on protein digestion of atrophic gastritis in humans appears to be minimal.

Bibliography

Anderson, N., Hansky, J., and Titchen, D. A. Effects on plasma pepsinogen, gastrin, and pancreatic polypeptide of *Ostertagia* spp. transferred directly into the abomasum of sheep. *Int J Parasitol* **15:** 159–165, 1985.

Barker, I. K., and Titchen, D. A. Gastric dysfunction in sheep infected with *Trichostrongylus colubriformis,* a nematode inhabiting the small intestine. *Int J Parasitol* **12:** 345–356, 1982.

Greaves, P., and Boiziau, J.-L. Altered patterns of mucin secretion in gastric hyperplasia in mice. *Vet Pathol* **21:** 224–228, 1984.

Hansen, O. H. *et al.* Relationship between gastric acid secretion, histopathology, and cell proliferation kinetics in human gastric mucosa. *Gastroenterology* **73:** 453–456, 1977.

Isaacson, P. Immunoperoxidase study of the secretory immunoglobulin system and lysozyme in normal and diseased gastric mucosa. *Gut* **23:** 578–588, 1982.

Krohn, K. J. E., and Finlayson, N. D. C. Interrelations of humoral and cellular immune responses in experimental canine gastritis. *Clin Exp Immunol* **14:** 237–245, 1973.

Lev, R., Siegel, H. I., and Glass, G. B. J. Effects of salicylates on the canine stomach: A morphological and histochemical study. *Gastroenterology* **62:** 970–980, 1972.

McNeil, P. L., and Ito, S. Gastrointestinal cell plasma membrane wounding and resealing *in vivo. Gastroenterology* **96:** 1238–1248, 1989.

Miller, H. R. P. Gastrointestinal mucus, a medium for survival and for elimination of parasitic nematodes and protozoa. *Parasitology* **94:** S77–S100, 1987.

Murray, M., Jennings, F. W., and Armour, J. Bovine ostertagiasis: Structure, function, and mode of differentiation of the bovine gastric mucosa and kinetics of the worm loss. *Res Vet Sci* **11:** 417–427, 1970.

Wallace, J. L. Increased resistance of the rat gastric mucosa to hemorrhagic damage after exposure to an irritant. Role of the "mucoid cap" and prostaglandin synthesis. *Gastroenterology* **94:** 22–32, 1988.

D. Pyloric Stenosis

Pyloric stenosis is a functional and sometimes anatomic problem, which in part represents probably the only anomaly of the stomach recognized in animals. It is relatively common in dogs, and rare in cats and horses.

Recurrent vomition and poor growth in recently weaned animals suggest the clinical diagnosis of a congenital lesion. Contrast radiographic studies will confirm delayed gastric emptying. There is limited critical functional information on this problem. In some dogs there may be hypertrophy of pyloric muscle, which appears grossly thickened. Tonic stenosis of the pyloric sphincter may occur in dogs, perhaps because of unconfirmed lesions of the myenteric plexus or of gastrin excess. In cats, no gross alteration in the diameter of the pylorus or the thickness of its muscle is recognized. An association with esophageal dilation has been made in the cat. Congenital pyloric stenosis in a foal was associated with signs of abdominal pain and reluctance to consume solid feed. In all species the clinical problem is usually abolished by pyloromyotomy.

Acquired functional pyloric obstruction may be a component of abomasal hypomotility, resulting in abomasal impaction, as discussed subsequently.

Acquired pyloric stenosis or obstruction due to physical causes occurs following ulceration, granulation, and stricture of the pyloric canal in any species, due to foreign bodies, as a complication of polyps and tumors in the area; and due to chronic hypertrophic pyloric gastropathy in dogs.

Chronic hypertrophic pyloric gastropathy is the term coined for a syndrome of pyloric obstruction in dogs, associated with mucosal hypertrophy, hypertrophy of circular smooth muscle, or a combination of the two. Mucosal hypertrophy alone is the most common lesion; muscular hypertrophy alone is the least common, though some degree of muscular hypertrophy is seen in about half the cases. A scoring system (I, II, III) for the type of lesions is used, but it is inconsistently applied in the literature. Affected animals are typically of small breeds, and middle-aged or older, suggesting that this is an acquired problem. Males outnumber females. The pathogenesis is speculative, and it is not clear whether muscular hypertrophy is primary, as it seems to be in some cases, or whether it is secondary, in response to obstruction related to excess mucosa. Since mucosal and muscular lesions can be present independently, they may have separate causes. The mucosal hypertrophy has features in common with hypertrophic gastritis described elsewhere. The cardinal presenting sign is chronic intermittent vomition, perhaps with weight loss, and with gastric distension in a few cases.

Gross examination, by gastroscopy, at gastrotomy, or at necropsy, in most cases reveals a pyloric mucosa thrown into irregular, prominent, sometimes polypoid, rugations, with a focal or diffuse distribution. This reflects hypertrophy of glands, which may involve foveolar or deeper glandular elements alone, or in combination, perhaps with cystic dilation of deeper portions of glands. There is usually a concomitant chronic inflammatory infiltrate in the mucosa and occasionally submucosa, and small erosions of the mucosal surface may occur. If there is muscular hypertrophy, this is reflected on the cut surface of the pylorus by irregular firm thickening of the circular muscle. Microscopically, smooth muscle fibers in affected fascicles are irregularly hypertrophic. Recognition of smooth muscle hypertrophy requires a full-thickness biopsy, which will not be obtained by endoscopy. Grossly, muscular hypertrophy may mimic the desmoplastic response often seen in gastric adenocarcinoma. However, in hypertrophic pyloric gastropathy, mucosal ulceration, which often accompanies gastric carcinoma, is absent.

Bibliography

Barth, A. D., Barber, S. M., and McKenzie, N. T. Pyloric stenosis in a foal. *Can Vet J* **21:** 234–236, 1980.

Bellenger, C. R. *et al.* Chronic hypertrophic pyloric gastropathy in 14 dogs. *Aust Vet J* **67:** 317–320, 1990.

Church, S., Baker, J. R., and May, S. A. Gastric retention associated with acquired pyloric stenosis in a gelding. *Equine Vet J* **18:** 332–334, 1986.

Happe, R. P., van der Gaag, I., and Wolvekamp, W. Th. C. Pyloric stenosis caused by hypertrophic gastritis in three dogs. *J Small Anim Pract* **22:** 7–17, 1981.

Matthiesen, D. T., and Walter, M. C. Surgical treatment of chronic hypertrophic pyloric gastropathy in 45 dogs. *J Am Anim Hosp Assoc* **22:** 241–247, 1986.

McGill, C. A., and Bolton, J. R. Gastric retention associated with a pyloric mass in two horses. *Aust Vet J* **61:** 190–191, 1984.

Morse, C. C., and Richardson, D. W. Gastric hyperplastic polyp in a horse. *J Comp Pathol* **99:** 337–342, 1988.

Pearson, H. Pyloric stenosis in the dog. *Vet Rec* **105:** 393–394, 1979.

Pearson, H. *et al.* Pyloric and oesophageal dysfunction in the cat. *J Small Anim Pract* **15:** 487–501, 1974.

Sikes, R. I. *et al.* Chronic hypertrophic pyloric gastropathy: A review of 16 cases. *J Am Anim Hosp Assoc* **22:** 99–104, 1986.

E. Gastric Dilation and Displacement

Gastric dilation in the horse is often a secondary effect of obstruction of the small bowel, or of colic with ileus, and is also part of the syndrome called grass sickness, discussed elsewhere in this chapter. Primary gastric dilation in horses is a sequel to consumption of excess fermentable carbohydrate, sudden access to lush pasture, or excessive intake of water. Dilation associated with intake of fermentable feed is probably analogous to grain overload in cattle. Ingesta may swell through absorption of saliva and gastric secretion. Evolution of gas and organic acids, including lactic acid, by bacterial fermentation of carbohydrate, occurs in the cranial portion of the stomach. An influx of water follows as the result of increased osmotic pressure in the stomach, contributing to increased distension and to systemic dehydration. Animals surviving for any time with acute gastric dilation of this type may develop laminitis. The contents of the stomach in gastric dilation may be fluid, especially in secondary dilation, and can smell fermented in primary dilation. **Gastric rupture** may follow primary or secondary dilation of the equine stomach; it may be idiopathic, in that no clear cause is identified. Gastric rupture is diagnosed in about 5% of horses with colic admitted to veterinary hospitals. Rupture usually occurs along the greater curvature, parallel to the omental attachment, releasing gastric content into the omental bursa or the abdominal cavity. Death ensues acutely as the result of shock and peritonitis. Often, tearing of the serosa and muscularis is more extensive than the laceration of the mucosa, which may be 10–15 cm long. The margins of the laceration show evidence of antemortem hemorrhage, which differentiates the lesion from postmortem rupture of a dilated stomach. There also may be congestion of the cervical esophagus and blanching of the thoracic esophagus, producing a prominent bloat line. This, and compression atelectasis of the lungs in some cases, attests to the tremendous increase in intra-abdominal and intrathoracic pressure exerted by the dilated stomach prior to rupture. Congestion of cervical and cranial soft tissues, and blanching of the abdominal organs also are found. Perforation, as distinct from rupture, of the stomach in the horse is rare, and is associated with parasitism, gastric ulcer, or neoplasia.

Gastric dilation and volvulus in the dog (Fig. 1.37) occur relatively commonly, and the condition has been reported in cats. In dogs, gastric dilation and volvulus is usually a problem associated with eating, and probably aerophagia, especially in the deep-chested breeds such as Great Danes, St. Bernards, Irish setters, wolfhounds, borzois, and

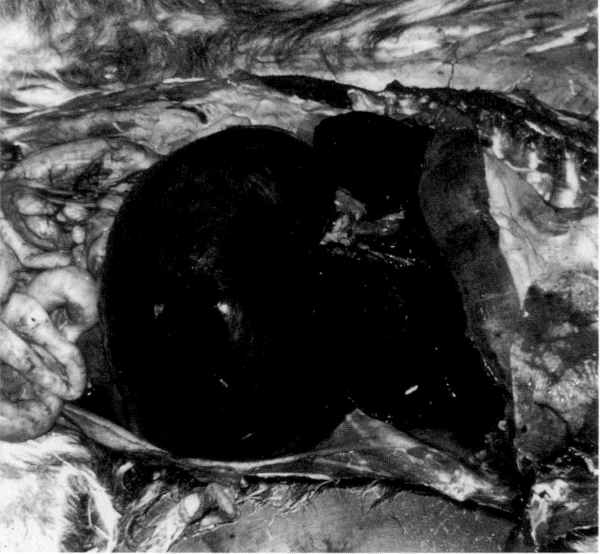

Fig. 1.37 Gastric volvulus in a dog. The stomach has undergone venous infarction due to strangulation of its vascular outflow, and is extremely distended and congested.

bloodhounds. Delayed gastric emptying has been hypothesized to predispose animals to the problem. Management, behavior, and type of feed appear not to contribute to the development of dilation.

The gas which contributes to the development of dilation is probably the result of aerophagia, and possibly the evolution of carbon dioxide by physiologic mechanisms. Inability to relieve the accumulation of food, fluid, and gas in the stomach causes the organ to dilate and alter its intra-abdominal position, so that its long axis rotates from a transverse left–right orientation to one paralleling that of the abdomen. In simple dilation, the esophagus is not physically completely occluded, the spleen remains on the left side, and the duodenum is only slightly displaced dorsally and toward the midline. The gastric mucosa at this stage is usually not infarcted, though the effects of dilation on venous return from the abdomen and on the systemic circulation may be substantial.

For reasons which are unclear, gastric dilation may be converted to gastric volvulus. Perhaps this is related to laxity or laceration of the gastrohepatic ligament, or to the development of violent antiperistalsis and abdominal contraction in vain attempts by the dog to vomit against a functionally or physically obstructed cardia. The stomach rotates about the esophagus in a clockwise direction, as viewed from the caudal aspect. The greater curvature of the distended organ moves ventrally and caudally, and then rotates dorsally and to the right. This forces the pylorus and terminal duodenum cranially to the right and clockwise around the esophagus. Ultimately they lie to the left of midline across and ventral to the esophagus, compressed between the esophagus and the dilated stomach.

Depending on the degree of volvulus, the spleen, which follows the gastrosplenic ligament, usually ends up lying in a right ventral position, between the stomach and liver or diaphragm. It is bent into a V shape by tension on its ligaments, becomes extremely congested, and may undergo torsion, infarction, and rupture. The esophagus becomes completely occluded in volvulus, which may involve rotation of 270–360°. Venous infarction of the gastric mucosa ensues, as volvulus progressively constricts outflow of blood from the stomach. The mucosa, and usually the full thickness of the gastric wall, are edematous and dark red to black, and there is bloody content in the lumen of the stomach. Ischemic mucosa becomes necrotic, and the stomach may rupture. Hemoperitoneum may occur, due to avulsion of gastric blood vessels. Reperfusion of ischemic mucosa during surgery may exacerbate tissue damage through generation of free radicals.

Obstruction of veins by volvulus, and pressure exerted by the distended stomach, result in decreased venous return via the portal vein and posterior vena cava, causing reduced cardiac output and circulatory shock. Endotoxemia is implicated speculatively in disseminated intravascular coagulation, and may contribute to shock. Increased intra-abdominal pressure impinges on the diaphragm and compromises respiration. A variety of acid–base and electrolyte abnormalities ensue in dogs with gastric dilation and volvulus, contributing to the physiologically precarious state. Cardiac arrhythmias as a sequel to gastric dilation and volvulus have been associated with putative release of myocardial depressant factor from an ischemic pancreas, and with myocardial necrosis, resulting from ischemia. Death is inevitable in dogs which are not treated early for acute gastric volvulus. Rare cases of chronic gastric volvulus are reported, with fixation of the spleen in the right side of the abdomen by omental adhesions.

In swine, gastric volvulus is a cause of sudden death in adult sows, perhaps with a brief premonitory period of anorexia, abdominal distension, dyspnea, and salivation. It is associated with excitement in anticipation of feeding among pigs which are fed at regular, often long, intervals, and may be a sequel to greedy ingestion of feed, water, and air. The twist may occur in either direction about the long axis of the stomach, though clockwise torsion predominates. The stomach is markedly distended, with large amounts of air and partly digested fluid ingesta. The gastric wall is congested, as is the spleen, if it has followed the rotation of the stomach.

Abomasal displacement and volvulus is a common clinical problem in high-producing, intensively managed dairy cattle, particularly around the time of parturition, but it also occurs in animals which are predominantly pasture fed. The displacement usually is ventrally and to the left of the rumen. Many affected animals have concurrent problems, including ketosis, hypocalcemia, metritis, and retained placenta. Abomasal atony and increased gas production are believed to be prerequisites for displacement of the organ. Influx of high concentrations of volatile fatty acids from the rumen, and hypocalcemia, may play a part in instigating hypomotility, whereas evolution of gas in the abomasum is directly related to the amount of concentrate in the ration. Left displacement of the gas-filled abomasum is amenable to treatment, and is rarely encountered at autopsy. Handling of an affected animal postmortem may correct displacements in any case. Other than possible scarring of the lesser omentum, the abomasum may be unremarkable. Abomasal fistulae, draining in the right paramedian area, may ensue if, during abomasopexy to prevent recurrent displacement, nonabsorbable sutures fixing the abomasum to the abdominal wall penetrate the abomasal mucosa. In calves, left abomasal displacement is associated with gastric ulceration.

Simple right displacement, which accounts for about 15% of abomasal displacements, is probably caused by similar agencies. But right displacement may be complicated in about a fifth of cases by progression to abomasal volvulus, which is clinically serious.

Abomasal volvulus is probably the sequel to rotation of a loop formed by a distended abomasum and attached omasum and duodenum, counterclockwise about a transverse axis through the lesser omentum, when viewed from the right side.

Rotation, buoyed by the gas-filled body of the abomasum, may be in the sagittal plane. With a 360° volvulus, the pylorus ends in the anterior right portion of the abdomen dorsal to the twisted omasum, with the duodenum trapped medial to the omasum and lateral to the partially rotated reticulum. Alternative modes of displacement and rotation are possible, but all may end in this relationship.

Obstruction of duodenal outflow in volvulus results in sequestration of chloride in the abomasal content and the development of metabolic alkalosis. Severe volvulus causes obstruction of blood vessels at the neck of the omasum, as well as causing trauma to the vagus nerves in the region. The abomasum becomes distended with bloodstained fluid and gas. Infarction of the deeply congested mucosa may result in ultimate abomasal rupture, often near the omasoabomasal orifice, and peritonitis. Damage to the vagal branches may prohibit return of normal abomasal motility in animals successfully withstanding surgery. Cases of abomasal torsion are also reported occasionally in preruminant calves; these are usually fatal.

Bibliography

Badylak, S. F., Lantz, G. C., and Jeffries, M. Prevention of reperfusion injury in surgically induced gastric dilatation–volvulus in dogs. *Am J Vet Res* **51:** 294–299, 1990.

Bolton, J. R. *et al.* Normal abomasal electromyography and emptying in sheep and the effects of intra-abomasal volatile fatty acid infusion. *Am J Vet Res* **37:** 1387–1392, 1976.

Breukink, H. J., and de Ruyter, T. Abomasal displacement in cattle: Influence of concentrates in the ration on fatty acid concentrations in ruminal, abomasal, and duodenal contents. *Am J Vet Res* **37:** 1181–1184, 1976.

Coppock, C. E. Displaced abomasum in dairy cattle: Etiological factors. *J Dairy Sci* **57:** 926–933, 1974.

Frazee, L. S. Torsion of the abomasum in a one-month-old calf. *Can Vet J* **25:** 293–295, 1984.

Fubini, S. L. *et al.* Right displacement of the abomasum and abomasal volvulus in dairy cows: 458 cases (1980–1987). *J Am Vet Med Assoc* **198:** 460–464, 1991.

Habel, R. E., and Smith, D. F. Volvulus of the bovine abomasum and omasum. *J Am Vet Med Assoc* **179:** 447–455, 1981.

Hall, J. A. Canine gastric dilatation–volvulus update. *Sem Vet Med Surg (Small Anim)* **4:** 188–193, 1989.

Hawkins, C. D. *et al.* Left abomasal displacement and ulceration in an eight-week-old calf. *Aust Vet J* **63:** 53–55, 1986.

Horne, W. A. *et al.* Effects of gastric distention–volvulus on coronary blood flow and myocardial oxygen consumption in the dog. *Am J Vet Res* **46:** 98–104, 1985.

Kiper, M. L., Traub-Dargatz, J., and Curtis, C. R. Gastric rupture in horses: 50 cases (1979–1987). *J Am Vet Med Assoc* **196:** 333–336, 1990.

Leib, M. S., Monroe, W. E., and Martin, R. A. Suspected chronic gastric volvulus in a dog with normal gastric emptying of liquids. *J Am Vet Med Assoc* **191:** 699–700, 1987.

Lippincott, C. L., and Schulman, A. J. Gastric dilatation–volvulus–torsion syndrome. *In* "Textbook of Veterinary Internal Medicine," S. J. Ettinger (ed.), Vol. 2, pp. 1270–1288. Philadelphia, Pennsylvania, Saunders, 1989.

Morin, M. *et al.* Torsion of abdominal organs in sows: A report of 36 cases. *Can Vet J* **25:** 440–442, 1984.

Muir, W. W. Acid–base and electrolyte disturbances in dogs with gastric dilatation–volvulus. *J Am Vet Med Assoc* **181:** 229–231, 1982.

Muir, W. W., and Weisbrode, S. E. Myocardial ischemia in dogs with gastric dilatation–volvulus. *J Am Vet Med Assoc* **181:** 363–366, 1982.

Parker, J. E., and Fubini, S. L. Abomasal fistulas in dairy cows. *Cornell Vet* **77:** 303–309, 1987.

Poulsen, J. S. D. Aetiology and pathogenesis of abomasal displacement in dairy cattle. *Nord Vet Med* **28:** 299–303, 1976.

Smith, D. F. Right-sided torsion of the abomasum in dairy cows: Classification of severity and evaluation of outcome. *J Am Vet Med Assoc* **173:** 108–111, 1978.

Strombeck, D. R., and Guilford, W. G. Gastric dilatation, gastric dilatation–volvulus, and chronic gastric volvulus. *In* "Small Animal Gastroenterology," 2nd Ed., pp. 228–243. Davis, California, Stonegate Publishing, 1990.

Todhunter, R. J., Erb, H. N., and Roth, L. Gastric rupture in horses: A review of 54 cases. *Equine Vet J* **18:** 288–293, 1986.

Van Kruiningen, H. J., Gregoire, K., and Meuten, D. J. Acute gastric dilatation: A review of comparative aspects, by species, and a study in dogs and monkeys. *J Am Anim Hosp Assoc* **10:** 294–324, 1974.

F. Gastric Foreign Bodies and Impaction

A variety of foreign bodies may be encountered in the stomach and, rarely, in the abomasum. Most are incidental findings, or at worst, associated with vomition; mild, acute, or chronic gastritis; or occasionally, with ulceration. Hair balls are often found in the stomach of long-haired cats, and in calves reared on diets low in roughage, where most are in the rumen, with a few in the abomasum. Phytobezoars and trichophytobezoars have been implicated as the cause of pyloric obstruction and death in young lambs on pasture and, in certain regions, in cattle grazing fibrous plants. Fine sand may accumulate in the abomasum in considerable amounts, usually with little apparent ill effect.

Gastric impaction by inspissated content in the horse is related to factors such as consumption of fibrous roughage, inadequate water intake, and poor mastication. It may cause anorexia and mild colic and loss of body condition, and is to be differentiated clinically and at autopsy from gastric impaction secondary to pyrrolizidine alkaloid poisoning, from dilation secondary to intestinal obstruction, and from primary gastric dilation.

Primary abomasal impaction in cattle may result from restricted water intake and coarse, high-roughage feed, such as wheat stubble or straw, as may occur in winter feeding of cattle in northern prairie areas. It may be potentiated by advanced gestation. Secondary abomasal impaction may follow pyloric stenosis, physical or functional, of any cause. It is perhaps most common as a functional abomasal stasis in one of the manifestations of vagus indigestion. Loss of abomasal motility may be the product of intrathoracic inflammatory or neoplastic vagal lesions; vagal involvement in adhesions following traumatic reticuloperitonitis; vagal trauma in surgically corrected abomasal volvulus; adhesions of the abomasum and omasum which may physically impair motility; or systemic disease which causes abomasal stasis.

The abomasum is impacted with thick porridgelike or inspissated coarse fibrous digesta, despite an apparently patent pylorus. Rupture of the abomasum may ensue, particularly in primary impaction associated with coarse feed, and results in diffuse peritonitis. Most commonly, the laceration is near the omasal–abomasal orifice, but it may be elsewhere. Abomasal ulcers, which may perforate, and perforation of necrotic mucosa, presumed to be due to ischemia resulting from pressure exerted by the impacted content, also may occur. Omasal dilation and ruminal distension also are found in many of these cases; omasa usually contain inspissated digesta, whereas rumen content tends to be fluid. Metabolic derangement due to sequestration of chloride in the rumen following regurgitation from the obstructed abomasum, and hypokalemia due to decreased intake in feed in the face of continued normal renal excretion, place these animals in perilous physiologic circumstances, often before inanition becomes a significant factor.

A syndrome known clinically as **abomasal dilation and emptying defect** occurs in sheep, especially Suffolks, in North America. The animals develop chronic inappetence and weight loss, and at necropsy they have a markedly distended abomasum containing digesta resembling rumen contents. No morphologic gross or microscopic lesions of the stomach, vagus nerve, or other organs have been found. The cause is unknown, though it does not seem familial within the breed, or related to quality of roughage fed. Though rumen chloride levels are elevated, few animals become hypochloremic and alkalotic, as cattle with abomasal impaction do. Scrapie, speculated to be associated with abomasal impaction of sheep in Britain, has not been implicated.

Bibliography

Ashcroft, R. A. Abomasal impaction of cattle in Saskatchewan. *Can Vet J* **24:** 375–380, 1983.

Kopcha, M. Abomasal dilatation and emptying defect in a ewe. *J Am Vet Med Assoc* **192:** 783–784, 1988.

Kuiper, R., and Breukink, H. J. Secondary indigestion as a cause of functional pyloric stenosis in the cow. *Vet Rec* **119:** 404–406, 1986.

Mitchell, K. J. Dietary abomasal impaction in a herd of dairy replacement heifers. *J Am Vet Med Assoc* **198:** 1408–1409, 1991.

Neal, P. A., and Edwards, G. B. Vagus indigestion in cattle. *Vet Rec* **82:** 396–402, 1968.

Njau, B. C., Kasali, O. B., and Scholtens, R. G. Abomasal impaction associated with anorexia and mortality in lambs. *Vet Res Com* **12:** 491–495, 1988.

Osborne, A. D. Hairballs in veal calves. *Vet Rec* **99:** 239, 1976.

Owen, Rh. ap Rh., Jagger, D. W., and Jagger, F. Two cases of equine primary gastric impaction. *Vet Rec* **121:** 102–105, 1987.

Ruegg, P. L, George, L. W., and East, N. E. Abomasal dilatation and emptying defect in a flock of Suffolk ewes. *J Am Vet Med Assoc* **193:** 1534–1536, 1988.

G. Circulatory Disturbances

Hyperemia of the gastric mucosa occurs with ingestion of chemicals, which usually also cause superficial erosion and necrosis, discussed later with chemical gastritis. Focal hyperemia may be related to local irritation of the mucosa by foreign bodies, and with focal acute viral lesions of the abomasum in cattle. Congestion of the mucosa can occur in conditions causing portal hypertension, including cirrhosis and shock in the dog.

Uremic gastritis, presenting as severe congestion of the body of the stomach, associated with signs of hematemesis and melena, is found in some dogs, and occasionally in cats and horses, with renal disease. In such animals, the mucosa is thickened and deep red-black. Lesions vary in severity from case to case, and premonitory changes without severe hemorrhage and necrosis are present in animals euthanized earlier in the course of disease. In such dogs there may be no gross gastric lesion, or variable edema and thickening of rugal mucosa, perhaps with focal ulceration, is evident.

Microscopically, the lamina propria between glands is edematous, and there are increased mast cells. Deposits of basophilic ground substance and mineral are found, especially on the basement membrane of vessels and glands, or on collagen fibrils and in degenerative smooth muscle. These changes occur particularly in the middle and deeper portions of the mucosa. Parietal cells in this area are usually mineralized as well. Such mineral deposits may be seen at autopsy in gross cross sections of mucosa. More extensive mineral deposition also involves the muscular coats and arterioles of the submucosa and serosa. Such vessels also show evidence of endothelial damage, medial necrosis, and in some cases, thrombosis. Severe mucosal congestion, edema, and necrosis are possibly related to ischemia secondary to the vascular lesions, though perhaps not directly associated with arterial thrombosis and obstruction, which is often not readily found. Microvascular lesions in the lamina propria, and systemic states in uremia, may be contributory. Impaired renal degradation and excretion of gastrin may promote hyperchlorhydria and exacerbate mucosal damage.

The cause of the vascular lesions may be a poorly characterized circulating toxic peptide associated with uremia. Mineral deposition is probably the product of altered systemic metabolism of calcium in renal failure, perhaps coupled with the local microenvironment resulting from bicarbonate moving across the basal border of secreting parietal cells. Membrane lesions in metabolically compromised parietal cells may also act as foci of mineral deposition. (See The Urinary System for discussion of uremia, Chapter 5, Section I,D of this volume). Mineralization is also a feature of vitamin D intoxication.

Gastric venous infarction is a common lesion in swine, and is also encountered in ruminants and horses. It is related to endothelial damage and thrombosis in venules, usually associated with endotoxemia or other bacterial or toxic damage. Salmonellosis and *Escherichia coli* septicemia in all species, and in addition, in swine, postweaning coliform gastroenteritis, erysipelas, swine dysentery, Glasser's disease, and hog cholera are associated with the lesion. The fundic mucosa is bright red or deep red-black and may have some excess mucus or perhaps fibrin on the surface. Occasionally the superficial mucosa is obviously necrotic, adopting a yellow-brown caseous appearance, and may lift off with the ingesta. In section there is thrombosis of venules in the mucosa and often at the mucosal–submucosal junction, usually with prominent fibrin plugs. Thrombosed capillaries and venules may be present at any level of the mucosa, along the base of the ischemic zone of superficial coagulation necrosis, with local hemorrhage and edema. There may be an acute inflammatory reaction delineating the necrotic area in the mucosa. Sometimes the full thickness of the gastric mucosa, focally or diffusely, may be necrotic.

Edema of the gastric rugae occurs with hypoproteinemia in any species, in portal hypertension, and is found in the abomasum of cattle poisoned by arsenic. Edema fluid collects in the submucosa of the folds, and is particularly obvious in the normally thin abomasal plicae. Edema may contribute to the thickening of rugae seen in gastritis. Edema of the submucosa of the stomach is a common and important lesion in edema disease of swine. It is best appreciated by making several slices through the serosa and external muscle to the submucosa on the greater curvature over the body of the stomach. Edema disease is considered fully in the section of Infectious and Parasitic Diseases of the Gastrointestinal Tract (Section VII of this chapter).

Bibliography

Cheville, N. F. Uremic gastropathy in the dog. *Vet Pathol* **16:** 292–309, 1979.

H. Gastritis

Gastritis is a term often applied to acute gastric injury with grossly visible hemorrhage or necrosis, when inflammatory processes, strictly speaking, are scarcely present. **Chemical gastritis or abomasitis,** reflected in diffuse gastric congestion, hemorrhage, necrosis, and ulceration, may be induced by chemicals such as arsenic, thallium, formalin, bronopol, aspirin, phosphatic fertilizers, and by the toxic principle in bitterweed (*Hymenoxon odorata*). Blister beetle (*Epicauta* spp.) intoxication in horses, induced by the cantharidin contained in these insects, may cause necrosis and ulceration of the distal esophagus and pars esophagea, and intense hyperemia of the glandular mucosa of the stomach. In some cases it is associated with ulcers or gastric rupture, in addition to enterocolitis, nephrosis, hemorrhages of the urinary bladder, and myocardial hemorrhage and necrosis. Zinc may cause acute mortality, in which the mucosa of the abomasum and duodenum is a distinctive lime green and necrotic, with an underlying congested, edematous submucosa. Microscopically, radiating crystals are evident in the necrotic tissue. Subacute zinc intoxication may be reflected in abomasal damage characterized by exfoliation of glandular epithelium, ablation of glands in some areas, and reparative proliferation of mucous neck cells, in addition to fibrosing pancreatitis and mild nephrosis.

Eosinophilic infiltrates occur in the squamous stomach of horses with an eosinophilic epitheliotropic syndrome, discussed with eosinophilic enteritis.

Acute and chronic inflammatory cells are uncommon in the lamina propria of the gastric fundic mucosa in normal domestic animals. Acute inflammatory infiltrates in the gastric wall are usually associated with subacute superficial irritation or erosion, a stable gastric ulcer, gastric venous infarction, clostridial and mycotic gastritis, or some systemic viral infections.

Chronic gastritis occurs with gastric trauma, abomasal and gastric parasitisms, and in some viral infections of large animals, where it may be associated with mucous metaplasia and hyperplasia of the fundic mucosa.

Chronic gastritis is also recognized in dogs, and occasionally cats, which are subjected to gastric biopsy for obscure gastrointestinal disease, usually involving vomition. **Chronic superficial gastritis** is a term applied in humans to a lesion with a chronic inflammatory infiltrate, and perhaps some increased fibrous stroma, confined to the interfoveolar propria; normal gastric glands are present, with minimal deep interstitial inflammatory infiltrate. Such an entity is seen relatively commonly in gastric biopsies in dogs, with no etiologic connotation.

Helicobacter (*Campylobacter*) *pylori,* or similar agents, have been associated with acute and chronic type B gastritis (always involving pyloric antrum, and fundus variably) in humans, other primates, and ferrets, and with peptic ulceration in humans. A spirillumlike bacterium in the gastric mucosa of dogs has been associated with the presence of mucosal lymphoid aggregates, but not rigorously. It, and a similar agent isolated from the feline stomach, and provisionally named *Helicobacter felis,* are often found in fundic glands, usually without any local inflammatory response. *Chlamydia* have been recognized in surface mucous cells of otherwise normal fundic mucosa in cats with no signs of disease. Experimental infection produced conjunctivitis, respiratory disease, but only mild gastritis. A thick band of amorphous collagen is seen sporadically on the luminal aspect of the muscularis mucosae in the stomach of cats. The cause and significance are unknown.

Chronic atrophic gastritis is not commonly encountered in small animals. The inflammatory infiltrate is diffusely distributed in the mucosa, or may form follicular lymphoid aggregates. In dogs, there is as yet no evidence that, with age, this entity progresses from chronic superficial gastritis, and proceeds to gastric atrophy, as it does in humans. Autoimmune gastritis, causing atrophy of parietal cell mass, and the development of pernicious anemia (human type A gastritis, which spares the pyloric antrum), is not known to occur spontaneously in animals, though it can be induced in dogs by immunization with gastric juice. However, in some dogs, chronic diffuse gastritis is associated with a reduction in mucosal thickness, loss of parietal cell mass, mucous metaplasia with shortening of glands, and encroachment and condensation of stroma in the area deep to and between fundic glands. Atrophy of glands may be marked, and achlorhydria may ensue, with responsive hypergastrinemia.

Chronic antritis with reduced gastrin secretion theoretically might result in atrophy of parietal cell mass. Duodenal reflux in dogs has been associated with a syndrome of vomition and gastric hyposecretion. Mononuclear cell infiltrates and follicle formation in the lamina propria of the antrum and fundus are found, with subjective atrophy of parietal cell mass. Intestinal metaplasia of the gastric mucosa, considered to be a sequel to chronic gastritis in humans, is rarely recognized in domestic animals.

Chronic hypertrophic gastritis, similar in many respects to Menetrier's disease of humans, occurs in dogs. Vomition and weight loss, in some cases associated with inappetence or diarrhea, are described in the history. The characteristic lesion is marked gastric rugal hypertrophy involving part or most of the fundic gland mucosa in the body of the stomach. Grossly thickened folds of mucosa over an area 4–10 or 12 cm in diameter are thrown up in a convoluted pattern, which may resemble cerebral gyri.

Microscopically, these areas are composed of hypertrophic/hyperplastic mucosa, which may or may not include secondary folds of muscularis mucosae and submucosa. Findings are variable in the few cases reported. There may be foveolar and glandular epithelial hyperplasia with progressive or total loss of parietal cells, which are replaced by mucous cells of varying degrees of differentiation. Marked cystic dilation of mucous glands may occur, which may be evident grossly. Mononuclear cells infiltrate the lamina propria between glands and near the muscularis mucosae, and the propria may be edematous, especially superficially. If the gross appearance of the mucosa in animals with hypertrophic gastritis is not seen by endoscopy or at surgery, biopsies which do not sample the full thickness of the mucosa may be diagnosed as chronic superficial or diffuse gastritis.

The cause of chronic hypertrophic gastritis is unknown, but in part it may be mediated by immune events in the mucosa. The condition in humans is associated with protein-losing gastropathy. Significantly, chronic gastritis and chronic hypertrophic gastritis have been reported in the basenji, a breed of dog in which a syndrome of protein-losing gastroenteritis and diarrhea is well recognized (see diseases of the intestine, Sections VI,J and VI,K of this chapter).

Chronic hypertrophic gastritis is to be differentiated from adenomatous polyps; from fundic mucosal hypertrophy due to the trophic effects of histamine excess in mastocytoma, or from gastrin excess in Zollinger–Ellison syndrome; from infiltrating lymphoid tumors; and in cats, from *Ollulanus tricuspis* gastritis.

Hypertrophic antritis, producing a thickened, sometimes convoluted, mucosa in the antrum, is part of the syndrome of chronic hypertrophic pyloric gastropathy, associated with pyloric stenosis in dogs, considered earlier. Etiologic factors are unknown.

Eosinophilic gastroenteritis occasionally may involve the stomach in dogs. Eosinophils infiltrate the mucosa and submucosa in large numbers, usually accompanied by a mixed chronic inflammatory cell population, and perhaps with some atrophy of glands, and interstitial fibrosis. Gastric disease is often associated with a syndrome of protein loss, eosinophilia and eosinophilic infiltrates in more distal gut (see diseases of intestine, Sections VI,J and VI,K of this chapter). Even rarer cases of scirrhous eosinophilic gastritis and arteritis, and of histiocytic gastritis in association with amyloidosis, are on record in dogs.

Braxy, or bradsot, is an acute abomasitis of sheep and less commonly, calves, due to infection with *Clostridium septicum* (Fig. 1.38). It is a sporadic disease of young animals, usually occurring in cooler climates. It is reported from Iceland, Scandinavia, Scotland, Canada, the northern United States, Tasmania, and Victoria, Australia. The factors initiating bacterial invasion are unknown, though local tissue damage in the abomasum is implicated. Cold weather is usually associated with the disease, but it is difficult to imagine feed being cold enough, by the time it attains the abomasum, to cause significant mucosal trauma or hypothermia and necrosis. Production of exotoxin by *C. septicum* causes the signs and death, which usually ensues quickly.

At autopsy there may be blood-tinged abdominal fluid, and the serosa of the abomasum may be congested or fibrin covered. Mucosal lesions may be diffuse, or involve demarcated foci of variable size and shape. Abomasal folds may be thickened, reddened, occasionally hemorrhagic or necrotic. Most notable is the presence of extensive gelatinous edema and emphysema in the submucosa. Diffuse edema, and extensive areas of suppurative infiltrate demarcating areas of coagulation necrosis, with prominent pockets of emphysema, are evident in tissue sections. These involve mainly submucosa, and extend into adjacent mucosa and external muscle. There may be

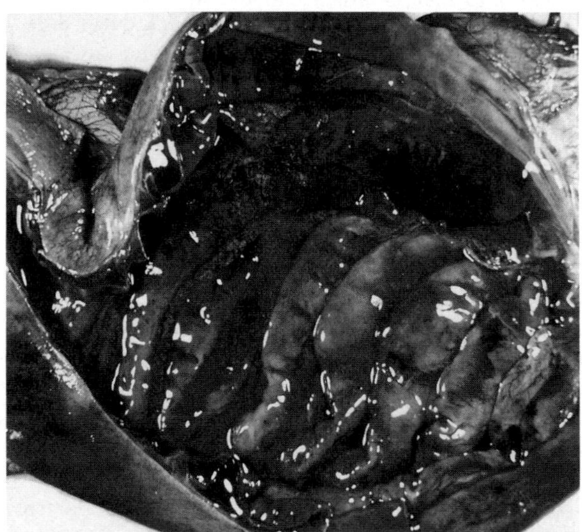

Fig. 1.38 Braxylike clostridial abomasitis (*C. septicum*). Calf. (Courtesy of M. Bergeland.)

venous thrombosis and hemorrhage. Gram-positive bacilli are usually evident as individuals or colonies in affected tissue. They may be identified as *C. septicum* by fluorescent antibody reaction or culture. Such lesions are occasionally complicated by other clostridia. Braxy must be differentiated from cellulitis of the abomasal wall due to mixed anaerobic flora without *C. septicum.*

Clostridium perfringens type A has been associated with a syndrome of tympany, abomasitis, and abomasal ulceration in calves in the western United States. Animals have abdominal tympany and pain, depression, or may die suddenly. Grossly, there is variable congestion, hemorrhage, erosion, and ulceration of the abomasal mucosa, usually in the fundic area. Circular or linear perforating ulcers may develop. In association with the expected microscopic changes in erosion or ulceration, there is exfoliation and necrosis of mucosal epithelium, edema of the submucosa, dilation and thrombosis of submucosal lymphatics, and mild acute inflammatory infiltrates in the submucosa. Gram-positive bacilli may be on the mucosal surface, or in inflamed submucosa. Proliferation of *C. perfringens* in the rumen of calves with overflow of milk from the reticular groove is believed to promote colonization of the abomasum, and production of necrotizing exotoxin.

Abomasitis associated with viral infection occurs in a number of the systemic viral diseases affecting the gastrointestinal tract, including infectious bovine rhinotracheitis in calves and rarely older animals, herpesvirus infections of small ruminants, mucosal disease, rinderpest, malignant catarrhal fever, and bluetongue. Abomasal lesions are rarely the sole manifestation of these diseases, but form part of a picture at autopsy which may suggest an etiologic diagnosis. The appearance and pathogenesis of abomasitis in these diseases varies with the conditions (see Infectious and Parasitic Diseases of the Gastrointestinal Tract, Section VII of this chapter).

Mycotic gastritis is a sporadic problem almost invariably secondary to insults which cause achlorhydria, or focal atrophy, necrosis, or ulceration under conditions in which mycotic colonization can occur. Compromised resistance, perhaps associated with neoplasia, endogenous or exogenous steroids, lympholytic viral disease, and altered gastrointestinal flora due to antibiotic therapy, may further promote mycosis. Fungal hyphae attaining the submucosa typically invade venules and arterioles, causing thrombosis and a hemorrhagic infarct. The agents involved are usually zygomycetes (phycomycetes) such as *Rhizopus, Absidia,* or *Mucor;* rarely, *Aspergillus* may be implicated.

Mycotic abomasitis in calves is secondary to gastrointestinal infectious bovine rhinotracheitis and to venous infarction of the mucosa in endotoxemia or septicemia with *E. coli* or *Salmonella.* Some cases in very young calves are thought to be secondary to mycotic placentitis. Mucosal disease and occasionally gastric ulcer provide conditions for mycotic invasion of the abomasum in older cattle. The lesions are areas of necrosis, with an intensely congested or hemorrhagic periphery, ranging in diameter from 1 to 2 cm, to confluence over much of the body of the stomach (Fig. 1.39A). Affected mucosa is thickened, red or pale in the necrotic zone, and may be covered by hemorrhage. Edema and hemorrhage are evident in the submucosa. The lesion may penetrate to the serosa, where it is typically seen as a roughly circular area of hemorrhage in the external muscle and subserosa. Hyphae, usually broad and nonseptate zygomycotic in type, are present in sections of the necrotic mucosa, submucosa, and invading vessels, where they initiate thrombosis (Fig. 1.39B,C). The associated inflammatory infiltrate is usually consistent with acute or subacute insult.

In dogs, rare cases of acute multifocal infarctive or granulomatous gastritis are reported, associated with zygomycetes. Mycosis of the glandular stomach of piglets is rare, and it is virtually unknown in horses. Candidiasis of the pars esophagea may occur in swine, often in association with preulcerative epithelial hyperplasia and parakeratosis. For an overview of mycosis of the digestive system, and its sequelae, see Infectious and Parasitic Diseases of the Gastrointestinal Tract (Section VII of this chapter).

Parasitic gastritis is generally of little significance in small animals. Members of the genera *Physaloptera* and *Gnathostoma* are found in dogs, where the former cause focal ulceration, and the latter are the cause of submucosal inflammatory cysts containing suppurative exudate and worms. In cats *Physaloptera* spp. may attach to mucosal ulcers, whereas *Gnathostoma* spp. and *Cylicospirura felineus* are found in nodules in the gastric wall. *Ollulanus tricuspis* is found on the mucosa of the stomach in cats, where it may cause mild to, rarely, severe chronic gastritis. *Cryptosporidium* infection of the gastric mucosa occurs rarely in cats, with uncertain significance.

In the horse, *Draschia megastoma* is found in inflammatory nodules in the submucosa of the cardiac zone, especially along the margo plicatus. *Habronema muscae* and *H. majus* are found on the mucosa and have been associated with mild ulceration. *Trichostrongylus axei* may cause chronic gastritis in the horse. Bots of the genus *Gasterophilus* are found attached to small erosions and ulcers in the esophageal and glandular mucosa.

In swine the spirurids *Ascarops* spp., *Physocephalus* spp., and *Simondsia* spp. are associated with mild gastritis in heavy infections. *Gnathostoma* may be embedded in inflammatory cysts in the submucosa. *Ollulanus tricuspis* may be encountered. *Hyostrongylus rubidus* can cause chronic gastritis and wasting in pigs.

In cattle, sheep, and goats, members of the genera *Haemonchus* and *Mecistocirrus* are large abomasal bloodsucking trichostrongyles, capable of causing severe anemia and hypoproteinemia. *Ostertagia* spp., related genera including *Camelostrongylus, Teladorsagia, Marshallagia,* and *Trichostrongylus axei,* in various ruminants, cause chronic abomasitis with mucous metaplasia, achlorhydria, diarrhea, and plasma protein loss. *Cryptosporidium* spp. occasionally cause subclinical abomasitis in cattle, associated with mucosal hypertrophy, attenuation of epithelium lining the neck of fundic glands, and dilation of glands. The small basophilic organisms are present on

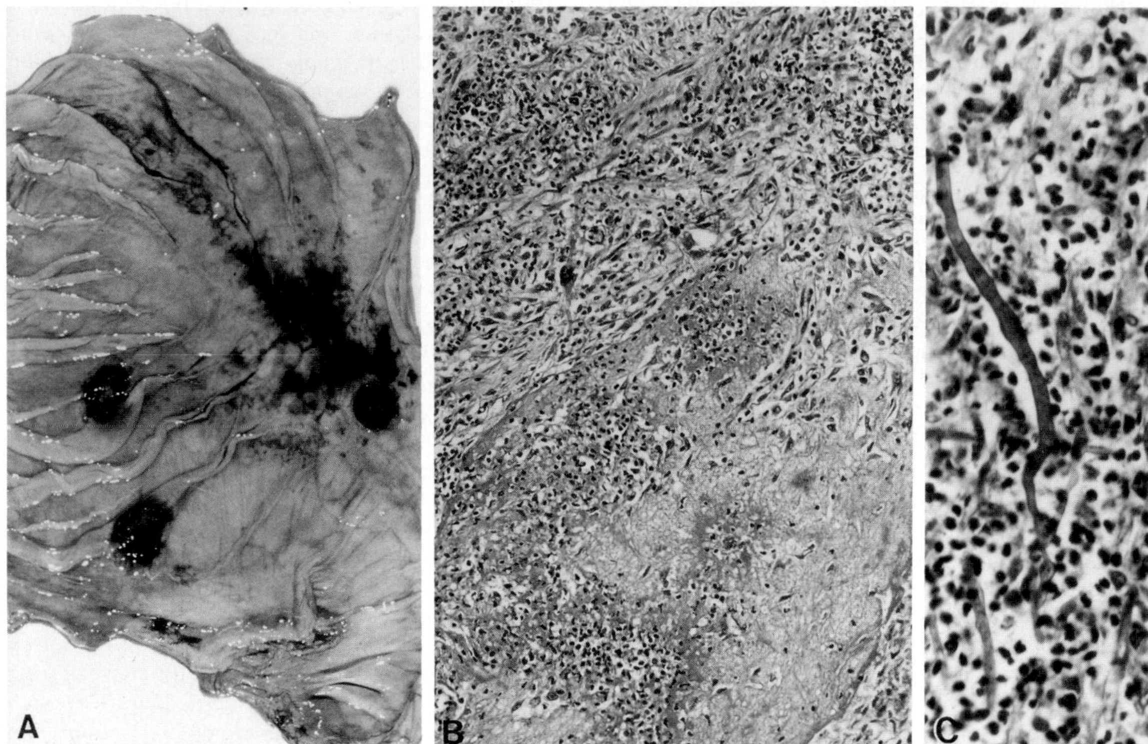

Fig. 1.39 Mycotic abomasitis. Calf. (A) Focal lesions surrounded by deep red areas of infarction and hemorrhage due to thrombosis of mucosal and submucosal vessels. (B) Thrombosis of a venule in submucosa of abomasum due to hyphal invasion. (C) Nonseptate hyphae of zygomycete invading the submucosa.

the surface of epithelium from the base of glands to the mucosal surface. Large schizonts of undetermined coccidia in sheep and goats produce harmless pinpoint pale foci in the abomasal mucosa; formerly the obsolete name *Globidium gilruthi* was applied. Gastric parasitism is considered with Infectious and Parasitic Diseases of the Gastrointestinal Tract (Section VII of this chapter).

Bibliography

Abdurahman, O. S., Hilali, M., and Jarplid, B. A light- and electron-microscopic study on abomasal globidiosis in Somali goats. *Acta Vet Scand* **28:** 181–187, 1987.

Allen, J. G. *et al.* Acute zinc toxicity in sheep. *Aust Vet J* **63:** 93–95, 1986.

Anderson, B. C. Abomasal cryptosporidiosis in cattle. *Vet Pathol* **24:** 235–238, 1987.

Barsanti, J. A., Attleberger, M. H., and Henderson, R. A. Phycomycosis in a dog. *J Am Vet Med Assoc* **167:** 293–297, 1975.

Breitschwerdt, E. B. *et al.* Hypergastrinemia in canine gastrointestinal disease. *J Am Anim Hosp Assoc* **22:** 585–592, 1986.

Buck, G. E. *Campylobacter pylori* and gastrointestinal disease. *Clin Microbiol Rev* **3:** 1–12, 1990.

Camp, B. J. The toxic principle of bitterweed (*Hymenoxon odorata*). *In* "Plant Toxicology," A. A. Seawright *et al.* (eds.), pp. 473–478. Yeerongpilly, Qld., Australia, Queensland Dept. of Primary Industries, 1985.

Dennis, R. *et al.* A case of hyperplastic gastropathy in a cat. *J Small Anim Pract* **28:** 491–504, 1987.

Dickson, J., and Mullins, K. R. Suspected superphosphate poisoning in calves. *Aust Vet J* **64:** 387–388, 1987.

Ellis, T. M., Rowe, J. B., and Lloyd, J. M. Acute abomasitis due to *Clostridium septicum* infection in experimental sheep. *Aust Vet J* **60:** 308–309, 1983.

Eustis, S. L., and Bergeland, M. E. Suppurative abomasitis associated with *Clostridium septicum* infection. *J Am Vet Med Assoc* **178:** 732–734, 1981.

Fox, J. G. *et al. Helicobacter mustelae*-associated gastritis in ferrets. *Gastroenterology* **99:** 352–361, 1990.

Gaillard, E. T. *et al.* Pathogenesis of feline gastric chlamydial infection. *Am J Vet Res* **45:** 2314–2321, 1984.

Hayden, D. W., and Fleischman, R. W. Scirrhous eosinophilic gastritis in dogs with gastric arteritis. *Vet Pathol* **14:** 441–488, 1977.

Henry, G. A. *et al.* Gastric spirillosis in beagles. *Am J Vet Res* **48:** 831–836, 1987.

Hindmarsh, M. Mortality in calves associated with the feeding of milk containing bronopol. *Aust Vet J* **67:** 309–310, 1990.

Kelly, D. G. *et al.* Giant hypertrophic gastropathy (Menetrier's disease): Pharmacologic effects on protein leakage and mucosal ultrastructure. *Gastroenterology* **83:** 581–589, 1982.

Kipnis, R. M. Focal cystic hypertrophic gastropathy in a dog. *J Am Vet Med Assoc* **173:** 182–184, 1978.

Lee, A. *et al.* A small animal model of human *Helicobacter pylori* active chronic gastritis. *Gastroenterology* **99:** 1315–1323, 1990.

MacLachlan, N. J. *et al.* Gastroenteritis of basenji dogs. *Vet Pathol* **25:** 36–41, 1988.

Mahanta, S., and Chaudhury, B. Prevalence, pathology and isolation studies on phycomycotic gastric ulcer in neonatal piglets. *Sabouraudia: J Med Vet Mycol* **23:** 395–397, 1985.

McLeod, C. G., Langlinais, P. C., and Brown, J. C. Ulcerative histiocytic gastritis and amyloidosis in a dog. *Vet Pathol* **18:** 117–120, 1981.

Neitzke, J. P., and Schiefer, B. Incidence of mycotic gastritis in calves up to 30 days of age. *Can Vet J* **15:** 139–144, 1974.

Roeder, B. L. *et al.* Experimental induction of abomasal tympany, abomasitis, and abomasal ulceration by intraruminal inoculation of *Clostridium perfringens* type A in neonatal calves. *Am J Vet Res* **49:** 201–207, 1988.

Ruhr, L. P., and Andries, J. K. Thallium intoxication in a dog. *J Am Vet Med Assoc* **186:** 498–499, 1985.

Sanford, S. E. Gastric zygomycosis (mucormycosis) in 4 suckling pigs. *J Am Vet Med Assoc* **186:** 393–394, 1985.

Schoeb, T. R., and Panciera, R. J. Pathology of blister beetle (*Epicauta*) poisoning in horses. *Vet Pathol* **16:** 18–31, 1979.

Smith, J. M. B. Mycoses of the alimentary tract of animals. *N Z Vet J* **16:** 89–100, 1968.

Strombeck, D. R., and Guilford, W. G. Chronic gastritis, gastric retention, gastric neoplasms and gastric surgery. *In* "Small Animal Gastroenterology," 2nd Ed., pp. 208–227. Davis, California, Stonegate Publishing, 1990.

Strombeck, D. R., Doe, M., and Jang, S. Maldigestion and malabsorption in a dog with chronic gastritis. *J Am Vet Med Assoc* **179:** 801–805, 1981.

van der Gaag, I. Hypertrophic gastritis in 21 dogs. *Zbl Vet Med (A)* **31:** 161–173, 1984.

van der Gaag, I. The histological appearance of peroral gastric biopsies in clinically healthy and vomiting dogs. *Can J Vet Res* **52:** 67–74, 1988.

van der Gaag, I., and Happe, R. P. Follow-up studies by peroral gastric biopsies and necropsy in vomiting dogs. *Can J Vet Res* **53:** 468–472, 1989.

Yardley, J. H. Pathology of chronic gastritis and duodenitis. *In* "Gastrointestinal Pathology," H. Goldman *et al.* (eds.), pp. 69–143. Baltimore, Maryland, Williams & Wilkins, 1990.

I. Gastroduodenal Ulceration

Gastroduodenal ulcer produces signs much less often in animals than in humans. The pathogenesis of peptic ulcer in humans or animals is by no means clear. However, in general it seems to resolve into a relative imbalance between the necrotizing effects of gastric acid and pepsin on one hand, and the ability of the mucosa to maintain its integrity on the other. Hypersecretion of acid, or impairment of mucosal integrity in the face of normal acid secretion, may be invoked as general mechanisms.

Factors implicated in hypersecretion of acid include abnormally high basal secretion, possibly associated with an expanded parietal cell mass, perhaps the result of increased trophic stimulation by gastrin. Gastrinomas cause Zollinger–Ellison syndrome, characterized by elevated gastric acid secretion and severe gastroduodenal ulceration. Increased histamine levels associated with mastocytosis or mastocytoma also cause acid hypersecretion and ulceration.

Ulceration due to compromise of mucosal protective mechanisms is attributed to nonsteroidal antiinflammatory agents such as aspirin, phenylbutazone, and indomethacin. The ulcerogenic properties of these drugs reside partly in direct toxicity to the gastric epithelium, and partly in their effects on prostaglandin metabolism, which is also their therapeutic mechanism. Orally administered nonsteroidal antiinflammatory agents which are weak organic acids, such as aspirin, have a direct deleterious effect on the stomach. In the acid gastric lumen, unionized lipid-soluble acetylsalicylic acid readily crosses the surface-cell membrane. At neutral pH within the cell it ionizes, damaging the cell metabolically, permitting back-diffusion of acid and incipient ulceration. Ulcer induction by these agents is secondarily attributable to depression of prostaglandin synthesis. This they block by interfering with the cyclooxygenase-catalyzed conversion of arachidonic acid to the prostaglandin (PG) endoperoxides PGG_2, PGH_2. In the stomach, prostaglandin-mediated vasodilation, modulation of histamine-induced acid secretion, and other protective effects may be impaired. Phenylbutazone may also have a direct toxic effect on vascular endothelium in the mucosa, which compromises circulation and precipitates ulcer.

In humans, antral gastritis associated with *Helicobacter* (*Campylobacter*) *pylori* infection, and duodenal colonization with this agent, may be associated with development of duodenal ulcer. *Helicobacter*-associated gastritis extending cranially in the stomach is associated with gastric ulcer. Though many infected humans do not have clinical disease, it is presumed that, in some, gastritis interferes with cytoprotective mechanisms at the mucosal surface of the duodenum and stomach, predisposing to back-diffusion of acid; but mechanisms are unclear. The *Spirillum*-like organisms found in the fundic glands of small animals, which tentatively have been included in the genus *Helicobacter,* and are discussed with chronic gastritis, have yet to be implicated in ulcer formation.

Reflux of duodenal contents containing bile salts has been implicated in the induction of gastritis and gastric ulcer. Under some experimental conditions, acid back-diffusion into the gastric mucosa, and morphologic damage, have been caused by application of bile salts. The effects are dependent on the pKa of the bile salt, which must be soluble at acid pH, and on the concentration of hydrogen ion. Lipid solubility of bile salts, and associated damage to surface-cell membranes, may mediate these effects. Alcohols, also lipid-soluble compounds, alter permeability of gastric mucosa and permit back-diffusion of acid. Lysolecithin, formed when pancreatic lipase hydrolyzes lecithin in bile, also increases gastric mucosal permeability.

Glucocorticoids and stress have been implicated in the genesis of ulcer, though the role of steroids is controversial. Experimentally, gastroduodenal hemorrhage and ulceration occur in some species of animals stressed by restraint or social factors, and they are a feature of trap-death syndrome in small mammals. Severe gastric hemorrhage or ulceration may occur following neurosurgery, trauma to the spinal cord, and burns, and it is considered by some to be stress related. However, the role of steroids, rather than changes in blood flow, autonomic, or central nervous effects, or other physiologic mechanisms, is not proven in these situations. Steroids decrease reparative gastric epithelial cell turnover, and by stabilizing membranes, may decrease the availability of arachidonic acid for prostaglandin synthesis. These effects may predispose to development of ulcer when combined with other insults. However, steroids have also been demonstrated to have a sparing effect on the challenged gastric mucosa.

Reduced mucosal perfusion or ischemia may be a principal factor interacting in stress-associated ulceration, and in that initiated by other modalities discussed previously. Reduced blood flow to the mucosa in local areas has been suspected, under a number of circumstances, to precede mucosal hemorrhage or erosion. Ischemia will result in hypoxemic compromise of surface cells. In combination with the effects of other insults, this may initiate mucosal permeability and back-diffusion of acid. Neutralization by blood-borne bicarbonate of acid diffusing into the mucosa also may be reduced in ischemia. Mechanisms of mucosal ischemia are obscure. Reduction in local prostaglandin concentration may contribute, as may local or systemic hypotension. Following mucosal damage and back-diffusion of hydrogen ions, vasodilation and hyperemia develop, perhaps the result of liberation of mucosal histamine. Microvascular disruption then results in hemorrhage. Ischemia may be more significant in the induction of fundic, rather than antral ulcers.

Whatever the cause, the results of a breach of the gastric glandular mucosa have the potential to follow a **common pathway to ulceration** in all species. Acute superficial lesions such as those associated with stress or following administration of aspirin are often seen as areas of reddening and hemorrhage, especially along the margins of rugae in the fundic mucosa. Acid treatment of hemoglobin gives blood on the surface or in the gastric lumen a red-brown or black color. In some species, severe stress-associated gastric hemorrhage may occur diffusely over the entire congested gastric mucosa, resulting in hypovolemic shock and anemia, with melena. In some instances melena, presumably the result of a recent episode of gastric bleeding, may be present in the lower intestine, with minimal gross evidence of hemorrhage or ulceration in the stomach. The microscopic lesion associated with hemorrhage of this type is often subtle, bleeding seemingly resulting from diapedesis, with minimal mucosal damage. Usually there is superficial erosion of the mucosa, often difficult to differentiate from autolysis, with granules of brown acid hematin in debris on the surface. Inflammation is usually absent. Evidence for healing mild gastric erosion is the presence of basophilic, poorly differentiated, flattened, cuboidal or low columnar cells on the mucosal surface, with mitotic cells in the upper neck of the glands.

Lesions of any genesis proceeding to gastric ulcer do so by progressive coagulation necrosis of the gastric wall. Ulcers vary in microscopic appearance depending on their aggression, and the point in their development at which they are intercepted. Acute gastric lesions appear as erosions with superficial eosinophilic necrotic debris and loss of mucosal architecture to the depths of the foveolae, or as a depression in the mucosal surface with necrotic debris at the base. Necrosis usually extends rapidly to the muscularis mucosae, causing ulceration. Once the superficial portion of the mucosa is destroyed, natural local buffering is lost, and the proliferative compartment of the gland, which is near the surface, is obliterated, preventing a local epithelial regenerative response. Ulcers attaining the submucosa impinge on arterioles of increasing diameter, multiplying the risk of significant gastric hemorrhage. The ulcer may progress through the muscularis and serosa, culminating in perforation of the gastric wall. Severe gastric hemorrhage or perforation are relatively common sequelae of gastroduodenal ulceration in domestic animals.

Ulcers which come into equilibrium with reparative processes may do so at any level of the gastric wall below the mucosa, but usually at the submucosa. Subacute to chronic ulcers have a base and sides composed of granulation tissue of varying thickness and maturity, infiltrated by a mixed inflammatory cell population, and overlain by a usually thin layer of necrotic debris. Chronic ulcers wax and wane. Depending on the relative dominance of reparative processes and aggressive ulceration, the layer of granulation tissue may be thick and mature, or thinner, less mature, and with superficial evidence of recent necrosis. There is mucous metaplasia and hyperplasia in glands at the periphery of the ulcer, which, with time, overhang the edge of the lesion. Under favorable conditions they gradually fill in the mucosal defect from the margins. Healed ulcers are usually depressed and may be somewhat puckered, with a scirrhous submucosa on cut section. The mucosa of healed ulcers, even in the fundic zone, is composed of mucous glands. Excessive scarring of healed ulcers strategically located near the pylorus may lead to pyloric obstruction in any species.

Duodenal ulcers, which usually occur proximal to the opening of the pancreatic and bile ducts, resemble gastric ulcer in their microscopic appearance (allowing for their intestinal location), evolution, and sequelae.

Peptic ulcer occurs commonly in cattle, less commonly in dogs, rarely in cats, and is unusual in horses and swine, where ulceration of the esophageal, rather than glandular, gastric mucosa is the rule. In most species the prevalence of ulcer is probably underestimated, since only lesions producing severe signs associated with pain, hemorrhage, or perforation come to attention.

Peptic ulcer in dogs is relatively infrequently reported in the literature, but is seen on a regular basis in veterinary clinics, usually in adult animals. Signs associated with peptic ulcer include variable appetite, abdominal pain, vomition, melena, and anemia. Ulcers, a few millimeters to 3–4 cm in diameter, are found most commonly in the pyloric antrum or proximal duodenum. The gross and microscopic appearance of ulcers varies with their aggressiveness and duration, as previously described. Thrombosed arterioles and venules cut by the ulcerative process are often seen, and should be sought in the bed of gastric and duodenal lesions associated with anemia or obvious hemorrhage.

Perforation of gastric or duodenal ulcers may lead to massive hemorrhage or release of gastric contents into the abdomen. Perforating duodenal ulcer may instigate pancreatitis. Some ulcers perforate silently, the serosal lesion healing by granulation, or adhesion by, and fibroplasia in, the omentum. The irritant nature of gastric contents released in these circumstances may lead to chronic inflammation, granulation, and thickening of the serosa, even when previous perforation cannot be appreciated. A search for microscopic particles of food such as plant material or muscle fibers in the serosal inflammatory response confirms perforation in this circumstance. Chronic peptic ulcers with thickened mucosal margins, scirrhous bases, and perhaps serosal thickening associated with perforation or near perforation, must be differentiated from gastric adenocarcinoma in the dog.

Syndromes clearly the result of hypersecretion of acid occur in dogs. **Mastocytoma is associated with peptic ulcer,** presumably due to histamine-stimulated acid hypersecretion and microvascular effects. The tumor and mastocytosis do not involve the stomach directly, and ulcers may occur in animals with solitary skin tumors. In one series of 24 dogs with recurrent or metastatic mastocytoma, gastric and duodenal erosions or ulcers, frequently multiple, were present in 20. In many cases such lesions are clinically silent, and they should be looked for at autopsy in animals with mastocytoma. Mast cell tumors have been associated rarely with gastric ulceration in the cow, and in the cat, where gastric ulcer is very uncommon.

Zollinger–Ellison syndrome, peptic ulcer due to gastrin-secreting pancreatic islet cell tumors or gastrinomas, has been reported in a few dogs and a cat. The history usually includes inappetence, vomition, weight loss, and possibly diarrhea or melena. Reflux esophagitis and gastric or duodenal ulcer are present in most cases. Small nodular masses histologically confirmed as islet cell tumors may be found in the pancreas, and in most animals, metastases to the liver, spleen, or hepatic lymph nodes are present. Hypertrophy of the fundic mucosa has been associated with a subjective increase in parietal cell mass. Peptic ulcer and reflux esophagitis in such cases result from gastrin-stimulated acid hypersecretion.

Firm diagnosis rests on demonstration of elevated serum gastrin levels by radioimmunoassay; by identification of gastrin-bearing cells in fixed or frozen tumor tissue by immunohistochemistry; or by demonstration of gastrin in extracts of frozen tumor. Other peptide hormones may also be present, and a similar syndrome in a dog has been associated with an islet cell tumor secreting pancreatic polypeptide and insulin, but apparently not gastrin.

The microscopic appearance of these islet cell tumors is not diagnostic for gastrinoma, nor is the ultrastructural appearance of tumor cells necessarily characteristic of the G cell. Pancreatic islet cell neoplasms may be difficult to find, and should be sought assiduously in suspect cases. In humans, some gastrinomas arise in the wall of the stomach or duodenum. The usual therapy in humans is medical suppression of gastric acid production, or removal of the target tissue by gastric resection, rather than ablation of often occult and disseminated islet cell tumor.

The cause in dogs of gastroduodenal ulcer possibly associated with decreased resistance to back-diffusion of acid is less clear. Hepatic disease is often present in dogs with gastric ulcer, but the basis for a causal association is obscure. Some ulcers are obviously associated with administration of glucocorticoids in high doses as antiinflammatory, immunosuppressive, or antineoplastic therapy. Nonsteroidal antiinflammatory drugs such as aspirin, naproxen, indomethacin, flunixin meglumine, and pyroxicam, sometimes given in excessive quantity, are also associated with spontaneous ulcers. Gastric hemorrhage and gastroduodenal ulceration are occasionally seen in dogs following trauma or major surgery. A syndrome of gastric hemorrhage, pancreatitis, and colonic ulceration and perforation is recognized in dogs following spinal trauma. The pathogenesis of this problem is obscure and undoubtedly complex. Endogenous and exogenous hyperglucocorticoidism appear to be implicated, in association with the stress of trauma and surgery, and putative neurogenic influences initiated by damage to the spinal cord. In dogs diffuse gastric hemorrhage due to reduced mucosal resistance to acid must be differentiated from the effects of heavy metal ingestion, uremic gastritis, coagulopathy especially due to warfarin or disseminated intravascular coagulation, and canine hemorrhagic gastroenteritis, among others.

Abomasal ulcers in cattle are common (Fig. 1.40); duo-

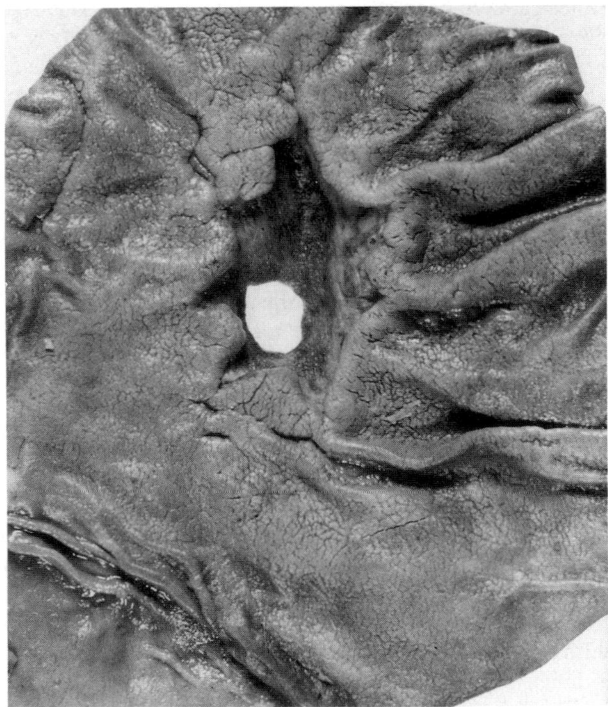

Fig. 1.40 Perforated abomasal ulcer. Calf.

denal ulcer is rarely encountered in this species. Acute ulcers or erosions considered to be the result of stress are frequently seen incidentally in animals, of any age, dying of a variety of causes. They are present usually as linear areas of brown or black hemorrhage or erosion along the margins of abomasal rugae, or as punctate hemorrhages and erosions scattered over the mucosa, especially of the fundus. Such lesions must be differentiated from foci of acute necrosis and ulceration due to systemic viral infections, and from gastric venous infarcts.

The causes of abomasal ulcer are usually unclear, but they are most common in young calves, dairy cows, and feedlot animals. Abomasal ulcer occurred in about 3–4% of feedlot cattle in one study, with about half the cases symptomatic, whereas there are reports of more than 6% of European dairy cows slaughtered with evidence of active or previous abomasal ulcers. A very high proportion, often in excess of 50%, of veal calves may have abomasal ulcers at slaughter. Ulcers often appear to be subclinical, and apparently without effect on growth or performance.

Ulcers often seem to occur under stressful circumstances, as in recently weaned and veal calves, postparturient cows, animals with concurrent disease such as abomasal displacement or mastitis, or after transportation. Lactic acid and histamine entering the abomasum from the forestomachs in animals poorly adapted to high-concentrate rations may contribute to mucosal damage. In veal calves, consumption of straw, shavings, or other roughage has been associated with an increased prevalence of ulcers, and there appears to be an increase in thickness, and altered mucus production in the pyloric mucosa. Abomasal ulcers in range calves in western North America have been associated with *C. perfringens* gastritis, consumption of roughage at pasture, and possibly copper deficiency. Abomasal stasis may play a part in animals with physical or physiological abomasal obstruction or displacement. Ulceration of the abomasal mucosa infiltrated by lymphosarcoma will occur, and it may be a sequel to ingestion of toxins such as arsenic.

Hemorrhage causing exsanguination, or perforation and septic peritonitis, are the usual cause of death due to abomasal ulcers. Ulcers are common in the pyloric region in cattle, and especially at the torus pyloricus in veal calves. Often more than one ulcer is present. Most are 2–4 cm in diameter and approximately circular, though some may be irregular or linear, and to 15 cm in size. Active ulcers may have a dirty brown or gray necrotic floor with some fibrin. Arteries may be visible in the base of bleeding lesions. Older ulcers are puckered by scarring, with an overhanging periphery. Abomasal rugae or plicae may be scalloped along their margins or perforated by active or healed ulcers, and in a study of pastured dairy cattle, most ulcers and scars were found in the fundic area.

Bleeding abomasal ulcer should be looked for in cattle with melena or anemia, and perforating abomasal ulcer in animals presenting with septic peritonitis, especially if digesta is in the abdominal cavity. Perforation may occur into the omental bursa, localizing contamination, whereas some points of perforation will be adherent to the abdominal wall, or occluded by superficially adherent omentum.

Abomasal stress ulcer in calves must be differentiated from lesions associated with infectious bovine rhinotracheitis, and mycotic abomasitis must be differentiated from ulcer in calves and older animals. Mycosis is a rare complication of peptic ulcer. In juvenile and adult cattle, focal abomasal lesions due to bovine virus diarrhea must be differentiated.

Gastric ulcer in swine is usually restricted to the pars esophagea; in a small proportion of affected pigs, lesions extend into the contiguous esophagus. Rarely are significant ulcers of the cardiac, fundic, or pyloric mucosa encountered in swine, sometimes in association with ulcer of the pars esophagea, occasionally with gastric parasitism or systemic disease. Venous infarcts in the body of the stomach in swine are not to be confused with gastric ulcer.

Under conditions of modern pig husbandry, the prevalence of ulcer and associated abnormalities of the pars esophagea is high. Weaned growers and feeders are commonly affected. Most lesions are subclinical; however, some prove fatal. Pigs die without premonition, or with a short history which may include anemia, weakness, inappetence, vomition, and melena. Other animals are affected chronically, with signs of anorexia, intermittent melena, and weight loss, which may culminate in death or slow recovery with runting. Despite its high subclinical prevalence, and occasional outbreaks of clinical disease or loss of individual valuable pigs, most studies indicate that the economic significance of gastric ulceration is marginal. Little or no effect on growth rate or feed efficiency is evident in most subclinically affected animals. There is little disagreement over the morphology of ulceration of the pars esophagea; its etiopathogenesis remains unresolved. Factors implicated in the etiology are many, and their mode of involvement, if any, is usually obscure. Stressful husbandry practices have been considered to contribute to development of ulcer, though glucocorticoid administration results in lesions of the fundus, not pars esophagea, in pigs. High dietary copper levels, feeding of whey, starchy diets low in protein, and high levels of dietary unsaturated fatty acids have been associated. Experimental infection with *Ascaris suum* has been implicated with ulcer, but natural infection is not considered causally associated. Experimentally, factors stimulating acid secretion, especially histamine, consistently cause ulcers of the pars esophagea, suggesting that gastric acidity may play an etiologic role. Repeatedly, finely ground rations have been found to be ulcerogenic and are the single most important contributing factor.

Squamous epithelium has no innate buffering capacity, and it is highly susceptible to attack by gastric acid, as occurs in reflux esophagitis. Similar events may initiate ulceration of the pars esophagea. Swine with gastric ulcer often have abnormally fluid stomach contents. In experimental studies there is slow gastric emptying with progressive declines in pH with time. Feeding of finely divided rations is associated experimentally with increased water in stomach content. Abnormally fluid gastric content fails to partition properly, and the pH gradient from esophagus to pylorus which occurs in the normal porcine stomach is not established. Relatively low pH occurs at the esophageal end of the stomach, whereas the pH at the pylorus is higher than normal. Under these conditions of prolonged gastric distension and relatively high antral pH, gastrin-stimulated acid secretion may be excessive. Fluidity and increased mixing of content may expose the pars esophagea, which should normally be in contact with material buffered to pH 5 or greater, to excess acid. This may initiate the epithelial changes described, which culminate in ulceration. Whey may in itself be acid, and would presumably cause an abnormally fluid gastric environment. This could explain its association with ulcer in swine. How other factors mentioned might be implicated in ulcerogenesis is less clear.

Lesions of the pars esophagea may involve only a small part, or virtually all, of the gastric squamous mucosa. The lesion evolves through parakeratosis, to fissuring and erosion, with ultimate ulceration in severe cases. All stages in this progression will be encountered at autopsy in pigs. The milder lesions are incidental findings. The epithelium of the pars esophagea often appears yellowish and is thickened, irregular, roughened, and may flake or peel off readily. This gross change is the result of microscopic thickening and parakeratosis, with nucleated cells present at the irregular mucosal surface. *Candida* may be present over the epithelial surface, with hyphae invading the parakeratotic epithelium, perhaps due to favorable cystine or glycogen levels. Rete pegs and proprial papillae are elongate. Neutrophils and eosinophils may be present at the tips of proprial papillae, and infiltrating into the epithelium, which appears hydropic and may erode over the tips of papillae.

Erosion of the epithelium progresses to ulceration and exposure of papillae and deeper propria, which bleed as small vessels are disrupted. Such lesions begin as fissures in the hyperplastic parakeratotic epithelium, but advance to ulcerate the entire pars esophagea. They usually spare only a microscopically visible margin of squamous epithelium adjacent to the cardiac gland mucosa. Ulcers of the pars esophagea, like peptic ulcer, have a floor of necrotic debris overlying exposed connective tissue (Fig. 1.41). Depending on the stage and aggression of the ulcer, there may be a well-developed inflammatory margin to the necrosis and a bed of granulation tissue. Fatal gastric hemorrhage often occurs, and thrombosed arterioles and venules cut by ulceration are exposed in the floor of the acute ulcer, often overlain by a blood clot. Ulcers of the pars esophagea usually involve only the submucosa, but they may advance to the muscularis externa and occasionally to the serosa. They rarely perforate.

Grossly, fully developed ulceration of the pars esophagea is apparent as a punched-out lesion with elevated rolled edges, obliterating the entire pars esophagea and obscuring the esophageal opening (Fig. 1.42). The floor of the ulcer may be so smooth that it is misinterpreted as normal by the inexperienced. Pigs with gastric ulcer at any stage of evolution tend to have fluid content in the stomach. Those with hemorrhagic ulcer may have red-brown gastric content, or massive hemorrhage into the stomach with large blood clots in the lumen, and thrombosed blood adherent to the base of the ulcer and its exposed bleeding points. Melenic content will often be in the intestine, and the colon may contain firm, black, pelleted feces. The carcasses of animals which bleed out

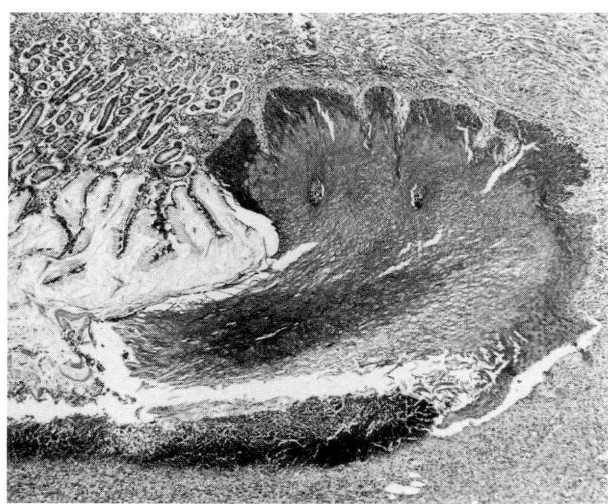

Fig. 1.41 Margin of ulcer. Pars esophagea. Pig. Cardiac glandular mucosa. A normal remnant of squamous and adjacent cardiac mucosa overhangs margin of ulcer.

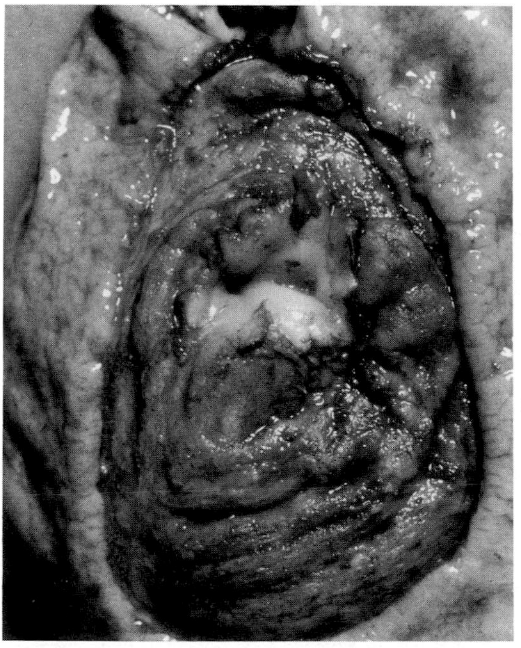

Fig. 1.42 Ulceration of the pars esophagea. Pig. Squamous mucosa is ulcerated, but adjacent cardiac glandular mucosa is unscathed.

with gastric ulcer are very pale. Blood in the intestine associated with gastric ulcer in pigs must be differentiated from mesenteric torsion and proliferative hemorrhagic enteropathy associated with *Campylobacter*. A few pigs with parakeratosis, erosion, and ulceration of the pars esophagea have esophageal lesions suggestive of gastric reflux.

Gastric ulcers in some pigs resolve by granulation, and they may become reepithelialized. Such lesions usually become scirrhous, puckered, and contracted as the ulcer closes from the periphery, and scarring may be visible from the serosa (Fig. 1.43). In these circumstances occlusion of the esophageal opening into the stomach may occur, and pigs with this problem can develop muscular hypertrophy of the distal esophagus. Swine which have suffered chronic gastric hemorrhage may have an enlarged spleen due to extramedullary hematopoiesis.

In horses, ulcers in the stomach of foals and adults are often found at autopsy incidental to some other disease process. Gastric ulcer as a clinical entity is less commonly recognized, though a syndrome of abdominal pain, in some cases associated with gastric reflux, has been described in foals, and appears to be increasing. Ulcers are most common in foals younger than 4 months; about half of a group of foals without symptoms of gastric disease had ulcers visible by endoscopy. They are often multiple, and although most frequent in the esophageal region, they

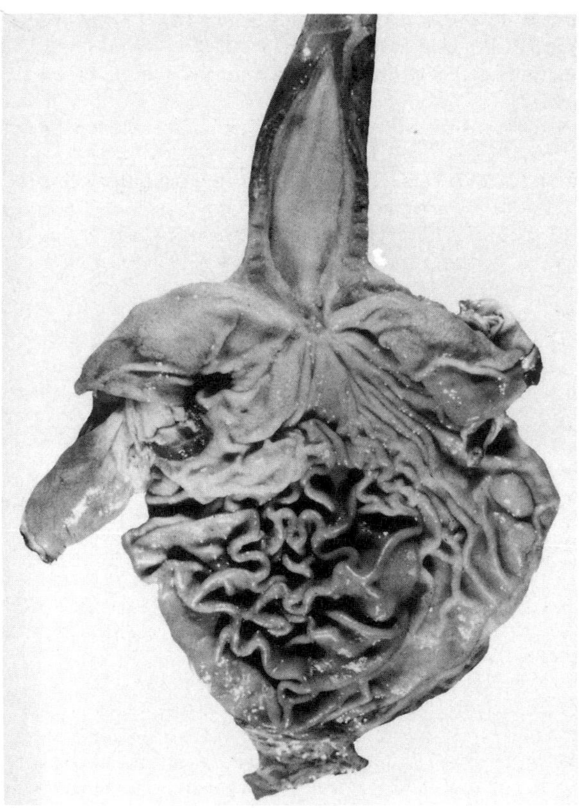

Fig. 1.43 Scarring of distal esophagus and pars esophagea following ulceration. Pig.

can simultaneously involve all four mucosal zones of the stomach, and the duodenum.

Ulcers of the esophageal zone are common. They are usually most severe at or adjacent to the margo plicatus, involving the edge of the squamous epithelium. They are often large and irregular in shape. There may be extensive fissuring, erosion, and ulceration of the squamous mucosa on the remainder of the pars esophagea. Often islands of thickened white proliferative mucosa are scattered as plaques on a predominantly ulcerated mucosa (Fig. 1.44A,B). Ulcers in the secretory stomach are less common, and occur most frequently in animals with clinical signs. These ulcers are also often large and multiple, though a full range from focal punctate to extensive deep lesions may be seen. Microscopically, gastric ulcers in horses follow the typical pattern previously described. *Candida* may colonize hyperkeratotic squamous mucosa of the esophageal portion of the stomach in some horses with ulcers. Lesions of the margo plicatus have been reported as a site colonized with *Clostridium botulinum* type B, implicated in toxicoinfectious botulism of horses.

Perforation may occur at any site of ulceration, and in one series, represented 1% of 600 autopsies on foals. Some foals may exsanguinate due to bleeding ulcers, and occasionally clotted blood will fill the stomach, forming a cast.

Pyloric and duodenal stenosis have been associated with healing ulcers in horses. Ulcerative lesions involving the circumference, or the antimesenteric mucosa, of the proximal duodenum have been associated with gastric ulcers in foals, and duodenal stricture may represent a more chronic phase of this process. Severe esophagitis occurs in foals with ulcer and gastric reflux.

The pathogenesis of gastric ulcers in horses is unclear. Many cases are associated with enteric disease, ileus, surgery, or other circumstances which can be considered stressful. *Candida* is considered contributory to ulceration by some, but it is often not present. It is unclear whether the ulcerative duodenitis seen in some cases is a product of peptic ulceration, or whether it represents a process such as proximal enteritis, which in turn results in stricture, and gastric reflux with ulceration. *Clostridium perfringens* has been considered as a potential cause of the associated duodenitis. Administration of steroids and analgesics such as flunixin meglumine and phenylbutazone is commonly associated with gastroduodenal ulcers, and lesions of the glandular and squamous stomach and pylorus, among other lesions, have been induced in horses intoxicated with phenylbutazone. Esophageal reflux and the severity of lesions in the esophageal portion of the stomach suggest that altered partitioning of fluid gastric content, and access of acid to squamous mucosa, in some cases perhaps associated with ileus or duodenal stricture, may explain lesions in the nonglandular gastric mucosa and esophagus. Hypersecretion of acid has not been confirmed, but some cases show subjective clinical response to the histamine-blocking agents, other inhibitors of gastric secretion, and protectants.

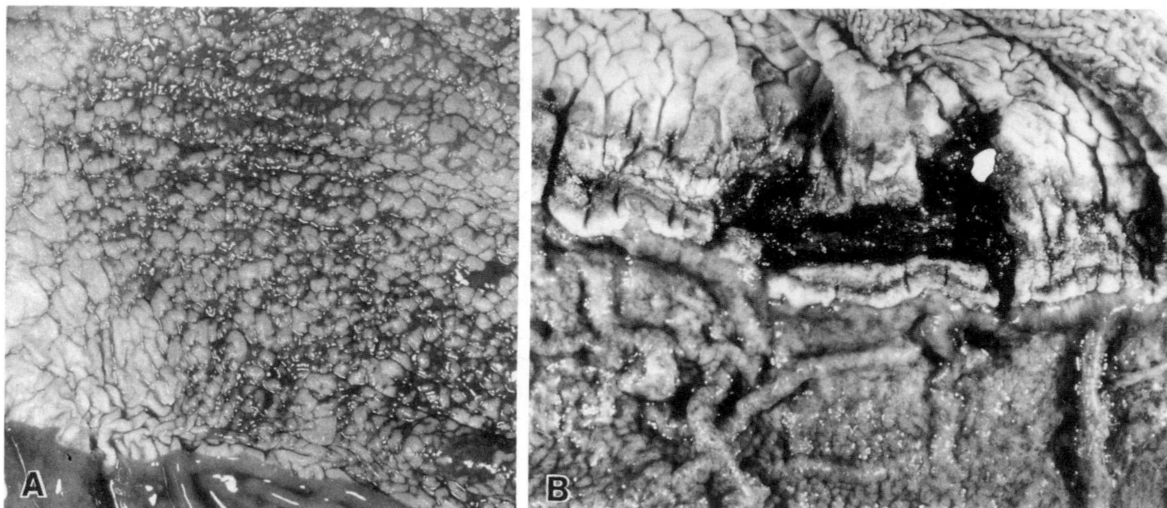

Fig. 1.44 Stomach. Foal. (A) Multiple confluent areas of ulceration of the squamous mucosa. Smooth nodular islands of surviving hyperplastic mucosa are scattered over the ulcerated area. (B) Ulceration with perforation of squamous gastric mucosa.

Bibliography

Acland, H. M., Gunson, D. E., and Gillette, D. M. Ulcerative duodenitis in foals. *Vet Pathol* **20:** 653–661, 1983.

Adair, H. M. Epithelial repair in chronic gastric ulcers. *Br J Exp Pathol* **59:** 229–236, 1978.

Ader, P. Penetrating gastric ulceration in a dog. *J Am Vet Med Assoc* **175:** 710–713, 1979.

Becht, J. L., and Byars, T. D. Gastroduodenal ulceration in foals. *Equine Vet J* **18:** 307–312, 1986.

Boosinger, T. R. *et al.* Multihormonal pancreatic endocrine tumor in a dog with duodenal ulcers and hypertrophic gastropathy. *Vet Pathol* **25:** 237–239, 1988.

Campbell-Thompson, M. L. *et al.* Gastroenterostomy for treatment of gastroduodenal ulcer disease in 14 foals. *J Am Vet Med Assoc* **188:** 840–844, 1986.

Carrig, C. B., and Seawright, A. A. Mastocytosis with gastrointestinal ulceration in a dog. *Aust Vet J* **44:** 503–507, 1968.

Daehler, M. H. Transmural pyloric perforation associated with naproxen administration in a dog. *J Am Vet Med Assoc* **189:** 694–695, 1986.

Dobson, K. J., Davies, R. L., and Cargill, C. F. Ulceration of the pars oesophagea in pigs. *Aust Vet J* **54:** 601–602, 1978.

Dodd, D. C. Hyostrongylosis and gastric ulceration in the pig. *N Z Vet J* **8:** 100–103, 1960.

Dow, S. W. et al. Effects of flunixin and flunixin plus prednisone on the gastrointestinal tract of dogs. *Am J Vet Res* **51:** 1131–1138, 1990.

English, R. V. *et al.* Zollinger–Ellison syndrome and myelofibrosis in a dog. *J Am Vet Med Assoc* **192:** 1430–1434, 1988.

Ewing, G. O. Indomethacin-associated gastrointestinal hemorrhage in a dog. *J Am Vet Med Assoc* **161:** 1665–1668, 1972.

Fatimah, I., Butler, D. G., and Physick-Sheard, P. W. Perforated duodenal ulcer in a cow. *Can Vet J* **23:** 173–175, 1982.

Gfeller, R. W, and Sandors, A. D. Naproxen-associated duodenal ulcer complicated by perforation and bacteria- and barium sulfate-induced peritonitis in a dog. *J Am Vet Med Assoc* **198:** 644–646, 1991.

Gross, T. L., and Mayhew, I. G. Gastroesophageal ulceration and candidiasis in foals. *J Am Vet Med Assoc* **182:** 1370–1373, 1983.

Hammond, C. J., Mason, D. K., and Watkins, K. L. Gastric ulceration in mature thoroughbred horses. *Equine Vet J* **18:** 284–287, 1986.

Hani, H., and Indermuhle, N. A. Esophagogastric ulcers in swine infected with *Ascaris suum*. *Vet Pathol* **16:** 617–618, 1979.

Happe, R. P., and van den Brom, W. E. Duodenogastric reflux in the dog, a clinicopathological study. *Res Vet Sci* **33:** 280–286, 1982.

Howard, E. B. *et al.* Mastocytoma and gastroduodenal ulceration. *Pathol Vet* **6:** 146–158, 1969.

Jensen, R. *et al.* Fatal abomasal ulcers in yearling feedlot cattle. *J Am Vet Med Assoc* **169:** 524–526, 1976.

Kauffman, G. Aspirin-induced gastric mucosal injury: Lessons learned from animal models. *Gastroenterology* **96:** 606–614, 1989.

Krauser, K. Untersuchungen zur Pathogenese der Pylorusulzera beim Mastkalb. *Berl Münch Tierärztl Wschr* **100:** 156–161, 1987.

Lev, R., Siegel, H. I., and Glass, G. B. J. Effects of salicylates on the canine stomach: A morphological and histochemical study. *Gastroenterology* **62:** 970–980, 1972.

Maxwell, C. V. *et al.* Use of tritiated water to assess, *in vivo,* the effect of dietary particle size on the mixing of stomach contents in swine. *J Anim Sci* **34:** 212–216, 1972.

Meschter, C. L. et al. The effects of phenylbutazone on the morphology and prostaglandin concentrations of the pyloric mucosa of the equine stomach. *Vet Pathol* **27:** 244–253, 1990.

Miller, T. A. Mechanisms of stress-related mucosal damage. *Am J Med* **83** (Suppl. 6A): 8–14, 1987.

Moore, R. W., and Withrow, S. J. Gastrointestinal hemorrhage and pancreatitis associated with intervertebral disk disease in the dog. *J Am Vet Med Assoc* **180:** 1443–1447, 1982.

Moreland, K. J. Ulcer disease of the upper gastrointestinal tract in small animals: Pathophysiology, diagnosis, and management. *Compend Cont Ed Pract Vet* **10:** 1265–1280, 1988.

Murray, M. *et al.* Peptic ulceration in the dog: A clinicopathological study. *Vet Rec* **91:** 441–447, 1972.

Murray, M. *et al.* Endoscopic evaluation of changes in gastric lesions of thoroughbred foals. *J Am Vet Med Assoc* **196:** 1623–1627, 1990.

O'Brien, J. J. Gastric ulcers. *In* "Diseases of Swine," A. D. Leman *et al.* (eds.). 5th Ed., pp. 632–646. Ames, Iowa, Iowa State University Press, 1981.

Palmer, J. E., and Whitlock, R. H. Perforated abomasal ulcers in adult dairy cows. *J Am Vet Med Assoc* **184:** 171–174, 1984.

Pearson, G. R., Welchman, D. deB., and Wells M. Mucosal changes associated with abomasal ulceration in veal calves. *Vet Rec* **121:** 557–559, 1987.

Peterson, W. L. *Helicobacter pylori* and peptic ulcer disease. *N Engl J Med* **324:** 1043–1048, 1991.

Pfeiffer, C. J., Keith, J. C., Jr., and April, M. Topographic localization of gastric lesions and key role of plasma bicarbonate concentration in dogs with experimentally induced gastric dilation. *Am J Vet Res* **48:** 262–267, 1987.

Phillips, B. M. Aspirin-induced gastrointestinal microbleeding in dogs. *Toxicol Appl Pharmacol* **24:** 182–189, 1973.

Pocock, E. F. *et al.* Dietary factors affecting the development of esophago-gastric ulcer in swine. *J Anim Sci* **29:** 591–597, 1969.

Rebhun, W. C., Dill, S. G., and Power, H. T. Gastric ulcers in foals. *J Am Vet Med Assoc* **180:** 404–407, 1982.

Schoen, R. T., and Vender, R. J. Mechanisms of nonsteroidal antiinflammatory drug-induced gastric damage. *Am J Med* **86:** 449–458, 1989.

Seawright, A. A., and Grono, L. R. Malignant mast cell tumor in a cat with perforating duodenal ulcer. *J Pathol Bacteriol* **87:** 107–111, 1964.

Shaw, D. H. Gastrinoma (Zollinger–Ellison syndrome) in the dog and cat. *Can Vet J* **29:** 448–452, 1988.

Silen, W. Experimental models of gastric ulceration and injury. *Am J Physiol* **255:** G395–G402, 1988.

Smith, D. F., Munson, L., and Erb, H. N. Abomasal ulcer disease in adult dairy cattle. *Cornell Vet* **73:** 213–224, 1983.

Sorjonen, D. C. *et al.* Effects of dexamethasone and surgical hypotension on the stomach of dogs: Clinical, endoscopic, and pathologic evaluations. *Am J Vet Res* **44:** 1233–1237, 1983.

Swerczek, T. W. Toxicoinfectious botulism in foals and adult horses. *J Am Vet Med Assoc* **176:** 217–220, 1980.

Thomas, N. W. Piroxicam-associated gastric ulceration in a dog. *Compend Cont Ed Pract Vet* **9:** 1004, 1006, 1030, 1987.

von Ritter, C. *et al.* Gastric mucosal lesions induced by hemorrhagic shock in baboons. Role of oxygen-derived free radicals. *Dig Dis Sci* **33:** 857–864, 1988.

Welchman, D. deB., and Baust, G. N. A survey of abomasal ulceration in veal calves. *Vet Rec* **121:** 586–590, 1987.

Wyatt, J. I. The role of *Campylobacter pylori* in the pathogenesis of peptic ulcer disease. *Scand J Gastroenterol* **24** (Suppl. 157): 7–11, 1989.

Zamora, C. S. *et al.* Effects of prednisone on gastric secretion and development of stomach lesions in swine. *Am J Vet Res* **36:** 33–39, 1975.

J. Gastric Neoplasia

Gastric neoplasms are uncommon in all species, and are very rare in some.

Adenocarcinoma of the stomach is most frequently reported in **dogs,** usually in animals younger than 10 years, and it is the most common gastric neoplasm in that species. Males predominate in the population with gastric cancer, and over half of gastric adenocarcinomas in dogs occur in the pyloric region. Grossly some gastric neoplasms appear as nonulcerating, firm thickenings involving most of the gastric wall and causing loss of the normal rugal pattern on the mucosal surface. Others are more localized, plaquelike thickenings which tend to obliterate rugae, and which ulcerate centrally. Ulceration occurs in over half of canine gastric adenocarcinomas. Surface proliferation or irregularity other than ulceration is very uncommon in gastric carcinoma in dogs. Cut sections through the stomach wall invaded by carcinoma reveal edema and pale, firm fibrous tissue. Induration or plaquelike pale masses may be evident on the serosa, where the outline of infiltrated lymphatics may be prominent. Widespread gastric mural fibrosis and thickening causes linitis plastica or the so-called leather bottle appearance. The scirrhous nature of most gastric carcinomas in the dog is the result of desmoplasia induced by the malignant epithelium.

These tumors adopt two basic microscopic forms. Most gastric adenocarcinomas in dogs are of the diffuse type, consisting of widespread infiltrates of neoplastic cells dispersed singly or in small clusters among supporting stromal elements. The cell type is usually relatively uniform within a single neoplasm, commonly consisting of poorly differentiated round or angular mucus-secreting epithelial cells. In many of these tumors, some cells adopt the hollow, mucus-filled signet ring appearance, and extracellular mucin may be present. Occasional tumors of this type have a more variable cell population, with some cells containing little cytoplasm, others with extensive eosinophilic cytoplasm, and large atypical nuclei. Other tumors will have scattered irregular glandlike structures. Desmoplasia is typically heavy in diffuse gastric carcinomas.

Adenocarcinomas of the tubular or intestinal type are encountered less commonly in the canine stomach. They are characterized by tubular glandular structures, with a lumen, and a relatively well differentiated and polarized lining epithelium. They retain this form with some variation as they infiltrate and metastasize, and they are relatively less scirrhous than the diffuse type. There may be papilliform infoldings of the epithelium of tubular adenocarcinomas; some form smaller acinar structures; others rarely adopt a more solid form of growth, with occasional acinar structures and a more anaplastic cytologic appearance. Cells may have eosinophilic cytoplasm, and many contain mucin. The better-differentiated tubular tumors resemble pyloric glands. Infiltrates of lymphocytes and plasma cells, sometimes with follicle formation, may occur in the primary site of all types of gastric carcinoma.

A single squamous cell carcinoma is reported arising from the pyloric gland mucosa in a dog, and carcinoids develop, very rarely, in the gastric mucosa.

Gastric carcinomas in dogs infiltrate the stomach wall aggressively, invading lymphatics, and they have usually metastasized to the local lymph nodes, and often to distant organs, particularly lung, liver, and adrenal, by the time they are diagnosed.

Benign adenomatous polyps or sessile proliferative lesions occur uncommonly in the pyloric stomach, in dogs (Fig. 1.45A). These have been alluded to previously as a potential cause of pyloric stenosis or obstruction, and as a possible hyperplastic sequel to chronic antritis. Their exact status, whether inflammatory hyperplasia, or benign neoplasia, is unclear. Although there are reports of malignant polypoid adenocarcinoma, it seems, on the basis of the relative frequency of adenomas *vis-à-vis* adenocarcinoma, that they are unlikely to be common precursors of gastric cancer. Grossly, these lesions appear as solitary or multiple raised, convoluted, nodular, sessile, or sometimes pedunculate, polypoid masses, usually 1–2 cm in size. Microscopically there is foveolar and glandular hyperplasia, with well-differentiated columnar mucous cells on the surface and in glands. Some mucus-filled glandular cysts may be present, and mononuclear cell infiltrates are often in the mucosal propria.

Mesenchymal tumors of the stomach in dogs are less common than are adenocarcinomas. Most are typical leiomyomas, which may produce nodular, sometimes polypoid, masses, several centimeters in size, which project into the gastric lumen, or protrude from the serosa. Leiomyosarcomas, lymphosarcomas, rare extramedullary plasmacytomas, and anaplastic sarcomas are also found in the canine stomach. These tumors may ulcerate the mucosa and, to that extent, mimic the behavior of adenocarcinoma. Their microscopic appearance is typical; extramedullary plasmacytoma may be associated with local amyloid deposition and hyalinization of arterial walls in the vicinity of the neoplasm.

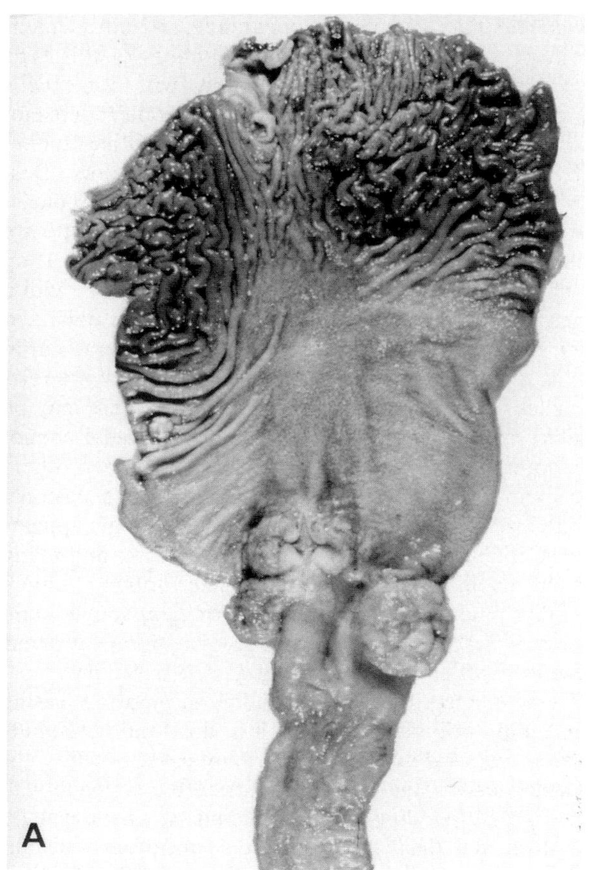

Fig. 1.45A Mucosal polyps at the pylorus and along the greater curvature of the stomach. Dog.

Tumors other than lymphosarcoma are rarely encountered in the stomach of **cats,** and even that is uncommon. Several cases of gastric adenocarcinoma are described, adopting tubular and diffuse patterns.

Gastric adenocarcinoma in **cattle** is exceptionally uncommon, but when it occurs it resembles similar tumors in other species, being scirrhous, invading the wall, and being capable of ulceration. Much more important in cattle is lymphosarcoma of the abomasum. Involvement of this organ is common in adult cattle. Diffuse mucosal and submucosal lymphocytic infiltrates or nodular proliferations may occur. Strategically placed pyloric tumor may cause obstruction. Diffuse lesions, thickening the gastric wall, frequently ulcerate, and hemorrhage from such ulcers, as melena, is a common sign. The lymphoid infiltrates are recognizable as firm gray-white tissue in the submucosa and mucosa. Involvement of abomasal lymph nodes is disproportionately slight. Gastric lymphosarcoma also occurs in swine, where it is usually diffuse. The wall of the stomach is thickened by submucosal lymphocytic infiltrates, which sometimes invade the mucosa locally in many areas, producing nodular elevations which may ulcerate.

In the **horse,** squamous cell carcinomas, derived from the esophageal mucosa, are the most common tumor; occasional adenocarcinomas originating in glandular epithelium, and leiomyomas, are also reported. Squamous cell carcinomas occur in middle-aged horses. They usually present in an advanced state, with a history of unexplained anorexia, occasionally dysphagia, and weight loss sometimes progressing rapidly to emaciation. At autopsy there may be peritoneal effusion, and there is usually evidence of the neoplasm as proliferative or scirrhous tissue on the serosa of the stomach. There also may be peritoneal implants, especially on intestine, testes, omentum, parietal abdominal surfaces, and diaphragm; direct extension to adjacent organs including liver, spleen, and diaphragm, with progression to the pleural space; and sometimes distant metastases, usually in liver and lung. The appearance of the tumor on serosal surfaces resembles mesothelioma, with smooth creamy plaques or nodules as large as 2–4 cm in diameter.

The origin of these lesions is usually a fungating cauliflowerlike mass 10–40 cm in diameter, with superficial fissures, projecting above the surface of the pars esophagea (Fig. 1.45B). Sometimes these lesions are superficially more ulcerative than proliferative. Necrosis and hemorrhage are evident in the tumor mass, which is usually well demarcated from adjacent normal squamous mucosa. Occasionally the tumor extends into the distal esophagus, and may obstruct it. Microscopically, these neoplasms are typical squamous cell carcinomas, invading in cords or

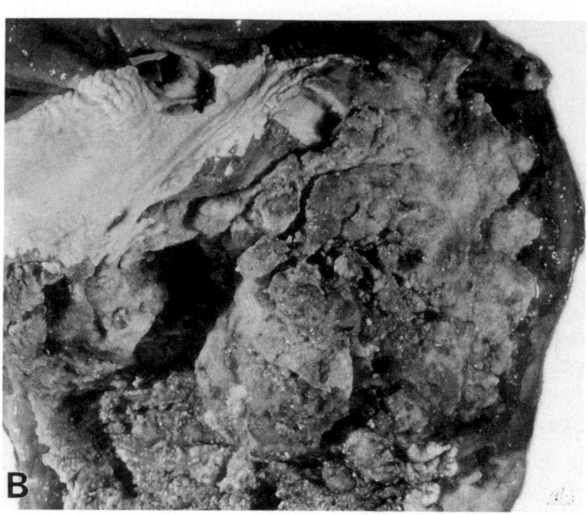

Fig. 1.45B Fungating and ulcerative squamous cell carcinoma arising from the gastric squamous mucosa. Horse.

nests of cells through the gastric wall. They induce desmoplasia, imparting a scirrhous, firm texture and appearance to the thickened gastric wall and to the peritoneal and pleural implants. One such tumor has been reported as a cause of pseudohyperparathyroidism in a horse.

Bibliography

Chapman, W. L., and Smith, J. A. Abomasal adenocarcinoma in a cow. *J Am Vet Med Assoc* **181:** 493–494, 1982.

Conroy, J. D. Multiple gastric adenomatous polyps in a dog. *J Comp Pathol* **79:** 465–467, 1969.

Cotchin, E. Some tumors of dogs and cats of comparative veterinary and human interest. *Vet Rec* **71:** 1040–1050, 1959.

Culbertson, R., Branam, J. E., and Rosenblatt, L. S. Esophageal/gastric leiomyoma in the laboratory beagle. *J Am Vet Med Assoc* **183:** 1168–1171, 1983.

Grundmann, E., and Schlake, W. Histological classification of gastric cancer from initial to advanced stages. *Pathol Res Pract* **173:** 260–274, 1982.

Happe, R. P. *et al.* Multiple polyps of the gastric mucosa in two dogs. *J Small Anim Pract* **18:** 179–189, 1977.

Hayden, D. W., and Nielsen, S. W. Canine alimentary neoplasia. *Zbl Veterinaermed (A)* **20:** 1–22, 1973.

Head, K. W. Tumors of the lower alimentary tract. *Bull WHO* **53:** 167–186, 1976.

Lingeman, C. H., Garner, F. M., and Taylor, D. O. N. Spontaneous gastric adenocarcinomas of dogs: A review. *J Nat Cancer Inst* **47:** 137–153, 1971.

MacEwen, E. G. *et al.* Extramedullary plasmacytoma of the gastrointestinal tract in two dogs. *J Am Vet Med Assoc* **184:** 1396–1398, 1984.

Meagher, D. M. *et al.* Squamous cell carcinoma of the equine stomach. *J Am Vet Med Assoc* **164:** 81–84, 1974.

Meuten, D. J. *et al.* Gastric carcinoma with pseudohyperparathyroidism in a horse. *Cornell Vet* **68:** 179–195, 1978.

Murray, M. *et al.* Primary gastric neoplasia in the dog: a clinicopathological study. *Vet Rec* **81:** 474–479, 1972.

Patnaik, A. K., and Lieberman, P. H. Gastric squamous cell carcinoma in a dog. *Vet Pathol* **17:** 250–253, 1980.

Patnaik, A. K., Hurvitz, A. I., and Johnson, G. F. Canine gastrointestinal neoplasms. *Vet Pathol* **14:** 547–555, 1977.

Patnaik, A. K., Hurvitz, A. I., and Johnson, G. F. Canine gastric adenocarcinoma. *Vet Pathol* **15:** 600–607, 1978.

Sautter, J. H., and Hanlon, G. F. Gastric neoplasms in the dog: A report of 20 cases. *J Am Vet Med Assoc* **166:** 691–696, 1975.

Sullivan, M. *et al.* A study of 31 cases of gastric carcinoma in dogs. *Vet Rec* **120:** 79–83, 1987.

Tennant, B. *et al.* Six cases of squamous cell carcinoma of the stomach of the horse. *Equine Vet J* **14:** 238–243, 1982.

Turk, M. A. M., Gallina, A. M., and Russell, T. S. Nonhematopoietic gastro-intestinal neoplasia in cats: A retrospective study of 44 cases. *Vet Pathol* **18:** 614–620, 1981.

Wester, P. W., Franken, P., and Hani, H. J. Squamous cell carcinoma of the equine stomach. *Vet Q* **2:** 95–103, 1980.

VI. The Intestine

A. Normal Form and Function

The microtopography of the **small bowel** is extensively modified, to increase its surface area, by spiral mucosal folds in some species, and by villi projecting into the lumen. The villi, projections of lamina propria covered by a layer of epithelium one cell thick, expand the absorptive surface of the small bowel 7- to 14-fold. In most species, villi are tallest in the duodenum, and decline somewhat in height toward the ileum. The length and shape of villi in normal animals varies with the species, age, intestinal microflora, and immune status. In general, villi in dogs, cats, neonatal piglets, and ruminants tend to be tall and cylindrical; those in horses and in young ruminants tend to be moderately tall and cylindrical; villi in weaned ruminants and swine may be cylindrical, leaf- or tongue-shaped, or rarely ridgelike, with their broad surface at right angles to the long axis of the gut.

Opening onto the mucosal surface around the base of each villus are several crypts of Lieberkühn. These are straight or somewhat coiled (depending on the species and the proliferative status) tubular glandlike structures, lined by a single layer of epithelium. The progenitor compartment of the enteric epithelium resides here, producing cells which differentiate and move up onto the surface of villi, mainly as absorptive enterocytes, ultimately to be extruded as effete cells from the tips of villi.

Stem cells are present at the base of the crypts, and they divide to produce cells of four main types. **Poorly differentiated cells,** which are cuboidal or low columnar, with relatively few, short microvilli, are the predominant type of cell lining crypts. Especially in the lower half of crypts, these cells form a population which cycles rapidly, undergoing amplification division. One of the ensuing daughter cells usually differentiates and moves into the functional compartment of absorptive enterocytes on the villus. Undifferentiated crypt epithelial cells also secrete electrolyte and water.

Oligomucous cells, derived by mitosis from the basal stem cells, also form a population undergoing amplification division. They contain mucous granules, and are intermediate in structure between undifferentiated crypt epithelium and goblet cells, into which they mature. Well-differentiated **goblet cells** are present in crypts and on the surface of villi, with varying prevalence and distribution at various levels of the intestine, and in the different species. They have basal nuclei and secrete mucus, apparently by exocytosis, from the luminal border of the cell. **Intestinal mucus** stains strongly for neutral, sialic acid- or ester sulfate-rich mucosubstances, depending on the species and cell of origin; its precise function is uncertain. It lubricates, and probably serves to insulate the surface from organisms, which it may entrap or immobilize. It contains lysozyme and IgA secreted into it by epithelium. Goblet cell hyperplasia and mucus secretion are promoted by a variety of noxious stimuli, by inflammatory mediators, and by cell-mediated immune events in the gut.

Paneth cells, a population of enigmatic cells turning over slowly in the base of crypts, are most obvious in horses, among the domestic animals. They are not found in dogs, cats, or swine, and they are not prominent in the intestine of ruminants. Eosinophilic secretory granules are present in the apical cytoplasm of Paneth cells. They contain lysozyme, which probably has an antimicrobial function in the crypt and in mucus through hydrolysis of peptidoglycans in bacterial cell wall. Other putative attributes include phagocytosis, IgA transport, and secretion of immunoregulatory peptides.

The fourth type of cell found in intestinal crypts is the **enteroendocrine** cell. They too are derived from crypt stem cells, and comprise a heterogeneous population of over a dozen amine- or peptide-secreting endocrine/paracrine cells. These are the cells variously recognized as enterochromaffin, argentaffin, or argyrophil; the specific cell type is defined by immunocytochemistry and the ultrastructure of secretory granules. Enteroendocrine cells are scattered singly among other cells on villi, and more commonly, in crypts. They tend to be located peripherally in the epithelial layer, with little luminal exposure, and contain, in the basal cytoplasm, scattered small secretory granules, the ultrastructural morphology of which is often unique to the cell type. Hormones with relatively clearly understood functions, such as secretin and cholecystokinin, as well as peptides or amines whose endocrine or paracrine implications are less certain, are secreted. Some undoubtedly integrate in function with similar neurohormones secreted by the enteric nervous system. With the exception of carcinoid tumors of serotonin-secreting cell origin, and rare functional neoplasms of other enteroendocrine cells in humans, the pathologic implications of this class of cells are still very poorly defined.

Scattered among the cells of the crypt and villus are specialized **caveolated or tuft cells.** These are flask-shaped cells tapering toward the luminal border, which are found also in other gastrointestinal and respiratory epithelial surfaces. They have an apical tubulovesicular system, from which they derive their name. The function of these cells is not known, though it is speculated that they may be chemoreceptors. Specialized **cup epithelial cells,** of unknown function, have been described also on villi in the ileum of several species.

The **enterocytes,** which are responsible for the final digestion and absorption of nutrients, electrolytes, and water, are by far the predominant cell type on intestinal villi. They are normally tall columnar cells, polygonal in cross section, with a regular basal nuclear polarity. A tight junction, which is nevertheless leaky to small molecules and water, joins the apical margins of adjacent cells. The barrier to transepithelial macromolecular movement is essentially maintained even at sites of extrusion of effete enterocytes at the tips of villi. Basal to the tight junction the lateral cell membranes interdigitate loosely, and a long, narrow potential space exists between enterocytes. The basolateral cell membrane is the site of sodium-potassium dependent adenosine triphosphatase (ATP), which drives the sodium pump, and of carrier systems exporting monosaccharides from the cell. Absorptive epithelial cells lie on a basal lamina, which they may, in part, produce.

The apical surface of normal enterocytes is highly modified into microvilli, about 0.5–1.5 μm long and 0.1 μm wide, which are regularly arrayed in close apposition to each other at right angles to the surface of the cell. They are visible as the brush border by conventional microscopy. Microvilli increase the surface area of absorptive epithelium by a factor of about 15–40 times. The plasmalemma of microvilli is studded with massive numbers of enzyme molecules, including aminopeptidases and disaccharidases involved in terminal digestion of peptides and carbohydrates. These protrude as minute knoblike structures into the glycoprotein glycocalyx, which coats the surface of microvilli. Proteins binding calcium ions, vitamin B_{12}, and water-soluble vitamins, and proteins involved in the transport into the cell of peptides, amino acids, glucose, galactose, and triglyceride, coupled with transport of sodium ion, are also embedded in the plasmalemma of microvilli. Clines in the distribution of microvillus-associated functions are present along the small intestine. The activities of alkaline phosphatase and most disaccharidases are greater in the anterior small bowel, whereas the receptor for vitamin B_{12}:intrinsic factor is concentrated in the ileum.

In neonatal swine and ruminants, vacuolation of absorptive enterocytes is normal, and the nucleus is often also displaced into the apical cytoplasm. In piglets vacuolation is usual in the ileum, but not in the duodenum, and seems to be a function of cell age. Such vacuolation should be differentiated from the presence of eosinophilic colostrum present in cytoplasmic vacuoles in the epithelial cells of neonates (Fig. 1.46).

The cytoplasm of absorptive enterocytes is stabilized at the apical border by the filaments of the terminal web. Smooth endoplasmic reticulum is most prominent in the upper half of cells, whereas cisternal elements of rough endoplasmic reticulum are more uniformly distributed. The Golgi zone lies above the nucleus. Free ribosomes and polyribosomes are numerous in differentiating cells of

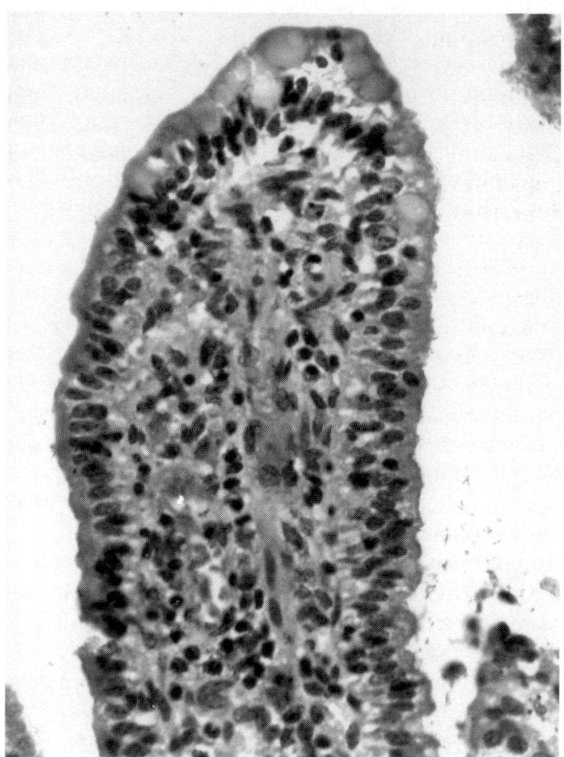

Fig. 1.46 Distended vacuoles containing eosinophilic colostral protein in apical cytoplasm of enterocytes at the tip of the villus of a 2-day-old calf.

the upper crypt and lower villus, and are relatively fewer in mature absorptive enterocytes.

The complex of endoplasmic membranes and Golgi apparatus is active particularly in handling absorbed lipid, which diffuses from micelles at the cell surface, through the apical membrane, in the form of long-chain fatty acids or monoglyceride. These are reesterified to triglyceride, appearing in the smooth endoplasmic reticulum, and are complexed with apoproteins produced in the rough endoplasmic reticulum, to be excreted, via the Golgi apparatus, through the basolateral cell membrane as chylomicrons. Chylomicrons enter the extracellular space, and leave the villus via the lacteal. Mitochondria are numerous in the metabolically active absorptive enterocyte. Vacuoles formed by endocytosis of macromolecules at the base of microvilli fuse with lysosomes in the subapical cytoplasm, and by this process of heterophagia, potentially noxious material is destroyed. In addition to lysosomes, acid phosphatase-containing vesicular bodies, and peroxisomes containing catalase, but of uncertain function, are also found in intestinal epithelium.

The **lamina propria,** a highly plastic mesenchymal stroma, supports the epithelium of the small intestinal mucosa. It is composed of loose fibrous tissue, through which course blood vessels, and in which smooth muscle, inflammatory, and immune-active cells are interspersed. Surrounding the crypt of Lieberkühn, and underlying the basal lamina of the epithelium of the villi is a sheath of mesenchymal cells, probably myofibroblasts. Their function is uncertain, but they may be contractile and secrete extracellular matrix. Proliferation of these sheath cells has been demonstrated, and tritiated thymidine-labeled mesenchymal cells appear to move in concert with overlying epithelium, up onto villi, though evidence for this is conflicting. They may ultimately undergo degeneration in the lamina propria at the villus tip. Here histiocytes containing nuclear fragments may be found, presumably phagocytosing effete sheath cells. These should not be mistaken for foci of necrosis in the lamina propria. Ceroid, hemosiderin, and bile pigment may also be present in histiocytes in the lamina propria at tips of villi, which are particularly prominent in horses.

Lymphocytes, neutrophils, and eosinophils are scattered in the lamina propria of villi and between crypts. Eosinophils are common in the intestine of ruminants and horses, with no specific pathologic connotation. Intraepithelial lymphocytes (theliolymphocytes) are frequently found between epithelial cells on villi, and less commonly, in crypt lining. Globule leukocytes may be found in the epithelium of crypts and low on villi, or sometimes in the lamina propria between crypts. Plasma cells normally are not numerous in villi, but are concentrated in the lamina propria between the upper portions of crypts.

The **vascular supply to the small intestinal mucosa** arises in submucosal arteries, which give off arterioles at right angles, some of which send branches to a capillary plexus around crypts of Lieberkühn. The majority pass up the centers of villi, arborizing near the villus tip into a dense capillary plexus which lies immediately beneath the basal lamina of the epithelium. Capillaries in villi have fenestrations facing the basal lamina, which may be more permeable than the remainder of the endothelium. One or more venules drain blood from the capillaries in villi and between crypts, and flow into larger veins in the submucosa, which drain into mesenteric veins and the hepatic portal circulation. At least in swine, there appear to be anastomoses between the capillary plexuses of villus and crypt. The lacteal, or central lymphatic vessel of the villus, is sufficiently permeable to permit the entry of macromolecules and chylomicrons, and is the main route of lipid transport from the villus.

Juxtaposition of arteriole and venule in the villus may result in a countercurrent multiplier system in the villus, establishing an increasing gradient of sodium concentration and a decreasing oxygen gradient, toward the tip of the villus, though this is in debate. Anastomoses between capillary plexuses surrounding the villi and crypts might provide a mechanism for shunting electrolyte and water, just absorbed in the villi, into the vicinity of crypts, where secretion is occurring. Thus a putative crypt–villus fluid and electrolyte circuit would be provided with a direct vascular arm.

The **cecum and colon** vary widely in anatomy and size among domestic animals, depending largely on the significance of microbial fermentation of carbohydrate in the hindgut. Production of volatile fatty acid from carbohydrate by colonic flora occurs in all species. In the horse this is a primary source of energy, and it is significant in swine and ruminants as well. Extensive movement of electrolytes and water occurs across the colonic wall. In the horse, a volume of fluid approaching that of the extracellular fluid space of the animal may be in the large bowel, which must maintain a fluid medium for microbial fermentation; daily fluid absorption from the hindgut may exceed the extracellular fluid volume. Absorption of electrolytes and water, an electrolyte conserving mechanism, is probably the major function of the colon in dogs and cats, and of the distal colon of herbivores.

The mucosa of the cecum and colon in all domestic species lacks villi, though there are ridges or folds on the mucosal surface. The surface of the hindgut is lined by a single layer of columnar **absorptive epithelial cells** with basal nuclei. These cells generally have more sparse and less regular microvilli in comparison with absorptive cells of the small bowel, and numerous glycoprotein-laden vesicles are in the apical cytoplasm in most species. Typical goblet cells are also interspersed on the colonic surface in variable numbers, depending on the species and a variety of other factors.

Colonic crypts or glands are straight tubular structures. The architecture of colonic glands and their cell population resembles somewhat that of small intestinal crypts. Stem cells are present in the base of the gland, and poorly differentiated mitotic columnar epithelium composed of an amplifier population is present in the basal two thirds of the gland, though its extent may vary considerably. These cells, which contain small glycoprotein-laden vesicles, differentiate progressively toward absorptive epithelium as they approach the surface. Oligomucous cells, derived from basal stem cells, form a second proliferative population in the lower half of the colonic gland. Well-differentiated goblet cells are usually present in the upper half of glands in the large bowel, as well as on the surface. Spirochetes have been found in colonic goblet cells in apparently normal dogs and cats, and in some laboratory animals. Enteroendocrine cells of about a half dozen types have been recognized, scattered in the cell column lining glands in the large bowel.

The **lamina propria** of the colon is minimal between closely packed glands. It contains a cell population similar to that in the small bowel. A myofibroblast sheath encloses the colonic glands, and appears to migrate with the epithelium. Normally, relatively few inflammatory and immune-active cells are present in the superficial mucosa in small animals, and young herbivores; most plasma cells and lymphocytes are between deeper portions of glands. Older herbivores may have somewhat heavier superficial proprial inflammatory infiltrates, and macrophages containing phagocytosed debris may be present below the surface epithelium between the mouths of glands, especially in the horse. In the equine colon, terminal arterioles which enter the mucosa branch at right angles from the submucosal plexus. Capillaries ramify to surround colonic glands, and form an anastomosing network at the luminal surface. Sparsely distributed venules drain the superficial capillary plexus.

The connective tissue of the **submucosa** lies between the mucosa and the **external muscle** of the gut, which comprises inner circular, and outer longitudinal layers, made up of fascicles of smooth muscle cells. An extensive **enteric nervous system,** with submucosal (Meissner's), and myenteric (Auerbach's) plexuses marked by ganglia, modulates external autonomic neural regulation and coordinates gastrointestinal motility and function. The neurons of the enteric system equal in number those in the spinal cord, and their ramifications sense and influence epithelial absorption and secretion, local endocrine/paracrine secretion, blood flow, immune events, and motility in the gut. Their effect is mediated by amine and peptide neurotransmitters, which in some cases are also produced by endocrine cells of the gut and pancreas. Some of these same peptides, acting centrally or at the level of the gut, have an effect on appetite and satiety, and are likely to be implicated in the inappetence which frequently accompanies gastrointestinal disease in animals. The complexity and mechanisms of the enteric neural system are incompletely understood, as is its influence on abnormal form and function in the gut. Disorders of motility associated with enteric neural lesions, such as the dysautonomias and grass sickness, are discussed with intestinal obstruction (Section VI,F of this chapter).

Interpretation of intestinal and colonic biopsies is often subjective, unless clear-cut diagnostic criteria can be met, by recognition of an etiologic agent, a specific cell type, a characteristic pattern of inflammation, or cytologic and morphologic abnormalities indicating malignancy. There are significant variations in the microscopic morphology of the gut among species and with age, at different levels of the small and large intestine within species, and as a result of factors influencing physiologic inflammation in the mucosa. Limited morphometric data are available, describing in a quantitative manner the normal morphology of the intestinal mucosa and its epithelial and inflammatory cell populations in domestic animals. Most are cited in succeeding sections. However, until more such information is available, and its application, particularly in the diagnosis of inflammatory bowel disease, is validated, pathologists would do well to expand their experience of normal intestinal morphology by critical examination of tissues from animals in which gastrointestinal disease is not indicated clinically.

Biopsy interpretation is enhanced by increased size of specimen; increased numbers of specimens; the sampling of all layers of the bowel wall; minimal trauma; rapid fixation; and optimal orientation. Sacrifice of any of these attributes increases the subjectivity with which a biopsy is interpreted; hence, in dealing with endoscopic and other small biopsies, care must be taken in handling to reduce traumatic artefact and to optimize orientation. Clinicians and pathologists dealing with endoscopic, capsule, and forceps biopsies must remember the limitations in interpretation imposed by small sample size; difficulties in orientation; the frequent failure to sample the deep mucosa; and the usual failure to sample the submucosa and muscularis. These costs are offset to some degree by the opportunity to obtain a greater number of samples than may be possible by other means, at arguably lower risk and cost, and possibly more focused on a lesion by direct endoscopic examination.

Bibliography

Argenzio, R. A. Functions of the equine large intestine and their interrelationship in disease. *Cornell Vet* **65:** 303–330, 1975.

Bellamy, J. E. C. *et al.* The vascular architecture of the porcine small intestine. *Can J Comp Med* **37:** 56–62, 1973.

Brown, P. J. *et al.* Histochemistry of mucins of pig intestinal secretory epithelial cells before and after weaning. *J Comp Pathol* **98:** 313–323, 1988.

Canfield, P. J. *et al.* Large intestinal biopsies from normal dogs. *Res Vet Sci* **28:** 6–9, 1980.

Dobesh, G. D., and Clemens, E. T. Effect of dietary protein on porcine colonic microstructure and function. *Am J Vet Res* **48:** 862–865, 1987.

Eade, M. N. *et al.* No evidence of a countercurrent multiplier in the intestinal villus of the dog. *Gastroenterology* **98:** 3–10, 1990.

Eastwood, G. L. Gastrointestinal epithelial renewal. *Gastroenterology* **72:** 962–975, 1977.

Egberts, H. J. A. *et al.* Biological and pathobiological aspects of the glycocalyx of the small intestinal epithelium. A review. *Vet Q* **6:** 186–199, 1984.

Figlewicz, D. P. *et al.* Gastroenteropancreatic peptides and the central nervous system. *Annu Rev Physiol* **49:** 383–395, 1987.

Fox, J. E. T. Control of gastrointestinal motility by peptides: Old peptides, new tricks—new peptides, old tricks. *Gastroenterol Clin North Am* **18:** 163–177, 1989.

Guilford, W. G. The enteric nervous system: Function, dysfunction, and pharmacologic manipulation. *Sem Vet Med Surg (Small Anim)* **5:** 46–56, 1990.

Hart, I. R. The distribution of immunoglobulin-containing cells in canine small intestine. *Res Vet Sci* **27:** 269–274, 1979.

Hart, I. R., and Kidder, D. E. The quantitative assessment of normal canine small intestinal mucosa. *Res Vet Sci* **25:** 157–162, 1978.

Henry, R. W. and Al-Bagdadi, F. K. Duodenal microanatomy of the domestic cat (*Felis catus*). *Histol Histopathol* **1:** 355–362, 1986.

Hintz, H. F. Digestive physiology of the horse. *J S Afr Vet Assoc* **46:** 13–16, 1975.

Holmes, R., and Lobley, R. W. Intestinal brush border revisited. *Gut* **30:** 1667–1678, 1989.

Hoskins, J. D. *et al.* Scanning electron microscopic study of the small intestine of dogs from birth to 337 days of age. *Am J Vet Res* **43:** 1715–1720, 1982.

Jodal, M., and Lundgren, O. Countercurrent mechanisms in the mammalian gastrointestinal tract. *Gastroenterology* **91:** 225–241, 1986.

Johnson, L. R. (ed.) "Physiology of the Gastrointestinal Tract," 2nd Ed. New York, Raven Press, 1987. [See chapters by H. J. Cooke (pp. 1307–1350), D. N. Granger *et al.* (pp. 1671–1697), M. Lipkin (pp. 255–284), J. L. Madara and J. S. Trier (pp. 1209–1249), M. E. Neutra and J. F. Forstner (pp. 975–1009), E. Solcia *et al.* (pp. 111–130).]

Keast, J. R. Mucosal innervation and control of water and ion transport in the intestine. *Rev Physiol Biochem Pharmacol* **109:** 1–59, 1987.

Keshav, S. *et al.* Tumor necrosis factor mRNA localized to Paneth cells of normal murine intestinal epithelium by *in situ* hybridization. *J Exp Med* **171:** 327–332, 1990.

LeFevre, M. E., *et al.* Macrophages of the mammalian small intestine. A review. *J Reticuloendothel Soc* **26:** 553–573, 1979.

Maala, C. P., and Cummings, J. F. Ultrastructural features of the bovine cecal mucosa. *Zbl. Vet Med C* **14:** 116–141, 1985.

Madara, J. L. Maintenance of the macromolecular barrier at cell extrusion sites in intestinal epithelium: Physiological rearrangement of tight junctions. *J Membrane Biol* **116:** 177–184, 1990.

Mebus, C. A. *et al.* Scanning electron, light, and transmission electron microscopy of intestine of gnotobiotic calf. *Am J Vet Res* **36:** 985–993, 1975.

Miller, H. R. P. Gastrointestinal mucus, a medium for survival and for elimination of parasitic nematodes and protozoa. *Parasitology* **94:** S77–S100, 1987.

Moon, H. W., and Joel, D. D. Epithelial cell migration in the small intestine of sheep and calves. *Am J Vet Res* **36:** 187–189, 1975.

Moon, H. W. *et al.* Vacuolation: A function of cell age in porcine ileal absorptive cells. *Lab Invest* **28:** 23–28, 1973.

Ochoa, R. *et al.* Hemosiderin deposits in the equine small intestine. *Vet Pathol* **20:** 641–643, 1983.

Pfeiffer, C. J., and MacPherson, B. R. Anatomy of the gastrointestinal tract and peritoneal cavity. *In* "The Equine Acute Abdomen," N. A. White, II, (ed.), pp. 2–24. Philadelphia & London, Lea & Febiger, 1990.

Pfeiffer, C. J. *et al.* The equine colonic mucosal granular cell: Identification and x-ray microanalysis of apical granules and nuclear bodies. *Anat Rec* **219:** 258–267, 1987.

Pout, D. The mucosal surface patterns of the small intestine of grazing lambs. *Br Vet J* **126:** 357–363, 1970.

Richman, P. I. *et al.* Colonic pericrypt sheath cells: Characterisation of cell type with new monoclonal antibody. *J Clin Pathol* **40:** 593–600, 1987.

Roberts, M. C. Carbohydrate digestion and absorption in the equine small intestine. *J S Afr Vet Assoc* **46:** 19–27, 1975.

Simmons, H. A., and Ford E. J. H. Liquid flow and capacity of the caecum and colon of the horse. *Res Vet Sci* **48:** 265–266, 1990.

Sjoqvist, A., and Beeuwkes, R. Villus sodium gradient associated with volume absorption in the feline intestine: An electron-microprobe study on freeze-dried tissue. *Acta Physiol Scand* **136:** 271–281, 1989.

Smith, M. W., and Jarvis, L. G. Growth and cell replacement in the new-born pig intestine. *Proc R Soc Lond (B)* **203:** 69–89, 1978.

Snyder, J. R. *et al.* Microvascular circulation of the ascending colon in horses. *Am J Vet Res* **50:** 2075–2083, 1989.

Spinato, M. T. *et al.* A morphometric study of the canine colon: Comparison of control dogs and cases of colonic disease. *Can J Vet Res* **54:** 477–486, 1990.

Staley, T. E. *et al.* Fine structure of duodenal absorptive cells in the newborn pig before and after feeding of colostrum. *Am J Vet Res* **30:** 567–581, 1969.

Strombeck, D. R., and Guilford, W. G. "Small Animal Gastroenterology," 2nd Ed., Davis, California, Stonegate Publishing, 1990.

Thomas, J., and Anderson, N. V. Interepithelial lymphocytes in the small intestinal mucosa of conventionally reared dogs. *Am J Vet Res* **43:** 200–203, 1982.

Thomson, A. B. R. *et al.* Intestinal aspects of lipid absorption: In review. *Can J Physiol Pharmacol* **67:** 179–190, 1989.

Thrall, D. E., and Leininger, J. R. Irregular intestinal mucosal margination in the dog: Normal or abnormal. *J Small Anim Pract* **17:** 305–312, 1976.

Tisserand, J.-L. Microbial digestion in the large intestine in relation to monogastric and polygastric herbivores. *Acta Vet Scand (Suppl.)* **86:** 83–92, 1989.

Tse, S.-K., and Chadee, K. The interaction between intestinal mucus glycoproteins and enteric infections. *Parasitol Today* **7:** 163–172, 1991.

Ulyatt, M. J. *et al.* Structure and function of the large intestine of ruminants. *In* "Digestion and Metabolism in the Ruminant," Proc. IV. Int. Symp. Rum. Physiol. Sydney, August 1974. I. W. Macdonald and A.C.I. Warner (eds.), pp. 119–133, Armidale NSW, Australia, University of New England, 1975.

Willard, M. D., and Leid, R. W. Nonuniform horizontal and vertical distributions of immunoglobulin A cells in canine intestines. *Am J Vet Res* **42:** 1573–1580, 1981.

Willard, M. D. *et al.* Number and distribution of IgM cells and IgA cells in colonic tissue of conditioned sex- and breed-related dogs. *Am J Vet Res* **43:** 688–692, 1982.

1. Electrolyte and Water Transport in the Intestine

Water movement in the bowel is passive, following osmotically the transport of electrolyte and nutrient solutes. The small intestinal mucosa is highly permeable to the passive movement of small ions and water and is therefore considered leaky, despite the presence of tight junctions at the apical margins of absorptive enterocytes. This ensures that the content of the small bowel is approximately isosmolal with the interstitial fluid space. The leaks in the small intestinal epithelium are paracellular, at the tight junctions, and act as water-filled spaces 0.3–0.8 nm in diameter. The permeability of junctional complexes appears to be sensitive to Starling forces, influenced by intravascular hydrostatic and oncotic pressure, so that fluid and solute actively absorbed may leak back into the lumen, thus modulating net absorption by the mucosa.

Sodium absorption takes place by a number of active transcellular mechanisms, which vary in importance at different levels of the gut, and with the physiologic circumstance. Fundamentally, Na^+ absorption depends on electrochemical forces established by the ATP-dependent Na^+ pump on the basolateral cell membrane of the absorptive enterocyte. This pump moves Na^+ up a concentration gradient from the cell into the lateral intercellular space, exchanging K^+ for Na^+, but not at an equal rate. One mechanism involves diffusional, or uncoupled electrogenic, Na^+ absorption. Sodium enters the cell from the luminal solution passively, down the electrostatic and concentration gradient established by the sodium pump at the basolateral membrane. It is then pumped into the lateral intercellular space. A second mechanism involves absorption of Na^+ into the epithelium by a process that exchanges it for H^+, which enters the lumen. In some situations, Na^+ and Cl^- are probably absorbed together by a neutral process, with exchange of H^+ and an anion such as HCO_3^-, which move out of the cell to the lumen. Absorption of Na^+ is also coupled to that of organic solutes such as amino acids and glucose.

The concentration of solute, especially Na^+ in the lateral intercellular space, causes water to follow from the intestinal lumen. Since cell membranes and junctional complexes are highly permeable to water, movement is rapid via both transcellular and paracellular routes, and differences in osmotic pressure between lumen and lateral intercellular space are small. Absorbed solute and water in isotonic proportions move into the interstitium of the villus, where within a few micrometers, they encounter a subepithelial capillary or lacteal. The tight junctions also appear to become permeable during Na^+-nutrient cotransport across the apical cell membrane, resulting in solvent drag of large nutrient molecules into the lateral intercellular space. The dilated lateral intercellular space is readily seen in sections of villus epithelium that were actively absorbing when fixed.

The colon of carnivores, the spiral colon of ruminants and swine, and the small colon of the horse is charged with the task of reducing the volume of electrolytes and water lost to the animal in the feces. In contrast to that of the small intestine, the colonic epithelium is relatively restrictive to the free movement of sodium and chloride, though not to potassium. Therefore it is capable of maintaining differences in osmotic pressure, ionic composition, and electrical potential between luminal and proprial surfaces, which makes it more efficient than the small bowel in absorbing some electrolytes and water. Ultimately, fecal water may be hypotonic with respect to plasma. Sodium absorption in the colon may involve electrogenic or coupled Na^+–Cl^- electroneutral mechanisms, similar to those in the small bowel; glucose- and amino acid-coupled Na^+ absorption does not occur. Absorption of volatile fatty acids also accounts for considerable water absorption from the colon. Potassium increases in concentration in colonic content as Na^+ concentration declines; this is due to an active secretory process, and a passive response to transepithelial electrochemical gradients.

The mucosa of the small and large intestine, under some conditions, also secretes chloride, potassium, bicarbonate, and water. This process, which appears to be a function mainly of the crypts, is important in some pathologic states; but it is also physiologic, and segmental, maintaining the fluidity and buffering capacity of the intestinal content. Chloride moves from the interstitial fluid, across the basolateral membrane of the cell, coupled to a Na^+–K^+ cotransporter, and driven by the gradient established by the Na^+ pump. It then moves from the cell to the lumen down an electrochemical gradient through Cl^- channels in the apical membrane, which control Cl^- secretion. Sodium and water follow via the paracellular path.

Solute movement across the intestinal epithelium is regulated by a number of hormones and neurotransmitters, which act through intracellular second messengers. Activation of adenylate cyclase and guanylate cyclase, and increased intracellular Ca^{2+}, all depress nutrient-independent absorption of Na^+ by enterocytes, and open Cl^- channels in crypt cells, promoting secretion. Some products of the intrinsic and extrinsic neurons, such as vasoactive intestinal polypeptide (VIP) and acetylcholine, may be secretory, whereas others, such as somatostatin and norepinephrine, are absorptive or antisecretory. Local paracrine effects are mediated by the products of enteroendocrine cells, such as somatostatin, and neurotensin (secretory). Serotonin is secretory, possibly directly, and also through stimulation of local prostaglandin production. Mesenchymal elements in the lamina propria, including lymphocytes, mast cells, macrophages, and other inflammatory and connective tissue cells also produce locally active substances with a direct or indirect effect on epithelial function. Histamine may be secretory. Kallikrein activates circulating kinins, which in turn stimulate epithelial secretion, and local production of prostaglandins and other eicosanoids. Eicosanoids may have a direct secretory effect, as well as stimulating neurotransmitter release through local neuronal reflexes. Circulating hormones also influence mucosal function. Aldosterone and glucocorticoids enhance Na^+ absorption by the colon, and the latter may inhibit local production of eicosanoids.

Hence, immunoinflammatory events are integrated with the systemic and local neural and hormonal regulation of intestinal absorption and secretion. Dysfunctions of absorption and secretion will be considered with the pathogenesis of diarrhea (Section VI,J,2 of this chapter).

Bibliography

Argenzio, R. A. Fluid and ion transport in the large intestine. *In* "Aspects of Digestive Physiology in Ruminants," A. Dobson and M. J. Dobson (eds.), pp. 140–155. Ithaca, New York, Comstock, 1988.

Argenzio, R. A. Physiology of digestive, secretory, and absorptive processes. *In* "The Equine Acute Abdomen," N. A. White II, (ed.), pp. 25–35. Philadelphia, Pennsylvania, Lea & Febiger, 1990.

Argenzio, R. A., and Liacos, J. A. Endogenous prostanoids control ion transport across neonatal porcine ileum *in vitro*. *Am J Vet Res* **51:** 747–751, 1990.

Bern, M. J. *et al.* Immune system control of rat and rabbit colonic electrolyte transport. Role of prostaglandins and enteric nervous system. *J Clin Invest* **83:** 1810–1820, 1989.

Field, M., Rao, M. C., and Chang, E. B. Intestinal electrolyte transport and diarrhea. Part 1. *N Engl J Med* **321:** 800–806, 1989.

Johnson, L. R. (ed.) "Physiology of the Gastrointestinal Tract," 2nd ed. New York, Raven Press, 1987. [See chapters by W. M. Armstrong (pp. 1251–1265), H. J. Binder and G. I. Sandle (pp. 1389–1417), D. W. Powell (pp. 1267–1305).]

Madara, J. L. Pathobiology of the intestinal epithelial barrier. *Am J Pathol* **137:** 1273–1281, 1990.

Murray, M. J. Digestive physiology of the large intestine in adult horses. Part I. Mechanisms of fluid, ions, and volatile fatty acid transport. *Compend Cont Ed Pract Vet* **10:** 1204–1210, 1988.

Turnberg, L. A. The small intestine: Prospects for therapeutic approaches in secretory diarrheal diseases. *Scand J Gastroenterol* **25** (Suppl. 175): 85–92, 1990.

2. Immune Elements of the Gastrointestinal Tract

The gastrointestinal tract is continually presented with antigens in food, ingested toxins, viruses, bacteria and their products, and parasites and their excretions and secretions. The epithelial barrier of the gut is but one cell thick and has enormous surface area. Therefore, it is not surprising that the epithelium and associated lymphoid and inflammatory cells in the mucosa and submucosa have evolved a complex system for blocking, sampling, tolerating, or neutralizing and eliminating antigens. Intestinal lymphoid tissue has been estimated to compose 25% of the mucosal mass, and to exceed that of the spleen in volume.

The epithelial cell of the neonate is capable of uptake and transport of macromolecules from the intestinal lumen to the basolateral cell surface. In all species of domestic animals, **colostral transfer of immunoglobulins** by this route provides the neonate with passive humoral immunity during the early postnatal period. The selectivity of macromolecular transfer varies with the species, being least specific in neonatal ruminants, piglets, and foals, which take up most macromolecules contacting the epithelium. Permeability of the gut to macromolecules is the result of energy-dependent pinocytosis by the apical cell membrane at the base of microvilli. Colostral protein is transferred in membrane-bound vacuoles in the cytoplasm to the basolateral membrane, where, by exocytosis, the contents are extruded, to find their way via the lacteals and lymphatics to the general circulation. The period of active uptake of macromolecules is short, usually only 24–48 hr in ungulates, and closure precludes further bulk transport of macromolecules. Closure is probably at least partly related to maturity of the epithelium, and involves failure of intracellular transport or exocytosis, possibly due to replacement of surface enterocytes by cells incapable of export of proteins. Cells containing eosinophilic protein-filled cytoplasmic vacuoles (Fig. 1.46), which may displace the nucleus toward the surface, persist longest in the distal small bowel.

Although bulk transport does not occur, nutritionally inconsequential amounts of macromolecules continue to be transferred by enterocytes in mature animals, via mechanisms analogous to those occurring in the neonate. For uptake to occur, molecules must escape intraluminal hydrolysis, and pinocytosis must exceed the rate of lysosomal degradation to permit molecules to be exported from the cell. Macromolecules gaining entry to the portal circulation are largely phagocytosed by Kupffer's cells in the liver. These cells form a second line of defense against macromolecules entering from the gut, and are important in clearing endotoxin from the portal blood. Fully differentiated small intestinal absorptive epithelial cells express on their basolateral membranes major histocompatibility complex (MHC) class II molecules, as do antigen-presenting macrophages and dendritic cells. Enterocytes are capable of directly presenting antigen to T cells, and they modulate the immune response through the release of cytokines, including prostaglandins. Significantly, in some intestinal parasitisms, and cell-mediated inflammatory bowel disease, crypt cells and immature surface enterocytes express MHC class II molecules, suggesting an increased capacity to influence immune events in response to luminal antigen.

In addition to the pinocytotic activity of absorptive enterocytes, specific epithelial cells called **M cells,** associated with Peyer's patches and intestinal lymphoid follicles, actively sample particulate matter and macromolecules impinging on the mucosal surface. M cells are interspersed among cells resembling absorptive enterocytes, on the surface of the dome in the mucosa overlying lymphoid aggregates in the submucosa. They often adopt an inverted cup shape, with one or more lymphocytes and occasional macrophages in the basal concavity, in contact with the membrane of the M cell. Material taken up by M cells is transmitted to the associated lymphocytes or macrophages. The M cell is a probable portal of entry to the mucosa for bacteria, perhaps including *Salmonella, Yersinia,* and *Listeria* in some species, and for some viruses. Neutrophils are seen transmigrating the epithelium of the dome, and in the lumen over the dome, in enteric bacterial infections of calves in particular. Neutrophils may also play a role in phagocytosis in the enteric lumen in pigs under some conditions.

The **aggregated lymphoid follicles,** or **Peyer's patches,** are scattered in the mucosa of the small intestine, and lymphoglandular complexes or solitary proprial lymphoid nodules may be grossly visible, studding the colonic mucosa. Peyer's patches are present throughout the length of the small intestine in all species, though they tend to be larger distally. They are grossly visible, usually as oval or elongate structures as wide as several centimeters, thickening the antimesenteric wall of the intestine. They may project slightly above the mucosal surface, or appear as depressions, which must not be mistaken for ulcers, especially in dogs. In neonates of some species, including swine, they may be poorly developed and not visible grossly. Elongate **continuous Peyer's patches** have been described in the distal ileum, involving the terminal 15–20% of the small intestine, in calves, lambs, and piglets. This structure is different morphologically and functionally from other gut-associated lymphoid tissue, and may be a primary site of B-cell generation. Continuous Peyer's patches involute as the animal matures.

Peyer's patches comprise follicular aggregates of B lymphocytes in the submucosa, underlying a discontinuous muscularis mucosae. Between the upper borders of adjacent lymphoid follicles are aggregates of T lymphocytes. Overlying the lymphoid follicles is a mixed population of T and B lymphocytes extending into the lamina propria in rounded mucosal projections, the domes, which lie between villi. Short crypts provide epithelium to domes and adjacent villi. Cell populations of Peyer's patches in newborns and gnotobiotes of most species tend to be sparser than those in older or bacterially colonized animals, though those in neonatal calves appear relatively well developed.

B and T immunoblasts gain access to Peyer's patches via permeable postcapillary venules (PCV), mediated by specific receptors in the PCVs. The major cell populations in Peyer's patches appear to be B lymphocytes committed mainly to IgA production, whereas among the T cells is a large proportion of T-helper cell precursors. Antigen is processed in Peyer's patches largely by **dendritic cells; macrophages** are less common in Peyer's patches than in lamina propria, and their role in the interaction among M cells and T and B lymphocytes is unclear. They probably play an effector role in cell-mediated reactions to bacteria entering via Peyer's patches, and certainly in response to agents such as *Mycobacterium a. paratuberculosis* and *Histoplasma capsulatum,* found in the lamina propria.

Macrophages and dendritic cells scattered in the lamina propria may play a role in presenting antigen to sensitize lymphocytes present in the propria, and in cytokine production. Interleukins regulate immune activity, whereas complement, eicosanoids, and interleukins influence inflammatory events. Cachectin (tumor necrosis factor) has systemic effects, producing anorexia and fever, and mediating endotoxic shock. In addition to functioning in defense against microorganisms, macrophages phagocytose inert particulate matter reaching the lamina propria from the lumen. They also sequester iron, inhibiting bacterial metabolism, and, by loss at the villus tip, may have some role in iron excretion. Bile pigment, perhaps derived from meconium, is seen sometimes in macrophages in the tips of villi in neonates. The involvement of macrophages in the phagocytosis of cells (enterocytes, theliolymphocytes, fibroblast sheath) in the subepithelial lamina propria at the tips of villi or between the openings of colonic glands has been alluded to previously. This process is most obvious in equine large and small intestine, where it should be distinguished from necrotic foci in the lamina propria.

IgA lymphoblasts leave the Peyer's patch for the mesenteric lymph node and, via the thoracic duct, the general circulation, whence they home on the intestinal mucosa and other mucosal surfaces, including the respiratory tract, mammary gland, and salivary glands. In the lamina propria of the intestine, they differentiate into IgA-secretory plasma cells, found mainly in close apposition to columnar epithelium of the upper crypt. Dimeric IgA binds via the J chain to glycoprotein secretory component present on the basolateral border of columnar crypt epithelial cells. With secretory component, it is transported in vesicles through the cytoplasm to be released from the apical border of the cell into the lumen of the crypt. It then spreads over the intestinal surface, partly bound to mucus. Dimeric IgA entering the circulation is selectively taken up by hepatocytes and is secreted into bile, in some rodents and lagomorphs.

Immunoglobulin A-secreting cells are the predominant class of plasma cell in the lamina propria in most species. However, **IgM-secreting plasma cells** are prevalent in young calves, swine, and dogs; IgM is also taken up by secretory component in some species and transported to the intestinal lumen. This may be significant in the young piglet and calf. Although IgA and IgM are secreted, IgG_1 is the major antibody class in intestinal secretion in cattle; it appears to be selectively secreted by the gut and in the bile in that species.

The function of IgA in the gut lumen probably lies mainly in blocking attachment by bacteria and viruses to epithelial cells, neutralizing intraluminal toxins, and in limiting absorption of antigens originating in food and produced by microorganisms in the gut. It thereby reduces the likelihood of reaginic and other forms of immune response in the propria. Secretion into the bile, by hepatocytes, of IgA complexed with antigen may, in the species in which it occurs, be a significant means of clearing the circulation of antigen absorbed from the gut. IgA deficiency is reported in beagle, German shepherd, and Shar-Pei dogs, where it is associated with increased susceptibility to parvovirus infection, and chronic small intestinal and respiratory disease.

Plasma cells containing IgG are relatively uncommon in the intestinal lamina propria in species other than ruminants. However, locally produced and systemically circulating IgG may assume significance when vascular permeability and inflammation occur, because of its ability to fix complement, facilitate antibody-dependent cell-mediated cytotoxicity, and to opsonize.

Plasmacytes producing IgE are present in the lamina propria, and this class of immunoglobulin has been implicated particularly in immune responses to some intestinal parasites. Its significance may be in IgE-dependent cytotoxicity by eosinophils and perhaps by mast cells, as well as in mediating immediate (type I) hypersensitivity reactions in the mucosa.

Intestinal mast cells differ histochemically and physiologically from mast cells in most other tissues. They are not so demonstrable after formalin fixation, in comparison with basic lead acetate or Carnoy's fluid. Proliferation of intestinal mast cells is T cell dependent, and is prominent in some parasitisms. Mast cells interact with the enteric nervous system, and undoubtedly play a central role in regulation of physiologic, immune, and inflammatory processes in the gut. The effects of histamine, serotonin, and other mediators released by mast cells, on vascular tone and permeability, motility, chemotaxis, and effector function of leukocytes, on immune-active cells, and possibly in mucus release, are many and complex.

Globule leukocytes are visible in hematoxylin and eosin-stained tissue sections as mononuclear cells with large eosinophilic cytoplasmic granules, in the epithelium of the crypt and lower villus, and sometimes in the lamina propria. They are probably derived from intestinal mast cells. Intestinal **eosinophils** probably do not differ functionally from eosinophils in other sites, being cytotoxic effector cells and modulators of local inflammation.

T cells are present in Peyer's patches, and distributed throughout the lamina propria, and are the great majority of the **intraepithelial lymphocyte** population. Lymphocytes may compose in excess of 10–20% of cells present in the epithelial layer of the small intestine. Some intraepithelial lymphocytes may be natural-killer cells. Many of the other intraepithelial lymphocytes may be cytotoxic or suppressor T cells, or may be under the influence of epithelial cells in regulating the response to luminal antigen. In contrast, a lower proportion of proprial T lymphocytes have markers characteristic of suppressor cells, and some may also be T-helper cells or pluripotential stem T cells. As might be expected, B lymphocytes are numerous in the lamina propria, and are most highly concentrated in Peyer's patches, where the greatest numbers of T-helper cells are also found.

T immunoblasts from the gut seem to follow a pathway similar to that of B lymphocytes, through mesenteric lymph node and the systemic circulation, before homing on the lamina propria or intraepithelial intercellular space. Intraepithelial lymphocytes increase in number in association with cell-mediated immune reactions in the intestinal mucosa. Understanding of the mechanisms of cell-mediated immunity in the intestine is still poor. They may be mediated by helper-T cell-promoted antibody production, by local direct cytotoxic effects, and by release of lymphokines. In intestinal parasitism, probably some food allergies, and celiac disease in humans, cytokines associated with cell-mediated immune events alter epithelial proliferation and differentiation, resulting in villus atrophy. T cells also regulate proliferation and differentiation of goblet cells and mast cells.

Immunoinflammatory events in the large bowel are less well understood than those in the small intestine. Presumably, similar principles prevail. **Lymphoglandular complexes,** consisting of submucosal follicular lymphoid aggregates penetrated by glands extending from the mucosa, occur in the cecum and proximal colon of the dog, in the porcine colon, and at the cecocolic junction, beginning of the spiral colon, and in the terminal rectum, in ruminants. Epithelium lining the glands is in close contact with lymphocytes. **Solitary mucosal lymphoid nodules,** normally without penetrating glands, and generally restricted to the lamina propria and superficial submucosa, are also scattered throughout the cecum and colon in all species. Plasma cells in the lamina propria principally produce IgA. Depending on the species, their location varies. In dogs most tend to be in the deeper portion of the lamina propria between glands.

Bibliography

Atkins, A. M., and Schofield, G. C. Lymphoglandular complexes in the large intestine of the dog. *J Anat* **113:** 169–178, 1972.

Bienenstock, J. *et al.* Nerves and neuropeptides in the regulation of intestinal immunity. *Adv Exp Med Biol* **257:** 19–26, 1989.

Bland, P. MHC class II expression by the gut epithelium. *Immunol Today* **9:** 174–178, 1988.

Brandtzaeg, P. *et al.* Immunobiology and immunopathology of human gut mucosa: Humoral immunity and intraepithelial lymphocytes. *Gastroenterology* **97:** 1562–1584, 1989.

Carlson, J. R., and Owen, R. L. Structure and functional role of Peyer's patches. *In* "Immunopathology of the Small Intestine," M. N Marsh (ed.), pp. 21–40. Chichester, England, John Wiley, 1987.

Chu, R. M., and Liu C. H. Morphological and functional comparisons of Peyer's patches in different parts of the swine small intestine. *Vet Immunol Immunopathol* **6:** 391–403, 1984.

Chu, R. M. *et al.* Granular mucosal lymphocytes in porcine small intestine. *Am J Vet Res* **49:** 1456–1459, 1988.

Huntley, J. F., Newlands, G., and Miller, H. R. P. The isolation and characterization of globule leukocytes: Their derivation from mucosal mast cells in parasitized sheep. *Parasite Immunol* **6:** 371–390, 1984.

Husband, A. J. Ontogeny of the gut-associated immune system. *In* "The Ruminant Immune System," J. E. Butler (ed.), pp. 633–647. New York, Plenum, 1981.

Husband, A. J. The intestinal immune system. *In* "Viral Diarrheas of Man and Animals," L. J. Saif and K. W. Theil (eds.), pp. 289–312. Boca Raton, Florida, CRC Press, 1990.

Jeffcott, L. B. Passive immunity and its transfer with special reference to the horse. *Biol Rev* **47:** 439–464, 1972.

Keren, D. F. Gastrointestinal immune system and its disorders. *In* "Gastrointestinal Pathology," H. Goldman *et al.* (eds.), pp. 247–285. Baltimore, Maryland, Williams & Wilkins, 1990.

Landsverk, T. *et al.* The intestinal habitat for organized lymphoid tissues in ruminants; comparative aspects of structure, function and development. *Vet Immunol Immunopathol* **28:** 1–16, 1991.

Lascelles, A. K. *et al.* The mucosal immune system with particular reference to ruminant animals. *In* "The Ruminant Immune System in Health and Disease," W. I. Morrison, (ed.), pp. 429–457. Cambridge, England, Cambridge University Press, 1986.

Liebler, E. M. *et. al.* Gut-associated lymphoid tissue in the large intestine of calves. I. Distribution and histology. *Vet Pathol* **25:** 503–508, 1988.

Marshall, J. S., and Bienenstock, J. Mast cells. *Springer Sem Immunopathol* **12:** 191–202, 1990.

McGuire, T. C. *et al.* Failure of colostral immunoglobulin transfer in calves dying from infectious disease. *J Am Vet Med Assoc* **169:** 713–718, 1976.

McGuire, T. C. *et al.* Failure of colostral immunoglobulin transfer as an explanation for most infections and deaths of neonatal foals. *J Am Vet Med Assoc* **170:** 1302–1304, 1977.

Miller, H. R. P. Immunity to internal parasites. *Rev Sci Tech Off Int Epiz* **9:** 301–313, 1990.

Morfitt, D. C., and Pohlenz, J. F. L. Porcine colonic lymphoglandular complex: Distribution, structure, and epithelium. *Am J Anat* **184:** 41–51, 1989.

Mowat, A. McI. The cellular basis of gastrointestinal immunity. *In* "Immunopathology of the Small Intestine," M. N. Marsh (ed.), pp. 41–72. Chichester, England, John Wiley, 1987.

Murata, H., and Namioka, S. The duration of colostral immunoglobulin uptake by the epithelium of the small intestine of neonatal piglets. *J Comp Pathol* **87:** 431–439, 1977.

Parsons, K. R. *et al.* Follicle-associated epithelium of the gut associated lymphoid tissue of cattle. *Vet Pathol* **28:** 22–29, 1991.

Porter, P. *et al.* Intestinal secretion of immunoglobulins in the preruminant calf. *Immunology* **23:** 299–312, 1972.

Salmon, H. The intestinal and mammary immune system in pigs. *Vet Immunol Immunopathol* **17:** 367–388, 1987.

Santos, L. M. B. *et al.* Characterization of immunomodulatory properties and accessory cell function of small intestinal epithelial cells. *Cell Immunol* **127:** 26–34, 1990.

Sawyer, M. *et al.* Passive transfer of colostral immunoglobulins from ewe to lamb and its influence on neonatal lamb mortality. *J Am Vet Med Assoc* **171:** 1255–1259, 1977.

Stead, R. H. *et al.* Mast cells are closely apposed to nerves in the human gastrointestinal mucosa. *Gastroenterology* **97:** 575–585, 1989.

Stokes, C., and Bourne, J. F. Mucosal immunity. *In* "Veterinary Clinical Immunology," R. E. W. Halliwell and N. T. Gorman (eds.), pp. 164–192. Philadelphia, Pennsylvania, W. B. Saunders, 1989.

Strobel, S. *et al.* Human intestinal mucosal mast cells: Evaluation of fixation and staining techniques. *J Clin Pathol* **34:** 851–858, 1981.

Strombeck, D. R., and Guilford, W. G. Gastrointestinal immune system. *In* "Small Animal Gastroenterology," 2nd Ed., pp. 22–43. Davis, California, Stonegate Publishing, 1990.

Torres-Medina, A. Morphologic characteristics of the epithelial surface of aggregated lymphoid follicles (Peyer's patches) in the small intestine of newborn gnotobiotic calves and pigs. *Am J Vet Res* **42:** 232–236, 1981.

Vellenga, L. *et al.* Biological and pathological aspects of the mammalian small intestinal permeability to macromolecules. *Vet Q* **7:** 322–332, 1985.

B. Gastrointestinal Microflora

After birth, no part of the gastrointestinal tract is sterile. Several hundred species of bacteria inhabit the stomach and intestine, forming an ecosystem of enormous complexity. Generally speaking, bacterial populations are least in the stomach and upper small intestine of ruminants and carnivores, being limited by the acid gastric environment and by peristalsis. The anaerobes and facultative anaerobes, mainly *E. coli,* increase to about 10^7 per gram of content in the lower small intestine, and total bacterial populations in excess of 10^{10} or 10^{11} per gram of content are present in the cecum and colon. Prominent among colonic bacteria are coliforms, *Lactobacillus,* and strict anaerobes, including *Bacteroides, Fusobacterium, Clostridium, Eubacterium, Bifidobacterium,* and *Peptostreptococci.* Spirochetes are found in swine and dogs. Anaerobic bacteria outnumber facultative anaerobes by a thousandfold in the large bowel.

The complex ecology of the gut flora imparts on it a considerable stability, and if disturbed, it tends to return toward the original state. It is relatively resistant to the intrusion of new inhabitants, and this is one of the major factors protecting against the establishment of pathogenic bacteria. It is no coincidence that bacterial diarrhea occurs most commonly in the neonate with a poorly established flora, or after changes in husbandry or antibiotic therapy, which may disturb the enteric bacterial population.

Normal flora acts as a barrier to colonization by pathogens through several means. The secretion of proteins such as colicins has little significance in modulating enteric bacterial populations; more important is the production of acetic and butyric acids by the anaerobes. Under the pH and anaerobic conditions in the large bowel, fatty acids are highly detrimental to members of the Enterobacteriaceae. The high population of lactobacilli in the gut of milk-fed animals probably reduces establishment of Enterobacteriaceae by this means. Facultative anaerobes are important in maintaining the redox environment for strict anaerobes, by scavenging oxygen. Competition for energy, and the effect of metabolites other than short-chain fatty acids produced by the native flora, militate against establishment by exogenous bacteria. Host factors influencing gut flora include composition of the diet; peristalsis, which continually flushes the small intestine of a large proportion of its bacterial population; lysozyme; lactoferrin; gastric acidity if unbuffered or undiluted; and in the abomasum of suckling calves, perhaps a lactoperoxidase–thiocyanide–hydrogen peroxide system.

The enteric microbial flora promotes the development of a population of immune and inflammatory cells in the lamina propria, by antigenic stimulation. Mucosal epithelial kinetics are also speeded up in conventional animals, in comparison with germ-free animals. In germ-free gut, the proliferative compartment in the crypts is smaller and less active, and epithelial transit times to the tips of villi are slower than in conventional animals. The effects of altered intestinal epithelial turnover and immune activity on normal flora are poorly defined, and probably minor as far as luminal bacteria are concerned. Secretion of IgA into the lumen probably influences populations close to the mucosa, and immune activity as a whole must limit establishment on and ingress by microorganisms and their products into the mucosa. Lactogenic immunity similarly has an inhibitory effect on enteric organisms to which specific antibody is present in ingested milk.

1. Mechanisms of Bacterial Disease Arising in the Intestine

Disequilibrium of the normal microflora, or a competitive advantage, may permit the establishment in the intestine of pathogenic strains of bacteria, or the abnormal proliferation by opportunistic pathogens of the resident flora.

An abnormal microflora, colonic in character, may develop in the small intestine. This bacterial overgrowth is due to achlorhydria, and physical or physiologic derangements resulting in gut stasis or loss of normal peristaltic flushing. Deconjugation of bile salts and fat malabsorption result in steatorrhea and other complications considered more fully later, with malabsorption and diarrhea.

Availability of abnormally large amounts of nutrient substrate may permit the proliferation of strains of toxigenic *Clostridium perfringens*. The toxins produced can have a local necrotizing effect in the gut, as occurs in lambs, piglets, and calves, and may be implicated in canine intestinal hemorrhage syndrome and perhaps colitis in horses. *Clostridium perfringens* type D produces epsilon toxin. It has no physical effect in the gut, but exemplifies the principle of enterotoxemic diseases by being absorbed and acting at a site or sites distant from the intestine. Verotoxin produced by strains of *E. coli* causing gut edema, or edema disease, also falls into this category.

Certain strains of *E. coli* have the capacity to attach to the epithelium of the small intestine by pili, permitting colonization. Production of secretory diarrhea by the local effect of a toxin which has a physiologic, but little or no physical, effect on the gut is characteristic of these strains; some strains of *Salmonella* may also be enterotoxic. *Salmonella,* however, is generally considered to be enteroinvasive, invading and traversing the epithelium. Enteroinvasive bacteria often stimulate acute inflammation and cause extensive mucosal damage, with erosion and effusion of tissue fluid, probably through local production of necrotizing verotoxins. Some strains of *E. coli* also have this capability.

Changes which are interpreted as increased epithelial proliferation, associated with superficial erosion, are characteristic of *Serpula* infection in swine dysentery, and some *Campylobacter*-like infections, particularly proliferative hemorrhagic enteropathy in pigs. The organisms penetrate the epithelial cells in the latter condition; spirochetes are essentially noninvasive in swine dysentery. The effect in both these diseases is to cause loss of absorptive function, and to permit effusion of tissue fluid. In proliferative hemorrhagic enteropathy, severe mucosal damage, by unknown mechanisms, may culminate in hemorrhage.

Mucosal invasion by mycobacteria will produce granulomatous enteritis, lymphangitis, and lymphadenitis, associated with villus atrophy and intestinal protein loss in Johne's disease. Localization of *Rhodococcus equi* largely in local lymphoid tissue in the gut, with ulceration, may progress to suppurative lymphadenitis. In domestic animals *Yersinia* may follow a similar route, which may culminate in caseous lymphadenitis and/or bacteremia.

The intestinal mucosa can be a site for embolic establishment by circulating bacteria, and subsequent ulceration, as occurs in *Haemophilus somnus* septicemia of cattle, and *Pasteurella* septicemia in lambs. More often, bacteria originating in the gut enter the lymphatics or portal drainage, gaining access to the circulation and causing bacteremia or septicemia. Bacteria causing Tyzzer's disease in foals, septicemic salmonellosis in some species, and probably some cases of *E. coli* septicemia in calves and lambs, arise in the gut. For details of the pathogenesis and pathology of disease caused by these agents see Infectious and Parasitic Diseases of the Gastrointestinal Tract (Section VII of this chapter).

Bibliography

Ducluzeau, R. Implantation and development of the gut flora in the newborn animal. *Ann Rech Vét* **14:** 354–359, 1983.

Evans, N. Bacterial toxins and their effect on the gut. *In* "Natural Toxins: Animal, Plant, and Microbial," J. B. Harris (ed.), pp. 212–236. Oxford, U.K., Oxford University Press, 1986.

Finlay, B. B., and Falkow, S. Common themes in microbial pathogenicity. *Microbiol Rev* **53:** 210–230, 1989.

Gedek, B. Intestinal flora and biogregulation. *Rev Sci Tech Off Int Epiz* **8:** 417–437, 1989.

Morris, J. A. Bacterial mechanisms in intestinal disease. *In* "Function and Dysfunction of the Small Intestine," R. M. Batt and T. L. J. Lawrence (eds.), pp. 247–264. Liverpool, England, Liverpool University Press, 1984.

Reiter, B., Marshall, V. M., and Phillips, S. M. The antibiotic activity of the lactoperoxidase–thiocyanate–hydrogen peroxide system in the calf abomasum. *Res Vet Sci* **28:** 116–122, 1980.

Strombeck, D. R., and Guilford, W. G. Microflora of the gastrointestinal tract and its symbiotic relationship with the host. *In* "Small Animal Gastroenterology," 2nd Ed., pp. 15–21. Davis, California, Stonegate Publishing, 1990.

Ward, G. E., and Nelson, D. I. Effects of dietary milk fat (whole milk) and propionic acid on intestinal coliforms and lactobacilli in calves. *Am J Vet Res* **43:** 1165–1167, 1982.

Yokoyama, M. T., and Johnson, K. A. Microbiology of the rumen and intestine. *In* "The Ruminant Animal: Digestive Physiology and Nutrition," D. C. Church (ed.), pp. 124–144. Englewood Cliffs, New Jersey, Prentice-Hall, 1988.

C. Congenital Anomalies of the Intestine

Congenital enzyme deficiencies of the intestinal absorptive epithelium, such as the specific disaccharidase deficiencies of humans, have not been reported in domestic animals. Membranous cytoplasmic bodies have been reported in duodenal epithelial cells, and in various cell types in the lamina propria, in cats with generalized congenital gangliosidosis (see The Nervous System, Volume 1, Chapter 3).

Segmental anomalies of the intestine are commonly encountered. In early embryonal life the intestine consists of a simple tube, the lumen of which is lined by epithelial cells of endodermal origin. An outer layer of connective tissue from the splanchnic ectoderm surrounds and supports the tube. As the intestines grow with the developing fetus, they form coiled loops, which herniate into the umbilicus. In later stages of fetal development, the intestines withdraw, in an anterior-to-posterior direction, from the umbilicus into the abdomen. The most plausible cause of segmental defects in intestinal continuity is ischemia of a segment of gut during early fetal life, resulting in necrosis of the affected area. In addition, there is an association between pressure on the amniotic vesicle during palpation of the embryo for pregnancy diagnosis prior to 42 days of gestation, and the development of atresia coli in calves. The mechanism of this effect is uncertain.

The segmental anomalies of the intestine may vary in degree. **Stenosis** implies incomplete occlusion of the lumen; complete occlusion is referred to as **atresia.** Atresia is further subdivided into membrane atresia, in which the obstruction is formed by a simple membrane or diaphragm; cord atresia, in which the blind ends of the gut are joined by a cord of connective tissue; and blind-end atresia, in which a segment of gut and possibly the corresponding mesentery are missing, leaving two blind ends. All types of segmental anomaly can be produced experimentally by ischemia to a portion of the fetal intestine.

Atresia coli is the most common segmental anomaly of the intestine in domestic animals. It is seen particularly in the spiral colon of Holstein calves, and in the large and small colon of foals; it occurs rarely in cats. Heritability of atresia coli in Holsteins has not been established; neither has an explanation for the apparent breed predisposition. A predisposition for male calves has been described, but this is not consistent among studies.

Atresia of the small intestine is less common. **Atresia ilei** is most prevalent in calves, and rare in foals, lambs, piglets, and pups. Atresia jejuni in Jersey cattle and atresia ilei in Swedish Highland cattle are claimed to be inherited as lethal autosomal recessive traits, but the data are weak. Atresia is rarely encountered in the duodenum. Occasionally, extensive defects in intestinal continuity, associated with lesions high in the mesenteric artery, are reported.

These obstructions prevent the normal movement of gut content and meconium in the fetus and neonate. Therefore, they lead to dilation of the anterior segment, with progressive abdominal distension, which may become so extensive prepartum as to cause dystocia. The bowel beyond the discontinuity is small in diameter, and devoid of content other than mucus and exfoliated cells. Animals fail to pass feces after birth.

Atresia ani (imperforate anus), overall, is the most common congenital defect of the lower gastrointestinal tract. It may affect all species, but is most often encountered in calves and in pigs, in which it is considered to be hereditary. The defect may consist only of failure of perforation of the membrane separating the endodermal hindgut from the ectodermal anal membrane, or both anus and rectum may be atretic. Atresia ani may be an isolated abnormality, or it may be associated with other malformations, especially of the distal spinal column (spinal dysraphia, sacral or coccygeal vertebral agenesis), of the genitourinary tract (rectovaginal fistula, renal agenesis, horseshoe kidney, polycystic kidneys, cryptorchidism, duplication of scrotum), and occasionally, with intestinal atresia or agenesis of the colon.

Short colon, probably the result of abnormal rotation of the midgut and failure to lengthen during fetal life, has been reported in several cats and dogs. Signs were mild, and possibly unrelated to the colonic lesion. The cecum was on the left side, and ascending, transverse, and descending colon were not demarcated on contrast radiographs. In several cases, anorectal or urogenital abnormalities were concurrent. **Anomaly of the colonic mesenteric attachments,** presumably congenital, has been associated with the development of colic in a horse, due to distortion and convolution of the large colon.

Hypoplasia of the small intestinal mucosa, with short villi and sparse crypts, has been reported in foals with failure of passive transfer of immunoglobulin. This may represent a defect in fetal organogenesis.

Congenital colonic aganglionsis, somewhat analogous to Hirschsprung's disease of humans, has been reported in white foals which are the offspring of overo-spotted parents. It has not been convincingly demonstrated in other species of domestic animals. Clinically, the foals, which are predominantly white with a few pigmented dots on the muzzle, abdomen, and hindquarters, develop colic, and die generally within 48 hr after birth. There is stenosis mainly of the small colon, but the entire colon and rectum may be involved. The intestine anterior to the stenotic segment is distended with gas and meconium. The descending colon is contracted but patent. Microscopically, ganglia of the myenteric plexus are absent in the walls of the terminal ileum, cecum, and colon, though occasional nerve fibres are evident. Except for the few pigmented spots, melanocytes are absent in the skin. The condition is similar in many respects to aganglionic colon in piebald and spotted mutant mouse strains. Cutaneous melanoblasts and the myenteric plexus are both derived from the neural crest, which may explain the association between unpigmented skin and lack of the myenteric ganglia. Megacolon associated with few myenteric ganglion cells in Clydesdale foals is not clearly congenital, and is discussed with intestinal obstruction, as is megacolon in other species.

Persistent Meckel's diverticulum is an uncommon anomaly of the lower small bowel, mainly in swine and horses. It is derived from the omphalomesenteric (vitelline) duct, which is the stalk of the yolk sac. This duct is normally obliterated before the end of the first third of pregnancy. Rarely, it may be retained in postnatal life as a patent tube extending from the antimesenteric side of the intestine to the umbilicus. More commonly, only that portion immediately adjacent to the intestine remains patent. This pouch or tubelike remnant is Meckel's diverticulum. Its mucosal lining is similar to that of the ileum. In swine it usually occurs as a tube, the width of the ileum, 5–30 cm in length (Fig. 1.47). In horses it is present as a short cone-shaped sac about 10 cm in diameter, which may be attached by mesodiverticular bands to the ventral abdominal wall. It is usually an incidental finding, although in horses it has been associated with impaction, and with strangulation of intestine herniating through the mesodiverticular bands.

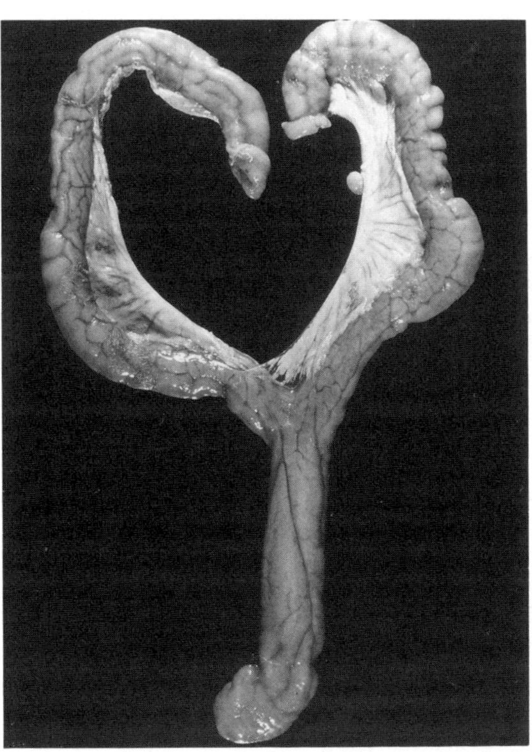

Fig. 1.47 Persistent Meckel's diverticulum. Midjejunum. Pig.

Intestinal diverticula, not always clearly remnants of the vitelline duct, occur rarely in dogs, cats, and horses. They may be incidental, or are associated with obstruction, diverticuloumbilical fistula, or with diverticulitis, perforation, and peritonitis. Intestinal adenocarcinoma, smooth muscle tumors, and heterotopic gastric fundic and pyloric mucosa may occur in the wall. Heterotopic gastric fundic gland tissue is also reported in the nondiverticular ileal mucosa of a beagle dog, as an incidental finding at necropsy.

Bibliography

Ablin, L. W. *et al.* Intestinal diverticular malformations in dogs and cats. *Compend Cont Ed Pract Vet* **13:** 426–430, 1991.

Anderson, W. I. *et al.* Segmental atresia of the transverse colon in a foal with concurrent equine herpesvirus-1 infection. *Cornell Vet* **77:** 119–121, 1987.

Blisard, K. S., and Kleinman, R. Hirschsprung's disease: A clinical and pathologic overview. *Human Pathol* **17:** 1189–1191, 1986.

Cho, D.-Y, and Taylor H. W. Blind-end atresia coli in two foals. *Cornell Vet* **76:** 11–15, 1986.

Constable, P. D. *et al.* Atresia coli in calves: 26 cases (1977–1987). *J Am Vet Med Assoc* **195:** 118–123, 1989.

Cork, L. C. *et al.* The pathology of feline GM_2 gangliosidosis. *Am J Pathol* **90:** 723–734, 1978.

Doughri, A. M. *et al.* Some developmental aspects of the bovine fetal gut. *Zbl Vet Med A* **19:** 417–434, 1972.

Dreyfuss, D. J., and Tulleners, E. P. Intestinal atresia in calves: 22 cases (1978–1988). *J Am Vet Med Assoc* **195:** 508–513, 1989.

Ducharme, N. G. *et al.* Colonic atresia in cattle: A prospective study of 43 cases. *Can Vet J* **29:** 818–824, 1988.

Fluke, M. H. *et al.* Short colon in two cats and a dog. *J Am Vet Med Assoc* **195:** 87–90, 1989.

Freeman, D. E. *et al.* Mesodiverticular bands as a cause of small intestinal strangulation and volvulus in the horse. *J Am Vet Med Assoc* **175:** 1089–1094, 1979.

Gonzalez-Licea, A. *et al.* Duodenal gangliosidosis in a cat: Ultrastructural study. *Am J Vet Res* **39:** 1342–1347, 1978.

Hooper, R. N. Small intestinal strangulation caused by Meckel's diverticulum in a horse. *J Am Vet Med Assoc* **194:** 943–944, 1989.

Hultgren, B. D. Ileocolonic aganglionosis in white progeny of overo spotted horses. *J Am Vet Med Assoc* **180:** 289–292, 1982.

Johnson, R. Intestinal atresia and stenosis: A review. *Vet Res Commun* **10:** 95–104, 105–111, 1986.

Jubb, T. F. Intestinal atresia in Friesian calves. *Aust Vet J* **67:** 382, 1990.

Kramme, P. M. Extensive intestinal atresia and forestomach distention in a full-term fetal calf. *Vet Pathol* **26:** 346–348, 1989.

McAfee, L. T., and McAfee, J. T. Atresia ani in a dog. *Vet Med Small Anim Clin* **71:** 624–627, 1976.

McCabe, L. *et al.* Overo lethal white foal syndrome: Equine model of aganglionic megacolon (Hirschsprung's disease). *Am J Med Genet* **36:** 336–340, 1990.

Nihleen, B., and Eriksson, K. A hereditary lethal defect in calves—atresia ilei. *Nord Vet-Med* **10:** 113–127, 1958.

Norrish, J. G., and Rennie, J. C. Observations on the inheritance of atresia ani in swine. *J Hered* **59:** 186–187, 1968.
Oikawa, M. *et al.* Villous hypoplasia of small intestine in neonatal foals. *Jpn J Vet Sci* **52:** 855–858, 1990.
Prieur D. J., and Dargatz, D. A. Multiple visceral congenital anomalies in a calf. *Vet Pathol* **21:** 452–454, 1984.
Rawlings, C. A., and Capps, W. F., Jr. Rectovaginal fistula and imperforate anus in a dog. *J Am Vet Med Assoc* **159:** 320–326, 1971.
Rest, J. R. Gastrointestinal anomalies in the dog—two case reports. *Vet Rec* **121:** 426–427, 1987.
Smart, M. E. *et al.* Congenital absence of jejunum and ileum in two neonatal Alaskan malamute pups. *Can Vet J* **19:** 22–23, 1978.
Suann, C. J., and Livesey, M. A. Congenital malformation of the large colon causing colic in a horse. *Vet Rec* **118:** 230–231, 1986.
Swartz, H. A. *et al.* Chromosomal evaluation of a ewe lamb with atresia ani vaginalis. *Am J Vet Res* **46:** 2145–2146, 1985.
Van Der Gaag, I., and Tibboel, D. Intestinal atresia and stenosis in animals: A report of 34 cases. *Vet Pathol* **17:** 565–574, 1980.
Vonderfecht, S. L. *et al.* Congenital intestinal aganglionosis in white foals. *Vet Pathol* **20:** 65–70, 1983.
Weaver, A. D. Massive ileal diverticulum: An uncommon anomaly. *Vet Med* **82:** 73–74, 1987.
West, H. J. *et al.* Volvulus of the intestines in a neonatal calf with two caeca, rectal stenosis, and a cardiac anomaly. *Vet Rec* **123:** 471–472, 1988.
Yovich, J. V., and Horney, F. D. Congenital jejunal diverticulum in a foal. *J Am Vet Med Assoc* **183:** 1092, 1983.

D. Miscellaneous Conditions of the Intestinal Tract

Intestinal lipofuscinosis is characterized grossly by brown discoloration of the intestinal muscularis (Fig. 1.48A). It may involve all areas of the gut, but is most common in the lower small intestine. The bladder, mesenteric, and peripheral lymph nodes may also be affected grossly. Although the lesion may be incidental, it is usually associated with chronic enteric and pancreatic disease. Lipofuscinosis has been reported in boxer dogs with histiocytic ulcerative colitis, but a definite correlation between the two conditions has not been established. A high prevalence of lipofuscinosis has also been reported in dogs that were fed rations high in polyunsaturated fats with a relative deficiency of vitamin E, and it is prevented by vitamin E supplementation. Any condition causing a reduction in the absorption of fats, and consequently of the fat-soluble vitamins, especially in the presence of polyunsaturated fatty acids in the diet, may predispose to lipofuscinosis.

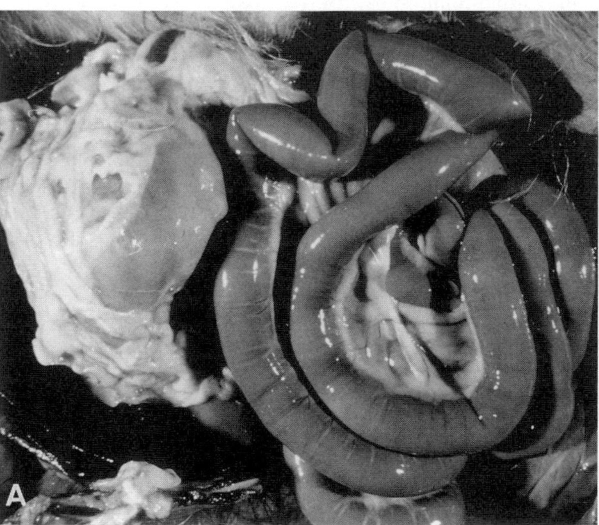

Fig. 1.48A Intestinal lipofuscinosis (brown gut), discoloring the small intestine to a tan hue. Dog.

The microscopic lesions of brown gut are gray to brown granules in the perinuclear regions of smooth muscle cells in both inner and outer muscle layers (Fig. 1.48B). The granules stain as lipofuscin (PAS positive, sudanophilic, weakly acid fast with Ziehl–Neelsen), and fluoresce dim yellow in paraffin section. The granules, termed leiomyometaplasts, are oxidized polymerized phospholipids which are highly resistant to further endophagocytic degradation. They are derived from excess cell membrane lipid peroxidation in vitamin E deficiency.

Muscular hypertrophy of the intestine was formerly a common finding in **swine,** but it appears to have diminished in prevalence in most areas. It may be found in apparently healthy animals at slaughter as a uniform thickening of the muscular coats of the terminal ileum. The segment involved always includes the most caudal portion, but it may extend a variable distance forward, usually between 25 and 50 cm. The affected area is thickened and has the turgid feel of a rubber hose. The lumen is small, and the mucosa is thrown into thick folds, but it is the muscle that thickens the wall. This condition must be differentiated from adenomatosis

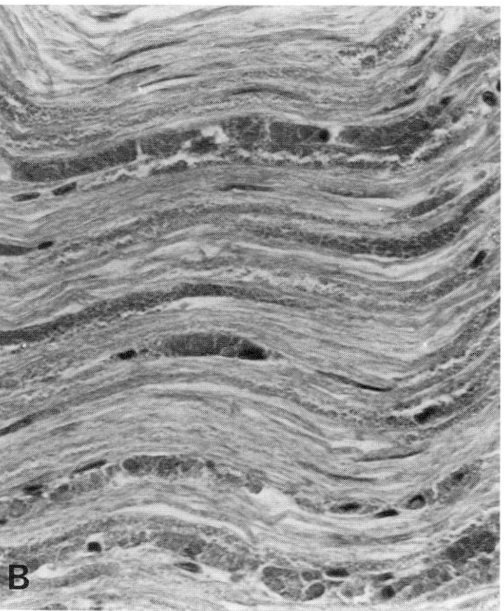

Fig. 1.48B Granular accumulations of ceroid–lipofuscin pigment (leiomyometaplasts) in smooth muscle cells. Small intestine. Dog. Intestinal lipofuscinosis.

and necrotic ileitis, manifestations of enteropathy associated with *Campylobacter*-like spp. in swine.

Rupture may occur, in association with impaction of dehydrated feed in the hypertrophic segment. The actual rupture may be a result of violent peristalsis, or diverticula may develop (Fig. 1.49A), the mucosa undergoing necrosis with secondary bacterial inflammation. Perforation occurs at these weakened areas.

Whereas the underlying basis of this condition is obscure, it is likely that the muscular hypertrophy is secondary to a functional obstruction of the ileocecal orifice.

Muscular hypertrophy of the small intestine, of uncertain cause, but sometimes associated with *Anoplocephala* spp. tapeworms at the ileocecal orifice, also occurs in **horses** (Fig. 1.49B). The lesions are similar to those described in swine, except that the affected segment may occur at any point along the small intestine, and occasionally in the large intestine, although the ileum is the most common site. Horses with this condition may have chronic mild colic or intermittent diarrhea with progressive loss of weight. Perforation is an unusual complication in the horse.

Diverticulosis of the small intestine is a rare lesion that is sometimes associated with muscular hypertrophy in pigs and horses. It is characterized by the presence of saccular dilatations, which are lined by intestinal mucosa,

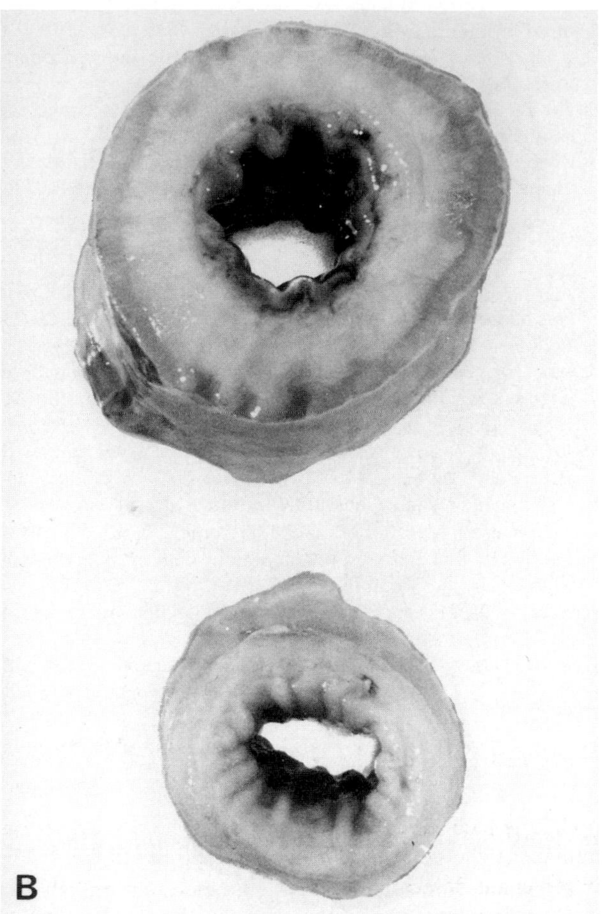

Fig. 1.49B Ileal muscular hypertrophy. Horse. (Normal equine ileum below.)

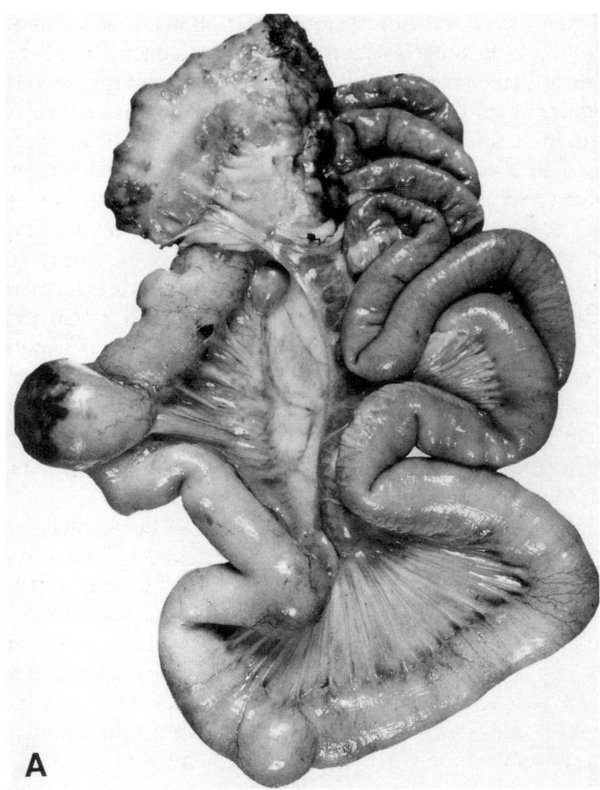

Fig. 1.49A Multiple saccular dilations with impending perforation in muscular hypertrophy of ileum. Pig. (Courtesy of S. Nielsen and the *Journal of the American Veterinary Medical Association*.)

in the muscularis and subserosa of the small intestine. The diverticula tend to follow the pathway of blood vessels and are mainly located adjacent to the mesenteric attachment. Rupture of the diverticula causes peritonitis.

In sheep, diverticulosis occurs independent of muscular hypertrophy, and the most common sites are the duodenum and ileum. Diverticula of mucosa between muscle layers is to be differentiated from congenital diverticula, which resemble intestine in having all layers of the bowel in cross section.

Intestinal emphysema in pigs is a rare condition found mainly in post-weaning pigs. The lesion is usually an incidental finding in slaughtered animals and has no economic significance. It is characterized by numerous thin-walled, gas-filled cystic structures, a few millimeters to several centimeters in diameter, in the gut wall and on the serosal surface (Fig. 1.50). These are located mainly in the small intestine, although the large intestine, mesentery, and mesenteric lymph nodes may be involved. Microscopically, the cystic structures appear to be dilated lymphatics, which are located in the lamina propria, submucosa, muscularis, subserosa, mesentery, and mesenteric lymph

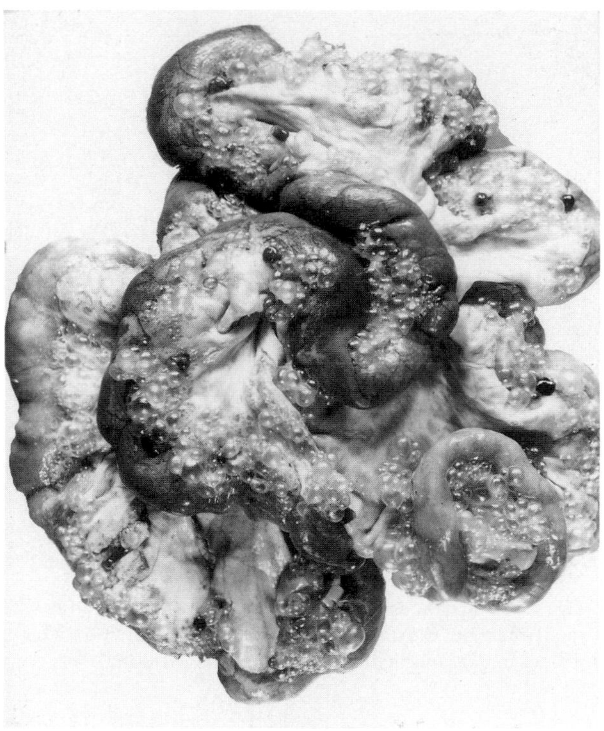

Fig. 1.50 Intestinal emphysema. Pig.

nodes. A pleocellular inflammatory reaction may be evident in the walls of the cysts. Although production of gas by bacteria has been implicated, the cause remains obscure.

Rectal prolapse most commonly occurs in swine, sheep, and cattle. It may occur in any animal which has prolonged episodes of tenesmus or straining, usually associated with colitis or urinary infection or obstruction. In pigs, rectal prolapse occurs as a herd problem when the ration contains zearalenone, an estrogenic mycotoxin produced by fungi of the genus *Fusarium*. The toxin causes marked swelling and congestion of the vulva and vaginal mucosa, which may be followed by vaginal prolapse. Affected pigs strain continuously, and rectal prolapse is a common complication. Rectal prolapse in sheep may be the consequence of ingestion of estrogenic pastures, and is accompanied by other signs of hyperestrogenism (see The Female Genital System, Volume 3, Chapter 4).

The prolapsed rectum is edematous, congested, and there may be necrosis and ulceration of the everted mucosa. These lesions are ischemic in origin because of interference with venous blood flow from the prolapsed section. Only the mucosa, or all layers, may be involved in the prolapse. In swine surviving slough or amputation of the prolapsed tissue, rectal stricture may ensue. Rectal stricture is discussed further with salmonellosis.

Bibliography

Cloutier, R. Intestinal smooth muscle response to chronic obstruction: Possible applications in jejunoileal atresia. *J Pediatr Surg* **10:** 3–8, 1975.

Cordes, D. O., and Dewes, H. F. Diverticulosis and muscular hypertrophy of the small intestine of horses, pigs, and sheep. *N Z Vet J* **19:** 108–111, 1971.

Cordes, D. O., and Mosher, A. H. Brown pigmentation (lipofuscinosis) of intestinal muscularis. *J Pathol Bacteriol* **92:** 197–206, 1966.

Hayes, K. C. *et al.* Vitamin E deficiency and fat stress in the dog. *J Nutr* **99:** 196–209, 1969.

Livesey, M. A., and Keller, S. D. Segmental ischemic necrosis following mesocolic rupture in postparturient mares. *Compend Cont Ed Pract Vet* **8:** 763–768, 1986.

Meyer, R. C., and Simon, J. Intestinal emphysema (pneumatosis cystoides intestinalis) in a gnotobiotic pig. *Can J Comp Med* **41:** 302–305, 1977.

Smith, B. H., and Welter, L. J. Pneumatosis intestinalis. *Am J Clin Pathol* **48:** 455–465, 1967.

E. Intestinal Obstruction

Clinically acute obstruction typically involves the upper or middle small intestine; chronic blockage usually involves the ileum and large bowel. Intestinal obstruction may be the sequel to a physical blockage of the lumen resulting from **stenosis** due to an intrinsic lesion involving the intestinal wall; **obturation** by an intraluminal mass; or **extrinsic compression.** Failure of the intestinal circular smooth muscle to contract blocks the peristaltic wave, causing **functional obstruction,** or pseudo-obstruction, in that there is no luminal occlusion. Ileus is a common sequel to peritoneal irritation, and pain; it occurs proximal to any form of mechanical obstruction. Circulatory embarrassment of a segment of bowel, through embolism or venous infarction, will also cause functional obstruction without a physical blockage. Many of the displacements of gut which produce obstruction, such as volvulus, incarceration, strangulation of a hernia, or intussusception, may cause ischemia. The term **strangulation obstruction** is applied to an event which simultaneously causes ischemia and physically blocks the intestine. Mucosal hypoxia may also be a sequel to venous occlusion resulting from distension of gut proximal to a site of obstruction; it may result from local pressure caused by an adjacent mass; or it may be a sequel to circulatory failure. Ischemia in any circumstance is a serious complication, the pathogenesis of which is dealt with later.

We shall consider first the evolution of the sequelae to intestinal obstruction, then return for a closer look at the various types of blockage. Proximal to the point of obstruction there is accumulation of fluid, derived from ingesta, gastric, biliary, pancreatic, and intrinsic intestinal secretion, and gas, swallowed or originating with bacterial activity in the gut. Intestinal distension results in sequestration of water and electrolyte in the intestinal lumen, edema of the mucosa, further secretion into the gut, and in extreme cases, transudation from the peritoneal surface. Secretion into obstructed gut is stimulated by distension and increased intraluminal pressure, which causes mucosal venous and lymphatic collapse, interstitial edema, and filtration secretion. Secretion may also be stimulated by neurogenic reflexes acting on the epithelium, perhaps through mediation of the secretagogue vasoactive intestinal polypeptide, and by products of bacterial overgrowth in the static bowel. Upper small bowel obstruction progresses rapidly to cause vomiting in those species which can vomit, with dehydration, hypochloremia, hypokalemia, and metabolic alkalosis due to loss of acid in vomitus, or sequestration of fluid in the forestomachs.

Obstruction of the lower small intestine may result in distension with dehydration. But there is usually less acute electrolyte and acid–base imbalance, since vomition is less severe, and absorption of fluid proximal to the obstruction may prevent serious distension and its associated secretion, for some time. Metabolic acidosis eventually ensues following dehydration and catabolism of fat and muscle due to cessation of food consumption and assimilation. Incomplete or slowly developing obstruction may be associated with compensatory muscular hypertrophy proximal to the offending lesion. Incomplete obstruction often becomes total due to progress of the primary lesion or the accumulation of solid digesta. Colonic obstruction may result in accumulation of large quantities of content in the bowel, with considerable abdominal distension.

If ischemia and its complications, including rupture, do not ensue, the animal with acute obstruction succumbs to the systemic effects of hypovolemia, electrolyte and acid–base disturbance. Lower intestinal or colonic obstruction may result in eventual metabolic acidosis and starvation following a chronic course. In the horse particularly, obstruction or impaction of the cecum or colon may result in local ischemia and rupture.

In obstruction the outstanding gross alteration in the bowel is distension proximal to the point of blockage, due to ileus and the accumulation of fluid contents and gas. The location, degree, and duration of the obstruction determines the segment and length of bowel involved and the degree of distension. As distension increases, interference with venous return may develop, and the mucosa and submucosa become congested. Devitalization of severely dilated gut, or pressure necrosis of the mucosa at the site of lodgement of intraluminal foreign bodies, may occur, leading to gangrene or perforation and peritonitis. Distal to the point of obstruction, the bowel is collapsed and empty.

1. Stenosis and Obturation

Intrinsic obstruction due to congenital segmental atresia and imperforations is considered under congenital anomalies of the intestine. **Acquired stenosis** due to pathological processes arising within the wall of the intestine may be partial or complete. The primary lesions include intramural abscesses, intramural hematomas, neoplasms (Fig. 1.51), and scarring following ulceration. Many of these develop slowly with a course as previously described for simple chronic obstruction.

Foreign bodies of all kinds are commonly found. Small, rounded foreign bodies and even some sharp-edged ob-

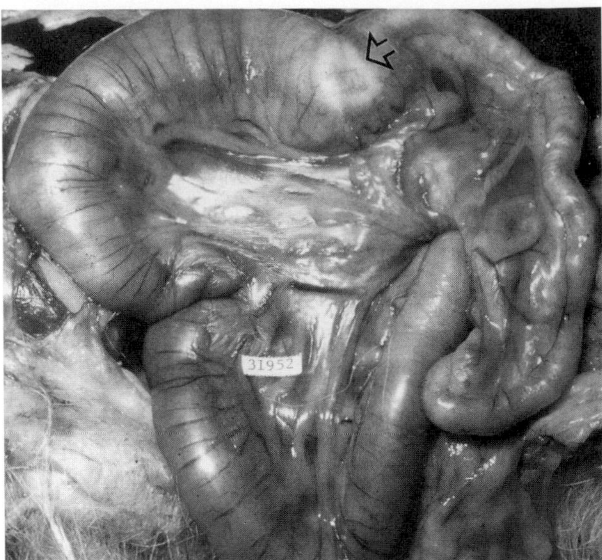

Fig. 1.51 Scirrhous adenocarcinoma (arrow) infiltrating wall of small intestine, causing obstruction. Dog. Dilation proximal to obstruction and contraction of empty distal intestine.

jects may pass through the intestines uneventfully, but for these and many large foreign bodies, the course is unpredictable. Some may reside in the intestine for long periods and produce no disturbance until they act as a nucleus for the development of an enterolith. Sharp-pointed foreign bodies may become impacted in the intestine and cause pressure necrosis with ulceration and possibly perforation. Blunt foreign bodies which become impacted cause acute or chronic obstruction depending on their size and location; often they cause local pressure necrosis, perforation occurring in some cases. **Linear foreign bodies,** such as strips of cloth or string, which are not infrequently ingested by dogs and cats, may pass through the intestine. However, if they become immobilized, they produce a typical lesion. One portion of a string becomes fixed, commonly around the base of the tongue, or by impaction at the pylorus. A free end then is stretched taut distally by peristaltic movements, which pleat the gut on the string (Fig. 1.52A). It progressively cuts into the lesser curvature of intestinal loops, causing first a puckering of the mesentery and finally perforation and peritonitis.

Enteroliths (mineral concretions) were common in the colon of horses in the past, and they seem to be reemerging as a problem in some areas, such as California and Florida. Arabs seem more susceptible than other breeds, and enteroliths usually occur in horses older than 4 years. They are rare in other species. The stones comprise magnesium ammonium phosphate deposited in concentric lamellae, at the center of which there is a nucleus—a foreign body such as a nail, wire, stone, or particle of feed. They vary greatly in size, some weighing as much as 10 kg, and there may be one or more large ones or many small ones. They are usually smooth and often spherical,

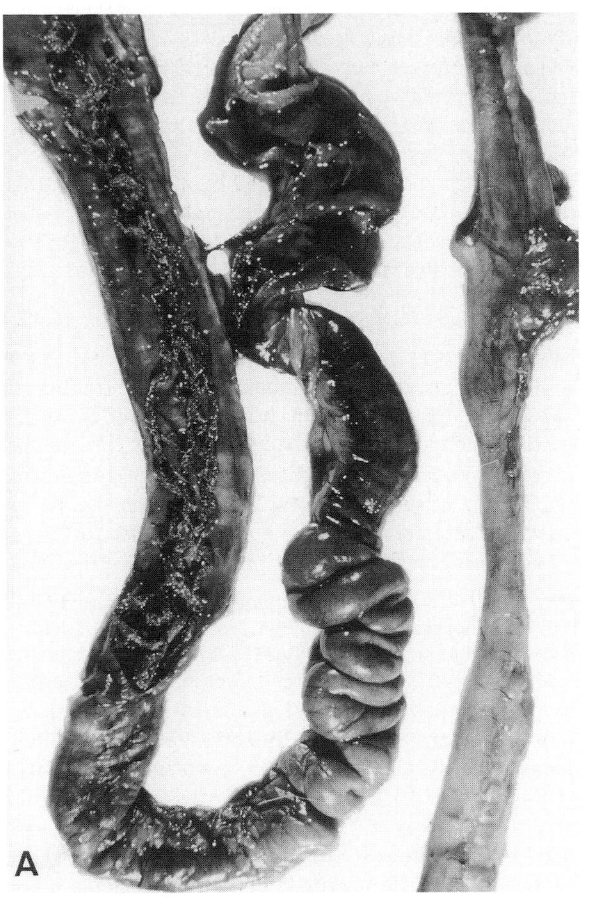

Fig. 1.52A Pleating of the small intestine along a linear foreign body in a cat. The lower segment of bowel is normal (right).

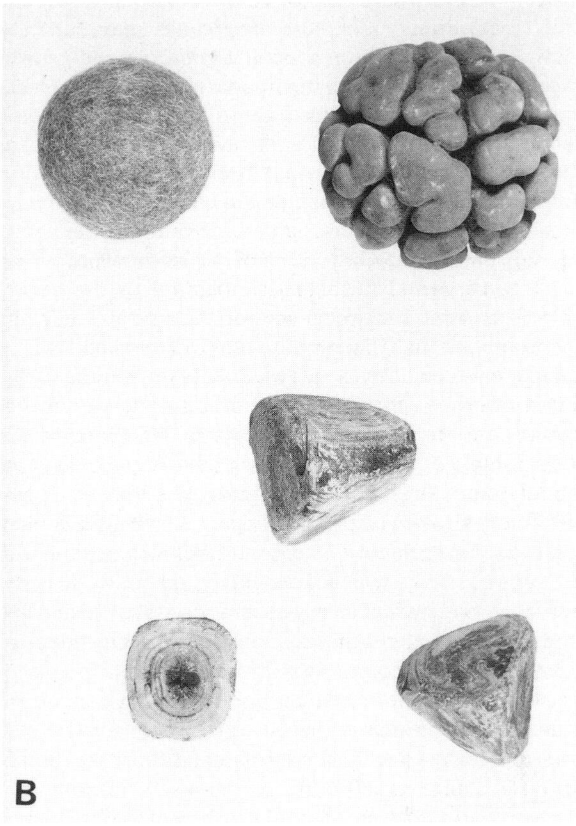

Fig. 1.52B Trichobezoar (top left). Phytobezoar (top right). Enteroliths (below).

but contact with other liths, and abrasion, may smoothly flatten some surfaces (Fig. 1.52B). Irregular mineralized masses may also occur, usually based on a fibrous nidus, such as twine, rope, or netting. The source of the magnesium phosphate is probably grain, bran, alfalfa, or alkaline water. The mineral salts deposit around a nidus under poorly understood circumstances, but colonic pH above 6.6 seems to contribute to their formation.

Fiber balls (**phytobezoars** or phytotrichobezoars), which consist largely of plant fibers impregnated with some phosphate salt, may be found in the colon of horses, especially. They are not as heavy as enteroliths, are moist, and have a velvety surface. They are usually round and smooth, but some are convoluted like the surface of the cerebrum (Fig. 1.52B). Hair balls (**trichobezoars**) sometimes occur in dogs and cats and in ruminants; in the latter they occur in the forestomachs and abomasum. They may obstruct the pylorus, but rarely cause problems in the intestine.

Enteroliths and bezoars in horses are usually not significant, and small ones may pass in the feces. Apparently they are moved about enough by peristalsis to avoid pressure necrosis. They may obstruct the gut when they are impacted, usually where the colon narrows, in the pelvic flexure and transverse or small colon.

Small intestinal obstruction may be caused by parasites, which can form ropelike tangled masses in the lumen. This is may occur in pigs and foals infested with large numbers of ascarids. It also occurs rarely in sheep heavily infested with tapeworms. Impaction of the equine small intestine has been caused by wood ingested by horses which crib, cracked corn, and high-fiber feed, such as Bermuda grass. Content in the affected region is relatively inspissated, and doughy to firm in consistency. The ileum is the common site of impaction obstruction in the equine small bowel, but any level may be involved.

Impaction of the colon, by feces in dogs and cats, and by digesta, fibrous foreign material, sand, or feces in horses, is not uncommon and causes a simple intestinal obstruction, complicated in the horse by intestinal tympany from fermentative gases if the obstruction is complete. In dogs, obstipation of the colon may be the result of voluntarily suppressed painful defecation, as in prostatic enlargement and inflammation of the anal sacs. Occasionally, it is due to an impaction with foreign bodies, especially hair or fine bones in the colon or rectum, or due to stenosis caused by tumors or strictures. It may also complicate trauma to the pelvic area, and paralyzing lesions of the spinal cord; it may occur in Manx cats due to sacral spinal cord anomalies. **Megacolon** may ensue, if the obstruction persists. In small animals, megacolon is frequently idiopathic, with no organic or physical explanation. Lesions of the myenteric plexus have not been convincingly implicated, and the physiologic integrity of the colonic nervous system has not been examined.

Impaction of the cecum or colon in horses may be precipitated by water deprivation, a change of diet from something soft and lush to hay or chaff, or poor dentition. In animals with dental problems, impaction of the cecum may be recurrent, and cecal smooth muscle may become hypertrophic. Abnormal motility due to altered colonic or cecal pacemaker activity may explain impaction in the absence of other predisposing causes. The acaricide amitraz may cause impaction in this way. In the colon, fibrous digesta usually impacts at the pelvic flexure, or transverse or small colon. Ingestion of indigestible synthetic fibers, in the form of rope, or pieces of conveyor belt, has been associated with colonic impaction. **Sand** may sediment in the colons of horses which have grazed on poorly covered sandy soils. Sand may cause a chronic colitis with diarrhea and weight loss, or it may accumulate at any level of the large or small colon, causing one or more points of impaction obstruction, often associated with concurrent displacement or torsion. Ingestion of large numbers of acorns and leaves may also cause impaction of the intestinal tract in ruminants. Rupture of the viscus may occur if impactions are not treated, and the bowel wall becomes ischemic and devitalized.

Cecal rupture in horses occurs as a complication of impaction, and of parturition in mares. Idiopathic cecal rupture, associated with overload of normal digesta, rather than impaction, is also reported, sometimes as a complication of general anesthesia. Also termed cecal dysfunction, cecal overload is differentiated from impaction by the more fluid consistency of the contents. The cecum is distended, and the mucosa may be hyperemic and somewhat thickened at surgery. Disordered motility with increased intracecal pressure has been invoked speculatively to explain subsequent cecal rupture. The lacerations of the cecum in this circumstance are reported on the medial aspect at some distance from the base, but this is not consistent.

2. *Extrinsic Obstruction*

Compression of intestine causing obstruction is rather common and is caused by tumors, abscesses, peritonitis, and fibrous adhesions. **Neoplasms** involve the intestine by extension from adjacent viscera, particularly pancreas. Therefore, many tumors involve the anterior dorsal part of the abdominal cavity and impinge on the duodenum. Inflammatory peritoneal **adhesions** are common, and fibrous bands may stretch from the wall of the bowel to some fixed point, or between two or more points along the bowel or mesentery; the obstruction develops gradually as scarring ties the bowel down or puts kinks in the mesentery. Large firm masses of **abdominal fat necrosis** cause compression stenosis of small intestine, coiled colon, and particularly descending colon and rectum of cattle. **Pedicles of some tumors,** especially mesenteric lipomas in older horses, occasionally become wound about loops of intestine and cause obstruction and strangulation. Similarly, the **suspensory ligaments of the ovary** may entrap the equine colon if the ovary is enlarged by neoplasia or other phenomena. Incarceration in hernias, discussed with other displacements of the bowel, is also a common cause of compression obstruction of the gut.

3. *Functional Obstruction*

Paralytic ileus is in itself not of specific interest to the pathologist but is a rather common condition. It frequently follows abdominal surgery in transient episodes, especially when the intestines are handled roughly, or traumatized. It also occurs in peritoneal irritation of any cause, especially in peritonitis. It is the result of neurogenic reflexes which interfere with control of the inhibitory neurons of the myenteric plexus. Continual tonic discharge by these neurons inhibits contraction of circular smooth muscle and prevents peristalsis.

The intestines are distended with a mixture of gas and fluid, and the wall is flaccid. The defect may be segmental, involving less than a meter of the intestinal length, but there may be many such segments involved, especially in diffuse peritonitis. Gastric rupture may occur in the horse as a complication of obstructive or postoperative ileus of the small intestine.

Pseudo-obstruction, a clinical syndrome in which there is no physical occlusion of the lumen of an impacted intestine, may result from segmental or diffuse neuromuscular dysfunction in the gut. It overlaps in part with paralytic ileus, and with elements of impaction and megacolon related to intestinal dysmotility, as previously discussed. Pseudo-obstruction associated with neuronal hypocellularity or ganglioneuritis involving autonomic ganglia in the gastrointestinal tract, systemic dysautonomia, and intrinsic disease of intestinal smooth muscle, are recognized among domestic animals, in addition to congenital aganglionosis of spotted foals, discussed earlier. Occasionally a segment of contracted bowel is noted, causing obstruction; more commonly, in neurogenic disease, affected bowel is dilated, flaccid, and incapable of maintaining tone.

Ganglioneuritis involving submucosal, myenteric, and other autonomic ganglia has been associated with disordered motility, usually pseudo-obstruction, but occasionally diarrhea, in cattle, horses, and dogs. In dogs, a syndrome resembling dysautonomia, described subsequently, is reported, rarely. The bowel is segmentally or diffusely dilated, flaccid and full of content of normal or somewhat inspissated consistency. The diagnosis is based on a mixed or mainly mononuclear inflammatory cell infiltrate, associated with degeneration and necrosis of neurons, in ganglia of the enteric autonomic plexuses, and often in other autonomic ganglia. In some animals, it is evident that autonomic dysfunction, and probably lesions, extend beyond the enteric nervous system; a thorough examination of the autonomic and central nervous system is warranted in suspect cases. The etiology is usually unidentified. In one outbreak in dogs, pseudorabies virus was implicated; in humans with similar syndromes associated with Chagas' disease and small-cell carcinoma of the lung, autoimmune phenomena are suspected. Since inflammatory processes may be transient, some cases of enteric hypoganglionosis may represent resolved ganglioneuritis.

Megacolon in Clydesdale foals, in association with hypoganglionosis of the myenteric plexus, has been reported from the United States and Australia in animals 4–9 months of age. The dorsal colons were markedly dilated, and the intestinal wall, thin. Small colon was patent but devoid of content. Ganglion cells of the myenteric plexus in the transverse and small colons were reduced or absent. There was variation in ganglion cell density in the dorsal colon; in two cases they were present, whereas in the third, they were markedly reduced in number. Inflammation was not noted. The time of clinical onset of these cases suggests that they may not have been congenital. The common breed suggests a possible genetic basis for the syndrome. If the lesion is acquired, the factors causing myenteric ganglion cell loss are unknown.

Grass sickness in horses, which seems to be the prototypic **dysautonomia** in domestic animals, occurs chiefly in parts of the United Kingdom and western Europe, usually in animals at pasture. Although horses of any age may be afflicted, the disease is more common in those 3–6 years of age. Affected animals are dull but show occasional bouts of colicky restlessness. In the acute disease, there is progressively severe tympany, swallowing is avoided, and saliva drools freely. Any attempt to swallow is apparently painful and stimulates reverse peristalsis in the esophagus. Fine muscular tremors develop over the shoulders, and there is sweating. The course in acute cases is from 12 to 72 hr. Some survive the acute phase to live much longer, but die in due course of the disease.

Lesions at necropsy are confined to the alimentary tract. The esophageal wall is sometimes edematous, and the mucosa may show longitudinal bands of congestion and ulceration, which may extend into the stomach. The stomach is distended with fluid (as much as 22 liters have been measured), often of khaki color and peasoup consistency, although sometimes more watery with fibrous material. This fluid is alkaline and mucinous. Sometimes the stomach is ruptured. There may also be a excess fluid in the small intestine. The large intestine is impacted with dry contents, and the fecal pellets in the small colon are small and dry. These masses may have a surface blackened by a small amount of exuded blood. In chronic cases, the volume of alimentary content is reduced to scant amounts in the stomach and small intestine, and the content of the large intestine is soupy.

The cause of grass sickness is speculative. Degenerative lesions, marked by often subtle chromatolysis, nuclear eccentricity, and neuronal necrosis, and the formation of perineuronal eosinophilic axonal spheroids, have been described in many autonomic ganglia, especially the celiacomesenteric, as well as in some central neuronal nuclei. Significant inflammation is not evident. Transfusion of whole blood from donor horses which show clinical signs of grass sickness, or injection of a putative neurotoxin, into ponies, results in lesions in the autonomic ganglia that are similar to those present in spontaneous cases. However, the ponies remain clinically normal. These observations suggest that relatively high plasma concentrations of the neurotoxic factor are required to cause clinical signs, or that the microscopic neuronal lesions are an epiphenomenon.

It is, however, difficult to avoid the conclusion that this disease is, in the final analysis, pseudo-obstruction due to dysautonomia. Its differentiation from primary colonic impaction may be difficult.

Feline dysautonomia, or Key–Gaskell syndrome, is a recently recognized autonomic dysfunction of unknown etiology, most common in the United Kingdom and Europe, with sporadic cases reported elsewhere. A similar syndrome has also been reported in a few dogs. All age groups are affected. Signs include depression, anorexia, reduced lacrimation and salivation, bradycardia, pupillary dilation with delayed pupillary light reflex, megaesophagus, constipation, and rarely, ileal impaction. Diarrhea is reported in some dogs with dysautonomia. The gastrointestinal signs suggest disordered motility, and animals often succumb to the effects of regurgitation, inanition, or aspiration pneumonia, among other problems.

Involvement of functions controlled by both sympathetic and parasympathetic divisions of the autonomic nervous system, and of some functions under voluntary control, is reflected in the distribution of neuronal lesions in ganglia of the autonomic system, and in cranial nerve nuclei III, V, VII, and XII, ventral horns of the spinal gray matter, and in dorsal root ganglia. Chromatolysislike lesions of affected neurons seen by light microscopy have a distinctive ultrastructural appearance in dysautonomia. Autophagocytic vacuoles, large cisternae, and complex stacks of smooth endoplasmic membranes are in the cytoplasm of affected cells. Neuronal lesions and subsequent drop-out may be transient, and in the later stages of the disease, diagnosis may need to be based on comparative cell counts in ganglia of affected and unaffected cats, unless neuronal loss has been obviously severe. Peptides secreted by neurons of the enteric nervous system, especially vasoactive intestinal polypeptide, are depleted in this condition, presumably reflecting autonomic dysfunction.

Intrinsic disease of intestinal smooth muscle may produce a syndrome of **intestinal sclerosis,** somewhat resembling that in progressive systemic sclerosis or scleroderma of humans. However, in dogs the lesions are restricted to the intestinal tract, where they usually appear to involve the small and large bowel diffusely. There is usually mild to obvious dilation of the bowel. In section, there is a mononuclear inflammatory infiltrate among smooth muscle fibers in the circular and longitudinal layers of the bowel wall. Associated with this is interstitial fibrosis, and atrophy of smooth muscle cells. In one case, sclerosis involved the smooth muscle of the muscularis mucosae, with fibrosis of the mucosa and superficial submucosa. The muscularis externa was not inflamed or sclerotic, the circular layer was hypertrophic, and the bowel appeared thickened grossly. The etiology is unknown, but the enteric nervous system seems not to be involved.

Bibliography

Adams, S. B. Recognition and management of ileus. *Vet Clin North Am: Equine Pract* **4:** 91–104, 1988.

Allen, D., Swanyne, D., and Belknap, J. K. Ganglioneuroma as a cause of small intestinal obstruction in the horse: A case report. *Cornell Vet* **79:** 133–141, 1989.

Allen, D. A. *et al.* Morphologic effects of experimental distention of the equine small intestine. *Vet Surg* **17:** 10–14, 1988.

Andrews, F. M., and Robertson, J. T. Diagnosis and surgical treatment of functional obstruction of the right dorsal colon in a horse. *J Am Vet Med Assoc* **193:** 956–958, 1988.

Baker, J. S. *et al.* Postpartum atony of the small and large intestine in a Holstein cow: A case of pseudo-obstruction. *Cornell Vet* **75:** 289–296, 1985.

Basson, M. D. *et al.* Does vasoactive intestinal polypeptide mediate the pathophysiology of bowel obstruction? *Am J Surg* **157:** 109–115, 1989.

Bertone, J. J. *et al.* Diarrhea associated with sand in the gastrointestinal tract of horses. *J Am Vet Med Assoc* **193:** 1409–1412, 1988.

Bohanon, T. C. Duodenal impaction in a horse. *J Am Vet Med Assoc* **192:** 365–366, 1988.

Boles, C. L., and Kohn, C. W. Fibrous foreign body impaction in young horses. *J Am Vet Med Assoc* **171:** 193–195, 1977.

Burns, G. A. *et al.* Equine myenteric ganglionitis: A case of chronic intestinal pseudo-obstruction. *Cornell Vet* **80:** 53–63, 1990.

Campbell, M. L. *et al.* Cecal impaction in the horse. *J Am Vet Med Assoc* **184:** 950–952, 1984.

Dimski, D. S. Constipation: Pathophysiology, diagnostic approach and treatment. *Sem Vet Med Surg (Small Anim)* **4:** 247–254, 1989.

Ducharme, N. G. *et al.* Small intestinal obstruction caused by a persistent round ligament of the liver in a cow. *J Am Vet Med Assoc* **180:** 1234–1236, 1982.

Dyke, T. M. *et al.* Megacolon in two related Clydesdale foals. *Aust Vet J* **67:** 463–464, 1990.

Edney, A. T. B. *et al.* Feline dysautonomia—an emerging disease. *J Small Anim Pract* **28:** 333–378, 1987.

Edwards, J. F., and Ruoff, W. W. Idiopathic cecal rupture in foals after anesthesia for gastric endoscopy. *J Am Vet Med Assoc* **198:** 1421–1422, 1991.

Evard, J. H. *et al.* Ovarian strangulation as a cause of small colon obstruction in a foal. *Equine Vet J* **20:** 217–218, 1988.

Gay, C. C. *et al.* Foreign body obstruction of the small colon in six horses. *Equine Vet J* **11:** 60–62, 1979.

Gilmour, J. S. Equine dysautonomia: Epidemiology and pathology. *J Small Anim Pract* **28:** 373–378, 1987.

Green, P., and Tong, J. M. Small intestinal obstruction with wood chewing in two horses. *Vet Rec* **123:** 196–198, 1988.

Guilford, W. G. The enteric nervous system: Function, dysfunction, and pharmacological manipulation. *Sem Vet Med Surg (Small Anim)* **5:** 46–56, 1990.

Hilbert, B. J. *et al.* Caecal overload and rupture in the horse. *Aust Vet J* **64:** 85–86, 1987.

Hintz, H. F. *et al.* Studies on equine enterolithiasis. *Proc Am Assoc Equine Pract* **34:** 53–59, 1989.

Hoskins, J. D. Managment of fecal impaction. *Compend Cont Ed Pract Vet* **12:** 1579–1585, 1990.

Howell, J. *et al.* Observations on the coeliaco-mesenteric ganglia of horses with and without grass sickness. *Br Vet J* **130:** 265–270, 1974.

Kelly, D. F. Pathological aspects of dysautonomia. *J Small Anim Pract* **28:** 407–416, 1987.

Krishnamurthy, S., and Schuffler, M. D. Pathology of neuromuscular disorders of the small intestine and colon. *Gastroenterology* **93:** 610–639, 1987.

Livingstone, E. H., and Passaro, E. P. Postoperative ileus. *Dig Dis Sci* **35:** 121–132, 1990.

Lloyd, K. *et al.* Enteroliths in horses. *Cornell Vet* **77:** 172–186, 1987.

Moore, R., and Carpenter, J. Intramural intestinal hematoma causing obstruction in three dogs. *J Am Vet Med Assoc* **184:** 186–188, 1984.

Moore, R., and Carpenter, J. Intestinal sclerosis with pseudo-obstruction in three dogs. *J Am Vet Med Assoc* **184:** 830–833, 1984.

Parks, A. H. *et al.* Ileal impaction in the horse: 75 cases. *Cornell Vet* **79:** 83–91, 1989.

Pinsent, P. J. N. Grass sickness of horses (grass disease: Equine dysautonomia). *Vet Ann* **29:** 169–174, 1989.

Platt, H. Caecal rupture in parturient mares. *J Comp Pathol* **93:** 343–346, 1983.

Richardson, D. W. Paraovarian–omental bands as a cause of small intestinal obstruction in cows. *J Am Vet Med Assoc* **185:** 517–519, 1984.

Rosin, E. *et al.* Subtotal colectomy for treatment of chronic constipation associated with idiopathic megacolon in cats: 38 cases (1979–1985). *J Am Vet Med Assoc* **193:** 850–853, 1988.

Ross, M. W. *et al.* Cecal perforation in the horse. *J Am Vet Med Assoc* **187:** 249–253, 1985.

Sellers, A. F., and Lowe, J. E. Review of large intestinal motility and mechanisms of impaction in the horse. *Equine Vet J* **18:** 261–263, 1986.

Sharp, N. J. H. Feline dysautonomia. *Sem Vet Med Surg (Small Anim)* **5:** 67–71, 1990.

Specht, T. E., and Colahan, P. T. Surgical treatment of sand colic in equids: 48 cases (1978–1985). *J Am Vet Med Assoc* **193:** 1560–1564, 1988.

Strombeck, D. R., and Guilford, W. G. "Small Animal Gastroenterology," 2nd Ed., Davis, California, Stonegate Publishing, 1990.

Swayne, D. E. *et al.* Sclerosing enteropathy in a dog. *Vet Pathol* **23:** 641–643, 1986.

van Wuijckhuise-Sjouke, L. A. Three cases of obstruction of the small colon by a foreign body. *Vet Q* **6:** 1–37, 1984.

White, N. A. (ed.) "The Equine Acute Abdomen." Philadelphia, Pennsylvania, Lea & Febiger, 1990.

Willard, M. D. *et al.* Diarrhea associated with myenteric ganglionitis in a dog. *J Am Vet Med Assoc* **193:** 346–348, 1988.

Wise, L. A.. and Lappin, M. R. A syndrome resembling feline dysautonomia (Key–Gaskell syndrome) in a dog. *J Am Vet Med Assoc* **198:** 2103–2106, 1991.

Wright, J. A., and Hodson, N. P. Pathological changes in the brain in equine grass sickness. *J Comp Pathol* **98:** 247–252, 1988.

F. Displacements of the Intestines

1. Eventration

Eventration is displacement of a portion of the gut, usually the small intestine, outside the abdominal cavity. This is commonly congenital as in schistosomus reflexus, patent umbilicus, and congenital diaphragmatic hernia. Acquired eventrations result from trauma, and therefore are varied. In some cases, the displaced intestine herniates into the abdominal muscle or subcutis, or it may be completely exteriorized. Vaginal evisceration may occasionally occur in females following trauma induced by breeding, parturition, or bestiality. The bowel may protrude through a lacerated vaginal fornix, or through a ruptured everted bladder.

2. Cecal and Colonic Dilation, Tympany, and Torsion

In **ruminants, cecal dilation and torsion** is an uncommon condition. It occurs mainly in animals fed high-concentrate rations, but it has been associated with late gestation, and ileus from other causes. It usually occurs within 2 months postpartum in cattle. It is rare in other ruminants. About 30% of the carbohydrates in the ration are digested in the cecum of ruminants. Sudden change from a roughage to a grain-based ration results in an increase in the concentration of volatile fatty acids, with only a slight decrease in pH of the cecal contents. An increase in the concentration of dissociated volatile fatty acids, especially butyric acid, causes atony of the cecum, and dilation follows. Once the cecum is dilated and distended with watery digesta, various degrees of clockwise or counterclockwise rotation can occur, which may incorporate adjacent viscera, particularly terminal ileum and a loop of distal jejunum. Obstruction ensues, and the cecum may become strangulated.

In **horses, cecal and colonic tympany** has a similar pathogenesis. Readily fermentable carbohydrate, following a sudden change in feed, results in an increase in volatile fatty acid production, which exceeds the buffering and absorptive capacity of the organ. As the pH drops, and fermentation shifts to production of the less well absorbed butyric and lactic acids, water is drawn into the lumen by the osmotic effect. The large bowel dilates with fluid digesta and gas, and motility is reduced by the effects of the volatile fatty acids. Severe abdominal distension, compression of intra-abdominal organs, reduced cardiac return due to postcaval compression, and reduced respiratory capacity due to compression of the diaphragm, may follow, with attendant severe pain. Death due to hypovolemia and acidosis may occur before the large bowel ruptures. In recovered horses, laminitis may occur, owing to absorption of endotoxin through the cecal mucosa, which becomes eroded and permeable as a result of local acidosis.

3. Displacements of the Equine Colon

The large colon of the horse comprises a loop of capacious bowel joined along its length by the short mesocolon, and folded upon itself at the sternal, pelvic, and diaphragmatic flexures. The loop is fixed only at its base, by the cecum, the transverse colon, and mesenteric root. Its volume and lack of attachment make the large colon prone to displacement or torsion.

Right dorsal displacement of the colon is of unknown etiology. It presumably results from displacement and wedging of the large colon due to tympany. The left colon may become displaced clockwise (in the standing animal viewed from above) to the right of the cecum as the pelvic flexure migrates cranial to the cecal root, caudad and to the left across the pelvic inlet, and craniad on the left side, coming to rest at the sternum. This is termed right dorsal displacement with flexion. Alternatively, the left colon may move in the opposite direction, caudal and to the right of the base of the cecum, with the pelvic flexure again lying at the sternum. This is termed right dorsal displacement with medial flexion. Some degree of torsion may also occur, and obstruction, with mild to severe colic, ensues. Surgery is required to correct the displacement.

Left dorsal displacement of the colon, variously known as entrapment of the colon by the nephrosplenic, renosplenic, or phrenicosplenic ligament, or by the suspensory ligament of the spleen, is also encountered as a cause of obstruction and colic in horses (Fig. 1.53A,B). The left dorsal and ventral colon move laterally and dorsally between the spleen and the left body wall, and become trapped, with the spleen to the left and below, the suspensory ligament of the spleen below, the left kidney on the medial aspect, and the abdominal wall dorsally. The sternal and diaphragmatic flexures may be in their normal position, ventral to the stomach, or they may have moved cranially and become displaced dorsal to the stomach. The colon caudal to the entrapment may become curved cranially, with the pelvic flexure rotated through 180°, because of tension on the taeniae. The stomach and spleen may be displaced caudally and ventromedially, if the flexures have become displaced dorsally into the space cranial to the stomach, in apposition with the left lobe of the liver. If the colon has moved dorsal to it, the stomach often becomes grossly distended, as a result of compression of the esophagus and the duodenal outflow by the incarcerated colon. Compression of the colon at the point of entrapment can cause local bruising or edema and partial ischemia of the displaced organ, and results in obstruction, which may be incomplete. The cecum and small intestine may be distended as a result of the colonic obstruction. The cause of left dorsal displacement is unknown, but may be related to an anatomic predisposition resulting from a large cleft between the spleen and the left kidney. Surgical intervention is frequently necessary for resolution, though some cases may be cured by rolling the anesthetized horse.

Abnormal flexion of the cecum and/or colon also may occur in the horse. The pelvic flexure may be displaced medially, laterally, or dorsally. The tip of the cecum may similarly bend upon itself. In displacement of both organs, there is the risk of vascular embarrassment and infarction due to kinking of the bowel.

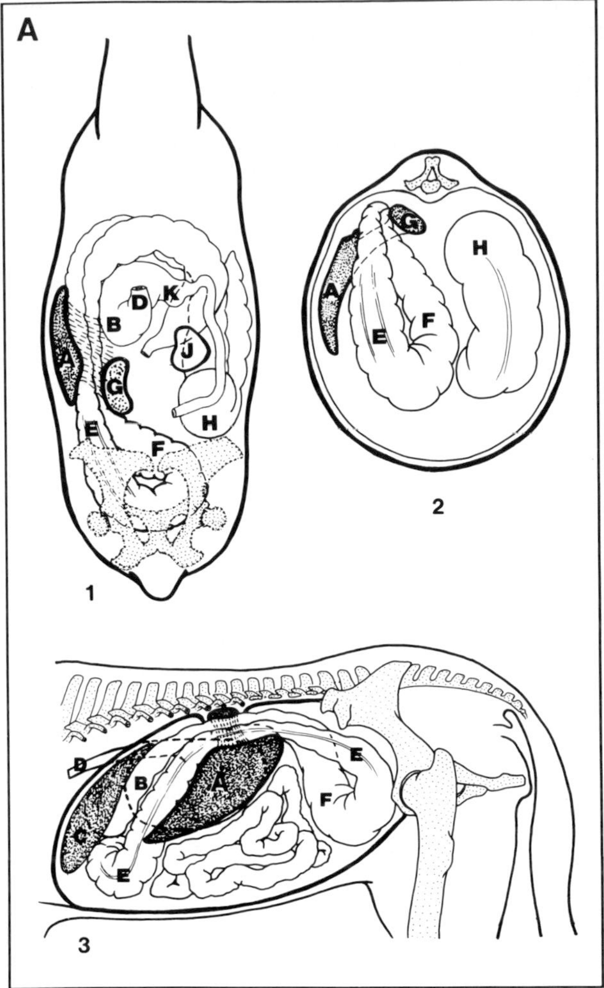

Fig. 1.53 Left dorsal displacement (nephrosplenic entrapment) of the equine colon. (A) 1, 2, 3, entrapment with the sternal and diaphragmatic flexures of the colon below the stomach.

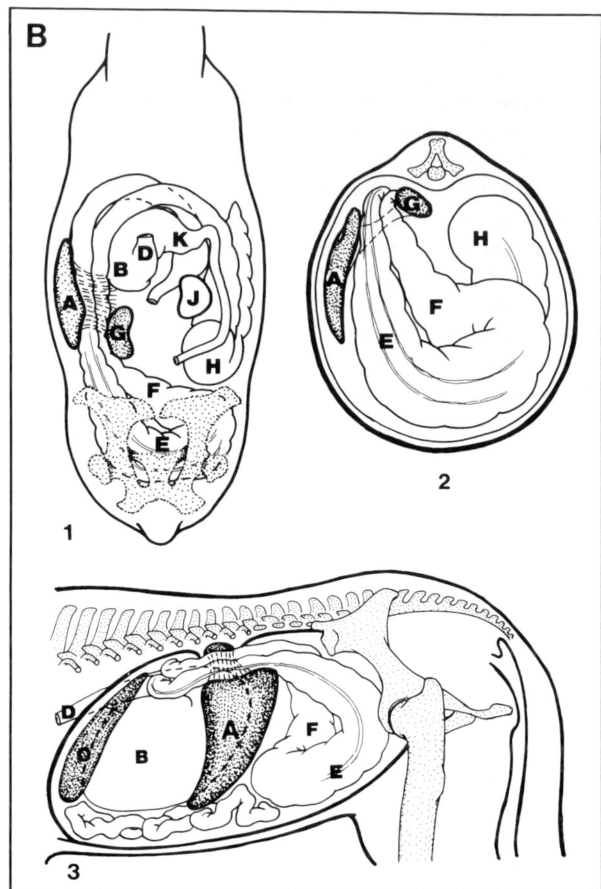

Fig. 1.53B 1, 2, 3, entrapment with the sternal and diaphragmatic flexures displaced dorsal to the stomach. A, spleen; B, stomach; C, liver; D, esophagus; E, left ventral colon; F, left dorsal colon; G, left kidney; H, base of cecum; J, right kidney; K, duodenum. (Reprinted with permission from M. A. Livesey *et al., Can Vet J* **29:** 135–141, 1988).

4. Internal Hernia

This is a displacement of intestine through normal or pathological foramina within the abdominal cavity without the formation of a hernial sac. It is uncommon.

Herniation through a natural foramen occurs mainly in horses. In right-to-left **incarceration in the epiploic foramen,** a portion of small intestine, usually distal jejunum and ileum, may pass down into the omental bursa and become incarcerated, if the normally short and slitlike epiploic foramen of Winslow is dilated for any reason. In these circumstances, the wall of the omental bursa often ruptures. Less commonly, the herniation occurs in a left-to-right direction, the gut carrying the omentum retrograde over the portal vein and out through the bursa to the right side, where it becomes incarcerated.

Omental hernia occurs when a loop of intestine passes through a tear in the greater or lesser omentum. **Mesenteric hernia** is due to passage of intestine through a tear in the mesentery. These are probably traumatic defects and usually involve the mesentery of the small intestine, but occasionally, that of the colon.

Pelvic hernia, sometimes referred to as gut-tie, occurs in young ruminants, and rarely in other species, following castration. During the operation, excessive traction on the spermatic cord may tear the peritoneal fold of the ductus deferens (mesoductus), which fixes the duct to the pelvic wall. A hiatus is formed between the ductus deferens and the lateral abdominal or pelvic walls and, through it, loops of intestine may become incarcerated.

Gut may also become incarcerated by passing through lacerations in the lateral ligament of the bladder, by the remnant of a persistent urachus, and by the gastrosplenic ligament, and mesodiverticular or vitelloumbilical bands in the horse.

5. External Hernia

External hernia typically consists of a hernial sac formed as a pouch of parietal peritoneum; a covering of skin and soft tissues; depending on the location of the hernia, a hernial ring; and the hernial contents. The hernial ring is an opening in the abdominal wall, and this may be acquired, or it may be natural as, for example, the vaginal ring at the inguinal canal. The hernia usually contains a portion of omentum, a freely mobile portion of the intestine, and occasionally, other viscera.

Ventral hernia of the abdominal wall occurs uncommonly in horses, rarely in cattle, and exceptionally in other species, except perhaps following blunt trauma in small animals. These hernias, through the abdominal musculature into the subcutaneous tissue, may be spontaneous in heavily pregnant females, or be a consequence of blunt trauma, horn injuries, surgical scars, or inflammations, which cause weakening or perforation of the muscle. In pregnant mares, they often occur in the lower flank lateral to the mammae, where there is only a single layer of muscle, the transverse abdominal. They may become very large in herbivores because of the weight of the alimentary viscera and pregnant uterus. The lesion must be differentiated from rupture of the prepubic tendon, and from postmortem rupture of abdominal muscle in bloated animals.

Umbilical hernia is common and is often present as a congenital and perhaps inherited defect. It is most frequent in pigs, foals, calves, and pups, and depends on persistent patency of the umbilical ring. The hernial sac is formed by peritoneum and skin; the contents depend on the size of the ring and of the sac. Incarceration of enclosed intestine is uncommon. **Parietal hernia,** in which only the antimesenteric portion of the circumference of the bowel is incarcerated, may convert to umbilical abscess or enterocutaneous fistula if the incarcerated bowel wall undergoes necrosis.

Inguinal hernia may evolve to **scrotal hernia** when the herniated viscera pass down the inguinal canal. The internal, or deep, inguinal ring remains patent in intact male animals, but its diameter and the tendency to herniation in the neonate may be inherited. Inguinal hernias are of several types, based on whether the herniated viscus passes down the inguinal canal within or outside the parietal vaginal tunic.

Indirect inguinal hernia is by far the most common form, occurring as a congenital problem in the young of many species, and as an acquired problem in older animals. Although size of the inguinal rings may be a factor in neonates, there is usually no apparent cause in acquired cases. The herniated viscus passes through the inguinal and vaginal rings within the vaginal sheath, coming to lie in the scrotum inside the cavity of the tunica vaginalis. If the hernia is scrotal, there may be degeneration of the testicles. Routine castration of such animals can lead to eventration through the scrotal incision, and closed castration may cause infarction of the herniated loop of gut.

Congenital inguinal hernia is rare in dogs; West Highland whites, Pekingese, and basenjis may be predisposed, and they are more common in males than females. However, overall, inguinal hernia is much more common in female dogs. The bitch differs from females of other species in having a patent inguinal ring and canal, through which the omentum and the uterus may pass. The herniated uterus may become incarcerated when pregnant, or if pyometra develops.

Direct, or false, inguinal hernias may also develop in males, especially horses. The displaced viscus does not pass within the cavity of the tunica vaginalis, but outside it, in a subcutaneous position. The rupture in the serosa may occur in the peritoneum and transverse fascia overlying the deep inguinal ring, causing an inguinal rupture, encountered occasionally in stallions. Alternatively, it may occur in the inguinal canal, as a complication of what was probably originally an indirect hernia, causing a ruptured inguinal hernia; this is usually seen in foals. Direct hernias are the result of increased intra-abdonimal pressure, and in foals in which ruptured inguinal hernia is recognized postpartum, the problem is probably initiated by the pressure in the birth canal.

Differentiation of indirect hernias and ruptured inguinal hernias is significant in the management and prognosis of the cases. Indirect hernias in neonatal foals are unlikely to strangulate, and usually self-reduce with time. Ruptured inguinal hernias are life-threatening. They cause necrosis of the overlying skin, which becomes edematous and friable, due to disruption of the blood supply. And they tend to become fixed in the subcutaneous tissues by adhesions, becoming irreducible, and more prone to strangulation.

Femoral hernias develop as an outpouching of peritoneum through the femoral triangle along the course of the femoral artery. They contain omentum and small intestine.

Perineal hernias occur principally in old male dogs in association with prostatic enlargement and obstipation. They are precipitated by abdominal straining and are probably predisposed to by weakening of perineal fascia and muscles from some unknown cause, possibly hormonal. They are very unusual in females. Retroperitoneal pelvic fat bulges through a defect between the coccygeus medialis muscle and the anterior border of the anal sphincter. Usually this is the only tissue to prolapse, and the lesion consists, essentially, of a loss of support on one side of the anal ring. Concomitant with the loss of pelvic support, the rectum deviates, and the prostate and the bladder may move into the pelvis. Further displacement may occur occasionally, and then the latter organs are forced through the ruptured perineal fascia, causing acute urethral obstruction. Perineal hernias are most commonly unilateral, but bilateral hernias may occur.

Diaphragmatic hernias are common. The defect in the diaphragm may be congenital, but most often it is acquired, generally as the result of increased abdominal pressure. Though abdominal viscera pass into the thoracic cavity, strangulation of displaced gut is rare. Congenital and acquired diaphragmatic hernias are considered more fully in the chapter on the peritoneal cavity (Chapter 4 of this volume).

The **sequelae of hernias** depend largely on their location and content, but some generalities apply to all. As long as the hernial contents remain freely movable and reducible, there may be no untoward sequelae. Fixation of the hernial contents (incarceration) is a serious development. Incarceration may result from stenosis or tension of the hernial ring, adhesion between the contents and the sac, or distension of the herniated viscus. This distension may be due to accumulated gas or ingesta in the intestine, urine in a herniated bladder, and fetuses or pus in a herniated uterus. The pressure which promotes incarceration is probably mainly the result of tension of the vaginal ring, rather than at the inner or outer inguinal rings, in indirect hernias. This pressure impairs venous drainage; the resulting edema increases the bulk of the tissue, so that it becomes incarcerated. Incarcerated intestine may become obstructed, undergo ischemic necrosis, and perforate, causing peritonitis. Small bowel fixed at one point by incarceration may be predisposed to volvulus.

Bibliography

Baird, A. N. *et al.* Renosplenic entrapment of the large colon in horses: 57 cases (1983–1988). *J Am Vet Med Assoc* **198:** 1423–1426, 1991.

Baxter, G. M. *et al.* Persistent urachal remnant causing intestinal strangulation in a cow. *J Am Vet Med Assoc* **191:** 555–558, 1987.

Cox, J. E. Hernias and ruptures: Words in the heat of the deeds. *Equine Vet J* **20:** 155–162, 1988.

Fubini, S. L. *et al.* Cecal dilatation and volvulus in dairy cows: 84 cases (1977–1983). *J Am Vet Med Assoc* **189:** 96–99, 1986.

Hackett, R. P. Nonstrangulated colonic displacement in horses. *J Am Vet Med Assoc* **182:** 235–240, 1983.

Hance, S. R. *et al.* Umbilical, inguinal, and ventral hernias in horses. *Compend Cont Ed Pract Vet* **12:** 862–871, 1990.

Hayes, H. M., Jr. Congenital umbilical and inguinal hernias in cattle, horses, swine, dogs, and cats: Risk by breed and sex among hospital patients. *Am J Vet Res* **35:** 839–842, 1974.

Kreuger, A. S. *et al.* Ultrastructural study of the equine cecum during onset of laminitis. *Am J Vet Res* **47:** 1804–1812, 1986.

Livesey, M. A. *et al.* Equine colic: Seventy-six cases resulting from incarceration of the large colon by the suspensory ligament of the spleen. *Can Vet J:* **29:** 135–141, 1988.

Modransky, P. D. *et al.* Cecal volvulus in a ewe. *J Am Vet Med Assoc* **194:** 1726–1727, 1989.

Strande, A. Inguinal hernia in dogs. *J Small Anim Pract* **30:** 520–521, 1989.

van der Velden, M. A. Ruptured inguinal hernia in new-born colt foals: A review of 14 cases. *Equine Vet J* **20:** 178–181, 1988.

Vasey, J. R. Incarceration of the small intestine by the epiploic foramen in fifteen horses. *Can Vet J* **29:** 378–382, 1988.

Weaver, A. D. Acquired incarcerated inguinal hernia: A review of 13 horses. *Can Vet J* **28:** 195–199, 1987.

Wolfe, D. F. *et al.* Incarceration of a section of small intestine by remnants of the ductus deferens in steers. *J Am Vet Med Assoc* **191:** 1597–1598, 1987.

Yovich, J. V., Stashak, T. S., and Bertone, A. L. Incarceration of small intestine through rents in the gastrosplenic ligament in the horse. *Vet Surg* **14:** 303–306, 1985.

G. Intestinal Ischemia and Infarction

Inadequate or interrupted circulation of blood to the gut is a common problem, particularly in the horse. Obstruction of the efferent veins, blockage of afferent arteries, and reduced flow through an open circulation cause hypoxic damage to the intestine. Whatever the initiating cause, the effect of hypoxia at the level of the mucosa is similar.

In the small intestine, within 5–10 min of the onset of ischemia, changes are observed at the tips of villi in tissue sections examined under the light microscope, and lesions are well advanced by 30 min. Separation of the epithelium from the basement membrane, beginning at the tip of the villus, and progressing with time toward the base, causes the formation of the so-called Gruenhagen's space. Epithelial cells appear relatively normal, but may separate from the villus in sheets. The core of the villus contracts toward the base. Within 1–3 hr, the villus is completely denuded of epithelium, and the mesenchymal core is disintegrating or collapsed and stumpy, with hemorrhage from capillaries.

That this lesion is largely a function of hypoxia is indicated by the mitigating effects of intraluminal oxygen perfusion. The putative countercurrent exchange of oxygen between the afferent arteriole and efferent venules in the villus, and an associated progressive decline in oxygen tension distally in the villus, may render the tip prone to early damage in hypoxia. Intraluminal enzymes, especially elastase, may contribute to epithelial damage by altering glycoproteins in the vicinity of the brush border, perhaps opening the way for further damage by other pancreatic enzymes, but this is debated. Villus smooth muscle contraction, exacerbating the epithelial exfoliation on the distal villus, may be mediated by sympathetic stimulation in ischemia.

Dissociation and necrosis of cells in the crypts of Lieberkühn begins about 2–4 hr after the initiation of ischemia, and within 4–5 hr, the epithelium appears completely necrotic or has sloughed, leaving a mesenchymal ghost of the mucosa. The muscularis mucosae may undergo necrosis, but the muscularis externa remains viable for 6–7 hr. During acute ischemia, there is initial hyperexcitability of muscle in affected areas, followed by progressive loss of contractility, which will fail to recover if ischemia persists beyond 4–6 hr. Mesothelial cells on the serosa undergo necrosis within 30–60 min of ischemia, and exfoliate; there is a local acute inflammatory response, which may predispose to the development of adhesions. The speed with which lesions develop in hypoxia emphasizes the significance of rapid fixation of intestinal mucosa if artefact is to be avoided.

The colon of the dog and horse seems less sensitive to short-term ischemia than does the small intestine. Mild morphologic damage, characterized by mild edema, and separation and exfoliation of surface epithelium between crypts, is found after 1 hr. However, by 3–4 hr, crypt epithelium is becoming necrotic, dissociating, and exfoliating, and from that point, events progress as in the small intestine.

Reperfusion injury may enhance the severity of the lesion, if hypoxia is only partial, or ischemia is transient, and reflow of blood raises the tissue oxygen tension. Reperfusion injury implies that the effects of the hypoxic episode have not progressed to complete necrosis of the mucosa, and that further damage is possible. Hence, there is a relatively short duration of hypoxia, and a concomitant mild-to-intermediate degree of mucosal damage, permissive of this phenomenon. In cases of enteric ischemic disease encountered in veterinary medicine, this threshold frequently may have been crossed by the time the animal is presented for therapy. Reperfusion injury will occur in the equine small bowel following 3 hr of arteriovenous occlusion, but was not demonstrable following venous infarction in the horse and rat. This may be a function of poor blood flow through damaged vessels after reestablishment of circulation. There is equivocal evidence for reperfusion injury in the equine colon rendered ischemic for as long as 2 hr.

Reperfusion injury is mediated by free radicals generated largely through xanthine oxidase mechanisms in the intestinal mucosa, and through nicotinamide adenine dinucleotide phosphate (NADPH) oxidase mechanisms in leukocytes, mainly neutrophils, which accumulate in the damaged tissue as part of the inflammatory response. Hypoxia stimulates the conversion of xanthine dehydrogenase to xanthine oxidase in epithelial cells. This enzyme system is concentrated in epithelial cells on villi, especially near the tips, but seems not to be present in colonic epithelium of the horse. Its distribution may, in concert with the putative cline in oxygen tension along the villus, explain the predisposition of the villus tip to damage in transient hypoxia. In the presence of xanthine oxidase, hypoxanthine accumulating from ATP degradation in hypoxia is converted to xanthine, and molecular oxygen is reduced, generating hydrogen peroxide, superoxide radical, and hydroxyl radical intermediates. The hydroxyl radical is probably most significant in damaging proteins and initiating a cascade of lipid peroxidation, which degrades cell membranes, resulting in metabolic and structural lesions culminating in cell death.

Short-term ischemia (maximally, ~ 3–4 hr), with preservation of at least the base of the crypts of Lieberkühn, will permit repair, as cells proliferating in the crypts reepithelialize the mucosal surface within 1–3 days. Normal architecture is reestablished after up to 1–2 weeks, though necrotic muscularis mucosae is not replaced. Effusion of tissue fluid and acute inflammatory cells prevails until epithelium extends to fully cover the eroded surface. Partial damage to the proliferative compartment initially results in dilatation of crypts, lined by flattened epithelium resembling that seen after radiation injury (Fig 1.55D). If the amplifier population of progenitor cells can be regenerated, hyperplastic basophilic cells will populate crypts until the mucosal architecture is reconstituted.

Ischemic necrosis of the full thickness of the mucosa will be bounded by an acute inflammatory reaction in the submucosa, which, under favorable conditions, evolves into a granulating ulcerated surface. Neutrophilic infiltration and effusion may be considerable if bacterial contamination of the lumen is heavy. Focal ulcerative lesions may ultimately heal by epithelial migration, over the bed of granulation tissue, from surviving crypts within the lesion and around the periphery.

Extensive mucosal ulcers which form following severe ischemia have little chance of resolution, due to their large surface area. Chronic ischemic ulcers in the small bowel tend to develop a depressed, fairly clean granulating surface, occasionally with some fibrinous exudate. Ischemic ulcers in the large bowel, especially of horses, develop a dirty yellow-gray fibrinonecrotic surface, perhaps due to the effects of anaerobic bacteria. If the animal does not succumb to the effects of malabsorption and protein loss from the defect, or to transmural bacterial invasion, scarring and stricture may occur. The sequelae of ischemia with reflow are seen mainly in strangulated segments of gut which have been reduced without, or with inadequate, resection, and in some cases of presumed thromboembolic infarction of the equine colon.

Persistent ischemia results in necrosis involving all mural elements. The full thickness of the gut wall ultimately becomes gangrenous, green-brown or black, flaccid, and friable.

The consequences of ischemic lesions are partly a function of the species, and of the level of bowel affected. Strangulation, volvulus, and similar lesions cause physical obstruction at the site, and ileus proximal to it. Reduced arterial perfusion or thromboembolism causes functional obstruction and ileus. Loss of mucosal integrity results in cessation of electrolyte and water absorption, and ultimately in effusion of tissue fluid and blood into the lumen. Proliferation of anaerobes occurs in the lumen of the stagnant ischemic area, with accumulation of gas, and extreme distension of the closed loop in strangulation obstruction. Toxin production by anaerobes, particularly clostridia, plays a large part in gangrene and ultimate rupture of ischemic gut, as well as having systemic effects. Absorption of endotoxin from the lumen may occur through devitalized mucosa via the portal flow, lymphatic return, or peritoneum. Toxins have a severe detrimental effect on cardiovascular function, contributing to the circulatory failure. If death from some other cause does not supervene, transmural invasion by enteric bacteria or perforation of the devitalized wall result in septic peritonitis, which is ultimately fatal.

1. Venous Infarction

Obstruction of efferent veins is by far the most common cause of intestinal ischemia. This is a sequel to incarceration of herniated loops of bowel; strangulation by pedunculated masses, such as lipomas in older horses; torsion (twist about long axis of the viscus); volvulus (twist across the long axis of the gut); and intussusception. In these circumstances compression of thin-walled veins tends to occur before the influx of arterial blood is obstructed.

Primary thrombosis of the mesenteric veins is rare, but may occur in animals, especially dogs, with disseminated intravascular coagulation. Local invasion of the mucosa by mycotic agents may result in focal or segmental thrombotic lesions due to hyphal invasion of submucosal veins.

In venous infarction, the affected tissue field, sometimes including involved mesentery, becomes intensely edematous, congested, and hemorrhagic, so that the hypoxic bowel wall is thickened and eventually assumes a deep red-black appearance (Fig. 1.54A). It has been estimated that 40 liters of fluid may accumulate in the wall of a horse colon that has undergone volvulus. Bloody fluid content and gas distend the lumen of the infarcted segment. As gangrene of the intestinal wall proceeds, the tissue becomes green-black, and septic peritonitis eventually ensues, with or without perforation of the bowel. Advanced venous infarction involves the full thickness of the intestinal wall, and the initiating intestinal accident is commonly evident, except in cases subjected to surgery. Even if a displacement, volvulus, or strangulation has been reduced, the limits of the infarcted segment are usually relatively sharply demarcated, and the affected bowel remains edematous and hemorrhagic.

Microscopically, severe transmural edema, congestion, distension of veins, sometimes venous thrombosis, and hemorrhage are present, initially most severe in the mucosa and submucosa. With time, the full thickness of the mucosa becomes necrotic, and the deeper layers of the muscular wall are also devitalized, with invading enteric flora present throughout. Lesions which have advanced to significant necrosis or effacement of the crypt epithelium are associated with failure of the animal to survive, either due to euthanasia on the grounds of the degree of damage, or systemic complications despite correction of the strangulation, or resection.

Displacements of intestine which may progress to incarceration or volvulus with strangulation and infarction have been discussed in the previous section. They are a common cause of colic and mortality in horses.

Torsion of the long axis of the mesentery occurs commonly in suckling ruminants and in swine, uncommonly in horses, and rarely in cats and dogs. In all species, the result is rapid death. The abdomen is distended, and on opening the cavity, tensely dilated deep red-to-black loops of bowel are usually immediately apparent.

In swine the mesentery of the small intestine and sometimes the large bowel is often involved in a torsion which usually is counterclockwise, when viewed from the ventrocaudal aspect. In torsion involving the small and large intestines, the apex of the cecum may be pointing cranial in the anterior left quadrant of the abdomen, reflecting the rotation of about 180°. In swine, mesenteric torsion may be due to gas production from a highly fermentable substrate in the colon, and its subsequent displacement, with progression to mesenteric torsion. Mesenteric torsion is a common cause of sporadic sudden death in swine but may occur as a recurrent problem in a herd. Many cases of so-called intestinal hemorrhage syndrome in that species are probably misdiagnosed mesenteric torsion. The presence of red-black or bloody content in the intestine of feeder swine, without torsion, may also signal bleeding gastric ulcer or proliferative hemorrhagic enteropathy associated with *Campylobacter*-like organisms.

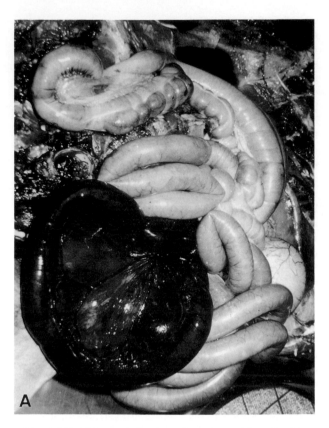

Fig. 1.54A Venous infarction of a segment of equine ileum which has undergone volvulus.

Death due to mesenteric torsion is common in suckling or artifically reared calves and lambs. In these species, vigorous ingestion of large amounts of feed over a short period may predispose to gas formation in the gut, or perhaps hypermotility, which induces torsion. Usually only the mucosa of the proximal duodenum and terminal ileum, cecum, and colon is spared from infarction, though occasionally volvulus is restricted to shorter segments of intestine. Similar lesions are occasionally encountered in other species.

In dogs, mesenteric torsion has been associated with ingestion of large quantities of food, and with pancreatic exocrine insufficiency in German shepherds. It is accompanied occasionally by gastric volvulus.

Volvulus of varying lengths of the small intestine may occur in any species, but is perhaps most prevalent in the horse, where it is a common cause of strangulation obstruction of the bowel.

Volvulus of the large colon of the horse is predisposed to by its lack of mesenteric anchorage, and potential mobility. It may be due to dorsomedial (ventral colon rotating dorsally and medially relative to the dorsal colon) or dorsolateral rotation of the colonic loop along its long axis. Rotation of the left colon commonly progresses to volvulus at the sternal and diaphragmatic flexures. The right colon may rotate in its middle, cranial to the level of the cecocolic fold. Part of the cecum may be incorporated in the volvulus, the right colon and cecum rotating in the region of attachment of the cecocolic fold, or almost the entire large colon and cecum may be involved in a rotation at the cecal base and transverse colon. The equine cecum alone rarely undergoes torsion, and if so, it may be related to hypoplasia of the cecocolic fold.

The most common direction of rotation of the right colon is dorsomedial. Sites of rotation vary among series; the least common seems to be at the mid-right colon. The direction and sites of rotation suggest that lesions may begin with tympany and dorsomedial torsion in the left colon, with progression of the twist, from left to right colon. The sternal/diaphragmatic flexures presumably provide some resistance to rotation, causing some twists to be found there. The first site of fixation of the large colon is the cecocolic fold, which may explain a tendency for twists to be localized there; progression beyond this level bases the twist at the mesenteric root of the large bowel. Clinical signs are associated with rotations of more than 180°, and torsions involving the cecal base are usually at least 360°.

At surgery or necropsy, the usual signs of strangulation obstruction are evident, including dilation and devitalization of the infarcted segment, and distension of the cecum, if it is not twisted. Postmortem rupture of the diaphragm or abdominal wall may occur, because of tympany.

Intussusception involves the telescoping of one segment of bowel into an outer sheath formed by another, usually distal, segment of gut. Any level of the gut with sufficient mesenteric mobility may be involved. The cause is usually not apparent, though linear foreign bodies, heavy parasitism, previous intestinal surgery, enteritis, and intramural lesions such as abscesses and tumors may be associated. The case implicating *Anoplocephala perfoliata* in intussusceptions involving the equine cecum is unproven. It also may be a terminal, agonal, or postmortem event. The history is that of partial or complete intestinal obstruction, perhaps with bloody feces, and it is most common in young animals.

Intussusception is common in dogs (Fig. 1.54B), where most frequently it is ileocolic. It is much less common in cats. Intussusception is also moderately common in lambs, calves, and young horses, where it may involve small intestine, cecum, and colon.

The progressive invagination of the leading edge of the intussusceptum into the posterior segment results in the wall of the intussusception being composed of three layers, the inner entering, and middle returning segment of invaginated bowel, and the outer wall of the receiving segment of gut. It is limited in length by the increasing tension on the mesentery drawn into the lesion, to about 10–12 cm in small animals, and about 20–30 cm in large animals. This tension along one edge of the gut may cause the mass to become bowed or spiraled.

Tension and compression of mesenteric veins causes the intussusceptum, or a portion of it, to undergo venous infarction. It swells, with edema and congestion, and the adjacent apposed serous surfaces become adherent as fibrin and inflammatory cells effuse from the affected bowel. Adhesion quickly renders the intussusception irreducible. Necrosis and gangrene of the invaginated intestine usually develop, but sometimes the intussusceptum will slough, and the remaining viable segments will maintain continuity of the gut, or rarely, will form two adjacent blind ends. Intestine above obstructing intussusceptions may be dilated, and that below, contracted and devoid of content. If obstruction is chronic or partial, there may be hypertrophy of the smooth muscle of proximal bowel. In horses, chronic ileocecal intussusception involves a relatively short (less than 10 cm) length of bowel. Incidental terminal, agonal, or postmortem intussusception is recognized by the relative absence of congestion, edema, and adhesion of the involuted segment of gut.

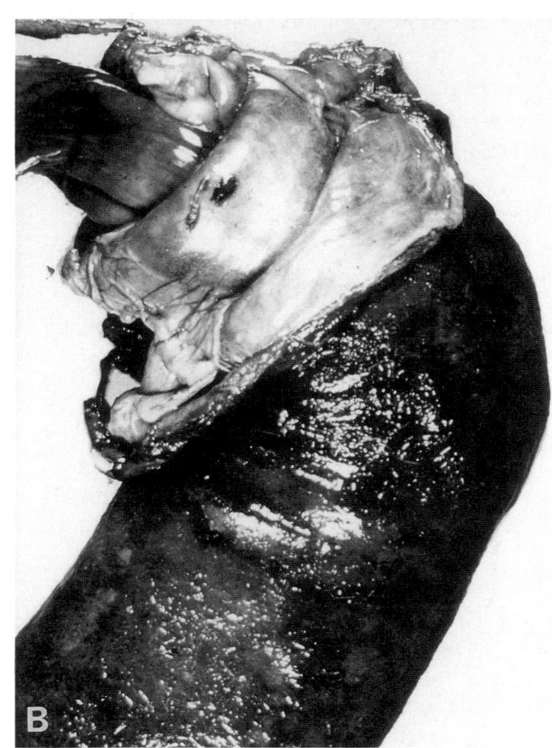

Fig. 1.54B Intussusception. Intestine. Dog. Outer intestinal layer has been cut away to expose the edematous and congested infarcted mucosa of strangulated portion of the intussusception.

Cecal inversion, and cecocolic intussusception in the horse, with inversion of the cecum into itself, or into the right ventral colon, may result in ischemia of the cecum and possibly part of the involved colon; if partial, ischemia usually involves the more distal cecum.

Segmental ischemic necrosis of the small colon may occur in pregnant or postpartum mares, because of mesenteric tension from intussusception and rectal prolapse of the distal large bowel, or perhaps due to laceration of the mesocolon and associated vessels by the feet of the foal during parturition. Obstruction, colic, and intestinal necrosis, rupture and peritonitis may follow.

2. *Arterial Thromboembolism*

Ischemia due to arterial thrombosis and embolism is rare in domestic animals other than the horse. Mucosal and occasionally transmural focal or segmental infarctive lesions are seen in *Pasteurella* septicemia in lambs and in *Haemophilus somnus* bacteremia in cattle.

In **horses** it is associated with **endoarteritis,** mainly at the root of the cranial mesenteric circulation, usually in animals younger than 3 years, caused by migrating larvae of *Strongylus vulgaris* (see The Cardiovascular System, Volume 3, Chapter 1). Suffice it to say here that endoarteritis due to this worm is most common in the cranial mesenteric circulation, sometimes at a number of sites a considerable distance distal to the usual location at the root of the artery. Although endoarteritis is common, in only a small minority of horses dying of intestinal accidents can the infarction be confidently attributed to *S. vulgaris*. This may be declining as advanced worm control programs are adopted.

Candidates for a diagnosis of nonstrangulating infarction are animals in which the anatomic distribution of an ischemic lesion is incompatible with volvulus or other strangulation, or in which physical evidence for incarceration or strangulation obstruction is not present in the surgical history or at autopsy. In the horse, animals in this category may have relatively localized mucosal or transmural damage, or extensive transmural lesions of the distal small intestine, cecum, and large colon, that is, in the circulatory field of the cranial mesenteric artery. Lesions limited essentially to the mucosa appear usually to be subacute, and are ulcerative or fibrinonecrotic, usually with an hyperemic margin. They may be tens to many hundreds of square centimeters in area.

Transmural lesions are of two types. The least common is a large irregular area of devitalized gut, sometimes involving most of the cecum or colon, with a dirty khaki-colored, flaccid, friable wall, which is not markedly thickened. Along the poorly defined margin of the necrotic tissue there may be transmural congestion, hemorrhage, and edema. The fluid content in the affected gut is foul-smelling, but not particularly blood-tinged. More commonly, irregularly demarcated areas of infarcted intestine have a thickened, edematous, congested wall, which appears deep red-black or green-black on both mucosal and serosal aspects. Gut content is blood-tinged. The peritoneal cavity may contain an excessive quantity of turbid yellow or blood-tinged fluid, and animals with both types of transmural lesions may progress to rupture of the bowel, with distribution of content throughout the abdomen.

Dissection of the cranial mesenteric artery and its ramifications is mandatory in such cases, and care should be taken at necropsy to preserve it intact for exploration. Whereas verminous arteritis is evident in large-caliber vessels in most affected animals, even an assiduous search reveals macroscopic thrombi in more peripheral arteries serving infarcted tissue in only a minority of cases.

We interpret devitalized gray-brown intestine of normal thickness to represent arterial obstruction without significant reflow, except along the boundary with viable tissue. Large edematous, congested, or hemorrhagic, full-thickness lesions, physically or anatomically inconsistent with strangulation, we interpret as severe arterial obstruction, with subsequent reflow either by relief of the obstruction or by way of collaterals. Ischemic damage to vessels of the mucosa, submucosa, and perhaps deeper structures results in hemorrhage and edema when blood flow returns (Fig. 1.55A). Ulcerative or fibrinonecrotic mucosal lesions are probably the result of transient ischemia, and superficial or mucosal damage, with subsequent reflow (Fig. 1.55B). Similar lesions may occur following relief of strangulation of short duration, and in salmonellosis, which itself may, in part, involve mucosal microthrombosis.

Infarction of the equine cecum and colon by arterial ligation is experimentally difficult, reflecting the extensive collateral communications. These are present between the dorsal and ventral colic arteries; along the rete mirabile surrounding the colic veins; between the caudal mesenteric arterial field and the middle and right colic arteries; and between the lateral and medial cecal arteries. Even then, ischemic lesions may be limited to the less well perfused watersheds at the periphery of circulatory fields—the pelvic flexure and the tip of the cecum, where lesions are sometimes present in spontaneous cases.

Evidence of reflow, and failure to find thrombi lodged in arteries in the infarcted area, may be explained in several ways. Fibrinolysis may have removed the obstructing thrombi; thrombi may be multiple and microscopic (sometimes they are found in arteries in sections of infarcted tissue); the lesions may be the result of diminished tissue perfusion due to obstructed flow caused by verminous endarteritis (but not thromboembolism) or by vascular spasm. In the latter case they may be the result of slow flow, discussed further subsequently.

3. *Reduced Perfusion*

Ischemia due to reduced perfusion of the intestinal vascular bed is a difficult and uncommon diagnosis. Circumstances in which it may be expected to occur include severe hypovolemic states, such as hemorrhagic shock in the dog, cat, and possibly other species; in animals, particularly dogs, with disseminated intravascular coagulation; in dogs with hepatic disease and portal hypertension; in hypotensive shock due to heart failure; and in animals with reduced mesenteric arterial perfusion, mainly horses with severe verminous endoarteritis.

In **shock gut** in dogs, and rarely, other species, associated terminally with heart failure, hemorrhage, hypovolemia, and disseminated intravascular coagulation, part or all of the mucosa of the small intestine is deeply congested, and the content is hemorrhagic.

The pathogenesis of the lesion is related to reflex vasoconstriction in the mucosa and submucosa, shunting of blood away from the mucosa, dilation of mucosal capillaries, and reduction in rate of flow of blood through the villus. Countercurrent transfer of oxygen from the afferent to efferent ves-

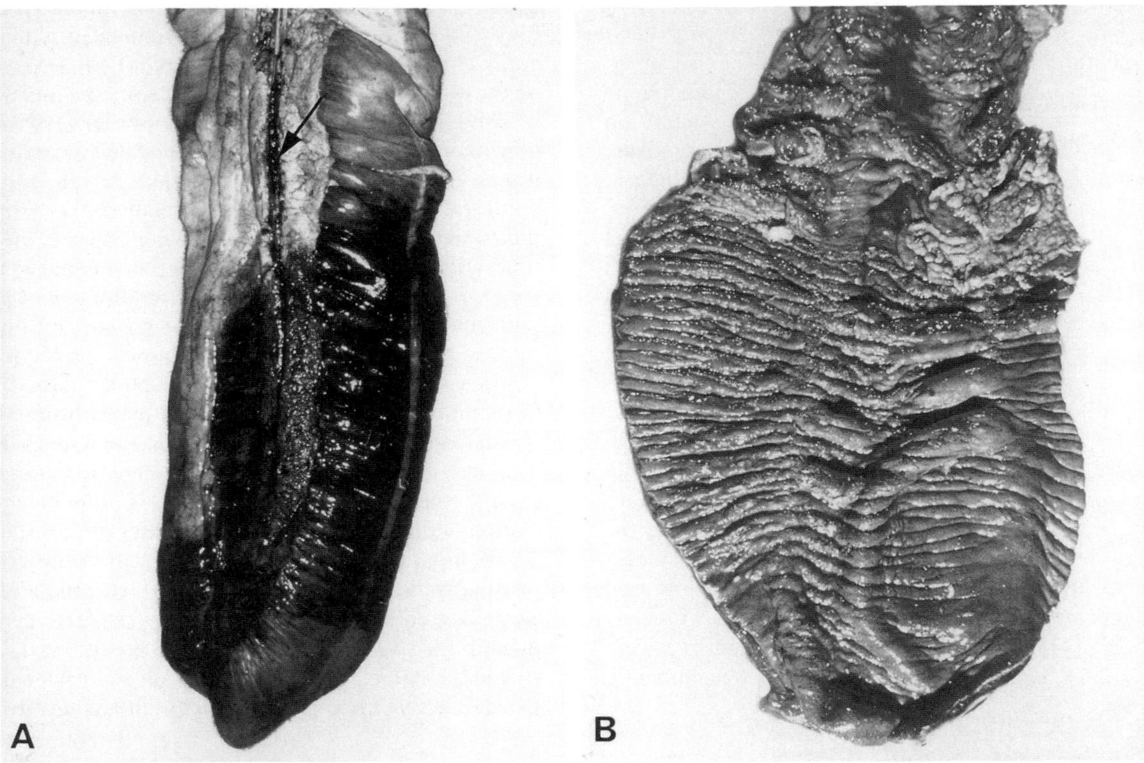

Fig. 1.55 (A) Infarction of pelvic flexure. Horse. Large colon: colic artery contains a thrombus (arrow). Hemorrhage and edema of serosa suggest that arterial thrombosis and infarction have been followed by reperfusion, with extravasation of blood from damaged vessels in the affected tissue. (B) Mucosa of equine cecum that has undergone ischemic necrosis due to reduced arterial perfusion. Subsequent reflow has occurred, and the infarcted mucosa is covered with fibrinonecrotic exudate. Irregular ulcers and foci of exudation are present on mucosa along proximal margin of the lesion (toward top).

sels in the villus aggravates hypoxemia in the villus by increased shunting of oxygen to the efferent venule. Splanchnic pooling of blood, systemic arterial hypotension, and intestinal vasoconstriction occur in endotoxic shock in dogs, causing similar mucosal lesions. Microthrombosis associated with sluggish flow, disseminated intravascular coagulation, and endotoxemia may contribute to mucosal ischemia by obstructing capillaries in the villi, and mucosal and submucosal venules. Microthrombi in these vessels in association with hemorrhagic mucosal necrosis suggests the possibility of ischemia due to slow flow.

Transient or incomplete reduction in perfusion due to obstruction of the arterial blood supply has a similar effect on the mucosa. The obstruction may be due to arteriospasm, perhaps induced by vasoactive mediators such as thromboxane. Mucosa devitalized by hypoxia will become hemorrhagic with continued blood flow. Since the primary problem may not involve a systemic state as complicated as severe shock, the animal may survive long enough to develop an effusive ulcerated or pseudomembranous mucosa, with some prospect of stabilization or repair, if the lesion is not widespread. Slow flow due to reduced arterial perfusion with inadequate collateral flow may be expected to affect the watershed of a circulatory field preferentially. In the horse this may be the explanation for mucosal lesions at the pelvic flexure and apex of the cecum in which thromboembolism cannot be implicated, but in which mural thrombi in the cranial mesenteric root could have caused significantly reduced perfusion.

Ischemia at the periphery of the circulatory field of the caudal mesenteric artery may possibly predispose to rectal perforation in horses. The precarious perfusion of the mucosa at this site may contribute to ischemic ulceration and the development of rectal stricture in swine. This condition in many cases appears to be associated with *Salmonella* infection, and it is discussed further with porcine salmonellosis.

Transient or noninfarctive slow flow has been proposed as a cause of intermittent colic due to verminous arteritis. It may also play a role in the development of functional obstruction and volvulus in horses with cranial mesenteric arterial lesions.

Acute acorn poisoning in the horse may cause severe gastrointestinal edema and focal hemorrhage, with infarction and ulceration in the cecum and colon. Microscopic lesions in the small and large intestine are consistent with an ischemic pathogenesis, and microthrombi have been associated with mucosal infarcts in the large bowel, as well as in other organs. **Mercury intoxication** is also associated with colonic ulceration in the horse.

Nonsteroidal antiinflammatory drugs cause ulceration of the upper small intestine and colon, as well as oral and gastric ulceration, which seems to be related to ischemia, in horses and dogs. In horses, phenylbutazone administered at doses greater than 8.8mg/kg causes ulcers on the lips, gingiva, palate, and tongue; pharyngeal tonsils; squamous and more commonly, glandular gastric mucosa; duodenum and proximal jejunum; cecum; and large colon, especially the right ventral colon. Renal papillary necrosis is often concurrent if animals are dehydrated. Animals may develop diarrhea and hypoproteinemia as a result of the extensive mucosal defects.

Lesions in the oral cavity are deep crateriform ulcers, with a clean granulating base; the tonsillar lesions seem to be based on coagulation necrosis of lymphoid tissue. Concurrent with punched-out ulcers in the glandular mucosa, there may be chronic gastritis and atrophy of the mucosa with loss of differentiation of the cells in the fundus. Hyperkeratosis and erosion may be evident in the squamous mucosa. In the upper small intestine, ulcers may be focal, linear, or segmental and annular, several centimeters long. Microscopic lesions which may precede ulceration of the small intestine include mild to severe atrophy of villi, epithelial necrosis, mucosal inflammation, and fibrin exudation. Lesions in the large intestine may be focal, linear, or extensive and segmental, involving the entire circumference of the bowel (Fig. 1.55C). Depending on the duration and severity of the lesion, the mucosa may be congested and edematous, with superficial necrosis and fibrin exudation, or extensively eroded and ulcerated, with fibrino-necrotic exudate. Early in the process, superficial epithelial necrosis and progressive mucosal necrosis and inflammation are evident. Damaged mucosa, in which many crypts have been effaced, may be covered by attenuated epithelium, or there may be erosion and ulceration with fibrin exudation and secondary bacterial colonization. Mucosal lymphoid follicles may be depleted.

Microvascular injury, with subsequent microthrombosis and ischemic ulceration, is considered by some to be the cause of the lesions in the stomach and intestine. This may be the result of direct phenylbutazone toxicity to the microvasculature. There is no clear association with altered levels of prostaglandins in tissue 48–96 hr after treatment. However, an initial effect on prostaglandin levels has not been ruled out, and PGE_2 administered with phenylbutazone is protective. Prostaglandin E_2 may promote blood flow, and it is cytoprotective in the colon. Vasoconstriction or depression of other cytoprotective effects, mediated by phenylbutazone inhi-

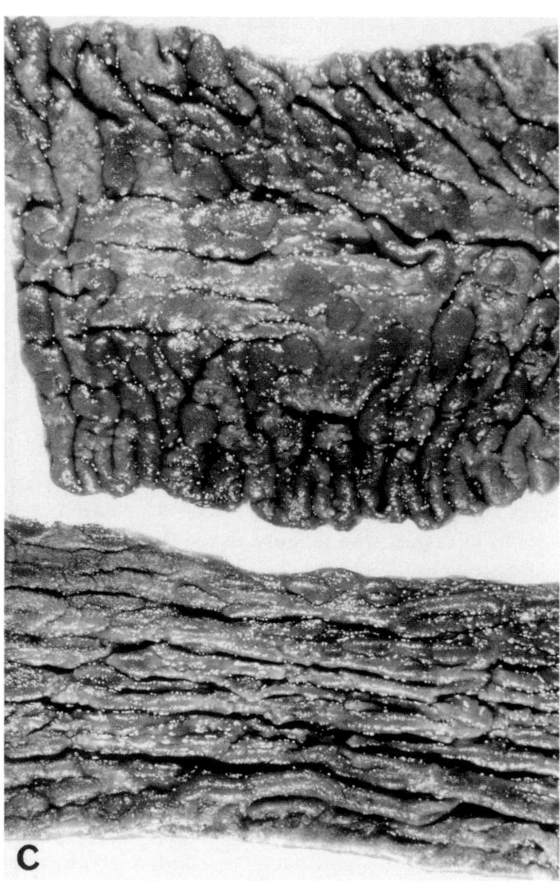

Fig. 1.55C Fibrinonecrotic enterocolitis in a foal treated heavily with non-steroidal antiinflammatory drugs.

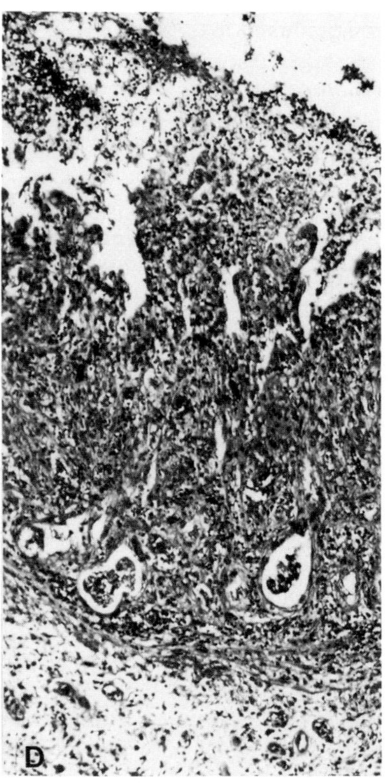

Fig. 1.55D Small intestine, sequel to transient ischemia 2 days previously. Ulcerated mucosa and dilated crypts lined by attenuated epithelium and containing necrotic debris. Inflammatory cells and fibrin exude from the mucosa, which is devoid of villi.

bition of prostaglandin synthesis, could be the cause of the lesions. Renal papillary necrosis is ischemic, due to prostaglandin inhibition. Muscular contractions may further compress already marginally compromised mucosa, taking it over the threshold for ischemic necrosis. This may cause the annular pattern of lesions in the duodenum, and the linear pattern on the surface of mucosal folds often seen in pyloric sphincter and the large bowel.

In foals, flunixin meglumine, another nonsteroidal antiinflammatory agent, will also cause diarrhea, associated with oral and gastric ulceration, and cecal petechial hemorrhage. In dogs, pyloric, duodenal, and colonic ulceration may be induced by administration of flunixin meglumine alone, or in combination with a glucocorticoid. Microscopically, the lesions in the duodenum and colon of dogs are very similar to those induced by phenylbutazone in horses, with villus atrophy or superficial mucosal necrosis, progressing to erosion or ulceration with obvious microthrombosis. Steroid administration potentiates the effects of flunixin meglumine. Flunixin meglumine does cause reduced mucosal perfusion on the equine duodenum, though under the conditions of the study, viability of the tissue was not compromised.

Some speculate that nonsteroidal antiinflammatory agents may be implicated in the pathogenesis of right dorsal colitis in horses, and in at least some cases of anterior (proximal) enteritis, a recently recognized syndrome of necrotizing duodenitis–jejunitis in foals and horses.

Bibliography

Angus, K. W., Coop, R. L., and Mapes, C. J. Pathological changes or postmortem changes in parasitic infections: The influence of slaughter methods on intestinal histopathology. *Int J Parasitol* **2:** 485–486, 1972.

Anderson, G. A. *et al.* Fatal acorn poisoning in a horse: Pathologic findings and diagnostic considerations. *J Am Vet Med Assoc* **182:** 1105–1110, 1983.

Arden, W. A. *et al.* Effects of ischemia and dimethyl sulfoxide on equine jejunal vascular resistance, oxygen consumption, intraluminal pressure, and potassium loss. *Am J Vet Res* **50:** 380–387, 1989.

Arden, W. A. *et al.* Morphologic and ultrastructural evaluation of effect of ischemia and dimethyl sulfoxide on equine jejunum. *Am J Vet Res* **51:** 1784–1791, 1990.

Argenzio, R. A., Henrikson, C. K., and Liacos, J. A. Effect of prostaglandin inhibitors on bile salt-induced mucosal damage of porcine colon. *Gastroenterology* **96:** 95–109, 1989.

Barclay W. P. *et al.* Chronic nongranulomatous arteritis (sic) in seven horses. *J Am Vet Med Assoc* **190:** 684–686, 1987.

Bounous, G. Pancreatic proteases and oxygen-derived free radicals in acute ischemic enteropathy. *Surgery* **99:** 92–94, 1986.

Brown, M. F. *et al.* The role of leukocytes in mediating mucosal injury of intestinal ischemia/reperfusion. *J Ped Surg* **25:** 214–217, 1990.

Carrick, J. B. *et al.* Clinical and pathological effects of flunixin meglumine administration to neonatal foals. *Can J Vet Res* **53:** 195–201, 1989.

Cawthorne, R. J. G., Taylor, S. M., and Purcell, D. A. Pathological changes in parasitic infections of the intestine of calves and lambs: A technique for avoiding postmortem artefacts. *Int J Parasitol* **3:** 447–449, 1973.

Chiu, G. J. *et al.* Intestinal mucosal lesion in low-flow states. I. A morphological, hemodynamic, and metabolic reappraisal. *Arch Surg* **101:** 478–483, 1970.

Collins, L. G., and Tyler, D. E. Experimentally induced phenylbutazone toxicosis in ponies: Description of the syndrome and its prevention with synthetic prostaglandin E_2. *Am J Vet Res* **46:** 1605–1615, 1985.

Dow, S. W *et al.* Effects of flunixin and flunixin plus prednisone on the gastrointestinal tract of dogs. *Am J Vet Res* **51:** 1131–1138, 1990.

Fell, B. F. Cell shedding in the epithelium of the intestinal mucosa: Fact and artefact. *J Pathol Bacteriol* **81:** 251–254, 1961.

Fenwick, B. W., and Kruckenberg, S. Comparison of methods used to collect canine intestinal tissues for histologic examination. *Am J Vet Res* **48:** 1276–1281, 1987.

Filez, L. *et al.* Influences of ischemia and reperfusion on the feline small-intestinal mucosa. *J Surg Res* **49:** 157–163, 1990.

Ford, T. S. *et al.* Ileocecal intussusception in horses: 26 cases (1981–1988). *J Am Vet Med Assoc* **196:** 121–126, 1990.

Freeman, D. E. *et al.* Early mucosal healing and chronic changes in pony jejunum after various types of strangulation obstruction. *Am J Vet Res* **49:** 810–818, 1988.

Gaughan, E. M., and Hackett, R. P. Cecocolic intussusception in horses: 11 cases (1979–1989). *J Am Vet Med Assoc* **197:** 1373–1375, 1990.

Gay, C. C., and Speirs, V. C. Parasitic arteritis and its consequences in horses. *Aust Vet J* **54:** 600–601, 1978.

Geor, R. J. *et al.* The protective effects of sucralfate and ranitidine in foals experimentally intoxicated with phenylbutazone. *Can J Vet Res* **53:** 231–238, 1989.

Hackett, M. S., and Hackett, R. P. Chronic ileocecal intussusception in horses. *Cornell Vet* **79:** 353–361, 1989.

Haglund, U. *et al.* Mucosal lesions in the human small intestine in shock. *Gut* **16:** 979–984, 1975.

Harrison, I. W. Equine large intestinal volvulus—a review of 124 cases. *Vet Surg* **17:** 77–81, 1988.

Harrison, I. W. Cecal torsion in a horse as a consequence of cecocolic fold hypoplasia. *Cornell Vet* **79:** 315–317, 1989.

Jodal, M., and Lundgren, O. Countercurrent mechanisms in the mammalian gastrointestinal tract. *Gastroenterology* **91:** 225–241, 1986.

Karcher, L. F. *et al.* Right dorsal colitis. *J Vet Intern Med* **4:** 247–253, 1990.

Lewis, D. D., and Ellison, G. W. Intussusception in dogs and cats. *Compend Cont Ed Pract Vet* **9:** 523–534, 1987.

Livesey, M. A., and Keller, S. D. Segmental ischemic necrosis following mesocolic rupture in postparturient mares. *Compend Cont Ed Pract Vet* **8:** 763–770, 1986.

Matushek, K. J., and Cockshutt, J. R. Mesenteric and gastric volvulus in a dog. *J Am Vet Med Assoc* **191:** 327–328, 1987.

Menge, H., Meyers, M., and Robinson, J .W. L. Early phase of jejunal regeneration after short-term ischemia in the rat. *Lab Invest* **40:** 25–30, 1979.

Meschter, C. L. *et al.* Histologic findings in the gastrointestinal tract of horses with colic. *Am J Vet Res* **47:** 598–606, 1986.

Meschter, C. L. *et al.* The effects of phenylbutazone on the intestinal mucosa of the horse: A morphological, ultrastructural, and biochemical study. *Equine Vet J* **22:** 255–263, 1990.

Meyers, K. *et al.* Circulating endotoxinlike substances and altered hemostasis in horses with gastrointestinal disorders: An interim report. *Am J Vet Res* **43:** 2233–2238, 1982.

Milne, E. M. *et al.* Caecal intussusception in two ponies. *Vet Rec* **125:** 148–151, 1989.
Moore, J. N. *et al.* Effect of intraluminal oxygen in intestinal strangulation obstruction in ponies. *Am J Vet Res* **41:** 1615–1620, 1980.
Moore, J. N. *et al.* Endotoxemia following experimental intestinal strangulation obstruction in ponies. *Can J Comp Med* **45:** 330–332, 1981.
Morin, M. *et al.* Torsion of abdominal organs in sows: A report of 36 cases. *Can Vet J* **25:** 440–442, 1984.
Nelson, A. W., Collier, J. R., and Griner, L. A. Acute surgical colonic infarction in the horse. *Am J Vet Res* **29:** 315–327, 1968.
Owen, Rh. ap Rh., Jagger, D. W., and Quan-Taylor, R. Cecal intussusceptions in horses and the significance of *Anoplocephala perfoliata*. *Vet Rec* **124:** 34–37, 1989.
Pablo, L. S. *et al.* Disseminated intravascular coagulation in experimental intestinal strangulation obstruction in ponies. *Am J Vet Res* **44:** 2115–2122, 1983.
Park, P. O. *et al.* The sequence of development of intestinal tissue injury after strangulation ischemia and reperfusion. *Surgery* **107:** 574–580, 1990.
Pearson, G. R., and Logan, E. F. The rate of development of postmortem artefact in the small intestine of neonatal calves. *Br J Exp Pathol* **59:** 178–182, 1978.
Penning, P. D., and Treacher, T. T. Intestinal haemorrhage syndrome in artificially reared lambs. *Vet Rec* **88:** 613–615, 1971.
Robinson, J. W. L. *et al.* Functional and morphological response of the dog colon to ischaemia. *Gut* **13:** 775–783, 1972.
Rochat, M. C. An introduction to reperfusion injury. *Compend Cont Ed Pract Vet* **13:** 923–930, 1991.
Ross, M. W., Stephens P. R., and Reimer J. M. Small colon intussusception in a broodmare. *J Am Vet Med Assoc* **192:** 372–374, 1988.
Schoenberg, M. H., and Beger, H. G. Oxygen radicals in intestinal ischemia and reperfusion. *Chem-Biol Interact* **76:** 141–161, 1990.
Schuh, J. C., Ross, C., and Meschter, C. L. Concurrent mercury blister and dimethyl sulfoxide (DMSO) application as a cause of mercury toxicity in two horses. *Equine Vet J* **20:** 68–71, 1988.
Slone, D. E. *et al.* Noniatrogenic rectal tears in three horses. *J Am Vet Med Assoc* **180:** 750–751, 1982.
Smart, M. E. *et al.* Intussusception in a Charolais bull. *Can Vet J* **18:** 244–246, 1977.
Snyder, J. R. *et al.* Morphologic alterations observed during experimental ischemia of the equine large colon. *Am J Vet Res* **49:** 801–809, 1988.
Snyder, J. R. *et al.* Strangulating volvulus of the ascending colon in horses. *J Am Vet Med Assoc* **195:** 757–764, 1989.
Stick, J. A *et al.* Effects of flunixin meglumine on jejunal blood flow, motility, and oxygen consumption in ponies. *Am J Vet Res* **49:** 1173–1178, 1988.
Sullins, K. E. *et al.* Pathologic changes associated with induced small intestinal strangulation obstruction and nonstrangulating infarction in horses. *Am J Vet Res* **46:** 913–916, 1985.
Todd, J. N. *et al.* Intestinal haemorrhage and volvulus in whey-fed pigs. *Vet Rec* **100:** 11–12, 1977.
Traub-Dargatz, J. L. *et al.* Chronic flunixin meglumine therapy in foals. *Am J Vet Res* **49:** 7–12, 1988.
Tulleners, E. P. Surgical correction of volvulus of the root of the mesentery in calves. *J Am Vet Med Assoc* **179:** 998–999, 1981.
Wagner, R., Gabbert, H., and Hohn, P. Ischemia and postischemic regeneration of the small intestinal mucosa. *Virchows Arch (Cell Pathol)* **31:** 259–276, 1979.
Westermarck, E., and Rimaila-Pärnänen, E. Mesenteric torsion in dogs with exocrine pancreatic insufficiency: 21 cases (1978–1987). *J Am Vet Med Assoc* **195:** 1404–1406, 1989.
White, N. A. Intestinal infarction associated with mesenteric vascular thrombotic disease in the horse. *J Am Vet Med Assoc* **178:** 259–262, 1981.
White, N. A. Thromboembolic colic in horses. *Compend Cont Ed Pract Vet* **7:** S156–S164, 1985.
White, N. A., Moore, J. N., and Trim, C. M. Mucosal alterations in experimentally induced small intestinal strangulation obstruction in ponies. *Am J Vet Res* **41:** 193–198, 1980.
Whitehead, R. The pathology of intestinal ischaemia. *Clin Gastroenterol* **1:** 613–637, 1972.
Yale, C. E., and Balish, E. The importance of clostridia in experimental intestinal strangulation. *Gastroenterology* **71:** 793–796, 1976.

H. Epithelial Renewal in Health and Disease

1. Small Intestine

a. Normal Form and Function The intestinal surface is lined by an extremely labile population of cells, ultimately derived from stem cells at the base of crypts or glands, but with its proximate source in amplifier populations of undifferentiated columnar or oligomucous cells in the lower half of the crypts. These cells lose their ability to undergo mitosis, and differentiate into goblet cells and the functional population of enterocytes as they move from the crypt to the villus. In most species, they are shed from the tips of villi in about 2–8 days. Relatively little definitive information is available on the transit time of epithelium moving from crypt to tip of villus in domestic animals. Generally, cells move off the villus more quickly in the ileum than in the duodenum, presumably related to the decline in height of villi with distance down the gut in most species. As well, in some species the number of crypts contributing cells to a single villus is lower in the ileum than in the duodenum.

Normally, the mass and topography of the mucosa are quite stable. This steady state is the product of a dynamic equilibrium between the rate of movement of cells out of crypts and onto villi, and the rate at which they are lost from the tips of villi. The stability of this equilibrium suggests that local feedback exists between the functional compartment on villi and the proliferative compartment in the crypts. Soluble chalones released from the functional compartment have been proposed as the effectors of a negative feedback mechanism acting on crypt cells, but they are poorly characterized. Inhibitors of replication, such as transforming growth factor-β, concentrated in epithelium at the villus tip, may be candidates. Experimental destruction of the functional epithelium on villi stimulates hyperplasia in the proliferative compartment serving affected villi, confirming that local feedback control is real.

In the young animal the intestine grows by generation of new crypts, and with them, new villi. As the bowel attains mature size, the number of villi stabilizes, and apparently remains relatively constant. The number of crypts also stabilizes, but some adaptive variation in the ratio of crypts to villi may occur. Adaptive responses to a variety of factors alter the size and rate of turnover of the proliferative and functional epithelial cell populations and with them the microtopography of the gut. The appearance of the small intestinal mucosa is a compromise, achieved by the equilibrium between the rate of cell production and rate of loss. At one extreme lies the intestine of the germ-free animal, with a short crypt containing a small proliferative compartment, and tall villi supporting a large functional compartment with a low rate of cell loss. At the other end of the spectrum is the animal suffering from severe intestinal helminthosis, with long crypts reflecting an increased proliferative compartment, yet a flat mucosal surface with relatively few functional enterocytes and an apparently high rate of cell loss.

Although quantitative description of epithelial kinetics is possible experimentally, in the diagnostic situation it is necessary to make a subjective or semiquantitative assessment of the status of the proliferative and functional compartments in tissue sections. The size of the proliferative compartment is reflected in the length and diameter of the crypts, and in the location of the uppermost mitotic cell. The prevalence of mitotic figures can be subjectively assessed, but beyond calculating a mitotic index, no inferences can be drawn about the proportion of the crypt cell population which is replicating, or the duration of the cell cycle.

There is obviously also some correlation between the length and profile of villi and the functional surface area, though the three-dimensional structure of an abnormal mucosa is often poorly reflected in section. Hence, it is highly desirable to correlate the histologic appearance with the microtopography of the mucosa as seen under the dissecting or scanning electron microscope. The degree of differentiation, and therefore, the functional status of enterocytes on villi, can be inferred from their appearance. Cytoplasmic basophilia; loss of regular basal nuclear polarity; low columnar, cuboidal, or squamous shape; and an ill-defined brush border all point to a poorly differentiated population of surface enterocytes, which is possibly turning over more rapidly than normal.

Fasting reduces the mucosal epithelial mass; the atrophy is related to prolongation of the postmitotic phase of the cell cycle in the proliferative compartment. Villi do not regress severely, however, since cells on the surface persist for twice as long, moving off the villus more slowly. The effect is reversed immediately by refeeding. Total parenteral nutrition does not abolish the effect of starvation. Surgical removal of a loop of bowel from the flow of digesta also causes atrophy of the epithelial population, which is reversed by restoration of continuity with the rest of the gut. Resection of a segment of gut causes hypertrophy of the mucosa remaining distal to the surgical site, which is reflected in dilation of the bowel, and thickening of the mucosa due to longer crypts and villi. Postresectional hypertrophy also occurs in the mucosa of separated loops of gut and in cross-circulated animals, suggesting a hormonal influence. Diversion of the opening of the pancreatic and bile ducts to the distal small bowel causes hypertrophy of the ileal mucosa, but does not result in atrophy of more proximal mucosa.

Many of these adaptive changes in experimental or surgical situations are interpreted as supporting the concept that exposure of enterocytes to nutrients is trophic, and an important factor in maintaining mucosal mass. Hormonal and possibly paracrine factors are also active. Gastrin is trophic for duodenal mucosa; growth hormone and glucocorticoids also have trophic effects on intestine under some circumstances, perhaps mediated through gastrin. Enteroglucagon is a prime candidate as a hormone trophic for the intestinal mucosa, and it is apparently elevated in calves with neonatal diarrhea, suggesting that it has a role in the adaptive response to mucosal damage in that and other species. However, its status as a trophic factor is uncertain. There is some evidence that other peptides, released from enteroendocrine cells and enteric nerves in the gut in response to a variety of luminal stimuli, may also influence epithelial proliferation. Epidermal growth factor, produced in the salivary glands and Brunner's glands, may also have a luminal trophic effect. Prostaglandins are trophic for the small intestine, where they may slow epithelial transit off the villus; apparently they are not trophic for the colon. Polyamines (putrescine, and its derivatives, spermidine and spermine), produced by the action of ornithine decarboxylase in enterocytes, or from ornithine decarboxylation by luminal bacteria, are possibly involved in regulation of intestinal epithelial proliferation. They are elevated in regenerating or replicative mucosa.

Restitution of epithelial integrity following minor loss of mucosal surface cells is by lateral migration of adjacent intact epithelium, and occurs within minutes. If epithelium on villi is obliterated, for instance by transient ischemia or by viral cytolysis, the villus core contracts, probably because of myofibroblast activity mediated by the enteric nervous system. Surviving epithelial cells become attenuated, and extend across the denuded intercrypt surface. The proliferative compartment then undergoes hyperplasia, generating new epithelium, and the three-dimensional architecture of the mucosa is rebuilt within a few days. Increased polyamine activity is essential for epithelial restitution and mucosal reconstitution. Extensive mucosal ulcers will form a bed of granulation tissue, and with time (weeks to months) may become covered by a neomucosa, with crypts and villi, which evolves following the centripetal immigration of flattened epithelium from the periphery of the lesion. A similar process repairs the mucosal gap in healing intestinal anastomosis.

b. VILLUS ATROPHY Atrophy of villi is a common pathologic change in the intestine of domestic animals. It results in malabsorption of nutrients, and sometimes is associated with increased plasma protein loss in the gut. Mucosa with short villi can be categorized morphologically into two broad types, recognition of which has implications with respect to pathogenesis and prognosis. The first category includes intestine with apparently normal, or hypertrophic crypts, associated with atrophy of villi to varying degrees. The second category is composed of gut with some evidence of damage to the proliferative compartment, and variable villus atrophy. The recognition, evolution, and interpretation of each will be considered in turn.

Villus atrophy with an intact or hypertrophic proliferative compartment takes two forms in domestic animals. A **primary increase in rate of loss of epithelium** from the surface of villi is one mechanism initiating such a lesion. This is the major pathogenetic action of a number of important virus diseases, including coronavirus and rotavirus infection; of coccidial infections which damage surface enterocytes predominantly; of some enteroinvasive bacteria; of transient ischemia, in which the effect is limited to the functional compartment; and, in some circumstances, of necrotizing toxins released by clostridia in the lumen of the bowel. The effect of these agents is to cause significantly increased loss of surface epithelium over a relatively short period. Villi contract as the size of the functional compartment is diminished, and they may become very stubby. If the animal survives the metabolic sequelae to the malabsorption which results from the damage to surface cells, compensatory expansion of the proliferative compartment in crypts permits complete recovery. Epithelium emerging from crypts regenerates villi, resulting in a normal mucosal topography within a few days, and full function returns.

The microscopic appearance of the mucosa depends partly on the number of functional cells lost, which determines the initial degree of villus atrophy, and partly on the amount of regeneration which has occurred by the time the gut is examined. During the early phase of cell loss, damaged epithelium may be seen exfoliating into the lumen of the gut, and villi are shorter or blunter than normal. Subsequently, the atrophic villi are covered by poorly differentiated, low columnar, cuboidal, or squamous cells. There may be fusion of the lateral surfaces or tips of villi in some areas. In severe atrophy there may be mild erosion if inadequate epithelium is available to cover even the much-reduced mucosal surface area. In the acute phase, crypts appear of normal size, but within 12–24 hr proliferative activity is noticeably increased. Crypts enlarge in diameter and length to accommodate more mitotic cells, which are basophilic, crowded, and obviously dividing, sometimes very close to the surface of the mucosa. The lamina propria appears moderately hypercellular, perhaps because of condensation, possibly due to a mild mononuclear cell infiltrate. As regeneration occurs, progressively longer villi with increasingly well-differentiated epithelium are evident, and hypertrophy of the proliferative compartment gradually subsides.

Atrophy of villi and hypertrophy of crypts also is associated with chronic processes such as nematode parasitism; chronic coccidial infection of surface epithelium; giardiasis in some species; response to dietary components in some species, including soybean protein in calves, kidney bean protein in pigs, and wheat in dogs; chronic inflammatory reactions in the lamina propria, such as Johne's disease and histoplasmosis; and idiopathic granulomatous enteritis or chronic enteritis characterized by heavy lymphocytic and plasmacytic infiltrates in the mucosa. The epithelial kinetics have not been investigated in most of these situations in domestic animals. However, they all have in common chronic antigenic exposure, parasitism, or an infectious process in the lumen, epithelium, or lamina propria, usually associated with a significant lymphocytic and plasmacytic infiltrate in the mucosa.

Cell-mediated immune events in the mucosa initiate cryptal hypertrophy and villus atrophy in experimental graft-versus-host reaction, intestinal trichinellosis, and giardiasis in mice. A similar pathogenesis in humans probably mediates intestinal allergy to some dietary antigens, causes celiac disease (gluten-sensitive enteropathy), and perhaps human immunodeficiency virus-related enteropathy; similar phenomena are likely to be active in domestic animals. In these conditions villus atrophy and loss of cells from the mucosal surface are not transient; they persist, despite obvious hyperplasia in the proliferative compartment.

In experimental mucosal lesions induced by cell-mediated immunity, hypertrophy of the proliferative compartment **precedes** the development of villus atrophy, and **is not a response to it.** This also occurs in *Nippostrongylus*-infected rats and *Eimeria acervulina*-infected chickens. In experimental intestinal trichostrongylosis, hypertrophy of crypts precedes villus atrophy; the epithelium emerging from hypertrophic crypts exfoliates soon after reaching the surface, rather than moving up the villus.

Evidence points to local stimulation of the proliferative compartment, and perhaps the associated myofibroblast sheath, by cytokines released by activated T lymphocytes in the mucosa. Cytotoxicity or damage to the functional compartment is apparently not a necessary precursor to hyperplasia by crypt cells, though it is not ruled out. Epithelial cells leaving the crypts usually do not differentiate fully. They exfoliate prematurely, low on the villus or near the crypt opening, and as the preexisting enterocytes are shed, villi undergo atrophy over a period of several days. Epithelium which reaches the surface subsequently fails to differentiate fully, and is rapidly lost into the lumen, matching the rate of cell production.

In villus atrophy of this type, the microtopography of the gut may vary from moderately short cylindrical villi, through short leaf or tongue shapes, to ridges on the mucosa. These would be interpreted in section as villi of varying height. More severely attenuated mucosal projections form convoluted intercrypt ridges, which in section may be misinterpreted as stumpy villi, with crypts opening directly onto the surface (subtotal villus atrophy). In extreme cases the mucosa becomes virtually flat, and crypt mouths project above the surface (total villus atrophy). In animals with moderate villus atrophy, the surface epithelium may appear relatively normal by light microscopy;

enterocytes which appear poorly differentiated or secrete mucus are usually present on more severely atrophic mucosa. In extreme atrophy, the epithelium may become squamous, and the surface may be eroded.

Hypertrophy of crypts is the early and outstanding change in this lesion, and is consistently present. In its milder forms the lesion may be better characterized by elongate crypts than by obvious atrophy of villi. The proliferative compartment is expanded and active, and mitotic figures are numerous. Elongation of crypts may be so great that even with severe atrophy of villi, the total mucosal thickness will not be much reduced from normal. The lamina propria often has a prominent population of lymphocytes, plasmacytes, and associated inflammatory cells, and intraepithelial lymphocytes are common. The etiologic agent, in the form of parasites, intracellular bacteria, or yeasts may be evident. Removal of the causal stimulus usually results in a return to normal within days or weeks.

Intestinal anaphylaxis, mediated by antigen–antibody reactions, may also be associated with mild villus atrophy and crypt hypertrophy. Circumstances in which this occurs in domestic animals are not well documented. Villus atrophy associated with some dietary antigens may speculatively be related to this mechanism.

Immune events have not been convincingly implicated in the development of postweaning villus atrophy in pigs, which seems in some cases to be associated initially with reduced crypt cell production, and to be mitigated by presenting the ration as a slurry, rather than dry. However, soy protein tends to be associated with a more severe and persistent postweaning villus atrophy in pigs than do other dietary proteins, and immune mechanisms may be implicated here, and in calves.

However it is induced, atrophy of villi with hypertrophy of crypts is associated with local malabsorption of nutrients and water; elongate crypts and perhaps poorly differentiated surface epithelium may secrete electrolyte and water; and if there is proprial inflammation and microerosion of the mucosa, effusion of tissue fluid may ensue. Increased turnover of epithelium may contribute to enteric loss of endogenous protein.

Villus atrophy associated with damage to the proliferative compartment is also seen commonly in domestic animals. It is the sequel to insults which cause necrosis of cells in crypts, or impair their mitotic capacity. The agents that produce these lesions usually have a propensity for damaging dividing cells in any tissue. Since ionizing radiation was recognized early as a cause of such lesions, they are often termed radiomimetic. Other causative agencies include cytotoxic chemicals and mitotic poisons, such as cancer chemotherapeutic agents, T-2 mycotoxin, and pyrrolizidine alkaloids in large doses; viruses which infect proliferating cells, particularly the parvoviruses, and bovine virus diarrhea and rinderpest viruses. Ischemia of sufficient duration to cause necrosis of some or all cells lining the crypts also causes a lesion in this category (Fig. 1.55D).

The microscopic appearance of affected mucosa depends on the severity and extent of the insult, and the interval since it occurred. The primary event is damage to the proliferative compartment, and except in ischemia, lesions will be evident in crypts well before significant atrophy of villi occurs. Apoptotic epithelial cells, and polymorphs may be present in the lumen of damaged crypts, which tend to dilate. If crypt cell necrosis is severe, remaining cells become extremely flattened in the course of attempting to maintain the integrity of the crypt lining. Following radiation, cytotoxic damage, and parvovirus infection, bizarre irregular epithelial cells with large nuclei and nucleoli may be present in crypts and will migrate on to the surface.

Preexisting surface epithelium continues to move off the tips of villi at an apparently normal rate, even though few or no new cells emerge from crypts. Villi eventually become atrophic or collapse as the surface cell population shrinks. If most proliferative and stem cells have been damaged, crypts stripped of epithelium will also collapse, or drop out, perhaps leaving a few scattered cystic remnants, lined by attenuated epithelium, in the deeper lamina propria. The overlying surface will be covered by squamous epithelial cells derived from surviving crypts, or will be eroded; it may eventually ulcerate, to be lined by granulation tissue. Crypts which have not been so severely damaged will undergo hypertrophy, as compensatory hyperplasia of lining cells occurs within a week or so of the original insult.

In viral diseases the severity and appearance of the lesion often vary considerably at different sites in the gut, and even within an individual tissue section. Lesions due to ischemia tend to be uniform in severity but may be localized; acute or subacute lesions are often hemorrhagic, if there has been reflow. Cytotoxic and radiation damage tend to be relatively uniform and more widespread, though some variation occurs because of differences in the proliferative activity, and therefore the susceptibility, of the epithelium at the time of insult. The inflammatory reaction depends on the availability of leukocytes, which may also have been diminished by the same insult which caused the epithelial necrosis. In the early stages, neutrophils and eosinophils may be in and around damaged crypts.

Extensive lesions due to crypt cell necrosis lead to erosion or ulceration, with severe malabsorption, and effusion of tissue fluid and hemorrhage. The mucosa is often invaded by the enteric flora. Local ulceration may lead to persistent plasma loss, and if circumferential, to stricture and stenosis. Small ulcers in areas where a few crypts have dropped out will heal as epithelium from adjacent crypts moves over the surface, but crypts may not regenerate for some time, and local villus atrophy will persist.

Villus atrophy occurs commonly **in association with alimentary lymphosarcoma.** Diffuse or focal infiltration of the lamina propria by neoplastic lymphocytes appears to separate and crowd out crypts. It also distorts the shape of villi, which become stubby, and are covered by low columnar or cuboidal epithelium. Presumably the atrophy of villi is related at least partially to a reduced density of crypts in the mucosa, and therefore fewer cells moving onto the surface per unit area. In severe cases, erosion of the epithelium will occur over lymphosarcomatous infiltrates.

2. Large Intestine

Epithelial turnover in the cecum and colon is fundamentally similar to that in the small intestine, though villi are not present on the surface. Cells lose the ability to divide after leaving the proliferative compartment in the lower part of the gland. In the upper portion of the gland they differentiate into goblet cells or columnar absorptive cells, which emerge and move out over the surface. They are lost into the lumen, probably within about 4–8 days of being produced, though no studies of colonic epithelial turnover have been made in domestic animals. Fasting reduces, and refeeding restores, proliferative activity in colonic glands in experimental animals, and physical distension and certain types of dietary fiber in the colon also appear to be trophic for the mucosa. Eicosanoids also may influence colonic epithelial proliferation. The colon of gnotobiotic animals has a small number of proliferative cells, limited to the lower portion of the glands. With conventionalization of the gut flora, the proliferative compartment expands.

Restitution of the epithelial integrity of the surface of the large bowel, following insult to, and exfoliation of, surface cells, resembles that in the small bowel. Within a few minutes of injury, surviving surface epithelium, and cells emerging from crypts, become attenuated and migrate at a rate of several micrometers per minute to extend over mucosal defects. Ulcers, surgical incisions, or anastomotic sites in the colon heal by immigration of a single layer of epithelium from the periphery of the defect, with gradual differentiation of crypts, and eventual restitution of normal mucosal architecture. In the horse, depending on the type of anastomosis, epithelium may take more than 2 weeks to bridge the granulation tissue in the gap in the mucosa, and restitution of mucosal architecture may require about 2 months. In adapting to compensate for extensive resection of the equine large colon, the intercrypt absorptive surface of the remaining colon increases slowly.

Lesions in the large bowel presumed to be associated with increased epithelial turnover include alterations in both surface and glandular epithelium. The number of goblet cells on the surface and in the upper portion of glands is diminished, and epithelium in these areas appears poorly differentiated, is more basophilic than normal, and may be low columnar, cuboidal, or squamous. In severe diseases, microerosion of the surface is present. The proliferative compartment in the gland may hypertrophy, causing glands to elongate and dilate. Crowded mitotic cells are present over a greater proportion of the length of the gland, sometimes virtually to the surface of the mucosa. Such changes may be associated with acute, chronic, or chronic active inflammation of the lamina propria. It is uncertain whether such changes are caused both by primary damage to surface epithelium, and by primary immune-mediated stimulation to the proliferative compartment. Experimentally, cell-mediated immune reactions increase crypt cell production. Colonic lesions consistent with increased epithelial cell turnover occur mainly in swine dysentery, proliferative hemorrhagic enteropathy in swine, trichuriasis, canine histiocytic ulcerative colitis, granulomatous colitis due to a variety of agents, and idiopathic colitis of dogs.

The proliferative compartment in the cecal and colonic glands is damaged by the same insults that attack cells in the crypts of the small bowel. However, cytotoxins and parvoviruses tend not to produce severe lesions so commonly in large bowel as they do in small intestine, perhaps because a lower proportion of the proliferative compartment is in mitosis at the time of maximal availability of drug or virus. Additions to the list of agents damaging the proliferative compartment in large intestine include coronavirus in calves, cattle, and dogs, and several species of coccidia in ruminants, which develop in the cells lining glands in the large bowel.

The evolution and sequelae of lesions resulting from damage to proliferative epithelium in the large intestine are similar to those in small bowel. Dilation of crypts containing necrotic debris, and lined by attenuated epithelium, indicates such damage. Severe lesions will lead to loss of glands, and erosion and ulceration of the mucosa, perhaps with hemorrhage. Stricture and stenosis may ensue. Following milder damage that spares some stem cells in each gland, the mucosa has the potential to recover fully after a period of reparative hyperplasia.

Bibliography

Angus, K. W., Coop, R. L., and Sykes, A. R. The rate of recovery of intestinal morphology following anthelmintic treatment of parasitised sheep. *Res Vet Sci* **26:** 120–122, 1979.

Argenzio, R. A. *et al.* Villous atrophy, crypt hyperplasia, cellular infiltration, and impaired glucose–Na absorption in enteric cryptosporidiosis of pigs. *Gastroenterology* **98:** 1129–1140, 1990.

Barker, I. K., and Ford, G. E. Development and distribution of atrophic enteritis in the small intestine of rabbits infected with *Trichostrongylus retortaeformis*. *J Comp Pathol* **85:** 427–435, 1975.

Barratt, M. E. J. *et al.* Immunopathology of intestinal disorders in farm animals. *In* "Immunopathology of the Small Intestine," M. N. Marsh, (ed.), pp. 253–281. Chichester, England, John Wiley, 1987.

Bennett, R. E. *et al.* The role of apoptosis in atrophy of the small gut mucosa produced by repeated administration of cytosine arabinoside. *J Pathol* **142:** 259–263, 1984.

Berthrong, M., and Fajardo, L. F. Radiation injury in surgical pathology. Part II. Alimentary tract. *Am J Surg Pathol* **5:** 153–178, 1981.

Bertone, A. L. *et al.* Alteration in intestinal morphological features associated with extensive large-colon resection in horses. *Am J Vet Res* **51:** 1471–1475, 1990.

Bloom, S. R. Gut hormones in adaptation. *Gut* **28:** 31–35, 1987.

Bone, D. L. *et al.* Evaluation of anastomoses of small intestine in dogs: Crushing versus noncrushing suturing techniques. *Am J Vet Res* **44:** 2043–2048, 1983.

Bristol, J. B., and Williamson, M. A. Nutrition, operations and intestinal adaptation. *J Parenteral Enteral Nutr* **12:** 299–309, 1988.

Buret, A. *et al.* Intestinal protozoa and epithelial cell kinetics, structure and function. *Parasitol Today* **6:** 375–380, 1990.

Bustamante, S. A., Forshult, M., and Lundgren O. Evidence for an intramural nervous control of epithelial cell migration in the small intestine of the rat. *Acta Physiol Scand* **135:** 469–475, 1989.

Chang, E. B. Transforming growth factors and intestinal epithelia: More questions than answers. *Gastroenterology* **97:** 1587–88, 1989.

Curtis, G. H. *et al.* Intestinal anaphylaxis in the rat. *Gastroenterology* **98:** 1558–1566, 1990.

Deprez, P. *et al.* Liquid versus dry feeding in weaned piglets: The influence on small intestinal morphology. *J Vet Med (B)* **34:** 254–259, 1987.

Dunsford, B. R. *et al.* Effect of dietary soybean meal on the microscopic anatomy of the small intestine in the early-weaned pig. *J Anim Sci* **67:** 1855–1863, 1989.

Feil, W. *et al.* Rapid epithelial restitution of human and rabbit colonic mucosa. *Gastroenterology* **97:** 685–701, 1989.

Ferguson, A. Models of immunologically driven small intestinal damage. *In* "Immunopathology of the Small Intestine," M. N. Marsh, (ed.), pp. 225–252. Chichester, England, John Wiley, 1987.

Fernando, M. A., and McCraw, B. M. Changes in the generation cycle of duodenal crypt cells in chickens infected with *Eimeria acervulina*. *Z Parasitenkd* **52:** 213–218, 1977.

Ferreira, R. C. *et al.* Changes in the rate of crypt epithelial cell proliferation and mucosal morphology induced by a T cell-mediated response in human small intestine. *Gastroenterology* **98:** 1255–1263, 1990.

Hall, G. A., and Byrne, T. F. Effects of age and diet on small intestinal structure and function in gnotobiotic piglets. *Res Vet Sci* **47:** 387–392, 1989.

Hanson, R. R. *et al.* Evaluation of three techniques for end-to-end anastomosis of the small colon in horses. *Am J Vet Res* **49:** 1613–1620, 1988.

Johnson, L. R. (ed.) "Physiology of the Gastrointestinal Tract," L. R. Johnson, (ed.). New York, Raven Press, 1987. [See chapters by L. R. Johnson (pp. 301–333), M. Lipkin (pp. 255–284).]

Kaur, P., and Potten, C. S. Cell-migration velocities in the crypts of the small intestine after cytotoxic insult are not dependent on mitotic activity. *Cell Tissue Kinet* **19:** 601–610, 1986.

Kelly, D. *et al.* Effect of creep feeding on structural and functional changes of the gut of early weaned pigs. *Res Vet Sci* **48:** 350–356, 1990.

Kik, M. J. L. *et al.* Pathologic changes of the small intestinal mucosa of pigs after feeding *Phaseolus vulgaris* beans. *Vet Pathol* **27:** 329–334, 1990.

Luk, G. D., and Yang, P. Polyamines in intestinal and pancreatic adaptation. *Gut* **28,** (Suppl. 1): 95–101, 1987.

MacDonald, T. T. The role of activated T lymphocytes in gastrointestinal disease. *Clin Exp Allergy* **20:** 247–252, 1990.

Mowat, A. McI., and Felstein, M. V. Experimental studies of immunologically mediated enteropathy. V. Destructive enteropathy during an acute graft-versus-host reaction in adult BDF1 mice. *Clin Exper Immunol* **79:** 279–284, 1990.

Perdue, M. H. *et al.* Intestinal mucosal injury is associated with mast cell activation and leukotriene generation during *Nippostrongylus*-induced inflammation in the rat. *Dig Dis Sci* **34:** 724–731, 1989.

Riecken, E. O. *et al.* Growth and transformation of the small intestinal mucosa—importance of connective tissue, gut-associated lymphoid tissue, and gastrointestinal regulatory peptides. *Gut* **30:** 1630–1640, 1989.

Rijke, R. P. C. *et al.* The effect of ischemic villus cell damage on crypt cell proliferation in the small intestine. Evidence for a feedback control mechanism. *Gastroenterology* **71:** 786–792, 1976.

Symons, L. E. A. Kinetics of the epithelial cells and morphology of villi and crypts in the jejunum of the rat infected by the nematode *Nippostrongylus brasiliensis*. *Gastroenterology* **49:** 158–168, 1965.

Thompson, J. S. Growth of neomucosa after intestinal resection. *Arch Surg* **122:** 317–319, 1987.

Thurman, J. D., Creasia, D. A., and Trotter, R. W. Mycotoxicosis caused by aerosolized T-2 toxin administered to female mice. *Am J Vet Res* **49:** 1928–1931, 1988.

Townsend, C. M., Jr. *et al.* Growth factors and intestinal neoplasms. *Am J Surg* **155:** 526–536, 1988.

Uribe, A., and Johansson, C. Initial kinetic changes of prostaglandin E_2-induced hyperplasia of the rat small intestinal epithelium occur in the villus compartments. *Gastroenterology* **94:** 1335–1342, 1988.

Van Dijk, J. E. *et al.* Gastrointestinal food allergy and its role in large domestic animals. *Vet Res Commun* **12:** 47–59, 1988.

Wang, J. Y., and Johnson, L. R. Polyamines and ornithine decarboxylase during repair of duodenal mucosa after stress in rats. *Gastroenterology* **100:** 333–343, 1991.

I. Pathophysiology of Enteric Disease

The effects of gastrointestinal diseases are mediated by a number of mechanisms that often interact. Common consequences of enteric disease include inability to eat or loss of appetite; reduced growth rate, weight loss, or cachexia; hypoproteinemia, and anemia, perhaps with obvious hemorrhage into the gut. Dehydration and acid–base imbalance are associated with reduced water consumption, obstruction, vomition, or diarrhea. Dysfunction of other organs, and of systemic homeostasis, may be caused by toxins, parasites, bacteria, or viruses originating in the gut.

Malassimilation of nutrients occurs commonly in animals with gastrointestinal disease. Failure to assimilate nutrients may result in a reduced growth rate, and in emaciation and cachexia if nutrient requirements for maintenance are not met. Malassimilation often occurs concurrent with enteric protein loss, and the contribution of these two factors, along with loss of appetite, to reduced growth rate or to cachexia, must be recognized and differentiated. Diarrhea is a common sign of malassimilation, but its pathogenesis is only partly explained by this mechanism.

Protein–energy malnutrition, due to intake of too little feed, or of feed deficient in quantity or quality of nutrients, results in depletion of fat and muscle mass, emaciation, and ultimately, death by starvation. It must be differentiated from the effects of endogenous conditions resulting in malassimilation, or protein-losing enteropathy, and from other problems which may result in recumbency.

In neonates, several factors predispose to death by starvation within the first few weeks of life. These include increased energy demands due to cold and exposure; fetal malnutrition with poor fat depots at birth; and post-partum hyponutrition, which in calves is often associated with poor quality or insufficient milk replacer. Piglets are born with negligible fat reserves and die quickly of hypoglycemia if not fed adequately. Neonatal ruminants usually have depots sufficient to compensate for longer periods of inanition (2–4 days for lambs; 6–10 days for calves), if cold stress is not severe. In the neonatal ruminant, fat depots in the omentum and mesentery are depleted first, whereas epicardial fat is mobilized last. In the adult, the marrow fat is the last to be depleted. The perirenal fat depot is the largest in the neonatal ruminant, and does not appear to be typical brown fat, in that it is not restricted to local thermogenesis, but can be mobilized for fatty acid oxidation elsewhere.

In animals which have died of inanition, muscle mass is reduced, because of mobilization of amino acids for gluconeogenesis. Fat in the bone marrow, coronary groove, on the pericardial sac, and around the kidneys is completely depleted, and has the gelatinous clear pink appearance of serous atrophy. The liver may appear small, with sharp margins, presumably due to reduced trophic stimuli. In extreme cachexia of starvation, there may be osteopenia. A diagnosis of starvation is supported by a history of conditions compatible with reduced quantity or quality of feed, and by steps to rule out problems causing malassimilation and protein-losing gastroenteropathy.

1. Malassimilation

Digestion and assimilation of nutrients have an intraluminal phase, mediated by the biliary and pancreatic secretions, and an epithelial phase, carried out by enzyme systems on the surface and in the cytoplasm of absorptive enterocytes. The final step is delivery of the nutrient by the enterocyte to the interstitial fluid, and its uptake into the blood or lymph.

Pancreatic exocrine insufficiency is the major cause of intraluminal maldigestion, and it is usually due to juvenile pancreatic atrophy in dogs, or to pancreatic fibrosis and atrophy following repeated episodes of pancreatic necrosis (see The Pancreas, Chapter 3 of this volume). It may be complicated by bacterial overgrowth of the small intestine. Bile salt deficiency is rarely seen as a cause of intraluminal maldigestion in domestic animals.

The **epithelial phase of digestion** is impaired by loss of functional epithelial surface area. This occurs in short-bowel syndrome following intestinal resection, in which greater than 75–85% of the small bowel has been lost, and more commonly, in villus atrophy. Congenital deficiencies of enzymes which are normally present on the microvilli are not recognized in domestic animals. However, neonates and ruminants have low levels of maltase; ruminants lack sucrase. In most species, lactase levels decline with age, and malabsorption in dogs fed milk has been attributed to low levels of lactase. The poorly differentiated surface epithelium present on atrophic villi may lack the full complement of enzymes on the brush border and in the cytoplasm necessary for nutrient digestion and assimilation. Lectins present in uncooked beans attach to and damage microvilli on enterocytes, which may explain the malabsorption and diarrhea associated with their use in feeds; lectins also promote bacterial adhesion and overgrowth in the small intestine. Delivery of nutrients, especially lipid, to the circulation, may be impaired in lymphangiectasia. The pathogenesis of malabsorption of the major classes of nutrients will be considered briefly.

Assimilation of fat is susceptible to interference at all three phases of digestion and absorption. Lipolysis is impaired if insufficient lipase is available. Most commonly this is a result of pancreatic atrophy or fibrosis. It may be due to failure by atrophic intestinal mucosa to release the cholecystokinin/pancreozymin necessary for pancreatic secretion. The availability of bile salts for micelle formation is reduced in intrahepatic cholestasis or biliary obstruction, and by depletion of the bile salt pool due to reduced ileal absorption following resection or atrophy. As a result, fatty acid and monoglyceride are not incorporated onto micelles and emulsified; they are, therefore, not so accessible to absorptive enterocytes. Reduced surface area for lipid uptake will contribute to malabsorption of fat. Poorly differentiated enterocytes on atrophic gut may be less able than normal epithelium to re-esterify long-chain fatty acids to triglyceride and to produce chylomicrons for export from the cell. In lymphangiectasia, granulomatous enteritis, and intestinal lymphosarcoma, lymphatic drainage may be obstructed, and with it the flow of chylomicrons to the systemic circulation.

Malabsorption of lipids may cause steatorrhea (excess fat in the feces). It is seen in monogastric animals, especially dogs, in which species fat often forms a large proportion of the daily caloric intake. Severe fat malabsorption may result in deficiencies of fat-soluble vitamins. Malabsorption of calcium, magnesium, and zinc occurs because of their sequestration in soaps formed by combination with malabsorbed luminal fatty acids. Increased absorption of oxalate, and consequent nephrolithiasis, may be a sequel to reduced concentrations of calcium in the lumen due to soap formation. Malabsorbed lipid may cause colonic diarrhea, by mechanisms which will be discussed subsequently.

Maldigestion of polysaccharides occurs if levels of pancreatic amylase are reduced; this is encountered most commonly in dogs with severe loss of functional exocrine tissue. Calves and older ruminants normally lack significant amounts of pancreatic amylase and digest starch poorly in the small intestine. Mucosal oligosaccharidase deficiency occurs in villus atrophy, with reduced mucosal surface area. Poor differentiation of enterocytes results in irregular, short, and sparse microvilli, and a reduced complement of oligosaccharidases. The result is impaired membrane digestion of disaccharide and malabsorption of carbohydrate, much of which is subsequently fermented by colonic flora. The osmotic effect of malabsorbed disaccharide augments intraluminal fluid accumulation in the small intestine, and this may be compounded by hydrolysis in the colon. Carbohydrate malabsorption is an important component of disease in neonatal diarrhea due to rotavirus and coronavirus, and in other conditions in which there is extensive villus atrophy in the small intestine.

Protein digestion in the lumen is reduced if pancreatic protease activity is decreased to ~ 10% of normal, as may occur with exocrine pancreatic insufficiency. Loss of gastric proteolytic activity is of little nutritional significance. In conditions with villus atrophy, reduced mucosal surface area and poor differentiation of enterocytes result in malabsorption of small peptides and particularly of amino acids by mechanisms similar to those involved in carbohydrate malabsorption. It is conceivable that atrophy of duodenal villi may result in reduced availability of the brush border enzyme enterokinase, which is necessary for the activation of pancreatic trypsinogen to trypsin, initiating the subsequent activation of other pancreatic proteases by trypsin. Some dogs with mucosal malabsorption do appear to have partial pancreatic insufficiency, perhaps for this reason. The influence of reduced protein digestion and assimilation on energy metabolism and anabolic activity must be differentiated from the effects of the loss of plasma and other endogenous protein into the lumen of the gut.

A reduction in absorption of minerals and vitamins may be intuitively expected in animals with reduced absorptive surface in villus atrophy, above and beyond specific mechanisms alluded to previously. If villus atrophy is relatively localized, the reserve capacity of more distal small bowel may offset the effects of local nutrient malabsorption, and there may not be net malabsorption over the full length of the small intestine.

Bibliography

Batt, R. M. The molecular basis of malabsorption. *J Small Anim Pract* **21:** 555–569, 1980.

Batt, R. M. New approaches to malabsorption in dogs. *Compend Cont Ed Pract Vet* **8:** 783–794, 1986.

Bird, P. H. *et al.* Carbohydrate malabsorption in dogs assessed using bioluminescence assays to measure simple sugars. *Aust Vet J* **67:** 341–342, 1990.

Bolton, J. R. *et al.* Normal and abnormal xylose absorption in the horse. *Cornell Vet* **66:** 183–197, 1976.

Craig, R. M., and Atkinson, A. J. D-Xylose testing: A review. *Gastroenterology* **95:** 223–231, 1988.

Gray, G. M. Carbohydrate digestion and absorption. *N Engl J Med* **292:** 1225–1230, 1975.

Jacobs, R. M. *et al.* Laboratory diagnosis of malassimilation. *Vet Clin North Am Small Anim Pract* **19:** 951–977, 1989.

Muir, P. *et al.* Evaluation of carbohydrate malassimilation and intestinal transit time in cats by measurement of breath hydrogen excretion. *Am J Vet Res* **52:** 1104–1109, 1991.

Nicholson, A., Watson, A. D. J., and Mercer, J. R. Fat malassimilation in three cats. *Aust Vet J* **66:** 110–113, 1989.

Oetzel, G. R., and Berger, L. L. Protein–energy malnutrition in domestic ruminants. Part I. Predisposing factors and pathophysiology. Part II. Diagnosis, treatment, and prevention. *Compend Cont Ed Pract Vet* **7:** S672–S680, 1985; **8:** S16–S22, 1986.

Riley, J. W., and Glickman, R. M. Fat malabsorption—Advances in our understanding. *Am J Med* **67:** 980–988, 1979.

Schoonderwoerd, M. *et al.* Protein–energy malnutrition and fat mobilization in neonatal calves. *Can Vet J* **27:** 365–371, 1986.

Sleisenger, M. H., and Kim, Y. S. Protein digestion and absorption. *N Engl J Med* **300:** 659–663, 1979.

Strombeck, D. R., and Guilford, W. G. Maldigestion, malabsorption, bacterial overgrowth, and protein-losing enteropathy. *In* "Small Animal Gastroenterology," 2nd Ed., pp. 296–319. Davis, California, Stonegate Publishing, 1990.

Sweeney, R. W. Laboratory evaluation of malassimilation in horses. *Vet Clin North Am: Equine Pract* **3:** 507–514, 1987.

Sykes, A. R., Coop, R. L., and Angus, K. W. Experimental production of osteoporosis in growing lambs by continuous dosing with *Trichostrongylus colubriformis* larvae. *J Comp Pathol* **85:** 549–559, 1975.

Tate, L. P. *et al.* Effects of extensive resection of the small intestine of the pony. *Am J Vet Res* **44:** 1187–1191, 1983.

Weinman, M. D. *et al.* Repair of microvilli in the rat small intestine after damage with lectins contained in the red kidney bean. *Gastroenterology* **97:** 1193–1204, 1989.

Weser, E., Fletcher, J. T., and Urban, E. Short bowel syndrome. *Gastroenterology* **77:** 572–579, 1979.

Whitenack, D. L., Whitehair, C. K., and Miller, E. R. Influence of enteric infection on zinc utilization and clinical signs and lesions of zinc deficiency in young swine. *Am J Vet Res* **39:** 1447–1454, 1978.

Yanoff, S. R., and Willard, M. D. Short bowel syndrome in dogs and cats. *Sem Vet Med Surg (Small Anim)* **4:** 226–231, 1989.

2. *Diarrhea*

Diarrhea is the presence of water in feces in relative excess in proportion to fecal dry matter. Diarrhea usually reflects increased absolute fecal loss of water, but may not, if absolute fecal dry matter excretion is markedly reduced. Loss of solute and water in diarrhea may lead to severe electrolyte depletion, acid–base imbalance, and dehydration, which are life-threatening if not corrected.

Large volumes of fluid derived from ingesta, and from gastric, pancreatic, biliary, and enteric secretion, enter the small bowel; in addition, considerable passive movement of water occurs into the upper small bowel from the circulation, in response to osmotic effects. Overall, the bulk of the fluid entering the small intestine is absorbed by the enterocytes, so that the volume leaving the ileum and entering the colon is but a small fraction of the total fluid flux through the small bowel. The large size of this flux implies that relatively small perturbations in unidirectional movement of electrolyte and water may have significant effects on the net movement of fluid.

The colon, in addition to its fermentative function, has the ultimate responsibility for conserving electrolyte and water by absorption from the digesta, thereby minimizing fecal loss. It has a finite capacity for absorption, and if this is exceeded by the rate at which content enters from the small bowel, diarrhea occurs. This is important in small-bowel diarrheas, in which the lesion is in the small intestine. Since the colon has reserve absorptive capacity, the excess volume entering from the ileum must be considerable for diarrhea to occur. The large capacity and fermentative function of the equine colon may mitigate to some extent the expression of small-bowel diarrhea in mature animals of that species.

Large-bowel diarrhea, on the other hand, reflects an intrinsically reduced capacity of the colon to handle even normal volumes of fluid and electrolyte presented to it by the small intestine.

Small-bowel diarrhea is classed as secretory, malabsorptive, and effusive, but the mechanisms are not mutually exclusive.

Secretory diarrhea is due to an excess of secretion over absorption of fluid in the small intestine, resulting from derangement of normal secretory and absorptive mechanisms. It is best exemplified by the effects of diarrheagenic bacterial enterotoxins. *Vibrio cholerae* and *E. coli* are the most important sources of such toxins, though only the latter occurs in domestic animals; some *Salmonella* serotypes, *Yersinia enterocolitica, Shigella* and *Campylobacter jejuni* also produce enterotoxin. Cholera, heat-labile *E. coli,* and *C. jejuni* enterotoxin act through the mediation of cyclic AMP (cAMP). In surface enterocytes, toxin-stimulated cAMP shuts down sodium chloride cotransport at the luminal cell membrane, reducing passive water absorption. Meanwhile, in crypt epithelium, cAMP-stimulated chloride secretion is promoted, and water follows. The resultant increase in secretion by crypts and decrease in absorption by villi increases the solute and water load passing from the small bowel to the colon. Heat-stable *E. coli* and *Y. enterocolitica* enterotoxins stimulate cyclic guanosine monophosphate (GMP)-mediated secretion by the mucosa.

In addition to bacterial enterotoxins, other factors may potentially cause secretory diarrhea. Prostaglandins, other eicosanoids, histamine, kinins, and various cytokines directly or indirectly stimulate secretion, and they may contribute to diarrhea in inflammatory bowel disease, though this is speculative. Vasoactive intestinal polypeptide secreted by pancreatic islet cell tumors causes severe diarrhea (pancreatic cholera) in humans with such tumors. Thyroid C cell tumors secrete calcitonin; carcinoids secrete serotonin, bradykinin, and substance P; whereas mast cell tumors secrete histamine, which is also diarrheagenic.

Malabsorptive diarrhea is exemplified by the osmotic retention of water in the gut lumen by poorly absorbed magnesium sulfate, used therapeutically as a laxative. Malabsorption commonly results from villus atrophy, no matter what the cause. Electrolyte and nutrient solute, malabsorbed as the result of reduced villous and microvillous surface area, are retained in the lumen of the bowel, along with osmotically associated water. The additional solute and water is passed on to the colon. A secretory component probably contributes to diarrhea due to villus atrophy, at least in transmissible gastroenteritis in pigs. Here, since the villous limb of the postulated crypt–villus fluid circuit is diminished or missing, fluid secreted by the crypts may not be absorbed. Poorly differentiated cells emerging onto the intestinal surface from crypts also may retain some secretory capacity. Malabsorptive diarrhea also occurs in short-bowel syndome, because of reduced absorptive surface.

Increased permeability of the mucosa may contribute to diarrhea by permitting increased retrograde movement of solute and fluid from the lateral intercellular space to the lumen, or by facilitating transudation of tissue fluid. **Filtration secretion** is characterized by increased fluid movement through the epithelial membrane via the paracellular route; the force for secretion is provided by the transepithelial hydrostatic pressure gradient. Elevated capillary hydrostatic pressure, or decreased plasma oncotic pressure in the villus, alter Starling forces, resulting in edema. This overrides the hydrostatic pressure in the interepithelial space, and permits leakage of interstitial fluid and large protein molecules through enlarged pores at the tight junctions. Portal hypertension or right-sided heart failure, hypoalbuminemia, and expansion of plasma volume establish such conditions. Effusion may occur in lymphangiectasia, and in inflamed lamina propria, with increased vascular permeability, proprial edema, and enteric plasma protein loss. Increased exfoliation of epithelium and transient microerosions may provide further potential sites for effusion of interstitial fluid.

Severe necrosis of the epithelium and vascular damage in the mucosa cause obvious malabsorption, and effusion of tissue fluid and blood, evident as fibrin and hemorrhage, in the lumen. *Clostridium difficile* produces enterocyte-lethal toxins, which increase intestinal permeability, and in animals, clostridial enterotoxemias and conditions such as salmonellosis might have similar effects.

Large-bowel diarrhea is due to a reduction in the innate capability of the colon to absorb the solute and fluid presented by the more proximal bowel. A reduction in net absorption by the colon that is relatively small in absolute terms may be sufficient to cause fluid feces. Colonic diarrhea is characterized by frequent passage of small amounts of fluid feces, perhaps with mucus and blood. Colonic dysfunction has not received the same attention as small-bowel disease, but secretory, malabsorptive, and effusive mechanisms are implicated here as well, and they frequently appear to act concurrently.

The colonic mucosa is not so leaky as the small intestinal mucosa, due to the nature of the tight junctions between epithelial cells. As a result, it resists alterations in permeability due to increased hydrostatic pressure in the propria, when compared with the small intestine. Ulceration or erosion may be expected to result in reduced colonic function due to loss of absorptive surface epithelium. Although effusion is anticipated in these states, abnormal macromolecular permeability was not demonstrated in *Salmonella* colitis or swine dysentery. However, in swine dysentery, net electrolyte and water absorption ceases. In colitis, inflammation and increased turnover of the epithelium, resulting in poorly differentiated cells on the surface, are associated with reduced epithelial electrolyte transport, and perhaps eicosanoid-mediated secretion.

Bile acids mediate diarrhea associated with ileal disease, and fatty acids are the cause of diarrhea in steatorrhea. The mechanisms of action of these agents appear to be similar; though both may affect the small bowel, the major effect is in the colon. Moderate ileal damage or resection results in the escape of excess bile acids to the colon. This loss is compensated by increased hepatic synthesis to maintain the size of the bile salt pool, but the increased load of bile salts entering the colon is converted to secondary bile acids by the colonic flora. Fatty acids enter the colon in increased quantities in steatorrhea, resulting from bile salt depletion. Both dihydroxy bile acids and long-chain fatty acids, especially hydroxy fatty acids produced by bacterial action, alter mucosal permeability and cause mild damage to the surface epithelium. They both also stimulate secretion by the colonic mucosa, perhaps by causing local prostaglandin release, or other mechanisms. The result is net fluid secretion by the colon, and diarrhea. This also is the mode of action of a number of laxatives, including senna, and castor oil, which contains the hydroxy fatty acid ricinoleic acid.

Although colonic secretion stimulated by bacterial enterotoxin is not clearly implicated in diarrhea, alterations in the flora in the large bowel may be detrimental to normal function. Absorption of volatile fatty acids produced by bacterial fermentation is responsible for considerable concurrent absorption of water in the large intestine. Reduced production or absorption of volatile fatty acids, secondary to imbalance of the bacterial flora in the cecum and colon, may explain some problems of wasting and diarrhea in horses in which no morphologic abnormality of the mucosa can be found.

Osmotic overload of the large bowel results from the delivery by the small bowel of a large volume of fermentable substrate. This may result from excessive intake, but usually is due to malabsorption in the small intestine. Of the malabsorbed nutrients, carbohydrate is the only one of significance in initiating colonic osmotic overload. Bacterial fermentation of carbohydrate results in the production of excess volatile fatty acid. This is readily handled by the colon under normal circumstances, by rapid absorption and by bicarbonate buffering. However, a heavy carbohydrate load may overwhelm the colonic buffering capacity, and cause a reduced pH. This results in an altered gut flora dominated by organisms producing lactic acid, which is absorbed at a slower rate than the volatile fatty acids. Further acidification causes mucosal permeability, permitting an influx of water and solute into the lumen from the tissue, as a result of the increased osmotic pressure generated by lactic acid in the lumen. Diarrhea follows.

Increased intestinal motility probably does not have a primary role in the pathogenesis of diarrhea. Often the small intestine of animals with diarrhea is flaccid and fluid filled, rather than hypermotile. Increased colonic motor activity is often segmental and antiperistaltic, and probably unrelated to increased transit. Hypermotility, if it does occur, may be in response to, rather than a cause of, increased volumes of fluid in the gut.

Bacterial overgrowth in the small bowel may be a consequence of ileus or hypomotility, partial small bowel obstruction, and radiation injury. Achlorhydria or hypochlorhydria and pancreatic exocrine insufficiency in the dog may also predispose to this problem. Aerobic bacterial overgrowth seems relatively innocuous, but stagnant-loop or blind-loop syndrome ensues if anaerobes proliferate in the lumen of the small intestine to levels approaching those in the large bowel. Mild or moderate villus atrophy may develop in the affected area, and bacteria will be seen on the mucosal surface in tissue sections, an unusual finding in the small bowel. Ultrastructural lesions and cytoplasmic lipid accumulation can be present in surface enterocytes, though the brush border may be intact. Deconjugation of bile acids by anaerobes results in free bile acids, many of which precipitate at the pH of the gut content and are lost to the recirculating pool. Some are absorbed passively, but dihydroxy secondary bile salts may be the cause of damage to enterocytes. Fat malabsorption occurs when conjugated bile acids fall below critical micellar concentrations, reducing emulsion and absorption. Malabsorption is further exacerbated by the toxic damage to cells. Steatorrhea results.

Protein digestion and absorption may not be affected by bacterial overgrowth; however, some amino acids may be deaminated by anaerobes and metabolized to ammonia, which is absorbed, converted to urea in the liver, and largely lost through the kidney. Plasma protein loss into the gut can also occur, as may impaired uptake of disaccharides. Binding of vitamin B_{12} by enteric flora prevents absorption in the ileum and may lead to deficiency. Dihydroxy bile acids and malabsorbed fatty acids promote secretion by the small bowel and colon, resulting in diarrhea.

Aerobic overgrowth of the small bowel in dogs results in depression of alkaline phosphatase in the brush border of enterocytes, in contrast to the findings in dogs with predominantly anaerobic overgrowth. Morphologic lesions are minor, though biochemical abnormalities have been detected. Antibiotic therapy resolved the biochemical lesions, as it did in anaerobic overgrowth as well. Replacement with pancreatic enzymes seems to resolve in most cases the mixed bacterial overgrowth encountered in dogs with exocrine pancreatic insufficiency.

Bibliography

Argenzio, R. A. Pathophysiology of neonatal calf diarrhea. *Vet Clin North Am: Food Anim Pract* **1:** 461–469, 1985.

Banwell, J. G. Pathophysiology of diarrheal disorders. *Rev Infect Dis* **12:** S30–S35, 1990.

Batt, R. M., McLean, L., and Riley, J. E. Response of the jejunal mucosa of dogs with aerobic and anaerobic bacterial overgrowth to antibiotic therapy. *Gut* **29:** 473–482, 1988.

Butler, D. G. *et al.*, Transmissible gastroenteritis: Mechanisms responsible for diarrhea in an acute viral enteritis in pigs. *J Clin Invest* **53:** 1335–1342, 1974.

Duffy, P. A., Granger, D. N., and Taylor, A. E. Intestinal secretion induced by volume expansion in the dog. *Gastroenterology* **75:** 413–418, 1978.

Field, M., Rao, M. C., and Chang, E. B. Intestinal electrolyte transport and diarrheal disease. *N Engl J Med* **321:** 879–883, 1989.

Isaacs, P. E. T., and Kim, Y. S. The contaminated small bowel syndrome. *Am J Med* **67:** 1049–1057, 1979.

Johnson, L. R. (ed.). "Physiology of the Gastrointestinal Tract," 2nd Ed., New York, Raven Press, 1987. [See chapters by H. J. Binder and G. I. Sandle (pp. 1389–1418), M. Donowitz and M. J. Welsh (pp. 1351–1388), G. L. Simon and S. L. Gorbach (pp. 1729–1747).

Johnson, S. E. Pancreatic APUDomas. *Sem Vet Med Surg (Small Anim)* **4:** 202–211, 1989.

Kertzner, B. *et al.* Transmissible gastroenteritis: Sodium transport and the intestinal epithelium during the course of viral enteritis. *Gastroenterology* **72:** 457–461, 1977.

King, C. E., and Toskes, P. P. Small intestinal bacterial overgrowth. *Gastroenterol* **76:** 1035–1055, 1979.

Kirsch, M. Bacterial overgrowth. *Am J Gastroenterol* **85:** 231–237, 1990.

Merritt, A. M., and Smith, D. A. Osmolarity and volatile fatty acid content of feces from horses with chronic diarrhea. *Am J Vet Res* **41:** 928–931, 1980.

Ooms, L., and Degryse, A. Pathogenesis and pharmacology of diarrhea. *Vet Res Commun* **10:** 355–397, 1986.

Sandle, G. I. *et al.* Cellular basis for defective electrolyte transport in inflamed human colon. *Gastroenterology* **99:** 97–105, 1990.

Simpson, K. W. *et al.* Effects of exocrine pancreatic insufficiency and replacement therapy on the bacterial flora of the duodenum in dogs. *Am J Vet Res* **51:** 203–206, 1990.

Sprouse, R. F., and Garner, H. E. Normal and perturbed microflora of the equine cecum. *In* "Proceedings of the Equine Colic Research Symposium," T. D. Byars *et al.* (eds.), pp. 53–61. Athens, Georgia, College of Veterinary Medicine, University of Georgia, 1982.

Strombeck, D. R., and Guilford, W. G. Maldigestion, malabsorption, bacterial overgrowth, and protein-losing enteropathy. *In* "Small Animal Gastroenterology," 2nd Ed., pp. 296–319. Davis, California, Stonegate Publishing, 1990.

Williams, D. A., Batt, R. M., and McLean, L. Bacterial overgrowth in the duodenum of dogs with exocrine pancreatic insufficiency. *J Am Vet Med Assoc* **191:** 201–206, 1987.

3. Protein Metabolism in Enteric Disease

Disorders of protein metabolism attributable to enteric disease are responsible for significant economic loss in the form of reduced weight gain, wool growth, and milk production. Severe derangement in any species may lead to cachexia, hypoproteinemia, and death. Nitrogen economy may be affected at three main points. Nitrogen intake may be reduced; there may be decreased protein digestion and assimilation; or increased catabolism and loss of endogenous nitrogen may occur. The metabolism and distribution of nitrogen in the system may vary depending on the way in which its economy is disrupted.

Decreased protein intake is the most obvious threat to the nitrogen economy, and it is probably the most important in many chronic gastrointestinal diseases. Subclinical inefficiency in production, reduced growth, and emaciation may be the product of varying degrees of inappetence. If the quality of the feed available is poor, the effect of reduced intake on production will be compounded. Painful prehension or mastication, dental attrition, chronic dysphagia, or recurrent vomition are all obvious causes of reduced feed intake.

A sharp decline in appetite, or anorexia, is a common sign of indigestion, obstruction, or systemic disease. In ruminants, loss of appetite to varying degrees is an important component of the pathogenicity of gastrointestinal parasites, including those infecting the abomasum (*Ostertagia*), small intestine (*Trichostrongylus*), and large bowel (*Oesophagostomum*). About 40–90% of the inefficiency in production in these parasitisms is attributable to reduced feed intake. The factors influencing satiety in diseased animals are uncertain and deserve greater attention. Among them may be the hormones gastrin and cholecystokinin, which are elevated in association with inappetence in parasitized sheep. They, and other peptides secreted locally in the gut, which act as neurotransmitters in the brain, also influence satiety. The bulk and particle size of the feed consumed influences distension of the reticulorumen and rate of throughput of digesta. Altered gastrointestinal motility or stasis, perhaps the result of elevated gastrin levels, will also detrimentally influence feed intake, as may reduced absorption of amino acids from the small intestine.

Malabsorption of peptides and amino acids may occur locally in the small intestine as a result of significant villus atrophy. However, unless the lesion is widespread, or low in the small bowel, net absorption of nitrogen over the length of the small intestine may not be reduced, due to the compensatory capacity of more distal normal mucosa. Overall, the contribution of malabsorption to disordered nitrogen metabolism appears to be minor in most situations.

Protein-losing gastroenteropathy, increased catabolism, and loss of endogenous nitrogen via the gastrointestinal tract is important in many diseases. Excess endogenous protein entering the intestine is derived from two main sources: increased turnover of cells lining the gut, and effusion of plasma protein into the lumen of the bowel. The contribution to endogenous nitrogen loss by increased turnover of enterocytes and secretion of mucoprotein has not been well defined. However, in conditions causing chronic villus atrophy, such as intestinal parasitism by *Trichostrongylus* and *Strongyloides,* it may be substantial.

Plasma protein loss into the gut presupposes abnormal permeability of the mucosa to large molecules. This may be the product of the bloodsucking activity of nematodes such as *Haemonchus, Ancylostoma,* and *Bunostomum,* or hemorrhage from sites of trauma in the mucosa caused by the feeding activity of worms such as *Oesophagostomum columbianum, Chabertia,* and *Strongylus.* Erosive lesions result in considerable loss of red blood cells and plasma protein. Such lesions may be due to infarction, severe cryptal necrosis, or acute inflammatory damage to the mucosa associated with bacteria, viruses, and coccidia, causing fibrinohemorrhagic enteritis. Microscopic leaks in the mucosa also permit plasma loss into the gut. These may result from increased exfoliation of enterocytes into the lumen in villus atrophy, as transient gaps in the mucosa at the site where the cell sloughs. In villus atrophy with a high rate of enterocyte turnover, temporary microerosions may develop when flattened cells fail to maintain the integrity of the surface epithelium. The permeability of tight junctions between epithelial cells may be sufficiently altered to permit transit of plasma protein molecules (**filtration secretion**) when the hydrostatic pressure in the proprial interstitium is elevated in congestive heart failure and portal hypertension; by decreased plasma oncotic pressure; by increased vascular permeability in acute or chronic inflammation; and in lymphatic obstruction or lymphangiectasia.

Plasma protein loss into the gut is nonselective. Albumin, immunoglobulins, clotting factors, and a variety of transport or carrier proteins, including transferrin, ceruloplasmin, and transcortin, are lost. The physiologic consequences of protein-losing enteropathy may reflect increased catabolism of any of these molecules, but are most obviously related to increased turnover of the albumin pool. Plasma albumin loss into the gut, when expressed as a proportion of the total body pool, will vary in absolute terms, depending on the size of the pool. This concept of **fractional catabolic rate** is essential to understanding the kinetics of plasma protein turnover.

In protein-losing enteropathy, albumin turnover may pass through three phases. During the first phase, the fractional catabolic rate increases and with it, the absolute amount of protein lost into the bowel; as the size of the circulating pool of albumin shrinks, so does the absolute rate of loss of protein, even though the fractional rate remains the same. During the second phase, the size of the circulating pool stabilizes as the rate of albumin synthesis by the liver increases to match in absolute terms the rate of loss. The plasma albumin pool is then in a state of hyperkinetic equilibrium; the pool is smaller, with a higher than normal fractional catabolic rate compensated by an increased rate of hepatic synthesis. Provided that the size of the loss does not exceed the synthetic capacity of the liver, this equilibrium may persist for a considerable period. In the third phase, hypoalbuminema develops as the fractional catabolic rate continues to increase so that it exceeds in absolute terms the synthetic capacity of the liver. Alternatively, hypoalbuminemia occurs in the third phase if the rate of synthesis declines, due to deficiency in amino acids derived from the diet and by catabolism of other body protein. The hypoalbuminemia in enteric plasma loss is often associated with hyperglobulinemia, since compensatory synthesis of immunoglobulin is remarkable. Several times more immunoglobulin than albumin may be lost into the gut as a result.

The progress and clinical manifestations of protein-losing enteropathy vary with the rate of onset of plasma loss and the fractional catabolic rate. A sudden onset of severe plasma protein loss may cause death during the first phase, before there is time for compensatory synthesis. If the fractional catabolic rate is gradually and only slightly increased, so that compensation occurs with the albumin pool in equilibrium at only a marginally reduced state (perhaps near or within the normal range), subclinical protein loss occurs. Though the fractional catabolic rate is only slightly elevated, the relatively large size of the albumin pool may mean that the absolute loss of protein exceeds that in a hypoalbuminemic animal with a higher fractional catabolic rate, but a smaller albumin pool.

Plasma protein leaking from the stomach or upper small intestine, and protein derived from exfoliated cells in villus atrophy with increased epithelial turnover, may be digested and absorbed in the small intestine. This is dependent on luminal proteolysis by pancreatic enzymes, and compensatory membrane digestion and absorption making up for any malabsorption by proximal atrophic mucosa. But the efficiency of protein digestion, even if it is not reduced, is not total. Therefore, a proportion of the increased endogenous protein entering the lumen will be added to the protein escaping digestion in the small bowel, and will enter the large intestine. Here, most of this protein may be converted to ammonia by the colonic flora and absorbed, so that in animals losing protein high in the gut, there may be little or no increase in fecal nitrogen excretion. On the other hand, much of the protein lost into the colon from lesions at that level is passed in the feces, often as protein, and is lost. Ammonia nitrogen absorbed from the colon is converted in the liver mainly to urea. Animals with increased endogenous protein loss into the stomach or small intestine tend to have slightly raised levels of blood urea nitrogen, and an elevated rate of urinary urea excretion.

Elevated hepatic synthesis of albumin due to increased turnover of the plasma albumin pool, and increased enteric protein synthesis in support of elevated epithelial turnover in conditions with chronic villus atrophy, is at the expense of anabolic processes elsewhere. Dietary amino acid is diverted to preferential synthesis of plasma and enteric protein. If protein intake is poor due to inappetence or a low-quality ration, or if the rate of protein loss is high, the animal moves into negative nitrogen balance. Catabolism of peripheral protein then assumes an increasingly important role in maintaining the pool of amino acids available for plasma and intestinal protein synthesis. This explains in part the reduced growth rate, decreased muscle mass, and depressed deposition of bone matrix in sheep with subclinical or mild parasitism, and the cachexia of severe parasitism. The additional metabolic cost of increased protein synthesis also causes inefficiency in energy utilization. These principles probably hold for all syndromes causing enteric loss of endogenous protein in any species.

Loss of enteric protein, and especially plasma, should be suspected in cachectic or hypoproteinemic animals. Diarrhea is often, but not invariably, present. The two major routes of occult abnormal plasma protein loss are the kidney in glomerular disease, and the gastrointestinal tract. Weeping skin lesions are another source. Anemia and hypoproteinemia may be due to external or internal hemorrhage. Advanced liver disease may cause hypoalbuminemia, in which case other signs of hepatic failure will probably be concurrent (see The Liver and Biliary System, Chapter 2 of this volume). Inanition also causes emaciation, usually without profound hypoalbuminemia. The cachexia of malignancy must also be differentiated.

The adequately hydrated hypoalbuminemic animal has subcutaneous, mesenteric, or gastric submucosal edema, perhaps with hydrothorax or ascites. Muscle wasting may be marked if the protein loss has been severe and chronic. Unlike starvation, protein-losing gastroenteropathy may be associated with the presence of internal fat depots, since assimilation of energy is not necessarily severely impaired.

The principles discussed in the kinetics of plasma albumin during enteric plasma loss may be applied also to the kinetics of the erythron and the development of anemia following loss of blood into the gastrointestinal tract.

Bibliography

Abbott, E. M., Parkins, J. J., and Holmes, P. H. The effect of dietary protein on the pathophysiology of acute hemonchosis. *Vet Parasitol* **20:** 291–306, 1986.

Castro, G. A. Gastrointestinal function in the parasitized host. *In* "Isotopes and Radiation in Parasitology IV," pp. 143–153. Vienna, Austria, International Atomic Energy Agency, 1981.

Dargie, J. D. The pathophysiological effects of gastrointestinal and liver parasites in sheep. *In* "Digestive Physiology and Metabolism in Ruminants," Y. Ruckebusch and P. Thivend (eds.), pp. 349–371. Lancaster, U.K., MTP Press, 1980.

Figlewicz, D. P., Lacour, F., and Sipols, A. Gastroenteropancreatic peptides and the central nervous system. *Annu Rev Physiol* **49:** 383–395, 1987.

Fossum, T. W. Protein-losing enteropathy. *Sem Vet Med Surg (Small Anim)* **4:** 219–225, 1989.

Fox, M. T. *et al.* Effects of omeprazole treatment on feed intake and blood gastrin and pepsinogen levels in the calf. *Res Vet Sci* **46:** 280–282, 1989.

Fox, M. T. *et al. Ostertagia ostertagi* infection in the calf: Effects of a trickle challenge on the hormonal control of digestive and metabolic function. *Res Vet Sci* **47:** 299–304, 1989.

Granger, D. N. *et al.* The microcirculation and intestinal transport. *In* "Physiology of the Gastrointestinal Tract," 2nd Ed., L. R. Johnson, (ed.), pp. 1671–1697. New York, Raven Press, 1987.

Poppi, D. P. *et al.* Nitrogen transactions in the digestive tract of lambs exposed to the intestinal parasite, *Trichostrongylus colubriformis*. *Br J Nutr* **55:** 593–602, 1986.

Rothschild, M. A., Oratz, M., and Schreiber, S. S. Albumin metabolism. *Gastroenterology* **64:** 324–337, 1973.

Rowe, J. B. *et al.* The effect of haemonchosis and blood loss into the abomasum on digestion in the sheep. *Br J Nutr* **59:** 125–139, 1988.

Symons, L. E. A. "The Pathophysiology of Endoparasitic Infection Compared with Ectoparasitic Infestation and Microbial Infection." North Ryde, NSW, Australia, Academic Press, 1989.

Titchen, D. A., and Reid, A. M. Putative roles of peptides in the genesis and control of parasitic diseases. *In* "Aspects of digestive physiology in ruminants," A. Dobson and M. J. Dobson, (eds.), pp. 217–237. Ithaca, New York, Comstock, 1988.

J. Malassimilation and Protein Loss in the Small Intestine

In dogs, and to a lesser extent in horses, cats and other species, idiopathic syndromes occur, variably signaled by chronic diarrhea, weight loss, hypoproteinemia, and malabsorption. Intestinal biopsy is usually necessary to make a diagnosis and establish a prognosis. These syndromes are usually characterized by abnormal infiltrates (eosinophils, lymphocytes and plasma cells, granulomatous inflammation, amyloid and lymphosarcoma) in the lamina propria, perhaps associated with villus atrophy. Lymphangiectasia may also produce a similar syndrome.

The limitations on interpretation of intestinal biopsies considered in the section on the normal intestine must be borne in mind. Neoplasia will be differentiated from inflammation. If inflammatory bowel disease is recognized, associated or complicating problems, such as *Giardia* infection and bacterial overgrowth of the bowel, should be sought. An attempt also should be made to seek associations with the dietary habits and history of the animal, since some syndromes may be associated with an inappropriate response to dietary antigen.

Bibliography

Barton, C. L. *et al.* The diagnosis and clinicopathological features of canine protein-losing enteropathy. *J Am Anim Hosp Assoc* **14:** 85–91, 1978.

Batt, R. M., and Hall, E. J. Chronic enteropathies in the dog. *J Sm Anim Pract* **30:** 3–12, 1989.

Lieb, M. S. (ed.) Inflammatory bowel disease. Sem Vet Med Surg (Sm Anim) **7(2):** 105–171, 1992.

Roberts, M. C. Malabsorption syndromes in the horse. *Compend Cont Ed Pract Vet* **7:** S637–S646, 1985.

Strombeck, D. W., and Guilford, W. G. Idiopathic inflammatory bowel disease. *In* "Small Animal Gastroenterology, 2nd ed.", pp. 357–390. Davis, Ca., Stonegate Publishing, 1990.

van der Gaag, I., and Happe, R. P. Follow-up studies by peroral small intestinal biopsies and necropsy in dogs with chronic diarrhea. *J Vet Med A* **37:** 561–568, 1990.

1. Lymphangiectasia

Lymphangiectasia is among the more common causes of malabsorption/protein-losing enteropathy in dogs. No breed predisposition is evident, other than in the Lundehund, a Norwegian spitz, in which lymphangiectasia is part of a syndrome of protein-losing enteropathy with inflammatory bowel disease, and perhaps in the Wheaten terrier. Lymphangiectasia is associated with chronic diarrhea, wasting, hypoproteinemia, lymphopenia, hypocalcemia, and hypocholesterolemia. Peripheral edema, ascites, and hydrothorax result from hypoalbuminemia.

The lesion in the small intestine is dilation of the lacteals, and often lymphatics of the submucosa, muscularis,

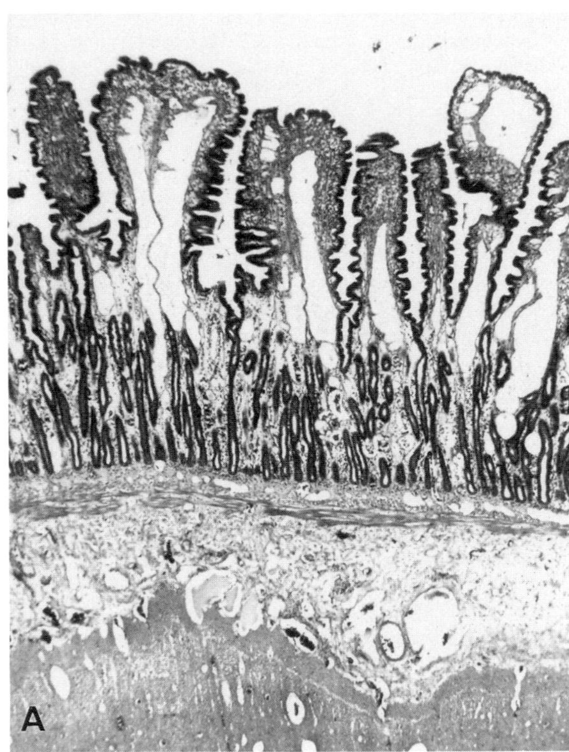

Fig. 1.56A Lymphangiectasia. Dog. Lacteals are dilated, lamina propria and submucosa are edematous, and lymphatics in submucosa and muscularis are open.

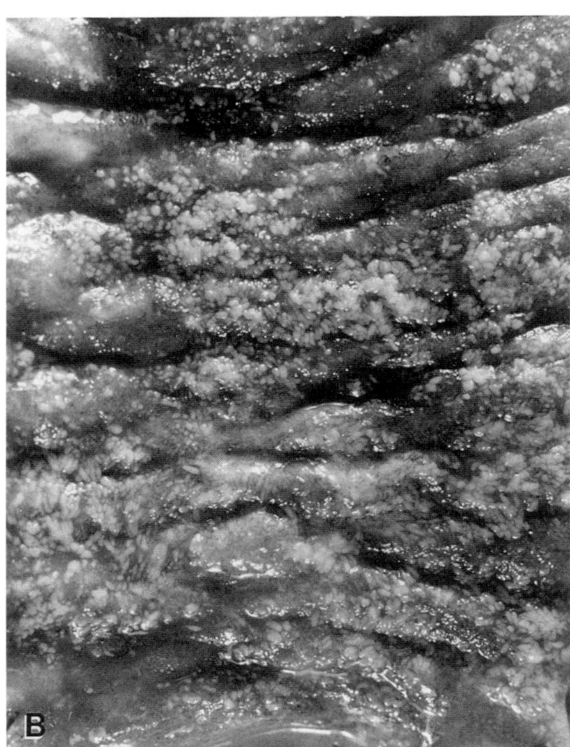

Fig. 1.56B Lymphangiectasia. Small intestine. Dog. Mucosa, thickened by edema, is thrown in folds. Many villi contain white chyle-filled lacteals.

serosa, and mesentery (Fig. 1.56A). Villi containing dilated chyle-filled lacteals may stand out grossly as white papillate foci in a thickened, transversely folded edematous mucosa (Fig. 1.56B). Serosal and mesenteric lymphatics may be prominent, white, and dilated. Nodular white masses as large as 5-10 mm may be present on the serosa at the mesenteric border and along lymphatics; rarely, they are found on the liver, diaphragm, other abdominal organs, and pleura.

In section, villi may be of normal length or somewhat blunt or stubby, with some hypertrophy of crypts. The surface epithelium may appear normal or perhaps slightly attenuated, and lateral interepithelial spaces are often dilated. The lacteals in many villi are distended, and lymphatics in deeper portions of the mucosa, submucosa, and muscularis usually are. Occasional lipid-laden macrophages are present in and around lacteals and lymphatics; large focal accumulations of lipophages around lymphatics, sometimes with a local granulomatous response to lipid or saponified fat, form the white masses which may be seen grossly. A similar reaction may be present in the draining lymph nodes. The lamina propria is edematous, and the submucosa and deeper portions of the gut wall usually are. The proprial inflammatory cell population may be normal, or the numbers of lymphocytes, plasma cells, and eosinophils may be increased.

The cause of lymphangiectasia is presumably lymphatic obstruction. Many cases appear to be acquired, and some may be due to lymphosarcomatous or granulomatous infiltrates obstructing flow in mesenteric lymph nodes. Lipogranulomas along the lymphatic drainage are not a constant feature of lymphangiectasia, and are probably in response to chronic leakage of lipid-laden chyle, rather than a cause of lymphatic obstruction. Usually, no congenital or acquired obstruction of the lymphatic system is obvious, though several dogs with lymphangiectasia have had chylothorax associated with thoracic duct obstruction. Experimental obstruction of mesenteric lymphatics produces hypoproteinemia and lymphangiectasia, but not diarrhea and weight loss, suggesting that the etiology of the clinical syndrome may be more complex than simple lymphatic obstruction.

Moderate malabsorption of lipid, and plasma protein loss into the gut, cause the signs associated with lymphangiectasia. Malabsorbed lipid may contribute to diarrhea via the effects of fatty acids on colonic secretion. Increased proprial hydrostatic pressure may cause net intestinal secretion and contribute to plasma protein loss. Dilated lacteals may rupture, releasing lymph into the lumen of the intestine. Hypocalcemia may be related to loss of the mineral bound to plasma albumin, and perhaps to vitamin D malabsorption, or formation of soaps with malabsorbed lipid in the gut lumen. Hypocholesterolemia is due to lipid malabsorption and effusion of plasma. Lymphopenia is thought to be the result of the loss of lymphocyte-rich lymph into the gut.

Bibliography

Banks, S. *et al.* The lymphatics of the intestinal mucosa. *Am J Dig Dis* **12:** 619–632, 1967.

Fossum, T. W. *et al.* Intestinal lymphangiectasia associated with chylothorax in two dogs. *J Am Vet Med Assoc* **190:** 61–64, 1987.

Frank, B. W., and Kern, F. Intestinal and liver lymph and lymphatics. *Gastroenterology* **55:** 408–422, 1968.

Granger, D. N., and Barrowman, J. A. Microcirculation of the alimentary tract. II. Pathophysiology of edema. *Gastroenterology* **84:** 1035–1049, 1983.

Landsverk, T., and Gamlem, H. Intestinal lymphangiectasia in the Lundehund. *Acta Pathol Microbiol Immunol Scand (A)* **92:** 353–362, 1984.

Meschter, C. L., Rakich, P. M., and Tyler, D. E. Intestinal lymphangiectasia with lipogranulomatous lymphangitis in a dog. *J Am Vet Med Assoc* **190:** 427–430, 1987.

Suter, M. M., Palmer D. G., and Schenk, H. Primary intestinal lymphangiectasia in three dogs: A morphological and immunopathological investigation. *Vet Pathol* **22:** 123–130, 1985.

Van Kruiningen, H. J. *et al.* Lipogranulomatous lymphangitis in canine intestinal lymphangiectasia. *Vet Pathol* **21:** 377–383, 1984.

Vardy, P. A., Lebenthal, E., and Shwachman, H. Intestinal lymphangiectasia: A reappraisal. *Pediatrics* **55:** 842–851, 1975.

2. *Chronic Inflammatory Disease*

Some animals, mainly dogs, but also cats and horses, showing signs consistent with malabsorption and/or plasma loss into the gut, have microscopic lesions in the small intestine described as **lymphocytic–plasmacytic enteritis.**

The cardinal finding is abnormally intense infiltrates of well-differentiated lymphocytes and plasma cells in the lamina propria of villi, between crypts, and sometimes in the submucosa. Normally, plasma cells are not numerous in the lamina propria of villi. A layer of lymphocytes, plasma cells, and perhaps neutrophils, eosinophils, and histiocytes, may be present in the deep mucosa, below the crypts and above the muscularis mucosae. Villi may be normal, clubbed, or moderately to severely atrophic, and occasionally fusion of villi may be prevalent (Fig. 1.57A,B). The surface epithelium may appear relatively normal, mucous metaplastic, or low columnar to cuboidal with an indistinct brush border; theliolymphocytes often are common. Crypts may be hypertrophic. There may be edema of the lamina propria and dilation of lacteals, suggesting concurrent lymphangiectasia, but usually the edema is not so severe as occurs with that lesion.

In this and other conditions with increased inflammatory infiltrates or edema in the lamina propria, including lymphangiectasia, crypts may be obstructed and dilated, and contain mucus and a few exfoliated epithelial cells. This has been termed cystic mucinous enteropathy; it is merely a severe variant of lymphocytic–plasmacytic enteritis, and we see no benefit in expanding the nomenclature in an already confused area. Occasionally, rupture of such crypts will be seen; lakes of mucus, reactive histiocytes, and occasional giant cells are present in the lamina

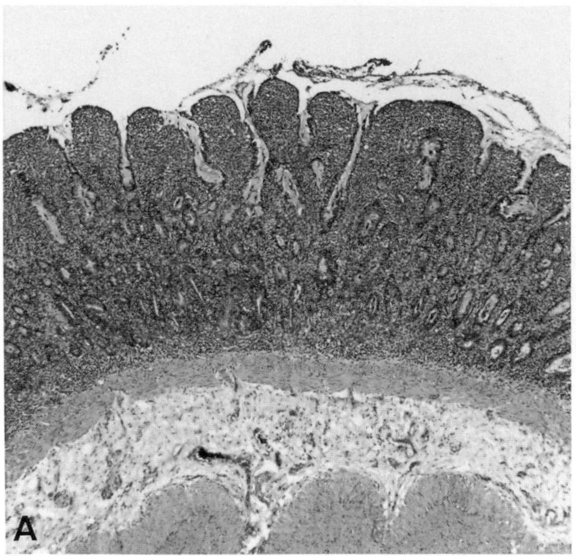

Fig. 1.57A Lymphocytic–plasmacytic enteritis. Dog. Villi are stumpy, club shaped, or fused. Excessive mononuclear infiltrate at all levels of the mucosa, including between the base of crypts and the muscularis mucosae.

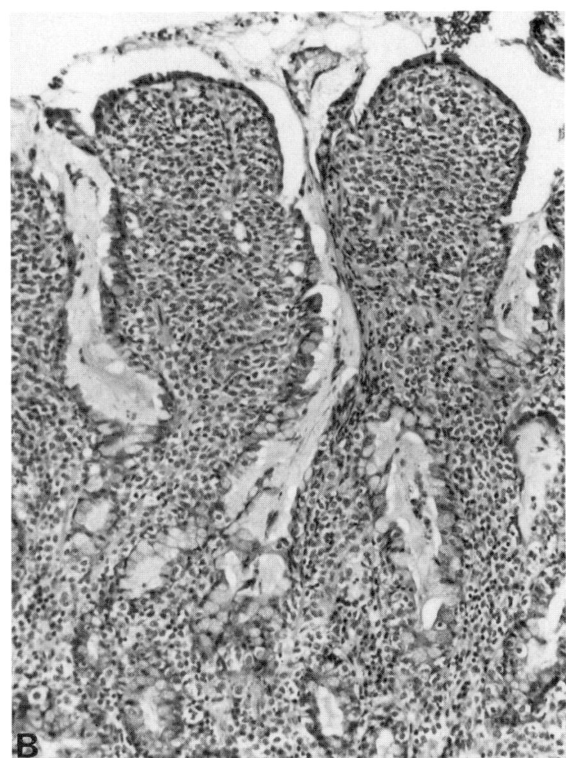

Fig. 1.57B Lymphocytic–plasmacytic enteritis. Dog. Blunt and club-shaped villi, cuboidal and attenuated surface epithelium, excess mucus secreted from crypts, and abnormal infiltrate of lymphocytes, plasma cells, and histiocytic cells in lamina propria.

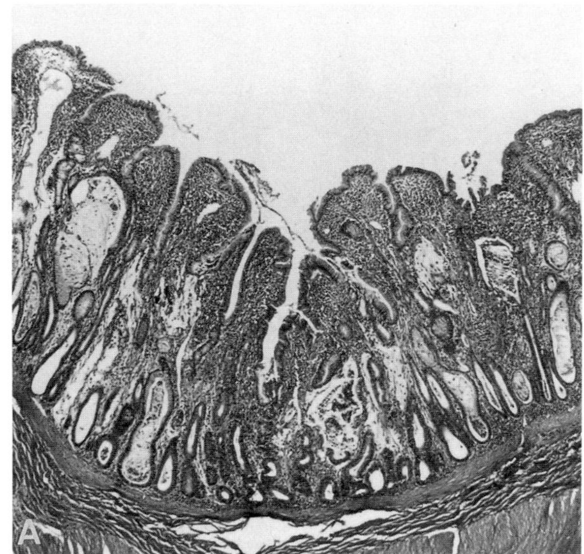

Fig. 1.58A Small intestine. Dog with malabsorption and intestinal protein loss. Blunt and occasionally fused villi, mononuclear cells in lamina propria, and elongate, dilated, and mucus-filled crypts. Some distended crypts have ruptured, releasing mucus into lamina propria.

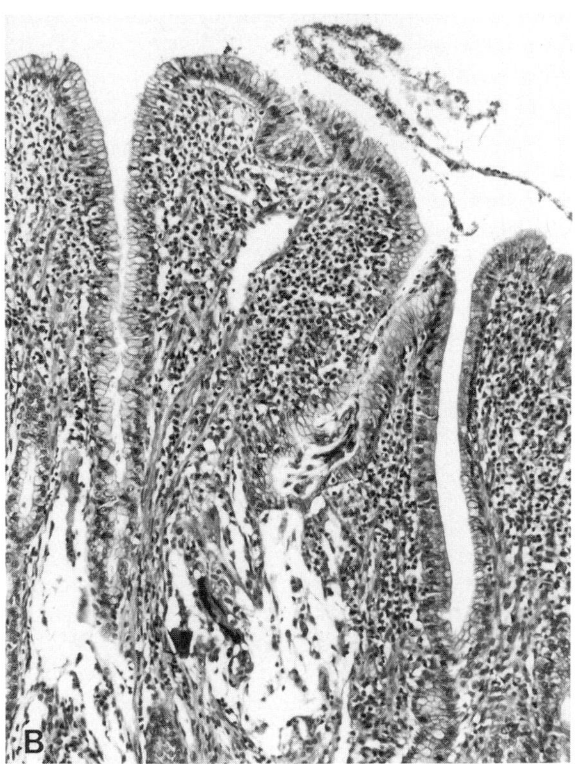

Fig. 1.58B Detail of (A) showing mucus in lamina propria due to rupture of a dilated crypt. Leak of cells and mucus from lamina propria and abnormal numbers of bacteria in lumen.

propria (Fig. 1.58A,B). Other distended crypts may contain casts of eosinophilic glycoprotein.

In the Lundehund and in basenji dogs, syndromes of hypoalbuminemia, chronic diarrhea, and wasting occur with high prevalence. They seem primarily attributable to the development of lymphocytic–plasmacytic enteritis, with lymphangiectasia in some dogs. In the basenji, chronic gastritis or hypertrophic gastritis may be associated, and malassimilation and plasma protein loss into the gut have been documented. Hypergammaglobulinemia occurs commonly in the late stages of the syndrome in basenjis, and lymphosarcoma develops in some affected animals. In this sense, the syndrome resembles immunoproliferative small intestinal disease (α-heavy chain disease, or Mediterranean lymphoma), which is a disorder of IgA immunoblasts in humans. Immunoglobulin A plasmacytes do not dominate in the basenji intestinal mucosa; though high circulating levels of IgA are present, it is not known whether they are associated with abnormal α-heavy chain protein. In dogs and horses, submucosal or transmural lymphoplasmacytic infiltrates may signal a precursor to lymphoma.

Animals with the gray collie syndrome (cyclic hematopoiesis) also may have lymphocytic–plasmacytic enteritis (see The Hematopoietic System, Volume 3, Chapter 2).

The etiopathogenesis of lymphocytic–plasmacytic enteritis is not understood in any species. The nature of the inflammatory infiltrate that gives it its name suggests that an inappropriate response to dietary antigen may be implicated. The common morphologic changes in the mucosa of cryptal hypertrophy, villus atrophy, and, in severe cases, mucous metaplasia of surface enterocytes, may be side effects of T cell-mediated activity in the mucosa. Similar lesions occur in humans with celiac disease (gluten-sensitive enteropathy), which appears to be T cell mediated, and lymphocytic–plasmacytic enteritis associated with familial sensitivity to wheat protein has been demonstrated in Irish setter but not in basenji dogs.

Bibliography

Cheville, N. F., Cutlip, R. C., and Moon, H. W. Microscopic pathology of the gray collie syndrome. *Pathol Vet* **7:** 225–245, 1970.

Clark, E. S. *et al.* Lymphocytic enteritis in a filly. *J Am Vet Med Assoc* **193:** 1281–1283, 1988.

Edwards, D. F., and Russell, R. G. Probable vitamin K-deficient bleeding in two cats with malabsorption syndrome secondary to lymphocytic–plasmacytic enteritis. *J Vet Intern Med* **1:** 97–101, 1987.

Flesja, K., and Yri, T. Protein-losing enteropathy in the Lundehund. *J Small Anim Pract* **18:** 11–23, 1977.

Ghermai, A. K. Chronisch-entzündliche Darmerkrankungen der Katze. *Tierärztl Prax* **17:** 195–199, 1989.

Hall, E. J., and Batt, R. M. Development of wheat-sensitive enteropathy in Irish setters: Morphologic changes. *Am J Vet Res* **51:** 978–982, 1990.

Hayden, D. W., and Van Kruiningen, H. J. Lymphocytic–plasmacytic enteritis in German shepherd dogs. *J Am Anim Hosp Assoc* **18:** 89–96, 1982.

Jacobs, G. *et al.* Lymphocytic–plasmacytic enteritis in 24 dogs. *J Vet Intern Med* **4:** 45–53, 1990.

Landsverk, T., and Gamlem, H. Scanning electron microscopy of the Lundehund enteropathy. *J Ultrastr Res* **69:** 153–154, 1979.
MacAllister, C. G. *et al.* Lymphocytic–plasmacytic enteritis in two horses. *J Am Vet Med Assoc* **196:** 1995–1998, 1990.
MacLachlan, N. J. *et al.* Gastroenteritis of basenji dogs. *Vet Pathol* **25:** 36–41, 1988.
Platt, H. Chronic inflammatory and lymphoproliferative lesions of the equine small intestine. *J Comp Pathol* **96:** 671–684, 1986.
Ross, L. A., Lamb, C. R., and Jakowski, R. M. Cystic mucinous enteropathy in a dog. *J Am Anim Hosp Assoc* **26:** 93–96, 1990.
Rutgers, H. C., Batt, R. M., and Kelly, D. F. Lymphocytic–plasmacytic enteritis associated with bacterial overgrowth in a dog. *J Am Vet Med Assoc* **192:** 1739–1742, 1988.
Tams, T. R. Chronic feline inflammatory bowel disorders. Part I. Idiopathic inflammatory bowel disease. *Compend Cont Ed Pract Vet* **8:** 371–376, 1986.

Conditions typified by abnormally heavy eosinophilic infiltrates of the gastrointestinal mucosa occur in dogs, cats, and horses.

Eosinophilic gastroenteritis in the dog is a regional or diffuse affliction, affecting one or more areas of the alimentary tract from stomach to rectum. Signs may vary from vomition associated with gastritis, to chronic small bowel diarrhea, or chronic large bowel diarrhea with hematochezia resulting from eosinophilic colitis. Diarrhea and weight loss suggest malabsorption and protein-losing enteropathy, and circulating eosinophilia is often present. The syndrome may occur in any breed.

At autopsy or laparotomy, aside from lesions attributable to cachexia and hypoproteinemia, there may be enlarged mesenteric lymph nodes. The affected segment of the alimentary tract is thickened, or the mucosa may be irregularly folded or nodular and perhaps hemorrhagic, eroded, or ulcerated. Gross lesions are associated with increased infiltrates of normal eosinophils in the mucosa, submucosa, and sometimes involving muscularis and serosa. Lymphoplasmacytic infiltrates in the mucosa may also be increased. The proportion of the infiltrate which must be eosinophils, or the absolute density of these cells in inflammatory bowel disease, for the case to qualify as eosinophilic gastroenteritis, is subjective. However, eosinophils are very rare in the normal gastric mucosa and the intestinal submucosa of dogs, and if they are present there, it adds credence to a diagnosis of eosinophilic gastroenteritis (Fig. 1.59A). Villi may be mildly to severely atrophic; the epithelium can appear relatively normal, or enterocytes may be low columnar or cuboidal. In the colon the epithelium may be eroded or the mucosa ulcerated in areas with heavy infiltrates of eosinophils. Eosinophils may be present in sinusoids throughout affected lymph nodes.

Eosinophilic granulomas also have been reported as a rare syndrome in dogs which had severe transmural disease, with gastric involvement or intestinal obstruction causing vomition or diarrhea. Eosinophilic granulomas may form large nodules resembling tumors in the mucosa/submucosa and muscularis, and they may partially efface or ulcerate the overlying mucosa. In one case, Splendore–Hoeppli bodies were evident in the center of the eosinophilic granulomas. There may be peripheral eosinophilia, and eosinophil infiltrates and granulomas in regional lymph nodes. Larvae of *Toxocara canis* were implicated as the cause of eosinophilic granulomas in gastrointestinal tissues and other organs of a series of German shepherds; this seems not to be a general cause of gastrointestinal eosinophilic granulomas in dogs. This syndrome has not been reported in Siberian huskies, in which oral eosinophilic granuloma occurs. Scirrhous eosinophilic gastritis and arteritis is also a unique, rare syndrome.

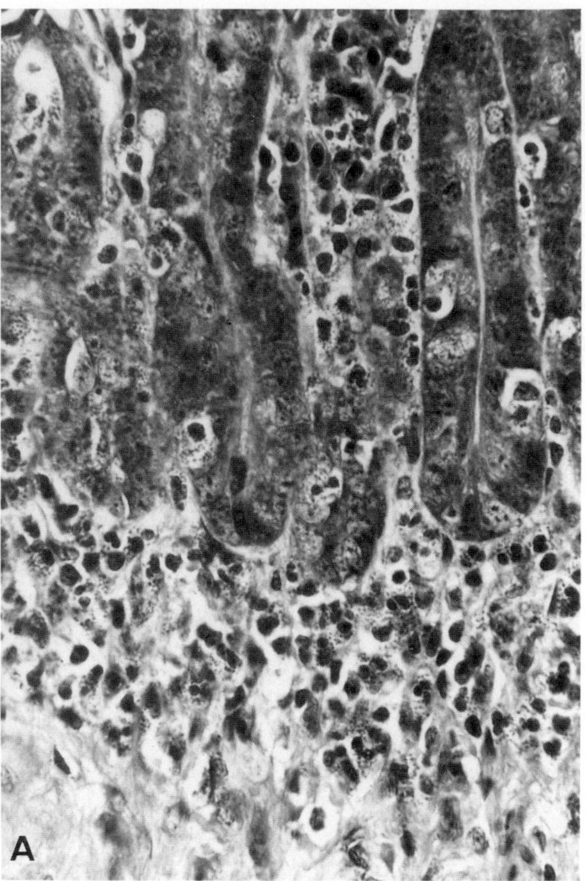

Fig. 1.59A Eosinophilic enteritis. Dog. Numerous eosinophils infiltrating the epithelium of small intestinal crypts, adjacent lamina propria, and between the base of crypts and underlying muscularis mucosae.

Eosinophilic enteritis in cats is rare, and appears to be one manifestation of a hypereosinophilic syndrome which may involve many organs in middle aged or older cats. It is much more severe than eosinophilic gastroenteritis in dogs. Diarrhea (sometimes bloody), vomition, loss of appetite, and loss of condition may occur. Clinically, intestinal thickening, hepato- and splenomegaly, and enlarged mesenteric lymph nodes may be present, in association with circulating eosinophilia and hyperplasia of the eosinophil series in the marrow.

The postmortem picture reflects the clinical findings. Enlargement of the various organs including liver, spleen, lymph nodes in many locations, and tan nodularities on the kidneys are associated with heavy infiltrates of usually well-differentiated eosinophils. In the small intestine the eosinophilic infiltrate may be transmural and is accompanied by grossly visible hypertrophy of the muscle layers (Fig. 1.59B). Eosinophilic colitis may occur in some cases. Lymph nodes may have hyperplastic follicles and many mature eosinophilis in sinusoids. Alternatively they may vary through eosinophilic lymphadenitis with fibrosis to complete obliteration of normal architecture and replacement by eosinophils in a fibrillar stroma extending through the capsule into surrounding tissue.

Chronic eosinophilic enteritis in horses has been described as part of a distinct multisystemic epitheliotropic syndrome, associated with eosinophilic granulomatous pancreatitis and eosinophilic dermatitis, among other lesions. Affected animals have weight loss, and diarrhea or unformed feces, associated with hypoalbuminemia, suggesting enteric loss of plasma protein. Reduced absorption of glucose occurs, but peripheral eosinophilia is absent. At autopsy, mucosal and sometimes transmural thickening may occur at any level of the alimentary tract from esophagus to rectum. Esophageal and gastric squamous mucosa is hyperkeratotic. Thickened mucosa is thrown into turgid transverse folds, or occasionally is fissured and roughened. Focal or diffuse ulcers may be present on the small and large intestine, and focal caseous lesions as large as 1.5 cm in diameter may be in the submucosa of the gut and common bile duct, as well as in an enlarged fibrotic pancreas.

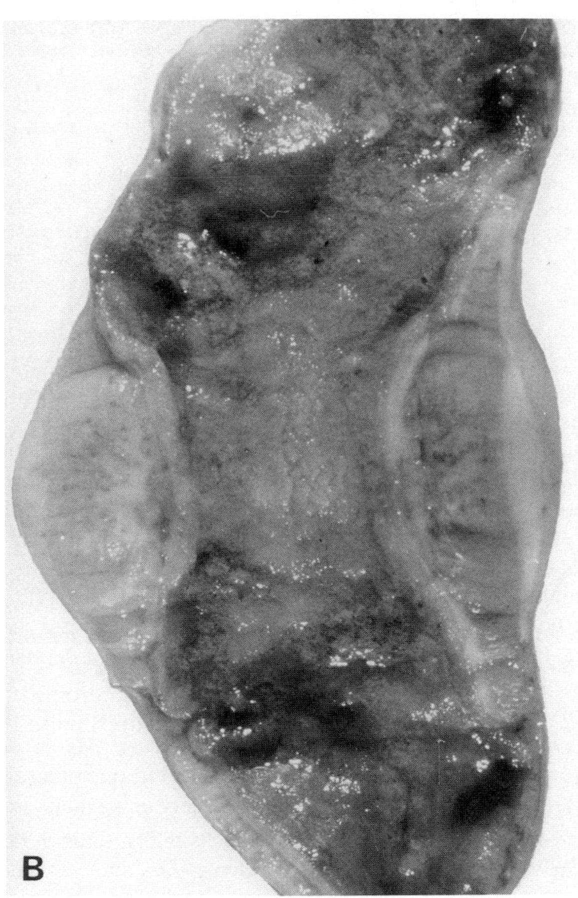

Fig. 1.59B Eosinophilic enteritis. Cat. Foci of mucosal congestion, and segmental transmural thickening and hypertrophy of smooth muscle in an area heavily infiltrated by eosinophils.

Microscopically there is diffuse infiltration of the mucosa, submucosa, and often deeper layers of the enteric wall by eosinophils, mast cells, macrophages, lymphocytes, and some plasma cells. Moderate to severe villus atrophy, fibroplasia in the lamina propria, and hypertrophy of the muscularis mucosae occur. Caseous foci in the mucosa and submucosa consist of central masses of eosinophils, sometimes surrounded by macrophages, giant cells, and occasionally fibrous tissue. Eosinophilic interstitial infiltrates and granulomas are described in the biliary and pancreatic ducts, pancreas, salivary glands, capsule and outer cortex of enlarged firm mesenteric lymph nodes, and near portal tracts in the liver. The skin may be thickened and hyperkeratotic and the limbus of the hoof, thickened and ulcerated. The eosinophilic dermatitis is described with The Skin and Appendages (Volume 1, Chapter 5).

Villus atrophy is common, but if large-bowel lesions are absent, there is no diarrhea. Chronic inflammation in the mucosa may explain protein loss and hypoalbuminemia. The cause of this syndrome is unknown; an immune-mediated etiology is suggested, and there is a clinical response to steroid therapy.

Bibliography

Alliah-Davis, R., and Batdorf, K. Eosinophilic granuloma complex in a dog. *Mod Vet Pract* **66:** 756, 1985.

Cello, J. P. Eosinophilic gastroenteritis—a complex disease entity. *Am J Med* **67:** 1097–1104, 1979.

Gibson, K. T., and Alders, R. G. Eosinophilic enterocolitis and dermatitis in two horses. *Equine Vet J* **19:** 247–252, 1987.

Griffin, H. E., and Meunier, L. D. Eosinophilic enteritis in a specific-pathogen-free cat. *J Am Vet Med Assoc* **197:** 619–620, 1990.

Hayden, D. W., and Fleischman, R. W. Scirrhous eosinophilic gastritis in dogs with gastric arteritis. *Vet Pathol* **14:** 441–448, 1977.

Hayden, D. W., and Van Kruiningen, H. J. Eosinophilic gastroenteritis in German shepherd dogs and its relationship to visceral larva migrans. *J Am Vet Med Assoc* **162:** 377–384, 1973.

Hendrick, M. A spectrum of hypereosinophilic syndromes exemplified by six cats with eosinophilic enteritis. *Vet Pathol* **18:** 188–200, 1981.

Nimmo Wilkie, J. S. *et al.* Chronic eosinophilic dermatitis: A manifestation of a multisystemic, eosinophilic, epitheliotropic disease in five horses. *Vet Pathol* **22:** 297–305, 1985.

Quigley, P. J., and Henry, K. Eosinophilic enteritis in the dog: A case report with a brief review of the literature. *J Comp Pathol* **91:** 387–392, 1981.

van der Gaag, I., Happe, R. P., and Wolvekamp, W. Th. C. Eosinophilic gastroenteritis complicated by partial ruptures and a perforation of the small intestine in a dog. *J Small Anim Pract* **24:** 575–581, 1983.

The presence of chronic inflammatory infiltrates including aggregates of histiocytes, and perhaps giant cells, in the lamina propria is the criterion for a diagnosis of **granulomatous enteritis.** Granulomatous enteritis occurs in all species. Johne's disease, other intestinal mycobacteriosis, and *Histoplasma* enteritis are specific examples (see Infectious and Parasitic Diseases of the Alimentary Tract, Section VII of this chapter). Often the cause is not identified.

Transmural granulomatous enteritis is seen occasionally in dogs and cats. It is generally segmental and perhaps discontinuous in distribution, usually affecting the lower ileum, colon, and draining lymph nodes; the term **regional enteritis** is often applied. Due to the extent of the attendant fibrosis, these lesions may be stenotic, and must be differentiated from invasive carcinoma. Idiopathic granulomatous enteritis as a cause of wasting and protein-losing enteropathy is most commonly seen as a sporadic problem in **horses.** Depending on the duration of the disease, animals may be markedly cachectic, have subcutaneous edema, especially of dependent areas, and there may be hydrothorax, hydropericardium, and ascites. Lesions in the horse usually affect the small intestine; stomach and large bowel are occasionally involved also. There may be thickened pale plaques or prominent lymphatics on the serosa of the bowel. The mucosa of the small intestine may be irregularly granular or thickened; there may be transverse corrugations of the mucosa; or raised, firm gray areas with hyperemic foci may be evident. Linear or extensive ulcers of small and large bowel have been described. Mesenteric lymph nodes are usually enlarged, edematous, with mottled firm gray areas, fibrotic nodules, or rarely caseous or mineralized foci on the cut surface. Granulomatous pale, caseous, or calcified foci may be scattered in the liver.

The microscopic lesion may be patchy, regional, or diffuse, and it may be mucosal, or transmural, ultimately gaining the draining lymph nodes. Transmural inflammation is characteristically granulomatous. Villi are mildly to markedly atrophic with hypertrophy of crypts. The epithelium may vary from apparently normal to low columnar or cuboidal with an indistinct brush border. There may be leaks between cells on the surface, or microerosions may be present, through which neutrophils and proteinaceous exudate pass into the lumen. The lamina propria is edematous and contains scattered aggregates of histiocytes and perhaps giant cells, or, less commonly, more organized granulomatous foci. Neutrophils and eosinophils are distributed diffusely throughout the lamina propria, and may be concentrated in or near granulomatous foci. A heavy population of lymphocytes and plasma cells inhabits the lamina propria, and the infiltrate and edema may separate crypts abnormally from each other.

In **dogs** with regional enteritis there may be marked necrosis in the centers of granulomas, and considerable fibrosis. The inflammatory reaction typically follows lymphatics into the submucosa and through the muscularis to the serosa. The submucosa is usually edematous, and lymphatics are prominent. Granulomas may be present in the submucosa or at intervals along lymphatics. The affected lymph nodes are hyperplastic, usually with prominent sinus histiocytosis. Giant cells may be present in sinusoids, or granulomatous foci of varying sizes may be evident. Sinusoids contain numerous neutrophils and perhaps eosinophils, and neutrophils may accumulate in the center of granulomas.

Rarely are agents isolated or identified in such lesions in horses and dogs. *Mycobacterium avium* or environmental mycobacteria are incriminated occasionally. Comparisons are drawn between granulomatous enteritis in horses and Crohn's disease in humans, the etiology of which is also uncertain, though *M. paratuberculosis* is incriminated by some. Focal pyogranulomatous aggregates associated with blood vessels are found in the submucosa and especially the subserosa of the intestine of cats with feline infectious peritonitis.

Bibliography

Cline, J. M. *et al.* Abortion and granulomatous colitis due to *Mycobacterium avium* complex infection in a horse. *Vet Pathol* **28:** 89–91, 1991.

DiBartola, S. P. *et al.* Regional enteritis in two dogs. *J Am Vet Med Assoc* **181:** 904–908, 1982.

Lindberg, R. Ultrastructure of granulomatous infiltrates in the small bowel in equine granulomatous enteritis. *J Vet Med (A)* **33:** 111–122, 1986.

Schumacher, J. *et al.* Effect of intestinal resection on two juvenile horses with granulomatous enteritis. *J Vet Intern Med* **4:** 153–156, 1990.

3. Amyloidosis

Amyloid deposition in the small intestine and stomach may be encountered occasionally, in animals with systemic amyloidosis. Sometimes the gastrointestinal lesions predominate and contribute to the clinical syndrome. Significant intestinal amyloidosis leads to signs consistent with malabsorption and enteric protein loss. Usually there is no gross indication of the deposition of amyloid in the intestine. However, occasionally focal ulceration or hemorrhage may be noted. Microscopically, amyloid is seen beneath the epithelium or throughout the propria in villi, and perhaps around or within vessels in the submucosa (Fig. 1.59C). It must not be mistaken for collagen deposition, which is most unusual in these locations, though a band of collagenous material is sometimes present at the base of the mucosa in cats. The pathogenic effects of amyloid in the intestine seem to involve either impaired movement of interstitial fluid into lacteals or perhaps increased permeability of capillaries, possibly explaining protein loss into the lumen.

Bibliography

Hayden, D. W. *et al.* AA amyloid-associated gastroenteropathy in a horse. *J Comp Pathol* **98:** 195–204, 1988.

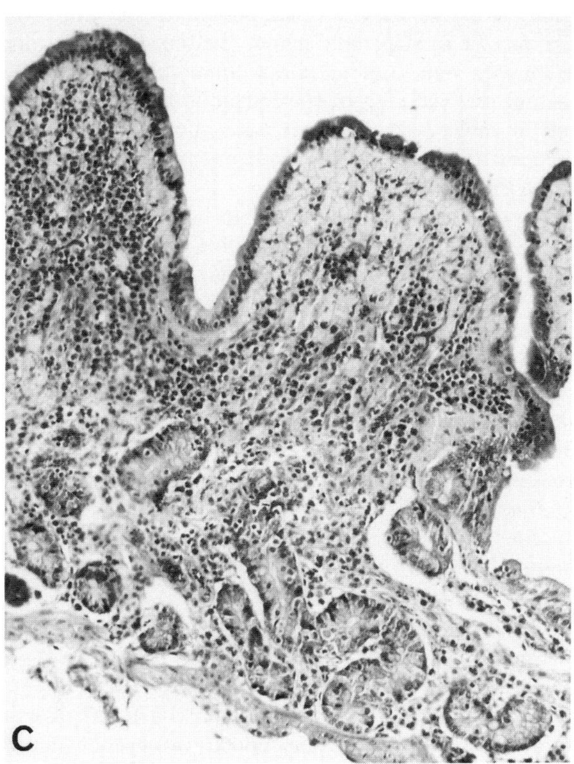

Fig. 1.59C Intestine. Goat. Deposits of pale amorphous amyloid beneath the epithelium on villi, and scattered in the lamina propria. (Courtesy of J. R. Duncan.)

K. Inflammation of the Large Intestine

The general reaction to injury of the cecal and colonic epithelium was considered earlier with Epithelial Renewal in Health and Disease (Section VI,I of this chapter).

Ischemia, obliteration of the proliferative epithelium by viruses or coccidia, severe inflammation in the mucosa, and perhaps necrotizing toxic insults from the lumen are responsible for the development of focal or diffuse ulceration of the large intestine. Inflammatory infiltrates in the lamina propria may be classified broadly as acute, chronic or chronic active, and granulomatous. They may be limited in distribution to the mucosa or be transmural, involving submucosa, muscularis, serosa, and frequently the draining lymph nodes. Typhlitis and colitis may be manifestations of a generalized or systemic disease; they may be part of an enterocolitis involving both small and large intestine; or they may be regional and limited to a segment of the intestine, often terminal ileum, cecum, and colon, or some shorter part of the large bowel.

The colonic mucosa may provide the portal of entry for systemic bacterial invasion and for uptake of toxins. Increased mucosal permeability in the colon may permit enteric loss of plasma protein or of blood. Disordered large bowel flora in hindgut fermenters may compromise uptake of volatile fatty acids and water. In any species, damage to the colonic mucosa may result in malabsorption of electrolytes and water, and perhaps net secretion. Colitis in each of the species will be considered in turn.

Colitis cystica profunda, the presence of dilated colonic glands protruding through the muscularis mucosae into the submucosa, is reported in several species. It is perhaps most often seen in swine, where it is an occasional finding, particularly associated with swine dysentery. The dilated glands may be grossly visible through the serosa and muscularis as nodular masses a few millimeters in diameter. Microscopically, a single, large flask-shaped gland, lined by columnar epithelium, and containing mucus and exfoliated cells or necrotic debris, may be present. Alternatively a cluster of glands appears to herniate into the submucosa, where one or more may become dilated by mucus and debris. The cause is unknown; the lesion may be a sequel to colitis and local damage to the muscularis mucosae, or it may represent herniation into the space left by an involuted submucosal lymphoid follicle. Though the lesion has been seen with colitis in a variety of circumstances, it may be found incidentally, with no specific etiologic association.

Bibliography

Ferguson, H. W., Neill, S. D., and Pearson, G. R. Dysentery in pigs associated with cystic enlargement of submucosal glands in the large intestine. *Can J Comp Med* **44:** 109–114, 1980.

Patton, N. M., and Blankevoort, M. Colitis cystica profunda in pygmy goats. *J Comp Pathol* **86:** 371–375, 1976.

1. Typhlocolitis in Dogs

Inflammation of the large bowel in dogs is usually associated with diarrhea, typically frequent, small in volume, mucoid or bloody, and often accompanied by tenesmus.

Severe acute necrotizing colitis and, less commonly, typhlitis, leading to **ulceration and perforation,** with subsequent peritonitis, has been associated with glucocorticoid administration, functional adrenal cortical tumors, and with trauma or surgery involving the spinal cord. Gastric ulceration may occur concurrently. The perforations usually occur in the antimesenteric border of the left colonic flexure or proximal descending colon, though they are reported from the cecum, and the ascending, transverse, and distal descending colon. The pathogenesis of the colonic lesions developing in these circumstances is unclear, but it does not seem to be associated with the interface between the cranial and sacral fields of autonomic nervous control, as has been proposed.

Ulcerative enterocolitis, with lesions apparently centered mainly on lymphoid tissue, as well as gastric ulcer, has been produced experimentally by administration of the analgesic drug **indomethacin** to dogs. Necrotizing colitis, ulceration, and perforation may occur rarely in dogs in **uremia.** The mechanism is uncertain, but colonic damage may be the effect of high concentrations of ammonia evolved by urease-producing colonic flora from urea diffusing into the gut from the blood. In **canine intestinal hemorrhage syndrome,** possibly associated with clostridial overgrowth in the gut, the colon may be involved, or at least contain hemorrhagic content. Severe ulcerative colitis speculatively associated with *C. difficile* has been reported in the dog.

Trichuris vulpis, the whipworm of dogs, may cause mucosal colitis, which rarely evolves into a granulomatous transmural condition. Clinical trichuriasis is generally associated with a population of worms which extends from the usual site of infection in the cecum and proximal ascending colon, into more distal parts of the large intestine. Rarely, trichuriasis may be complicated by infection with *Balantidium coli,* which possibly contributes to the development of mucosal erosion or ulceration. Ulcerative colitis in dogs is also caused rarely by ***Entamoeba histolytica.*** An ulcerative, granulomatous transmural colitis is more common as one of the enteric manifestations of **histoplasmosis.** ***Prototheca*** also is a cause of distinctive but rare enterocolitis in dogs, and colitis characterized by a heavy mucosal infiltrate of macrophages, in which the agent may be found, is reported in **leishmaniasis. Canine parvovirus** causes colonic damage, but virtually never without lesions elsewhere. **Canine coronavirus** has also been implicated as a cause of colonic as well as small intestinal lesions. These conditions are discussed fully in the section on Infectious and Parasitic Diseases of the Gastrointestinal Tract (Section VII of this chapter).

Spirochetes may be present in the canine colon, and although they are generally considered nonpathogenic, they may be embedded in the microvillous border of surface epithelium and may be associated with mild mucosal colitis. *Anaerobiospirillum* sp. has been isolated from the feces of dogs, and is associated with enteric disease in people. ***Campylobacter jejuni*** is isolated from dogs with diarrhea, but its possible relationship to colitis in clinical cases is currently unclear. The association of giardiasis and colitis in dogs is considered to be fortuitous. The role of antigens gaining the mucosa is unknown. If they are significant, their identity, origin, and the factors predisposing to their entry are obscure.

Idiopathic mucosal (lymphocytic–plasmacytic) colitis is the commonest form recognized in dogs. It is etiologically nonspecific, presenting as chronic or chronic–active lymphocytic–plasmacytic mucosal inflammatory disease; eosinophilic enterocolitis and histiocytic ulcerative colitis are the two distinctive patterns differentiated from it on microscopic grounds.

Mild acute mucosal colitis, reflecting a grossly reddened friable surface, is characterized by congestion of superficial capillaries and venules, and proprial edema. Neutrophils infiltrate the superficial lamina propria around vessels, and transmigrate or pass between surface epithelial cells into the lumen. The population of lymphocytes and plasma cells in the lamina propria may not differ from normal, but there is generally a moderate increase in mononuclear cells between glands. There is usually a reduced number of goblets on the surface and in glands, probably due to mucous discharge, rather than cell loss. Surface epithelium may be basophilic, low columnar or cuboidal (Fig. 1.60A,B). Hyperplasia of epithelium in glands may be evident, and glands dilated. Inflammatory cells, mainly neutrophils, may accumulate excessively along the mucosal side of the muscularis mucosae. The lesions in mild acute colitis often seem out of proportion to the severity of the clinical syndrome, which may be the result of irritation and tenesmus.

The spectrum of inflammation in colitis grades from acute toward an increasingly chronic infiltrate, which, along with edema, separates colonic glands and may accumulate deep in the mucosa between glands and muscularis mucosae. Neutrophils and eosinophils may be scattered in the propria and in glandular epithelium. Globule leukocytes may be prevalent. Accumulation of granulocytes and necrotic debris in the lumen of glands forms so-called crypt abscesses.

Greater severity of the lesion is reflected in attenuation and exfoliation of surface epithelium, and the development of microerosions on the mucosal surface (Fig. 1.60C). Inflammatory cells, mainly neutrophils, and tissue fluid effuse into the lumen through defects in the epithelium. Persistent erosion, or previous erosion in a healed mucosa, is marked by the development of a thin, horizontally arrayed layer of connective tissue in the superficial lamina propria. With increasing chronicity in colitis of mild or moderate degree, there may be deposition of a collagenous stroma, throughout which inflammatory cells are interspersed, which separates glands abnormally throughout the mucosa (Fig. 1.60D). Downgrowth of glands into submucosal lymphoid follicles may occur in chronic colitis.

Severe erosion and ulceration is usually associated with local acute inflammation and with a heavy, mainly mononuclear cell infiltrate in the lamina propria, and often in the submucosa. The ulcerated areas extend usually no farther than the muscularis mucosae, and have a base of granulation tissue infiltrated heavily by neutrophils, which effuse into the lumen of the bowel. The margin of surviving mucosa may overhang the ulcer. Crypt abscesses may be present in remaining mucosa, and all degrees of erosion and partial ulceration may be present. Idiopathic ulcerative colitis is uncommon, and does not seem so severe as histiocytic ulcerative colitis of boxers; it rarely comes to autopsy. Severely affected dogs may be cachectic, probably in part because of enteric loss of plasma protein. The mucosa in ulcerative colitis is usually deep red, swollen, folded, and granular because of edema and cellular infiltrates; the depressions may be punctate or up to several centimeters across, roughly round or oval, irregular or elongate. Their margins may be tattered or puckered. Colonic lymph nodes may be enlarged and edematous.

In canine colitis there is a broad three-dimensional spectrum: in chronicity and density of the inflammatory infiltrate; in the distribution of the infiltrate within the wall of the bowel; and in the severity of the epithelial and mucosal change. Generally, milder lesions of superficial epithelium are associated with mild or moderate mucosal inflammation, which may be acute or chronic. In many cases of mild chronic mucosal colitis, the glands do not appear

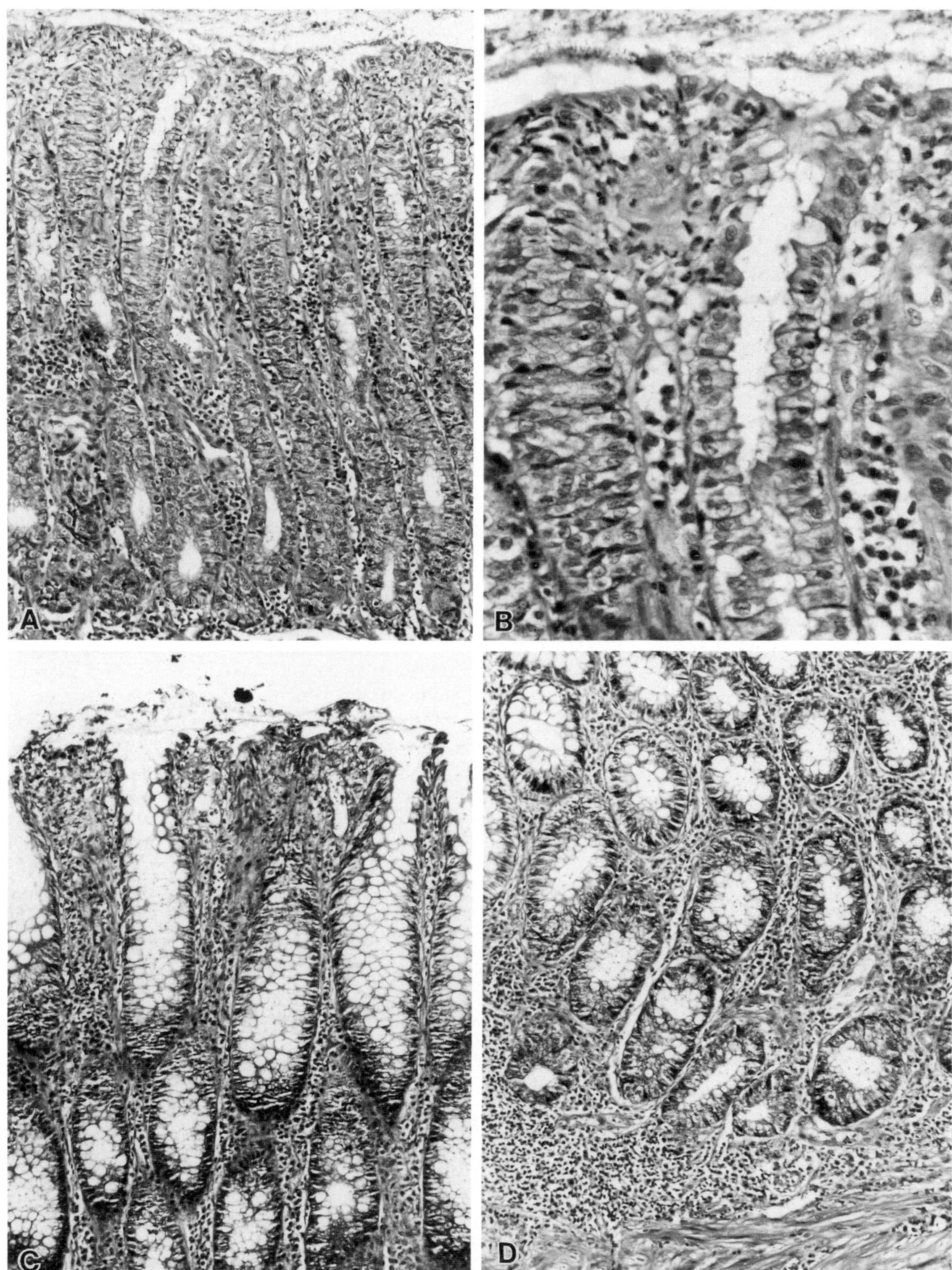

Fig. 1.60 Mild acute idiopathic mucosal colitis: (A) Goblet cells are sparse or absent in glands and on surface. Superficial epithelium is cuboidal and exfoliating in focal areas. (B) Epithelium in glands is hyperplastic and crowded. The superficial lamina propria is edematous. Chronic erosive colitis: (C) Hypertrophic glands are lined by goblet cells. The mucosal surface has widespread erosion and effusion of tissue fluid and neutrophils. (D) Edema of lamina propria. Deeper in mucosa there is a moderately increased population of mononuclear cells and increased fibrous stroma. Cells extend between base of glands and muscularis mucosa.

particularly hyperplastic. Severe erosion and ulceration is usually related to a more intense or heavy chronic inflammatory process, which may be limited to the mucosa, but which can extend into the submucosa. Truly granulomatous colitis is uncommon; when fully developed, perhaps as a component of a regional enteritis involving the ileocecocolic area, it is ulcerative and transmural. Occasionally, a granulomatous response to barium, or to other foreign material breaching the epithelium, may be observed in the mucosa and submucosa. Atrophic colitis, in which the mucosa is markedly thinned, with relatively inactive crypts and modest chronic or chronic–active interstitial inflammation, perhaps with notable interstitial fibrosis, is encountered occasionally.

Eosinophilic colitis forms part of the syndrome of eosinophilic gastroenteritis discussed with inflammatory disease of the small intestine. It usually conforms to the general description of idiopathic colitis, with the exception that eosinophils form a prominent part of the cellular infiltrate in the mucosa and superficial submucosa. Eosinophil infiltrates do not seem to be clearly associated with the activity or severity of the lesion. The separation of eosinophilic colitis from idiopathic mucosal colitis is subjective, based on the degree and significance of the eosinophil infiltrate. The presence of eosinophils in gastric mucosal biopsies in the same animal, or other evidence of significant eosinophil infiltrates higher in the gut, lends credence to diagnosis of eosinophilic colitis as part of the syndrome eosinophilic gastroenteritis.

Histiocytic ulcerative colitis is a distinctive histologic syndrome, which has been recognized only in boxers and the related French bulldog. It is a chronic transmural ulcerative colitis characterized by the presence of large numbers of macrophages containing PAS-positive granules, in the deep mucosa and submucosa, and in lymph nodes receiving drainage from the colon. Clinically affected animals are usually younger than 2 years. This condition causes typical large-bowel diarrhea, with mucus and blood; weight loss occurs, and chronic cases may become cachectic, probably because of protein loss into the gut.

Grossly, thc colon of dogs with advanced disease is variably thickened, folded, and perhaps dilated and shortened, with some segmental or focal areas of scarring and stricture. Lesions on the mucosa may vary from patchy, punctate red ulcers to more extensive irregular, circular, or linear lesions, which may coalesce, leaving only a few islands of persistent mucosa on a granulating colonic surface (Fig. 1.61A).

Early microscopic lesions are those of mild nonspecific inflammation. Goblets disappear from the surface and glands. Microerosion of epithelium in the upper glands and on the surface is associated with local acute inflammation, migration of neutrophils into the epithelium, and effusion of neutrophils and tissue fluid into the lumen. Macro-

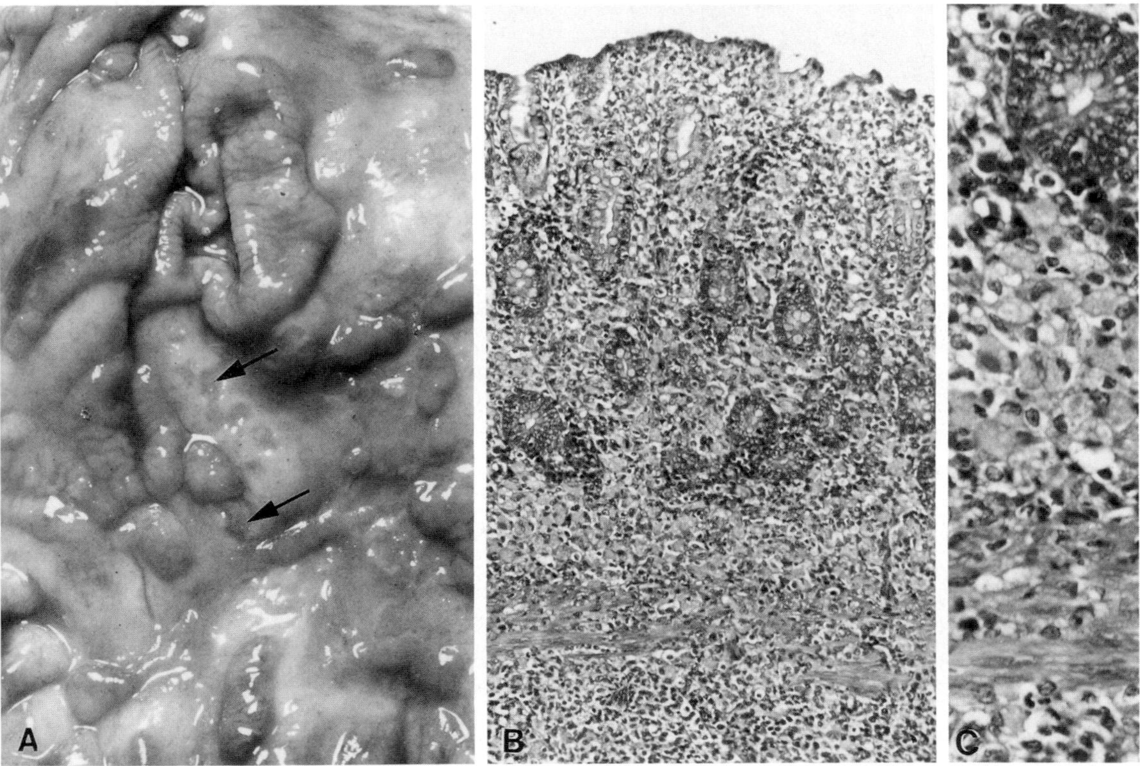

Fig. 1.61 Histiocytic ulcerative colitis. Boxer dog. (A) Mucosa is thickened and edematous. There are numerous erosions (arrows). (B) Accumulation of macrophages with abundant cytoplasm throughout mucosa, between base of glands and muscularis mucosae and in submucosa. (C) Detail of macrophages in mucosa deep to crypts.

phages in these areas may contain phagocytized necrotic debris and bacteria. In some areas the mucosa is thinned, and glands are relatively shortened, though lining epithelium appears hyperplastic. Macrophages with cytoplasmic vacuoles, which contain PAS-positive material, are mainly deep in the lamina propria, raising the base of crypts from the muscularis mucosae, and in the submucosa (Fig. 1.61B,C). Sometimes they may be relatively sparse in the mucosa, and may be missed in small biopsy specimens if the submucosa is not sampled. These same cells may be found about lymphatics in the muscularis and the serosa, and they may be numerous in subcapsular, cortical, and medullary sinuses in the draining lymph nodes. The cecum is often involved, to a lesser degree, with similar lesions. True granulomatous foci and giant cells are rarely encountered.

Ulceration seems to progress from the superficial epithelial erosion and destruction of the basement membrane seen in early lesions. Ulcers usually do not progress beyond the submucosa, and they are lined by granulation tissue. The bed of the ulcer is necrotic, and numerous neutrophils and erythrocytes may be passing into the lumen.

The cause of the condition is unknown, as is the origin of the material in the characteristic vacuoles in macrophages. Ultrastructural study suggests that these are digestion vacuoles containing mainly remnants of phospholipid membranes. The material being digested may be phagocytized cell debris and microorganisms picked up in the superficial lamina propria and carried in constipated macrophages to deeper structures. Certainly, bodies resembling microorganisms have been found in macrophages, and the involvement of chlamydia, rickettsia, and mycoplasmas has been postulated. It seems that a defect in lysosomal function may exist in some boxer dogs, which can lead to the accumulation of partially digested phospholipid membrane in macrophages, since similar histocytes do not accumulate in ulcerative colitis in other breeds of dogs.

Bibliography

Dvorak, J., Willard, M. D., and Floyd, E. Panfibrinonecrotic colitis in a dog treated by subtotal colectomy. *J Am Vet Med Assoc* **198:** 264–266, 1991.

Ferrer, L. *et al.* Chronic colitis due to *Leishmania* infection in two dogs. *Vet Pathol* **28:** 342–343, 1991.

Gomez, J. A. *et al.* Canine histiocytic ulcerative colitis. An ultrastructural study of the early mucosal lesion. *Dig Dis* **22:** 485–496, 1977.

Hudson, L. C. Horseradish peroxidase study of the location of extrinsic efferent and afferent neurons innervating the colon of dogs. *Am J Vet Res* **51:** 1875–1881, 1990.

Kraft, W., Ghermai, A. K., and von Bomhard, D. Zwei Fälle von Colitis cystica profunda beim Hund. *Tierärztl Prax* **17:** 299–302, 1989.

Leib, M. S. *et al.* Plasmacytic lymphocytic colitis in the dog. *Sem Vet Med Surg (Small Anim)* **4:** 241–246, 1989.

LeVeen, E. G. *et al.* Urease as a contributing factor in ulcerative lesions of the colon. *Am J Surg* **135:** 53–56, 1978.

Levine, D. S., and Haggitt, R. C. Normal histology of the colon. *Am J Surg Pathol* **13:** 966–984, 1989.

Moore, M. P., and Robinette, J. D. Cecal perforation and adrenocortical adenoma in a dog. *J Am Vet Med Assoc* **191:** 87–88, 1987.

Prescott, J. R. *et al. Campylobacter jejuni* colitis in gnotobiotic dogs. *Can J Comp Med* **45:** 377–383, 1981.

Roth, L. *et al.* Comparisons between endoscopic and histologic evaluation of the gastrointestinal tract in dogs and cats: 75 cases (1984–1987). *J Am Vet Med Assoc* **196:** 635–638, 1990.

Roth, L. *et al.* A grading system for lymphocytic plasmactyic colitis in dogs. *J Vet Diagn Invest* **2:** 257–262, 1990.

Salzmann, J. L. *et al.* Morphometric study of colonic biopsies: A new method of estimating inflammatory diseases. *Lab Invest* **60:** 847–851, 1989.

Spinato, M. T., Barker, I. K., and Houston, D. M. A morphometric study of the canine colon: Comparison of control dogs and cases of colonic disease. *Can J Vet Res* **54:** 477–486, 1990.

Stewart, T. H. M. *et al.* Ulcerative enterocolitis in dogs induced by drugs. *J Pathol* **131:** 363–378, 1980.

Strombeck, D. R., and Guilford, W. G. Idiopathic inflammatory bowel diseases. *In* "Small Animal Gastroenterology, 2nd Ed.", pp 357–390. Stonegate Publishing, 1990.

Toombs, J. P. *et al.* Colonic perforation in corticosteroid treated dogs. *J Am Vet Med Assoc* **188:** 145–150, 1986.

Turek, J. J., and Meyer, R. C. Studies on a canine intestinal spirochete: Scanning electron microscopy of canine colonic mucosa. *Infect Immun* **20:** 853–855, 1978.

van der Gaag, I. The histological appearance of large intestinal biopsies in dogs with clinical signs of large bowel disease. *Can J Vet Res* **52:** 75–82, 1988.

van der Gaag, I., and Happé, R. P. Follow-up studies by large intestinal biopsies and necropsy in dogs with clinical signs of large bowel disease. *Can J Vet Res* **53:** 473–476, 1989.

van der Gaag, I., and van der Linde-Sipman, J. S. Eosinophilic granulomatous colitis with ulceration in a dog. *J Comp Pathol* **97:** 179–185, 1987.

van der Gaag, I. *et al.* Regional eosinophilic coloproctitis, typhlitis, and ileitis in a dog. *Vet Q* **12:** 1–6, 1990.

Watson, A. D. J. Giardiosis and colitis in a dog. *Aust Vet J* **56:** 444–447, 1980.

2. Colitis in Cats

Colitis in cats is uncommon. **Idiopathic mucosal colitis,** similar to that described in dogs, occurs occasionally in cats.

Feline panleukopenia causes colonic lesions in about half the cases. They are similar to, but rarely as severe or widespread as, the lesions found in the small intestine. The relative paucity and mildness of lesions in the colon is related to the lower rate of epithelial proliferation in comparison with that of the small intestine. Panleukopenia is considered with Infectious and Parasitic Diseases of the Gastrointestinal Tract (Section VII of this chapter).

Mycotic colitis is found occasionally in cats. These are associated with a hemorrhagic ulcerative colitis, in which focal or diffuse mucosal invasion by *Candida,* zygomycetes or *Aspergillus* has occurred, sometimes causing microvascular thrombosis. These are mainly secondary to colonic damage and leukopenia caused by panleukopenia.

Necrotic colitis is reported mainly in older animals, as a cause of chronic foul, and sometimes bloody diarrhea. The colon and rectum are thickened, rough and congested, or hemorrhagic. The microscopic change is mucosal erosion or ulceration associated with severe damage to colonic glands (Fig. 1.62). Crypt-lining cells are cuboidal or flattened, and necrotic debris may be in the lumen of glands. Some glands may be collapsed because of complete epithelial necrosis. The lesion resembles that of panleukopenia but is generally more hemorrhagic and necrotic. Possibly the colitis is secondary to transient ischemia.

Feline leukemia virus infection is associated with cryptal necrosis in small intestine; whether it causes similar lesions in large bowel is unclear.

Bacillus piliformis was the cause of mild mucosal colitis in several kittens with soft feces and vague central nervous disorder. The lesions were characterized by hypertrophy of crypts; exfoliation of epithelium into the lumen of crypts, which were dilated and lined by flattened epithelium; and a moderate chronic interstitial inflammatory infiltrate. Vegetative forms and spores of *B. piliformis* were recognized ultrastructurally in crypt epithelium. Lesions were not evident elsewhere.

Transmural acute ulcerative colitis, with a heavy neutrophil infiltrate, is the hallmark of ***Salmonella typhimurium*** infection in cats, considered more fully with salmonellosis in the section on Infectious and Parasitic Diseases of the Gastrointestinal Tract (Section VII of this chapter).

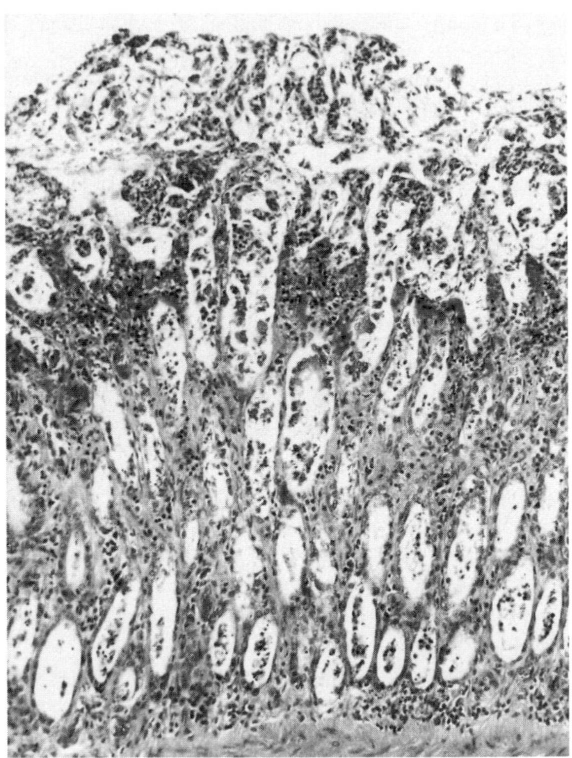

Fig. 1.62 Necrotic colitis. Cat. Active necrosis on surface of mucosa. Glands are dilated, contain necrotic cellular debris, or are lined by extremely flattened epithelium. (Courtesy of J. S. Nimmo Wilkie.)

Ulcerative colitis, grossly and microscopically similar to idiopathic ulcerative colitis of the dog, occurs very rarely in cats. Granulomatous or pyogranulomatous foci in the subserosa or submucosa may cause regional enterocolitis, characterized by fibrosis and serosal nodularity of affected segments, usually without severe mucosal defects. Fibrinoid arteritis causing hemorrhage and edema in the colonic submucosa, and ischemic necrosis of the mucosa, is also reported. The granulomatous syndrome is attributed to feline infectious peritonitis, and there may be characteristic lesions in other organs.

Bibliography

Nelson, R. W., Dimperio, M. E., and Long, G. G. Lymphocytic–plasmacytic colitis in the cat. *J Am Vet Med Assoc* **184:** 1133–1135, 1984.

Nimmo-Wilkie, J. S. Necrotic colitis in two cats—description of the lesions. *Can Vet J* **23:** 197–199, 1982.

Nimmo-Wilkie, J. S., and Barker, I. K. Colitis due to *Bacillus piliformis* in two kittens. *Vet Pathol* **22:** 649–652, 1985.

Van Kruiningen, H. J., Ryan, M. J., and Shindell, N. M. The classification of feline colitis. *J Comp Pathol* **93:** 275–294, 1983.

3. Typhlocolitis in Horses

The diagnosis of acute colitis in horses resolves into the differentiation of peracute and acute salmonellosis, and, where it occurs, Potomac horse fever (equine monocytic ehrlichiosis), from a similar condition, colitis X. Colitis also must be differentiated from the sequelae of intestinal accidents and thromboembolism involving the large bowel.

Colitis X is a sporadic acute disease, usually, but not always, associated with profuse foul-smelling, but rarely bloody, diarrhea. Some horses may die without having diarrhea. The remainder of the clinical syndrome is a reflection of the profound shock which occurs. At autopsy the animal is dehydrated, and there may be subcutaneous and serosal petechial hemorrhage. The blood is dark and clots poorly. Enteric lesions are virtually limited to the large bowel, which is distended with abnormally fluid content. The serosa of the cecum and large colon may appear cyanotic from congestion and hemorrhage in the mucosa (Fig. 1.63) and perhaps submucosa. The deeper tissues of the intestinal wall are not themselves compromised, as is the case usually in volvulus and often in thromboembolic infarction. The mucosa and submucosa are commonly markedly edematous, and edema is often present at the mesenteric attachment of the gut and in the cecal and colic lymph nodes. The mucosa may appear brown and necrotic with focal fibrinohemorrhagic exudate on the surface. More commonly it is deeply congested with focal hemorrhage, but blood is rarely present to significant degree in the contents. Gross lesions in other organs are those consistent with circulatory or endotoxic shock.

The microscopic lesions in the large bowel include su-

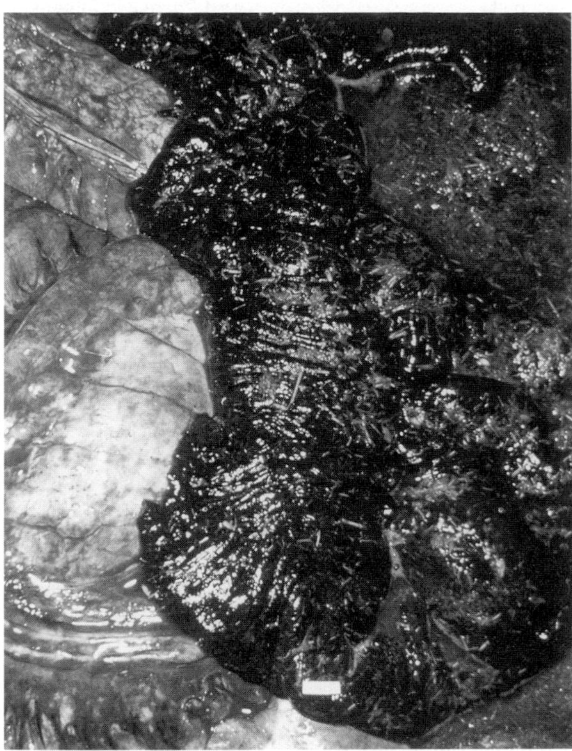

Fig. 1.63 Acute colitis (colitis X). Horse. The mucosa is very congested and edematous.

perficial or full-thickness necrosis of the mucosa, associated with dilation and perhaps thrombosis of small mucosal and submucosal venules. There is hemorrhage and edema in the mucosa, and the submucosa is markedly edematous, with dilated lymphatics. Some neutrophils may be evident in the mucosa or submucosa, and fibrin may be effusing from the damaged mucosal surface in less advanced cases. Submucosal lymphoid follicles show evidence of recent severe lymphocytolysis. Congestion, microvascular thrombosis, and hemorrhage may be found in a variety of other organs, especially the adrenal cortex.

The diagnosis of colitis X is, in large measure, one of exclusion. Failure to isolate *Salmonella* from the colonic mucosa and content differentiates it from peracute–acute salmonellosis. Potomac horse fever is usually not so acute, and organisms may be demonstrated in epithelium and macrophages of the colonic mucosa.

The pathogenesis of colitis X is uncertain and may be multifactorial. It seems likely that it, probably salmonellosis, and some even less well defined chronic diarrheas in horses, are the result of dysbacteriosis of the large bowel. Animals developing these conditions frequently have a recent history of change in feed, hard training, shipment, surgery, antibiotic (especially tetracycline) therapy, or other intervention.

Endotoxin plays a role, either by absorption through a mucosa already damaged by previous insult, or by release of abnormal amounts following a change in the flora in the large intestine. Systemic effects of endotoxin may contribute to shock, and to the microthrombosis and disseminated intravascular coagulation that often occurs.

Proliferation of toxigenic *Clostridium* species as a result of disruption of the bacterial ecosystem in the large bowel is hypothesized to be a cause of colitis X. The precedent for clostridial toxin- or endotoxin-mediated typhlocolitis following disruption of the gut flora lies in similar antibiotic-induced lesions in rabbits, guinea pigs, hamsters, and humans. Lincomycin-associated colitis resembling colitis X has been reported in horses. Overgrowth and exotoxin production by an organism resembling *C. cadaveris* has been implicated as the mechanism of colitis induced experimentally by clindamycin and/or lincomycin treatment of horses, and the organism has been recovered from a horse with colitis X. Experimental infection with *C. perfringens* type A, which is apparently an uncommon inhabitant of the equine bowel, also has been associated with the development of signs consistent in some cases with colitis X.

Subacute and chronic diarrhea in horses almost always involves the large intestine, with or without concomitant small-bowel involvement. ***Salmonella*** typhlocolitis must be suspected in such cases. Salmonellosis in horses may have an extremely variable course and pathologic manifestations (see Infectious and Parasitic Diseases of the Gastrointestinal Tract, Section VII of this chapter). **Potomac horse fever** usually results in diarrhea which does not exceed 10 days in duration; at necropsy there is congestion and ulceration of the mucosa of the large bowel, and enlargement of mesenteric lymph nodes. Suppurative ulcers involving lymphoid tissue in the typhlocolic mucosa, and cecal and colic lymphadenitis, characterize enteric infection with ***Rhodococcus equi*** in foals. **Histoplasmosis** has been reported once in a horse with salmonellosis and ulcerative colitis. Extensive mucosal involvement by **larval cyathostomes and strongyles** and rarely, ulcerative typhlitis due to **anoplocephalid tapeworms,** also may cause diarrhea and wasting; they are discussed with specific parasitisms.

Ciliate protozoa may be seen in the colonic mucosa of animals dead of a variety of enteric and nonenteric problems; there is rarely, if ever, an inflammatory response, and the tissues involved are frequently autolytic. They are terminal or postmortem invaders.

Chronic diarrhea and possibly cachexia may also result from persistent ulceration of the cecum or colon due to **ischemic mucosal lesions.** These may be the product of arterial thromboembolism and slow flow, or less likely, corrected strangulation with reflow. **Phenylbutazone** also has been associated with cecal and colonic ulceration and plasma protein loss. **Right dorsal colitis,** in which ulcerative lesions are limited to the named part of the large bowel, may be associated with colic, and acute or chronic diarrhea. It also may be related to use of nonsteroidal antiinflammatory agents in animals with reduced water intake. This syndrome and others associated with use of nonsteroidal antiinflammatory agents are considered with ischemia due to reduced perfusion (see Intestinal Ischemia and Infarction, Section VI,H of this chapter).

The specific cause of extensive ulceration may be difficult to determine. Smaller chronic ulcers and widespread subacute erosion and ulceration are most likely the result of salmonellosis, rather than ischemia. A history of administration of nonsteroidal antiinflammatory drugs, and the presence of lesions in the renal papilla, mouth, and upper alimentary tract, suggest intoxication by those agents.

Granulomatous and eosinophilic typhlocolitis in horses are extensions of the lesions considered previously with syndromes in the small bowel causing diarrhea and protein-losing enteropathy. Basophilic enterocolitis has been described in an animal with fibrinous and chronic ulcerative typhlocolitis. Basophils were prominent in a mixed inflammatory infiltrate, which was present in the ileal submucosa, and in the cecal and colonic mucosa and submucosa.

Chronic diarrhea occurs which does not appear to be related to morphologic lesions in the mucosa of the gut. Affected horses have a history of unformed cow-pat-like feces, or overt diarrhea, which may persist for weeks, months, and occasionally, years, with only periodic temporary remission. Examination of the feces may reveal none of the normal ciliate protozoan fauna, but often many flagellates, especially *Tritrichomonas* are present. It seems likely that the large numbers of these flagellate protozoa, and the paucity of ciliates, reflect gross alterations in the microenvironment and flora in the large bowel. If these changes also cause altered fermentation of carbohydrate and perhaps reduced production and absorption of volatile fatty acids, the diarrhea, and gradual reduction in body condition which often occurs, might be explained. These horses will show transient response to therapeutic agents which affect anaerobic bacteria and protozoa, but they usually regress when medication is withdrawn. The response to implants of cecal or colonic content is variable and usually discouraging.

Bibliography

Damron, G. W. Gastrointestinal trichomonads in horses: Occurrence and identification. *Am J Vet Res* **37:** 25–27, 1976.

Goetz, T. E., and Coffman, J. R. Ulcerative colitis and protein-losing enteropathy associated with intestinal salmonellosis and histoplasmosis in a horse. *Equine Vet J* **16:** 439–441, 1984.

Greatorex, J. C. Diarrhea in horses associated with ulceration of the colon and caecum resulting from *S. vulgaris* larval migration. *Vet Rec* **97:** 221–225, 1975.

Kirkpatrick, C. E., and Saik, J. E. Ciliated protozoa in the colonic wall of horses. *J Comp Pathol* **98:** 205–212, 1988.

Murray, M. J. Digestive physiology of the large intestine in adult horses. Part II. Pathophysiology of colitis. *Compend Cont Ed Pract Vet* **10:** 1309–1316, 1988.

Ochoa, R., and Kern, S. R. The effects of *Clostridium perfringens* type A enterotoxin in Shetland ponies—clinical, morphologic and clinicopathologic changes. *Vet Pathol* **17:** 738–747, 1980.

Pass, D. A., Bolton, J. R., and Mills, J. N. Basophilic enterocolitis in a horse. *Vet Pathol* **21:** 362–364, 1984.

Prescott, J. F. *et al.* A method for reproducing fatal idiopathic colitis (colitis X) in ponies and isolation of a clostridium as a possible agent. *Equine Vet J* **20:** 417–420, 1988.

Raisbeck, M. F., Holt, G. R., and Osweiler, G. D. Lincomycin-associated colitis in horses. *J Am Vet Med Assoc* **179:** 362–363, 1981.

Roberts, M. C. Acute equine colitis: Experimental and clinical perspectives. *Vet Ann* **30:** 1–11, 1990.

Schiefer, H. B. Equine colitis x, still an enigma. *Can Vet J* **22:** 162–165, 1981.

Staempfli, H. R., Townsend, H. G. G., and Prescott, J. F. Prognostic features and clinical presentation of acute idiopathic enterocolitis in horses. *Can Vet J* **32:** 232–237, 1991.

3. Typhlocolitis in Swine

The differential diagnosis of typhlocolitis in swine revolves mainly around identifying swine dysentery, *Salmonella* enterocolitis, and the large-bowel manifestations of the **intestinal adenomatosis complex** in weaned pigs. The latter condition is readily recognized by the consistent concurrent involvement of the terminal ileum by adenomatosis, with or without hemorrhage, or by necrotic ileitis. Mucosal thickening is reflected in the presence of the characteristic cerebriform folding of the serosal aspect of the bowel, which is commonly seen. Lesions in the large bowel are present in a minority of cases and involve the cecum and proximal colon; they resemble the ileal lesions in being either adenomatous or necrotic.

Swine dysentery involves only the cecum and spiral colon. It is a catarrhal to mildly fibrinohemorrhagic erosive mucosal typhlocolitis. The colonic content is fluid and usually blood-tinged. *Salmonella* enterocolitis, mainly due to *S. typhimurium,* is a fibrinous, erosive to focally ulcerative condition, mainly of the cecum and colon, but perhaps involving the small intestine, especially terminal ileum. The content is fluid but usually not bloody. Mesenteric lymph nodes are prominent. Button ulcers or necrotic enteritis in the lower intestine may occur in chronic salmonellosis, in subacute to chronic forms of **hog cholera,** and perhaps in **African swine fever.**

Campylobacter-like organisms associated with intestinal adenomatosis are readily identified in smears of affected mucosa stained with carbolfuchsin, and the large spirochetes causing swine dysentery may also be identified in mucosal scrapings at necropsy.

Postweaning colibacillosis is characterized by catarrhal to mild fibrinohemorrhagic enterocolitis in piglets after weaning, and intestinal adenomatosis may also occur in older suckling and in weanling piglets.

Fibrinohemorrhagic typhlitis is caused by heavy infestations with ***Trichuris suis,*** especially in weaned pigs with access to pastures and yards. Under similar circumstances ***Eimeria*** infection rarely may cause ileotyphlocolitis.

Rectal stricture appears to be a product of ischemic proctitis, probably related in many cases to infection with *S. typhimurium*. Details of these conditions are discussed in the section on Infectious and Parasitic Diseases of the Gastrointestinal Tract (Section VII of this chapter).

Mucous hyperplasia and obstruction of glands associated with lymphoid aggregates in the vicinity of the ileocecal orifice in pigs may cause grossly visible lesions. There may be a superficial accumulation of mucus and inspissated content over the glands, which contain white-to-green, moist-to-dry content, which may be manually expressed. Microscopically, the glands, lined by goblet cells, contain mucus, food particles, exfoliated epithelium, bacteria, and neutrophils. Occasionally, glands rupture, inciting a local acute inflammatory reaction. Concurrent disease is not evident.

Bibliography

Harper, P. A. W., and Christie, B. M. Mucoid hyperplasia and plugging of the glands of the ileocaecal opening of the pig. *Aust Vet J* **63:** 349–350, 1986.

5. Typhlocolitis in Ruminants

Diagnostic considerations in cattle older than 2–3 months with acute to subacute fibrinohemorrhagic typhlocolitis include salmonellosis, mucosal disease, rinderpest (in enzootic areas or populations at risk), coccidiosis, malignant catarrhal fever, adenovirus infection, and winter dysentery (coronavirus). Lesions of the oral cavity and upper alimentary tract may be expected, but are not necessarily present, in **mucosal disease, rinderpest,** and **malignant catarrhal fever;** in the latter, lymphadenopathy and lesions of the trachea, bladder, parenchymatous organs, eye, and brain may also be present. Lesions affecting Peyer's patches in the small intestine strongly suggest mucosal disease or rinderpest. **Coronavirus** causes microscopic lesions in colonic crypts in cattle with winter dysentery. A mild fibrinous typhlocolitis may be seen grossly. **Salmonellosis** affects all age groups from neonate to adult and may frequently involve both small and large intestine in catarrhal to fibrinohemorrhagic enteritis; mesenteric lymph nodes are usually enlarged. **Coccidiosis** may involve ileum and large intestine; it usually can be diagnosed by mucosal scraping at autopsy. **Adenovirus** infection may cause severe hemorrhagic colitis, with few lesions elsewhere, as may malignant catarrhal fever on occasion. **Arsenic,** other **heavy metals,** and **oak or acorn poisoning** may also cause hemorrhagic typhlocolitis and dysentery. Rarely, **trichuriasis** causes a hemorrhagic mucosal typhlitis in calves. Chronic fibrinous or ulcerative typhlocolitis may occur in salmonellosis, bovine virus diarrhea, and coccidiosis.

Granulomatous typhlocolitis associated with chronic diarrhea and wasting may occur in **Johne's disease,** concurrently with granulomatous ileitis and mesenteric lymphadenitis. The mucosa of the large bowel in these cases is thickened and rugose. Impressions of affected mucosa or ileocecal lymph node will contain acid-fast bacilli. Johne's disease in sheep and goats is associated usually with wasting but not with diarrhea. The large bowel may be involved in a minority of cases; the ileum is consistently affected.

In **sheep,** hemorrhagic typhlocolitis may be present in animals with **bluetongue** and ***peste des petits ruminants;*** it is rarely the only lesion. ***Heavy-metal intoxication*** is the only other significant cause of hemorrhagic typhlocolitis and dysentery in older animals. **Salmonellosis** may cause fibrinohemorrhagic enteritis in lambs and pregnant ewes, and **trichuriasis** will occur rarely. **Coccidiosis** may be implicated in hemorrhagic ileotyphlocolitis in lambs and kids, though the small intestine is usually more commonly and severely involved. In goats, enterotoxemia due to *C. perfringens* type D may cause a mild to moderately severe fibrinohemorrhagic typhlocolitis.

L. Hyperplastic and Neoplastic Diseases of the Intestine

In domestic animals, tumors of the intestine, whether benign or malignant, are uncommon. Malignant neoplasms are more common than benign tumors, and most are of epithelial origin. Polyps are generally hyperplastic or regenerative rather than neoplastic. The exceptions are rectal polyps in dogs, which are adenomas or carcinomas. Highly malignant scirrhous adenocarcinomas of the intestine occur in all species. The prevalence of this tumor in sheep is high in certain areas of the world.

Lymphosarcoma is the most common malignant tumor of mesenchymal origin in most species; it is most prevalent in the cat. Lymphosarcoma may arise in the gut, although involvement of this area is more often part of multicentric disease (see The Hematopoietic System, Volume 3, Chapter 2).

A hyperplastic condition of intestinal crypts in the ileum and colon in swine and some other species, called intestinal adenomatosis, or proliferative ileitis, is described with proliferative hemorrhagic enteropathy.

1. Colorectal Polyps in Dogs

These tumors are most common at the anal–rectal junction in middle-aged dogs. Tenesmus, prolapse of the polyp, rectal bleeding following defecation, chronic dyschezia, and diarrhea are the most common signs. Some but not all surveys indicate that this tumor is more common in males.

Macroscopically, the tumor is usually sessile or slightly pedunculated (Fig. 1.64); it may be firm or friable and hemorrhagic. The mucosal surface is often ulcerated. It varies from one to several centimeters in diameter. The tumors may be located 0–10 cm cranial to the anal–rectal margin, and they are usually single.

Microscopically, the polyp may have a predominantly tubular or papillary growth pattern (Fig. 1.65). In well-oriented specimens, the tubular pattern is characterized by branching crypts lined by well-differentiated columnar to cuboidal epithelial cells. These are supported by the lamina propria. The papillary type consists of villuslike projections of proprial connective tissue, which are covered by a pseudostratified layer of columnar epithelial cells. There may be loss of nuclear polarity, and nucleoli are prominent in epithelium in both types of polyps. The number of mitotic figures varies, often within the same tumor. The stalk of the tumor is highly vascular and

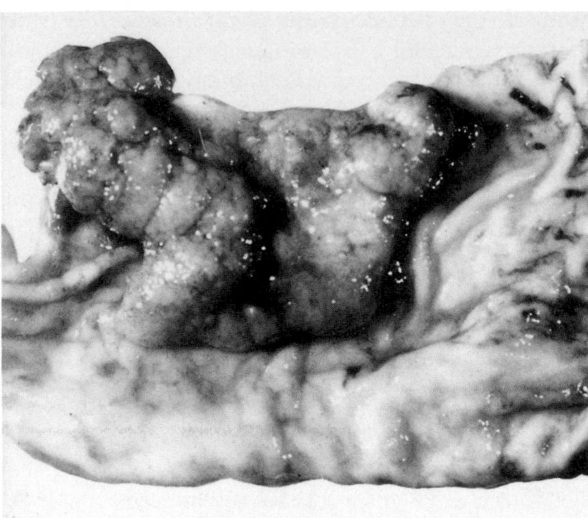

Fig. 1.64 Rectal polyp. Dog.

is continuous with the lamina propria or submucosa of the rectum. The tumors are generally well demarcated from the adjacent normal mucosa. The amount of mucin in the epithelium varies considerably, and it is often absent, especially in more dysplastic cells. Some polyps have a malignant appearance histologically. These are characterized by the presence of anaplastic epithelial cells *in situ* in the mucosa, and, in some cases, invading the propria and adjacent submucosa (Fig. 1.66).

There is little information on the biological behavior of these tumors. Adequate surgical removal usually results in complete recovery. In dogs, polyps which are more than 1.0 cm in diameter tend to have a more anaplastic appearance and appear to recur more commonly. Carcinoma *in situ* has been reported. Deep biopsies of these polyps are essential to rule out local invasion or infiltration of lymphatics, which should be sought in specimens with malignant epithelial morphology.

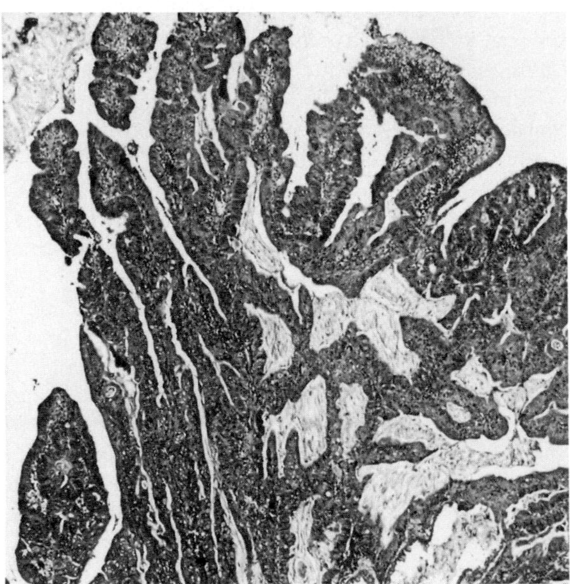

Fig. 1.65 Tubulopapillary colorectal polyp. Dog.

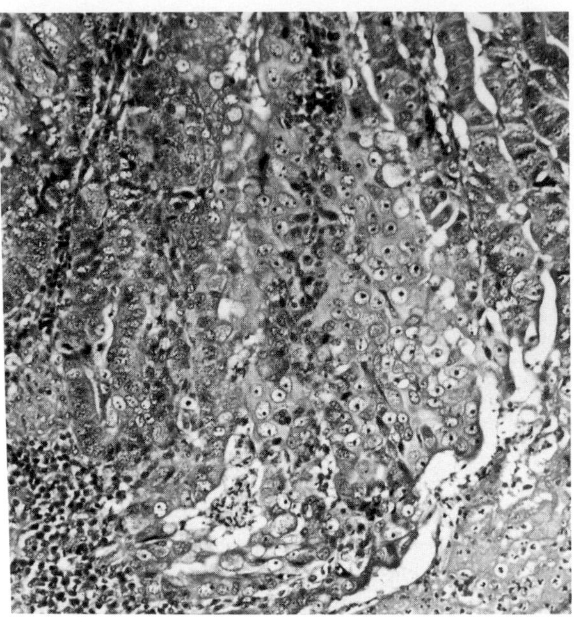

Fig. 1.66 Invasive carcinoma arising from the base of a tubulopapillary colorectal polyp in a dog.

Bibliography

Holt, P. E., and Lucke, V. M. Rectal neoplasia in the dog: A clinicopathological review of 31 cases. *Vet Rec* **116:** 400–405, 1985.

Seiler, R. J. Colorectal polyps of the dog: A clinicopathologic study of 17 cases. *J Am Vet Med Assoc* **174:** 72–75, 1979.

2. Polypoid Tumors In Other Species

Polypoid masses varying in diameter from one to several centimeters may be found at any level of the intestine in other species, especially cattle. They are usually an incidental finding, except in those cases in which they are large enough to cause partial obstruction. The tumors are raised, often pedunculated, gray to brown masses on the mucosal surface. They may occur singly, in grapelike clusters, or they may be scattered. Microscopically they resemble benign rectal polyps in the dog.

A high prevalence of intestinal adenomas, and, to a lesser extent, adenocarcinomas in cattle has been reported in upland areas in Scotland and northern England. These tumors often coexist with papillomas and squamous cell carcinomas of the upper alimentary tract (see Neoplasia of the Esophagus and Forestomachs, Section IV,I of this chapter). Three types of adenomas are recognized in the intestine of affected cattle in these endemic areas: a sessile plaque, an adenomatous polyp, and a more proliferative adenoma of the ampullae where the bile and pancreatic ducts open into the duodenum. Adenomatous polyps frequently occur in sheep with intestinal carcinoma. Hyperplastic polyps occur in the small intestines of lambs and goats with chronic coccidiosis (See Infectious and Parasitic Diseases of the Gastrointestinal Tract, Section VII of this chapter).

Bibliography

Ross, A. D., and Day, W. A. Intestinal polyps in a lamb. *N Z Vet J* **27:** 172N173, 1979.

Tontis, A., and Häfeli, W. Darmpolypen bei kleinen Ruminanten mit chronischer Kokzidiose. *Schweiz Arch Tierheilk* **127:** 401–405, 1985.

van Niel, M. H. F., van der Gaag, I., and van den Ingh, T.S.G.A.M. Polyposis of the small intestine in a young cat. *J Vet Med A* **36:** 161 165, 1989.

3. Intestinal Adenocarcinoma

Intestinal adenocarcinomas are uncommon in **dogs,** and they occur most frequently in the colon and rectum of animals averaging 8–9 years old. Some investigators have reported a slightly higher prevalence of intestinal carcinomas in male dogs, with a breed predisposition in boxers, collies, poodles, and German shepherds. Weight loss, persistent vomiting, anorexia, emaciation, and abdominal distension are the most common signs when the tumor is located in the small intestine. Dogs with colorectal tumors have tenesmus, hematochezia, and dyschezia. Many dogs with intestinal carcinomas are anemic.

Macroscopically, the tumors appear as gray-white, firm, sometimes annular, stenotic areas, which commonly affect the entire thickness of the intestinal wall (Fig. 1.51). These tumors often do not ulcerate, and they usually do not project into the lumen of the gut. The papillary or polypoid type of intestinal adenocarcinomas do form intraluminal masses, which tend to involve larger segments of the intestine, suggesting horizontal spread. There is dilation of the gut anterior to stenotic and obstructive tumors, and there may be hypertrophy of the intestinal muscularis proximal to such neoplasms.

On the basis of the microscopic appearance, intestinal carcinomas in dogs have been divided into four types, which may overlap. The acinar type is characterized by irregular glandular structures which obliterate the normal mucosa and infiltrate into submucosa and muscularis. The epithelial cells lining the acini are basophilic, cuboidal to columnar, and have small hyperchromatic nuclei in the basilar area of the cell. Amorphous eosinophilic material often fills the lumen of the glandular structures. Mucin is rarely found in this type of tumor. There is usually extensive necrosis with marked inflammation and fibrosis in the gut wall of the affected areas. At the periphery of these tumors, there may be hyperplasia of cryptal and villus epithelial cells.

In the solid undifferentiated type of intestinal carcinoma, the mucosa and gut wall are extensively infiltrated by nests and sheets of anaplastic epithelial cells. These have only a slight tendency to differentiate to acinar structures. The tumor cells have abundant amphophilic to basophilic cytoplasm and large vesicular nuclei with prominent nucleoli. There are some signet ring cells and a few lakes of mucin.

In the mucinous type of carcinoma, the anaplastic epithelial cells have pale eosinophilic cytoplasm. There are many signet ring cells. Large pools of extracellular mucin are evident in the stroma.

The papillary type consists of papilliferous projections into the lumen, which are covered by columnar, often highly anaplastic, epithelial cells. The mitotic index tends to be high. There is goblet cell hyperplasia of both crypts and villi. This type usually is only locally invasive when detected.

With the exception of papillary adenocarcinomas, desmoplasia is a prominent feature of these neoplasms, explaining their common tendency to cause stricture and obstruction of the intestine.

All types, except possibly the papillary type, metastasize widely, mainly via the lymphatics to the regional nodes (Fig. 1.67A). Involvement of the small intestine leads to metastases mainly in the mesenteric lymph nodes, less commonly to other abdominal nodes, liver, spleen, and lungs. Colonic adenocarcinomas metastasize to colic, iliac, and other pelvic and abdominal nodes. Metastases may also occur in most abdominal organs and the lungs. Implantation on serosal surfaces may result in obstruction

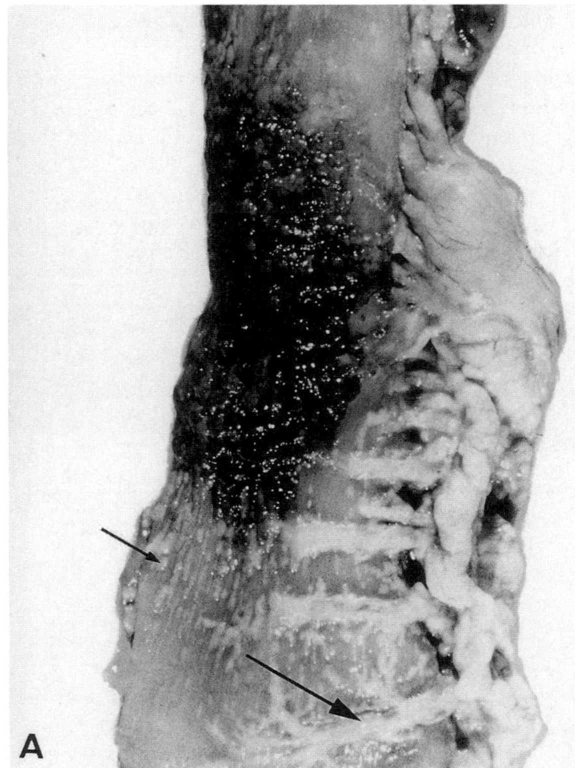

Fig. 1.67A Adenocarcinoma of rectum. Dog. Serosal hemorrhage, and plaque-like masses of desmoplastic fibrous tissue and neoplastic cells on the serosa (short arrow) and along serosal lymphatics draining to the mesentery (arrow).

of lymphatics followed by ascites. In a few cases malignant cells may show retrograde spread in the lymphatics of the abdomen and pelvic limbs, causing edema of the abdominal wall and legs. Dogs with annular colorectal carcinomas have a shorter survival period compared to dogs that have a single, pedunculated polypoid tumor in this location (<1.6 versus 32 months).

Intestinal adenocarcinoma rivals lymphosarcoma as the most common intestinal tumor in **cats.** The prevalence of intestinal carcinomas is lower in cats than in dogs. They are more common in Siamese cats than in other breeds. As in dogs, a higher prevalence of this tumor has been reported in males than females. The mean age of cats with intestinal carcinomas is 10–11 years, with a range of 4–14 years.

The ileum is the most common site affected, followed by the jejunum. When the tumor is located at the ileocecal junction, both the large and small intestine are usually involved. Intestinal carcinomas in cats rarely arise in the large intestine. The clinical signs and gross appearance are similar to those in dogs.

With some minor variations, the morphologic types of intestinal carcinomas described for dogs also occur in cats (Fig. 1.67B). Osteochondroid metaplasia of the stroma is a frequent feature of all types of intestinal adenocarcinoma in the cat. The rare carcinomas involving the large intestine have been mainly of the papillary type. They tend to be better differentiated and less scirrhous than carcinomas involving the small intestine.

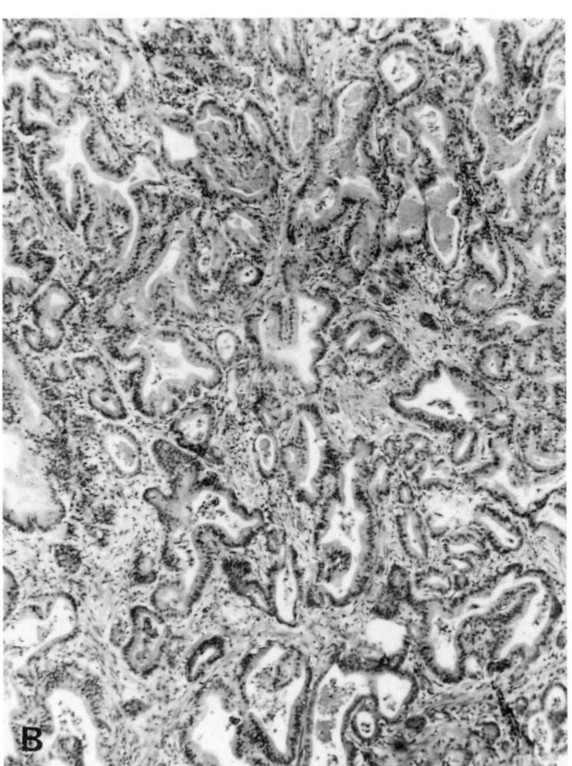

Fig. 1.67B Well differentiated intestinal adenocarcinoma. Cat.

The biological behavior of intestinal carcinomas in cats is similar to that in dogs. Some cats survive for several months even with advanced lesions.

Bibliography

Birchard, S. J., Guillermo Couto, C., and Johnson, S. Nonlymphoid intestinal neoplasia in 32 dogs and 14 cats. *J Am Anim Hosp Assoc* **22:** 533–537, 1986.

Church, E. M., Mehlhaff, C. J., and Patnaik, A. K. Colorectal adenocarcinoma in dogs: 78 cases (1973–1984). *J Am Vet Med Assoc* **191:** 727–730, 1987.

Cribb, A. E. Feline gastrointestinal adenocarcinoma: A review and retrospective study. *Can Vet J* **29:** 709–712, 1988.

Gibbs, C., and Pearson, H. Localized tumors of the canine small intestine: A report of twenty cases. *J Small Anim Pract* **27:** 507–519, 1986.

Kosovsky, J. E., Matthiesen, D. T., and Patnaik, A. K. Small intestinal adenocarcinoma in cats: 32 cases (1978–1985). *J Am Vet Med Assoc* **192:** 233–235, 1988.

Lingeman, C. H., Garner, F. M., and Taylor, D. O. N. Spontaneous adenocarcinomas of dogs: A review. *J Nat Cancer Inst* **47:** 137–153, 1971.

Patnaik, A. K., Liu, S.-K., and Johnson, G. F. Feline intestinal adenocarcinoma. A clinicopathologic study of 22 cases. *Vet Pathol* **13:** 1–10, 1976.

Pfeil, C., and Loupal, G. Tumoren im Darmtrakt des Hundes. *Zbl Vet Med (A)* **31:** 146–159, 1984.

Turk, M. A. M., Gallina, A. M., and Russell, T. S. Nonhematopoietic gastrointestinal neoplasia in cats: A retrospective study of 44 cases. *Vet Pathol* **18:** 614–620, 1981.

Intestinal adenocarcinoma is relatively common in **sheep** in New Zealand, Britain, Iceland, Scotland, Norway, and in southeastern Australia. The cause of the high prevalence in these areas is unknown but may be related to exposure to bracken fern or other unidentified carcinogens. In New Zealand and Australia there is a high prevalence in breeds used for fat lamb production. Other associations such as heavy use of certain fertilizers, and pastures with the weed *Cynosaurus cristatus,* have been reported from New Zealand. Tumors occur mainly in animals 5 years of age or older. Clinically, affected sheep lose weight and have abdominal distension due to ascites. Most cases are incidental findings at slaughter.

The tumors are usually located in the middle or lower areas of the small intestine, rarely in the colon (Fig. 1.68A,B). They are dense, firm, white masses, 0.5 cm to several centimeters long and as much as 1 cm thick, which may form annular constrictive bands at the affected site. Cauliflowerlike growths may be evident on the serosal surface. Polyps or plaques may protrude into the lumen, but ulceration of the mucosa is uncommon. The distal edge of the tumor is generally well demarcated. There is dilation of the intestine proximal to the lesion.

Metastasis occurs along the serosal lymphatics to the mesenteric lymph nodes. Implantations on serosal surfaces are common, and these appear as opaque to white plaques or diffusely thickened areas, which must be differ-

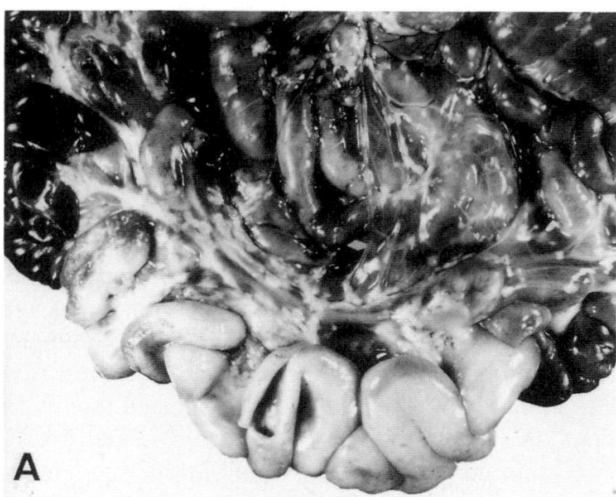

Fig. 1.68A White areas of scirrhous intestinal adenocarcinoma invading ileum. Sheep.

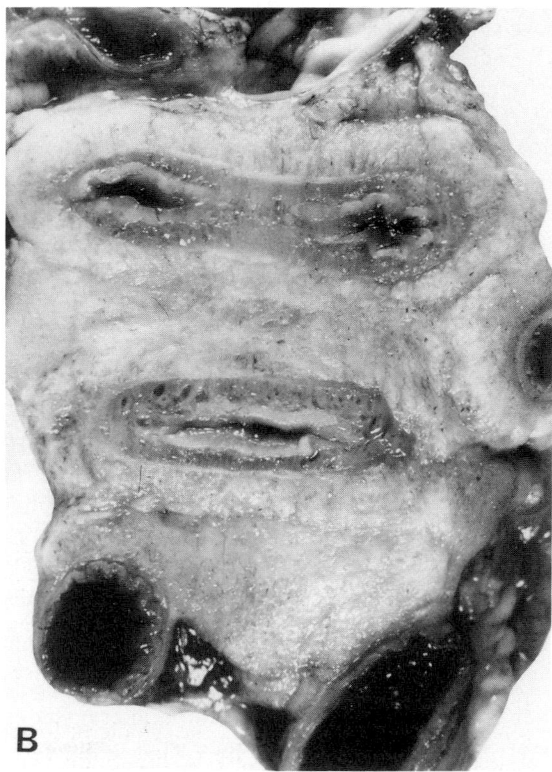

Fig. 1.68B White areas of scirrhous intestinal adenocarcinoma invading colon. Sheep.

entiated from mesothelioma. Obstruction of serosal lymphatics by tumor emboli may lead to ascites. Lung and liver metastases are rare.

Microscopically, the tumor is characterized by solid sheets or nests of well-differentiated to highly anaplastic polyhedral, cuboidal, or columnar epithelial cells, which may form irregular acinar structures. Neoplastic cells may be distributed singly, or in small aggregates, and are often

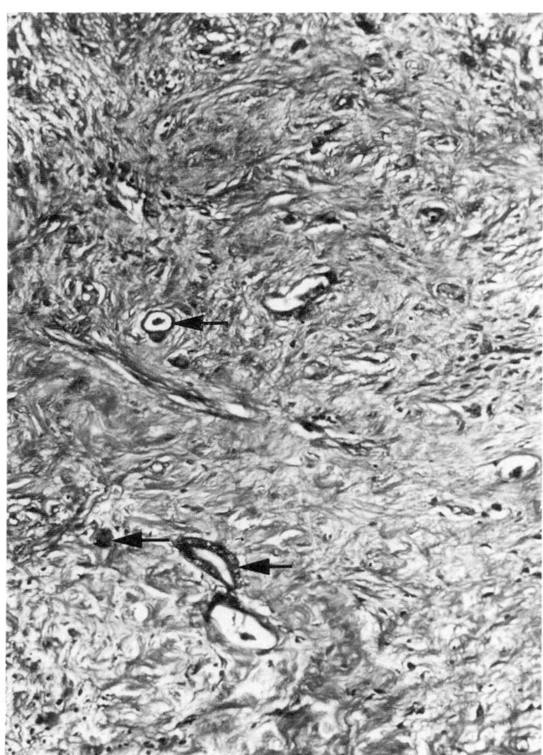

Fig. 1.69 Intestinal adenocarcinoma. Sheep. Islands of neoplastic epithelium (arrows) scattered in extensive desmoplastic reaction.

difficult to detect in the heavy fibrous desmoplastic response. Mitotic figures and acinar differentiation are infrequent. The neoplastic cells infiltrate the submucosa and the muscularis, along lymphatics, vessels, and nerve trunks, through to the serosal surface whence they spread via the lymphatics to the mesenteric lymph nodes. This is apparently followed by retrograde lymphogenous metastasis to the gut wall proximal to the primary tumor. These secondary tumors are particularly responsible for constriction of the gut lumen. The infiltrating tumor cells are invariably accompanied by a marked scirrhous reaction (Fig. 1.69). Sclerotic masses with anaplastic epithelial cells, many of which are PAS positive, are located on the serosal surfaces of the abdominal organs but rarely infiltrate the parenchyma. Argentaffin cells may form part of some intestinal carcinomas, especially in lymph node metastases. Mineralization and osseous metaplasia may develop in the stroma. The neoplastic cells appear to originate from undifferentiated cryptal epithelial cells.

Bibliography

Dodd, D. C. Adenocarcinoma of the small intestine of sheep. *N Z Vet J* **8:** 109–112, 1960.

Georgsson, G., and Vigfusson, H. Carcinoma of the small intestine of sheep in Iceland. A pathological and epizootiological study. *Acta Vet Scand* **14:** 392–409, 1973.

Ross, A. D., and Day, W. A. An ultrastructural study of adenocar-

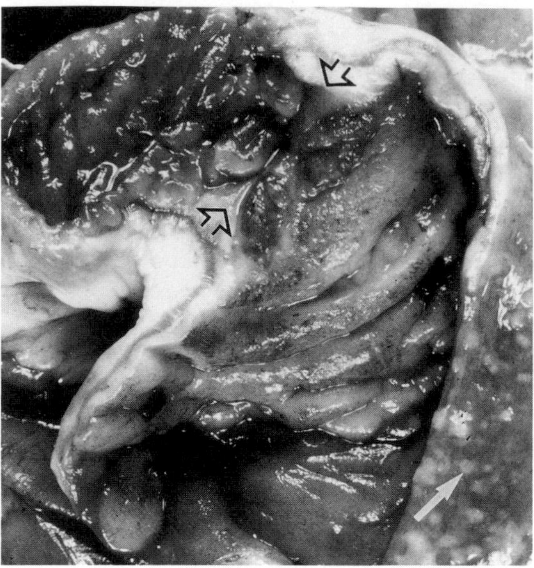

Fig. 1.70 Intestinal carcinoma. Cow. There is annular thickening of intestine (open arrows) with carcinomatous serosal plaques (arrow).

cinoma of the small intestine in sheep. *Vet Pathol* **22:** 552–560, 1985.

Ulvund, M. J. Occurrence of intestinal adenocarcinomas in sheep in the southwestern part of Norway. *N Z Vet J* **31:** 177–178, 1983.

Intestinal carcinomas generally are rare in **cattle, goats, horses,** and **swine** (Fig. 1.70), with the exception of those associated with bracken fern, papillomavirus, and upper alimentary cancer in cattle in certain parts of the United Kingdom, mentioned previously. There are reports of a higher prevalence of intestinal carcinomas in cattle in New Zealand where bracken fern and alimentary papillomatosis also occur. The prevalence of intestinal carcinomas in that country is high in humans, sheep, and possibly cattle, and it has been postulated that all three species may be exposed to similar dietary carcinogens that are activated by the gastrointestinal flora.

Intestinal carcinomas are usually an incidental finding at meat inspection. The location, morphology, and routes of metastasis are similar to those described for sheep, except that serosal lesions are less obvious. Hematogenous spread to the liver, lung, kidney, uterus, and ovaries may occur in cattle.

Bibliography

Haibel, G. K. Intestinal adenocarcinoma in a goat. *J Am Vet Med Assoc* **196:** 326–328, 1990.

Ross, A. D. Small-intestinal adenocarcinoma in cattle. *N Z Vet J* **32:** 98–99, 1984.

Rottman, J. B., Roberts, M. C., and Cullen, J. M. Colonic adenocarcinoma with osseous metaplasia in a horse. *J Am Vet Med Assoc* **198:** 657–659, 1991.

Vitovec, J. Carcinomas of the intestine in cattle and pigs. *Zbl Vet Med A* **24:** 413–421, 1977.

4. Carcinoid Tumors of the Intestine

Carcinoid tumors, also called enterochromaffin, argentaffin, Kulchitsky and amine precursor uptake and decarboxylation (APUD), arise from endocrine or paracrine cells located in the mucosal lining of a wide variety of organs, including the stomach and the intestine. These cells secrete vasoactive amines, which are responsible for the argentaffinic and argyrophilic tinctorial properties of the tumors. The cells are considered to be part of the APUD system. Functional derangements from excessive production of amines have not been reported in animals.

Carcinoid tumors of the gastrointestinal tract are rare in domestic animals. They have been reported mainly in aged dogs and occur rarely in the cat, cow, and horse. In dogs, carcinoids are mainly located in the duodenum, colon, and rectum. Clinically, they may cause intestinal obstruction, and anemia due to hemorrhage from ulcers. Rectal carcinoids may protrude from the anus and resemble adenomatous polyps.

Macroscopically, carcinoids are usually lobulated, firm, dark red to cream colored masses in the wall of the intestine. The tumor may result in submucosal or subserosal nodule formation and ulceration of overlying mucosa. Microscopically, carcinoids have a distinct endocrine appearance. Round or oval to polyhedral cells have abundant finely granular eosinophilic or vacuolated cytoplasm and vesiculate nuclei with prominent nucleoli. They form nests, ribbons, rosettes, or diffuse sheets in the mucosa, submucosa, and muscularis. A fine vascularized stroma divides the tumor masses into pseudoalveolar arrangements. Amyloid may be present in intercellular and perivascular spaces. Multinucleate giant cells are occasionally seen.

Confirmation of the diagnosis requires special stains to reveal argentaffinic and argyrophilic properties. These histochemical reactions may be negative, especially in rectal carcinoids. They may also be lost during fixation in formalin or by autolysis prior to fixation. Electron-microscopic examination helps to differentiate carcinoids from intestinal mast cell tumors. Carcinoid tumor cells have dense, round to oval, membrane-bound secretory granules in the cytoplasm, which vary in diameter from 75 to 300 nm. They have abundant rough endoplasmic reticulum, and the plasma membrane forms interdigitating processes. The ultrastructural characteristics of intestinal mast cell tumors are described subsequently. Carcinoid tumors are Schiff negative and do not show metachromasia with Giemsa stains.

Data on biological behavior of intestinal carcinoids in dogs are limited. The few cases reported were malignant. There may be extensive invasion of the gut wall and veins with metastasis especially to the liver. In this respect their behavior is similar to that of intestinal carcinoids in humans. The few cases that have been described in other species have features similar to those described in dogs. Goblet-cell carcinoids (adenocarcinoids, mucinous carcinoids) have features of carcinoids and adenocarcinomas, and these tumors are more commonly found in the appendix of humans. There is a single case report of this type of tumor in the rectum of a dog. Microscopically goblet-cell carcinoids have distinct areas of mucinous adenocarcinoma and carcinoid that may merge. The carcinoid component is most prominent in the primary tumor and the metastases.

Bibliography

Cho, D.-Y., and Archibald, L. F. Carcinoid tumor in the colon of a cow. *Vet Pathol* **22:** 639–641, 1985.

Orsini, J. A. *et al.* Intestinal carcinoid in a mare: An etiologic consideration for chronic colic in horses. *J Am Vet Med Assoc* **193:** 87–88, 1988.

Patnaik, A. K., Lieberman, P. H. Canine goblet-cell carcinoid. *Vet Pathol* **18:** 410–413, 1981.

Sykes, G. P., and Cooper, B. J. Canine intestinal carcinoids. *Vet Pathol* **19:** 120–131, 1982.

5. *Intestinal Mast Cell Tumors*

These tumors are uncommon. They occur mainly in aged cats, and rarely in dogs. They resemble carcinoids under the light microscope, and a definitive diagnosis requires histochemical and ultrastructural examination of tumor cells. They appear to be more common than intestinal carcinoid tumors in cats. Abnormal mast cells do not appear in circulation.

Intestinal mast cell tumors are mainly located in the small intestine, and rarely in the colon. Affected areas in the gut are tan-colored, firm, thickened, and may be one to several centimeters in length. Nests, cords, and whorls of pleomorphic mast cells infiltrate the mucosa and adjacent areas of the gut wall. These cells are unlike those in mastocytomas involving the skin and other organs. The latter are round and have an intensely eosinophilic granular cytoplasm with distinct cytoplasmic borders and central oval nuclei. In contrast, cells in intestinal mastocytomas are polygonal to spindle shaped. They have a finely granular or vacuolated cytoplasm with indistinct cytoplasmic borders and oval, hyperchromatic, eccentrically located nuclei. The degree of metachromatic staining varies considerably, and there is a marked variation in the number of eosinophils in the tumor.

Ultrastructurally, the cells in most respects resemble typical degranulated mast cells. The cytoplasm contains many membrane bound granules, which appear as single or fused vesicles. Fine fibrillar material forms a loose network within these vesicles. A few tumor cells contain electron-dense fibrillar granules or intermediate forms. None of the tumor cells contains the crystalline electron-dense granules which are present in normal mast cells and in mastocytomas in other sites.

Metastases occur most often in the mesenteric lymph nodes, followed by the liver, spleen, and rarely, the lungs. Ulceration of the gastrointestinal mucosa occurs commonly with systemic mast cell tumors in cats and large cutaneous mastocytomas in dogs. Mucosal ulceration is not a feature of intestinal mast cell tumors in the cat. This may be due to low levels of histamine in the cells in intestinal tumors.

Bibliography

Alroy, J. *et al.* Distinctive intestinal mast cell neoplasms of domestic cats. *Lab Invest* **33:** 159–167, 1975.

Garner, F. M., and Lingeman, C. H. Mast cell neoplasms of the domestic cat. *Pathol Vet* **7:** 517–530, 1970.

6. *Other Mesenchymal Intestinal Tumors*

Leiomyomas and **leiomyosarcomas** (Fig. 1.71) are probably more common than other types of mesenchymal tumors except lymphosarcoma. In dogs, these tumors occur most commonly in the small intestine and cecum, where they cause obstruction. Signs associated with leiomyosarcoma include weight loss, lethargy, anorexia, anemia due to intestinal hemorrhage, abdominal pain, diarrhea, vomition, and dehydration. The tumor is most common in old dogs, but it may occur in young animals. Some surveys report a higher prevalence in males than in females, whereas others mention the opposite. The neoplasm tends to be nodular rather than diffuse, and ulcerates and cavitates on the luminal surface. Invading microorganisms from the gut lumen may result in abscessation of the tumor and a secondary septic peritonitis. Leiomyosarcomas are slow to metastasize, usually only to the mesenteric nodes, giving these tumors a more favorable prognosis after complete resection than other malignant neoplasms.

In old horses, smooth muscle tumors of the intestine may cause intermittent bouts of colic that become more frequent with time. They may occur in the small intestine as well as encapsulated, firm, pale yellow masses on the serosal surface or pedunculated tumors protruding into the lumen of the rectum. These tumors are rare in other species. The histologic appearance is similar to that of smooth muscle tumors in other sites.

Gastrointestinal lymphomas occur in most species and

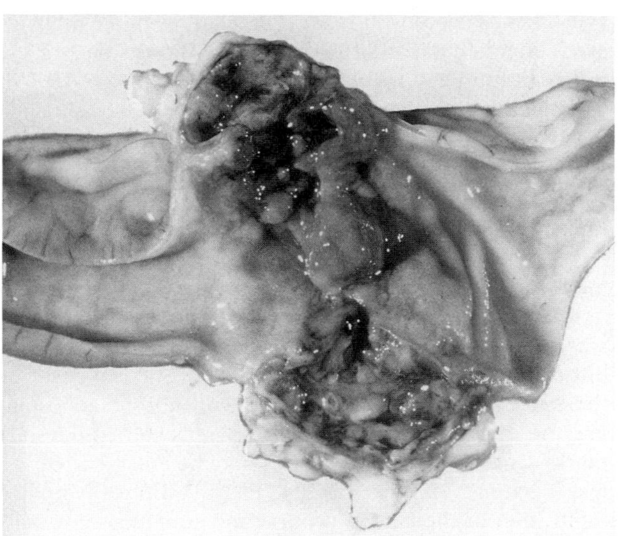

Fig. 1.71 Annular ulcerating leiomyosarcoma. Cat

are common in cats. These neoplasms may be primary, or part of the systemic or multicentric form of the neoplasm. There is disagreement on the definition of primary lymphoma of the intestine. Our preference is to include only animals with lymphomatous lesions in the intestine with or without involvement of the abdominal organs or bone marrow. If there are lesions in the thorax or peripheral sites accompanying those in the gut, the lesions in the latter location are considered to be part of the multicentric form of lymphoma.

In **dogs,** the majority of intestinal lymphomas appear to be primary. The reported age range is 19 months to 13 years (mean 6.7 years). There is a higher prevalence in male dogs. Signs may be acute or seen over a period of weeks to months. Hypoproteinemia, probably associated with enteric protein loss, occurs in ~30% of the affected dogs.

The tumors are located in the small intestine, stomach, and colon in that order of frequency. They are soft to firm, cream-colored masses located in the submucosa, and may protrude into the gut lumen. The overlying mucosa may or may not be ulcerated. The masses may be nodular to diffuse, and several sections of the gut are usually affected. The mesenteric nodes are often enlarged. Microscopically, the lamina propria and submucosa are diffusely infiltrated by noncleaved lymphoid cells that show marked anisocytosis. The neoplastic cells may infiltrate transmurally to the serosa. There is frequent involvement of the regional nodes, liver, and less often the marrow.

Some workers report a marked lymphoplasmacytic enteritis adjacent to or distant from the tumor. It has been suggested that lymphoplasmacytic enteritis in the dog, particularly the basenji, may represent a prelymphomatous stage similar to immunoproliferative small intestinal disease in humans. The latter is characterized by a diffuse lymphoplasmacytic infiltration of the small intestinal mucosa that results in malabsorption, and predisposes to the development of primary enteromesenteric lymphoma. Full-thickness biopsies from several areas of the intestine are recommended to differentiate lymphoplasmacytic enteritis from intestinal lymphoma.

The alimentary form of lymphoma is a relatively common tumor in the **horse**. It occurs mainly in young adults. Affected horses lose condition, probably due to malabsorption and protein loss; in addition, they may be anemic, icteric, and have mild intermittent bouts of colic. Diarrhea is inconsistent. Serum albumin is often decreased, but they are often hypergammaglobulinemic.

Macroscopic lesions in horses are usually located in the small intestine, and these are characterized by local to diffuse thickening of the gut wall with prominent rugae on the mucosa. Nodules or plaques with fibrous adhesions may be evident on the serosa. The mesenteric nodes are markedly enlarged. Other nodes may be enlarged but to a lesser extent. Microscopically, there is diffuse lymphoid infiltration of the lamina propria and submucosa, usually extending transmurally to the serosa. There is marked villus atrophy to the point of complete loss of villi and crypts. Plasmacytoid cells are regularly present in the lamina propria but less numerous in the submucosa. Similar lymphoid cell infiltration involves the mesenteric nodes and the perinodal connective tissue. Other lymph nodes are involved in about half the cases. A plasmacytoid or plasmacytic reaction and occasional giant cells are also present in the nodes.

The neoplastic lymphoid cells are probably of B-cell origin and home into the gut-associated lymphoid tissue and the lamina propria of the small intestine. An immune-mediated type of dermatitis has been associated with both chronic, inflammatory (granulomatous and eosinophilic enteritides) and lymphomatous lesions in the gut in horses (see The Skin and Appendages, Volume 1, Chapter 5).

Alimentary lymphoma in **cats** may be primary, which is most common, or secondary, as part of the multicentric form. The small intestine, especially the jejunum and ileum, are the most common locations in the primary form. Similar to that in the other species, the mesenteric nodes are usually involved. In **cattle and sheep,** alimentary lymphomas are generally part of the adult multicentric form of the disease.

Extramedullary plasmacytomas have been described previously in the section on oral tumors. These tumors have also been reported in the stomach, colon, and rectum of dogs and the duodenum of a cat. This neoplasm must be differentiated from plasmacytic inflammatory cell reactions of the gastrointestinal mucosa.

Other rare mesenchmal intestinal tumors that have been reported are fibromas and fibrosarcomas; osteosarcomas; schwannomas; ganglioneuromas in dogs, the latter also in a sow, horse, and a kitten; and neoplasms of globule leukocytes in cats.

Bibliography

Allen, D., Swayne, D., and Belknap, J. K. Ganglioneuroma as a cause of small intestinal obstruction in the horse: A case report. *Cornell Vet* **79:** 133–141, 1989.

Bruecker, K. A., and Withrow, S. J. Intestinal leiomyosarcomas in six dogs. *J Am Anim Hosp Assoc* **24:** 281–284, 1988.

Chen, H. C. *et al.* Duodenal leimyosarcoma with multiple hepatic metastases in a dog. *J Am Vet Med Assoc* **184:** 1506, 1984.

Clem, M. F., DeBowes, R. M., and Leipold, H. W. Rectal leiomyosarcoma in a horse. *J Am Vet Med Assoc* **191:** 229–230, 1987.

Couto, G. C. *et al.* Gastrointestinal lymphoma in 20 dogs. A retrospective study. *J Vet Intern Med* **3:** 73–78, 1989.

Fairley, R. A., and McEntee, M. F. Colorectal ganglioneuromatosis in a young female dog (Lhasa Apso). *Vet Pathol* **27:** 206–207, 1990.

Hawkins, E. C., Feldman, B. F., and Blanchard, P. C. Immunoglobulin A myeloma in a cat with pleural effusion and serum hyperviscosity. *J Am Vet Med Assoc* **188:** 876–878, 1986.

Head, K. W. Tumors of the intestine. *In* "Tumors in Domestic Animals," 3rd Ed., J. E. Moulton (ed.), pp. 416–420. Berkeley, California, University of California Press, 1990.

Holt, P. E., and Lucke, V. M. Rectal neoplasia in the dog: A clinico-pathological review of 31 cases. *Vet Rec* **116:** 400–405, 1985.

Honor, D. J. *et al.* A neoplasm of globule leukocytes in a cat. *Vet Pathol* **23:** 287–292, 1986.

Livesey, M. A., Hulland, T. J., and Yovich, J. V. Colic in two horses associated with smooth muscle intestinal tumors. *Equine Vet J* **18:** 334–337, 1986.

MacEwen, E. G. *et al.* Extramedullary plasmacytoma of the gastrointestinal tract in two dogs. *J Am Vet Med Assoc* **184:** 1396–1398, 1984.

Pardo, A. D. *et al.* Primary jejunal osteosarcoma associated with a surgical sponge in a dog. *J Am Vet Med Assoc* **196:** 935–938, 1990.

Platt, H. Alimentary lymphomas in the horse. *J Comp Pathol* **97:** 1–10, 1987.

Ribas, J. L., Kwapien, R. P., and Pope, E. R. Immunohistochemistry and ultrastructure of intestinal ganglioneuroma in a dog. *Vet Pathol* **27:** 376–379, 1990.

Une, Y. *et al.* Multiple ganglioneuroma derived from intramural plexus of jejunum in a sow. *Jpn J Vet Sci* **46:** 247–250, 1984.

Wilson, R. G. *et al.* Alimentary lymphosarcoma in a horse with cutaneous manifestations. *Equine Vet J* **17**: 148–150, 1985.

VII. Infectious and Parasitic Diseases of the Gastrointestinal Tract

A. *Viral Diseases*

1. Foot-and-Mouth Disease

Foot-and-mouth disease (aphthous fever) is a highly contagious viral infection of ruminants and swine and of at least 70 species of wild animals. It is a problem of worldwide concern, being enzootic in large areas of Africa, Asia, Europe, and in South America, except the Guyanas and Chile. Between these areas are other countries periodically visited by the virus and in whose susceptible populations the disease spreads rapidly. Some other areas, notably Japan, Australia, New Zealand, North and Central America including the Caribbean Islands, Scandinavia, Iceland, Ireland, and Great Britain are currently free because of geographic isolation and quarantine restrictions. Many outbreaks in Europe have been associated with vaccines that contained incompletely inactivated virus.

Foot-and-mouth disease is an acute febrile condition of cloven-hoofed animals characterized by the formation of vesicles in and around the mouth, on the feet, teats, and mammary glands. The disease is not notable for high mortality, except in sucklings, but morbidity is very high. In an affected population, productivity is reduced substantially, and the disease can cause severe economic loss because it usually leads to trade restrictions.

The virus of foot and mouth disease belongs to the genus *Aphthovirus* (aphtha, ulcer) in the Picornaviridae. The virus is highly resistant under many circumstances, but is inactivated by direct sunlight, because of drying and increase in temperature, and by moderate acidity (pH <5.0). The acid production which accompanies rigor mortis in carcasses and meat inactivates the virus. However, the alteration in pH is not dependable, and the virus survives in offal, viscera, lymph nodes, and bone marrow for an indefinite period under refrigeration. Next to the movement of infected animals, contaminated animal products are likely to be the most common mechanism of spread. The virus may survive on hay and other fomites for several weeks. Wind-borne spread may occur over considerable distances under favorable conditions. Spread of an outbreak in Brittany, France to the Isle of Wight and Jersey Island in 1981 was apparently due to wind-borne virus.

The resistance of the virus is of epidemiologic significance, especially where control policies involve slaughter rather than vaccination. The importance of a carrier state in the epidemiology of foot-and-mouth disease is uncertain. The carrier state has been observed in cattle, sheep, goats, and African buffalo (*Syncerus caffer*), but not in pigs. The carrier state may persist for as long as 2 years postinfection in cattle and 9 months in sheep. The virus is carried mainly in the oropharynx, probably in the tonsils. The carrier state exists even in animals with a significant level of serum-neutralizing antibody. Virus recovered from carrier animals can infect susceptible animals by means of inoculation. Sheep and goats are considered to be a frequent inapparent source of dissemination of the virus by some, but not all, investigators. African buffalo can carry foot-and-mouth disease (FMD) virus for at least 5 years. Field outbreaks have been associated with buffalo–cattle contact in Africa, but these appear to be rare. Although Asian water buffaloes (*Bubalus arnee*) may be affected in FMD outbreaks, it is not known whether they remain carriers. Restriction in the movement of domestic and feral animals is the most effective method of controlling further spread.

Of equal importance to the persistence of the virus is its antigenic heterogeneity and instability. There are seven principal antigenic serotypes, namely, the classical A, O, and C types, SAT-1, SAT-2, SAT-3, and Asia-1. These can be distinguished by serologic tests, although there are various degrees of overlap. Six of the seven serotypes (O, A, C, SAT-1, SAT-2, SAT-3) are known to occur in Africa; four (O, A, C, Asia 1), in Asia; and three (O, A, C), in Europe and South America. These serotypes are sufficiently different immunologically that infection with one type does not confer resistance to the other six. Within these seven major types there are antigenic subtypes, each different, to variable degrees, from the parent type. Generally, the subtypes cross-immunize to a useful degree, but exceptions do arise and become recognizable, especially when vaccination fails. Antigenic drift can also be demonstrated experimentally; new subtypes can be produced by passing the virus in immune or partially immune animals, or by growing the virus *in vitro* in the presence of immune serum. There are presently at least 63 distinct antigenic strains of the virus of natural origin and no reason to think that the possibility of recombination of subtypes is limited. The capsid protein VP-1 appears to be mainly responsible for the antigenic and immunogenic properties of the FMD virus. This protein is involved in the process of virus attachment to cells.

As well as differences and variability in antigenic characters, strains of the virus differ in virulence, and a given strain is probably able to vary in virulence. Certainly, comparing different outbreaks, there is considerable variation in the severity of the disease produced in a given host species. Virulence also varies between species. Some strains, for example, will infect pigs but not cattle, and others are pathogenic for cattle and not for pigs. A similar relationship pertains for sheep and goats, but, in general, virus strains are intermediate between these extremes. There can be little doubt, however, that adaptation to a host species does occur, and that this adaptive relationship may establish a reservoir of infection.

In addition to the domestic hosts, humans can become infected, but not importantly, either clinically or epidemiologically. The hedgehog, coypu, and some marsupials are highly susceptible to infection and could be important in the transmission of the disease. Some laboratory animals are also susceptible, the white mouse in particular. Suckling mice inoculated intraperitoneally are susceptible enough to be used for detection of small amounts of virus. They consistently develop spastic paraplegia with degeneration of skeletal musculature, and in ~50% there is myocardial degeneration and, in a variable percentage, pancreatic necrosis. Young adult guinea pigs regularly develop pancreatic necrosis with some necrosis of skeletal and cardiac muscle. In terms of evolution and epithelial lesions, the disease in guinea pigs is similar to that in cattle.

The main portal of entry and primary site of viral multiplication is the mucosa and the lymphoid tissues of the pharyngeal/tonsillar region. The ability of the virus to establish in this area is not affected by the presence of circulating antibodies. The incubation period varies between 3 and 8 days. Primary multiplication is followed by a viremic stage of 4–5 days. After the viremia there is a secondary phase of replication of virus in organs such as lymph nodes, mammary gland, thyroid, adrenals, kidneys, and sites where characteristic vesicles develop, referred to later. *In situ* hybridization techniques in guinea pigs have shown FMD virus in epidermal and visceral tissues very early in infection, well before the onset of clinical signs and lesions. The lungs are infected at this stage, and it has been suggested that alveolar macrophages transport inhaled virus into the circulation. Virus is also present in exhaled air, especially in pigs.

Virus is excreted in high titers in the vesicular fluid, and all body secretions and excretions, during the acute phase of the infection. Virus persists in the sites of lesions for 3–8 days after the appearance of significant neutralizing titers in serum, but seldom persists in lesions beyond day 11 of clinical illness. Virus may persist in the oropharynx for a considerable period in some species, as mentioned earlier. High titers of virus develop in all areas of skin, not necessarily related to lesions, and in several visceral tissues, including pancreas and hypophysis. Here they have been related to persistent aftereffects of natural and experimental infections.

Within a week of the development of neutralizing antibody, the titer of virus declines. Ordinarily, serum antibody titers decline progressively and fairly rapidly. The duration of persistence of antibody is correlated with the initial titer. In general, animals are resistant to reinfection with homologous strains by natural exposure for about 2–4 years; susceptibility increases as the antibody titer declines.

The characteristic lesions of foot and mouth disease are seen only in those animals which are examined at the height of disease. Later, the lesions heal or are obscured by secondary bacterial infection. Lesions develop mainly in areas subject to trauma: the oral mucosa, especially the tongue; the interdigital cleft; and the teats in lactating animals. In **cattle,** there is appreciable loss of weight, and the buccal cavity may contain much saliva. In the living animal, there is diffuse buccal hyperemia and mild catarrhal stomatitis, but the hyperemia disappears at death. Vesicles form on the inner aspects of the lips and cheeks, the gums, hard palate, dental pad, and especially on the sides and anterior portion of the dorsum of the tongue. Sometimes they form on the muzzle and exterior nares. The primary vesicles are small, but coalesce to produce bullae, which may be 5–6 cm across; these bullae rupture in 12–14 hr, leaving an intensely red, raw, and moist base to which shreds of epithelium may still adhere (Fig. 1.72A). A seropurulent exudate develops on the base of the erosion, and this coagulates to a scab, which in turn is replaced by regenerated epithelium in less than 2 weeks. Secondary infection may complicate this course.

Foot lesions occur in the majority of cases. There is inflammatory swelling of skin of the interdigital space, coronet, and heels a day or so before vesicles form. The swellings persist until the vesicles rupture and the resultant erosions heal; healing may be considerably delayed

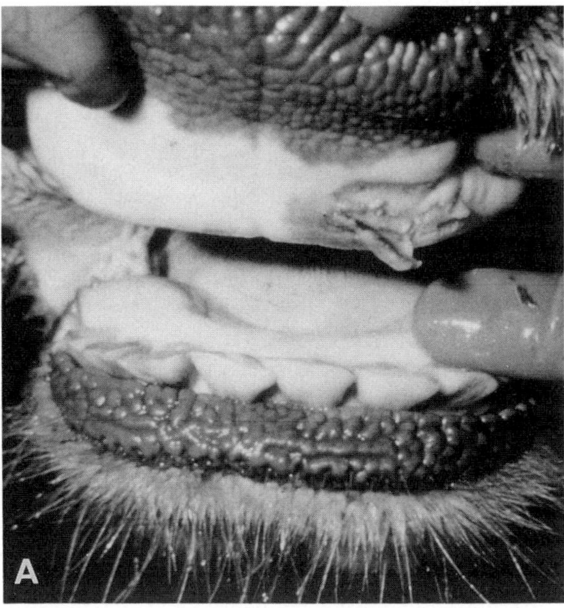

Fig. 1.72A Foot-and-mouth disease. Ruptured vesicle on the dental pad of a cow. (Courtesy of C. C. Brown, Foreign Animal Disease Diagnostic Laboratory, USDA.)

on the feet. Vesicles may also occur in the other sites, but much less frequently. When the teats and udder are involved, there is severe swelling.

Fluorescent antibody studies indicate that there is infection of individual cells in the stratum spinosum, adjacent to the papillae on mucosal surfaces, or in the follicular sheath in skin. The papilla serves as a bridge for transport of the virus from the vascular lamina propria to the squamous epithelium. Immunofluorescence occurs in mononuclear cells of the lamina propria before there is evidence of virus in the epithelial cells. The infected epithelial cells progressively swell, develop eosinophilia of the cytoplasm, and undergo acantholysis. There is extensive spongiosis of the stratum spinosum, and this, along with the necrosis of keratinocytes, results in the formation of vesicles. Superficial lesions may be formed in the stratum corneum. These vesicles tend to rupture as soon as they develop, with leakage of vesicular fluid followed by desiccation. The cells in this type of lesion remain spherical and adhere to each other by proteinaceous material. The early microvesicles coalesce and become macroscopically visible, and these in turn may form bullae. The base of the vesicle is formed by the basal germinative layer of epithelium, which is not usually breached, and the underlying dermis or lamina propria, which is infiltrated by inflammatory cells and is intensely hyperemic.

The virus replicates in the secretory epithelium of the bovine mammary gland. Acinar lesions are the direct result of virus replication. The initial damage to the epithelial cells is close to the basement membrane, which is the site of virus production. This progresses to focal areas of necrosis that increase in size and number with time. The acini and ducts in the necrotic areas contain mainly sloughed epithelial cells, cellular debris and small numbers of leukocytes. There is a moderate inflammatory cell reaction in the interstitium, consisting of macrophages and neutrophils, but inflammation is minimal in contrast to the degree of tissue injury.

Large amounts of virus are present in milk 7 days postinfection. Affected acini involute during the vesicular stage of the infection and this is probably responsible for the marked drop in milk production. Repair of acini, with poorly differentiated cells, is evident at 15 days postinfection.

In addition to the lesions of the oral cavity, skin, and mammary gland, there may be catarrhal inflammation of the respiratory passages. In animals dying of the disease, erosive and ulcerative lesions may be found on the ruminal pillars, and there are petechial hemorrhages of the abomasum and intestine, with congestion and diapedesis into the lumen. The abomasal hemorrhages quickly develop to ulcers. Pulmonary edema, modest splenomegaly, and hydropericardium with petechiae on the epicardium are nonspecific changes in this disease.

A malignant form of the disease, without vesiculation, does occur in young animals. In these, death is common, probably because of the myocarditis which develops. Poorly defined pale foci of varying size are seen in the wall of the ventricles and in the papillary muscle. This lesion is referred to as tiger-heart, on account of the striping and mottling. The myocarditis is acute, and hyaline degeneration and necrosis of muscle fibers is accompanied by a principally mononuclear cell infiltrate that varies in intensity. Similar lesions occur in skeletal muscle.

Prolonged convalescence or residual illness is frequently referred to in cattle, but is difficult to evaluate. Residual bacterial infections are common complications, especially in the oral cavity and mammary glands, and on the feet. Additionally, syndromes are described of panting and hypertrichosis; disturbances of the regulation of body temperature, of lactation and fertility, including abortion; and of emaciation or obesity. Such disturbances result from involvement of the hypothalamic–hypophyseal axis and endocrine organs in which nonspecific changes may be found. Diabetes mellitus is reported as a complication of the experimental and natural disease. The pancreatic islets may disappear almost completely, and the pancreas also shows acinar necrosis, inflammation, atrophy, and regeneration, the latter evident as proliferation of tubular structures. Clinical myocardial disease is frequent in convalescent cattle and is ascribed to degeneration of the myocardium and the conduction system.

Sheep are, in general, less susceptible than cattle, and the infection runs a milder course, though there may be exceptions. The incubation period in sheep is commonly 3–8 days, with fever lasting about 4 days. Lesions may not develop. When they do, the dental pad is the preferred site in the oral cavity. Lingual lesions tend to occur on the posterior dorsal portion as underrunning necrotic erosions rather than vesicles. These are small and easily missed, and they heal within a few days. Lameness is prominent in acute outbreaks. Typical vesicles develop in the interdigital cleft, on the coronet, and on the bulb of heel. They may occasionally involve all of the coronet and lead to eventual shedding of the hoof. Vesicles also occasionally occur on the teats, vulva, prepuce, and on the pillars of the rumen. Abortions have been reported in some outbreaks. The peracute form with myocardial necrosis may occur in lambs.

The disease in **goats** is, in general, similar to that described for sheep. According to some workers, both species may be inapparent carriers.

In **pigs** there is also considerable variability in virulence of strains and the acuteness of the disease. The incubation period is somewhat longer than that in cattle and may extend for a week or more. Lesions occur in the usual sites, although more commonly on the feet than in the mouth. They may be present on the snout and behind its rim (Fig. 1.72B), and on the teats of lactating sows. Abortion and stillbirth of infected piglets is recorded. The peracute form, with high mortality due to myocarditis, occurs in sucklings, often before vesicle formation is noticed in sows.

Foot and mouth disease must be differentiated from other viral vesicular diseases such as vesicular stomatitis, vesicular exanthema, and swine vesicular disease in sus-

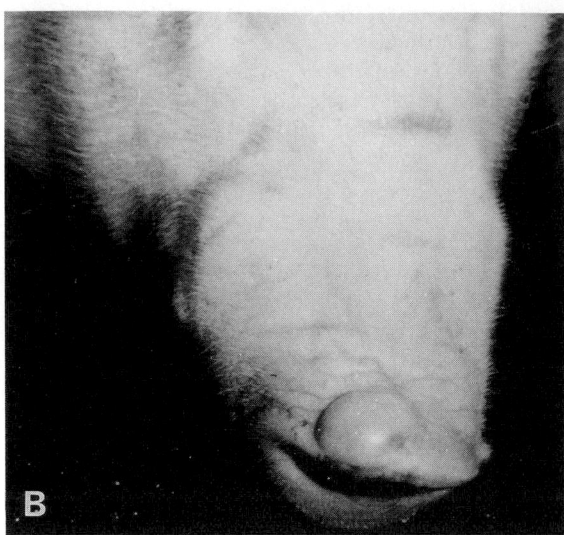

Fig. 1.72B Foot-and-mouth disease. Vesicle on snout. Pig. (Courtesy of C. C. Brown, Foreign Animal Disease Diagnostic Laboratory, USDA.)

ceptible species, and in the latter stages, from diseases producing erosive/ulcerative lesions of the oral cavity. The disease must be considered in the differential diagnosis in cases of sudden death among cloven-footed animals, especially the young.

Bibliography

Acharya, R. *et al.* The structure of foot-and-mouth disease virus: implications for its physical and biological properties. *Vet Microbiol* **23:** 21–34, 1990.

Anderson, E. C. The pathogenesis of foot and mouth disease in the African buffalo (*Syncerus caffer*) and the role of this species in the epidemiology of the disease in Kenya. *J Comp Pathol* **89:** 541–549, 1979.

Barboni, E., Manocchio, I., and Asdrubali, G. Observations on diabetes mellitus associated with experimental foot and mouth disease in cattle. *Vet Ital* **17:** 362–368, 1966.

Blackwell, J. H., and Wool, S. H. Destruction and repair of mammary gland parenchyma of cows infected with foot-and-mouth disease. *J Comp Pathol* **96:** 227–234, 1986.

Brown, C. C., Olander, H. J., and Meyer, R. F. A preliminary study of the pathogenesis of foot-and-mouth disease virus using *in situ* hybridization. *Vet Pathol* **28:** 216–222, 1991.

Burrows, R. Studies on the carrier state of cattle exposed to foot-and-mouth disease virus. *J Hyg (Camb)* **64:** 81–90, 1966.

Burrows, R. *et al.* The pathogenesis of natural and simulated natural foot-and-mouth disease infection in cattle. *J Comp Pathol* **91:** 599–609, 1981.

Carrillo, C. *et al.* Comparison of vaccine strains and the virus causing the 1986 foot-and-mouth disease outbreak in Spain: Epizootiological analysis. *Virus Res* **15:** 45–56, 1990.

Donaldson, A. I., Ferris, N. P., and G. A. H. Wells. Experimental foot-and-mouth disease in fattening pigs, sows, and piglets in relation to outbreaks in the field. *Vet Rec* **115:** 509–512, 1984.

Ferris, N. P. *et al.* Experimental infection of eland (*Taurotragus oryx*), sable antelope (*Ozanna grandicomis*), and buffalo (*Syncerus caffer*) with foot-and-mouth disease virus. *J Comp Pathol* **101:** 307–316, 1989.

Gailiunas, P., and Cottral, G. E. Presence and persistence of foot-and-mouth disease virus in bovine skin. *J Bacteriol* **91:** 2333–2338, 1966.

Hedger, R. S., and Condy, J. B. Transmission of foot-and-mouth disease from African buffalo virus carriers to bovines. *Vet Rec* **117:** 205, 1985.

Kitching, R. P. *et al.* Development of foot-and-mouth disease virus strain characterisation—a review. *Trop Anim Health Prod* **21:** 153–166, 1989.

Lubroth, J. *et al.* Foot-and-mouth disease virus in the llama (*Lama glama*): Diagnosis, transmission, and susceptibility. *J Vet Diagn Invest 2:* 197–203, 1990.

Paine, G. D. Susceptibility of African buffaloes and Asiatic water buffaloes to foot-and-mouth disease. *Aust Vet J* Vol. 67. N24–N25, 1990.

Pay, T. W. F. Foot-and-mouth disease in sheep and goats: A review. *Foot and Mouth Dis Bull* **26:** 2–13, 1988.

Perl, S. *et al.* Pathological changes in mountain gazelles challenged with FMD virus, with special reference to pancreatic lesions. *Rev Sci Tech Off Int Epiz* **8:** 765–769, 1989.

Platt, H. The localization of lesions in experimental foot-and-mouth disease. *Br J Exp Pathol* **41:** 150–159, 1960.

Scott, R. W., Cottral, G. E., and Gailiunas, P. Persistence of foot-and-mouth disease virus in external lesions and saliva of experimentally infected cattle. *Am J Vet Res* **27:** 1531–1536, 1966.

Sutmoller, P., McVicar, J. W., and Cottral, G. E. The epizootiological importance of foot-and-mouth disease carriers. I. Experimentally produced foot-and-mouth disease carriers in susceptible and immune cattle. *Arch Virus* **23:** 227–235, 1968.

Yilma, T. Morphogenesis of vesiculation in foot-and-mouth disease. *Am J Vet Res* **41:** 1537–1542, 1980.

2. Vesicular Stomatitis

Vesicular stomatitis affects horses, cattle, and pigs, and it is transmissible experimentally to a number of laboratory animals, including guinea pigs and mice. The disease is important because it causes a loss in production, especially in dairy herds, and it must be differentiated from foot-and-mouth disease in cattle and pigs. Vesicular stomatitis is the only vesicular disease naturally occurring in horses. Sheep and goats do not appear to be susceptible to the disease. Several wildlife species such as white-tailed deer, raccoons, and feral swine are susceptible to vesicular stomatitis. In humans, the virus may cause an inapparent infection or a mild influenzalike condition.

The virus of vesicular stomatitis belongs to the Rhabdoviridae, genus *Vesiculovirus*. It is an enveloped single-stranded RNA virus, rod-shaped, and about 80 × 120 nm. Apart from being inactivated by pasteurization temperatures, it shares qualities of resistance with the aphthoviruses. There are two serologically and immunologically distinct types of virus based on epitopes of the surface glycoproteins. The more common and more virulent New Jersey serotype has only one strain. The Indiana serotype has three strains. There is variation in virulence for different species between serotypes and strains within serotypes. The New Jersey serotype is responsible for most major epizootics, and swine are less commonly involved than are cattle and horses in these outbreaks. In contrast to foot-and-mouth disease, animals infected with vesicular stomatitis virus do not appear to become chronic carriers.

Vesicular stomatitis is enzootic in Central and South America and occurs sporadically elsewhere in the Americas. It has a seasonal occurrence, outbreaks occurring in the warmer seasons and ceasing usually with the onset of cold weather, although one major epizootic in the western United States continued to spread during the winter months. The seasonal nature of the disease suggests that it is transmitted by insects; however, insect transmission is not essential. The virus has been isolated from both biting and nonbiting insects. Biting insects most likely become infected from feeding on lesions rather than blood, since the viremic phase appears to be short-lived. Nonbiting insects act as mechanical carriers of the virus. It is not known how the virus spreads from one geographic area to another. The New Jersey serotype extends farthest north into more temperate zones, and subclinical infection with this serotype is enzootic in certain areas of the southern United States. The intact mucosa is resistant to infection, but abrasions in a susceptible site readily result in infection when contaminated with saliva or exudate from a lesion. Environmental factors that increase the chance of causing abrasions to the skin, teats, or oral mucosa may predispose to infection. Examples are arthropod bites; coarse, hard feed; rough feed troughs; rough flooring; and poor milking practices. Inter-pen movement of cattle may increase the rate of infection in dairy cattle.

Morbidity in lactating dairy cows may be as high as 100%, although only about 60% of the affected animals drool or froth around the mouth. The lesions of vesicular stomatitis occur mainly on the oral mucosa; occasionally they do occur elsewhere, including on the feet, and in swine, foot lesions are common. This is by no means a dependable feature, and outbreaks of the disease in cattle have been described in which the lesions were predominantly on the teats.

The incubation period following exposure by abrasion is 24–72 hr,and the viremic phase seems to be short-lived, because the virus cannot be cultured from blood. Secondary lesions are rare. In cattle, intramuscular injections will not initiate the disease, a useful distinguishing feature from foot and mouth disease. After experimental infection of swine, infectious viral particles can be recovered from a wide variety of tissues within 6 hr post-infection, including salivary gland, tonsils, snout, skin, and lymph nodes. However, infective virus, viral antigens, and nucleic acids cannot be demonstrated 6 days postinfection.

Specific serum-neutralizing antibodies persist for months in swine and years in cattle. There is no evidence that animals with persistent antibodies may act as a source of infection to herd mates. Animals are immune to the homologous but not the heterologous strains of the virus.

The lesions of vesicular stomatitis are indistinguishable from those of foot-and-mouth disease (Fig. 1.73A). Initially, in cattle, there is a raised, flattened, pale pink to blanched papule a few millimeters in diameter in or near the mouth. These papules rapidly become inflamed and hyperemic. In the course of a day or so, they develop into vesicles 2–3 cm in diameter, and by coalescence may involve large areas. The shallow erosions which follow rupture of vesicles heal within 1–2 weeks unless secondary infections occur; in the mouth, the latter are common. Oral lesions heal rapidly in swine, but coronary band lesions often become secondarily infected to the point where the claw may separate and slough. Serous rhinitis, with the development of tags of necrotic mucosa, has been described in experimentally infected swine.

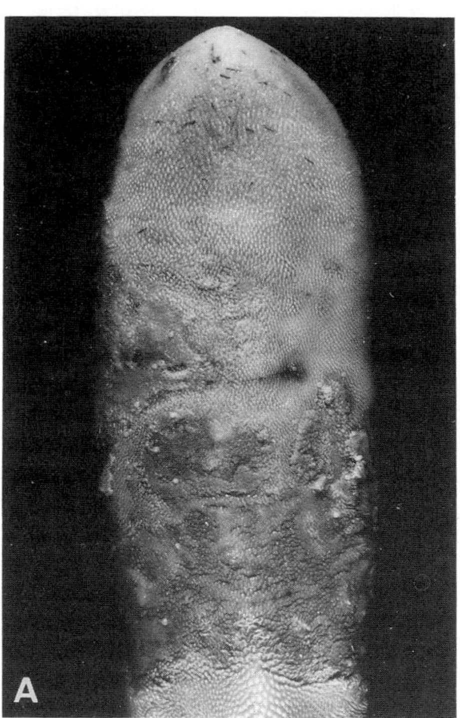

Fig. 1.73A Vesicular stomatitis. Erosion of vesicular lesions in tongue at 4 days postinoculation. (Courtesy of H. R. Seibold and the *American Journal of Veterinary Research*.)

The first microscopic changes are seen in the deeper layers of the stratum spinosum, where the virus replicates. Increasing prominence of the intercellular spaces and stretching of the desmosomes is accompanied by a reduction in volume of the cell cytoplasm (Fig. 1.73B). This dissociation of cells proceeds to distinct intercellular edema (spongiosis) followed by further cytoplasmic retraction until the affected epithelial cells float freely in enlarging vacuoles, which in turn are loculated by strands of cytoplasmic debris (Fig. 1.74). There is no hydropic degeneration of the epithelial cells, and the nuclei until now remain normal. There are no inclusion bodies. With the onset of epithelial cell necrosis there is a pleocellular inflammatory reaction in the mucosa and underlying lamina propria. Electron-microscopic examination of epithelial cells adjacent to the vesicles confirms the intercellular edema and keratinocyte necrosis seen under the light mi-

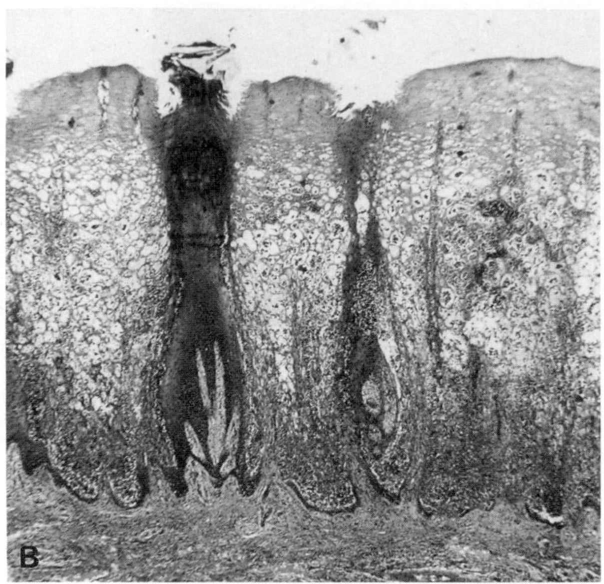

Fig. 1.73B Vesicular stomatitis. Intraepithelial vesicle formation in vesicular stomatitis. (Courtesy of H. R. Seibold and the *American Journal of Veterinary Research.*)

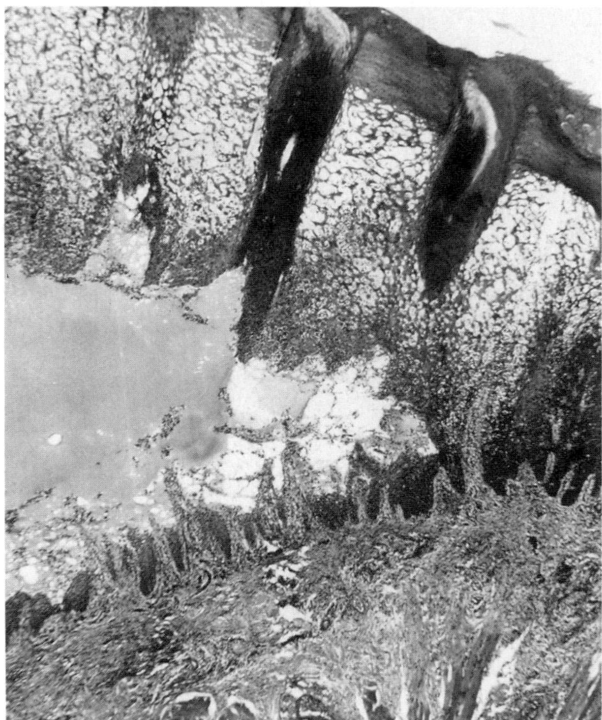

Fig. 1.74 Vesicular stomatitis. Edge of gross vesicle. (Courtesy of H. R. Seibold and the *American Journal of Veterinary Research.*)

croscope. The microscopic appearance of the lesions is not diagnostic.

Virions bud from the cytoplasmic membrane and are located in the dilated intercellular spaces. From there they infect adjacent epithelial cells. There is marked reduplication of desmosomes, and normal desmosomes are evident in the cytoplasm. These appear to be due to endocytosis of plasma membranes or adjacent damaged epithelial cells, and formation of desmosomes on invaginations of plasma membranes with subsequent migration into the cytoplasm of keratinocytes.

The severity of vesicular stomatitis in swine approximates that of foot-and-mouth disease, but in other species it tends to be milder. In light of its similarity to other vesicular diseases in cattle and swine, laboratory confirmation of vesicular stomatitis is essential. Vesicular fluid and mucosa from the tongue are good sources of the virus. Virus isolation in tissue culture or embryonated eggs, fluorescent antibody techniques, complement fixation to identify viral antigen, and inoculation of suckling mice are procedures that are currently used in diagnosis.

Bibliography

Carbrey, E. A. Vesicular stomatitis virus. *In* "Virus Infections of Porcines," M. B. Pensaert (ed.), pp. 211–218. Amsterdam, Elsevier Science Publishers, 1989.

Corn, J. L. *et al.* Isolation of vesicular stomatitis virus New Jersey serotype from phlebotomine sand flies in Georgia. *Am J Trop Med Hyg* **42:** 476–482, 1990.

Erickson, G. A. *et al.* Vesicular stomatitis in swine: Pathogenicity of an epizootic bovine strain versus an enzootic swine strain. *Proc Annu Mtg US Anim Health Assoc* **87:** 543–549, 1989.

Fenner, F. *et al.* Vesicular stomatitis. *In* "Veterinary Virology," pp. 541–544. Orlando, Florida, Academic Press, 1987.

Francy, D. B. *et al.* Epizoötic vesicular stomatitis in Colorado, 1982: Isolation of virus from insects collected along the Northern Colorado Rocky Mountain Front Range. *J Med Entomol* **25:** 343–347, 1988.

Hanson, R. P. Vesicular stomatitis: Introduction and overview. *In* "Proceedings of an International Conference on Vesicular Stomatitis," J. Mason (ed.), pp. 347-361. Mexico–U.S. Commission for the Prevention of Foot-and-Mouth Disease, Mexico City, 1986.

Proctor, S. J., and Sherman, K. C. Ultrastructural changes in bovine lingual epithelium with vesicular stomatitis virus. *Vet Pathol* **12:** 362–377, 1975.

Redelman, D. *et al.* Experimental vesicular stomatitis virus infection of swine: Extent of infection and immunological response. *Vet Immunol Immunopathol* **20:** 345–361, 1989.

Siebold, H. R., and Sharp, J. B. A revised concept of the tongue lesions in cattle with vesicular stomatitis. *Am J Vet Res* **21:** 35–51, 1960.

Thurmond, M. C. *et al.* Vesicular stomatitis virus (New Jersey strain) infection in two California dairy herds: An epidemiologic study. *J Am Vet Med Assoc* **191:** 965–970, 1987.

Van Der Maaten, M. J. Attempts to identify sites of vesicular stomatitis virus persistence in cattle and swine. *In* "Proceedings of an International Conference on Vesicular Stomatitis," pp. 347–361. Mexico–U.S. Commission for the Prevention of Foot-and-Mouth Disease, Mexico City, 1986.

3. Vesicular Exanthema

Vesicular exanthema is an acute, febrile disease of swine that is characterized by formation of vesicles on the snout, mouth, nonhaired skin and feet. It was first diagnosed in California in the 1930s and eventually spread to most swine-producing states in the United States of America. There was one outbreak of the disease in Iceland in 1955. The last reported outbreak of vesicular exanthema was in New Jersey in 1956.

The virus which causes vesicular exanthema belongs to the Caliciviridae, genus *Calicivirus*. It has a single-stranded RNA genome and has only one major polypeptide. It is about 35–40 nm in diameter, and characteristic cup-shaped structures (calyces) are evident in electron-microscopic preparations. There are 13 immunologically distinct serotypes, which vary in virulence.

In 1973, a virus which is biophysically and morphologically similar to vesicular exanthema virus was recovered from sea lions (*Zalophus californianus*) with vesicles on their flippers, off the coast of California near San Miguel Island. Several strains of this virus, called San Miguel sea lion virus, produce milder but otherwise identical lesions to those of vesicular exanthema when inoculated into swine. It has been suggested that the different serotypes of swine vesicular exanthema virus and San Miguel sea lion virus represent immunological variants of a single calicivirus agent whose natural reservoir resides in the ocean (Pacific basin). The host range of San Miguel sea lion virus is very broad. It includes marine and terrestrial mammals, amphibians, reptiles, ocean fish, and insects. One serotype, SMSV-7, has been isolated from opal-eye fish (*Girella nigricans*), and it produces lesions identical to vesicular exanthema when inoculated into swine, with horizontal transmission to contact swine. It is now thought that opal-eye fish are the primary host of the calicivirus, that may be passed on to pinnipeds and swine. Some serotypes of San Miguel sea lion virus are infective for other domestic species including horses, donkeys, cattle, sheep, dogs, and mink, in addition to swine.

Most outbreaks of vesicular exanthema have been associated with feeding of raw garbage containing pork waste. Therefore, the disease may be transmitted by direct contact and fomites. Spontaneous outbreaks of vesicular exanthema in swine due to San Miguel sea lion virus have not been documented. Vesicular exanthema disappeared with the introduction of a law in the United States requiring the cooking of garbage fed to swine.

After inoculation, there is an incubation period of about 18–72 hr, followed by fever, anorexia, lethargy, and development of vesicles on the snout, lips, tongue, on the mucosa of the oral cavity, and on the sole of the hoof, coronary band, dew claws, and interdigital skin. In some outbreaks, foot lesions are prominent; in others, they are minor. Occasionally, they are present on the teats of nursing sows and on the skin of the metacarpus and metatarsus. Pregnant sows may abort. The vesicles increase in size with time, and 4 days after experimental inoculation, most

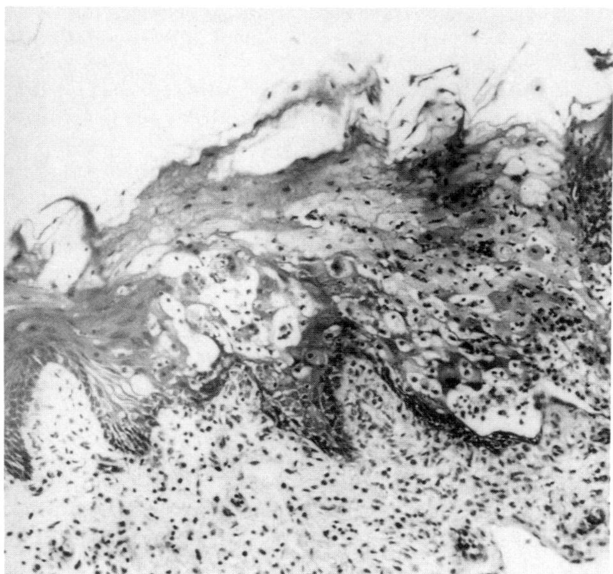

Fig. 1.75 Vesicular exanthema. Margin of vesicle. Pig.

vesicles have ruptured. Erosive and ulcerative lesions that are covered by red-brown crusts are evident until 7 days postinfection. After 10 days most of the lesions on the snout and the tongue have healed, but hooves may separate from the feet at the coronary band, usually the result of secondary bacterial infections, which are common.

In tissue section, numerous widely separated epithelial cells, some of which are shown to contain viral antigen by fluorescent antibody, are in microvesicles within 24 hr after inoculation. When infected cells rupture, adjacent cells become infected. Microvesicles coalesce to form grossly visible vesicles that may contain a few neutrophils and other inflammatory cells (Fig. 1.75). The lesions radiate upward into the skin from the epidermal–dermal junction. Virus replication is limited to the cytoplasm, and virus is released into the environment with rupture of the vesicles. Healing erosions are covered by fibrinocellular exudate, and epithelial cell regeneration progresses from the edges of the lesions. There is a marked perivascular inflammatory cell reaction in the underlying dermis. Viremia appears to occur early after inoculation and is short-lived. The virus may be isolated from several tissues for about 7 days after experimental infection. Mild encephalitis may be seen. There is no evidence that carriers occur. Serum neutralizing antibodies peak in 7–10 days, and animals are immune to the homologous strain of the virus.

The vesicular lesions are indistinguishable from those of vesicular stomatitis, swine vesicular disease, and foot-and-mouth disease.

Bibliography

Barlough, J. E. *et al.* The marine calicivirus story. Parts I & II. *Compend Cont Ed Pract Vet* **8:** F5–F14 and F75–F82, 1986.

Berry, E. S. *et al.* New marine calicivirus serotype infective for swine. *Am J Vet Res* **51:** 1184–1187, 1990.

Edwards, J. F. *et al.* Vesicular exanthema of swine virus: Isolation and serotyping of field samples. *Can J Vet Res* **51:** 358–362, 1987.

Gelberg, H. B., and Lewis, R. M. The pathogenesis of vesicular exanthema of swine virus and San Miguel sea lion virus in swine. *Vet Pathol* **19:** 424–443, 1982.

Gelberg, H. B., Mebus, C. A., and Lewis, R. M. Experimental vesicular exanthema of swine virus and San Miguel sea lion virus infection in phocid seals. *Vet Pathol* **19:** 406–412, 1982.

Gelberg, H. B., Dieterich, R. A., and Lewis, R. M. Vesicular exanthema of swine and San Miguel sea lion virus: Experimental and field studies in otarid seals, feeding trials in swine. *Vet Pathol* **19:** 413–423, 1982.

Madin, S. H. Vesicular exanthema virus. *In* "Virus Infections of Porcines," M.B. Pensaert (ed.), pp. 267–271. Amsterdam, Elsevier Science Publishers, 1989.

4. Swine Vesicular Disease

This is a highly contagious viral disease of pigs, which is characterized by formation of vesicles around the coronary bands and heels of the feet, and to a lesser extent on the mouth, lips, tongue, and teats.

The disease was first recognized in Italy in 1966, and it has since been reported from Hong Kong, the United Kingdom, continental Europe, and Asia. The economic importance of swine vesicular disease is related to losses in production and the fact that it is difficult to differentiate from other vesicular diseases in swine, including foot-and-mouth disease.

The cause of swine vesicular disease is a small RNA virus which belongs to the Picornaviridae, genus *Enterovirus*. It may be a porcine strain of human Coxsackie B5 enterovirus and occasionally infects humans, but not other domestic species. Swine vesicular disease virus is highly resistant to environmental factors. Unlike foot-and-mouth disease virus, it is not inactivated at the low pH in muscle commonly associated with rigor mortis.

Most outbreaks of swine vesicular disease appear to originate by feeding raw garbage containing pork products. Transmission within affected herds is by direct contact, especially during the early stages of the disease. The portal of entry is through damaged epithelium, and this is most likely to occur on the feet and to a lesser extent in the oral cavity. The tonsils and lower gastrointestinal tract may be routes of entry, but only when infective doses are high. Virus replicates at the site of entry and from there disperses via the lymphatics into the circulation. Viremia lasts for 2–3 days. Fluorescent studies and virus isolation have shown that swine vesicular disease virus has a strong affinity for the epithelial cells of the coronary band, tongue, snout, lips, lymphoid follicles of the tonsils, myocardial cells, and brain. Virus titers in tissue decrease with the appearance of circulating antibodies, which peak after 2–3 weeks and apparently persist for years. Secretions and excretions have high viral titers for a period of 12–14 days. Feces may contain virus as long as 3 months, but titers are apparently not sufficiently high to transmit disease. Carriers have been reported by some investigators but not by others; however, lesions may remain infective for a considerable time.

Clinically, vesicles are most common on the feet. Oral lesions occur only in about 10% of affected pigs. The foot lesions appear first at the junction between the heel and the coronary band. Initially, there is a 5.0 mm wide, pale, swollen area that encircles the digit. A dark red to brown zone 2–3 mm wide surrounds the pale zone on both sides. In later stages a 1.0 cm wide band of necrotic skin is located along the coronet. Well-demarcated areas of necrosis, resembling superficial abrasions, extend to the metacarpus, metatarsus, and interdigital cleft. Vesicles on the mouth, lips, and tongue occur in clusters, and they are small, ~2.0 mm in diameter, white, and opaque. They coalesce and rupture within 36 hr and may be covered by a pseudodiphtheritic membrane due to secondary bacterial infections. Affected pigs usually recover in 2–3 weeks.

The development of vesicles tends to follow a similar course as that reported for foot-and-mouth disease. The virus infects individual epithelial cells in the stratum spinosum, which leads to focal areas of keratinocyte degeneration and vesicle formation. Frequently, the necrosis involves the entire thickness of the epithelium including the basal layer. There is an intense leukocytic reaction in the necrotic areas, which is mainly neutrophilic. Spongiosis is less prominent in swine vesicular disease, compared to vesicular stomatitis, although this depends to some extent on the location of the vesicle. Intra- and intercellular edema may be extensive in the snout lesions.

After 1 week there are indications of epithelial regeneration. These consist of an increase in mitotic figures, and long, flat epithelial cells at the periphery of the erosion. In contrast to lesions of foot-and-mouth disease, which tend to heal in an orderly fashion, in swine vesicular disease, long cords of epithelial cells proliferate parallel and perpendicular to the skin surface. A moderate mononuclear cell reaction and fibroplasia may be evident in the underlying dermis. Necrosis and inflammation involve the external root sheath of hair follicles and the subepithelial glands, especially of the mouth.

The early lesions in the tonsils are characterized by degeneration of the squamous epithelial cells, which are replaced by large droplets of foamy basophilic, PAS-positive material. The tonsillar crypts are plugged with exudate. Similar changes are found in the inter- and intralobular collecting ducts of the salivary glands and pancreas. There is degeneration and hypertrophy of the renal pelvic epithelium. Foci of necrosis with a mild interstitial mononuclear cell reaction may be found in the myocardium. There is necrosis and depletion of lymphocytes in most lymphoid tissues.

Nervous signs and lesions have been reported in field outbreaks and reproduced experimentally in swine vesicular disease. The characteristic lesions are those of a nonsuppurative meningoencephalitis involving most areas in the brain. Some reports indicate that the lesions are more severe in the brain stem. Others indicate that the olfactory lobes have the first and most consistent and severe lesions, suggesting that in some cases this may be the site of entry of the virus into the brain from the mucosal epithelial cells of the ethmoid conchae. This hypothesis is further supported by the finding of a large amount of virus in nasal swabs. Nonviral, intranuclear, amphophilic inclusion bodies may be found in the capsule cells of the trigeminal and dorsal root ganglia.

Bibliography

Baker, K. B. Swine vesicular disease. *Vet Ann* **22:** 135–139, 1982.
Chu, R. M., Moore, D. M., and Conroy, J. D. Experimental swine vesicular disease; pathology and immunofluorescence studies. *Can J Comp Med* **43:** 29–38, 1979.
Hedger, R. S., and Mann, J. A. Swine vesicular disease virus. *In* "Virus Infections of Porcines," M. B. Pensaert (ed.), pp. 241–250. Amsterdam, Elsevier Science Publishers, 1987.
Lai, S.S. *et al.* Pathogenesis of swine vesicular disease in pigs. *Am J Vet Res* **40:** 463–468, 1979.
Lenghaus, C., and Mann, J. A. General pathology of experimental swine vesicular disease. *Vet Pathol* **13:** 186–196, 1976.
Lenghaus, C. *et al.* Neuropathology of experimental swine vesicular disease in pigs. *Res Vet Sci* **21:** 19–27, 1976.
Mann, J. A., and Hutchings, G. H. Swine vesicular disease: Pathways of infection. *J Hyg* **84:** 355–363, 1980.

5. *Bovine Virus Diarrhea–Mucosal Disease*

Virus diarrhea, as originally described in New York State in 1946, is an acute, highly contagious disease, which is rarely fatal, characterized by fever, diarrhea, mucosal lesions, and leukopenia.

Mucosal disease was described in 1953 in the United States of America as a disease with a morbidity of 2–50%, which was almost uniformly fatal. It was characterized by an initial febrile reaction, mucoid nasal discharge, anorexia, constant or intermittent watery diarrhea with feces often containing blood, rapid dehydration, and death. Erosions, ulcerations, and hemorrhages were always found in the alimentary canal.

For many years, the severe fatal syndrome of mucosal disease had seldom, if ever, been reproduced experimentally. An advance in the understanding of the pathogenesis of mucosal disease came with the discovery that transplacental infection of the fetus by a noncytopathic biotype of bovine virus diarrhea (NCP-BVD), during the first 4 months of gestation, may result in a persistently infected, specifically immunotolerant carrier animal. These animals may develop fatal mucosal disease when superinfected with an antigenically closely related cytopathic (CP-BVD) strain of the virus.

Infection with bovine virus diarrhea virus results in a spectrum of signs which are compatible with both clinical syndromes, that is, virus diarrhea and mucosal disease. The causative agent of bovine virus diarrhea–mucosal disease is a small, enveloped RNA virus, of the genus *Pestivirus*. Other antigenically and biologically related pestiviruses are hog cholera (classical swine fever virus) in pigs and Border disease virus in sheep. It has been suggested that a collective generic name be given to all three of these viruses. There is only one serotype of BVD virus, but strain variants are detectable by cross-neutralization and monoclonal antibody panels.

Noncytopathic and cytopathic biotypes of BVD virus are recognized, based on their behavior *in vitro,* with considerable significance in the pathogenesis of disease in infected animals. Another notable difference between the two biotypes is the ability of CP-BVD virus to synthesize an 80-kDa polypeptide that is absent in cells infected with NCP-BVD virus. This protein is apparently closely related to a 120-kDa polypeptide that is present in both biotypes. Glycoprotein analysis has identified different strains of virus that have marked heterogeneity in each biotype.

The virus is worldwide in distribution, and in some countries it is considered the most important virus infection of cattle. Other countries report a low seroprevalence. In addition to cattle, BVD virus naturally infects a variety of species, including pigs, sheep, goats, and several wild ruminants or those kept in zoos or on game farms. Most of these infections are subclinical, except for Border disease in sheep, and sporadic outbreaks in swine and captive wild ruminants. Subclinical infections in swine are of particular concern, especially in countries free of hog cholera, since they may interfere with the serologic diagnosis of the latter. There is limited evidence in diarrheic humans of infection with a pestivirus that is serologically related to BVD virus.

Transmission appears to be by direct contact with infected cattle, other infected species, or possibly fomites. There is little information on the survival of BVD virus in the environment, but hog cholera virus can survive in manure for about 2 weeks. The NCP-BVD virus has been transmitted, under experimental conditions, from a persistently infected animal to healthy BVD seronegative animals by blood-feeding flies (*Stomoxys calcitrans* and *Haematopota pluvialis*). The virus is present in a wide variety of excretions, secretions, body fluids, and tissues, including nasal excretions, saliva, urine, feces, semen, vaginal discharges, blood, amniotic fluid, and placenta. The virus titer in feces is usually low except in animals with mucosal disease. Aerosol transmission of the virus has been documented experimentally, and the portal of entry is likely to be the oronasal mucosa.

Primary replication occurs in the tonsil, especially the cryptal epithelial cells, and the oropharyngeal lymphoid tissues. Virus is taken up and transported by phagocytic cells to the draining lymph nodes. The final outcome of the infection depends on the strain and virulence of the infecting virus, the immune status of the host, whether or not the animal is pregnant, and the stage of pregnancy.

a. Bovine Virus Diarrhea Infection of immunocompetent, seronegative, nonpregnant animals usually results in subclinical infection. The animals develop a slight fever, leukopenia, and specific neutralizing antibodies. Of BVD virus infections, 70-90% apparently follow this course. In a small percentage of episodes, animals, mainly older than 6 months, develop a more severe infection, with a high morbidity and low mortality. The infecting agent is usually a NCP-BVD virus, but may be a cytopathic strain. After an incubation period of 5–7 days, the affected animals develop a fever, leukopenia, and viremia, which may persist as long as 15 days. The virus is present in leukocytes (buffy coat), especially lymphocytes and monocytes, and in serum. There is a transient decrease in the number of B and T lymphocytes and a decline in responsiveness to mitogen stimulation.

Clinically, the disease is characterized by lethargy, anorexia, mild oculonasal discharge, and occasional mild oral erosions and shallow ulcers. Diarrhea may occur. In dairy herds there is a transient drop in milk production. Affected animals develop neutralizing antibodies which peak in 10–12 weeks and persist for life. Continual antigenic stimulation may be due to noninfectious viral antigens that persist in lymphoid tissues.

This condition is referred to as **acute bovine virus diarrhea.** Whether or not this type of infection may, under certain circumstances, be associated with severe clinical disease remains controversial; it is likely that the relationships of this virus to the several hosts is still evolving. Experimental primary infection with some strains of CP- and NCP-BVD virus produces clinical disease similar to the more severe form of acute bovine virus diarrhea reported under natural conditions. Infection with some NCP-BVD viruses may produce a syndrome of thrombocytopenia and hemorrhage, discussed later.

b. Persistent Infection The epidemiology of the virus depends on persistent infections of the host, which is the outcome of transplacental infection of the fetus. Transplacental infection may occur during the viremic phase of acute bovine virus diarrhea in immunocompetent seronegative cows, or in persistently infected animals. Contaminated fetal calf serum in embryo transfer fluids, and modified live virus vaccine administered during pregnancy may also result in fetal infection. It apparently rarely occurs in seropositive animals. The outcome of fetal infection is primarily dependent on the stage of gestation. The most serious consequences occur if a NCP-BVD virus crosses the placental barrier during the first 4 months of gestation. It may result in fetal resorption, mummification, abortion, or a persistently infected calf. If the calf survives, it remains viremic for life, and it is also immunotolerant to the homologous strain of the infecting NCP-BVD virus. Immunotolerance develops because of failure of the immature fetal immune system to recognize the NCP-BVD virus antigens as nonself or foreign.

Persistently infected calves may be clinically normal, weak, or undersized at birth. They may remain normal, but often become unthrifty. The prevalence of these calves in a herd is usually less than 2%, but this figure may become as high as 25–30% in those herds in which a large number of naive cows, in the first 4 months of pregnancy, are exposed to NCP-BVD virus. Most of the persistently infected calves succumb to mucosal disease, usually between the ages of 6 months and 2 years. The offspring of the few animals that reach sexual maturity and become pregnant are also persistently infected. This may result in chronically infected families. These animals are viremic and constant shedders of NCP-BVD virus, acting as the most important source of virus to other susceptible animals and the environment.

In persistently infected animals, viral antigen is demonstrable in a wide variety of tissues, but the amount of virus is less than in cases of mucosal disease.

Lesions in persistently infected animals are minimal and subclinical, in spite of the widespread infection of tissues.

c. Mucosal Disease Persistently infected, NCP-BVD-viremic immunotolerant seronegative animals, exposed to a CP-BVD virus that is antigenically similar to the noncytopathic biotype, usually develop fatal mucosal disease. This phenomenon is referred to as superinfection, and it seems to be unique in virology. The origin of the superinfecting cytopathic biotypes in natural mucosal disease remains unclear. They may originate from mutation or recombination of NCP strains. This concept is further supported by the finding of considerable antigenic similarity, based on monoclonal antibody analyses, between pairs of CP and NCP biotypes isolated from fatal cases of mucosal disease. Recombination between viral and host cell RNA has recently been proposed as a model for the pathogenesis of mucosal disease. In this model the NCP-BVD virus mutates to a cytopathic biotype by taking up coding sequences, especially for ubiquitin, from the host cell. The superinfecting cytopathic biotype may also originate from other animals in the herd, or other animal sources mentioned earlier.

Some persistently infected animals that develop neutralizing antibodies to a superinfecting heterologous cytopathic strain may develop mucosal disease long after the challenge. There is some preliminary evidence to suggest that the interval between superinfection with the cytopathic biotype and the onset and duration of mucosal disease may be related to the degree of antigenic similarity between the pair of infecting biotypes. This interval appears to be shorter, and the disease more acute, when the pair of infecting biotypes are antigenically similar. When the cytopathic super-infecting strain is less closely related to the NCP virus, chronic mucosal disease may ensue. Complete heterology between the pair of biotypes usually does not cause disease.

As to the pathogenesis of mucosal disease, the following mechanisms have been proposed, based on the distribution of viral antigens and lesions. Many tissues may be infected; however, the distribution and titer of virus infection in mucosal disease are typically greater than those for persistent infections. Circulating precursor cells of macrophages take up virus from the mucosal cells in the respiratory tract and tonsils, and transport it intracellularly to the lymphoid tissues and to the subepithelial connective tissues of the dermis and the gastrointestinal tract, whence it spreads to overlying epithelial cells. Specific immunotolerance in the NCP-BVD virus-infected animal may allow a closely related cytopathic biotype to freely infect, replicate, and destroy cells. The chronic effects of the NCP virus on the cells may also enhance the replication of the superinfecting cytopathic virus.

Mucosal disease is almost invariably fatal. Whereas deaths may occur within a few days of illness, and almost always within 2 weeks, some cases remain clinically affected for months. The incubation period after experimental infection with a CP strain in an animal persistently infected with a NCP-BVD is usually 7–14 days, but may be considerably longer, depending on the degree of homology between the pair of viruses and probably other factors mentioned earlier. The morbidity under natural conditions is usually <5% but may be as high as 30%.

Acute fulminant mucosal disease closely resembles rinderpest. The onset is febrile, with serous to mucoid nasal discharge. Discrete oral lesions are preceded by an acute stomatitis and pharyngitis, the mucosae being hyperemic and pink and covered by a thin gray film of catarrhal exudate. White necrotic foci 1–2 mm in size surrounded by a margin of hyperemia then appear on the muzzle and the buccal mucosa. These erode or ulcerate and expand irregularly; the margins remain fairly discrete except for those on the soft palate and pharyngeal mucosa. There is severe diarrhea and tenesmus with feces containing little or no blood or mucus. Affected animals become lethargic, anorexic, and dehydrated; they have ptyalism, polypnea, and tachycardia, and may die quickly.

In chronic mucosal disease the development of the oral lesions is like that found in acute cases; however, by the time chronic cases die there is usually some evidence of healing. The watery diarrhea of the early phase gradually gives way to feces that are passed frequently, are scant in volume, and contain a large proportion of mucus flecked with blood. Late in the clinical course, there is lethargy, emaciation, ruminal stasis, and frequent attempts at defecation accompanied by severe tenesmus. Interdigital dermatitis, coronitis, and laminitis affecting all four feet may be present in chronically affected animals (Fig. 1.76A), resulting in lameness. In these too, the skin is dry and scurfy, especially over the neck, withers, back, perineal and preputial areas, and vulva, whereas that on the medial aspect of the thighs and forelegs becomes moist and discolored a dirty yellow.

At necropsy, the gross lesions of mucosal disease vary considerably, especially in acute cases, in which either upper alimentary or intestinal lesions may be absent, and less so in the chronic disease, in which a broader pathologic picture is often present, perhaps partially obscured by healing or evolution of lesions.

Crusts, erosions, and shallow ulcers are present on the muzzle and nares of many affected cattle. The anterior edges of the lower lip and its cutaneous junction are similarly affected. A similar loss of epithelium from much of the oral cavity is common. Diffuse hyperemia of the mucosa may persist after death. The most conspicuous oral erosions are on the palate, on the tips of the buccal papillae (Fig. 1.76B) and on the gingiva. Many, especially on the papillae and in the pharynx, are ulcers and expose a de-

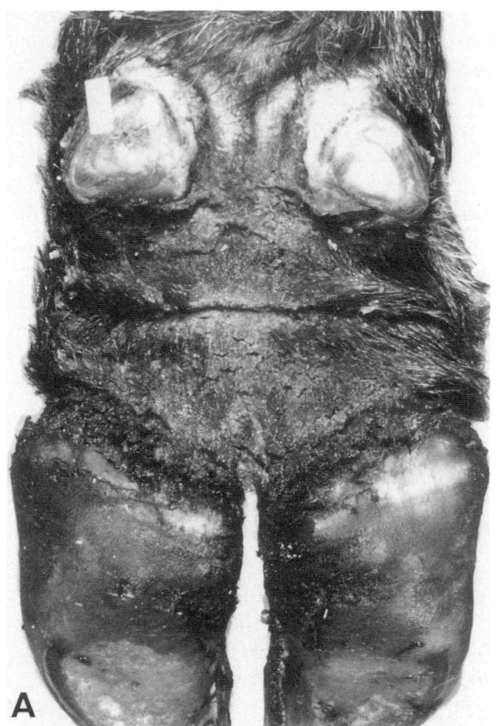

Fig. 1.76A Mucosal disease. Coronitis and erosive–ulcerative dermatitis of pastern.

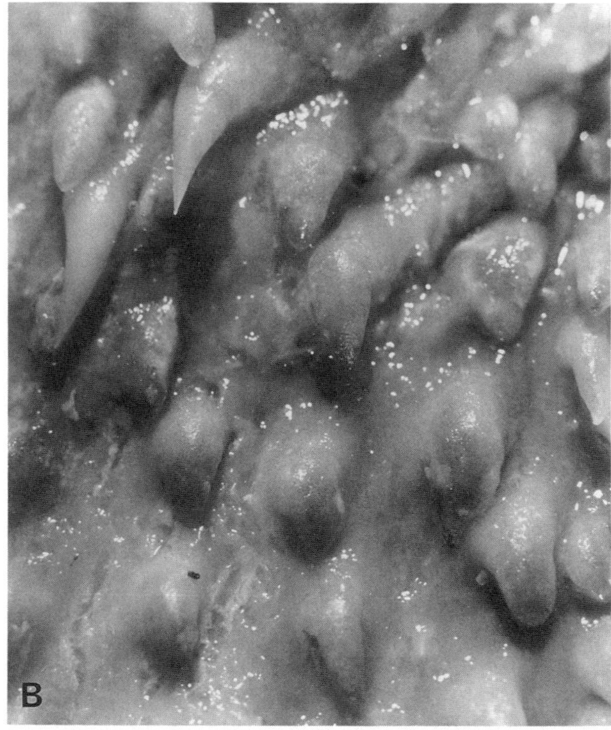

Fig. 1.76B Mucosal disease. Blunting of papillae on the buccal mucosa due to necrosis induced by virus infection. A few remaining normal papillae are long with sharp points.

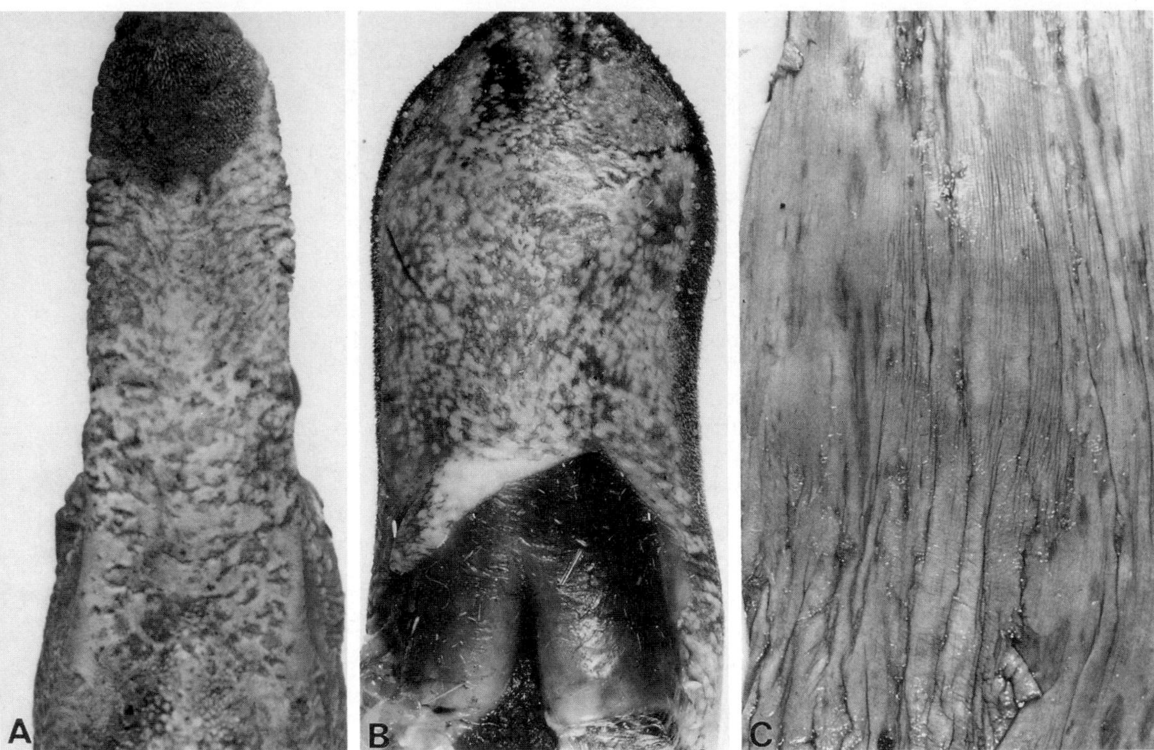

Fig. 1.77 Mucosal disease. (A) Dorsal surface of tongue showing multiple confluent ulcers. (B) Elevated surface of tongue showing multiple confluent ulcers. (C) Longitudinal erosions and ulcers on the esophagus.

nuded, intensely hyperemic lamina propria. The tongue is not always affected. When present, lesions may be evident on all surfaces (Fig. 1.77A,B). Those on the smooth lateral surfaces are typically erosive and irregular, although in some early cases the degenerate epithelium may remain attached, to form flat white plaques, which may be scraped off. On the anterior half of the dorsum, the degenerate epithelium may accumulate and develop deep irregular crevices and pits, or ulcerate to denude the greater portion of the surface.

In some cases the oral lesions are sharp, punched-out ulcers. These occur on the dental pad, palate, ventral and lateral surfaces of the tongue, the gums about the incisors, and the inside of the cheeks and pharynx. In some lesions of longer duration, the defect is being filled in from the margin by thickened white proliferative epithelium.

Esophageal lesions are usually present. They are common in the upper third of the esophagus. In some acute cases, the lesions are shallow erosions, rather than ulcers. The erosions are more or less linear but otherwise irregular, have a dirty brown base, and little or no reactive hyperemia (Fig. 1.77C). Shreds of adherent, necrotic epithelium give the surface a rough, worn, tattered appearance in animals which have not been swallowing. In more advanced cases, discrete ulcerations occur. In many chronically affected animals, the ulcers are beginning to heal and have yellowish-white, slightly elevated plaques of proliferative epithelium at the periphery of the mucosal defect.

Lesions are found in the ruminoreticulum and omasum, but not in the esophageal groove. The ruminal content in chronically affected animals with prolonged anorexia is usually scant and dry. The surface of the ingesta is frequently blackened, and the villi of the ruminal wall are thick, black, and dry. In most acute cases the ruminal content is unusually liquid and putrid. The lesions on the wall of the rumen resemble those present elsewhere in the upper alimentary tract and, although they occur anywhere, they are best seen on the pillars and other smooth or nonvillous portions of the mucosa (Fig. 1.78). The omasal lesions are most numerous along the edges of the leaves, sometimes causing a scalloped margin or perforation.

The morphogenesis of the lesions in the squamous mucosa of the upper alimentary tract begins with necrosis of the epithelium (Fig. 1.79). Individual cells and groups of cells deep in the epithelium are eosinophilic and swollen, with pyknotic nuclei. These foci enlarge progressively and form areas of necrosis which extend to, and may involve, the basal layer. In the early stages there is little or no inflammation of the lamina propria, but leukocytes infiltrate the necrotic epithelium. These small necrotic foci are elevated above the surface and form the pale, friable plaques described earlier on the squamous mucosae. They enlarge progressively and by coalescence, and may form small cleavage vesicles along the proprial–epithelial junction (Fig. 1.80A). If the necrotic epithelium is abraded, erosions and ulcers develop.

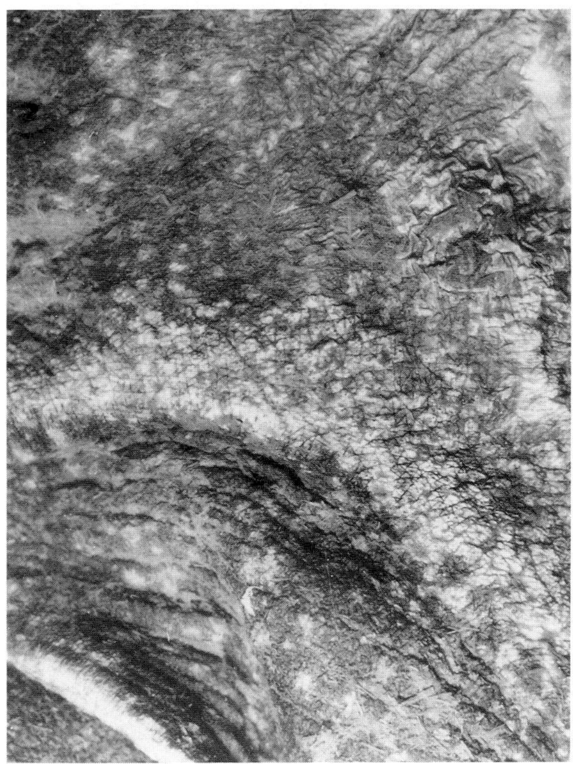

Fig. 1.78 Mucosal disease. Focal and confluent often preulcerative, plaquelike lesions on mucosa of dorsal sac of rumen.

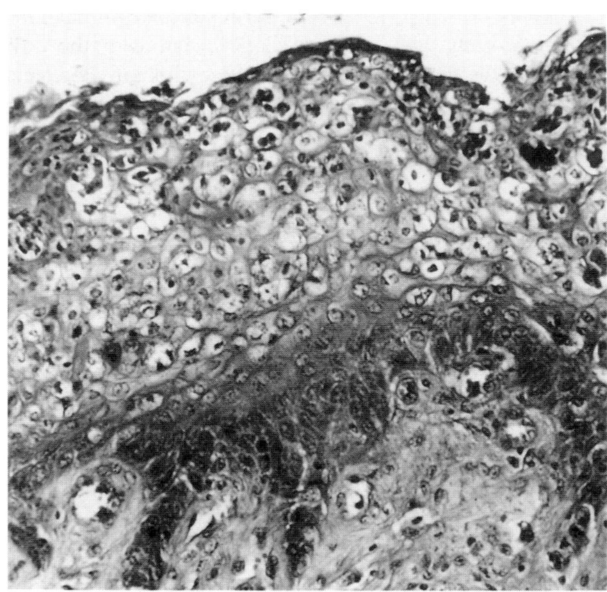

Fig. 1.79 Mucosal disease. Histologic appearance of early esophageal lesion.

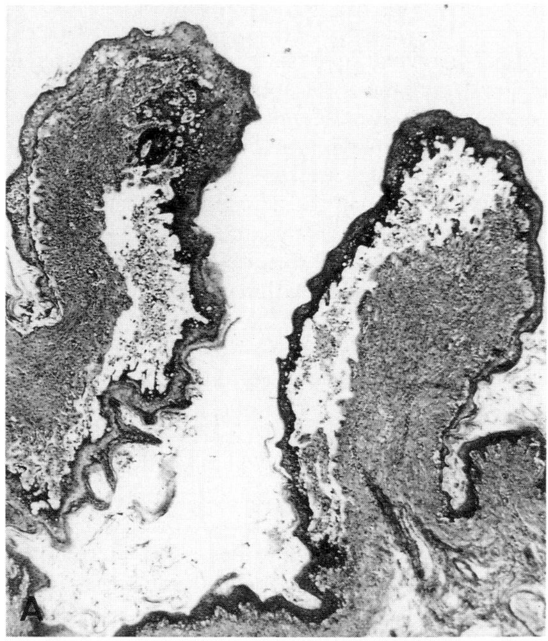

Fig. 1.80A Mucosal disease. Cleavage vesicles in rumen papillae.

The ulcerations of the squamous epithelium of the upper alimentary tract are accompanied by inflammation in the lamina propria, especially where this forms papillae (Fig. 1.80B). Capillaries are congested, the lymphatics are dilated, there is edema of the stroma, and a pleocellular in-

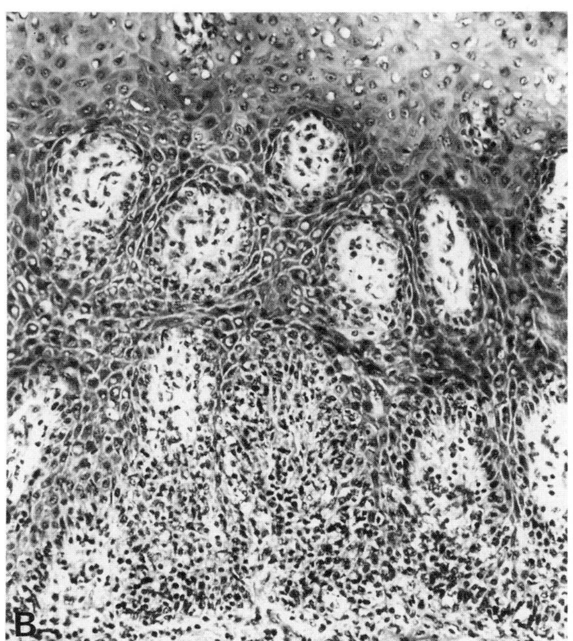

Fig. 1.80B Mucosal disease. Early lesion. Edema of proprial papillae, acute focal inflammation of papilla and propria. There is necrosis of scattered cells deep in the epithelium.

flammatory infiltrate is present. Focal hemorrhages may occur.

Changes are regularly present in the abomasum. The sides of the rugae bear what appear grossly to be ulcers, which may be punctate to 1 cm or more in diameter (Fig. 1.81). They are lesions with raised margins and a distinct pale halo; there may also be some peripheral hemorrhage. The histologic changes in the glandular epithelium of the abomasum are characterized by epithelial necrosis, mainly in the depths of the glands. The necrotic cells fragment and slough, and may cause dilation of affected glands. The mucosa is locally infiltrated by a variety of leukocytes, and is edematous. In some affected foci the glandular epithelium loses its differentiated appearance, becoming cuboidal, basophilic, and apparently mucus-secretory. These glands too may be dilated with a small quantity of contained epithelial and leukocytic debris. In some abomasa, mucous metaplasia may be patchy but widespread and may reflect inflammation in the mucosa. There is some edema, hemorrhage, and modest leukocytic infiltration of the submucosa. Some necrotic foci in the abomasal glands appear to be associated with necrosis of adjacent mucosal lymphoid follicles.

The mucosa of the small intestine often appears normal over much of its length. There may be inspissated mucoid material in the lumen. In some cases the mucosa of the small intestine may have patchy or diffuse congestion. In rare cases fibrin casts may be in the lumen of the small bowel. The wall is atonic but not dilated and may be greatly thickened by submucosal and subserosal edema, which may give a ground-glass appearance to the serosal surface, especially in the cecum and proximal colon.

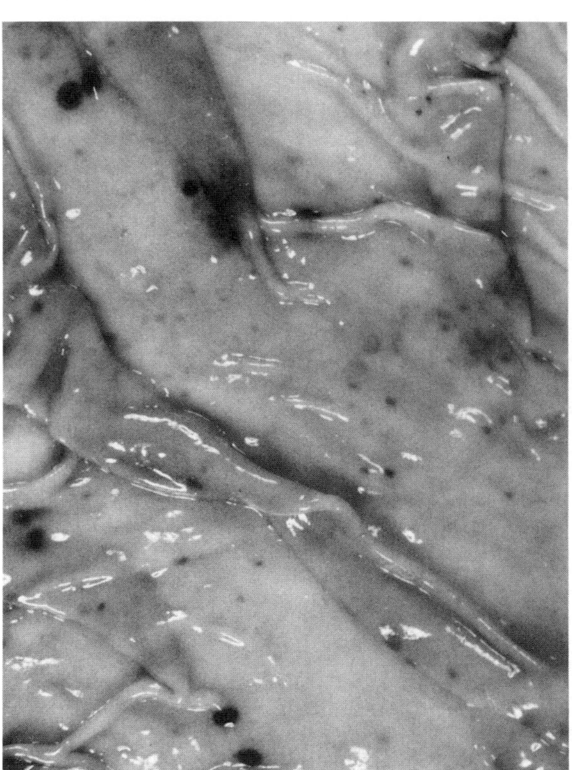

Fig. 1.81 Mucosal disease. Hemorrhage and ulceration. Abomasum.

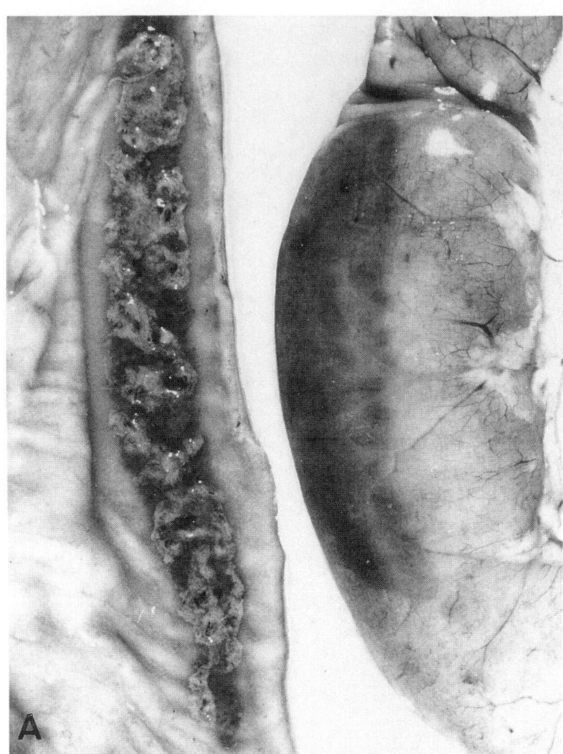

Fig. 1.82A Mucosal disease. Fibrinohemorrhagic exudate over Peyer's patch in the ileum (left). Deep red Peyer's patch visible through serosa of small intestine (right).

In acute cases, it is usual to find coagulated blood and fibrin overlying and outlining Peyer's patches, the covering of which is eroded. This, when present, is a very distinctive lesion that is paralleled only in rinderpest. Severely affected Peyer's patches are often obvious through the serosa as red-black oval areas as long as 10–12 cm on the antimesenteric border of the gut (Fig. 1.82A). Less acutely affected Peyer's patches may be overlain by a diphtheritic membrane, whereas in milder or more chronic cases, the patches may be depressed and covered by tenacious mucus. In chronic cases exudate may not be evident over Peyer's patches, which become less obvious or sunken, resembling an ulcer. Mesenteric lymph nodes may or may not be enlarged.

Lesions in the large bowel are highly variable. The mucosa may be congested, often in a tiger-stripe pattern following the colonic folds. In acute cases there may be fibrinohemorrhagic typhlocolitis (Fig. 1.82B). In more chronic cases, fibrinous or fibronecrotic lesions and focal or extensive ulceration may be present at any level of the large bowel, but particularly in the cecum and rectum.

The characteristic microscopic lesion in the intestinal mucosa is destruction of the epithelial lining of the crypts

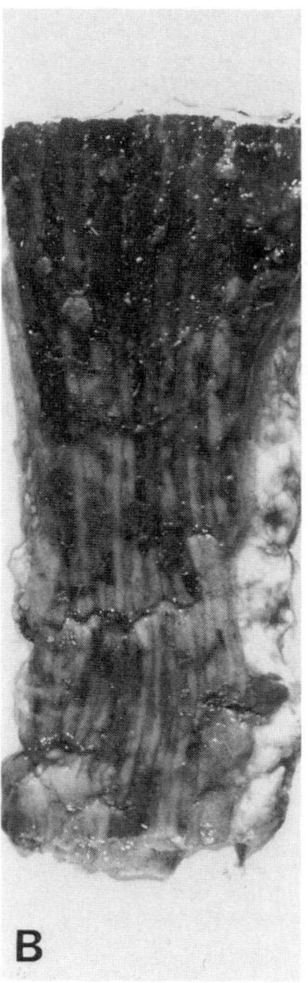

Fig. 1.82B Mucosal disease. Fibrinohemorrhagic colitis.

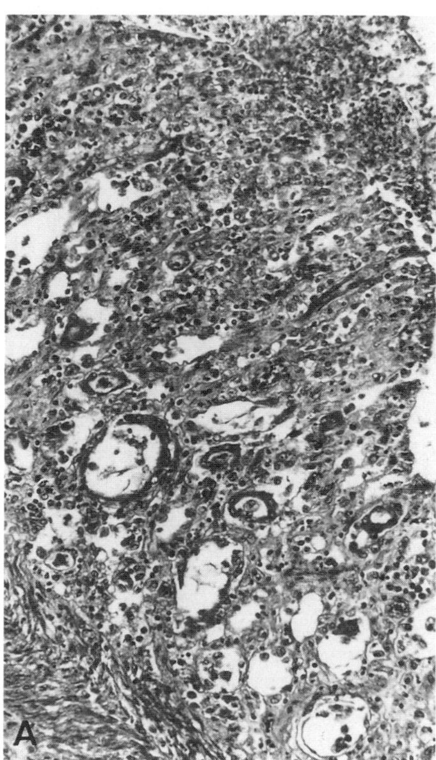

Fig. 1.83A Mucosal disease. Colon. Dilated and denuded glands, collapse of lamina propria and pseudomembrane formation.

of Lieberkühn. In the duodenum, a few crypts only are affected, but more crypts are affected more severely in the lower reaches of the small intestine and in the cecum and colon. Affected crypts are dilated and filled with mucus, epithelial debris, and leukocytes. Remaining crypt-lining cells are attenuated in an attempt to cover the basement membrane. Reparative hyperplasia of crypt lining is rarely encountered. Crypt drop-out may be evident microscopically. In the cecum and colon extensive damage to crypts and attendant collapse of the lamina propria is the probable cause of ulceration seen grossly (Fig. 1.83A). Congestion of mucosal capillaries, and in acute or ulcerated cases, effusion of fibrin and neutrophils from the mucosal surface may be evident. Macrophages predominate among the mainly mononuclear inflammatory cell reaction in the lamina propria, which is particularly prominent in chronic cases of mucosal disease.

The microscopic lesions of Peyer's patches are distinctive in bovine virus diarrhea, comparable lesions being caused only by rinderpest. In the acute phase of the disease severe acute inflammation in the mucosa over Peyer's patches accompanies almost complete destruction of the underlying glands, collapse of the lamina propria, and lysis of the follicular lymphoid tissues. The NCP biotype has a particular tropism for the gutassociated lymphoid tissues, and sequential studies have shown that this virus homes to the Peyer's patches. Later in the course of the disease, dilated crypts, lined, at least in part, by cuboidal epithelium and filled with necrotic epithelial cells, mucus, and inflammatory cells appear to herniate into the submucosal space previously occupied by involuted lymphoid follicles (Fig. 1.83B). Peyer's patches should be sought assiduously at autopsy since their gross and microscopic appearance may provide useful evidence for diagnosis.

An important microscopic lesion, which may have been previously overlooked, is hyaline degeneration and fibrinoid necrosis of submucosal and mesenteric arterioles (Fig. 1.84A). A mild to moderate mononuclear inflammatory cell reaction is frequently present in the walls of the vessels and in perivascular areas. The vascular lesions are not limited to the intestine, but may be present in a variety of other organs such as the heart, brain, and adrenal cortices, which may make it difficult to differentiate the disease from malignant catarrhal fever. The vascular lesions in acute mucosal disease are less consistently present and usually are milder. Multiple foci of lymphocytes, plasma cells, and eosinophils may be found in the adrenal and renal cortices, portal triads of the liver, and gallbladder submucosa. Cytoplasmic vacuolation of the ganglion cells of the myenteric plexus may be seen.

In the acute disease, the lymph nodes of the head and neck are often enlarged and discolored reddish black by congestion and hemorrhage. Microscopically the mesenteric and sometimes other lymph nodes show a diminished population of lymphocytes and necrosis of germinal cen-

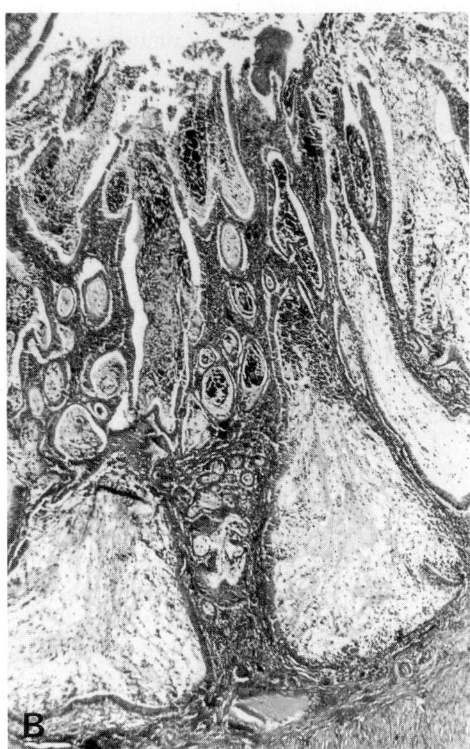

Fig. 1.83B Mucosal disease. Herniation of crypts of Lieberkühn into the submucosa replacing necrotic lymphoid follicles in Peyer's patch. Mucus and inflammatory exudate are in the cystic glands and on the surface of the mucosa.

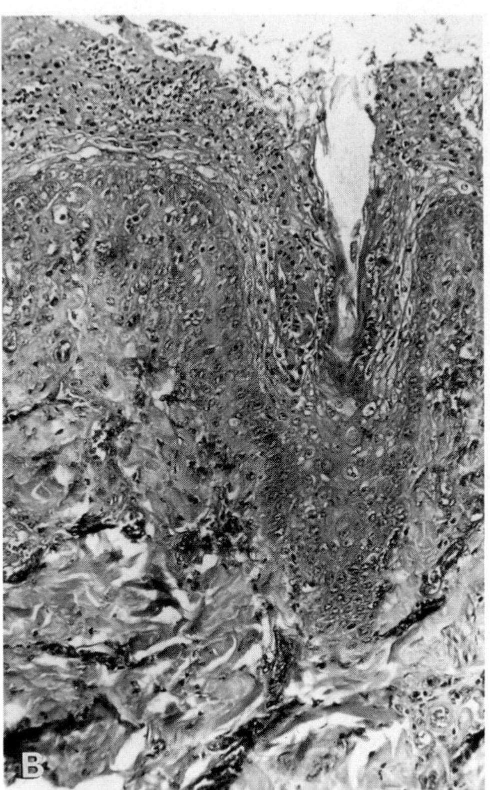

Fig. 1.84B Mucosal disease. Skin. Superficial epidermal necrosis extending into hair follicle. Hyperplasia, stratum germinativum.

ters. Similar lesions may be seen in the splenic lymphoid follicles, but they are not consistent and are difficult to interpret. There is marked thymic atrophy.

Coronitis may extend completely around the coronary band with some separation of the skin–horn junction causing disturbance and overgrowth of the horn (Fig. 1.76). Dermatitis may extend from the coronet up the back of the pastern. Milder dermatitis is generalized, with scurfiness

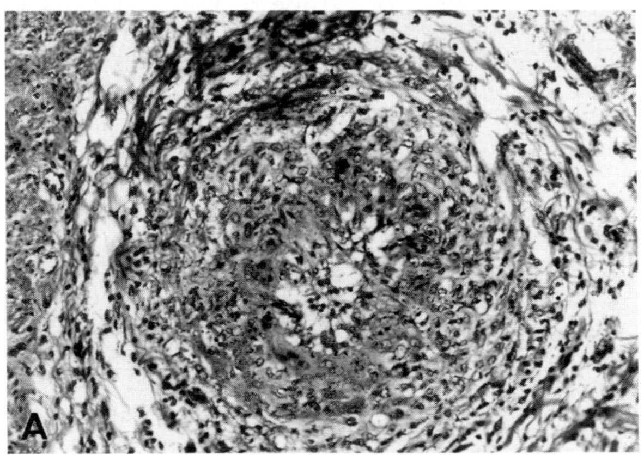

Fig. 1.84A Mucosal disease. Fibrinoid necrosis and mild periarteritis of a mesenteric arteriole, colon.

especially from the ears to the withers. In sections of the skin of animals with chronic mucosal disease, there is hyper- and parakeratosis with focal accumulations of necrotic epithelium with intense hyperemia of the adjacent superficial dermis. The epithelial lesions are basically similar to those in the squamous mucosa of the upper alimentary tract (Fig. 1.84B). Necrosis often extends deeply to or through the basal layers; it results in minute erosions or ulcerations. There is massive infiltration of macrophages, Langerhans-type cells, and some lymphocytes in the underlying dermis. These deeper lesions occur in the inner aspects of the legs and the perineum, and there is an exudation of serum in these areas. The overlying degenerate epithelium becomes disorderly and eventually is lifted off.

Some animals with chronic disease develop mycotic infections secondary to lesions in the forestomachs, abomasum, and Peyer's patches. The lesions are areas of hemorrhagic necrosis involving the mucosa, submucosa, and sometimes deeper layers of the wall. Fungal hyphae are found invading the stroma and causing thrombosis in venules.

d. Bovine Virus Diarrhea and Secondary Infections Bovine virus diarrhea infection suppresses interferon production, impairs lymphocyte function, monocyte proliferation and chemotaxis, humoral antibody production, neutrophil function, and bacterial clearance. These changes are transient in acute bovine diarrhea, but more persistent in chronically infected animals and in animals with mucosal disease. The failure of immunogenic response may be associated with immunotolerance, or destruction of immunocompetent cells, which is reflected in lymphopenia. In addition to a lack of humoral antibody response, there is also depression of cell-mediated immunity as indicated by a poor response of cultured peripheral lymphocytes to various mitogens. The impairment of polymorphonuclear cell function in cattle infected with BVD virus may explain in part the observation that such cattle appear to be more susceptible to secondary bacterial infections. Persistently infected cattle seem to have acceptable serum concentrations of immunoglobulins, though significant reductions in IgG have been reported in some persistently infected animals, and in animals with mucosal disease.

The exact mechanisms and consequences of impaired peripheral leukocyte function on immune responsiveness are still poorly understood. Many reports suggest that the virus enhances or potentiates the pathogenesis of both bacterial and viral infections. Mixed infections of BVD virus and infectious bovine rhinotracheitis, malignant catarrhal fever, rinderpest, bovine leukemia viruses, bovine papular stomatitis, bovine respiratory syncytial virus, bovine rota- and coronaviruses, *P. haemolytica, Salmonella* infections, and possibly Johne's disease, have been reported. The viruses may vary in their pneumopathogenicity. Experimental infections have shown that some cytopathic strains produce more severe lung lesions when inoculated with *P. haemolytica* than do noncytopathic strains.

e. Bovine Virus Diarrhea-Induced Thrombocytopenia Severe thrombocytopenia with extensive hemorrhage has been reported in primary BVD infection in calves, and rarely in adults, associated with certain strains of NCP-BVD virus. The disease has been reproduced experimentally. It is characterized by fever, severe thrombocytopenia, leukopenia, anemia, and diarrhea. There are extensive hemorrhages in the subcutis, oral mucosa, and most serosal surfaces. The hemorrhages tend to be massive on the serosa of the small intestine and mesentery. Characteristic lesions of mucosal disease in the upper and lower alimentary tract are not seen. Platelet counts may be $<5000/\mu l$ 3–11 days postinfection, and the thrombocytopenia may persist for 6 weeks. Animals may die of anemia associated with hemorrhage. Destruction and/or sequestration of thrombocytes may be due to the direct effect of the virus, which may be recovered from the platelets. Immunoglobulins are not bound to infected platelets, so immune-mediated thrombocytopenia is unlikely. The thrombocytopenia in swine infected with the antigenically related hog cholera virus probably has a similar mechanism. Platelets increase in number, corresponding to a rise in serum neutralizing antibodies, in calves that recover.

f. Teratogenic Effects of Bovine Virus Diarrhea Infections of seronegative immunocompetent dams during gestation (usually between 90 and 120 days) may result in a wide spectrum of teratogenic lesions, including microencephaly, cerebellar hypoplasia and dysgenesis, hydranencephaly, hydrocephalus, and defective myelination of the spinal cord. Ocular lesions such as microphthalmia, cataracts, retinal degeneration, atrophy, and dysplasia, and optic neuritis have all been associated with fetal infections by the virus (see The Nervous System, Volume 1, Chapter 3; The Eye and Ear, Volume 1, Chapter 4; and The Female Genital System, Volume 3, Chapter 4). Infections of the immunocompetent calf, usually after 135 days of gestation, result in antibody production that is detectable in precolostral serum samples of the newborn calf.

Alimentary tract lesions of the disease may be observed in the fetus. Punctate hemorrhages with ulcers 1–3 mm in diameter may be profuse in the oral cavity, excepting the dorsum of the tongue, and in the esophagus, larynx, trachea, conjunctiva, and abomasum. The fetal lesions of squamous epithelium evolve in somewhat the same manner as to those described earlier, with focal hemorrhages in the lamina propria and epithelial necrosis beginning in the basal layer.

Bibliography

Bielefeldt Ohmann, H. BVD virus antigens in tissues of persistently viraemic, clinically normal cattle: Implications for the pathogenesis of clinically fatal disease. *Acta Vet Scand* **29:** 77–84, 1988.

Bielefeldt Ohmann, H. *In situ* characterization of mononuclear leukocytes in skin and digestive tract of persistently bovine viral diarrhea virus-infected clinically healthy calves and calves with mucosal disease. *Vet Pathol* **25:** 304–309, 1988.

Bistner, S. I., Rubin, L. F., and Saunders, L. Z. The ocular lesions of bovine viral diarrhea—mucosal disease. *Pathol Vet* **7:** 275–286, 1970.

Bolin, S. R., McClurkin, A. W., and Coria, M. F. Effects of bovine viral diarrhea virus on the percentages and absolute numbers of circulating B and T lymphocytes in cattle. *Am J Vet Res* **46:** 884–886, 1985.

Bolin, S. R. *et al.* Severe clinical disease induced in cattle persistently infected with noncytopathic bovine viral diarrhea virus by superinfection with cytopathic bovine viral diarrhea virus. *Am J Vet Res* **46:** 573–576, 1985.

Bolin, S. R. *et al.* Response of cattle persistently infected with noncytopathic bovine viral diarrhea virus to vaccination for bovine viral diarrhea and to subsequent challenge exposure with cytopathic bovine viral diarrhea virus. *Am J Vet Res* **46:** 2467–2470, 1985.

Bolin, S. R., Matthews, P. J., and Ridpath, J. F. Methods for detection and frequency of contamination of fetal calf serum with bovine viral diarrhea virus and antibodies against bovine viral diarrhea virus. *J Vet Diagn Invest* **3:** 199–203, 1991.

Brock, K. V. Bovine viral diarrhea virus. *In* "Viral Diarrheas of Man and Animals," L. J. Saif and K. W. Theil (eds.), pp. 263–276. Boca Raton, Florida, CRC Press, 1990.

Brownlie, J. Pathogenesis of mucosal disease and molecular aspects of bovine virus diarrhoea virus. *Vet Microbiol* **23:** 371–382, 1990.

Brownlie, J., and Clarke, M. C. (eds.). Bovine virus diarrhea. *Rev Sci Tech Off Int Epiz* **9:** 13–229, 1990.

Castrucci, G. *et al.* A study of some pathogenetic aspects of bovine viral diarrhea virus infection. *Comp Immun Microbiol Infect Dis* **13:** 41–49, 1990.

Corapi, W. V. *et al.* Thrombocytopenia and hemorrhages in veal calves infected with bovine viral diarrhea virus. *J Am Vet Med Assoc* **196:** 590–596, 1990.

Cutlip, R. C., McClurkin, A. W., and Coria, M. F. Lesions in clinically healthy cattle persistently infected with the virus of bovine viral diarrhea—glomerulonephritis and encephalitis. *Am J Vet Res* **41:** 1938–1941, 1980.

Donis, R. O., and Dubovi, E. J. Differences in virus-induced polypeptides in cells infected by cytopathic and noncytopathic biotypes of bovine virus diarrhea–mucosal disease virus. *Virology* **158:** 168–173, 1987.

Hewicker, M. *et al.* Kidney lesions in cattle persistently infected with bovine viral diarrhoea virus. *J Vet Med B* **34:** 1–12, 1987.

Hewicker, M. *et al.* Immunohistological detection of bovine viral diarrhoea virus antigen in the central nervous system of persistently infected cattle using monoclonal antibodies. *Vet Microbiol* **23:** 203–210, 1990.

Kirkland, P. D. *et al.* Replication of bovine viral diarrhoea virus in the bovine reproductive tract and excretion of virus in semen during acute and chronic infections. *Vet Rec* **128:** 587–590, 1991.

Lambert, G., McClurkin, A. W., and Fernelius, A. L. Bovine viral diarrhea in the neonatal calf. *J Am Vet Med Assoc* **164:** 287–289, 1974.

Larsson, B. Increased suppressor cell activity in cattle persistently infected with bovine virus diarrhoea virus. *J Vet Med (B)* **35:** 271–279, 1988.

Liess, B. Bovine viral diarrhea virus. *In* "Virus Infections of Ruminants," Z. Dinter and B. Morien (eds.), pp. 247–266. Amsterdam, Elsevier Science Publishers, 1990.

Liess, B. *et al.* Embryotransfer und BVD-Virusinfektion bei Rindern. *Dtsch Tierärztl Wschr* **94:** 506–508, 1987.

Meyers, G. *et al.* Viral cytopathogenicity correlated with integration of ubiquitin-coding sequences. *Virology* **180:** 602–616, 1991.

Moennig, V. *et al.* Reproduction of mucosal disease with cytopathogenic bovine viral diarrhoea virus selected *in vitro*. *Vet Rec* **127:** 200–203, 1990.

Roberts, D. H. *et al.* Response of cattle persistently infected with bovine virus diarrhoea virus to bovine leukosis virus. *Vet Rec* **122:** 293–296, 1988.

Roeder, P. L., Jeffrey, M., and Cranwell, M. P. Pestivirus fetopathogenicity in cattle: Changing sequelae with fetal maturation. *Vet Rec* **118:** 44–48, 1986.

Roth, J. A., Bolin, S. R., and Frank, D. E. Lymphocyte blastogenesis and neutrophil function in cattle persistently infected with bovine viral diarrhea virus. *Am J Vet Res* **47:** 1139–1141, 1986.

Tarry, D. W., Bernal, L., and Edwards, S. Transmission of bovine virus diarrhoea virus by blood-feeding flies. *Vet Rec* **128:** 82–84, 1991.

Thoen, C. O., and Waite, K. J. Some immune responses in cattle exposed to *Mycobacterium paratuberculosis* after injection with modified-live bovine viral diarrhea virus vaccine. *J Vet Diagn Invest* **2:** 176–179, 1990.

Wilhelmsen, C. L. *et al.* Experimental primary postnatal bovine viral diarrhea viral infections in six-month-old calves. *Vet Pathol* **27:** 235–243, 1990.

Wilhelmsen, C. L. *et al.* Lesions and localization of viral antigen in tissues of cattle with experimentally induced or naturally acquired mucosal disease, or with naturally acquired chronic bovine viral diarrhea. *Am J Vet Res* **52:** 269–275, 1991.

Xue, W., Blecha, F., and Minocha, H. C. Antigenic variations in bovine viral diarrhea viruses detected by monoclonal antibodies. *J Clin Microbiol* **28:** 1688–1693, 1990.

g. Bovine Virus Diarrhea Virus Infection in Pigs The prevalence of naturally occurring antibodies to BVD virus in swine in different countries varies between 2 and 40%. The antibodies may complicate the diagnosis of hog cholera, especially in those countries considered to be free of this disease. Cattle, and modified live virus vaccines containing contaminated fetal bovine serum, are considered to be common sources of infection for swine. There are sporadic reports of disease associated with BVD virus infection, including stillbirth, and poorly viable piglets, some showing tremors. Some 2- to 4-week-old pigs in infected herds are anemic, have a rough hair coat, growth retardation, wasting, and diarrhea. Affected pigs fail to develop neutralizing antibodies to the infecting homologous BVD virus. Littermates that remain normal develop neutralizing antibodies. The suggestion is that the infections are congenital. Experimental *in utero* BVD virus infection of sows may result in prenatal and perinatal deaths, persistently infected, immunotolerant, or normal pigs. Many of these conditions resemble the effects of *in utero* infection with NCP-BVD virus in cattle.

Macroscopic lesions are characterized by hypertrophy and ulceration of the mucosa, especially of the stomach, cecum, and colon with formation of button ulcers in the latter. Other lesions reported include necrotic tonsillitis, excess fluid in the body cavities, polyserositis, and thymic atrophy. The clinical signs and macroscopic lesions resemble those of chronic hog cholera. Unfortunately, detailed descriptions of the microscopic lesions of the affected pigs are not available.

Bibliography

Carbrey, E. A. *et al.* Natural infection of pigs with bovine viral diarrhea virus and its differential diagnosis from hog cholera. *J Am Vet Med Assoc* **169:** 1217–1219, 1976.

Terpstra, C., and Wensvoort, G. Natural infections of pigs with bovine viral diarrhea virus associated with signs resembling swine fever. *Res Vet Sci* **45:** 137–142, 1988.

Wensvoort, G., and Terpstra, C. Bovine viral diarrhea virus infections in piglets born to sows vaccinated against swine fever with contaminated vaccine. *Res Vet Sci* **45:** 143–148, 1988.

h. Border Disease Border disease is a congenital infection of sheep and goats, usually with a NCP biotype of pestivirus that is antigenically related to BVD virus and hog cholera virus. The disease is characterized by embryonic and fetal death, abortion, mummification, and birth of weak lambs or kids. The affected animals have an abnormal body conformation, long hairs, clonic rhythmic tremors (hairy shakers), unthriftiness and poor viability (see

The Skin and Appendages, Volume 1, Chapter 5; The Nervous System, Volume 1, Chapter 3; and The Female Reproductive System, Volume 3, Chapter 4). The disease was first reported in lambs from border areas between England and Wales.

A syndrome resembling mucosal disease has been reported in lambs that survived the initial Border disease; they were persistently infected with a NCP-BVD virus, and superinfected with a homologous strain of cytopathic virus. The disease has been reproduced experimentally. Clinically the affected sheep develop chronic diarrhea, wasting, nasal discharge, and polypnea. Macroscopic lesions are particularly present in the cecum and colon, and in a few sheep, also the terminal ileum. There is marked thickening of the gut wall due to subserosal and mucosal edema and diffuse polypoid hyperplasia of the mucosa, which is hemorrhagic and focally ulcerated.

The microscopic lesions in the gut are similar to those described for mucosal disease in cattle. Lymphoid cell reactions are evident in the choroid plexus, portal triads of the liver, kidney, myocardium, thyroids, lungs, spleen, and lymph nodes. In addition, some lambs have marked hypertrophy and edema of the muscularis of the terminal ileum. The lesions in the terminal ileum resemble terminal ileitis, and BVD virus should be considered a possible cause of that syndrome.

The pathogenesis of fetal infections, resultant Border disease, and related enteric lesions in sheep, appear to be similar to the multitude of conditions associated with NCP-BVD virus prenatal infections in cattle. Seronegative ewes infected before 80 days of gestation may produce persistently infected, immunotolerant, chronically viremic lambs.

Bibliography

Ames, T. R. *et al.* Border disease in a flock of Minnesota sheep. *J Am Vet Med Assoc* **180:** 619–621, 1982.

Barlow, R. M., Gardiner, A. C., and Nettleton, P. F. The pathology of a spontaneous and experimental mucosal disease-like syndrome in sheep recovered from clinical border disease. *J Comp Pathol* **93:** 451–461, 1983.

Chalmers, G. A., Nation, P. N., and Pritchard, J. Border disease—a cause of terminal ileitis in lambs? *Can Vet J* **31:** 611, 1990.

Kelling, C. L. *et al.* Genetic comparison of ovine and bovine pestiviruses. *Am J Vet Res* **51:** 2019–2024, 1990.

Loken, T., Bjorkas, I., and Hyllseth, B. Border disease in goats in Norway. *Res Vet Sci* **33:** 130–131, 1982.

Niemi, S. M. *et al.* Border disease virus isolation from postpartum ewes. *Am J Vet Res* **43:** 86–88, 1982.

Parsonson, I. M. *et al.* The effects of bovine viral diarrhea–mucosal disease (BVD) virus on the ovine foetus. *Vet Microbiol* **4:** 279–292, 1979.

Plant, J. W., Gard, G. P., and Acland, H. M. A mucosal disease virus infection of the pregnant ewe as a cause of a border diseaselike condition. *Aust Vet J* **52:** 247–249, 1976.

Potts, B. J., Osburn, B. I., and Johnson, K. P. Border disease: Experimental reproduction in sheep, using a virus replicated in tissue culture. *Am J Vet Res* **43:** 1464–1466, 1982.

Terpstra, C. Border disease: A congenital infection of small ruminants. *Prog Vet Microbiol Immun* **1:** 175–198, 1985.

6. Rinderpest

Otherwise known as cattle plague, rinderpest is an acute or subacute, highly contagious disease of cattle, characterized by erosive or hemorrhagic lesions of all mucous membranes. The distribution of the disease is progressively shrinking, but it is still enzootic in tropical Africa, the Middle East, and the Orient, to which places it is restricted by limitations on animal movement and the use of highly efficacious vaccine. Pandemics have occurred in the Middle East, sub-Saharan and equatorial Africa, and some of these were apparently related to a relaxation in vaccination programs.

The virus which causes rinderpest belongs to the Paramyxoviridae, genus *Morbillivirus.* It is a highly pleomorphic, usually spherical but sometimes filamentous, single-stranded RNA virus with a core diameter of 120–300 nm and a spiked envelope. It is antigenically and morphologically closely related to the viruses causing *peste des petits ruminants,* canine distemper, and human measles (rubeola). The four viruses have immunologically identical nucleocapsids and shared envelope antigens. The virus is highly fragile under ordinary environmental conditions; it is incapable of surviving more than a few hours outside the animal body under normal circumstances.

It may be isolated in tissue cultures from a variety of organs from domestic ruminants, including renal or testicular cells, bovine thyroid cells, and pulmonary macrophages. The virus also replicates in primary cell cultures from tissues of infected animals. Once adapted, it grows readily in a large number of cell lines, and on the chorioallantoic membrane of the developing chick embryo. Characteristic cytoplasmic and nuclear inclusions are seen in syncytial cells in tissue culture. The syncytia are probably due to the action of virus-specific fusion protein, rather than abnormal nuclear division. The virus can be adapted to rabbits, although strains differ in the ease with which this is accomplished. Once adapted, the virus causes fever and characteristic grayish-white granular, necrotic patches in the intestinal lymphoid tissue.

Probably all cloven-hoofed animals are naturally susceptible to infection, but the expression of infection varies considerably. Natural infections tend to be milder or subclinical in sheep and are often associated with outbreaks in cattle. Goats are more severely affected than sheep. The disease must be differentiated from *peste des petits ruminants,* in countries where the latter infection is enzootic. Goats and sheep do respond, but inconsistently, to experimental inoculations of rinderpest virus. Infection in Asiatic pigs may be severe, but it tends to be mild in European breeds.

Although different strains of rinderpest virus vary considerably in their pathogenicity, they are grouped in a single serotype and, when suitably modified, make effective vaccines.

Control of the disease in endemic areas is impeded by

difficulties inherent in systems of husbandry and by the coexistence of cattle with large populations of susceptible ungulate wildlife. However, the infection usually flows from domestic to wild species. The lability of the virus is such that the spread of infection from endemic areas is most likely to be by live animals with mild or subclinical disease.

The disease in cattle may be mild, especially in endemic areas, but probably will be acute or peracute and severe in new foci. The different degrees of severity are in part due to real differences in virulence of strains, and largely due to differences in susceptibility of breeds or races of cattle. Such variations are well documented and apply also to modified vaccine strains which, although quite safe in some breeds of cattle, cause high mortality in others.

The nasopharyngeal mucosa appears to be the main portal of entry in rinderpest. The virus localizes and replicates in the palatine tonsils and regional lymph nodes. This is followed after an 8- to 11-day incubation by a 2- to 3-day period of viremia that coincides with the fever seen clinically. In circulation, the virus is located mainly in lymphocytes. After the viremic stage, the virus replicates in all lymphoid tissues, the bone marrow, and the mucosa of the upper respiratory tract and the gastrointestinal tract. Nasal and oral secretions and the feces contain high titers of the virus. In general, excretion of virus ceases by about the ninth day of the clinical disease with the onset of neutralizing antibodies. Recovered animals do not appear to be carriers, although there are reports to the contrary.

Fever and its attendant signs usher in the clinical syndrome, with early leukopenia, probably due to the lymphotropism of the virus. Fever reaches its peak in about 3 days and falls with the onset of diarrhea, which may be bloody. There is severe abdominal pain, anorexia, ocular and nasal discharge, tachypnea, fetid breath, occasional cough, lethargy, severe dehydration and emaciation, and prostration. Death occurs in 6–12 days. Explosive outbreaks with high morbidity and mortality are more likely to occur in naive populations. Vaccinated or recovered animals usually have a life-long immunity, with some exceptions, noted earlier. Naturally infected cattle also have IgA in the mucosa and mucus of the upper respiratory tract. Secondary bacterial, viral, protozoal, and rickettsial infections are common. Synergistic infections of rinderpest and bovine virus diarrhea viruses have been reported.

The gross morbid anatomical changes in rinderpest are characteristic but not pathognomonic, and are similar to mucosal disease (Fig. 1.85A,B). The lesions in the upper alimentary tract are necrotizing and erosive–ulcerative.

The virus of rinderpest has an affinity for the alimentary epithelium, which it gains hematogenously. Oral lesions are not invariably present in cattle and are often absent in sheep and goats. The oral lesions typically involve the inner side of the lower lips, the buccal papillae at the commissures, and the ventral surface of the free portion of the tongue. In severe cases, however, all mucous surfaces of the mouth may be involved (Fig. 1.85A) with the regular exception of the dorsal surface of the tongue. In

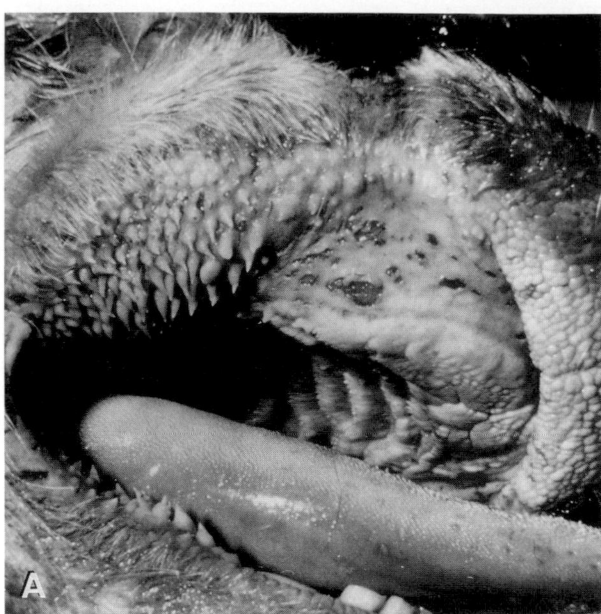

Fig. 1.85A Rinderpest. Ulcers on the buccal mucosa, and small incipient ulcers on the underside of the tongue. Cow. (Courtesy of C. C. Brown, Foreign Animal Disease Diagnostic Laboratory, USDA.

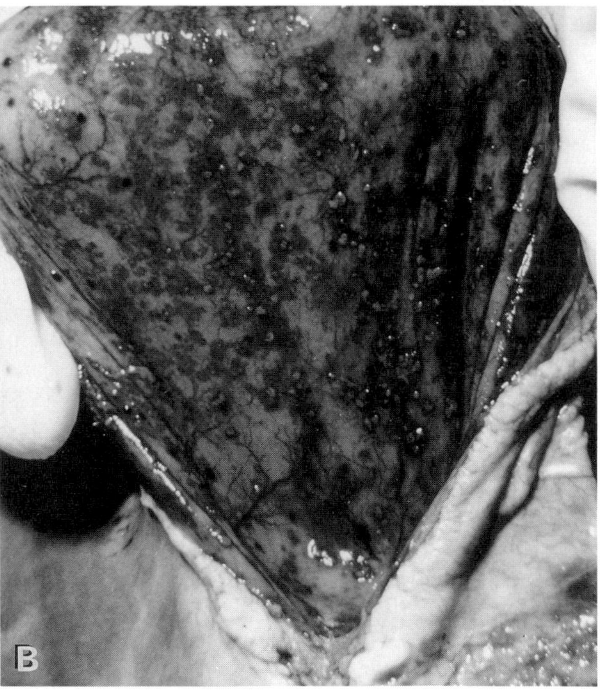

Fig. 1.85B Rinderpest. Multifocal to coalescing fibrinohemorrhagic colitis. Cow. (Courtesy of C. C. Brown, Foreign Animal Disease Diagnostic Laboratory, USDA.)

nonfatal cases there is rapid regeneration of the oral mucosal lesions. Esophageal erosions are usually mild and affect the anterior portion. The forestomachs rarely exhibit any lesions. When they do occur, the omasal leaves are involved.

The lesions of stratified squamous epithelium originate in the basal layer. Many epithelial cells undergo necrosis, the nuclei become pyknotic and fragmented, and the cytoplasm, coagulated and eosinophilic, but true vesicles do not develop. Multinucleate syncytia form in the epithelium (Fig. 1.86A,B,C), and these may have cytoplasmic and nuclear inclusions. The necrotic foci produce, initially, white pinpoint papules. Abrasion causes the necrotic tissue to lift off and produce shallow erosions. This occurs so readily that erosions are usually the first lesions observed. Their margins are sharp, and the bases are reddened by the underlying congested capillaries. The initial minute erosions enlarge and coalesce to form extensive defects. Ulceration may supervene.

The abomasum is usually involved in this disease, its pyloric mucosa most consistently and severely. The lesions of the fundus are linear on the margins of the mucosal folds, and in the pylorus they are more rounded. The mucosa becomes necrotic and grayish in affected foci and then sloughs, leaving sharply marginated irregular erosions, the bases of which are intensely hyperemic and ooze blood. Ulcers sometimes do occur. There usually is profuse submucosal edema, which thickens the fundic plicae.

Lesions in the small intestine are less severe than those elsewhere, but are similar, streaks of congestion and erosion developing on the margins of mucosal folds. They are best developed in the upper duodenum and in the ileum. The ileocecal valve and surrounding cecal mucosa are congested and eroded. The colon and rectum are more severely affected as a rule than the rest of the intestine (Fig. 1.85B). The linear lesions of the mucosal folds are well developed in the large bowel, resulting in a zebra-stripe appearance. Occasionally, the red foci are so numerous as to appear as diffuse hemorrhage, although they are, in reality, severely congested vessels of the lamina propria.

The Peyer's patches and other gastrointestinal lymphoid follicles, especially at the cecocolic junction, become hemorrhagic and necrotic (Fig. 1.87A), and this may be extensive enough to cause necrosis of the overlying mucosa, leaving lesions resembling deep ulcers.

Microscopically, the cryptal epithelium in the small intestine may become necrotic, and syncytia may form in crypts. Associated villi may be somewhat atrophic. Small hemorrhages occur from the intensely congested blood vessels. There is diffuse edema of the submucosa, but little leukocytic infiltration.

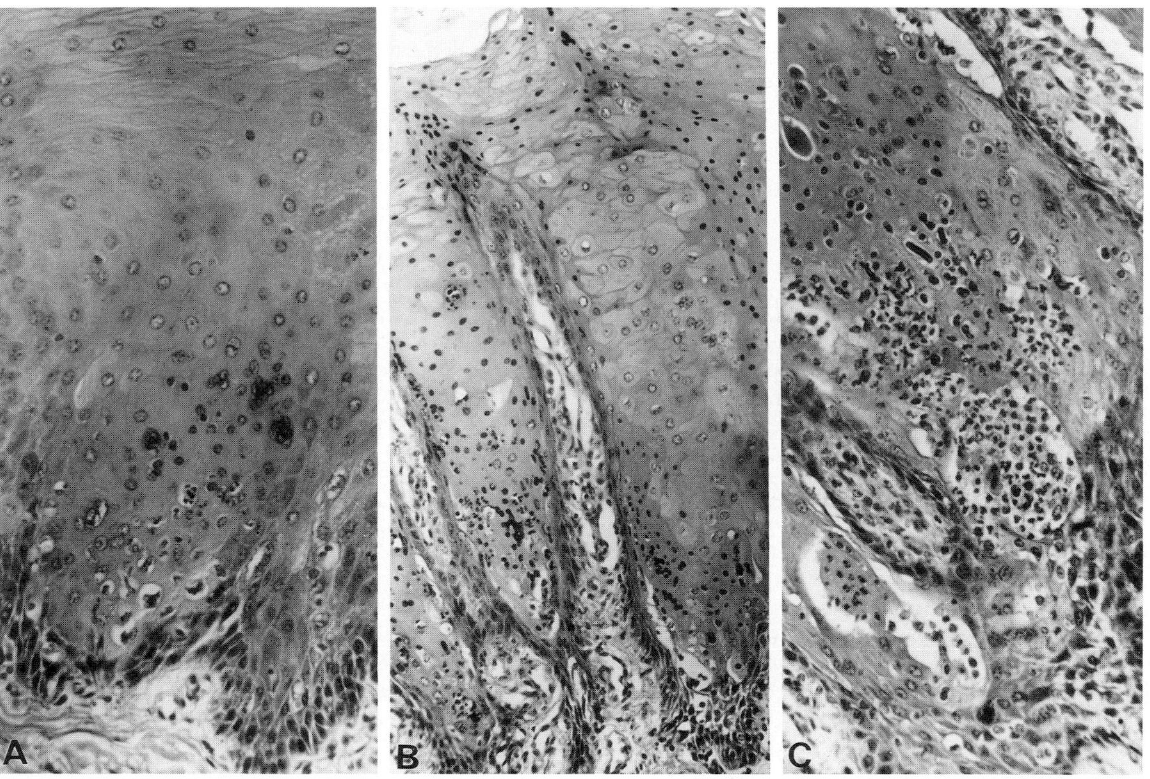

Fig. 1.86 Rinderpest. Ox. A.F.I.P. acc 625840. (A) Early stage of oral lesion showing disorganization of epithelium above the basal layer and formation of syncytial cells. Tongue. (B and C) Slightly later stage of (A) with beginning separation sparing basal cells.

The rinderpest virus is tropic for lymphoid tissues. Necrosis of lymphocytes is extreme, but gross inspection, which reveals little abnormality of nodes, is misleading. There is no hemorrhage or inflammation of lymph nodes, although they may be edematous. The necrosis begins in the germinal centers and proceeds until virtually all mature lymphocytes are lost in individual follicles, leaving only a reticular mesh (Fig. 1.87B). Multinucleate cells, similar to those in the mucosa, form in the lymph and hemolymph nodes. All or only some follicles may be involved, and there is often an increase of other leukocytes in the sinuses. Similar lesions occur in the spleen, tonsils, and as already noted, in the Peyer's patches.

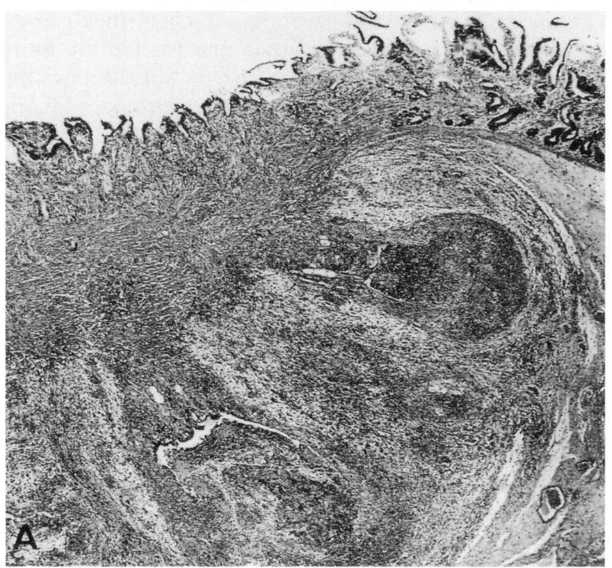

Fig. 1.87A Rinderpest. Ox. A.F.I.P. acc 625840. Necrosis of Peyer's patch. Ileum.

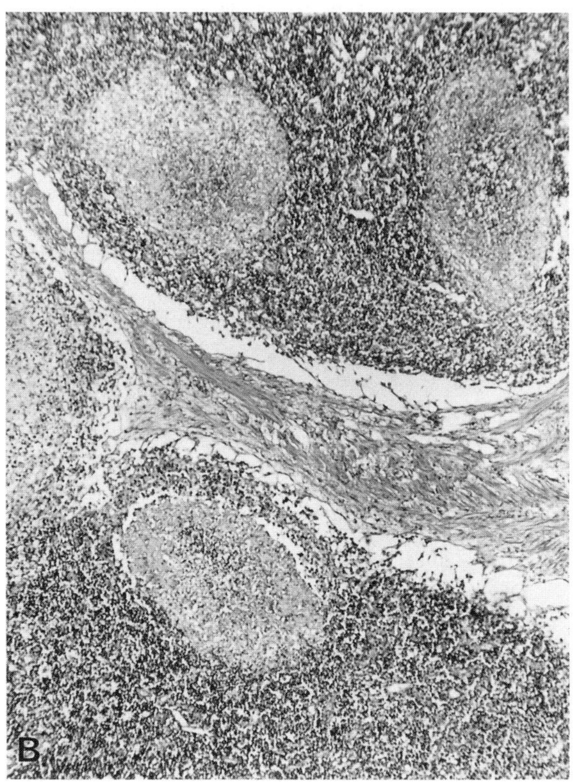

Fig. 1.87B Rinderpest. Ox. A.F.I.P. acc 623162. Necrosis of germinal centers. Lymph node.

Acute congestion and edema of the conjunctiva may be followed by purulent conjunctivitis and corneal ulceration. Petechiae are common in the mucosa of the upper respiratory tract, which is usually covered with mucopurulent exudate. Small erosions may develop on the larynx. Hemorrhages beneath the epicardium and endocardium are common but nonspecific, and there may be mild nonspecific myocardial degeneration. Mild erosive lesions develop in the mucosa of the bladder and vagina. Skin lesions have been described, especially in buffalo, but are considered rare. A moist eczematous lesion of the udder, scrotum, inner aspect of thighs, neck, and flank may develop, in which viral antigen may be demonstrated. Animals with such lesions usually die, but, if recovery occurs, the dried scabs of exudate peel off, removing the superficial epithelium and hair.

Bibliography

Anderson, E. C. *et al.* Observations on the pathogenicity for sheep and goats and the transmissibility of the strain of virus isolated during the rinderpest outbreak in Sri Lanka in 1987. *Vet Microbiol* **21:** 309–318, 1990.

Appel, M. J. G. *et al.* Morbillivirus diseases of animals and man. *In* "Comparative Diagnosis of Viral Diseases," E. Kurstak and C. Kurstak (eds.), Vol. IV, pp. 235–297. New York, Academic Press, 1981.

Liess, B., and Plowright, W. Studies on the pathogenesis of rinderpest in experimental cattle. I. Correlation of clinical signs, viraemia and virus excretion by various routes. *J Hyg (Camb)* **62:** 81–100, 1964.

Maurer, F. D. *et al.* The pathology of rinderpest. *Proc 92nd Annu Mtg Am Vet Med Assoc,* 201–211, 1956.

Plowright, W. Rinderpest. *Vet Rec* **77:** 1431–1438, 1965.

Rossiter, P. B. *et al.* Continuing presence of rinderpest virus as a threat in East Africa, 1983–1985. *Vet Rec* **120:** 59–62, 1987.

Scott, G. R. Rinderpest in the 1980s. *Prog Vet Microbiol Immunol* **1:** 145–174, 1985.

Shanthikumar, S. R., and Atilola, M. A. O. Outbreaks of rinderpest in wild and domestic animals in Nigeria. *Vet Rec* **126:** 306–307, 1990.

7. Peste des Petits Ruminants

This is an acute viral disease of sheep and goats, which closely resembles rinderpest and is also known as kata, stomatitis pneumoenteritis complex, goat plague, and pseudorinderpest. The causative agent is closely related to rinderpest virus, with which it shares common antigenic determinants. The virus cross-reacts with rinderpest virus in the immunodiffusion and complement fixation tests. It may be differentiated from rinderpest virus using monoclonal antibody techniques and complementary DNA (cDNA) probes. *Peste des petits ruminants* (PPR) virus is now considered a fourth member of the *Morbillivirus* genus. The disease was first recognized in West Africa. It is now distributed in sub-Saharan Africa, the Arabian Peninsula, and India. There are strain differences between African and Arabian isolates of the virus, based on neutralization tests and polyacrylamide gel analysis.

The clinical signs, pathogenesis, and lesions of the disease in sheep and goats are similar to those of rinderpest (Fig. 1.88A,B), except that the disease is more acute in onset, especially in goats, and follows a more rapid course. Another difference is the marked involvement of the respiratory tract; affected animals have dyspnea, hyperpnea, and cough. There is also a marked serous to mucopurulent nasal and ocular discharge. The macroscopic pulmonary lesions are characterized by consolidation, atelectasis, and dark red discoloration of the anteroventral lobes. Some animals have a fibrinous pleuritis (see The Respiratory System, Chapter 6 of this volume). Microscopically, there is a mild multifocal tracheitis, bronchitis, necrotizing bronchiolitis, and diffuse proliferative interstitial pneumonia, with formation of alveolar syncytial cells. Cytoplasmic and nuclear eosinophilic inclusions are present in the epithelial cells of the air passages, type II pneumocytes, and syncytial cells. Viral antigen may be demonstrated in the same cells with appropriate immunohistochemical techniques. The primary viral lesions are often complicated by secondary bacterial infections. The pulmonary lesions of PPR are similar to pneumonia due to distemper virus in dogs and measles virus infections in humans.

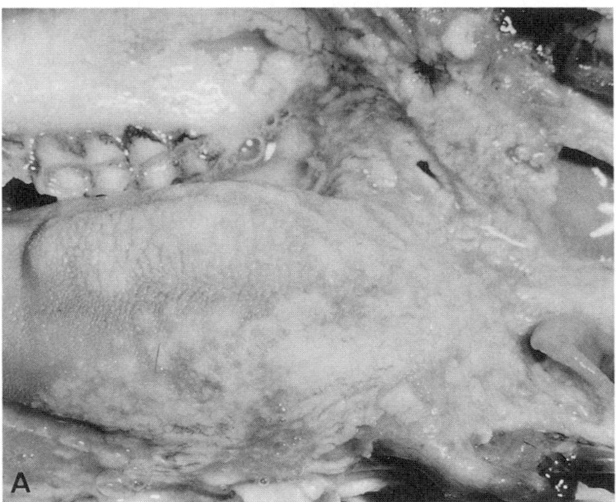

Fig. 1.88A *Peste des petits ruminants*. Goat. Palatine ulcers, and raised plaques on the mucosa of the side of the tongue and oropharynx.

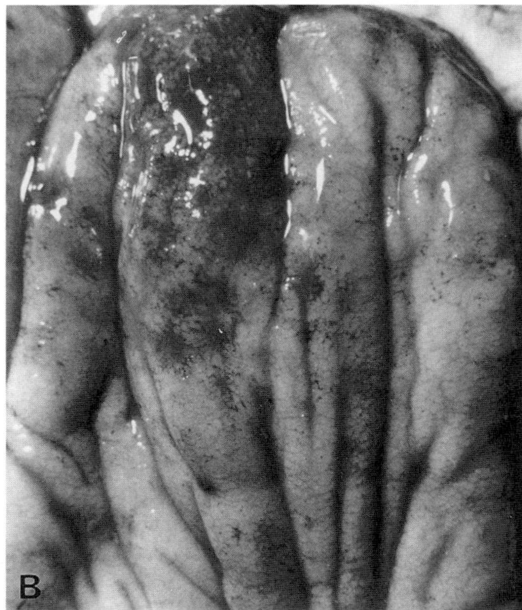

Fig. 1.88B *Peste des petits ruminants*. Goat. Diffuse edema, and focal congestion and ulceration of the cecal mucosa. (A and B courtesy of C. C. Brown, Foreign Animal Disease Diagnostic Laboratory, USDA.)

Experimental inoculation of PPR virus into cattle and pigs does not produce clinical disease, but these animals will resist subsequent challenge with rinderpest virus. These species are considered to be dead-end hosts, since they do not seem to spread the infection to other species. Natural infection or vaccination of sheep and goats with rinderpest virus will protect them against PPR virus.

A zoo outbreak of PPR that involved several species of wild ungulates has been reported. The distribution of the virus in free-ranging ungulate wildlife has not been investigated.

Bibliography

Brown, C. C., Mariner, J. C., and Olander, H. J. An immunohistochemical study of the pneumonia caused by *peste des petits ruminants* virus. *Vet Pathol* **28:** 166–170, 1991.

Bundza, A. *et al.* Experimental *peste des petits ruminants* (goat plague) in goats and sheep. *Can J Vet Res* **52:** 46–52, 1988.

Furley, C. W., Taylor, W. P, and Obi, T. U. An outbreak of *peste des petits ruminants* in a zoological collection. *Vet Rec* **121:** 443–447, 1987.

Hamdy, F. M. *et al.* Etiology of the stomatitis, pneumoenteritis complex in Nigerian dwarf goats. *Can J Comp Med* **40:** 276–284, 1980.

Liebermann, H. Die pest der kleinen Wiederkäuer (Ubersichtsreferat). *Mh Vet-Med* **42:** 269–272, 1987.

Obi, T. U. *et al. Peste des petits ruminants* (PPR) in goats in Nigeria: Clinical, microbiological, and pathological features. *Zbl Vet Med (B)* **30:** 751–761, 1983.

Rowland, A. C., Scott, G. R., and Hill, D. H. The pathology of an erosive stomatitis and enteritis in West African dwarf goats. *J Pathol* **98:** 83–87, 1969.

Shaila, M. S. *et al. Peste des petites ruminants* in sheep in India. *Vet Rec* **125:** 602, 1989.

Taylor, W. P., Al Busaidy, S., and Barrett, T. The epidemiology of *peste des petits ruminants* in the Sultanate of Oman. *Vet Microbiol* **22:** 341–352, 1990.

8. Malignant Catarrhal Fever

Malignant catarrhal fever (MCF) is a pansystemic infectious disease of domestic cattle and wild ruminants also known as malignant head catarrh, and snotsiekte. The disease is characterized by lymphoproliferation, vasculitis, and erosive–ulcerative mucosal and cutaneous lesions.

Malignant catarrhal fever is of worldwide distribution. It is generally sporadic, although severe herd outbreaks have been reported in feedlot, dairy and range cattle, and in zoos and game farms. Among the Cervidae, all species except fallow deer are probably susceptible. Other susceptible species of ungulates include bison, banteng, Cape buffalo, and greater kudu. Mortality in susceptible species approaches 100%. Although transmissible, it is apparently not contagious among cattle by direct contact. There are two forms of the disease: the African form, which occurs in animals associated with wildebeest (WA-MCF), and the sheep-associated form (SA-MCF).

The cause of WA-MCF is a cell-associated lymphotropic herpesvirus, provisionally assigned to the subfamily Gammaherpesvirinae, strain alcelaphine herpesvirus-1 (AHV-1), formerly known as bovine herpesvirus-3. The blue, brindled, or white-bearded wildebeest (*Connochaetes taurinus*), a member of the subfamily Alcelaphinae, carries AHV-1 as a latent infection. Wildebeest calves become infected during the first 2–3 months of life, when they are also viremic and shed cell-free AHV-1 in nasal and ocular secretions. Most wildebeest older than 7 months are serologically positive for AHV-1. *In utero* infections have also been reported. Viruses that are antigenically closely related to AHV-1 have been isolated from Coke's hartebeest *(Alcelathus buselaphus cokei)* and topi (*Damaliscus korrigum*). Antibody which reacts with AHV-1 can be detected in several species of three subfamilies of Bovidae, namely Alcelaphinae, Caprinae, and Hippotraginae. With the exception of the wildebeest, the other species do not seem to spread clinical MCF in the field. The hartebeest virus can be transmitted experimentally to cattle, but there is no evidence that this occurs under natural conditions. The native gammaherpesviruses of each of these species perhaps should be considered distinct viruses, rather than subtypes of AHV-1. Although wildebeest-associated virus produces MCF in many captive exotic species of ruminants, apparently most species which are exposed in their native habitat do not develop disease. Alcelaphine herpesvirus-1 has been transmitted and adapted to domestic rabbits, hamsters, rats, and guinea pigs, in which it produces MCF-like lesions.

The viral cytopathic effects in tissue cultures of bovine origin are characterized by formation of nuclear, basophilic (Cowdry type A) inclusions and syncytia, but these have not been observed in tissues of animals affected with MCF. Freezing of infected tissues destroys most of the virus; however, infected cell cultures can be stored at −70°C. The morphology and viral replication of AHV-1 are similar to those of other herpesviruses. Both naked and enveloped virus particles may be seen in infected cells of tissue cultures. Enveloped particles are 140–220 nm in diameter and have a loose, irregular external membrane that encloses a 85- to 100-nm central capsid, with a nucleoid about 40 nm in diameter, composed of hollow capsomeres. During viral replication, nucleic acids and nucleocapsids are synthesized in the nucleus. The nucleocapsids are enclosed within several concentric dark-staining rings. The nuclei of most infected cells have marked margination of chromatin, and uniformly distributed nucleocapsids and aggregates of immature virions. These probably represent the Cowdry type A nuclear inclusions seen in tissue cultures. Envelopes are acquired by budding through membranes of the Golgi apparatus, endoplastic reticulum, and plasma membranes.

The etiologic agent of SA-MCF has never been isolated from sheep, in spite of numerous attempts. There is mounting circumstantial, albeit sometimes conflicting, evidence that a gammaherpesvirus antigenically related to AHV-1 is widespread in sheep. A high percentage of domestic sheep, as well as exotic breeds of sheep and goats, have antibodies to AHV-1 on the basis of the indirect immunofluorescence (IIF) test. Immunoblotting techniques confirm that most sheep sera react with many of the components recognized by wildebeest sera in the same test. Some sera from gnotobiotic and specific pathogen-free lambs also have antibodies to AHV-1 by the IIF test, suggesting transplacental infection with a viral antigen related to AHV-1. Efforts to demonstrate neutralizing antibodies to AHV-1 in sheep sera have produced inconsistent results. The inconsistencies have been attributed to differences in techniques used to test for neutralizing antibodies. The putative sheep gammaherpesvirus seems antigenically less closely related to AHV-1 than the similar viruses in other Bovidae. Since some outbreaks of MCF in cattle and deer have not been clearly associated with sheep, other sources of virus may exist.

Several viruses have been isolated from cattle affected with SA-MCF, including morbillivirus, bovine syncytial virus, parvovirus, enterovirus, and herpesviruses. Except for one herpesvirus, the other viruses were probably coincidental infections. A herpesvirus morphologically and immunologically similar to AHV-1 has been identified in cell cultures infected with material from a cow with SA-MCF from an outbreak in dairy cattle in Minnesota. Initial attempts to induce clinical disease by experimental inoculation failed, but cattle immunized with this isolate survived a challenge with lethal doses of AHV-1. More recently, a MCF-like syndrome was produced by repeated inoculations of steers with this Minnesota isolate, which was presumed to be of sheep origin. Virus could not be recovered from the animals that died of MCF, but it was reisolated from a single animal that survived. All three steers developed virus-neutralizing antibodies. Attempts to reproduce MCF in cattle by inoculating sheep tissues and secretions have been unsuccessful, but MCF-like disease can be induced in rabbits, hamsters, and guinea pigs by transfer of lymphocytes or T-lymphoblast cell lines derived from MCF-affected cattle and deer. The domestic rabbit is the most commonly used model to study the pathogenesis of both forms of MCF.

There is considerable variation in the susceptibility of

various ruminant species to SA-MCF. The domestic cattle species *Bos taurus* and *B. indicus* appear to be relatively resistant, requiring high levels of exposure to induce disease. Bali cattle or banteng (*Bos javanicus*), the domestic water buffalo (*Bubalus bubalis*), and most species of deer, with the exception of fallow deer (*Dama dama*), seem to be highly susceptible. Sheep-associated MCF is considered to be one of the most serious diseases in farmed deer in New Zealand, Australia, and the United Kingdom. Multiple case outbreaks have also been reported in captive North American cervids. There is some concern that game ranching of exotic ruminants may result in WA-MCF becoming more prevalent in domestic cattle and game-ranched ruminants.

Wildebeest are infected for life and transmit AHV-1 to their calves without showing clinical signs. The calves are considered to be the main source of infection for cattle. They may shed infective cell-free virus, in nasal and ocular secretions, for several days. Transmission to cattle may occur even without intimate contact, suggesting aerosol spread. Viremia apparently ceases with the development of active neutralizing antibodies in animals >6 months old. It may be reactivated during late pregnancy or periods of stress, e.g., transportation. Sheep-associated MCF occurs where cattle and deer are kept in close contact with sheep. The highest risk of transmission seems to be during the peripartum period for both forms of the disease.

The mucosa of the upper respiratory tract and/or the tonsil are the most likely route of entry for AHV-1. Both forms of MCF can be transmitted with large volumes of whole blood or lymphoid tissues, but not by cell-free filtrates. This indicates that the agents are cell associated, probably with lymphocytes. It is more difficult to experimentally transmit SA-MCF than WA-MCF from animal to animal, and the former is more readily transmitted between deer than between cattle. Natural transmission between cattle does not seem to occur, probably because only cell-associated AHV-1 is shed by infected animals.

The pathogenesis, clinical signs, and lesions are similar for both forms of MCF. In spite of considerable research on the pathogenesis of MCF, the mechanisms involved in the development of the lesions remain poorly understood.

Viremia in WA-MCF usually starts about 7 days before the onset of fever, and persists throughout the course of the disease. Primary viral replication occurs mainly in small and medium-sized lymphocytes. Among lymphoid tissues, the spleen and lymph nodes have the highest virus titers. The exact mechanisms involved in the pathogenesis from this point remain somewhat speculative.

A number of mechanisms have been proposed for the main components of MCF-related lesions, which include proliferation of T lymphocytes and lymphoblasts, vasculitis, and tissue necrosis. The destructive lesions are probably immune mediated. However, typical antigen–antibody deposits have thus far not been demonstrated, and although the vasculitis is reminiscent of the Arthus reaction, its pathogenesis is unknown. The contribution of infarction to the necrotizing lesions is uncertain, but probably minor, perhaps with the exception of lesions in the kidney, and other solid organs. Malignant catarrhal fever is characterized by a marked T-lymphocyte hyperplasia. A population of large granular lymphocytes appears to be latently infected and transformed by AHV-1. These cells probably have T-suppressor cell and natural-killer cell activity. Dysfunction of this cell population may result in derepression of T-lymphocyte replication, permitting lymphoproliferation; deranged natural-killer activity may result in the tissue necrosis which is a feature of MCF.

Analogies have been drawn between MCF and lymphomas caused by other gammaherpesviruses, such as Marek's disease virus in poultry, *Herpesvirus ateles* of spider monkeys, *Herpesvirus saimiri* of squirrel monkeys, *Herpesvirus sylvilagi* of cottontail rabbits, and Epstein–Barr virus of humans. These viruses are highly cell associated, infect lymphocytes, and the related lesions are characterized by lymphocytic and lymphoblastic proliferation and infiltration. Lymphomalike lesions have been reported in AHV-1-infected rats, and in certain species of deer. However, in typical cases of MCF, the lymphoid-cell reaction in various tissues appears to be hyperplastic rather than neoplastic, and the normal architecture of lymphoid organs is generally retained. This does not preclude the possibility that the lymphoid cell responses may represent a preneoplastic lesion, but on epidemiologic grounds, this seems unlikely.

Low titers of neutralizing antibodies against AHV-1 can be detected in cattle with either form of MCF. Few serologic studies have been done on cattle with SA-MCF, and some of these have significant titers against AHV-1. The development of antibodies does not prevent the fatal outcome of the disease. The few animals that recover from experimental WA-MCF may have viremia for a period of 6 months, but these animals are immune to all strains of AHV-1.

The incubation period of both forms of malignant catarrhal fever is usually 2–8 weeks, but may, on occasion, be much longer than this. Initially, there is high fluctuating fever and depression, accompanied by an absolute increase in circulating medium-sized and large lymphocytes, followed by eosinopenia in the terminal stages.

There is potentially wide variation in the presenting clinical syndromes. Quite consistently, affected animals have enlarged lymph nodes, and there is usually some degree of ocular and oral disease, and exudative dermatitis. There is edema of the eyelids and palpebral conjunctivae and congestion of the nasal and buccal mucosae. Photophobia is accompanied by copious lacrimation. There is conjunctivitis and an increasing rim of corneal opacity, starting at the limbus and progressing centripetally. Corneal ulceration occurs in some cases, but in those which die quickly, the infiltration of the filtration angle may be all that is seen, and this is easily overlooked. Hypopyon may be seen. In some cases there are nervous signs, such as hyperesthesia, head pressing, trembling, nystagmus, incoordination, and behavioral changes. Other animals may have gastroenteritis with diarrhea, which may in acute cases be bloody. This is most commonly seen in deer. The disease may take an acute course of about 1–3 days, particularly in animals with hemorrhagic enteritis. Those with less severe gastroenteritis, central nervous signs, or generalized disease may linger for as long as 9–10 days.

Gross morbid changes may not be present in occasional animals which die of peracute malignant catarrhal fever, and in these the diagnosis must rest on the detection of the characteristic histologic changes and positive results of transmission experiments. With the sheep-associated disease, diagnosis is based usually on the microscopic findings. Bearing in mind the wide variation in the development and severity of lesions, the changes described in succeeding sections may be seen in any case.

The carcass is dehydrated, and may be emaciated if the course has been prolonged. Conjunctivitis as described may be evident. The muzzle and nares are heavily encrusted and, if wiped, often reveal irregular raw surfaces, although in some cases there may be only a slight serous discharge. Cutaneous lesions, especially in SA-MCF, are common, but often overlooked. Affected areas include the thorax, abdomen, inguinal regions, perineum, udder, and occasionally the head. There may be, acutely, a more or less generalized exanthema with sufficient exudation to wet and mat the hair, and to form detachable crusts; in unpigmented skin there is obvious hyperemia. The crusts may become several millimeters thick, and there is patchy loss of hair. Sometimes these cutaneous changes begin locally about the base of the hooves and horns, the loin, and perineum; they may remain localized or become generalized. In severe cases, the horns and hooves may slough.

The respiratory system may show minor or severe lesions (Fig. 1.89A). When the course is short, the nasal mucosa may show congestion and slight serous exudation only. Later, there is a copious discharge. The mucosa is then intensely hyperemic and edematous, and erosions of a few millimeters' diameter are common. These are irregular in shape with a hemorrhagic base. Occasionally, dirty brown pseudomembranes form and, if these are removed, raw surfaces remain. Lesions of severity similar to those on the septum and turbinates may develop in the sinuses. The pharyngeal and laryngeal mucosae are hyperemic and swollen and later develop multiple erosions or ulcerations and are often covered in part by grayish-yellow pseudomembranes. The tracheobronchial mucosa is hyperemic and usually petechiated, but ulceration may occur, and in a small percentage of cases, a pseudomembranous tracheobronchitis is present (Fig. 1.89B). The lungs are usually edematous and emphysematous, but in peracute cases they may appear perfectly healthy. A nonspecific bronchopneumonia may complicate chronic cases. The respiratory lesions are reportedly more severe in WA-MCF compared to the sheep-associated disease.

The lower alimentary mucosae may show no significant lesions in the peracute disease, although oral lesions are present in most cases of WA-MCF. Minor erosions are first observed on the lips adjacent to the mucocutaneous junction. Sometimes apparently normal epithelium on the

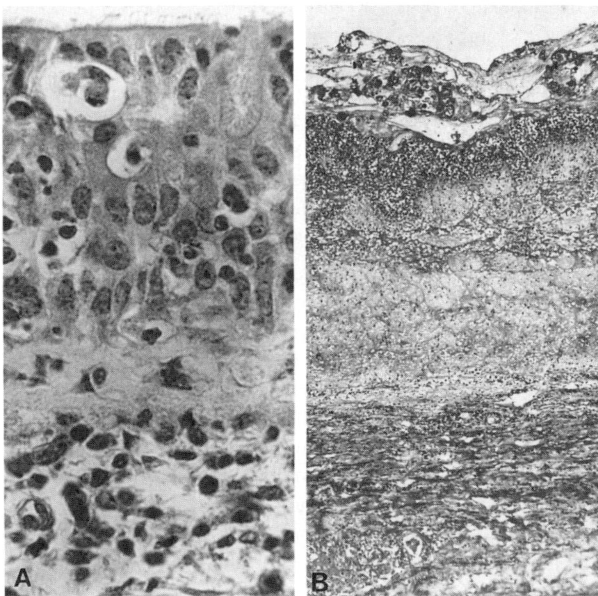

Fig. 1.89 Malignant catarrhal fever. (A) Nasal mucosa. Degeneration of epithelium and infiltration of lymphocytic cells in uncomplicated rhinitis. (B) Pseudomembranous tracheitis.

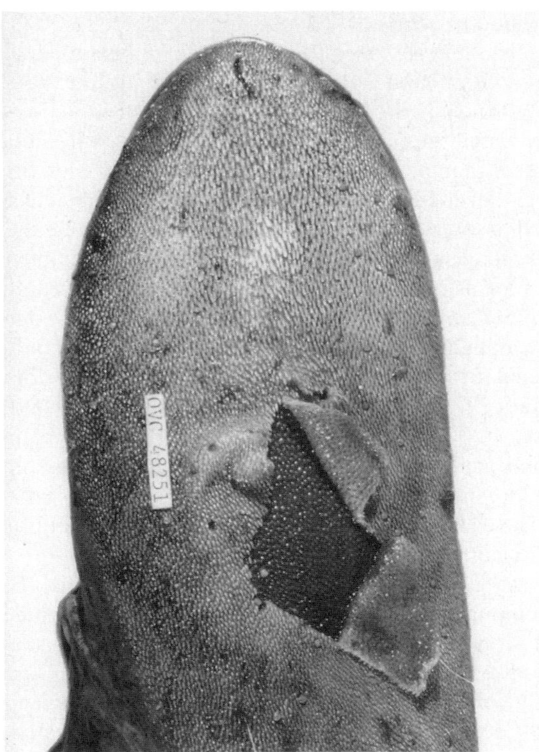

Fig. 1.90 Malignant catarrhal fever. Ox. Separation of necrotic lingual epithelium from underlying propria.

surface of the tongue peels off in sheets (Fig. 1.90). Later, erosive and ulcerative lesions may involve a large area of oral mucosa frequently occurring on all surfaces of the tongue, the dental pad, the tips of the buccal papillae, gingivae, both areas of the palate, and the cheeks. In some areas, the cheesy or tattered necrotic epithelium may not be sloughed at the time of inspection. Esophageal erosions, similar to those that occur in the other diseases causing ulcerative stomatitis, occur in malignant catarrhal fever, and, as in rinderpest, are most consistent in the anterior portion. Lesions of the same sort are present in the forestomachs.

The abomasal mucosa is hyperemic and edematous, diffusely or in patches, and is sprinkled with petechiae. Hemorrhagic ulcerations may be present, especially on the margins of the plicae and along the greater curvature. The wall of the small intestine may be firm and thickened by edema. The serosa is dull, very finely granular, and often peppered with fine petechiae. Intestinal content may be mucoid or hemorrhagic, and the mucosa thickened, perhaps with petechial hemorrhages and minor erosions. Similar lesions occur in the large intestine and rectum, but are more obvious; there are lines of congestion along the longitudinal mucosal rugae, and severe ulceration and hemorrhage may be present. The contents of the large intestine are scant and may be dry and pasty or bloody. The intestinal lesions tend to be more severe in deer, extending from the duodenum to the rectum.

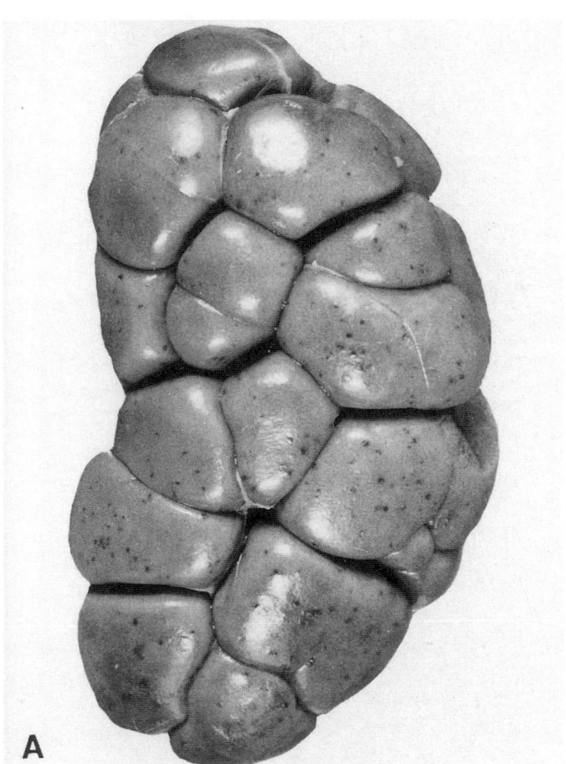

Fig. 1.91A Malignant catarrhal fever. Focal nonsuppurative interstitial nephritis.

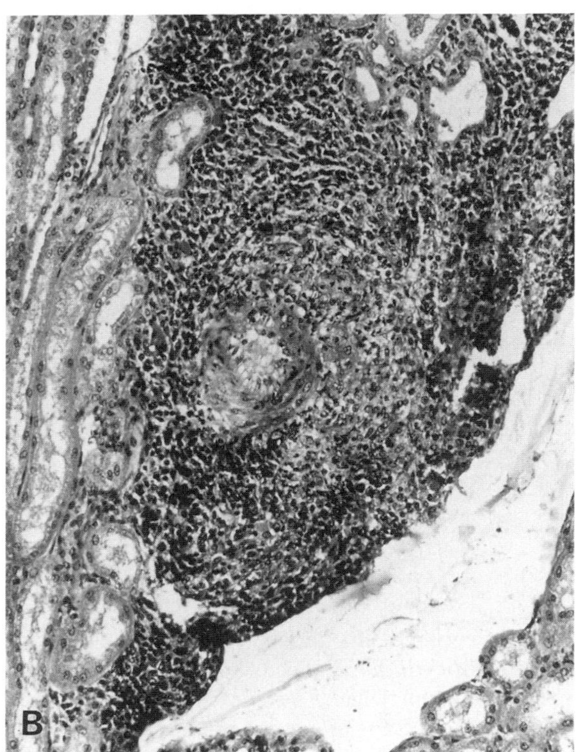

Fig. 1.91B Malignant catarrhal fever. Ox. Extensive cuff of mononuclear cells, and fibrinoid necrosis in the wall of a small arteriole. Kidney.

Rather characteristic lesions may occur in the urinary system. Renal changes are not always present. They are infarcts or 2- to 4-mm foci of nonsuppurative interstitial nephritis (Fig. 1.91A,B). They may be numerous enough to produce a mottled appearance. These foci may form slight rounded projections from the capsular surfaces. The pelvic and ureteral mucosa frequently have petechial and ecchymotic hemorrhages. Similar lesions are present on the mucosa of the urinary bladder, or there may be more severe hemorrhage associated with erosion and ulceration of the epithelium, and hematuria (Fig. 1.92). Superficial lesions occur in the vagina, similar to those of the oral cavity and skin.

The liver is slightly enlarged; close inspection will reveal, in some cases, a diffuse mottling with white foci, which are periportal accumulations of mononuclear cells (Fig. 1.93). There may be numerous small hemorrhages and a few erosions of the mucous membrane of the gallbladder.

Enlargement of lymph nodes is a characteristic lesion of malignant catarrhal fever. All nodes may be involved, or some may appear grossly normal. Affected nodes may be many times the normal size, and some, including hemolymph nodes, which are usually too small to recognize, may become quite obvious. There is edema of the affected nodes and the pericapsular connective tissue. On cross

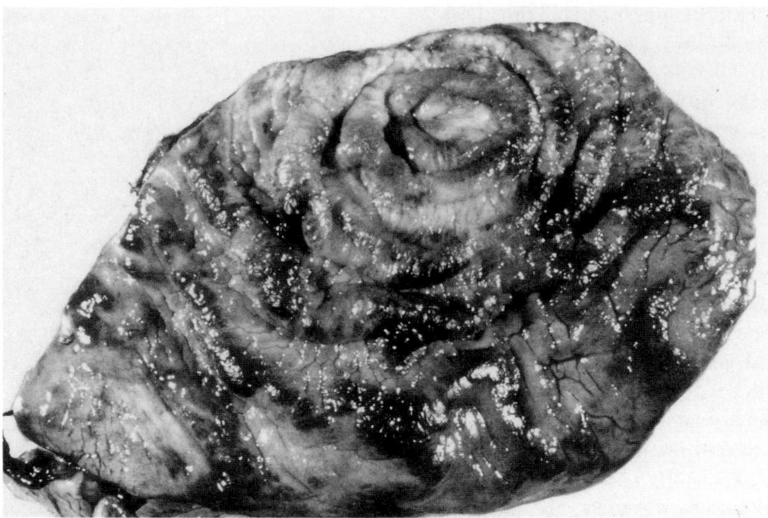

Fig. 1.92 Malignant catarrhal fever. Hemorrhages in mucosa of urinary bladder.

section it is apparent that much of the increase in size is due to lymphocytic hyperplasia. Some of the nodes are congested or hemorrhagic. The spleen is slightly enlarged, and the lymphoid follicles are prominent.

There is an excess of cerebrospinal fluid, which contains much protein and moderate numbers of mononuclear cells (Fig. 1.94). The meninges are wet, and there is some cloudiness in the subarachnoid space of the sulci. There

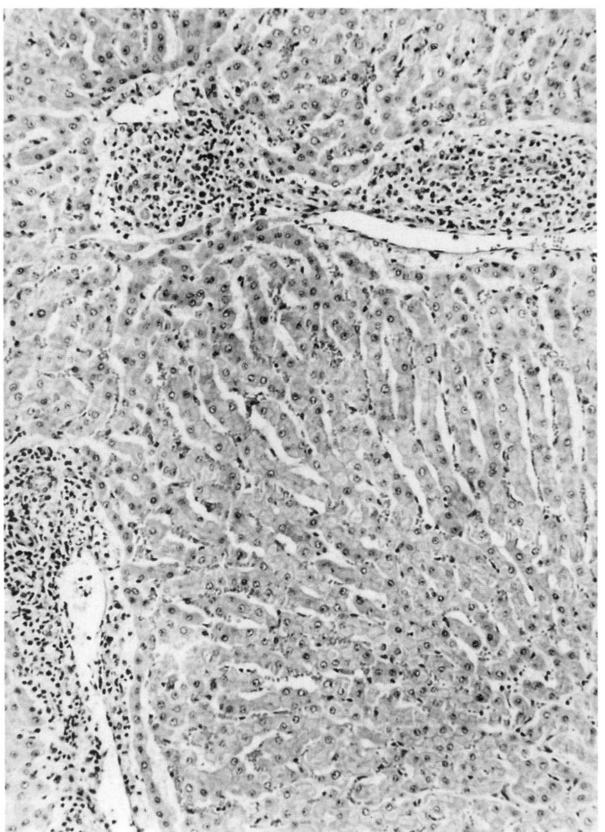

Fig. 1.93 Malignant catarrhal fever. Accumulations of lymphocytic cells in portal triads.

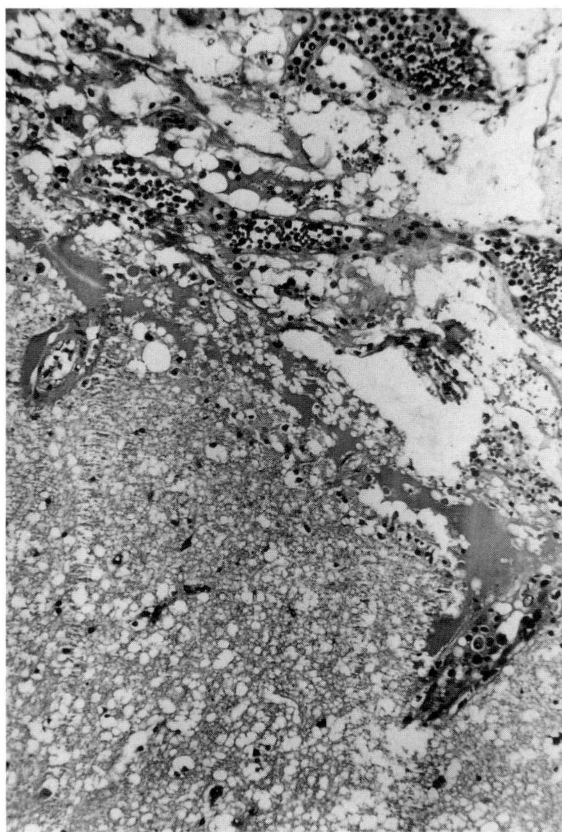

Fig. 1.94 Malignant catarrhal fever. Meningeal exudate and vasculitis.

also may be scattered petechial hemorrhages in the meninges. These lesions are usually most concentrated in the cerebellar leptomeninges.

Gross changes usually are not visible in the heart and larger blood vessels. Polyarthritis, characterized by increased amounts of cloudy synovial fluid and red swollen synovial membranes, has been reported in experimentally infected cattle.

The histologic changes usually must be relied on for the diagnosis of malignant catarrhal fever, and its differentiation from similar diseases. The characteristic histologic changes are found in lymphoid tissues and in the adventitia and walls of medium-sized vessels, especially arteries in any organ, and these will be described before other lesions. The vascular lesions are an accumulation of mainly mononuclear cells in the adventitia, and fibrinoid necrotizing vasculitis (Figs. 1.91B, 1.95A,B, 1.96). These changes may be focal or segmental, and may involve the full thickness of the wall, or be confined more or less to one of the layers. When the intima is involved, there is often endothelial swelling. Thrombi are difficult to demonstrate in damaged vessels. The media may be selectively affected, or perhaps the adventitia alone. Severely affected segments of vessel are replaced by a coagulum of homogeneous, eosinophilic material, in which nuclear remnants are seen. The altered nuclei are small, distorted, and fragmented. The perivascular accumulation of cells is particularly characteristic. They are mainly lymphoid cells with large open nuclei and prominent nucleoli; occasionally small lymphocytes and plasma cells may be present.

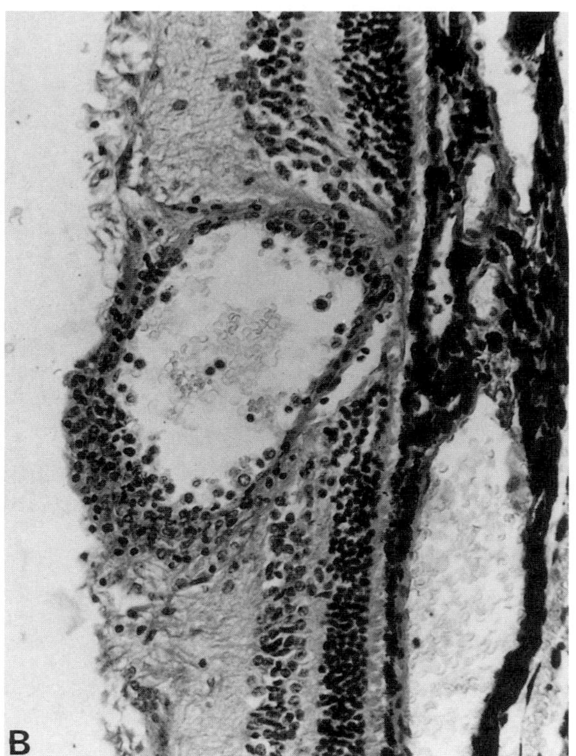

Fig. 1.95B Malignant catarrhal fever. Vasculitis in retina.

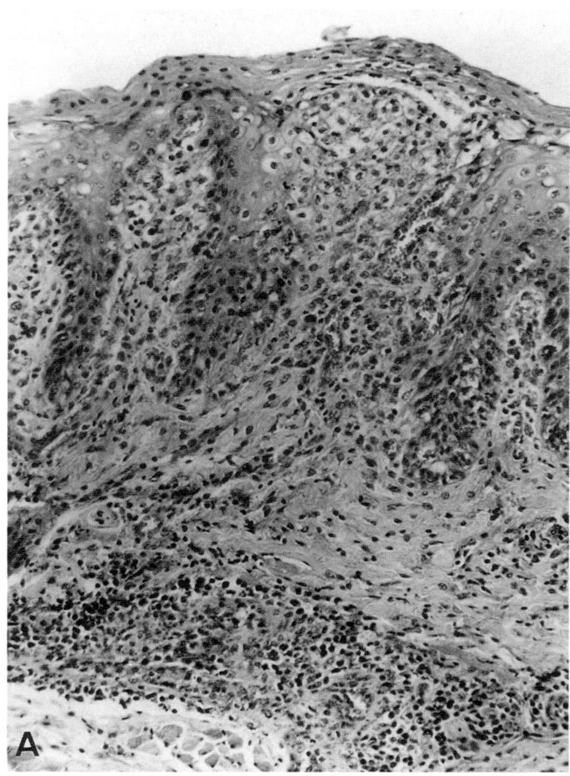

Fig. 1.95A Malignant catarrhal fever. Ox. Tongue. Vasculitis, infiltration of lamina propria by lymphocytic cells with developing ulcer over papilla.

In some forms of the experimental disease, fibrinoid necrosis, endothelial cell hyperplasia, and thrombosis are not prominent. Electron-microscopic studies in these cases have shown that the endothelial reaction consists primarily of lymphocytes and macrophages rather than endothelial cells. The degree of the mononuclear cell reaction in the vessel walls and the medial necrosis increase with progression of the disease.

These changes in the blood vessels strongly suggest malignant catarrhal fever; however, arteritis may be seen in mucosal disease, mainly in the submucosa in the lower alimentary tract. Fortunately for diagnostic purposes, arteritis is present in all cases of malignant catarrhal fever, whether peracute, acute, or mild with recovery, but it may be necessary to examine many sections to find it. The best organs to examine for vascular lesions are the brain and leptomeninges, carotid rete, kidney, liver, the adrenal capsule and medulla, salivary gland, and any area of skin or alimentary tract showing gross lesions.

Several hypotheses have been proposed to explain the pathogenesis of the vascular lesions, but none of these is well substantiated. The lack of circulating antibody and viral antigen, and absence of antigen–antibody complexes and complement in vessel walls, are inconsistent with immune-mediated vasculitis. However, some suggest that conglutinin, which is consistently present in cattle with

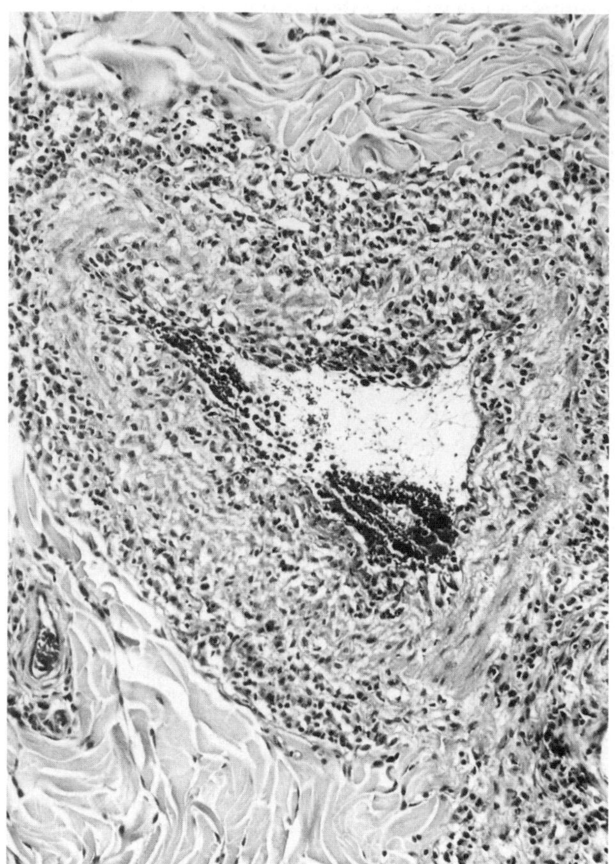

Fig. 1.96 Malignant catarrhal fever. Periarteritis in the deep dermis. Cow. (Courtesy of J. A. Yager.)

WA-MCF, may mask immunoglobulins, and that both of these proteins may hide antigens. The cellular reaction in MCF-related vasculitis is characterized by lymphoid cells in contrast to immune-mediated vasculitis, which consists primarily of neutrophils and plasmacytes. For further discussion of vasculitis see The Cardiovascular System (Volume 3, Chapter 1).

In lymph nodes there is active proliferation of lymphoblasts, which form extensive homogeneous populations of cells in the T cell-dependent areas of the interfollicular cortical and paracortical zones. Mitosis may be increased. There is usually concomitant necrosis of small mature lymphocytes, especially in the follicles. Focal areas of hemorrhage and necrosis associated with arteritis may be seen in all areas of the nodes. A marked lymphoid and macrophage reaction are evident in the medullary sinuses. Lymphoid cell infiltration and edema are usually seen in the pericapsular connective tissue. The lymphoid reaction in the spleen varies from marked lymphoid cell hyperplasia, in the periarteriolar sheaths, to atrophy and depletion of lymphocytes. In addition, there is marked proliferation and infiltration of lymphocytic and lymphoblastic cells, mainly perivascular in distribution, in a variety of organs. The lymphoreticular proliferation may become so severe in some organs that it is difficult to determine whether it is hyperplastic or neoplastic. The mechanisms possibly involved in the proliferation of lymphoid cells are noted earlier.

Microscopic arteritis similar to that present in other organs occurs in the nervous system of many cases. Necrotizing arteritis, plasma exudation into the meninges or Virchow–Robin space (Fig. 1.94), and the predominantly adventitial lymphocytic response are, in the brain of cattle, unique to malignant catarrhal fever, and allow it to be differentiated from other nonsuppurative encephalitides. Degenerative changes in nervous parenchyma can be explained on the basis of the vascular changes.

The lesions in skin and squamous mucosae of the alimentary tract are histologically similar. The dermis or propria and often the epithelium is diffusely infiltrated with a mainly lymphocytic cell population (Fig. 1.97). The dermis, especially its superficial portion, is edematous, and typical arteritis, involving small and medium-sized vessels, is present. Epithelial changes are related to the presence of a diffuse lymphocytic infiltrate, and to arteritis in the underlying dermis or propria. Groups of epithelial cells become necrotic, with swollen, strongly acidophilic cytoplasm; ultimately the full thickness of epithelium in affected areas undergoes necrosis and erodes (Fig. 1.97). Large areas of epithelium may thus be detached or lost, and there is not much acute leukocytic reaction in the exposed propria or dermis.

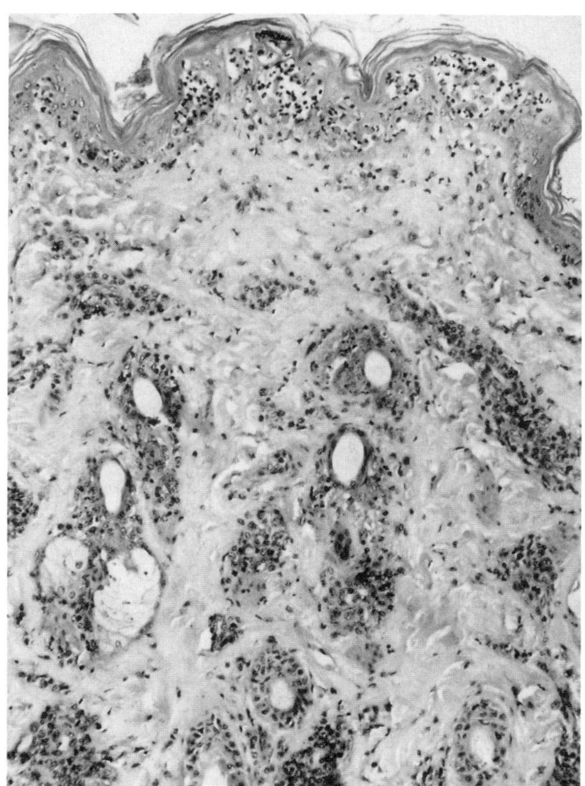

Fig. 1.97 Malignant catarrhal fever. Necrosis of epithelium. Skin.

The severity of the lesions in the oral squamous mucosa is, in experimental cases at least, related to the degree of lymphoid cell infiltration in the mucosa and underlying lamina propria, rather than to the vascular thrombosis, which is minimal.

These changes in the epithelium and its lamina propria account for the macroscopic lesions in the vagina, the prepuce, the bladder, and, although there is often much less hemorrhage, in the oral cavity, the nasal mucosa, the esophagus, and the forestomach. Although gross lesions are not present in the salivary glands, there are microscopic degenerative changes in the epithelium of the interlobular and excretory ducts, with multiple foci of parenchymal necrosis associated with arteritis.

The mucosa of the stomach and small and large intestine is also densely infiltrated focally and/or diffusely with large lymphocytes. Mucosal infiltrates and necrosis are associated with inflammation of arterioles in the underlying submucosa. In the abomasum, the glandular epithelium in affected areas becomes basophilic, cuboidal, or flattened mucous in type; eventually necrosis and focal ulceration occur. In the small intestine and large bowel, the lesion resembles ischemic damage. The superficial mucosa undergoes necrosis, and there is erosion and hemorrhage. Surviving crypts and glands are lined by flattened basophilic epithelium. In mucosa in which the epithelium is completely destroyed, the collapsed proprial stroma and mononuclear infiltrate is left resting on the muscularis mucosa (Fig. 1.98). The full thickness of the intestinal wall is edematous, and there is often mesenteric arteritis.

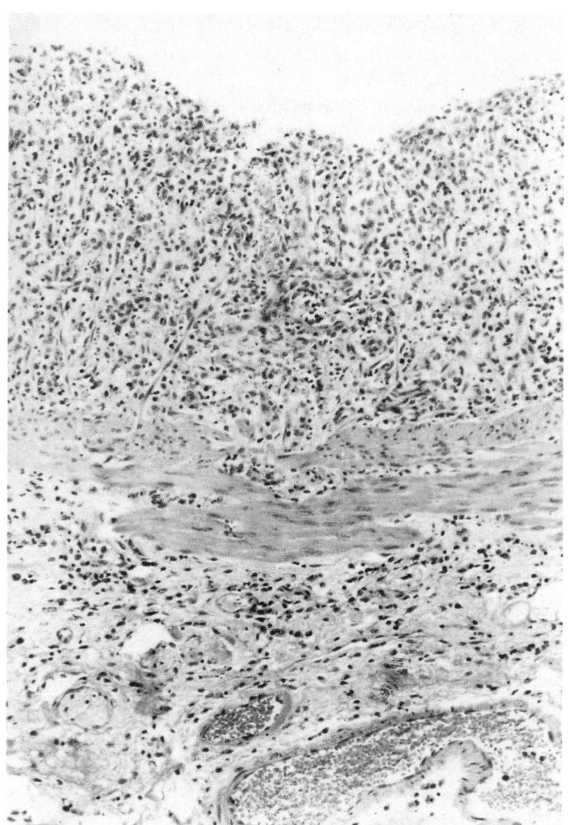

Fig. 1.98 Malignant catarrhal fever. Colitis with collapse of glands and edema of submucosa.

The mottling of liver and the focal nephritis seen grossly are due to the accumulation of mononuclear cells in the portal triads of the liver (Fig. 1.93) and in the cortices of the kidney. In the liver, these cuffs may be very large and invest the branches of the hepatic artery, which may undergo fibrinoid necrosis. Microscopic lesions are rather consistently present in the kidneys, even though gross lesions are not; they consist of vasculitis involving the smaller arteries and afferent arterioles. Extensive diffuse lymphocytic infiltrates disrupt the normal renal cortical architecture, and in some cases, infarcts appear to be associated with vasculitis involving arcuate arteries.

The microscopic lesions in the joints are characterized by a marked, mainly lymphocytic, reaction in the synovial membrane and underlying connective tissue, especially in perivascular areas. Focal areas of necrosis and desquamation may be evident over regions which are heavily infiltrated by lymphocytes. Fibrinous exudate may cover the necrotic areas. Joint lesions have been reported only in experimental cases of malignant catarrhal fever.

This completes a description of the histologic changes which are the basis of the gross lesions. However, these same changes may be found in any tissue, even in the absence of gross lesions. Rather constantly, there are vascular lesions of this sort in the neurohypophysis, but not the adenohypophysis, and in the adrenal glands. The adre-

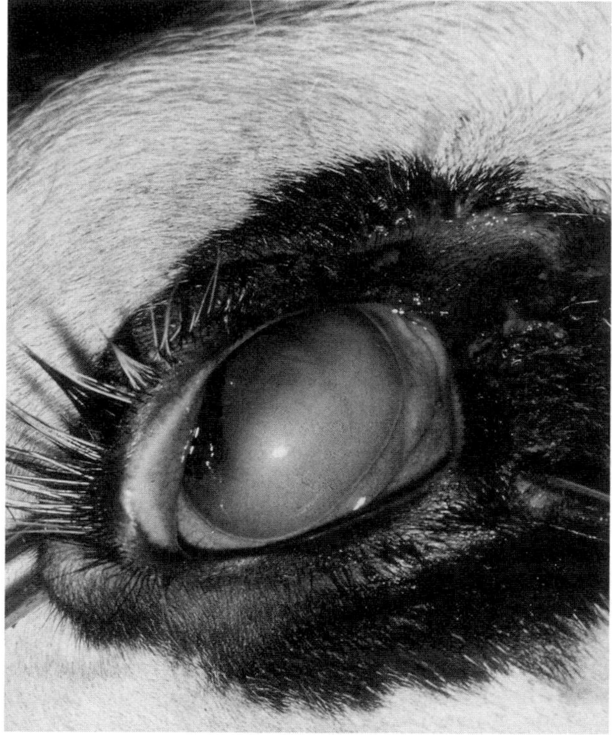

Fig. 1.99 Malignant catarrhal fever. Edema of cornea.

nal changes are in the capsule and its vessels and trabeculae, and in the medullary vessels. There may be minor focal necrosis of the cortex, and more often there is disorganization of the medulla and a diffuse lymphocytic infiltrate.

Ophthalmitis often occurs, and its presence is a useful differential criterion from other ulcerative diseases of the alimentary tract. All portions of the globe may be affected, and the lesions are characterized by a lymphocytic infiltration of various structures. Rather consistently there is fibrinocellular exudation from hyperemic ciliary processes, and the accumulation of this exudate in the filtration angle is responsible for the rim of opacity observed clinically. Later and as a result of conjunctivitis and inflammation of the limbic vessels, there is corneal edema with degeneration of the epi- and endothelial cells that may lead to ulceration and vascularization. The exudate in the anterior chamber consists mainly of mononuclear cells and fibrin, which may adhere to the corneal endothelial lining (Fig. 1.99). There is a retinal vasculitis and, in some cases, hemorrhagic or inflammatory detachment of the retina in focal areas. Lymphocytic optic neuritis and meningitis may be seen (see The Eye and Ear, Volume 1, Chapter 4).

In Bali cattle, MCF must be differentiated from Jembrana disease, a condition of unknown etiology, possibly due to an *Ehrlichia* sp. and characterized by fever, lymphadenopathy, and ulcerative oral lesions. Although some state that vascular, ocular, and brain lesions are not found in Jembrana disease, they are described by others. Jembrana disease is not always fatal.

Bibliography

Blake, J. E., Nielsen, N. O., and Heuschele, W. P. Lymphoproliferation in captive wild ruminants affected with malignant catarrhal fever: 25 cases (1977–1985). *J Am Vet Med Assoc* **196:** 1141–1143, 1990.

Buxton, D. *et al.* The pathology of "sheep-associated" malignant catarrhal fever in the hamster. *J Comp Pathol* **98:** 155–166, 1988.

Castro, A. E., and Daley, G. G. Electron microscopic study of the African strain of malignant catarrhal fever virus in bovine cell cultures. *Am J Vet Res* **43:** 576–582, 1982.

Castro, A. E. *et al.* Malignant catarrhal fever in an Indian Gaur and Greater Kudu: Experimental transmission, isolation, and identification of a herpesvirus. *Am J Vet Res* **43:** 5–11, 1982.

Castro, A. E. *et al.* Ultrastructure of cellular changes in the replication of the alcelaphine herpesvirus-1 of malignant catarrhal fever. *Am J Vet Res* **46:** 1231–1237, 1985.

Coulter, G. R., and Storz, J. Identification of a cell-associated morbillivirus from cattle affected with malignant catarrhal fever: Antigenic differentiation and cytologic characterization. *Am J Vet Res* **40:** 1671–1677, 1979.

Heuschele, W. P., and Castro, A. E. Malignant catarrhal fever. *In* "Comparative Pathobiology of Viral Diseases," R. G. Olsen, S. Krakowka, and J. R. Blakeslee, Jr. (eds.), pp. 115–125. Boca Raton, Florida, CRC Press, 1985.

Hoffman, D., and Young, M. P. Malignant catarrhal fever. *Aust Vet J* **66:** 405–406, 1989.

Jacoby, R. O., Buxton, D., and Reid, H. W. The pathology of wildebeest-associated malignant catarrhal fever in hamsters, rats, and guinea-pigs. *J Comp Pathol* **98:** 99–109, 1988.

Kalunda, M., Dardiri, A. H., and Lee, K. M. Malignant catarrhal fever. I. Response of American cattle to malignant catarrhal fever virus isolated in Kenya. *Can J Comp Med* **45:** 70–76, 1981.

Kalunda, M. *et al.* Malignant catarrhal fever. III. Experimental infection of sheep, domestic rabbits, and laboratory animals with malignant catarrhal fever virus. *Can J Comp Med* **45:** 310–314, 1981.

Katz, J., Seal, B., and Ridpath, J. Molecular diagnosis of alcelaphine herpesvirus (malignant catarrhal fever) infections by nested amplifiction of viral DNA in bovine blood buffy coat specimens. *J Vet Diagn Invest* **3:** 193–198, 1991.

Liggitt, H. D., and DeMartini, J. C. The pathomorphology of malignant catarrhal fever. I. Generalized lymphoid vasculitis. *Vet Pathol* **17:** 58–72, 1980.

Liggitt, H. D., and DeMartini, J. C. The pathomorphology of malignant catarrhal fever. II. Multisystemic epithelial lesions. *Vet Pathol* **17:** 73–83, 1980.

Liggitt, H. D., McChesney, A. E., and DeMartini, J. C. Experimental transmission of bovine malignant catarrhal fever to a bison (*Bison bison*). *J Wildl Dis* **16:** 299–304, 1980.

Metzler, A. E., and Burri, H.-R. Zur Aetiologie und Epidemiologie des bösartigen Katarrhalfiebers—Ein Übersicht. *Schweiz Arch Tierheilk* **132:** 161–172, 1990.

Mirangi, P. K., and Rossiter, P. B. Malignant catarrhal fever in cattle experimentally inoculated with a herpesvirus isolated from a case of malignant catarrhal fever in Minnesota, USA. *Br Vet J* **147:** 31–41, 1991.

Pierson, R. E. *et al.* Clinical and clinicopathologic observations in induced malignant catarrhal fever of cattle. *J Am Vet Med Assoc* **173:** 833–837, 1978.

Plowright, W. Malignant catarrhal fever virus. *In* "Virus Infections of Ruminants," Z. Dinter and B. Morein (eds.), pp. 123–150. Amsterdam, Elsevier Science Publishers, 1990.

Reid, H. W., and Buxton, D. Malignant catarrhal fever and the gammaherpesvirinae of bovidae. *In* "Herpesvirus Diseases of Cattle, Horses, and Pigs," G. Wittmann (ed.), pp. 116–162. Dordrecht, Netherlands, Kluwer Academic Publishers, 1989.

Reid, H. W. *et al.* Malignant catarrhal fever: Experimental transmission of the "sheep-associated" form of the disease from cattle and deer to cattle, deer, rabbits, and hamsters. *Res Vet Sci* **41:** 76–81, 1986.

Reid, H. W., Pow, I., and Buxton, D. Antibody to alcelaphine herpesvirus-1 (AHV-1) in hamsters experimentally infected with AHV-1 and the "sheep-associated" agent of malignant catarrhal fever. *Res Vet Sci* **47:** 383–386, 1989.

Rossiter, P. B. Immunology and immunopathology of malignant catarrhal fever. *Prog Vet Microbiol Immun* **1:** 121–144, 1985.

Seal, B. S. *et al.* Prevalence of antibodies to alcelaphine herpesvirus-1 and nucleic acid hybridization analysis of viruses isolated from captive exotic ruminants. *Am J Vet Res* **50:** 1447–1453, 1989.

Selman, I. E. *et al.* Transmission studies with bovine malignant catarrhal fever. *Vet Rec* **102:** 252–257, 1978.

Sharpe, R. T., Bicknell, S. R., and Hunter, A. R. Concurrent malignant catarrhal fever and bovine virus diarrhoea virus infection in a dairy herd. *Vet Rec* **120:** 545–548, 1987.

Soeharsono, Malignant catarrhal fever as compared with the diseases of Bali cattle, with special reference to Jembrana disease. *In* "Malignant Catarrhal Fever in Asian Livestock," P. W. Daniels, Sudarisman, and P. Ronohardjo (eds.), pp. 73–76. Canberra, Australia, Aust Cent for Int Agr Res, 1988.

Soesanto, M. *et al.* Studies on experimental Jembrana disease in Bali cattle. II. Clinical signs and haematological changes. *J Comp Pathol* **103:** 61–70, 1990.

Teuscher E., Ramachandran, S., and Harding, H. P. Observations on the pathology of Jembrana disease in Bali cattle. *Zbl Vet Med A* **28:** 608–622, 1981.

Westbury, H. A. Malignant catarrhal fever. *In* "Deer Refresher Course," Proc No. 72 Sydney, NSW, Univ Sydney Post Grad Com Vet Sci, pp. 417–424, 1984.

Whiteley, H. E. *et al.* Ocular lesions of bovine malignant catarrhal fever. *Vet Pathol* **22:** 219–225, 1985.

9. *Bluetongue and Related Diseases*

Bluetongue is caused by a Reovirus of the genus *Orbivirus*. There are at least 24 recognized serotypes of bluetongue virus, distinguished by serum neutralization tests, though they may represent not so much distinct types as points in a spectrum of antigenicity brought about by recombination of the segmented orbivirus genome. Immunity to one serotype does not confer resistance against another, and may cause sensitization, with a more severe syndrome following infection by a second type. Apparently, not all serotypes are pathogenic.

Epizootic hemorrhagic disease of deer is caused by a virus which represents another serogroup of *Orbivirus*. The virus causing Ibaraki disease, recognized in cattle in Japan, is a variant of epizootic hemorrhage disease virus; seropositive animals also have been found in Taiwan, Indonesia, and an identical virus has been isolated in Australia. Most other serogroups of orbiviruses, with the exception of the African horse-sickness serogroup, are not associated with disease.

Bluetongue, epizootic hemorrhagic disease, and related viruses are spread by *Culicoides* spp., known variously as midges, gnats, or sandflies. The virus multiplies by a factor of 10^3–10^4 in the *Culicoides* within a week of the infected blood meal being ingested, and transmission can occur, following infection of the salivary glands, 10–15 days after the initial blood meal. Transovarial transmission of virus in *Culicoides* does not occur.

Bluetongue virus circulates in a broad belt across the tropics and warm temperate areas, from about latitude 40°N to 35°S, with incursions or recrudescence during the *Culicoides* season, annually, or at irregular longer intervals, in cooler temperate areas. The condition is enzootic or seasonally epizootic in most of Africa, the Middle East, the eastern Mediterranean basin, the Indian subcontinent, the Caribbean, and the United States of America. It has appeared sporadically in the Iberian peninsula and in the Okanagan Valley of western Canada. A number of bluetongue serotypes have been isolated in Australia, but spontaneous disease seems rare, since as yet the range of efficient vectors does not overlap areas of intensive sheep raising.

Sheep, goats, and cattle are the susceptible domestic species, wherever bluetongue occurs. Sheep are the domestic species most highly susceptible to bluetongue, but there is considerable variation in expression of the disease, depending on the breed, age, and immune status of the sheep, the environmental circumstances under which they are held, and the strain of virus. Typically, indigenous breeds seem more resistant to clinical disease than do exotics. Goats, though susceptible to infection, rarely show signs; however, disease has occurred in goats in the Middle East and India. Infection in cattle usually produces only inapparent infection or mild clinical disease. In Africa, a wide variety of nondomestic ungulates and some small mammals may be inapparently infected; mortality has occurred in naturally or experimentally infected topi, cape buffalo, and kudu. In North America, wildlife species, particularly white-tailed deer, black-tailed or mule deer, elk (wapiti), bighorn sheep, and pronghorn antelope are also infected. Bluetongue is responsible for significant mortality in all these species except elk, which usually develop mild or inapparent infection.

Epizootic hemorrhagic disease serogroup virus has been isolated in Nigeria, but the natural vertebrate hosts there are not known. In North America, white-tailed deer, black-tailed or mule deer, pronghorn antelope, and elk are susceptible to infection. The white-tailed deer is extremely susceptible, and widespread epizootics have occurred among this species in the United States of America. A single outbreak has been recognized in Alberta, Canada. The rate of survival is much higher among black-tailed deer and pronghorn antelope, and elk are only very mildly affected. Clinical disease similar to that produced by bluetongue may occur rarely in cattle. Though sheep are not considered to develop disease when infected with this virus, occasional mild clinical signs and lesions resembling bluetongue have been reported in sheep inoculated with some Australian isolates. In Japan, the closely related virus of Ibaraki disease produces a clinical syndrome resembling bluetongue in cattle, but not in sheep.

The viruses of bluetongue and epizootic hemorrhagic disease circulate together in North America. Both viruses may be involved simultaneously in outbreaks of hemorrhagic disease in wild ruminants, and both have been isolated from *Culicoides* in a single locality at the same time. The role of cattle as reservoirs of bluetongue is uncertain. Although some suggest that prenatal vertical transmission may result in seronegative, tolerant, virus shedders among the offspring, results of research on this issue are conflicting.

The pathogenesis of bluetongue, epizootic hemorrhagic disease, and Ibaraki disease is fundamentally similar in all species in which disease is seen. Primary viral replication following insect bite occurs in regional lymph nodes and spleen. Viremia about 4–6 days after inoculation results in secondary infection of endothelium in arterioles, capillaries, and venules throughout the body, with microscopic lesions, fever, and lymphopenia beginning a day or so later, about a week after inoculation. Bluetongue virus in the blood appears to be closely associated with, or in, both leukocytes and erythrocytes, and it may cocirculate with antibody.

Endothelial damage caused by virus infection initiates local microvascular thrombosis and permeability. This is reflected microscopically by the presence of swollen endothelium, and fibrin and platelet thrombi in small vessels, with edema and hemorrhage in surrounding tissue. These lesions in turn mediate the full spectrum of gross findings. These are fundamentally ischemic necrosis of many tissues; edema due to vascular permeability; and hemorrhage resulting from vascular damage compounded, in severe cases, by consumption coagulopathy due to thrombocytopenia and depletion of soluble clotting factors.

Bluetongue in sheep is highly variable; it may cause inapparent infection or an acute fulminant disease. Typically, leukopenia and pyrexia occur, even in mild infections, coincident with viremia. The degree and duration of fever do not correlate with the severity of the syndrome otherwise. In the early phase there is hyperemia of the oral and nasal mucosa, salivation, and nasal discharge within a day or two of the onset of fever. Hyperemia and edema of the eyelids and conjunctiva may occur, and edema of lips, ears, and the intermandibular area becomes apparent. Hyperemia may extend over the muzzle and the skin of much of the body, including the axillary and inguinal areas. Focal hemorrhage may be present on the lips and gums, and the tongue may become edematous and congested or cyanotic, giving the disease its name. Infarcted epithelium thickens and becomes excoriated; erosions and ulcerations develop along the margins of the tongue opposite the molars, and the mucosa of much of the tongue may slough. Excoriation and ulceration also occur on the buccal mucosa, the hard palate, and dental pad. Affected areas of skin may also become encrusted and excoriated with time, and a break in the wool can result in parts or much of the fleece being tender or cast. The coronet, bulbs, and interdigital areas of the foot may become hyperemic. Coronary swelling and streaky hemorrhages in the periople may be evident as a result of lesions in the underlying sensitive laminae. These hemorrhages may persist in the hoof as brown lines which move down the hoof as it grows. A defect parallel to the coronet may also be evident in the growing hoof in recovered cases.

Internally, in acute cases, there is subcutaneous and intermuscular edema, which may be serous or suffused with blood. Superficial lymph nodes are enlarged and juicy. Bruiselike gelatinous hemorrhages and contusions, which may be small and easily overlooked if not numerous, are often present in the subcutis and intermuscular fascial planes. Focal or multifocal pallid areas of streaky myodegeneration may be present throughout the carcass, perhaps partly obscured by petechial or ecchymotic hemorrhage. Resolving muscle lesions may be mineralized or fibrous. Stiffness, reluctance to move, and recumbency seen clinically are due to these muscle lesions.

Necrosis may be present deep in the papillary muscle of the left ventricle, and elsewhere in the myocardium. The lesion which is perhaps most consistent and closest to pathognomonic for bluetongue is focal hemorrhage, petechial or to 1.0 cm wide × 2–3 cm long, in the tunica media at the base of the pulmonary artery. These hemorrhages are visible from both the internal and adventitial surfaces, and may be present in clinically mild cases with few other lesions. Petechial hemorrhage may also be present at the base of the aorta and in subendocardial and subepicardial locations over the heart.

There may also be edema and petechial or ecchymotic hemorrhage in the pharyngeal and laryngeal area. In severe cases the lungs may assume a purplish hue, with marked edematous separation of lobules, and froth in the tracheobronchial tree, probably due to pulmonary microvascular damage and heart failure. Animals with pharyngeal or esophageal myodegeneration suffer from dysphagia, or regurgitate, and may succumb to aspiration pneumonia.

Hyperemia, occasionally marked hemorrhage, or in advanced cases, ulceration of the mucosa may occur on rumen papillae, the pillars of the rumen, and the reticular plicae. In convalescent animals, stellate healing ulcers or scars on the wall of the forestomachs may be apparent. Petechial hemorrhage may be present in the abomasal mucosa, with congestion of the subserosa at the pylorus. The remainder of the intestinal mucosa may be congested, and occasionally there may be hemorrhage, particularly in the large bowel. Petechial hemorrhage of the mucosa of the gallbladder may also be seen.

The kidneys are commonly congested, and there may be petechial hemorrhage of the mucosa of the urinary bladder, urethra and vulva, or prepuce.

Microscopically, acute lesions are characterized by microvascular thrombosis, and edema and hemorrhage in affected sites recognized at autopsy. In squamous mucosa and skin, capillaries of the proprial and dermal papillae are involved, resulting in vacuolation and necrosis of overlying epithelium. There is a mild, local neutrophilic infiltrate acutely, and a similarly mild mononuclear reaction in the dermis or propria in uncomplicated chronic lesions, which may granulate if widely or deeply ulcerated. Similar microvascular lesions are associated with necrosis and fragmentation of infarcted muscle. Muscle during the reparative phase follows the usual course of regeneration of fibers or fibrous replacement, depending on whether or not the sarcolemma retains its integrity.

In **cattle,** clinical bluetongue is rarely apparent; in endemic areas it may never be evident. Mortality is low, and often it is attributed to secondary infection. Clinical disease may be a function of hypersensitivity in previously exposed animals, and disease in experimentally infected animals is poorly defined. Fever, loss of appetite, and leukopenia are usually seen after an incubation period of 6–8 days, and there may be a drop in milk production in dairy cattle. There is reddening of the epithelium of the mucous membranes, and of thin exposed skin, especially notable on the udder and teats. Edema of the lips and conjunctiva may be present. Salivation may become profuse, and as the disease progresses over the next several days, hyperemia and congestion of the mucosae become more intense. Ulcerations of the gingival, lingual, or buccal mucosa occur, most consistently on the dental pad. There may be necrosis of epithelium on the muzzle. Muscle stiffness is a feature of the disease in some animals. Laminitis, characterized by hyperemia and edema of the sensitive laminae at the coronet, may be apparent, and in some cases, hooves on affected feet may eventually slough. Sloughing or cracking of crusts of necrotic epithelium also may occur on affected parts of the skin, but the ulcerative or erosive defects heal readily. Viral antigen and thrombosis are present in small vessels in affected tissues during the acute phase.

The signs and lesions of **Ibaraki disease** are similar to those of bluetongue in cattle, though more severe in some cases. As well as the signs and lesions described in cattle with bluetongue, there may be difficulty in swallowing in 20–30% of clinically affected animals, and the swollen tongue may protrude from the mouth. At autopsy, in addition to the lesions observable externally, there may be congestion, erosion, or ulceration of the mucosa of the abomasum, and less commonly, the esophagus and forestomachs. Ischemic necrosis and hemorrhage of the striated muscle in the tongue, pharynx, larynx, and esophagus cause the difficulty in swallowing seen clinically, and similar changes are seen in other skeletal muscles. Necrotizing aspiration pneumonia is a sequel to dysphagia in some animals.

The hemorrhagic diseases in bighorn sheep, pronghorn antelope, and white-tailed and black-tailed or mule deer in North America resemble bluetongue in sheep. White-tailed deer may develop a particularly severe and fulminant hemorrhagic disease, with high mortality. There may be necrosis of velvet antler, and hooves may slough in survivors. Bluetongue in goats, though usually inapparent, can resemble bluetongue in sheep.

Bluetongue in sheep must be differentiated from foot-and-mouth disease, *peste des petits ruminants,* contagious ecthyma, and photosensitization in particular. In cattle, the condition must be differentiated from foot-and-mouth disease, vesicular stomatitis, bovine virus diarrhea, rinderpest, malignant head catarrh, and photosensitivity. In Japan, Ibaraki disease must in addition be differentiated, at least clinically, from ephemeral fever, and this would be the case in parts of Australia were bluetongue to produce clinical disease.

In addition to the systemic disease described, abortion, perhaps unobserved, and birth of progeny with various congenital defects, may follow bluetongue infection of pregnant sheep and cattle. In sheep, bluetongue infection of ewes early in gestation may result in hydranencephaly. Anomalous calves produced by bluetongue-infected cattle have excessive gingiva, an enlarged tongue, anomalous maxillae, dwarflike build, and rotations and contractures of the distal extremities. Porencephaly, hydranencephaly, and arthrogryposis are also reported in calves infected *in utero* with bluetongue. Antibody may be sought in neonates which have not sucked, and attempts should be made to isolate virus, since some prenatally infected animals may have immune tolerance, and persistent infection. The anomalies of the brain are considered further with The Nervous System (Volume 1, Chapter 3).

Bibliography

Anderson, G. A. *et al.* Subclinical and clinical bluetongue disease in cattle: Clinical, pathological, and pathogenic considerations. *In* "Bluetongue and Related Orbiviruses," T. L. Barber and M. M. Jochem (eds.), pp. 103–107. New York, Alan R. Liss, 1985.

Baldwin, C. A. *et al.* An outbreak of disease in cattle due to bluetongue virus. *J Vet Diagn Invest* **3:** 252–255, 1991.

Castro, A. E., and Rodgers, S. J. Congenital anomalies in cattle associated with an epizootic of bluetongue virus (Serotype 11). *Bov Pract* **19:** 87–91, 1984.

Erasmus, B. J. Bluetongue in sheep and goats. *Aust Vet J* **51:** 165–170, 228–232, 1975.

Fletch, A. L., and Karstad, L. H. Studies on the pathogenesis of experimental epizootic hemorrhagic disease of white-tailed deer. *Can J Comp Med* **35:** 224–229, 1971.

Forman, A. J., Hooper, P. T., and Le Blanc Smith, P. M. Pathogenicity for sheep of recent Australian bluetongue virus isolates. *Aust Vet J* **66:** 261–262, 1989.

Gorman, B. M. The bluetongue viruses. *Curr Top Microbiol Immunol* **162:** 1–19, 1990.

Hoff, G. L., and Trainer, D. O. Hemorrhagic diseases of wild ruminants. *In* "Infectious Diseases of Wild Mammals," J. W. Davis, L. H. Karstad, and D. O. Trainer (eds.), pp. 45–53. Ames, Iowa, Iowa State University Press, 1981.

Howerth, E. W., Greene, C. E., and Prestwood, A. K. Experimentally induced bluetongue virus infection in white-tailed deer: Coagulation, clinical pathologic, and gross pathologic changes. *Am J Vet Res* **49:** 1906–1913, 1988.

Inaba, Y. Ibaraki disease and its relationship to bluetongue. *Aust Vet J* **51:** 178–185, 1975.

Karstad, L., and Trainer, D. O. Histopathology of experimental bluetongue disease of white-tailed deer. *Can Vet J* **8:** 247–254, 1967.

Kitano, Y., Yamashita, S., and Fukuyama, T. Pathological observations on cattle died of Ibaraki disease. *J Jap Vet Med Assoc* **41:** 884–888, 1988.

Luedke, A. J., and Jones, R. H. Bluetongue: Diagnosis and significance in the bovine animal. *Bov Pract* **19:** 79–86, 1984.

Luedke, A. J. *et al.* Clinical and pathologic features of bluetongue in sheep. *Am J Vet Res* **25:** 963–970, 1964.

MacLachlan, N. J. *et al.* Bluetongue virus-induced encephalopathy in fetal cattle. *Vet Pathol* **22:** 415–417, 1985.

MacLachlan, N. J. *et al.* The pathogenesis of experimental bluetongue virus infection of calves. *Vet Pathol* **27:** 223–229, 1990.

Mahrt, C. R., and Osburn, B. I. Experimental bluetongue virus infection of sheep; effect of vaccination: Pathologic, immunofluorescent, and ultrastructural studies. *Am J Vet Res* **47:** 1198–1203, 1986.

Omori, T. Ibaraki disease: A bovine epizootic disease resembling bluetongue. *Nat Inst Anim Health Q Tokyo* **10** (Suppl.): 45–55, 1970.

Parsonson, I. M. Pathology and pathogenesis of bluetongue infections. *Curr Top Microbiol Immunol* **162:** 119–141, 1990.

Uren, M. F. Clinical and pathological responses of sheep and cattle to experimental infection with five different viruses of the epizootic haemorrhagic disease of deer serogroup. *Aust Vet J* **63:** 199–201, 1986.

Uren, M. F., and Squire, K. R. E. The clinicopathological effect of bluetongue virus serotype 20 in sheep. *Aust Vet J* **58:** 11–15, 1982.

10. Parapoxvirus Infections

a. Bovine Papular Stomatitis Papular stomatitis of cattle occurs worldwide. It generally is an insignificant infection, but needs to be differentiated from other more serious diseases affecting the oral cavity and skin. It is caused by a member of the genus *Parapoxvirus,* which is closely related, but not identical, to the paravaccinia virus which causes pseudocowpox in cattle, and milker's nodules in humans. It is morphologically similar to, and shares antigens with, the virus of contagious ecthyma (orf, contagious pustular dermatitis) of sheep and goats (see the following, and Viral Diseases of Skin, in Volume 1, Chapter 5). However, analysis of the genome indicates that these viruses are distinct.

Bovine papular stomatitis virus is relatively host specific; it grows on tissue cultures and produces cytoplasmic, acidophilic inclusions in infected epithelial cells. Neutralizing antibody is not readily demonstrated. Infection does not confer significant immunity, and successive crops of lesions and relapses can occur. The disease is more common in calves than in older animals, although the susceptibility of, or recrudescence in, the latter may be increased by intercurrent debility, disease such as bovine virus diarrhea, infectious bovine rhinotracheitis, or other stressors.

The papular lesions of this disease occur on the muzzle and in the anterior nares, on the gums, the buccal papillae, the dental pad, the inner aspect of the lips, the hard palate (Fig. 1.100A), the floor of the oral cavity behind the incisors, the ventral and lateral (not dorsal) surfaces of the tongue, and, occasionally in the esophagus (Fig. 1.100B) and forestomach. The lesions may be few or many; they may be transient, or repeated crops of them may take a course of several months.

The initial lesions, which are likely to be detected on the muzzle or lips, are erythematous macules, ~2 mm to 2 cm in diameter. Shortly, the central portion becomes elevated as a low papule, although the elevation is not easy to see, and by the second day a grayish central zone of epithelial hyperplasia has developed on which there is superficial scaliness and necrosis. The lesions expand slowly to assume a coin-shape, maintaining a hyperemic thickened periphery and grayish center; the central necrotic area may slough to form a shallow craterous defect surrounded by a slightly raised red margin. Lesions may coalesce. The course of individual lesions is about a week.

Histologically, there is focal but intense hyperemia and edema in the papillae of the lamina propria, with the accumulation of a few mononuclear leukocytes. The epithelium is thickened, sometimes to twice its normal depth, by hyperplasia and ballooning degeneration in the deeper layers (Fig. 1.100C). The cytoplasm of affected cells is clear, and the nucleus may be shrunken. Dense eosinophilic inclusion bodies lie in the vacuolated cytoplasm, especially in cells at the active margin of the lesion. In the central, more advanced part of the lesion, a mainly neutrophilic infiltrate into the superficial propria and epithelium

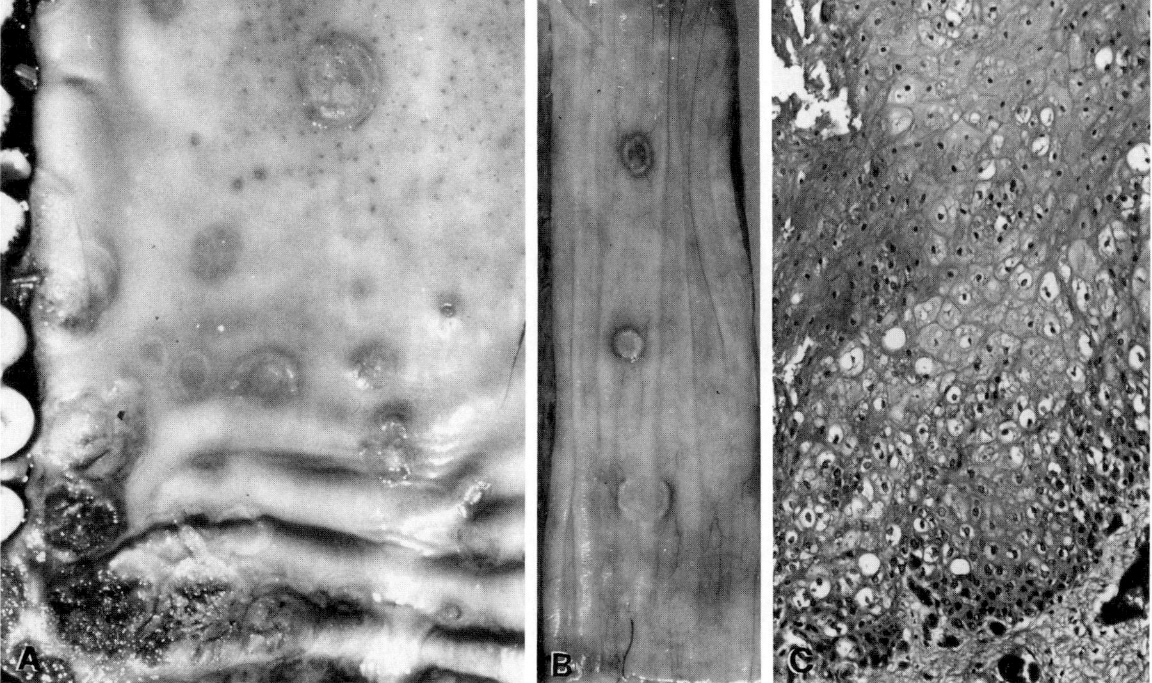

Fig. 1.100 Bovine papular stomatitis. (A) Lesions at various stages of evolution in palate. (B) Lesions in esophagus. (C) Thickened epithelium at the margin of a lesion, with ballooning degeneration of cells in the deeper layers.

is associated with erosion of the upper layers of necrotic cells. The basal layer survives and may be very flattened in eroded areas. Vesicles do not form.

Papular stomatitis is probably more common and widespread than reports indicate. Variation in the extent and gross appearance of the lesions is to be expected, depending on the usual host–parasite factors and the nature of superimposed infections. They may predispose to the development of necrotic stomatitis, and must be differentiated from the lesions of bovine virus diarrhea, alimentary infectious bovine rhinotracheitis, and other causes of ulcers and erosions in the upper alimentary tract. The infection can be transmitted to humans to produce small papules which may persist for several weeks on the skin, usually of the fingers or forearms.

Rapid diagnosis is readily accomplished by demonstration of characteristic parapoxvirus particles, resembling a ball of yarn or a coil of rope—the "clew" morphology—in negatively stained material from lesions examined under the electron microscope.

b. CONTAGIOUS ECTHYMA Contagious ecthyma, also called orf or contagious pustular dermatitis, is a parapoxviral disease of sheep and goats, characterized mainly by proliferative scabby lesions on the lips, face, and feet (see Viral Diseases of Skin, in Volume 1, Chapter 5). Lesions may extend into the oral cavity, involving the tongue, gingiva, dental pad, and palate. Involvement of the esophagus and forestomachs occurs, but is very unusual. In general the evolution of the lesions is similar to that of papular stomatitis of cattle, though they are more exudative and usually much more proliferative. Morbidity may be high, and death can occur in suckling animals. In the upper alimentary tract, lesions may consist of focal red, raised areas, which coalesce to form papules followed by pustules. The latter rupture, and on the muzzle and in the mouth they may become covered by a gray to brown scab, although scab formation may not occur in the mucosa of the upper alimentary tract. Diagnosis is by demonstration or isolation of parapoxvirus.

Bibliography

Baxby, D. Poxvirus infections in domestic animals. *In* "Virus Diseases in Laboratory and Captive Animals," G. Darai (ed.), pp. 17–35. Boston, Massachusetts, Martinus Nijhoff Publishers, 1988.

Carson, C. A., and Kerr, K. M. Bovine papular stomatitis with apparent transmission to man. *J Am Vet Med Assoc* **151:** 183–187, 1967.

Cheville, N. F., and Shey, D. J. Pseudocowpox in dairy cattle. *J Am Vet Med Assoc* **150:** 855–861, 1967.

Crandell, R. A., and Gosser, H. S. Ulcerative esophagitis associated with poxvirus infection in a calf. *J Am Vet Med Assoc* **165:** 282–283, 1974.

Griesemer, R. A., and Cole, C. R. Bovine papular stomatitis. III. Histopathology. *Am J Vet Res* **22:** 482–486, 1961.

Mayr, A., and Büttner, M. Bovine papular stomatitis virus. *In* "Virus Infections of Ruminants," Z. Dinter and B. Morein (eds.), pp. 23–28. Amsterdam, Elsevier, 1990.

Mayr, A., and Büttner, M. Ecthyma (Orf) virus. *In* "Virus Infections of Ruminants," Z. Dinter and B. Morein (eds.), pp. 33–42. Amsterdam, Elsevier, 1990.

Mazur, C., and Machado, R. D. Detection of contagious pustular dermatitis virus of goats in a severe outbreak. *Vet Rec* **125:** 419–420, 1989.

McKeever, D. J. *et al.* Studies of the pathogenesis of orf virus infection in sheep. *J Comp Pathol* **99:** 317–328, 1988.

Robinson, A. J., and Balassu, T. C. Contagious pustular dermatitis (orf). *Vet Bull* **51:** 771–782, 1981.

11. Infectious Bovine Rhinotracheitis

Bovine herpesvirus type 1 (BHV-1) has been associated with a wide range of clinicopathologic syndromes in cattle. These include necrotizing rhinotracheitis, infectious pustular vulvovaginitis and balanoposthitis, vesicular lesions of the udder, abortions, and latent infection (see appropriate chapters).

A systemic form of the disease, which usually involves the alimentary tract, may occur spontaneously in neonatal calves (in which it may be congenital, or acquired shortly after birth) and in feedlot cattle. It has been reproduced experimentally in young calves.

The pathogenesis of systemic infection with BHV-1 is poorly understood. Colostrum-deprived calves are especially susceptible, and the disease can be prevented by feeding colostrum from actively immunized dams. The virus probably spreads from the mucosa of the upper respiratory tract to other tissues by circulating leukocytes. Experimental infection of calves with noncytopathic bovine virus diarrhea virus (NCP-BVD) followed by BHV-1 inoculation results in dissemination of the latter to a variety of tissues. Bovine virus diarrhea virus impairs cell-mediated immunity, and this may allow BHV-1 to escape from the respiratory tract and lead to a systemic infection. Dual infections of BVD-virus and BHV-1 occur under field conditions, but coinfection of these two viruses is not a

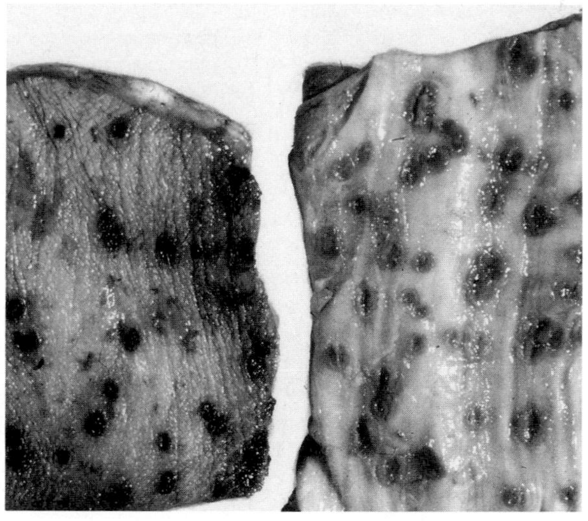

Fig. 1.101 Infectious bovine rhinotracheitis. Foci of necrosis on mucosa of esophagus (right) and rumen (left). Neonatal calf.

prerequisite for the disease to develop. It is suggested that this form of IBR may be due to an antigenic variant of BHV-1. Restriction endonuclease DNA fingerprints have shown that some herpesviruses isolated from encephalitic cases are distinct from BHV-1. However, encephalitis is not commonly part of the systemic syndrome.

Clinically affected animals have fever, leukocytosis, excessive salivation, nasal discharge, inspiratory dyspnea, depression, and often diarrhea. The oral and nasal mucosae are hyperemic, and focal areas of necrosis, erosion, and ulceration from a few millimeters to 3 cm in diameter are located on the nares, dental pad, gums, buccal mucosa, palate, and the caudal, ventral, and dorsal surfaces of the tongue. Characteristically, the lesions tend to be punctate with a slightly raised margin; the necrotic areas are covered by grayish-white layer of fibrinonecrotic exudate, which leaves a raw red base when removed.

The lesions may extend into the esophagus, usually only the upper third, and the forestomachs. In the esophagus, the erosions and ulcers may be irregular, circular, or linear, and often they have a punched-out appearance and a hyperemic border (Fig. 1.101). The ruminal lesions, which are most commonly located in the dorsal and anterior ventral sacs, vary considerably. The earliest lesions consist of foci of necrosis and hemorrhage, a few millimeters in diameter. In some cases, the necrosis may involve almost the entire surface of the ruminal mucosa, which becomes covered by a thick, dirty gray layer of exudate, resembling curdled milk, that adheres tightly to the wall (Fig. 1.102A). Similar lesions may be evident in the reticulum. Focal areas of necrosis result in the formation of holes, as large as 1.5 cm in diameter, in the leaves of the omasum. In addition, these calves may have focal areas of necrosis in the abomasal mucosal folds, which may coalesce to form areas of necrosis 2–3 cm in diameter. The intestines are red and dilated, and the serosal surface may be covered by a thin layer of fibrinous exudate.

The enteric lesions may be accompanied by changes in the upper respiratory tract. When present, the respiratory lesions are similar to those described for older cattle, although they are milder and generally limited to the nasal mucosa, larynx, and upper third of the trachea (see The Respiratory System, Chapter 6 of this volume).

Gray to yellow necrotic foci 2–5 mm diameter may be evident macroscopically on the capsular and cut surfaces of the liver, the adrenal cortices, the spleen, and in Peyer's patches.

Microscopically, the lesions in the squamous mucosa are characterized by focal areas of necrosis (Fig. 1.102B), erosion, and ulceration. A marked leukocytic reaction, predominantly neutrophilic, is evident in the

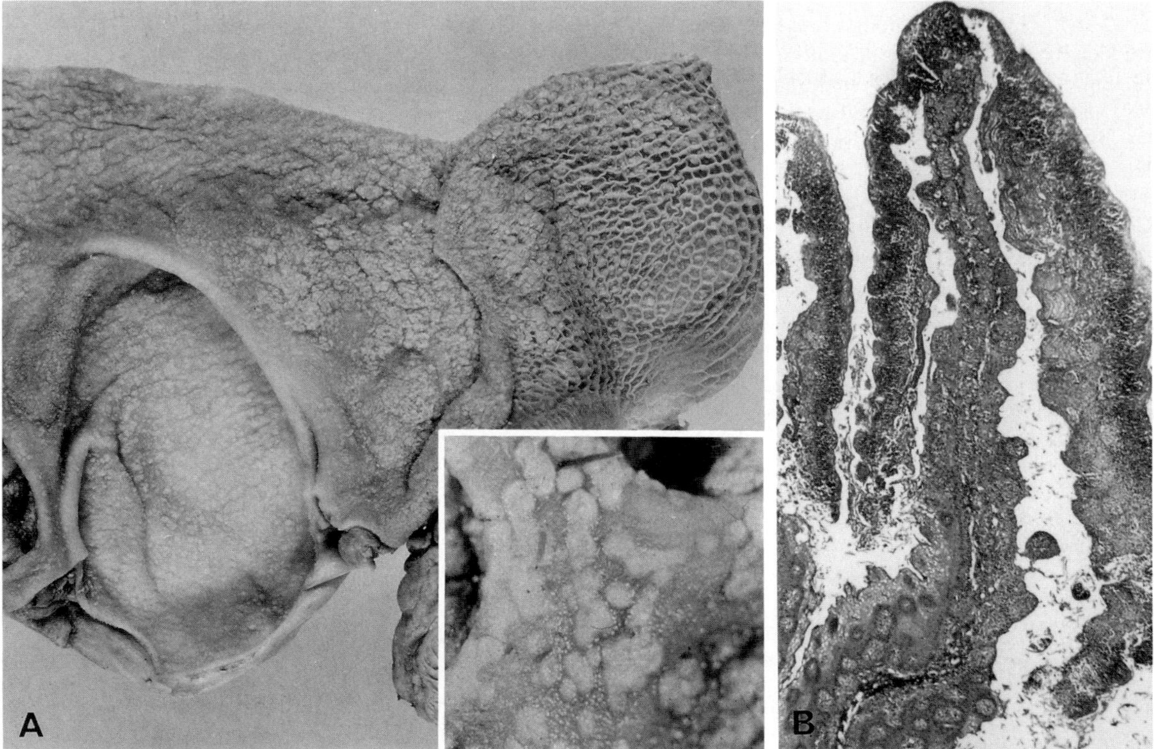

Fig. 1.102 A&B Infectious bovine rhinotracheitis. Neonatal calf. (A) Cheesy necrotic debris in rumen and reticulum. (Inset) Detail of rumen lesion. (B) Necrosis of omasal fold.

basilar areas of the lesions, extending from the underlying lamina propria. The epithelial cells at the periphery of the lesions are markedly swollen, and the cytoplasm is vacuolated. Severe necrosis may involve the entire papilla or mucosa more diffusely. Nuclear inclusions may be present in epithelial cells in the periphery of the lesion, although these are an inconsistent finding. They are more likely to be found if tissues are collected in the early stages of the disease and fixed in Bouin's fluid. The abomasal lesions consist of necrosis of glandular epithelial cells. Affected glands are dilated, and filled with necrotic debris. Focal necrotic lesions involving crypts and lamina propria may be present in both the small intestine (Fig. 1.103) and large bowel. Abomasal and intestinal lesions may predispose to the development of secondary mycosis, which is a common complication.

Foci of coagulation necrosis may occur in the liver, lymph nodes, thymus, Peyer's patches, spleen, and adrenal cortices. Typically, there is little inflammation associated with the necrosis. Herpes inclusions are inconsistently seen in cells at the periphery of the necrotic foci.

The lesions in the upper alimentary tract of cattle associated with bovine herpesvirus infection must be differentiated from those of calf diphtheria, bovine papular stomatitis, and bovine virus diarrhea. Bovine herpesvirus type 1 may be demonstrated in the lesions by means of electron-microscopic examination, fluorescent antibody technique, and tissue culture in a wide variety of systems. The ruminal lesions must be differentiated from those of bovine adenovirus infection and nonspecific rumenitis described elsewhere in this chapter. The liver lesions may be confused with focal necrosis associated with septicemias, for example, listeriosis or salmonellosis (see The Liver and Biliary System, Chapter 2 of this volume).

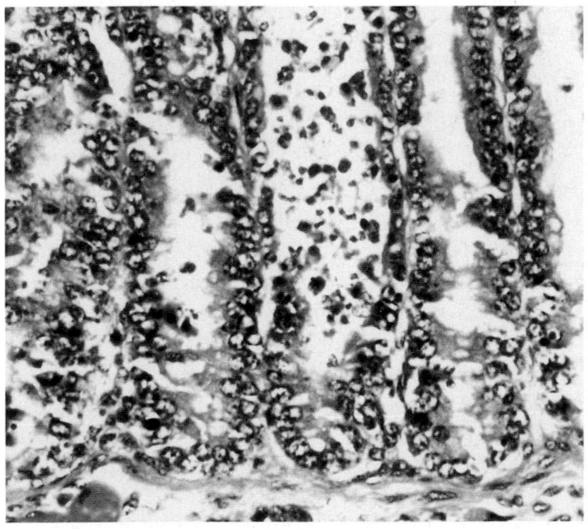

Fig. 1.103 Infectious bovine rhinotracheitis. Necrosis of epithelium in the crypts of Lieberkühn. Small intestine. Neonatal calf.

Bovine herpesvirus-4 (BHV-4), a cytomegalovirus, has been associated with a spectrum of lesions similar to those seen with BHV-1 infection, including enteritis, without a direct cause-and-effect relationship being established. This virus too, has been seen as a concomitant infection with other agents including bovine virus diarrhea virus, sheep-associated malignant catarrhal fever, vesicular stomatitis virus, and Johne's disease. It is thought to have an immunosuppressive effect. Bovine herpesvirus-4 is more difficult to isolate than BHV-1, but immunohistologic techniques and nucleic acid probes may clarify the significance of the former in enteritic lesions of calves. At this time, BHV-4 is considered to be only mildly or nonpathogenic for cattle.

Bibliography

Ehrensperger, F., and Polenz, J. Infektiose Bovine Rhinotracheitis bei Kalbern. *Schweiz Arch Tierheilkd* **121:** 635–642, 1979.

Evermann, J. F., and Henry, B. E., II. Herpetic infections of cattle: A comparison of bovine cytomegalovirus and infectious bovine rhinotracheitis. *Compend Cont Ed Pract Vet* **11:** 205–215, 1989.

Guy, J. S. *et al.* Isolation of bovine herpesvirus-1 from vesicular lesions of the bovine udder. *Am J Vet Res* **45:** 783–785, 1984.

Higgins, R. J., and Edwards, S. Systemic neonatal infectious bovine rhinotracheitis virus infection in suckler calves. *Vet Rec* **119:** 177–178, 1986.

Mechor, G. D. *et al.* Protection of newborn calves against fatal multisystemic infectious bovine rhinotracheitis by feeding colostrum from vaccinated cows. *Can J Vet Res* **51:** 452–459, 1987.

Miller, R. B., Smith, M. W., and Lawson, K. F. Some lesions observed in calves born to cows exposed to the virus of infectious bovine rhinotracheitis in the last trimester of gestation. *Can J Comp Med* **42:** 438–445, 1978.

Pálfi, V., Glávits, R., and Hornyák, A. The pathology of concurrent bovine viral diarrhoea and infectious bovine rhinotracheitis virus infection in newborn calves. *Acta Vet Hung* **37:** 89–95, 1989.

Potgieter, L. N. D. *et al.* Effect of bovine viral diarrhea virus infection on the distribution of infectious bovine rhinotracheitis virus in calves. *Am J Vet Res* **45:** 687–690, 1984.

Reed, D. E., Bicknell, E. J., and Bury, R. J. Systemic form of infectious bovine rhinotracheitis in young calves. *J Am Vet Med Assoc* **163:** 753–755, 1973.

Rogers, R. J. *et al.* Bovine herpesvirus-1 infection of the upper alimentary tract of cattle and its association with a severe mortality. *Aust Vet J* **54:** 562–565, 1978.

Thiry, E. *et al.* Bovine herpesvirus-4 (BHV-4) infections of cattle. *In* "Herpesvirus Diseases of Cattle, Horses, and Pigs," G. Wittmann (ed.), pp. 96–115. Boston, Massachusetts, Kluwer Academic Publishers, 1989.

12. Caprine Herpesvirus

A herpesvirus that shares some antigens with, but on the basis of restriction endonuclease analysis is distinct from, bovine herpesvirus-1, has been isolated from neonatal goat kids in California, New Zealand, Australia, Fiji, and Switzerland. The nomenclature for this virus is confusing. The sheep and goat herpesviruses belong to the bovid herpesviridae but are excluded from the subfamily bovine herpesvirus 2. Taxonomically, the sheep and goat herpesviruses have been designated as caprine herpesvirus 1 and 2, respectively. More recently, the goat herpesvirus has been referred to as caprine herpesvirus 1, and that designation is preferred here. This virus causes severe systemic disease with erosions and ulcerations of the alimentary tract in neonatal goats. Adult goats may be latent carriers, or develop vulvovaginitis or balanoposthitis (see The Female Genital System, Volume 3, Chapter 4). Experimental infection of pregnant does causes abortion. The virus is nonpathogenic for calves and lambs.

The disease in neonatal kids is characterized clinically by fever, conjunctivitis, ocular and nasal discharges, dyspnea, anorexia, abdominal pain, weakness, and death, usually within 1–4 days after onset of clinical signs. Affected kids have leukopenia and hypoproteinemia.

Macroscopic lesions are most obvious throughout the entire alimentary tract. Round or longitudinal erosions, which have a hyperemic border, are evident in the oral mucosa. These are particularly prominent on the gums around the incisor teeth and to a lesser extent in the pharynx and esophagus. Focal red areas of necrosis, which may be slightly elevated above the surrounding mucosa, occur in the rumen. In the abomasum numerous longitudinal, red erosions are located in the mucosa. The most severe lesions occur in the cecum and ascending colon, which are dilated, with a thickened wall, and contain focal to large areas of mucosal necrosis and ulceration, frequently covered by a pseudodiphtheritic membrane. The contents are yellow and mucoid. Hemorrhagic foci may be visible in the bladder mucosa.

Microscopically, the lesions in the upper alimentary tract are typical areas of necrosis and erosion of the squamous epithelial cells. The epithelial cells at the periphery of the necrotic areas are swollen and vacuolated, and these may contain herpes inclusions. There is marked inflammatory reaction in the underlying lamina propria. The abomasal lesions consist of acute foci of mucosal necrosis. Inclusions are particularly evident in this area. Lesions in the cecum and colon are more extensive and consist of large areas of mucosal ulceration and necrosis, which may involve the entire thickness of the wall. The submucosa is edematous and markedly infiltrated by inflammatory cells. The mesenteric nodes are edematous, and the germinal centers are depleted of lymphoid cells. Focal areas of necrosis with a mild inflammatory cell reaction are evident in the bladder mucosa.

The alimentary lesions in goat kids in many respects resemble the lesions in calves infected with bovine herpesvirus type 1. Focal areas of necrosis, which are often present in other organs, such as liver, spleen, and adrenal glands, in calves, are not reported in goats.

The virus may be isolated on various tissue cultures, including bovine turbinate, fetal lung, and caprine choroid plexus. Virus may be demonstrated in tissues and cell cultures with immunohistochemistry and electron microscopy.

Bibliography

Berrios, P. E., McKercher, D. G., and Knight, H. D. Pathogenicity of a caprine herpesvirus. *Am J Vet Res* **36:** 1763–1769, 1975.

Brake, F., and Studdert, M. J. Molecular epidemiology and pathogenesis of ruminant herpesviruses including bovine, buffalo, and caprine herpesviruses 1 and bovine encephalitis herpesvirus. *Aust Vet J* **62:** 331–334, 1985.

Mettler, F. *et al.* Herpesvirus-infektion bei Zicklein in der Schweiz. *Schweiz Arch Tierheilk* **121:** 655–662, 1979.

Mohanty, S. B., and Hyllseth, B. Other herpesviruses. *In* "Virus Infections of Ruminants," Z. Dinter and B. Morein (eds.), pp. 151–157. Amsterdam, Elsevier Science Publishers, 1990.

Saito, J. *et al.* A new herpesvirus isolate from goats: Preliminary report. *Am J Vet Res* **35:** 847–848, 1974.

Scott, F. M. M. Bovine herpesvirus 2 infections. *In* "Herpesvirus Diseases of Cattle, Horses, and Pigs," G. Wittmann (ed.), p. 80. Boston, Massachusetts, Kluwer Academic Publishers, 1989.

Tisdall, D. J. *et al.* New Zealand caprine herpesvirus: Comparison with an Australian isolate and with bovine herpesvirus type 1 by restriction endonuclease analysis. *N Z Vet J* **32:** 99–100, 1984.

13. Other Herpesviruses

Canine herpesvirus causes a systemic disease of neonatal puppies, which is characterized by foci of necrosis and hemorrhage in a wide variety of organs, especially the lungs and renal cortices (see Herpesvirus Infections of the Fetus and Newborn, in the Female Genital System, Volume 3, Chapter 4). Focal areas of necrosis may occur in the intestine as part of the systemic syndrome.

Feline viral rhinotracheitis virus (feline herpesvirus-1) causes alimentary tract lesions (see Erosive and Ulcerative Stomatitides, Section I,C,4,d of this chapter). Viruses antigenically related to feline herpesvirus-1 have been isolated from dogs with diarrhea, but descriptions of lesions are not available.

Natural infections with **Aujeszky's disease virus** often result in necrotizing tonsillitis. Experimental infection of pigs with this virus may cause a necrotizing enteritis of the distal small intestine. The enteric lesions are characterized by focal areas of necrosis of the cryptal mucosa, muscularis mucosae, and tunica muscularis, and necrosis of the neurons of Meissner's and Auerbach's plexuses. Nuclear inclusions may be found in cryptal epithelial cells and neurons of the autonomic plexuses.

Necrotizing enterocolitis in adult horses may occur because of **equine herpesvirus-1.** At necropsy, there are multiple areas of hemorrhage, necrosis, and ulceration, some several centimeters in diameter, of the mucosa in both small and large intestine. Microscopically, these lesions consist of erosions and ulcerations of the mucosa, and necrosis of cryptal epithelial cells in adjacent areas. Cryptal epithelial cells and some proprial mononuclear cells may have acido- and amphophilic nuclear inclusions.

Ultrastructurally, there are numerous herpesvirus particles in the nuclei.

Bibliography

Evermann, J. F. *et al.* Diarrheal condition in dogs associated with viruses antigenically related to feline herpesvirus. *Cornell Vet* **72:** 285–291, 1982.

Narita, M. *et al.* Necrotizing enteritis in piglets associated with Aujeszky's disease virus infection. *Vet Pathol* **21:** 450–452, 1984.

Pensaert, M. B., and Kluge, J. P. Pseudorabies (Aujeszky's disease). *In* "Virus Infections of Porcines," M.B. Pensaert (ed.), pp. 39–70. Amsterdam, Elsevier Science Publishers, 1989.

14. Adenovirus Enteritis

The adenoviruses which have been associated with enteric infections in humans, cattle, swine, horses, sheep, and dogs belong to the Adenoviridae, genus *Mastadenovirus*. Serologic surveys show that widely divergent serotypes occur both within and between host species, and their distribution is worldwide. All serotypes are morphologically similar; the virus consists of a nonenveloped icosahedral capsid, 70–80 nm in diameter, that has 252 capsomeres. Virus neutralization tests are used to distinguish serotypes. *In vivo* and *in vitro* infection of cells results in the formation of both Cowdry type A and B nuclear inclusions. Adenoviruses are relatively heat resistant and can survive for several days at room temperature. Most adenoviruses are transmitted by feces, aerosols, or possibly fomites, to susceptible, usually suckling or recently weaned, animals. Infected animals may remain carriers for weeks.

Adenoviruses are highly host specific. Infections in both humans and animals appear, in general, to be subclinical, and disease seems to occur more commonly in immunologically compromised individuals. Most infections are systemic; certain strains have a tropism for the respiratory tract, and others, for the alimentary tract, vascular endothelial cells, or hepatocytes. Their enteric manifestations will be considered here.

Bibliography

Benfield, D. A. Enteric adenovirus infections of animals. *In* "Viral Diarrheas of Man and Animals," L. J. Saif and K. W. Theil (eds.), pp. 115–135. Boca Raton, Florida, CRC Press, 1990.

a. BOVINE ADENOVIRUSES There are nine different serotypes of bovine adenovirus that are divided into two antigenically distinct subgroups on the basis of replication in tissue cultures. Infection has been mainly associated with keratoconjunctivitis and respiratory disease. Many strains have been isolated from normal cattle. Serotypes 1–8 have all been associated with a pneumoenteritis complex. Experimental infection with most strains usually produces only a mild respiratory infection, and Koch's postulates have not been fulfilled for the enteric form of the disease. It appears that after an initial viremic stage, the virus localizes in the endothelial cells of vessels in a variety of organs, resulting in thrombosis with subsequent focal areas of ischemic necrosis.

Clinically, enteric infections with bovine adenovirus occur sporadically in 1- to 8-week-old calves and in feedlot animals. Affected animals have fever, and diarrhea which may contain blood. They are dehydrated, and the mucous membranes of the muzzle and mouth are congested. Dry, encrusted exudate may cover the muzzle, and there may be serous to mucopurulent ocular and nasal discharges.

The macroscopic lesions may be present in the forestomachs, abomasum, and intestine. Those in the forestomachs are characterized by irregular, raised, red to gray necrotic areas, 2–4 mm in diameter on the mucosa of both the dorsal and ventral sacs of the rumen. In some cases the areas of necrosis coalesce to give rise to a diffuse necrotizing rumenitis. Ulcers as large as 1.5 cm in diameter may be located on the ruminal pillars, and these may be visible through the serosa. Similar lesions may be evident in the omasum. The abomasal mucosal folds are edematous and congested, with focal necrosis and ulceration in the mucosa which, like those in the forestomachs, may be visible on the serosal surface.

The intestinal lesions vary from slight dilation and distension with excessive fluid to severe multifocal or diffuse necrosis, which may be covered by a pseudodiphtheritic membrane. In young calves, the lesions are most severe in the jejunum and ileum, especially over the Peyer's patches. In feedlot cattle the lesions may be most prominent in the colon. The mucosa is dark red (Fig. 1.104), and there is marked edema of the mesocolon. The mesenteric lymph nodes are enlarged and edematous.

Microscopically, large basophilic to amphophilic inclusions completely or partially fill the nuclei of endothelium in the vessels of the lamina propria and submucosa of affected areas of the rumen, abomasum, and intestine. The endothelial cells are swollen and necrotic, and some veins and lymphatics contain thrombi. Foci of ischemic necrosis are evident in the overlying mucosa, and in more advanced lesions, the necrosis extends across the muscularis mucosae. Fibrinocellular exudate often covers the mucosal surface (Fig. 1.105A,B). Intestinal crypts are dilated, lined by flat epithelial cells, and usually contain necrotic debris. There is usually marked submucosal edema, congestion, and fibrinous exudation. Foci of necrosis are evident in the lymphoid follicles of the Peyer's patches, which are also depleted of lymphocytes.

Typical inclusions may also be found in endothelial cells of vessels and sinusoids of the adrenal glands, mesenteric lymph nodes, liver, spleen, glomeruli and interstitial capillaries in the kidney, and in the mucosa of the urinary bladder. Ultrastructurally, adenovirus particles are located in large numbers in the nuclei of endothelial cells.

Confirmation of enteric bovine adenovirus infection depends on the demonstration of the typical intranuclear

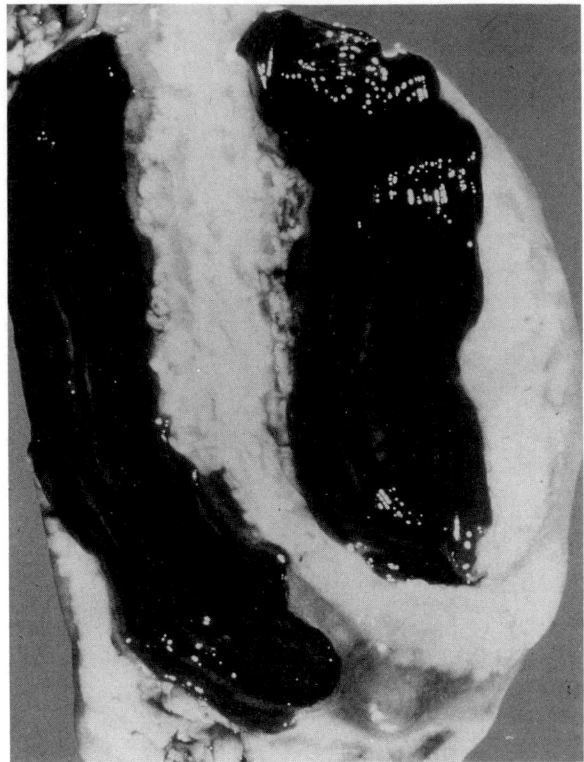

Fig. 1.104 Bovine adenovirus infection. Congested and hemorrhagic colon.

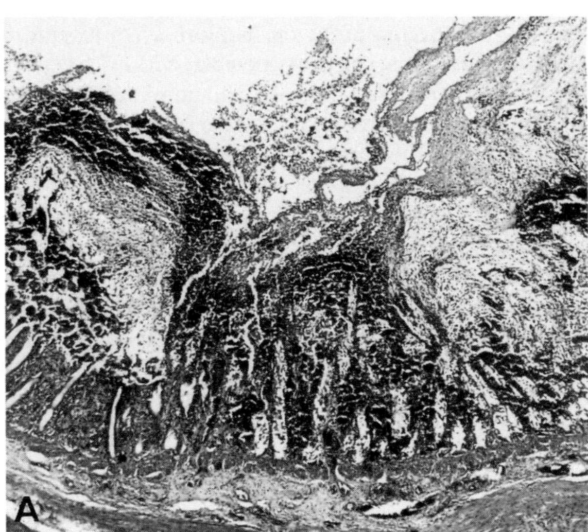

Fig. 1.105A Bovine adenovirus infection. (A) Infarctive necrosis and hemorrhage.

inclusions in endothelial cells, the ultrastructural presence of virus particles, and isolation of the virus in tissue cell cultures. The latter is often difficult because different serotypes and strains of the virus require specific tissue cell cultures, and several blind passages may be required before cytopathic changes are evident.

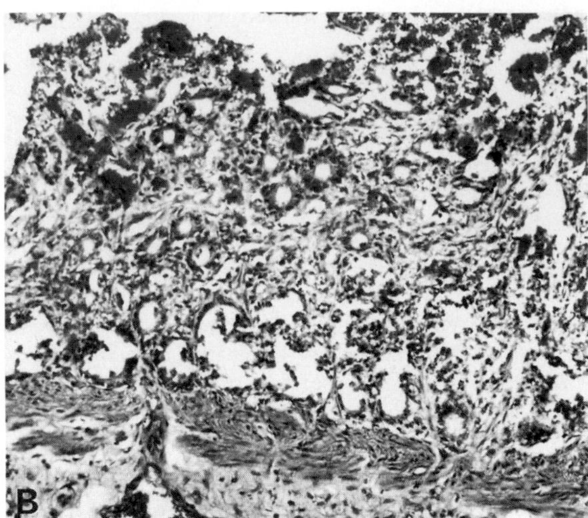

Fig. 1.105B Bovine adenovirus infection. (B) Infarctive necrosis and hemorrhage. Colon.

Bibliography

Bulmer, W. S., Tsai, K. S., and Little, P. B. Adenovirus infection in two calves. *J Am Vet Med Assoc* **166:** 233–238, 1975.

Horner, G. W., Hunter, R., and Thompson, E. J. Isolation and characterization of a new adenovirus serotype from a yearling heifer with systemic infection. *N Z Vet J* **28:** 165–167, 1982.

Mattson, D. E. Adenovirus infection in cattle. *J Am Vet Med Assoc* **163:** 894–896, 1973.

Mattson, D. E. Naturally occurring infection of calves with a bovine adenovirus. *Am J Vet Res* **34:** 623–629, 1973.

Mattson, D. E., Norman, B. B., and Dunbar, J. R. Bovine adenovirus type-3 infection in feedlot calves. *Am J Vet Res* **49:** 67–69, 1988.

Orr, J. P. Necrotizing enteritis in a calf infected with adenovirus. *Can Vet J* **25:** 72–74, 1984.

Reed, D. E., Wheeler, J. G., and Lupton, H. W. Isolation of bovine adenovirus type 7 from calves with pneumonia and enteritis. *Am J Vet Res* **39:** 1968–1971, 1978.

Scanziani, E. *et al.* Adenoviral fibrinous enteritis in calves. *Dtsch Tierarztl Wschr* **96:** 165–168, 1989.

Smyth, J. A. *et al.* Adenovirus-associated enterocolitis in a bullock. *Vet Rec* **119:** 574–576, 1986.

Thompson, K. G., Thomson, G. W., and Henry, J. N. Alimentary tract manifestations of bovine adenovirus infections. *Can Vet J* **22:** 68–71, 1981.

b. Porcine Adenovirus There are four different serotypes of adenoviruses in swine, which, according to serological surveys, are all common. Serotype 4 appears to be the most widely distributed strain of the virus in Europe and North America. Asymptomatic infections are most common in swine, and the virus may be isolated from feces of normal pigs.

The importance of adenoviruses as a cause of enteric disease in the field remains controversial. In Belgium, serotype 3 has been associated with diarrhea, occasional vomiting, dehydration, and reduced growth rate in 2- to 3-week-old pigs. Experimental oronasal infection of

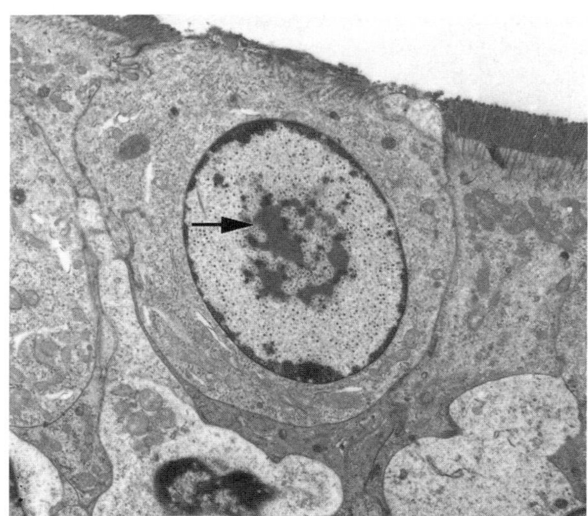

Fig. 1.106 Porcine adenovirus infection. Adenovirus-infected cell in epithelium of dome over Peyer's patch. Note inclusion (arrow). (Courtesy of D. M. Hoover and S. E. Sanford.)

hysterotomy-derived, colostrum-deprived pigs with this same serotype produces nonfatal diarrhea, after an incubation period of about 3–4 days. Diarrhea has also been produced experimentally with serotype 4 and other strains of the virus. Other lesions produced with serotype 4 are interstitial pneumonia, nonsuppurative meningoencephalitis, and focal interstitial nephritis. In general these lesions do not appear to cause clinical disease.

The macroscopic lesions in the intestine consist of excessive yellow watery to pasty contents and moderate enlargement of the mesenteric lymph nodes, which cannot be differentiated from other causes of diarrhea in neonatal pigs.

In contrast to the situation in calves, where the inclusions are located in the nuclei of endothelial cells, in pigs the inclusions are in enterocytes in the distal jejunum and ileum, where primary viral replication probably occurs. In experimentally inoculated animals, viral antigens may be demonstrated on enterocytes as early as 24 hr postinfection. Initially, the inclusions are amphophilic to basophilic and fill the entire nucleus, and the nuclear membrane is thickened. In later stages of the infection, the inclusions are smaller and are surrounded by a halo. The infected nuclei are enlarged, round, and displaced to the apical portion of the cell. The inclusions are mainly located in cells on the tips and sides of the villi, which may be short and blunt. They are often seen in epithelium, and occasionally associated lymphocytes, on the dome over Peyer's patches. They may persist as long as 45 days postinfection. There may be a moderate mononuclear cell reaction in the lamina propria. Inclusions are also found in the squamous epithelial cells of the tonsils.

Ultrastructurally, infected nuclei of enterocytes are round and swollen and contain numerous typical adenovirus particles (Fig 1.106). Affected enterocytes are cuboidal, and the apical portion protrudes slightly into the lumen. The cell membrane and microvilli are irregular, and the terminal web is absent. The rough endoplasmic reticulum shows local distension with formation of large multivesicular bodies. Eventually, there is complete loss of microvilli, and the cell membrane ruptures with the release of cell contents and virus particles into the gut lumen.

The presence of inclusions in enterocytes must be interpreted with caution. A survey in Canada revealed that 4.4% of 5-day-old to 24-week-old pigs had adenovirus inclusions in enterocytes, mainly in the ileum. More than 50% of the pigs had diarrhea; however, other enteropathogens were found in most of these animals. Enteric adenovirus infection may be an incidental infection, and more research is needed to determine the prevalence and significance of adenovirus infections in swine.

Bibliography

Abid, H. N., Holscher, M. A., and Byerly, C. S. An outbreak of adenovirus enteritis in piglets. *Vet Med Small Anim Clin* **79:** 105–107, 1984.

Coussement, W. *et al.* Adenovirus enteritis in pigs. *Am J Vet Res* **42:** 1905–1911, 1981.

Coussement, W. *et al.* Adenovirus enteritis bij varkens, een pathologische en epizootiologische studie. Adenovirus infection in swine, a pathological and epizootiological study. *VLAAMS Diergeneeskundig Tijdschrift* **52:** 167–176, 1983.

Derbyshire, J. B. Porcine adenovirus. *In* "Virus Infections of Porcines," M. B. Pensaert (ed.), pp. 73–80. Amsterdam, Elsevier Science Publishers, 1989.

Ducatelle, R., Coussement, W., and Hoorens, J. Sequential pathological study of experimental porcine adenovirus enteritis. *Vet Pathol* **19:** 179–189, 1982.

Sanford, S. E., and Hoover, D. M. Enteric adenovirus infection in pigs. *Can J Comp Med* **47:** 396–400, 1983.

c. Equine Adenovirus Two adenovirus serotypes have been identified in horses. Equine adenovirus serotype 1 has a worldwide distribution. Subclinical infections are common. Clinical disease occurs mainly as an upper respiratory infection in foals younger than 3 months. The infection is particularly important in Arabian foals with combined immunodeficiency, in which intestinal involvement is common. The virus is capable of replication in the intestinal epithelium and produces duodenal villus atrophy after experimental infection.

Another adenovirus, proposed to be a prototype of equine adenovirus serotype 2, has been isolated in Australia from foals with diarrhea. Rotavirus was also identified in the feces of these foals. A serologic survey showed that 77% of adult horses in the area had neutralizing antibodies to this particular serotype.

There is a single case report of an unidentified alimentary tract adenovirus infection in an Arabian foal which did not have lesions of combined immunodeficiency. The foal had diarrhea and progressive weight loss over a 2-month period. The macroscopic lesions consisted of ulcers in the distal esophagus and nonglandular mucosa of the stomach. The intestine contained soft to semifluid ingesta. Histologically, there was necrosis and ulceration of the esophageal and gastric squamous mucosa. Typical adenoviral inclusions were found at all levels of the small intestine. These were most commonly located in the villous epithelial cells, less often in the crypts, and only occasionally in the submucosal glands. There was focal to diffuse villus atrophy through the small intestine.

Bibliography

Corrier, D. E., Montgomery, D., and Scutchfield, W. L. Adenovirus in the intestinal epithelium of a foal with prolonged diarrhea. *Vet Pathol* **19:** 564–567, 1982.

Gleeson, L. J., Studdert, M. J., and Sullivan, N. D. Pathogenicity and immunological studies of equine adenovirus in specific-pathogen-free foals. *Am J Vet Res* **39:** 1636–1642, 1978.

Studdert, M. J., and Blackney, M. H. Isolation of an adenovirus antigenically distinct from equine adenovirus type 1 from diarrheic foal feces. *Am J Vet Res* **43:** 543–544, 1982.

d. ADENOVIRUSES IN OTHER SPECIES Six serotypes of adenovirus have been isolated from **sheep.** Serotypes 1, 2, and 3 have been recovered from feces of normal sheep, and lambs with enteritis and pneumoenteritis. Serotype 1 has been isolated, in France, from feces of a diarrheic lamb, which also had coccidiosis. Experimental inoculation of specific pathogen-free lambs with serotype 4 did not cause disease, but the virus was reisolated from feces and nasal secretions for several days postinfection. Colostrum-deprived lambs inoculated with serotype 5 developed diarrhea and nasal discharge, but lesions were confined to the respiratory tract. Serotypes 4, 5, and 6 have been associated mainly with respiratory disease. Some serotypes may replicate and persist in the alimentary tract of sheep, but there is no information on the pathogenesis and lesions associated with the virus in this site. Ovine adenoviruses and bovine adenovirus-2 have been associated with fatal cases of pneumoenteritis in fattening lambs in eastern Europe.

Two distinct but serologically related adenoviruses have been isolated from **dogs.** Canine adenovirus-1 infection is usually subclinical, but it may cause infectious hepatitis, and diarrhea may be present in these cases. The virus has a particular tropism for hepatocytes and endothelial cells. The serosal hemorrhages in the gastrointestinal tract and possibly the diarrhea may be related to vascular damage in the serosa and mucosa respectively (see The Liver and Biliary System, Chapter 2 of this volume). Canine adenovirus-2 (Toronto A26/61) is usually associated with upper respiratory infections in dogs (see The Respiratory System, Chapter 6 of this volume). Viruses serologically similar to canine adenovirus-2 have been isolated from feces of diarrheic dogs. DNA fingerprinting of two of these isolates indicated that they are distinct from canine adenovirus-2.

It may be that the fecal isolates are due to swallowing of virus originating from upper respiratory tract infections, or small changes in the DNA sequence which allow the virus to replicate in the alimentary tract. Further experimental infections are required to determine the significance of these isolates in dogs with enteric disease.

Bibliography

Belák, S. Ovine adenoviruses. *In* "Virus Infections of Ruminants," Z. Dinter and B. Morein (eds.), pp. 171–185. Amsterdam, Elsevier Science Publishers, 1990.

Hamelin, C., Jouveene, P., and Assaf, R. Genotypic characterization of type-2 variants of canine adenovirus. *Am J Vet Res* **47:** 625–630, 1986.

Macartney, L., Cavanagh, H. M. A., and Spibey, N. Isolation of canine adenovirus-2 from the faeces of dogs with enteric disease and its unambiguous typing by restriction endonuclease mapping. *Res Vet Sci* **44:** 9–14, 1988.

Sharp, J. M., Rushton, B., and Rimer, R. D. Experimental infection of specific pathogen-free lambs with ovine adenovirus type 4. *J Comp Pathol* **86:** 621–628, 1976.

15. Enteric Coronavirus Infections

Coronaviruses cause disease affecting a number of organ systems in a variety of species, many of which are outside our scope. Among domestic mammals they cause mainly enteric infections; the major exceptions are feline infectious peritonitis, hemagglutinating encephalomyelitis virus of swine, respiratory strains of transmissible gastroenteritis virus of pigs (which do not infect gut significantly), and bovine coronavirus (which infects both gut and respiratory tract). Replication of enteric coronaviruses in the oronasopharyngeal mucosa may produce large doses of virus, which infect the gut when swallowed.

Coronavirus is the only genus in the Coronaviridae. These viruses have a single-stranded RNA genome. They are pleomorphic or roughly spherical and vary in size from about 70–200 nm in diameter, averaging ~100–130 nm. They have a phospholipid-bearing envelope, probably derived in part from host cell membrane. They gain their name from the characteristic corona of petal- or droplet-shaped radial surface projections (peplomers) visible under the electron microscope in negatively stained preparations.

The coronaviruses infecting each species of host appear to be distinctive; some species are infected by more than one type of coronavirus. There are antigenic relationships among viruses from various hosts, and experimental cross infection will occur between some host species, usually without pathologic consequences. Transmissible gastroenteritis virus, feline infectious peritonitis virus, feline enteric coronavirus, and canine coronavirus are in one antigenic group. Bovine coronavirus is antigenically related to hemagglutinating encephalomyelitis virus of swine, mouse hepatitis virus, and rat coronavirus, among others. Persistent infections can occur.

Virus replication in the intestinal epithelium by coronaviruses is similar in all the species studied. Coronavirus infects and replicates in the apical cytoplasm of absorptive enterocytes on the tips and sides of intestinal villi. Virions are probably taken up by the apical border of the cell, by fusion with the plasmalemma. Replication and maturation appear to involve budding of virions from the cytosol through the membrane and into the lumen of vacuoles or cisternae in the smooth endoplasmic reticulum, where they accumulate. Virions are found in tubules of the Golgi apparatus. They may exit via that route from infected cells, by exocytosis at the apical cell membrane, or on the lateral cell surface, since virus particles are often seen lined up between microvilli or in the lateral intercellular space between infected cells. Virus may also be released by lysis of infected cells. Coronaviruses will also infect some mesenchymal cells in villi and probably mesenteric lymph nodes.

Changes in the infected cell occur by about 12–24 hr after infection. Mitochondria in virus-infected cells swell, cisternae of smooth and rough endoplasmic reticulum dilate, the cytoplasm of infected cells loses its electron density, and cells lose their columnar profile. The terminal web is fragmented; microvilli swell and become irregular, perhaps in association with blebbing of the apical membrane. Damaged epithelium may lyse *in situ*, releasing virus retained in cytoplasmic vacuoles, or it may exfoliate into the lumen. Profuse diarrhea usually begins about the time that early cytologic changes are becoming apparent, but before there is extensive epithelial exfoliation.

Exfoliation of damaged epithelium may be massive over a relatively short period, leading to the development of villus atrophy, the severity of which largely reflects the degree of initial viral damage. Villi may appear fused along their sides or tips, and during the exfoliative phase, some villi with denuded tips may be present. The enterocytes present on villi shortly after the initial exfoliative episode are mainly poorly differentiated low columnar, cuboidal, or squamous cells, with stubby irregular microvilli. Within 2–3 days, villi begin to regenerate, and the epithelium becomes progressively more columnar, though still lacking a well-developed brush border and its complement of enzymes. Defective fat absorption is reflected in the accumulation of lipid droplets in the cytoplasm of enterocytes on villi. This is particularly marked over the period of about 2–5 days after experimental inoculation.

With progressive epithelial regeneration from the crypts, the villus fusion, which may be the result of adhesion of temporarily denuded lamina propria of adjacent villi, regresses. Separation begins along the basal margins of the adhesions and progresses toward the tips of the villi. There may be focal acute inflammation in the lamina propria of temporarily denuded villi, and a mild mononuclear infiltrate in the stroma of collapsed villi. Though several cycles of virus replication may occur, poorly differentiated enterocytes appear relatively refractory to infection, and the virus titer falls, presumably as local immune mechanisms also come into play. Hyperplasia of epithelium in crypts usually results in eventual resolution of the villus atrophy, restoring normal function.

The diarrhea that occurs is a result of electrolyte and nutrient malabsorption, with some contribution by secretion from cells in crypts, and probably by poorly differentiated surface epithelium in the reparative phase. Mechanisms of diarrhea in villus atrophy are discussed with the Pathophysiology of Diarrhea (Section VI,J,2 of this chapter). Remission of signs occurs within about 4–6 days as regeneration of villi occurs, provided the animal survives the dehydration, electrolyte depletion, and acidosis brought about by diarrhea.

Bibliography

Möstl, K. Coronaviridae, pathogenetic and clinical aspects: An update. *Comp Immunol Microbiol Infect Dis* **13:** 169–180, 1990.

Saif, L. J. Comparative aspects of enteric viral infections. *In* "Viral Diarrheas of Man and Animals," L. J. Saif and K. W. Theil (eds.), pp. 9–31. Boca Raton, Florida, CRC Press, 1990.

Saif, L. J, and Heckert, R. A. Enteropathogenic coronaviruses. *In* "Viral Diarrheas of Man and Animals," L. J. Saif and K. W. Theil (eds.), pp. 185–252. Boca Raton, Florida, CRC Press, 1990.

a. SWINE Three coronaviruses cause gastrointestinal signs in swine. Hemagglutinating encephalomyelitis virus causes vomiting and wasting disease in suckling piglets; this is a condition mediated mainly by infection of the central and peripheral nervous system (see The Nervous System, Volume 1, Chapter 3). Transmissible gastroenteritis virus and porcine epidemic diarrhea virus (coronavirus 777) both cause syndromes of acute diarrheal disease in all age groups, and chronic diarrhea and runting in weaned pigs. In some areas, coronaviruses, especially transmissible gastroenteritis, are the major cause of diarrhea in neonatal swine.

Transmissible gastroenteritis (TGE) may affect swine of any age, causing vomition, severe diarrhea, and, in piglets, high mortality. The disease is recognized throughout most of the world, including the United Kingdom, Europe, all of North America, Central and South America, and the Far East. Australia and New Zealand seem to be free.

The epizootiology of TGE depends on the overall immune status of the herd and of the various age groups within the herd. Introduction of virus into a naive herd results in a rapid spread of disease with high morbidity affecting all age groups. Sows and older pigs will show transient inappetence, possibly diarrhea, and perhaps vomition. Signs may be more severe in sows exposed to high virus challenge from infected baby pigs. Agalactia may occur in recently farrowed sows, perhaps related to TGE infection of the mammary gland. Suckling piglets develop severe diarrhea, and mortality may approach 100% in piglets younger than 10–14 days. Older pigs usually develop less severe signs and have lower mortality. In herds with enzootic infection, high piglet mortality may occur in the offspring of recently introduced naive sows,

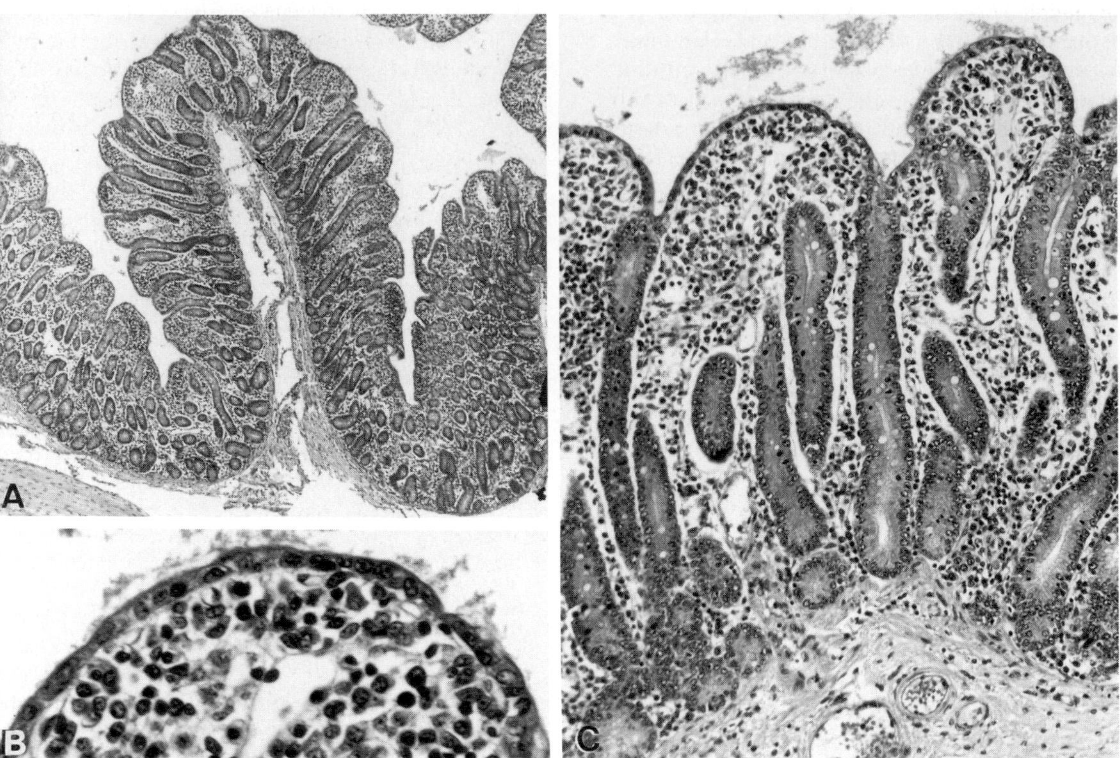

Fig. 1.107 Transmissible gastroenteritis. Pig. (A) Atrophy of villi in small intestine. (B) Enterocytes on surface of atrophic villus. (C) Atrophy of villi, with hypertrophy of crypts of Lieberkühn. Surface epithelium is cuboidal or flattened.

and diarrhea with lower mortality may occur in piglets older than about 2–3 weeks as milk intake and concomitant lactogenic immunity wane. Infected pigs in the late suckling or weanling age group may runt. Transmissible gastroenteritis is more prevalent in the winter months, perhaps because the virus is not resistant to summer environmental conditions of warmth and sunlight. Baby pigs which are chilled also seem less able to survive the effects of infection.

The severity of disease in baby pigs is related partly to their inability to withstand dehydration, due to their small size, and to their susceptibility to hypoglycemia. Probably as significant is the differentiation, and low rate of turnover, of small intestinal epithelium in the neonate. Villi in piglets younger than about 5 days are very tall, about 700–1200 μm long, with a villus : crypt ratio of about 7–9 : 1. The surface epithelium is mature and has an extensive vesicular network in the apical cytoplasm associated with uptake of macromolecules and colostrum during the first day or two after birth. Crypts are short and relatively inactive. The population of epithelium susceptible to infection on each villus is therefore large, and the capacity to regenerate new enterocytes is small. By about 3 weeks of age, villi are about 400–700 μm long, crypts are longer, and their epithelium is actively proliferative, so that the villus : crypt ratio is of the order of 3 : 1 or 4 : 1. Virus production by infected enterocytes in older pigs seems less efficient, and replacement of cells lost to infection is more rapid, contributing to the relative resistance seen in swine older than 3 weeks.

Piglets with TGE have the nonspecific gross appearance at necropsy of undifferentiated neonatal diarrhea. The stomach may contain a milk curd or bile-stained fluid. The small bowel is flaccid and contains yellow frothy fluid with flecks of mucus; chyle is not usually evident in mesenteric lymphatics since there is fat malabsorption.

The microscopic lesions are those of villus atrophy due to exfoliation of surface enterocytes (Fig. 1.107A,B,C), the severity of which is a function of the age of the pig and the stage of the disease. The lesions are most severe about the time of the onset of diarrhea, in young piglets. In later phases or in older pigs, there may be subtotal to moderate atrophy, and the mucosa may be lined by cuboidal to low columnar epithelium, with irregular nuclear polarity and an indistinct brush border. Severe atrophy is readily recognized at necropsy of neonatal piglets, by examination of the mucosa under a dissecting microscope. Lesions are most common in the middle and lower small intestine, and villi in the duodenum are usually tall and cylindrical. Lesions may be patchy, and several areas of lower small intestine must be examined before atrophy is considered not to be present. In animals beyond the neonatal age group, atrophy may not be so severe and readily recognized under the dissecting microscope, and the contrast with the normally shorter villi in the duodenum of older pigs is not so marked. Histologic assessment of the gut is essential.

The **respiratory variant of TGE** (porcine respiratory coronavirus) is genetically and antigenically extremely close to enteric TGE virus. It cross-reacts serologically; whether it induces local immunity against enteric infection is in dispute. It is widespread in Europe and England, and a similar agent has been detected in the United States. The virus is spread by inhalation, and infects lining cells of the upper respiratory tract, the tracheobronchial tree, and alveoli, as well as alveolar macrophages; intestinal replication is slight, and villus atrophy does not occur. It may be a minor primary respiratory pathogen. Mild bronchointerstitial pneumonia results from experimental infection, and the agent has been associated with outbreaks of respiratory disease.

Porcine epidemic diarrhea virus (PED; coronavirus 777), antigenically distinct from TGE, is reported from England, Europe, China, and Taiwan. It causes disease essentially similar to transmissible gastroenteritis in epidemiology, pathogenesis, and lesions, but is milder. In addition to infection of epithelium low on villi and occasionally in crypts in small bowel, PED may also cause mild exfoliative lesions in colonic crypts. It is differentiated from TGE by its distinct viral antigenicity.

Bibliography

Bohl, E. H. Transmissible gastroenteritis virus (classical enteric variant). *In* "Virus Infections of Porcines," M. B. Pensaert (ed.), pp. 139–153, 158–165. Amsterdam, Elsevier, 1989.

Chu, R. M., Glock, R. D., and Ross, R. F. Changes in gut-associated lymphoid tissues of the small intestine of eight-week-old pigs infected with transmissible gastroenteritis virus. *Am J Vet Res* **43:** 67–76, 1982.

Coussement, W. *et al.* Pathology of experimental CV777 coronavirus enteritis in piglets. I. Histological and histochemical study. *Vet Pathol* **19:** 46–56, 1982.

Ducatelle, R. *et al.* Pathology of experimental CV777 coronavirus enteritis in piglets. II. Electron microscopic study. *Vet Pathol* **19:** 57–66, 1982.

Haelterman, E. O. On the pathogenesis of transmissible gastroenteritis of swine. *J Am Vet Med Assoc* **160:** 534–540, 1972.

Kerzner, B. *et al.* Transmissible gastroenteritis: Sodium transport and the intestinal epithelium during the course of viral enteritis. *Gastroenterology* **72:** 457–461, 1977.

Larson, D. J. *et al.* Mild transmissible gastroenteritis in pigs suckling vaccinated sows. *J Am Vet Med Assoc* **176:** 539–542, 1980.

Moon, H. W. *et al.* Age-dependent resistance to transmissible gastroenteritis of swine. III. Effects of epithelial cell kinetics on coronavirus production and on atrophy of intestinal villi. *Vet Pathol* **12:** 434–445, 1975.

Morin, M., and Moorehouse, L. G. Transmissible gastroenteritis in feeder pigs: Observations on the jejunal epithelium of normal feeder pigs and feeder pigs infected with TGE virus. *Can J Comp Med* **38:** 227–235, 1974.

Moxley, R. A., and Olson, L. D. Lesions of transmissible gastroenteritis virus infection in experimentally inoculated pigs suckling immunized sows. *Am J Vet Res* **50:** 708–716, 1989.

Olson, D. P., Waxler, G. L., and Roberts, A. W. Small intestinal lesions of transmissible gastroenteritis in gnotobiotic pigs: A scanning electron microscopic study. *Am J Vet Res* **34:** 1239–1245, 1973.

O'Toole, D. *et al.* Pathogenicity of experimental infection with "pneumotropic" porcine coronavirus. *Res Vet Sci* **47:** 23–29, 1989.

Pensaert, M. B. Transmissible gastroenteritis virus (respiratory variant). *In* "Virus Infections of Porcines," M. B. Pensaert (ed.), pp. 154–165. Amsterdam, Elsevier, 1989.

Pensaert, M. B. Porcine epidemic diarrhea virus. *In* "Virus Infections of Porcines," M. B. Pensaert (ed.), pp. 167–176. Amsterdam, Elsevier, 1989.

Pospischil, A., Hess, R. G., and Bachmann, P. A. Light microscopy and ultrahistology of intestinal changes in pigs infected with epizootic diarrhoea virus (EVD): Comparison with transmissible gastroenteritis (TGE) virus and porcine rotavirus infections. *Zbl Vet Med (B)* **28:** 564–577, 1981.

Shepherd, R. W. *et al.* The mucosal lesion in viral enteritis. Extent and dynamics of the epithelial response to virus invasion in TGE in piglets. *Gastroenterology* **76:** 770–777, 1979.

Shimizu, M., and Shimizu, Y. Demonstration of cytotoxic lymphocytes to virus-infected target cells in pigs inoculated with transmissible gastroenteritis virus. *Am J Vet Res* **40:** 208–213, 1979.

Thake, D. C. Jejunal epithelium in transmissible gastroenteritis of swine. An electron microscopic and histochemical study. *Am J Pathol* **53:** 149–168, 1968.

Thake, D. C., Moon, H. W., and Lambert, G. Epithelial cell dynamics in transmissible gastroenteritis of neonatal pigs. *Vet Pathol* **10:** 330–341, 1973.

van Nieuwstadt, A. P., and Pol, J. M. A. Isolation of a TGE virus-related respiratory coronavirus causing fatal pneumonia in pigs. *Vet Rec* **124:** 43–44, 1989.

Wesley, R. D., Woods, R. D., and Cheung, A. K. Genetic analysis of porcine respiratory coronavirus, an attenuated variant of transmissible gastroenteritis virus. *J Virol* **65:** 3369–3373, 1991.

Woods, R. D., Cheville, N. F., and Gallagher, J. E. Lesions in the small intestine of newborn pigs inoculated with porcine, feline, and canine coronaviruses. *Am J Vet Res* **42:** 1163–1169, 1981.

b. CATTLE **In neonatal calves,** coronavirus infection is a common cause of diarrhea, either alone or in combination with other agents, particularly rotavirus and *Cryptosporidium*. The virus is capable of infecting absorptive epithelium in the full length of the small intestine, and in the large bowel. Viral antigen is also found in macrophages in the lamina propria of villi and in mesenteric lymph nodes. In field infections, microscopic le-

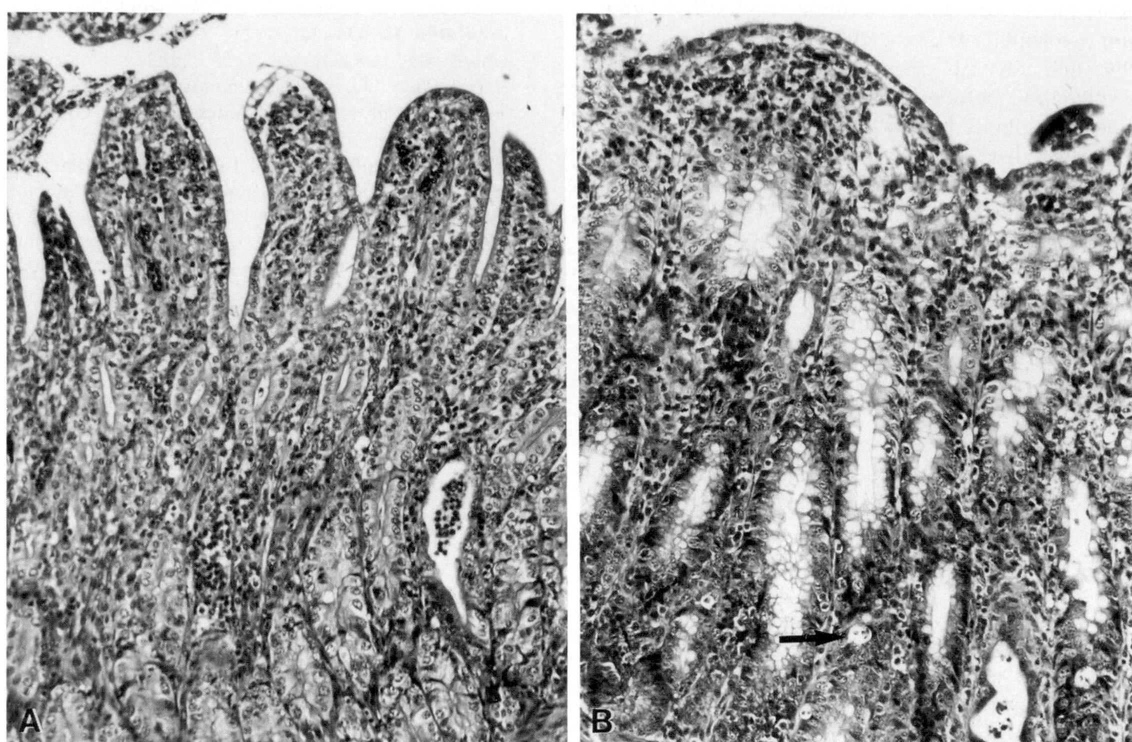

Fig. 1.108 Bovine coronavirus infection. (A) Blunt, fused villi with cuboidal surface epithelium. Small intestine. (B) Attenuation of surface epithelium and necrosis of gland epithelium (arrow). Colon. (Courtesy of M. Morin.)

sions are most consistently found in the lower small intestine and colon. Calves with coronavirus infection usually develop mild depression, but continue to drink milk despite developing profuse diarrhea. With progressive dehydration, acidosis, and hyperkalemia, the animals become weak and lethargic, death ensuing as a result of hypovolemia, hypoglycemia, and potassium cardiotoxicosis. Diarrhea in survivors resolves in 5–6 days.

At autopsy, affected animals have the nonspecific lesions of undifferentiated neonatal calf diarrhea. Rarely, mild fibrinonecrotic typhlocolitis is recognized at necropsy in calves with coronavirus infection. Mesenteric lymph nodes may be somewhat enlarged and wet.

The microscopic lesions of coronavirus infection in calves vary with the severity and duration of the infection; villus atrophy in combination with mild colitis is typical (Fig. 1.108A,B). In the small intestine, villus atrophy is rarely as severe as that seen in neonatal swine with TGE. Rather, villi are moderately shortened, or have subtotal atrophy, with a villus : crypt ratio of about 1 : 1 or 2 : 1. Villi are stumpy, club shaped, or pointed at the tips, and villus fusion may be common. In the early phase of the clinical disease, villi are often pointed, and covered by cuboidal to squamous epithelium. Exfoliation of epithelium and microerosion may be evident. Later, the epithelium is cuboidal to low columnar, basophilic, with irregular nuclear polarity and an indistinct brush border. Cryptal epithelium is hyperplastic. The lamina propria may contain a moderate infiltrate of mainly mononuclear inflammatory cells, some of which may have pyknotic or karyorrhectic nuclei. In the early stages of infection, necrosis of cells in mesenteric lymph nodes is associated with viral replication. Peyer's patches in animals examined after 4–5 days of clinical illness often appear involuted, and are dominated by histiocytic cells. Whether this is the result of viral activity or the effect of endogenous glucocorticoids is unclear.

In the colon during the early phase of infection, surface epithelium may be exfoliating, flattened, and squamous, or eroded in patchy areas; some colonic glands lined by flattened epithelium will contain exfoliated cells and necrotic debris. A moderate mixed inflammatory reaction is present in the lamina propria, and neutrophils may be in damaged glands or effusing into the lumen through superficial microerosions. Later in infection, some dilated debris-filled colonic glands will remain, but other glands will be lined by hyperplastic epithelium, and the surface epithelium will be restored to a cuboidal or low columnar cell type. Goblet cells are usually relatively uncommon. Colonic lesions may be recognizable in tissues from animals submitted dead, though postmortem change has obscured changes in the small intestine.

Live calves in the early stages of clinical disease are the best subjects for confirmation of an etiologic diagnosis. In calves younger than 4–5 days becoming ill, enterotoxigenic *E. coli* is the main alternative diagnosis. Rotavirus, *Cryptosporidium,* and combined infections must be considered in calves 5–15 days of age. Infectious bovine rhinotracheitis, salmonellosis, and bovine virus diarrhea must also be considered. Both salmonellosis and bovine virus diarrhea may be associated with depletion of Peyer's patches and colitis, which can be confused with that of coronavirus infection; neither is common in the strictly neonatal age group (younger than 7–14 days).

Respiratory tract infection also occurs in calves infected with bovine coronavirus. The virus replicates in the epithelium of the nasal turbinates and tracheobronchial tree, and respiratory infection may precede, be concurrent with, or follow enteric infection. Mild nasal discharge, cough, and increased respiratory rate are associated. Respiratory infections may play a role in maintaining the virus within a herd, and significant, but poorly characterized, pneumonia has been reported in some experimentally infected calves. Virus may be identified in tissue or nasal secretions by immunofluorescence.

Winter dysentery in adult cattle may also be attributable to coronavirus infection, though Koch's postulates have yet to be fulfilled. This syndrome has been recognized in association with coronavirus in New Zealand, Japan, France, the United States, and Canada. Animals develop a blood-tinged diarrhea, nasolacrimal discharge or cough, anorexia, and drop in milk production. Mortality is virtually unknown. The colon of affected animals has linear congestion and hemorrhage along the crests of mucosal folds. Coronaviruses are commonly demonstrated in the feces of cattle with winter dysentery; seroconversions occur, and seroprevalence increases in affected herds; and coronavirus antigen is found in the colonic glands of affected animals, in which there is necrosis and exfoliation of epithelial cells.

Bibliography

Doughri, A. M., and Storz, J. Light and ultrastructural pathologic changes in intestinal coronavirus infection of newborn calves. *Zbl Vet Med (B)* **24:** 367–385, 1977.

Heckert, R. A. *et al.* Epidemiologic factors and isotype-specific antibody responses in serum and mucosal secretions of dairy calves with bovine coronavirus respiratory tract and enteric tract infections. *Am J Vet Res* **52:** 845–851, 1991.

Jactel, B. *et al.* An epidemiological study of winter dysentery in fifteen herds in France. *Vet Res Commun* **14:** 367–379, 1990.

Kapil, S. *et al.* Experimental infection with a virulent pneumoenteric isolate of bovine coronavirus. *J Vet Diagn Invest* **3:** 88–89, 1991.

Langpap, T. J., Bergeland, M. E., and Reed, D. E. Coronaviral enteritis of young calves: Virologic and pathologic findings in naturally occurring infections. *Am J Vet Res* **40:** 1476–1478, 1979.

Lewis, L. D., and Phillips, R. W. Pathophysiologic changes due to coronavirus-induced diarrhea in the calf. *J Am Vet Med Assoc* **173:** 636–642, 1978.

Mebus, C. A. *et al.* Pathology of neonatal calf diarrhea induced by a coronaviruslike agent. *Vet Pathol* **10:** 45–64, 1973.

Morin, M., Lariviere, S., and Lallier, R. Pathological and microbiological observations made on spontaneous cases of acute neonatal calf diarrhea. *Can J Comp Med* **40:** 228–240, 1976.

Saif, L. J. A review of evidence implicating bovine coronavirus in the etiology of winter dysentery in cows: An enigma resolved? *Cornell Vet* **80:** 303–311, 1990.

Saif, L. J. *et al.* Winter dysentery in dairy herds: Electron microscopic and serological evidence for an association with coronavirus infection. *Vet Rec* **128:** 447–449, 1991.

Storz, J., Doughri, A. M., and Hajer, I. Coronaviral morphogenesis and ultrastructural changes in intestinal infections of calves. *J Am Vet Med Assoc* **173:** 633–635, 1978.

Van Kruiningen, H. J. *et al.* Calfhood coronavirus enterocolitis: A clue to the etiology of winter dysentery. *Vet Pathol* **24:** 564–567, 1987.

c. DOGS A coronavirus was first associated with diarrhea in military dogs in Germany, and with diarrhea in a kennel in Great Britain. Subsequent reports of coronavirus in normal canine feces, or associated with diarrhea, in Australia, North America, and Europe, have emerged. Although dogs of all ages appear to be susceptible to infection by coronavirus, the condition is probably most important as a rare, transient, generally nonfatal, diarrhea in puppies. Coronaviruses were at first associated with the pandemic of diarrhea in dogs in 1978, which was subsequently demonstrated to be due to canine parvovirus. Coronavirus is widely prevalent in the dog population, but causes diarrhea in only a minority of animals. Very few dogs with lesions consistent with coronavirus infection are submitted to biopsy or come to autopsy. Canine coronavirus is antigenically related to TGE virus, which will also infect dogs, subclinically.

Viral replication occurs in the enterocytes of the small intestine, and in experimental infections in neonatal puppies, the lesions resembles the villus atrophy associated with coronavirus infection in other species. Diarrhea begins as early as 1 day after inoculation and in most animals by 4 days. Onset of signs coincides with the development of moderate villus atrophy and fusion. Enterocytes on villi become cuboidal, contain lipid vacuoles, and have an indistinct brush border. Lesions are most consistent and severe in the ileum. Resolution of villus atrophy within 7–10 days is associated with remission of signs.

Colonic infection by canine coronavirus was not demonstrated by immunofluorescence in experimental animals, though mild colonic lesions were described, including loss of sulfomucins from goblet cells and some epithelial shedding. However, in the only published report of lesions due to spontaneous canine coronavirus infection, colonic infection and lesions were demonstrated. There was watery content in the lumen of the small and large intestine, and in the cecum and colon, fibrin mixed with some blood was evident. Mesenteric lymph nodes were enlarged and edematous. Villus atrophy in the jejunum was inconsistent, but there was necrotic debris in many glands in the cecum and colon. Virus-infected cells were exfoliating into the lumen.

A modified live coronavirus vaccine, which was briefly marketed in the United States, was associated with sudden death, neurologic signs, infertility, and the development of fetal monsters in vaccinates. Mild fibrinous polyserositis, nonsuppurative meningoencephalitis, chronic interstitial pancreatitis, and nephritis were described in some cases. The etiology was not ascertained, but interacting infections with other viruses could not be clearly implicated, and coronaviral antigen was demonstrated in the brain, lung, and pancreas of some dogs. Lesions were analogous in some respects with those of feline infectious peritonitis, which is caused by a coronavirus.

Bibliography

Appel, M. Canine coronavirus. *In* "Virus Infections of Carnivores," M. J. Appel (ed.), pp. 115–122. Amsterdam, Elsevier, 1987.

Binn, L. N. *et al.* Recovery and characterization of a coronavirus from military dogs with diarrhea. *Proc 78th Annu Meet U S Anim Health Assoc* Roanoke, Va., pp. 359–366, 1974.

Keenan, K. P. *et al.* Intestinal infection of neonatal dogs with canine coronavirus 1-71: Studies by virologic, histologic, histochemical, and immunofluorescent techniques. *Am J Vet Res* **37:** 247–256, 1976.

Martin, M. L. Canine coronavirus enteritis and a recent outbreak following modified live virus vaccination. *Compend Cont Ed Pract Vet* **7:** 1012–1017, 1985.

Schnagl, R. D., and Holmes, I. H. Coronaviruslike particles in stools from dogs, from some country areas of Australia. *Vet Rec* **102:** 528–529, 1978.

Takeuchi, A. *et al.* Electron microscope study of experimental enteric infection in neonatal dogs with a canine coronavirus. *Lab Invest* **34:** 539–549, 1976.

Vandenberghe, J. *et al.* Coronavirus infection in a litter of pups. *Vet Q* **2:** 136–141, 1980.

Wilson, R. B., Holladay, J. A., and Cave, J. S. A neurologic syndrome associated with use of a canine coronavirus–parvovirus vaccine in dogs. *Compend Cont Ed Pract Vet* **8:** 117–124, 1986.

d. Cats and Other Species Our understanding of the enteric implications of the coronavirus infections of cats is still incomplete. Feline infectious peritonitis is caused by a coronavirus that cross reacts with the virus of transmissible gastroenteritis in swine. Equivocal lesions, including mild villus atrophy, are described in cats with feline infectious peritonitis, but intestinal signs are not a feature of the disease. A morphologically similar virus, which is very closely related to feline infectious peritonitis virus, has been associated with diarrhea in cats. The infection is usually inapparent. Diarrhea, when it occurs, is usually mild or moderate, perhaps with some blood, and kittens are most susceptible. There is a single report of mortality, but feline panleukopenia cannot be ruled out as a co-infection in that case. Viral antigen is in cells on the tips of villi, and mild villus atrophy has been illustrated. A third coronavirus, with distinctive peplomer morphology, also has been described in the feces of cats, but is not antigenically cross-reactive and seems to be nonpathogenic.

Coronaviruses have been recovered from the feces of sheep with transient diarrhea, and they have been associated with severe villus atrophy in several spontaneous outbreaks of diarrhea. No experimental confirmation of the pathogenicity of coronavirus in sheep is available.

Coronavirus infection may also be associated with diarrhea in foals, but again, experimental confirmation of pathogenicity is lacking.

Bibliography

Bass, E. P., and Sharpee, R. L. Coronavirus and gastroenteritis in foals. *Lancet* **II:** 822, 1975.

Dea, S., Roy, R. S., and Elazhary, M. A. S. Y. Coronavirus-like particles in the feces of a cat with diarrhea. *Can Vet J* **23:** 153–155, 1982.

Grahn, B. H. The feline coronavirus infections: Feline infectious peritonitis and feline coronavirus enteritis. *Vet Med* **86:** 376–393, 1991.

Hayashi, T. *et al.* Enteritis due to feline infectious peritonitis virus. *Jpn J Vet Sci* **44:** 97–106, 1982.

Hoshino, Y., and Scott, F. W. Coronaviruslike particles in the feces of normal cats. *Arch Virol* **63:** 147–152, 1980.

Hoskins, J. D. Coronavirus infection in cats. *Compend Cont Ed Pract Vet* **13:** 567–586, 1991.

Huang, J. C. M., Wright, S. L., and Shipley, W. D. Isolation of coronaviruslike agent from horses suffering from acute equine diarrhoea syndrome. *Vet Rec* **113:** 262–263, 1983.

Pass, D. A. *et al.* Intestinal coronaviruslike particles in sheep with diarrhoea. *Vet Rec* **111:** 106–107, 1982.

Pedersen, N. C. Feline enteric coronavirus. *In* "Virus Infections of Carnivores," M. J. Appel (ed.), pp. 261–266. Amsterdam, Elsevier, 1987.

Pedersen, N. C. *et al.* An enteric coronavirus infection of cats and its relationship to feline infectious peritonitis. *Am J Vet Res* **42:** 368–377, 1981.

Pedersen, N. C. *et al.* Pathogenicity studies of feline coronavirus isolates 79-1146 and 79-1683. *Am J Vet Res* **45:** 2580–2585, 1984.

Reynolds, D. J., and Garwes, D. J. Virus isolation and serum antibody responses after infection of cats with transmissible gastroenteritis virus. *Arch Virol* **60:** 161–166, 1979.

Tzipori, S. *et al.* Enteric coronaviruslike particles in sheep. *Aust Vet J* **54:** 320–321, 1978.

16. Rotavirus Infection

Members of the genus *Rotavirus,* in the Reoviridae, infect the gastrointestinal tract of most mammals and birds. In the earlier literature they are frequently referred to as reoviruslike. Currently, five serogroups of rotaviruses are recognized, designated groups A–E; group A is most commonly implicated in diarrhea in domestic animals. A number of serotypes are recognized within serogroups. Nongroup A rotaviruses have been previously referred to as pararotaviruses or rotaviruslike viruses. Group A rotaviruses infect all species of domestic animals, as well as humans, and many species of laboratory animals and wildlife. Nongroup A rotaviruses infect pigs and ruminants, among domestic animals.

The ability to infect cells, and the serotype specificity of rotaviruses, are conferred by elements of the outer capsid layer. Some strains of rotaviruses isolated from one species can be transmitted successfully to other species, sometimes producing significant lesions and disease in experimental infections. The factors influencing viral host specificity and virulence, and their epizootiologic connotations, are unclear. The viruses are probably generally host specific, with little significant zoonotic potential. However, if epidemiologic circumstances are favorable, cross-species transmission may occur.

Rotaviruses infect the absorptive enterocytes and occasionally goblet cells on the tips and sides of the distal half or two thirds of villi in the small intestine. Virus production and the pathogenesis of infection is similar in all species studied. Rotaviruses adhere to cell receptors, and inner capsid components are internalized into the cell. Granular viroplasm containing incomplete virions is seen in the apical cytoplasm of infected cells, and virions acquire their complete capsid after budding into dilated cisternae of endoplasmic reticulum, where they accumulate. Elongate tubular structures are found in the nuclei and rough endoplasmic reticulum of some infected cells.

Virus-infected cells are most prevalent 18–24 hr after experimental infection, and they tend to diminish in number rapidly, so that by 3–4 days after infection, few cells containing viral antigen are present. Infected enterocytes lose cytoplasmic electron density, and mitochondria swell, as does the cell generally. Microvilli become irregular and somewhat stunted, and there may be some blebbing of membranes. Infected cells exfoliate into the intestinal lumen, and virus is released by lysis of damaged epithelium prior to or after exfoliation.

The pathogenesis of rotavirus infection resembles that of coronavirus. Group A rotaviruses infect cells on the apical half (ruminants) or the entire villus (pigs), mainly in the jejunum and ileum. Group B rotaviruses have a more patchy distribution near the tips of villi, and typically induce formation of epithelial syncytia. They were formerly known as intestinal syncytial virus. Since in pigs some group A rotavirus may also occasionally cause syncytia, this is not a criterion for diagnosis of the serogroup. Group C rotavirus in pigs resembles group A in distribution along the gut and villus. The diarrhea induced by group A and C rotaviruses is typically more severe than that induced by group B, presumably due to more extensive damage to enterocytes.

Exfoliation of infected epithelium over a relatively short period results in villus atrophy. The mucosal surface is covered by cuboidal, poorly differentiated epithelium, which has an ill-defined microvillous border and which may contain lipid droplets in the cytoplasm. Diarrhea is mediated probably by electrolyte and nutrient malabsorption, perhaps exacerbated by the effect of cryptal secretion. It begins about the time of early viral cytopathology 20–24 hr after infection, and may persist for a variable period, from a few hours to a week or more. Regeneration of the mucosa by epithelium emerging from crypts, and differentiating on reformed villi, is associated with remission of signs in animals surviving the effects of diarrhea.

Rotaviruses are widespread, if not ubiquitous, among populations of most species, and they are relatively resistant to the external environment. Protection against infection in neonates is apparently conferred largely by the presence of lactogenic immunity. Probably many individuals in a population undergo inapparent infection. Disease is seen in the various species when viral contamination of the environment is heavy, perhaps as a result of intensive husbandry practices, and lactogenic immunity is waning or absent. Though rotavirus infection is usually associated with younger age groups, and viral receptors on cells diminish with age in some species, naive older animals may become infected, sometimes with the development of diarrhea.

a. CATTLE Rotavirus infection is implicated mainly in diarrhea of neonatal beef and dairy calves, both suckled and artificially reared, though there are reports of its association with diarrhea in adult cattle. Diarrhea may be produced in calves by rotavirus infection alone, but the condition is usually considered to be relatively mild or transient in comparison with that induced by enterotoxigenic *E. coli* or coronavirus. Combinations of agents including rotavirus are frequently involved in outbreaks of diarrhea in neonatal calves. Rotavirus may be implicated in animals developing signs at any time before about 2–3 weeks of age, and it is more commonly encountered in animals older than 4–5 days.

The gross lesions of rotaviral infection are the nonspecific findings of undifferentiated neonatal diarrhea in calves. Microscopic lesions in the small intestine cannot be differentiated from those of coronavirus infection. They may vary somewhat, depending on the severity of the initial viral damage and the stage of evolution of the sequelae. Blunt club-shaped villi, mild or moderate villus atrophy, and perhaps villus fusion may be present (Fig. 1.109A,B). Villi are covered by low columnar, cuboidal, or flattened surface epithelium with a poorly defined brush border. There is usually a moderate proprial infiltrate of mononuclear cells and eosinophils or neutrophils, and hypertrophic crypts may be evident. The distribution of lesions may vary between animals and perhaps with time after infection within an individual animal, since the onset of maximal viral damage may not occur synchronously throughout the full length of the intestine. Lesions and viral antigen always should

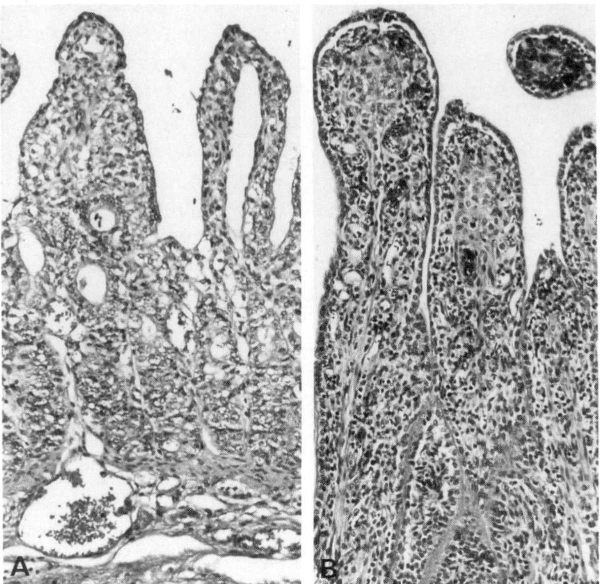

Fig. 1.109 Bovine rotavirus infection. (A) Stumpy villi with severely attenuated surface epithelium. (B) Club-shaped villi with cuboidal or flattened epithelium. (Courtesy of M. Morin.)

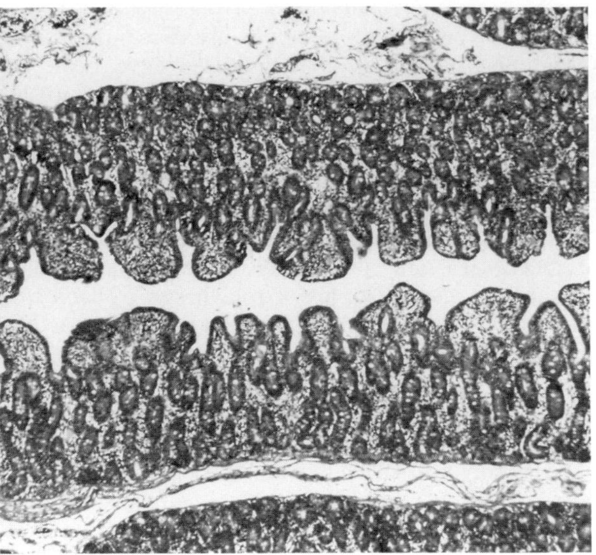

Fig. 1.110 Porcine rotavirus infection. Atrophy of villi. Small intestine of 3-week-old piglet.

be sought in the distal small intestine, and preferably at several sites along its length. Rotavirus does not cause gross or microscopic lesions in the colon, in contrast to coronavirus.

b. Swine Rotavirus infection is widespread and enzootic in most swine herds, and subclinical infection of piglets is common. It assumes particular importance as a cause of diarrhea in pigs with reduced lactogenic immunity, either as a result of removal of piglets from the sow at an early age, or following normal weaning. High environmental levels of virus may result in disease in piglets suckling the sow, but in these circumstances the signs are usually relatively mild. Rotavirus may be a cause of 3-week, white, or postweaning scours in piglets 2 to 7 or 8 weeks of age.

The signs may resemble those of transmissible gastroenteritis, although rotavirus infection is considered to be less severe. Vomition is less commonly encountered than with transmissible gastroenteritis, but depression, diarrhea, and dehydration are usual. The character of the feces varies with the diet. Steatorrhea occurs in white scours of suckling piglets. Rotavirus infection in swine may be associated with other causes of diarrhea, including *E. coli,* coccidiosis, adenovirus infection, and *Strongyloides*.

The gross and microscopic lesions, and pathogenesis of rotavirus infection in pigs resemble those of transmissible gastroenteritis (Fig. 1.110). As in TGE, severity of lesions seems inversely related to age.

c. Other Species **Neonatal lambs** have proven a useful model for the demonstration of the importance of lactogenic immunity in preventing disease due to rotavirus. Rotavirus may cause diarrhea in neonatal lambs alone or in combination with enterotoxigenic *E. coli* and *Cryptosporidium*. The pathogenesis and lesions of rotavirus infection in lambs are like those caused in other species, with the exception that viral infection of the colon may occur.

In **foals** younger than 3–4 months, diarrhea may be associated with rotavirus infection, though mortality is rare. Outbreaks have been reported in the United Kingdom, United States, Japan, Australia, and New Zealand. The natural and experimental disease resembles that seen in other species, with significant viral infection limited to enterocytes in the small intestine, where villus atrophy occurs.

In young **puppies,** especially those younger than 1–2 weeks, diarrhea, occasionally fatal, may be caused by rotavirus infection. In experimentally infected pups, green fluid content filled the lower small bowel and colon, and moderate villus atrophy was induced by exfoliation of epithelium from the distal half of villi.

Rotavirus has also been associated with diarrhea in an orphaned **kitten** being hand reared, and appears to be potentially pathogenic based on limited experimental evidence.

Rotavirus infection should be sought in cases of diarrhea in young animals of any species, and it should particularly be suspected in animals with villus atrophy in the small intestine. Rotavirus is part of the syndrome of undifferentiated neonatal diarrhea in any species.

Bibliography

Benfield, D. A. *et al.* Combined rotavirus and K99 *Escherichia coli* infection in gnotobiotic pigs. *Am J Vet Res* **49:** 330–337, 1988.

Chasey, D. *et al.* Atypical rotavirus and villous epithelial cell syncytia in piglets. *J Comp Pathol* **100:** 217–222, 1989.

Conner, M. E., and Darlington, R. W. Rotavirus infection in foals. *Am J Vet Res* **41:** 1699–1703, 1980.

Debouck, P., and Pansaert, M. Experimental infection of pigs with Belgian isolates of the porcine rotavirus. *Zbl Vet Med (B)* **26:** 517–526, 1979.

Ellis, G. R., and Daniels, E. Comparison of direct electron microscopy and enzyme immunoassay for the detection of rotaviruses in calves, lambs, piglets, and foals. *Aust Vet J* **65:** 133–135, 1988.

Fahey, K. J. *et al.* IgG_1 antibody in milk protects lambs against rotavirus diarrhoea. *Vet Immunol Immunopathol* **2:** 27–33, 1981.

Gelberg, H. B. *et al.* Multinucleate enterocytes associated with experimental group A porcine rotavirus infection. *Vet Pathol* **27:** 453–454, 1990.

Hall, G. A. *et al.* Effects of dietary change and rotavirus infection on small intestinal structure and function in gnotobiotic piglets. *Res Vet Sci* **47:** 219–224, 1989.

Hardy, M. E. *et al.* Analysis of serotypes and electropherotypes of equine rotaviruses isolated in the United States. *J Clin Microbiol* **29:** 889–893, 1991.

Hoskins, Y., Baldwin, C. A. and Scott, F. W. Isolation and characterization of feline rotavirus. *J Gen Virol* **54:** 313–323, 1981.

Hoskins, Y. *et al.* Isolation and characterization of a canine rotavirus. *Arch Virol* **72:** 113–125, 1982.

Janke, B. H., Morehouse, L. G., and Solorzano, R. F. Single and mixed infections of neonatal pigs with rotaviruses and enteroviruses: Clinical signs and microscopic lesions. *Can J Vet Res* **52:** 364–369, 1988.

Johnson, C. A. *et al.* A scanning and transmission electron microscopic study of rotavirus-induced intestinal lesions in neonatal gnotobiotic dogs. *Vet Pathol* **23:** 443–453, 1986.

McAdaragh, J. P. *et al.* Pathogenesis of rotaviral enteritis in gnotobiotic pigs: A microscopic study. *Am J Vet Res* **41:** 1572–1581, 1980.

Mebus, C. A. *et al.* Pathology of neonatal calf diarrhea induced by a reolike virus. *Vet Pathol* **8:** 490–505, 1971.

Morin, M., Magar, R., and Robinson, Y. Porcine group C rotavirus as a cause of neonatal diarrhea in a Quebec swine herd. *Can J Vet Res* **54:** 385–389, 1990.

Narita, M., Fukusho, A., and Shimizu, Y. Electron microscopy of the intestine of gnotobiotic piglets infected with porcine rotavirus. *J Comp Pathol* **92:** 589–597, 1982.

Pearson, G. R., and McNulty, M. S. Ultrastructural changes in small intestinal epithelium of neonatal pigs infected with pig rotavirus. *Arch Virol* **59:** 127–136, 1979.

Saif, L. J. Comparative aspects of enteric viral infections. *In* "Viral Diarrheas of Man and Animals," L. J. Saif and K. W. Theil, (eds.), pp 9–31. Boca Raton, Florida, CRC Press, 1990.

Saif, L. J. Nongroup A rotaviruses. *In* "Viral Diarrheas of Man and Animals," L. J. Saif and K. W. Theil, (eds.), pp 73–95. Boca Raton, Florida, CRC Press, 1990.

Shaw, D. P., Morehouse, L. G., and Solorzano, R. F. Experimental rotavirus infection in three-week-old pigs. *Am J Vet Res* **50:** 1961–1965, 1989.

Shaw, D. P., Morehouse, L. G., and Solorzano, R. F. Rotavirus replication in colostrum-fed and colostrum-deprived pigs. *Am J Vet Res* **50:** 1966–1970, 1989.

Snodgrass, D. R., Angus, K. W., and Gray, E. W. A rotavirus from kittens. *Vet Rec* **104:** 222–223, 1979.

Snodgrass, D. R. *et al.* Small intestine morphology and epithelial cell kinetics in lamb rotavirus infection. *Gastroenterology* **76:** 477–481, 1979.

Studdert, M. J., Mason, R. W., and Patten, B. E. Rotavirus diarrhoea of foals. *Aust Vet J* **54:** 363–364, 1978.

Svensmark, B. *et al.* Epidemiological studies of piglet diarrhoea in intensvely managed Danish sow herds. IV. Pathogenicity of porcine rotavirus. *Acta Vet Scand* **30:** 71–76, 1989.

Theil, K. W. Group A rotaviruses. *In* "Viral Diarrheas of Man and Animals," L. J. Saif and K. W. Theil, (eds.), pp. 35–72. Boca Raton, Florida, CRC Press, 1990.

Torres-Medina. A. Effect of combined rotavirus and *Escherichia coli* in neonatal gnotobiotic calves. *Am J Vet Res* **45:** 643–651, 1984.

Torres-Medina, A., and Underdahl, N. R. Scanning electron microscopy of intestine of gnotobiotic piglets infected with porcine rotavirus. *Can J Comp Med* **44:** 403–411, 1980.

Tzipori, S. *et al.* Enteritis in foals induced by rotavirus and enterotoxigenic *Escherichia coli. Aust Vet J* **58:** 20–23, 1982.

Vonderfecht, S. L. *et al.* Identification of a bovine enteric syncytial virus as a nongroup A rotavirus. *Am J Vet Res* **47:** 1913–1918, 1986.

17. Parvoviral Enteritis

The Parvoviridae, so named because of their small size, are non-enveloped viral particles about 18–26 nm in diameter, with icosahedral symmetry and a short, single-stranded DNA genome. They replicate in the nucleus of infected cells, usually producing inclusion bodies there. Members of the genus *Parvovirus* infect many species of laboratory and domestic animals. Among syndromes associated with parvovirus infection are disease in cats, dogs, and mink dominated clinically by enteritis; diarrhea in neonatal calves; and reproductive wastage in swine.

Feline panleukopenia virus (FPV), mink enteritis virus (MEV) and canine parvovirus-2 (CPV-2), the agent causing parvovirus enteritis in dogs, are considered host-range variants of the feline parvovirus subgroup within the genus *Parvovirus*. These viruses are biologically distinct, varying in their hemagglutination characteristics, *in vitro* host cell ranges, infectivity, and virulence in experimentally inoculated hosts. There are subtle antigenic differences among them, detected by monoclonal antibodies; these, and differences in host specificity, are conferred by variations in only very small segments of the viral genome. Based on the nucleotide sequence in the gene for capsid proteins VP-1/VP-2, FPV, and MEV are very closely related to each other, and somewhat less related to CPV-2. The latter virus is distinct from minute virus of canines (MVC, or canine parvovirus-1), which is poorly defined as a pathogen.

Though autonomous parvoviruses may infect cells at any phase of the cell cycle, replication is dependent on cellular mechanisms functional only during nucleoprotein synthesis prior to mitosis; hence, the effects of parvovirus infection are greatest in tissues with a high mitotic rate. These may include a variety of tissues during organogenesis in the fetus and neonate. In older animals, the proliferative elements of the enteric epithelium, hematopoietic, and lymphoid tissue are particularly susceptible. At the time of virus assembly, large basophilic or amphophilic Feulgen-positive nuclear inclusions may be found in infected cells, especially in Bouin's-fixed tissues. Parvovirus is demonstrated in these inclusions by electron microscopy. The chromatin in inclusion-bearing nuclei is usually clumped at the nuclear membrane. Inclusions are most prevalent late in the incubation period, prior to extensive exfoliation or lysis of infected cells; hence, they are not commonly encountered in animals submitted for autopsy after a period of clinical illness culminating in death. Large nucleoli, seen in proliferative cells encountered in the intestine of parvovirus-infected animals, should not be confused with intranuclear inclusions.

The pathogenesis of FPV and of CPV-2 infection is sufficiently similar for them to be considered together here, followed by separate discussions of the specific diseases. Oronasal exposure results in uptake of virus by epithelium over tonsils and Peyer's patches. Infection of draining lymphoid tissue is indicated by isolation of virus from mesenteric lymph nodes 1–2 days after experimental inoculation. Release of virus into lymph, and dissemination of infected lymphoblasts from these sites, may result in infection of other central and peripheral lymphoid tissues, including thymus, spleen, lymph nodes, and Peyer's patches, 3–4 days after infection. Lymphocytolysis in these tissues releases virus, reinforcing cell-free viremia. Viremia is terminated when neutralizing antibody appears in circulation about 5–7 days after infection. Moderate pyrexia occurs at about this time.

Infection of the gastrointestinal epithelium is a secondary event, following dissemination of virus by circulating lymphocytes and cell-free viremia. Peyer's patches are consistently infected at all levels of the intestine, and epithelium in crypts of Lieberkühn over or adjacent to Peyer's patches usually becomes infected a day or so later. Infection of gastrointestinal epithelium at other sites in the gut is less consistent, but is usually more severe in the lower small intestine. It may be the result of virus free in circulation, or carried by infected lymphocytes homing to the mucosa. Maximal infection of cryptal epithelium occurs during the period about 5–9 days after infection.

The occurrence and severity of enteric signs is determined by the extent of damage to epithelium in intestinal crypts. This seems to be a function of two main factors. The first is the availability of virus, which is influenced by the rate of proliferation of lymphocytes, and therefore their susceptibility to virus replication and lysis. The second factor influencing the degree of epithelial damage is the rate of proliferation in the progenitor compartment in crypts of Lieberkühn. If many cells are entering mitosis, large numbers will support virus replication and subsequently lyse. Destruction of cells in the crypts of Lieberkühn, if severe enough, ultimately results in focal or widespread villus atrophy and perhaps mucosal erosion or ulceration. The recognition, evolution, and sequelae of radiomimetic insult to the intestine, such as that caused by parvovirus, are described elswhere (see Epithelial Renewal in Health and Disease, Section VI,I of this chapter).

Regeneration of cryptal epithelium and partial or complete restoration of mucosal architecture will occur, if undamaged stem cells persist in most affected crypts, and the animal survives the acute phase of clinical illness. In some survivors, focal villus atrophy is associated with persistent dilated crypts containing cellular debris, and with local drop-out of crypts completely destroyed by infection. In rare animals recovered from acute disease, chronic malabsorption and protein-losing enteropathy are associated with persistent areas of ulceration caused by more extensive loss of crypts and collapse of the mucosa.

The low rate of replication of intestinal epithelium in germ-free cats explains failure to produce significant intestinal lesions and clinical panleukopenia in experimentally infected animals. In spontaneous cases, the lower prevalence of parvoviral lesions in the colon and stomach, in comparison with the small intestine, reflects the relatively lower rate of epithelial proliferation in those tissues. The consistency of epithelial lesions in the mucosa over Peyer's patches probably results from high local concentrations of virus derived from infected lymphocytes in the dome and follicle. This may be coupled with local stimulation of epithelial turnover by cytokines released by T lymphocytes in the vicinity. Variations in the rate of epithelial proliferation related to age, starvation and refeeding, or concomitant parasitic, bacterial, or viral infections (particularly coronavirus in dogs), may also influence the susceptibility of crypt epithelium to infection, and therefore affect the extent and severity of intestinal lesions and signs. It is difficult to duplicate fatal parvovirus infection experimentally.

Diarrhea in parvovirus infections is mainly the result of reduced functional absorptive surface in the small intestine. Effusion of tissue fluids and blood from a mucosa at least focally denuded of epithelium probably also contributes to diarrhea. Dehydration and electrolyte depletion are the result of reduced fluid intake, enteric malabsorption, effusion of tissue fluid, and in some animals, vomition. Hypoproteinemia is common, and anemia may occur because of enteric blood loss; both are exacerbated by rehydration. Anemia reflects hemorrhage into the gut.

Proliferating cells in the bone marrow are also infected during viremia. Lysis of many infected cells is reflected in hypocellularity of the marrow caused by depletion of myeloid and erythroid elements, particularly the former. Megakaryocytes also may be lost, but seem the least sensitive cell population in the marrow. The number of neutrophils in circulation drops quickly in severely affected animals. This is due to failure of recruitment from the damaged marrow, and peripheral consumption, especially in the intestine. Transient neutropenia, of about 2–3 days' duration, occurs consistently in cats, and less commonly in dogs. In surviving animals, regeneration of depleted myeloid elements from remaining stem cells restores the circulating population of granulocytes within a few days. Neutrophilia with left shift may occur during recovery.

Lymphopenia, relative or absolute, results from viral lymphocytolysis in all infected lymphoid tissue. Relative lymphopenia is more consistently observed in dogs than is neutropenia. When lymphopenia and neutropenia occur together, the combined leukopenia may be profound in both dogs and cats. In dogs surviving the lymphopenic phase, circulating lymphocytes return to normal numbers within 2–5 days, as regenerative hyperplasia occurs in lymphoid tissue throughout the body. Lymphocyte numbers increase rapidly, sometimes producing lymphocytosis in recovering dogs. However, there may be transient immunosuppression in gnotobiotic pups subclinically infected with CPV-2. Transient depression of T-cell response to mitogens occurs in cats a week after experimental infection with feline panleukopenia virus, but immunosuppression by these agents appears to be of little clinical significance.

Most infected cats and dogs do not develop clinical disease. When it occurs, signs usually begin during the late viremic phase, about 5–7 days after infection. Severe enteric damage is the major cause of mortality. Shedding of infective virus in feces begins about 3–5 days after infection, when Peyer's patches and cryptal epithelium first become infected. Virus shedding persists until coproantibody appears to neutralize virus entering the gut, about 6–9 days after infection. Virus-infected cells still may be detected in crypts and Peyer's patches at this time, and virus complexed with antibody may be found in feces or intestinal content by direct electron microscopy. However, attempts to demonstrate virus in tissues or feces after several days of clinical disease, or at death, are often thwarted by the fact that virus is neutralized by antibody present in tissue fluids. Persistent or sporadic shedding of virus by recovered animals may be the result of virus replication in cells entering mitosis days or weeks after they were infected during the viremic phase.

Infection of the fetus during late prenatal life by FPV causes anomalies of the central nervous system, mainly hypoplasia of the cerebellum. A syndrome of generalized parvovirus infection may occur rarely in neonatal dogs with CPV-2. Infection of proliferating cardiac myocytes in young puppies with CPV-2 results in a nonsuppurative myocarditis and sequelae of acute or chronic heart failure, discussed with The Cardiovascular System (Volume 3, Chapter 1). Similar syndromes are very rarely associated with spontaneous FPV infection; anomalies of the central nervous system have not been reported in puppies with CPV-2.

Bibliography

Appel, M. J. G. Does canine coronavirus augment the effects of subsequent parvovirus infection? *Vet Med* **83:** 360–366, 1988.

Bestetti, G., and Zwahlen, R. Generalized parvovirus infection with inclusion-body myocarditis in two kittens. *J Comp Pathol* **95:** 393–397, 1985.

Boosinger, T. R. *et al.* Bone marrow alterations associated with canine parvoviral enteritis. *Vet Pathol* **19:** 558–561, 1982.

Brunner, C. J., and Swango, L. J. Canine parvovirus infection: Effects on the immune system and factors that predispose to severe disease. *Compend Cont Ed Pract Vet* **7:** 979–988, 1985.

Carlson, J. H., and Scott, F. W. Feline panleukopenia. II. The relationship of intestinal mucosal cell proliferation rates to viral infection and development of lesions. *Vet Pathol* **14:** 173–181, 1977.

Carlson, J. H., Scott, F. W., and Duncan, J. R. Feline panleukopenia. I. Pathogenesis in germ-free and specific pathogen-free cats. *Vet Pathol* **14:** 79–88, 1977.

Carlson, J. H., Scott, F. W., and Duncan, J. R. Feline panleukopenia. III. Development of lesions in the lymphoid tissues. *Vet Pathol* **15:** 383–392, 1978.

Carman, P. S., and Povey, R. C. Pathogenesis of canine parvovirus-2 in dogs: Haematology, serology, and virus recovery. *Res Vet Sci* **38:** 134–140, 1985.

Carman, P. S., and Povey, R. C. Pathogenesis of canine parvovirus-2 in dogs: histopathology and antigen identification in tissues. *Res Vet Sci* **38:** 141–150, 1985.

Jacobs, R. M. *et al.* Clinicopathologic features of canine parvoviral enteritis. *J Am Anim Hosp Assoc* **16:** 809–814, 1980.

Kahn, D. E. Pathogenesis of feline panleukopenia. *J Am Vet Med Assoc* **173:** 628–630, 1978.

Kilham, L., Margolis, G., and Colby, E. D. Cerebellar ataxia and its congenital transmission in cats by feline panleukopenia virus. *J Am Vet Med Assoc* **158:** 888–906, 1971.

Larsen, S., Flagstad, A., and Aalback, B. Experimental feline panleukopenia in the conventional cat. *Vet Pathol* **13:** 216–240, 1976.

Macartney, L. *et al.* Canine parvovirus enteritis 2: Pathogenesis. *Vet Rec* **115:** 453–460, 1984.

Martyn, J. C., Davidson, B. E., and Studdert, M. J. Nucleotide sequence of feline panleukopenia virus: Comparison with canine parvovirus identifies host-specific differences. *J Gen Virol* **71:** 2747–2753, 1990.

McAdaragh, J. P. *et al.* Experimental infection of conventional dogs with canine parvovirus. *Am J Vet Res* **43:** 693–696, 1982.

Meunier, P. C. *et al.* Experimental viral myocarditis: Parvoviral infection of neonatal pups. *Vet Pathol* **21:** 509–515, 1984.

Meunier, P. C. *et al.* Pathogenesis of canine parvovirus enteritis: Sequential virus distribution and passive immunization studies. *Vet Pathol* **22:** 617–624, 1985.

O'Sullivan, G. *et al.* Experimentally induced severe canine parvoviral enteritis. *Aust Vet J* **61:** 1–4, 1984.

Parrish, C. R. Emergence, natural history, and variation of canine, mink, and feline parvoviruses. *Adv Vir Res* **38:** 403–450, 1990.

Pollock, R. V. H. Experimental canine parvovirus infection in dogs. *Cornell Vet* **72:** 103–119, 1982.

Rice, J. B. *et al.* Comparison of systemic and local immunity in dogs with canine parvovirus gastroenteritis. *Infect Immun* **38:** 1003–1009, 1982.

Schultz, R. D., Mendel, H., and Scott, F. W. Effect of feline panleukopenia virus infection on development of humoral and cellular immunity. *Cornell Vet* **66:** 324–332, 1976.

a. Panleukopenia (Infectious Feline Enteritis)

The virus of panleukopenia infects all members of the Felidae, as well as mink, raccoons, and some other members of the Procyonidae. Panleukopenia virus is ubiquitous in environments frequented by cats, and infection is common, though generally subclinical. The disease usually occurs in young animals exposed after decay of passively acquired maternal antibody, but it may occur in naive cats of any age. Clinical signs of several days' duration, including pyrexia, depression, inappetence, vomition, diarrhea, dehydration, and perhaps anemia may be evident in the history. However, many cases, particularly poorly observed animals or those prone to wander, may present as sudden death. The pathogenesis of panleukopenia has been considered above. Lesions of the central nervous system in kittens are considered with The Nervous System (Volume 1, Chapter 3).

At autopsy, external evidence of diarrhea may be present, the eyes may be sunken, and the skin is usually inelastic, with a tacky subcutis reflecting dehydration. Rehydrated animals may have edema, hydrothorax, and ascites due to hypoproteinemia. There is pallor of mucous membranes, fat, and internal tissues in anemic animals. Gross lesions of internal organs most consistently involve the thymus and the intestine. The thymus is markedly involuted and reduced in mass in young kittens. Enteric lesions may be subtle and are easily overlooked; hence, it is mandatory that intestine be examined microscopically despite the apparent absence of gross change.

The intestinal serosa may appear dry and nonreflective, with an opaque ground-glass appearance. Uncommonly in cats there may be petechiae or more extensive hemorrhage in the subserosa, muscularis, or submucosa of the intestinal wall. The small bowel may be segmentally dilated and can acquire a hoselike turgidity in places, perhaps due to submucosal edema. However, turgidity is difficult to assess in the intestine of the cat. The content is usually foul smelling, scant and watery, and yellowish gray at all levels of the intestine. The mucosa may be glistening gray or pink, with petechiae, perhaps covered by fine strands of fibrin (Fig. 1.111). Patchy diphtheritic lesions may be present, especially over Peyer's patches in the ileum. Flecks of fibrin, and sometimes casts, may be in the content in the lumen. Formed feces are not evident in the colon. Lymph nodes may be prominent at the root of the mesentery. Gross lesions elsewhere in the carcass are usually restricted to pulmonary congestion and edema in some animals, and pale gelatinous marrow in normally active hemopoietic sites.

Microscopic changes are consistently found in the intestinal tract in fatal cases, and are usual in lymphoid organs and in bone marrow. The intestinal lesions vary with the severity and duration of the disease. Their interpretation may be obscured by autolysis. Lesions may be patchy, and several levels of gut should be examined, preferably including ileum and, if possible, Peyer's patches. During the late incubation period and early phase of clinical disease, crypt-lining epithelium is infected. Intranuclear inclusions may be found, and damaged epithelium containing inclusions exfoliates into the lumen of crypts. Crypts are dilated and lined by cuboidal or more severely attenuated cells. The lamina propria between crypts contains numerous neutrophils and eosinophils at this time, and some emigrate into the lumen of crypts, where they join the epithelial debris.

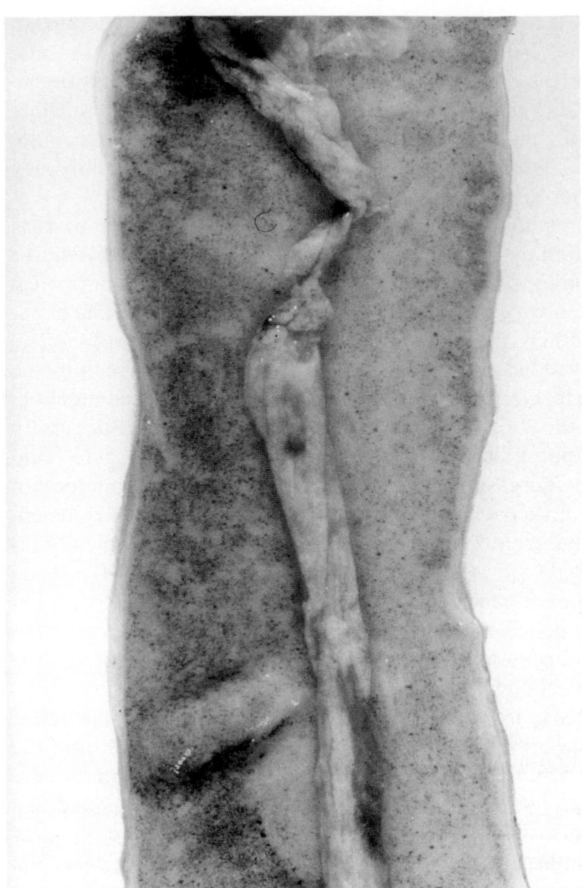

Fig. 1.111 Feline panleukopenia. Petechiae and fibrin cast on mucosa. Small intestine.

Subsequently, severely damaged crypts may be lined by extremely flattened cells, and by scattered large bizarre cells with swollen nuclei and prominent nucleoli (Fig. 1.112A). Enterocytes covering villi are not affected, but as they progress off the villus, they are replaced by a few cuboidal, squamous, or bizarre epithelial cells, so that villi in affected areas undergo progressive collapse. If cryptal damage is severe and widespread, the mucosa becomes thin and eroded or ulcerated, with effusion of tissue fluids, fibrin, and erythrocytes. Inflammatory cells are usually sparse in the gut of such animals, and superficial masses of bacteria may be present, occasionally accompanied by locally invasive fungal hyphae. In less severely affected animals with disease of longer duration, corresponding to about 8–10 days after infec-

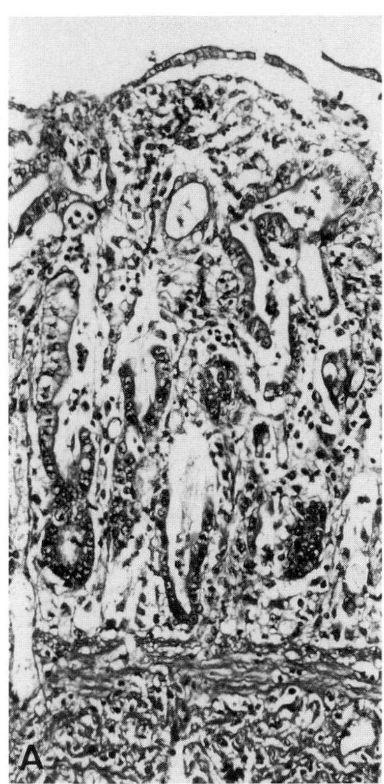

Fig. 1.112A Parvovirus infections. Severe atrophy of villi associated with damage to crypts of Lieberkühn. Cat. Attenuation of surface epithelium and depletion of proprial inflammatory infiltrate.

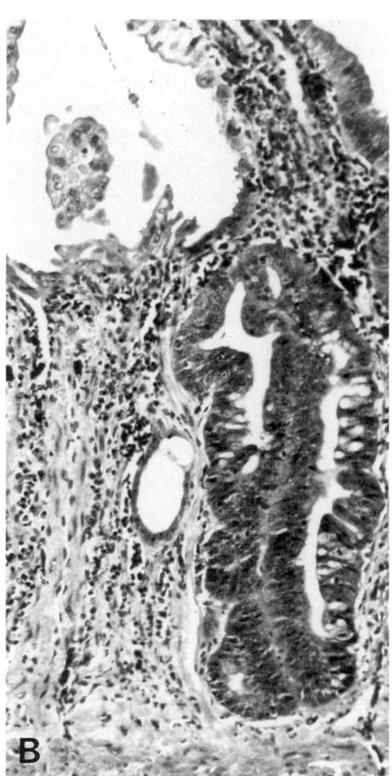

Fig. 1.112B Parvovirus infections. Loss of crypts and collapse of proprial stroma. Gland is lined by hyperplastic epithelium. (Mink virus enteritis.)

tion, scattered focal drop-out of crypts, or focal mucosal collapse and erosion or ulceration, may be evident. In these animals, remaining crypts recovering from milder viral damage show regenerative epithelial hyperplasia (Fig. 1.112B). Mucosal lesions are often most marked in the vicinity of Peyer's patches.

Lesions in the colon generally resemble those found in the small bowel, though they are often less severe or more patchy in distribution. Colonic lesions are present in about half of fatal cases of panleukopenia. Gastric lesions resulting from damage to mitotic epithelium are relatively uncommon in cats. They are recognized by flattening of basophilic cells lining the narrowed isthmus of gastric fundic glands, with some reduction in number of parietal cells in the upper portion of the neck of glands.

Lesions of lymphoid organs during the early phase of the disease consist of lymphocytolysis in follicles and paracortical tissue in lymph nodes, in the thymic cortex and splenic white pulp, and in gut-associated lymphoid tissue. Infected cells rarely contain inclusion bodies. Lymphocytes are markedly depleted in affected tissue, and large histiocytes are prominent, often containing the fragmented remnants of nuclear debris. Follicular hyalinosis, the presence of amorphous eosinophilic material in the center of depleted follicles, may be seen. Erythrophagocytosis by sinus histiocytes may occur in lymph nodes, especially those draining the gut. Severely depleted Peyer's patches may be difficult to recognize microscopically. Later in the course of clinical disease, corresponding to the period beyond about 7–8 days after infection, prominent regenerative lymphoid hyperplasia may be found.

In severely affected animals at the nadir of the leukopenia, virtually all proliferating elements in the bone marrow may be depleted. The extremely hypocellular, moderately congested marrow is populated only by scattered stem cells. Milder lesions affect mainly the neutrophil series, generally sparing megakaryocytes and the committed erythroid elements. During the later phases of the disease, marked hyperplasia of stem cells, and eventually of amplifier populations in the various cell lines, is evident.

In the liver, dissociation and rounding up of hepatocytes, and perhaps some periacinar atrophy and congestion, may be evident. This is probably associated with dehydration and anemia. Pancreatic acinar atrophy is also common, reflecting inappetence. The lung may be congested and edematous. In leukopenic animals, few white cells are seen in circulation in any organ.

A diagnosis of feline panleukopenia may be made on the basis of the characteristic microscopic intestinal lesions, in association with evidence of involution or regenerative hyperplasia of lymphoid and hematopoietic tissues. Inclusions may be sought in these tissues, but are usually present in significant numbers only during the late incubation and early clinical period. Application of fluorescent antibody or immunoperoxidase techniques may identify viral antigen in tissue as late as 8–10 days after infection, and isolation may be performed in tissue culture. Cryptal necrosis is reported also in the intestines of some cats with feline leukemia virus infection, which must be differentiated.

Bibliography

Doi, K. *et al.* Histopathology of feline panleukopenia in domestic cats. *Natl Inst Anim Health Q* **15:** 76–85, 1975.

Langheinrich, K. A., and Nielsen, S. W. Histopathology of feline panleukopenia: A report of 65 cases. *J Am Vet Med Assoc* **158:** 863–872, 1971.

Pollock, R. V. H. The parvoviruses. Part I. Feline panleukopenia virus and mink enteritis virus. *Compend Cont Ed Pract Vet* **6:** 227–237, 1984.

Reinacher, M. Feline leukemia virus-associated enteritis—a condition with features of panleukopenia. *Vet Pathol* **24:** 1–4, 1987.

Stokes, R. Intestinal mycosis in a cat. *Aust Vet J* **49:** 499–500, 1973.

b. Canine Parvovirus-2 Infection This virus presumably resulted by mutation of FPV or a closely related virus. It appeared spontaneously and virtually simultaneously in populations of dogs on several continents in 1978, and rapidly spread worldwide. Retrospective serologic studies suggest that it was circulating unnoticed in western Europe by 1976. In addition to domestic dogs, several species of wild canids, including coyotes, bush dogs, crab-eating foxes, raccoon dogs, and maned wolves are susceptible to infection.

Enteric disease due to this virus was epizootic for several years in naive populations of dogs, affecting animals of all ages. As the prevalence of antibody due to natural infection and vaccination increased, the problem subsided to one of an enzootic disease. It now affects those animals with reduced levels of passively acquired maternal immunity, or scattered naive individuals.

During the epizootic period, nonsuppurative viral myocarditis due to CPV-2 was prevalent in the offspring of naive bitches unable to protect pups with maternal antibody during the first 15 days of life, when replicating myocardial cells are susceptible to parvoviral damage. Myocardial disease in pups due to CPV-2 is now extremely rare, as most bitches have antibody. Enteric and myocardial disease rarely occur together in the same individual or cohort of animals. Occasional cases of generalized parvovirus infection are reported in susceptible neonates. Necrosis and inclusion bodies are found in organs such as kidney, liver, lung, heart, gut, and vascular endothelium. They are presumably related to mitotic activity during organogenesis. Necrotizing cerebral vasculitis, resulting in malacia and nervous signs, has been associated with CPV-2 infection in a 7-week-old pup.

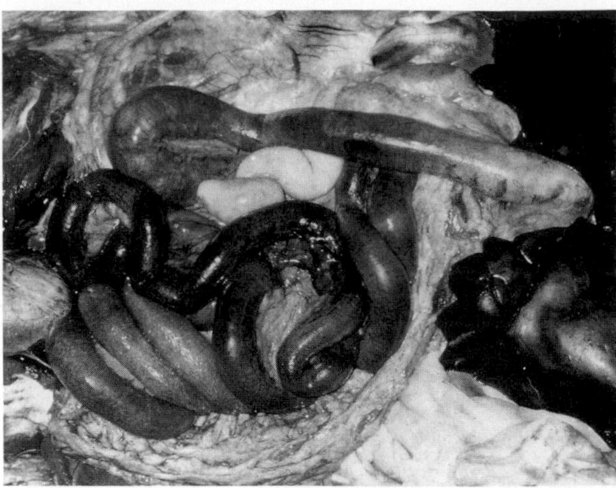

Fig. 1.113 Canine parvovirus infection. Segmental subserosal hemorrhage and mild fibrinous exudation on intestinal serosa.

Dogs with typical disease due to CPV-2 become anorectic and lethargic, may vomit and develop diarrhea, perhaps in association with transient moderate pyrexia. Relative or absolute lymphopenia or leukopenia of 1–2 days' duration may occur. Diarrhea may be mucoid or liquid, sometimes bloody, and is malodorous. After a period of 2–3 days, dogs either succumb to the effects of dehydration, hypoproteinemia, and anemia, or begin to recover.

Gross findings at autopsy of fatal cases are those of dehydration, accompanied by enteric lesions characteristic of the disease. There is often segmental or widespread subserosal intestinal hemorrhage, which may extend into the muscularis and submucosa. The serosa frequently appears granular due to superficial fibrinous effusion (Fig. 1.113). Peyer's patches may be evident from the serosal and mucosal aspects as deep red oval areas several centimeters long. The intestinal contents may be mucoid or fluid; sometimes they look like tomato soup, because of hemorrhage. The mucosa is usually deeply congested and glistening, or covered by a patchy fibrinous exudate. Severe mucosal lesions may be widespread or segmental, and their distribution is irregular; thus tissues from several levels of the small intestine should be selected for microscopic examination. Gross changes in the colon are similar, but less common. The stomach may have a congested mucosa and contain scant bloody or bile-stained fluid. Mesenteric lymph nodes may be enlarged, congested, and wet, or be reduced in size. Thymic atrophy is consistently present in young animals, and the organ may be so reduced in size as to be difficult to find. The lungs often appear congested, and have a rubbery texture.

The microscopic lesions in stomach, small intestine (Fig. 1.114A,B), colon, lymphoid tissue, and bone marrow due to canine parvovirus-2 infection do not differ significantly from those described in cats with panleukopenia. Gastric lesions are perhaps more frequently en-

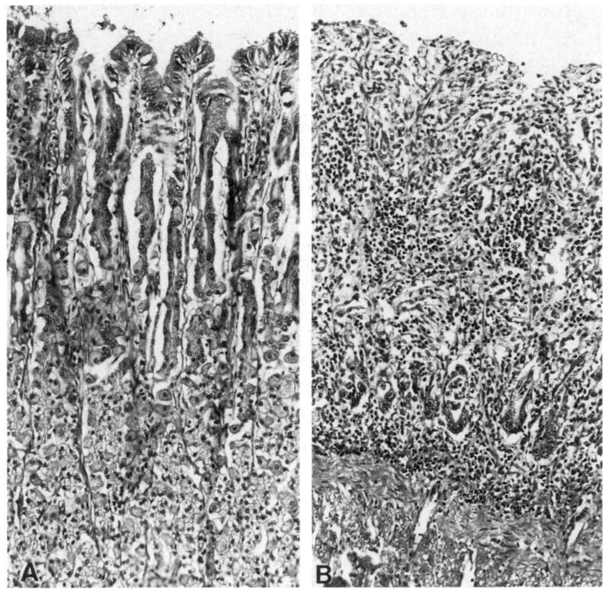

Fig. 1.114 Parvovirus infection. Dog. (A) Attenuation of epithelium lining isthmus and upper neck of fundic gastric glands. (B) Loss of crypts of Lieberkühn and collapse of proprial stroma in small intestine. Remnants of crypt-lining epithelium persist deep in lamina propria.

countered in dogs with parvovirus infection. Small-intestinal lesions are invariably severe in fatal cases. The colon is involved in a minority of animals. Pulmonary lesions such as alveolar septal thickening by mononuclear cells, congestion, and effusion of edema fluid and fibrin into the lumina of alveoli may be related to terminal Gram-negative sepsis and endotoxemia, which is common in fatal cases. Periacinar atrophy and congestion in the liver are attributable to anemia, hypovolemia, and shock, and prominent Kupffer's cells probably reflect endotoxemia.

The diagnosis of parvoviral enteritis in dogs follows the principles described for that of panleukopenia in cats. The disease must be differentiated from canine coronavirus infection, which very rarely is fatal, and from canine intestinal hemorrhage syndrome, shock gut, intoxication with heavy metals or warfarin, infectious canine hepatitis, and other causes of hemorrhagic diathesis. Involution of gut-associated lymphoid tissue and cryptal necrosis caused by parvovirus must be differentiated from similar lesions occasionally seen in canine distemper.

Bibliography

Carpenter, J. L. *et al.* Intestinal and cardiopulmonary forms of parvovirus infection in a litter of pups. *J Am Vet Med Assoc* **176:** 1269–1273, 1980.

Cooper, B. J. *et al.* Canine viral enteritis. II. Morphologic lesions in naturally occurring parvovirus infection. *Cornell Vet* **69:** 134–144, 1979.

Hayes, M. A., Russell, R. G., and Babiuk, L. A. Sudden death in young dogs with myocarditis caused by parvovirus. *J Am Vet Med Assoc* **174:** 1197–1203, 1979.

Lenghaus, C., and Studdert, M. J. Generalized parvovirus disease in neonatal pups. *J Am Vet Med Assoc* **181:** 41–45, 1982.

Meunier, P. C. *et al.* Canine parvovirus in a commercial kennel: Epidemiologic and pathologic findings. *Cornell Vet* **71:** 96–110, 1981.

Nelson, D. T. *et al.* Lesions of spontaneous canine viral enteritis. *Vet Pathol* **16:** 680–686, 1979.

Pollock, R. V. H. The parvoviruses. Part II. Canine parvovirus. *Compend Cont Ed Pract Vet* **6:** 653–664, 1984.

Robinson, W. F., Huxtable, C. R., and Pass, D. A. Canine parvoviral myocarditis: A morphologic description of the natural disease. *Vet Pathol* **17:** 282–293, 1980.

Turk, J. *et al.* Coliform septicemia and pulmonary disease associated with canine parvoviral enteritis: 88 cases (1987–1988). *J Am Vet Med Assoc* **196:** 771–773, 1990.

c. Minute Virus of Canines Minute virus of canines (MVC) is distinct from members of the feline panleukopenia subgroup, and antibody to it is widespread among dogs. It may be an occasional cause of mild diarrhea in pups, but its significance is poorly defined.

Experimental oral–nasal infection is clinically inapparent, but virus replicates in lymphoid tissues, and, in neonatal pups, in the duodenal crypts, where inclusion bodies may be found. Transient thymic atrophy, and lymphocytolysis in thymus, cortex of lymph nodes, and in gut-associated lymphoid tissue are reported.

The virus seems capable of transplacental transmission to the fetus, and exposure of pregnant dogs was associated with fetal resorption, or birth of dead or weak pups, depending on gestational stage at exposure. Anasarca and myocarditis are reported in dead or poorly viable pups. Spontaneous reproductive failure associated with MVC is not reported.

Bibliography

Carmichael, L. E., Schlafer, D. H., and Hashimoto, A. Pathogenicity of minute virus of canines (MVC) for the canine fetus. *Cornell Vet* **81:** 151–171, 1991.

Macartney, L. *et al.* Characterization of minute virus of canines (MVC) and its pathogenicity for pups. *Cornell Vet* **78:** 131–145, 1988.

d. Bovine Parvovirus Infection The antigenically distinct bovine parvovirus has been recognized for many years and occurs widely in cattle populations on all continents. A single serotype is known. It has been isolated from the feces of normal and recently diarrheic calves as well as from conjunctiva, and from aborted fetuses. The status of bovine parvovirus as an enteric pathogen is unclear. Virus shedding is not always associated with diarrhea, and it may be part of a mixed infection in diarrheic animals. It is rarely diagnosed as a cause of death, and unless sought specifically by culture or direct electron microscopy, would be missed as a cause of clinical diarrhea. Its significance may be greatest in neonatal calves and animals exposed while passive maternal antibody levels are waning, or in animals in the postweaning period.

The pathogenesis of infection with bovine parvovirus resembles that in carnivores. Initial virus replication following oral inoculation is in tonsils and gut, with spread to systemic lymphoid tissues, resulting in transient lymphopenia. Viral antigen has been identified in the nuclei of epithelium in intestinal crypts and in cells in thymus, lymph nodes, adrenal glands, and heart muscle. Transient lymphocytolysis in infected tissues, and exfoliation of epithelium in crypts of the small and large intestine, with moderate villus atrophy, depletion of colonic goblets, and mixed inflammatory cell infiltration of the mucosa, have been seen experimentally. Intranuclear inclusions are present when lesions are prevalent. Gross lesions other than abnormally fluid content in the gut are subtle, or absent. Intravenous inoculation of bovine parvovirus into young calves causes severe watery diarrhea and prostration. Milder diarrhea occurs in calves infected orally. The severity of the disease may be potentiated by concurrent infection with other enteric pathogens, or other factors which may increase intestinal epithelial proliferation.

Bibliography

Bridger, J. C. Small viruses associated with gastroenteritis in animals. *In* "Viral Diarrheas of Man and Animals," L. J. Saif and K. W. Theil (eds.), pp. 161–182. Boca Raton, Florida, CRC Press, 1990.

Durham, P. J. K., Johnson, R. H., and Parker, R. J. Exacerbation of experimental parvoviral enteritis in calves by coccidia and weaning stress. *Res Vet Sci* **39:** 16–23, 1985.

Durham, P. J. K., Lax, A., and Johnson, R. H. Pathological and virological studies of experimental parvoviral enteritis in calves. *Res Vet Sci* **38:** 209–219, 1985.

Storz, J. Bovine parvoviruses. *In* "Virus Infections of Ruminants," Z. Dinter and B. Morein (eds.), pp. 203–214. Amsterdam, Elsevier, 1990.

B. Bacterial Diseases

1. Escherichia coli

Escherichia coli has several virulence attributes which result in disease in animals. Principally, these promote **colonization or adhesion** to the mucosa; they cause **metabolic dysfunction or death of enterocytes;** they **affect the local or systemic vasculature;** or they promote **invasion and septicemia.** Disease syndromes caused by *E. coli* in domestic animals can be related to the combinations of virulence attributes expressed. Many terms and acronyms have been applied to the mechanisms of action of *E. coli;* some are obsolete; some apply mainly to *E. coli* in laboratory animals and humans, and are not directly applicable to domestic animals; others are synonyms.

Enterotoxigenic *E. coli* (ETEC) cause secretory small bowel diarrhea stimulated by enterotoxins produced by *E. coli* colonizing the mucosa of the small intestine. This condition is an important, common cause of diarrhea in neonatal animals of many species.

Enteropathogenic *E. coli* (EPEC) in humans may colonize the mucosa of the intestine by a mechanism involving adhesion-effacement [**entero-adherent** *E. coli* (EAEC)]. Some do not produce recognized toxins, but are associated with villus atrophy; they are an uncommon cause of disease in domestic animals. But other strains of *E. coli* which are attaching-effacing, in addition secrete cytotoxins (verotoxins), which have an effect locally or systemically. Depending on the location and manifestation of this effect, such *E. coli* have been categorized as **attaching-effacing** (AEEC); **verotoxigenic** (VTEC); or **enterohemorrhagic** (EHEC). The EHEC cause hemorrhagic enterocolitis in calves younger than a month.

Verotoxigenic infections in swine, which are not attaching-effacing, are associated with postweaning *E. coli* enteritis and also cause edema disease, which is a systemic toxemia.

Enteroinvasive *E. coli* (EIEC) are poorly documented in domestic animals.

Septicemic colibacillosis is another, and common, manifestation of disease caused by this organism. The intestine is not necessarily the portal of entry, and there may not be alimentary disease. The signs of *E. coli* septicemia are referable mainly to bacteremia, endotoxemia, and the effect of bacterial localization in a variety of tissue spaces throughout the body.

Bibliography

Holland, R. E. Some infectious causes of diarrhea in farm animals. *Clin Microbiol Rev* **3:** 345–375, 1990.

Levine, M. M. *Escherichia coli* that cause diarrhea: Enterotoxigenic, enteropathogenic, enteroinvasive, enterohemorrhagic, and enteroadherent. *J Infect Dis* **155:** 377–389, 1987.

a. Enterotoxigenic Colibacillosis Enterotoxigenic colibacillosis caused by ETEC is one of the major causes of diarrhea in neonatal pigs, calves, and lambs, as well as in humans.

Two major attributes confer virulence on these strains of *E. coli.* These are the ability to colonize the intestine, and the capacity to produce toxins which stimulate secretion of electrolyte and water by the intestinal mucosa. Colonization and enterotoxin production must occur together for disease to ensue. The diarrhea produced by enterotoxigenic *E. coli* is accompanied by relatively minor microscopic evidence of inflammation, and by little or no architectural change in the mucosa. As a result, overt enteritis usually is not evident at autopsy, and the disease is part of the syndrome of undifferentiated diarrhea of neonatal animals.

Intestinal colonization results from the adhesion of *E. coli* to the surface of enterocytes on villi in the small intestine, and proliferation there (Fig. 1.115A). By adhering to the mucosa, bacteria are able to resist the normal peristaltic clearance mechanisms. Large numbers of or-

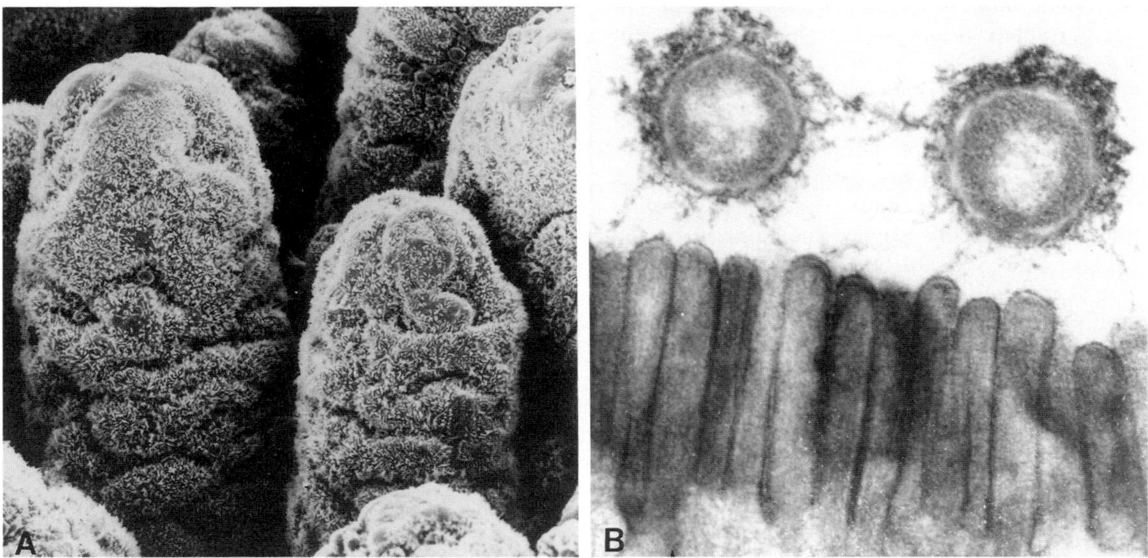

Fig. 1.115 (A) Scanning electron micrograph. *Escherichia coli* adherent to the surface of villi. Calf. (B) Transmission electron micrograph. Fimbriate *E. coli* adherent to microvilli. Small intestine. Calf. (Courtesy of J. J. Hadad and C. L. Gyles.)

ganisms, of the order of 10^7 or more per gram of mucosa, or 20–30 per enterocyte, line the surface of villi. The ability to attach to enterocytes is conferred on enterotoxigenic strains of *E. coli* by pili, and may be enhanced by the presence of a capsule.

Pili, or **fimbriae** [also known as **colonization factor antigens (CFA)**] are rodlike or filamentous projections from the cell wall of *E. coli* which attach to specific glycoconjugate receptors on the surface of enterocytes (Fig. 1.115B). They are distinct from type 1 fimbriae, which do not promote colonization of the gut. Pili are polymers of protein (pilin) subunits, which are coded by plasmid (K88 = F4, K99 = F5) or chromosomal (987P = F6, F17, F41) DNA. They are antigenically distinct, permitting recognition by specific antibody. Pilus adhesins tend to be associated with specific O serotypes of *E. coli,* and they tend to be relatively host specific, though some are functional in several hosts.

Pilus adhesins include **K99** in calves, lambs, and pigs; **F41, F17** = **F(Y)** in calves and pigs; **K88, 987P** in pigs. Combinations of adhesins may be expressed by the same strain of ETEC; typically, F41 is expressed by strains also expressing K99, and seems to be of minor importance. Bacteria possessing K88 colonize the entire small bowel, whereas those with K99 or 987P adhere mainly in the jejunum and ileum. Low pH suppresses K99 expression, but not that of K88, suggesting that the acidity of the environment in the proximal small intestine, not the availability of receptors, governs the distribution of *E. coli* with K99 pili.

Three types of K88 antigenic variants, K88ab, K88ac, and K88ad, are recognized. Swine vary in the expression of receptors on their enterocytes to these pili, such that some swine are refractory to adhesion of any K88 pili, whereas others have receptors to one or more of the K88 pilus phenotypes. Resistance to K88 adhesion is a recessive trait in pigs, but resistant pigs are susceptible to other pilus adhesins; a pattern of resistance to K99 adhesion has not been detected in swine. Variation in K88 receptor expression may explain variations in susceptibility of litters of pigs in outbreaks of ETEC diarrhea.

Susceptibility to bacterial pilus adhesins, especially K99 and 987P, appears to be somewhat age related; the ability of pilus-bearing *E. coli* to colonize the small intestine is greatest in animals only a few days old. K99 receptors on enterocytes decline in availability with age. In contrast, receptors for 987P are shed into the lumen in older pigs, facilitating clearance of bacteria from the mucosa, and interfering with colonization. Stimulation of maternal immunity to appropriate pilus antigens causes antibody secretion in the milk, which combines with adhesins and prevents colonization of the gut of suckling animals.

Enterotoxigenic strains of *E. coli* produce two types of plasmid-encoded toxins, which act locally in the intestine to alter secretion and absorption of electrolyte and water by enterocytes.

Heat-labile toxin (LT) is a large immunogenic molecule, antigenically similar to cholera toxin, and comprising a small A and a larger pentamer of five B subunits. The B subunits bind to ganglioside receptors on the enterocyte surface; the toxin complex then dissociates, and the A subunit is internalized into the cell. It operates via an adenylate cyclase pathway to cause chloride secretion by crypt cells, sodium and water following osmotically from the mucosa. Cotransport of sodium chloride by enterocytes, and associated water uptake, is probably also shut down at the same time. Labile toxin has a latent period prior to the development of secretion, but the effects are relatively irreversible.

Heat-stable toxins (ST) are small polypeptide molecules which exist in several forms, with different physical and functional characteristics. This is reflected in variations in host and age-group susceptibility to the various types of ST. The **STa** causes chloride and water secretion in the intestine of several species, including mice and neonatal pigs. The **STb,** on the other hand, causes bicarbonate secretion in the small intestine of pigs of all ages; in the presence of protease inhibitors, it will also stimulate secretion in some other species. Two genes for STa production are known: STaP occurs in ETEC infecting pigs, calves, and humans; STaH is not found in ETEC infecting animals. Although STa acts via the guanylate cyclase pathway to promote secretion, and possibly to inhibit Na–Cl cotransport and water absorption in villus enterocytes, crypt epithelium is not targeted by STa, and is not the source of secretion. With a different and unrelated amino acid structure, STb does not activate guanylate cyclase; its mode of action is unknown. When both toxins are expressed by a single strain of *E. coli,* the action of STa predominates. The effects of ST are rapid in onset, but require persistence of toxin. In addition to causing electrolyte and water secretion, ST may also slow intestinal transit, promoting colonization. In pigs, STb is capable of causing exfoliation of surface enterocytes, resulting in some atrophy of villi (about 20% reduction in 6- to 8-week-old pigs).

Enterotoxigenic colibacillosis is among the commonest causes of diarrhea in **pigs** from a few hours to about a week of age. Commonly, serogroups O8, O45, O138, O141, O147, O149, and O157, expressing K88, are involved in enterotoxigenic colibacillosis in piglets, though the prevalence of K88-bearing strains may be declining due to vaccination of sows. Less commonly, 987P, K99, and F41 pilus adhesins are involved. The most common toxin produced by porcine ETEC is STb; when LT is found, it is in association with STb, which may be encoded on the same plasmid. In strains of ETEC in swine, STa also occurs alone, or in combination with other enterotoxins.

At necropsy, enterotoxigenic colibacillosis cannot be separated readily from the other common causes of undifferentiated neonatal diarrhea without laboratory assistance. Generally there is dehydration, usually with evidence of diarrhea, or a history of its occurrence in the herd. Other than the presence of characteristic fluid content in the flaccid small and large bowel, usually with clotted milk still in the stomach, the internal findings are unremarkable.

In contrast to the viruses and *Isospora,* enterotoxigenic *E. coli* usually does not cause significant villus atrophy (Fig. 1.116A). Small clumps, or a continuous layer of bacteria may be found on the surface of enterocytes on villi in mucosal sections, most consistently in ileum (Fig. 1.116B). Some neutrophils may be present in the proprial

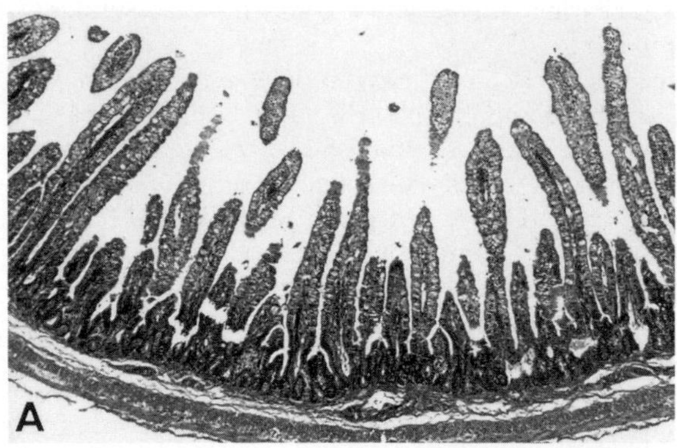

Fig. 1.116A Enterotoxigenic colibacillosis. Piglet. Villi are tall and crypts are short, as is expected in a 2 to 3-day-old animal.

core of villi, and transmigrating the epithelium into the lumen. However, inflammation is not marked, and epithelial lesions and erosion generally are not seen in well-fixed tissue in enterotoxic colibacillosis. Rare cases of villus atrophy associated with *E. coli* infection do occur in neonatal swine. These may be related to the toxic effects of STb on surface enterocytes, or to the presence of EIEC or uncharacterized AEEC, discussed subsequently.

The involvement of enterotoxigenic *E. coli* in postweaning diarrhea of pigs older than 3 weeks, and distinct from postweaning colibacillosis caused by AEEC and VTEC, discussed subsequently, is poorly documented, but may be related to colonization of intestine in weaned pigs in which rotavirus infection, changes in diet, or villus atrophy associated with dietary hypersensitivity, provide

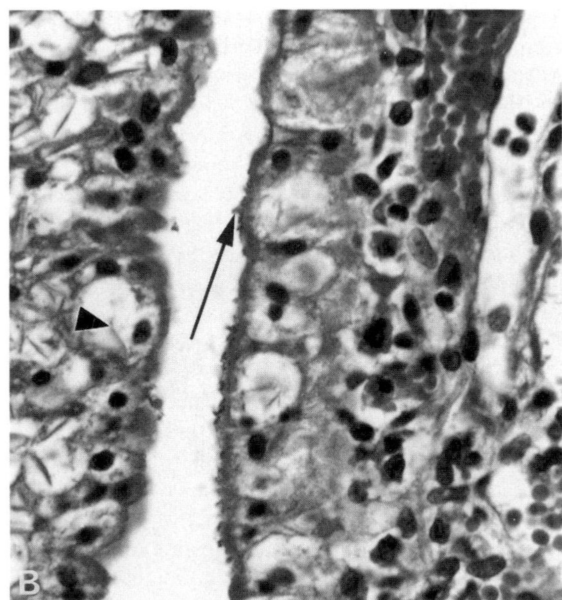

Fig. 1.116B Enterotoxigenic colibacillosis. Piglet. Bacteria are present on surface of enterocytes (arrow). Cytoplasmic vacuoles containing eosinophilic spicules (arrowhead) are normal in the ileal mucosa of young piglets.

adhesin-bearing *E. coli* with a competitive advantage. It is rarely fatal.

In **calves,** most ETEC produce K99 pilus adhesin, with STa, and have an O8, O9, O20, O26, O101, or O141 somatic antigen. Both K99 and STa are commonly coexpressed, since their DNA is sometimes in the same plasmid; LT and STb are not prevalent in ETEC infecting calves and lambs. Organisms of O9 and O101 serogroups may also express K41 pilus adhesin in addition to K99, and occasionally, virulent *E. coli* bearing only K41 adhesin are recognized.

Enterotoxigenic colibacillosis accounts for many cases of undifferentiated neonatal diarrhea in calves; depending on the locality and circumstances, as many as 20–30% may be due to ETEC. The infections typically occur within the first 2–3 days of life, probably because of the resistance of enterocytes in older calves to K99 adhesin. They cause profuse yellow diarrhea, and severe dehydration, with a high mortality in untreated animals.

Enteric colibacillosis must be differentiated from the other major causes of undifferentiated diarrhea in neonatal calves: coronavirus, rotavirus and *Cryptosporidium*. Enterotoxigenic *E. coli* is not uncommonly found in combination with coronavirus or rotavirus infection. Experimental evidence suggests that prior or concomitant infection with rotavirus may permit or promote establishment by enterotoxic *E. coli* in calves older than 2 days. Combined infection may enhance the severity of disease in calves younger than, and in some cases older than, 2 days.

The gross findings in calves with enterotoxigenic colibacillosis are the nonspecific appearance of diarrhea and dehydration. The infection is differentiated in tissue sections from the other infectious causes of this syndrome in calves by the absence of severe villus atrophy (Fig. 1.117) and by the presence of bacteria on the surfaces of villi in the distal small intestine. As in piglets, application of a variety of presumptive or specific tests for the presence of enterotoxigenic *E. coli* in the intestine confirms the diagnosis.

Enterotoxigenic *E. coli* are not considered to induce diarrhea by villus atrophy and malabsorption, in contrast to attaching-effacing *E. coli* and the significant viruses and *Cryptosporidium*. However, rarely, in the jejunum and ileum of some calves, where bacterial colonization of the surface of enterocytes is heavy, stumpiness, lateral corrugation and contraction, or moderate atrophy of villi may be present. Transmigration of neutrophils from the lamina propria to the lumen is present in colonized areas of gut, especially in the vicinity of the domes over Peyer's patches (Fig. 1.118).

Enterotoxigenic colibacillosis should be suspected in neonatal calves having large numbers of Gram-negative rods in smears of ileal scrapings. Though enterotoxigenic

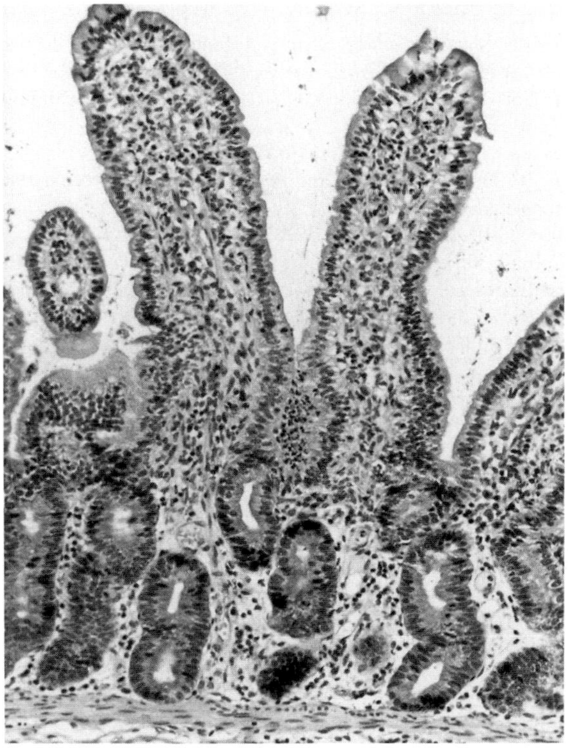

Fig. 1.117 Enterotoxigenic colibacillosis. Calf. Mild neutrophil infiltrate in lamina propria and between base of villi. Atrophy of villi not evident; surface epithelium normal. (Courtesy of J. J. Hadad and C. L. Gyles.)

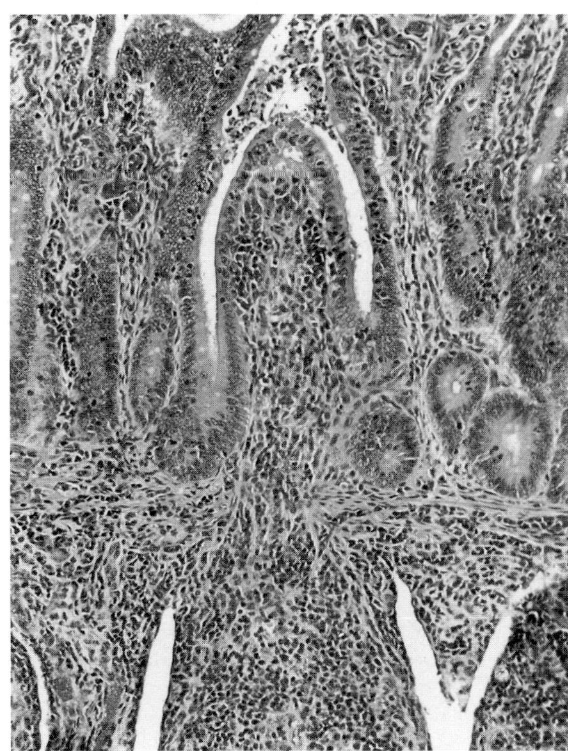

Fig. 1.118 Enterotoxigenic colibacillosis. Calf. Neutrophil effusion into lumen over dome of Peyer's patch. (Courtesy of J. Bellamy.)

E. coli may be isolated from mesenteric lymph nodes or other parenchymatous tissues at necropsy, systemic invasion is not a significant component of the disease. Enterotoxigenic colibacillosis must be differentiated from enteric colibacillosis in calves due to AEEC and EHEC, and from septicemic colibacillosis.

Enterotoxigenic colibacillosis is a significant problem in **lambs** in some areas. The serotypes involved, pathogenesis, and diagnosis of the condition are similar to those in calves. Synergism with rotavirus infection may occur.

There are several reports of ETEC isolated from **foals** with diarrhea. The organisms have pili, probably F41, and secrete LT or STa. However, their capacity to produce disease in foals is unproven. Diarrhea has not ensued in foals inoculated with K88 bearing *E. coli,* despite the presence of K88 receptors on enterocytes, and it seems that ETEC has little significance in this species.

Strains of *E. coli* have been associated with diarrhea in neonates of other species of animals, but their enterotoxigenicity and other attributes of virulence usually have not been well described.

Bibliography

Acres, S. D. Enterotoxigenic *Escherichia coli* infections in newborn calves: A review. *J Dairy Sci* **68:** 229–256, 1985.

Ansari, M. M., Renshaw, H. W., and Gates, N. L. Colibacillosis in neonatal lambs: Onset of diarrheal disease and isolation and characterization of enterotoxigenic *Escherichia coli* from enteric and septicemic forms of the disease. *Am J Vet Res* **39:** 11–14, 1978.

Bellamy, J. E. C., and Acres, S. D. Enterotoxigenic colibacillosis in colostrum-fed calves: Pathologic changes. *Am J Vet Res* **40:** 1391–1397, 1979.

Dean, E. A., Whipp, S. C., and Moon, H. W. Age-specific colonization of porcine intestinal epithelium by 987P-piliated enterotoxigenic *Escherichia coli. Infect Immun* **57:** 82–87, 1989.

Duchet-Suchaux, M. *et al.* Experimental *Escherichia coli* diarrhoea in colostrum-deprived lambs. *Ann Rech Vet* **13:** 259–266, 1982.

Evans, M. G., Waxler, G. L., and Newman, J. P. Prevalence of K88, K99, and 987P pili of *Escherichia coli* in neonatal pigs with enteric colibacillosis. *Am J Vet Res* **47:** 2431–2434, 1986.

Fairbrother, J. M., Larivière, S., and Johnson, W. M. Prevalence of fimbrial antigens and enterotoxins in nonclassical serogroups of *Escherichia coli* isolated from newborn pigs with diarrhea. *Am J Vet Res* **49:** 1325–1328, 1988.

Francis, D. H. Use of immunofluorescence, Gram's staining, histologic examination, and seroagglutination in the diagnosis of porcine colibacillosis. *Am J Vet Res* **44:** 1884–1888, 1983.

Francis, D. H., Allen, S. D., and White, R. D. Influence of bovine intestinal fluid on the expression of K99 pili by *Escherichia coli. Am J Vet Res* **50:** 822–826, 1989.

Hadad, J. J., and Gyles, C. L. Scanning and transmission electron microscopic study of the small intestine of colostrum-fed calves infected with selected strains of *Escherichia coli. Am J Vet Res* **43:** 41–49, 1982.

Harel, J. *et al.* Detection of genes for fimbrial antigens and enterotoxins associated with *Escherichia coli* serogroups isolated from pigs with diarrhea. *J Clin Microbiol* **29:** 745–752, 1991.

Hirsh, D. C. Fimbriae: Relation of intestinal bacteria and virulence in animals. *Adv Vet Sci Comp Med* **29:** 207–238, 1985.

Holland, R. E., Sriranganathan, N., and DuPont, L. Isolation of enterotoxigenic *Escherichia coli* from a foal with diarrhea. *J Am Vet Med Assoc* **194:** 389–391, 1989.

Klemm, P. Fimbrial adhesins of *Escherichia coli. Rev Infect Dis* **7:** 321–340, 1985.

Lintermans, P. F. *et al.* Characterization and purification of the F17 adhesin on the surface of bovine enteropathogenic and septicemic *Escherichia coli. Am J Vet Res* **49:** 1794–1799, 1988.

Mainil, J. G. *et al.* Hybridization of bovine *Escherichia coli* isolates with gene probes for four enterotoxins (STaP, STaH, STb, LT) and one adhesion factor (K99). *Am J Vet Res* **47:** 1145–1148, 1986.

Mainil, J. G. *et al.* Prevalence of four enterotoxin (STaP, STaH, STb, and LT) and four adhesin subunit (K99, K88, 987P, and F41) genes among *Escherichia coli* isolates from cattle. *Am J Vet Res* **51:** 187–190, 1990.

Moon, H. W. Protection against enteric colibacillosis in pigs suckling orally vaccinated dams: Evidence of pili as protective antigens. *Am J Vet Res* **42:** 173–177, 1981.

Moon, H. W. Colonization factor antigens of enterotoxigenic *Escherichia coli* in animals. *In* "Bacterial Adhesins," K. Jann and B. Jann (eds.), pp. 147–165. Current Topics in Microbiology 151. Berlin, Springer-Verlag, 1990.

Moon, H. W. *et al.* Pathogenic relationships of rotavirus, *Escherichia coli,* and other agents in mixed infections in calves. *J Am Vet Med Assoc* **173:** 577–583, 1978.

Moon, H. W., Schneider, R. A., and Moseley, S. L. Comparative prevalence of four enterotoxin genes among *Escherichia coli* isolated from swine. *Am J Vet Res* **47:** 210–212, 1986.

Mouricout, M. A., and Julien, R. A. Pilus-mediated binding of bovine enterotoxigenic *Escherichia coli* to calf small intestinal mucins. *Infect Immun* **55:** 1216–1223, 1987.

Olson, P., Hedhammar, A., and Wadström, T. Enterotoxigenic *Escherichia coli* infection in two dogs with acute diarrhea. *J Am Vet Med Assoc* **184:** 982–983, 1984.

Pearson, G. R., and Logan, E. F. Ultrastructural changes in the small intestine of neonatal calves with enteric colibacillosis. *Vet Pathol* **19:** 190–201, 1982.

Rapacz, J., and Hasler-Rapacz, J. Polymorphism and inheritance of swine small intestinal receptors mediating adhesion of three serological variants of *Escherichia coli*-producing K88 pilus antigen. *Anim Genet* **17:** 305–321, 1986.

Rose, R., Whipp, S. C., and Moon, H. W. Effects of *Escherichia coli* heat-stable enterotoxin b on small intestinal villi in pigs, rabbits, and lambs. *Vet Pathol* **24:** 71–79, 1987.

Runnels, P. L. *et al.* Effects of microbial and host variables on the interaction of rotavirus and *Escherichia coli* infections in gnotobiotic calves. *Am J Vet Res* **47:** 1542–1550, 1986.

Sivaswamy, G., and Gyles, C. L. Characterization of enterotoxigenic bovine *Escherichia coli. Can J Comp Med* **40:** 247–256, 1976.

Snodgrass, D. R., Smith, M. L., and Kraitil, F. L. Interaction of rotavirus and enterotoxigenic *Escherichia coli* in conventionally reared dairy calves. *Vet Microbiol* **7:** 51–60, 1982.

Tzipori, S. The relative importance of enteric pathogens affecting neonates of domestic animals. *Adv Vet Sci Comp Med* **29:** 103–206, 1985.

Tzipori, S. *et al.* Diarrhea in lambs: Experimental infections with

enterotoxigenic *Escherichia coli,* rotavirus, and *Cryptosporidium* sp. *Infect Immun* **33:** 401–406, 1981.
Tzipori, S. *et al.* Intestinal changes associated with rotavirus and enterotoxigenic *Escherichia coli* infection in calves. *Vet Microbiol* **8:** 35–43, 1983.
Ward, A. C. S. *et al.* Isolation of piliated *Escherichia coli* from diarrheic foals. *Vet Microbiol* **12:** 221–228, 1986.
Whipp, S. C. Intestinal responses to enterotoxigenic *Escherichia coli* heat-stable toxin b in nonporcine species. *Am J Vet Res* **52:** 734–737, 1991.
Whipp, S. C. *et al.* Effect of virus-induced destruction of villous epithelium on intestinal secretion induced by heat-stable *Escherichia coli* enterotoxins and prostaglandin E_1 in swine. *Am J Vet Res* **46:** 637–642, 1985.
Whipp, S. C., Moseley, S. L., and Moon, H. W. Microscopic alterations in jejunal epithelium of 3-week-old pigs induced by pig-specific, mouse-negative, heat-stable *Escherichia coli* enterotoxin. *Am J Vet Res* **47:** 615–618, 1986.
Whipp, S. C. *et al.* Functional significance of histologic alterations induced by *Escherichia coli* pig-specific, mouse-negative, heat-stable enterotoxin (ST_b). *Vet Res Commun* **11:** 41–55, 1987.
Wilson, R. A., and Francis, D. H. Fimbriae and enterotoxins associated with *Escherichia coli* serogroups isolated from pigs with colibacillosis. *Am J Vet Res* **47:** 213–217, 1986.

b. ENTEROPATHOGENIC COLIBACILLOSIS Some diarrheagenic *E. coli,* classed as enteropathogenic in humans, adhere to the mucosa by means other than pili, and may produce cytotoxins; analogous strains cause disease in domestic animals.

A nonpilus adhesin, involved in attachment of some enteropathogenic *E. coli* (EPEC), has been termed **EPEC adhesive factor (EAF),** and is encoded in the plasmid pMAR-2. This factor, which has been characterized *in vitro* using HEp-2 cells, results in **localized adherence (LA),** involving small areas of the cell surface. In contrast, **diffuse adherence (DA)** involves the whole cell surface, and is not medicated by pMAR-2. Localized adherence is characteristic of class I EPEC. Class II EPEC are EAF negative, though some are DA positive. The LA EAF is probably a 94-kDa outer membrane protein which binds with a glycoprotein receptor, possibly including fibronectin, on the cell surface. The nature of the DA adhesin is not well defined. Pili of undefined type may also be involved in adhesion of some EPEC.

Many enteropathogenic strains of *E. coli* efface microvilli, subsequently attaching intimately to the enterocyte and promoting exfoliation (**att-eff** virulence attribute, which is chromosomally encoded); they are known as **entero-adherent (EAEC)** or **attaching-effacing *E. coli* (AEEC).** This process may occur in two stages, the first involving nonintimate attachment facilitated by EAF, or possibly by pili or fimbriae (FY = Att25 in some species). The second stage results in effacement of microvilli and intimate attachment of bacteria to the apex of the enterocyte, and is not dependent on the first stage. Microvilli degenerate into small vesicular structures, which are released into the lumen of the bowel. A pedestal of cytoplasm protrudes from the cell surface, with a cup on the

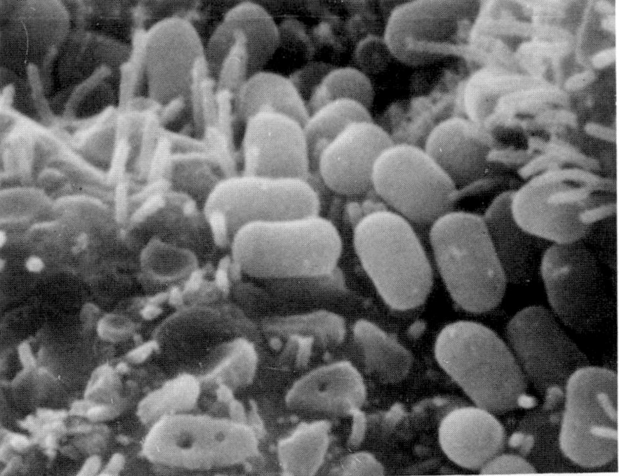

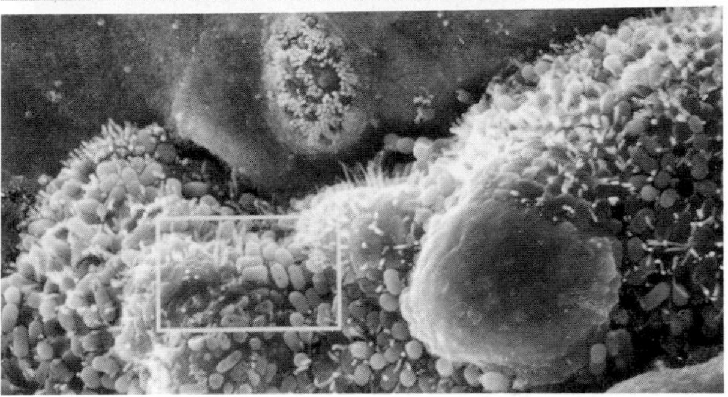

Fig. 1.119 Scanning electron micrograph. Colon. Calf. Enterohemorrhagic *E. coli* infection. (Lower) Note irregularity of microvilli on cells infected by adherent-effacing *E. coli,* in comparison with microvilli on uninfected cells in background. Outline indicates field illustrated in upper photo. Adherent bacteria are on pedestals projecting from the surface of enterocytes. Occasional bacteria have been lost artefactually, exposing underlying mushroomlike pedestals. (Courtesy of M. Schoonderwoerd and R. Clarke.)

end, to which the bacterial cell is closely attached (Figs. 1.119,1.120). The terminal web at the luminal end of the enterocyte is lost. The ultrastructural appearance of *E. coli* adherent by the att-eff mechanism is characteristic.

In animals and humans, some strains of **attaching-effacing *E. coli*** are pathogenic despite failure to secrete enterotoxins or cytotoxins. Adhesion is by att-eff, with or without the involvement of plasmid-encoded EAF. Disease in humans, rabbits, pigs, lambs, and dogs, associated with att-eff$^+$, LT, ST, and VT negative, *E. coli* has been documented, and it can be reproduced experimentally in pigs using EPEC of porcine and human origin. Diarrhea of varying degree, without blood, occurs in animals infected with AEEC.

A heavy layer of plump coccobacilli may be found over the luminal aspect of enterocytes on villi throughout the small intestine, and on the surface of the large intestine. The degree of diarrhea seems related to the extent of bacterial colonization, which is most consistent in lower small intestine and large bowel. Enterocytes to which

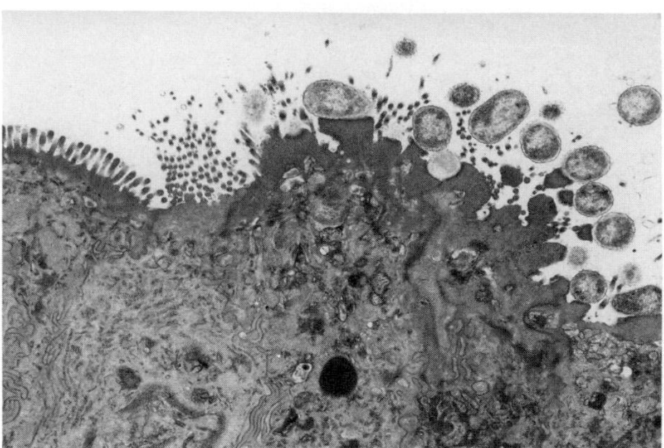

Fig. 1.120 Calf infected with enterohemorrhagic *E. coli*. Transmission electron micrograph. Enterocytes. Colon. Enterocyte adherent-effacing *E. coli* are on pedestals projecting from surface of infected cells. Microvilli are irregular and effaced on infected cells. Normal cell (left). (Reprinted with permission from Schoonderwoerd, M. *et al. Can J Vet Res* **52:** 484–487, 1988).

bacteria are adherent round up or contract, and exfoliate from the mucosa singly or in clumps, resulting in mild to severe atrophy of villi in the small bowel, and attenuation of surface cells, or microerosions, in the large intestine. Fusion of villi may occur in small intestine, and goblet cell numbers are depleted in both large and small bowel. There is moderate mucosal congestion, and local infiltration by neutrophils.

Diarrhea is presumably related to maldigestion and malabsorption of nutrients and electrolytes in small intestine, overloading the colon, the absorptive ability of which is also compromised by damage to surface cells. Microscopic diagnosis is based on recognition of AEEC on the mucosal surface. Among agents colonizing the brush border, AEEC are plumper than ETEC, and smaller, more regular in size, and usually more numerous than *Cryptosporidium*. Electron microscopy may confirm AEEC by demonstrating the characteristic attachment mechanism. Viruses such as coronavirus and rotavirus, which may cause villus atrophy, and in the case of coronavirus, colonic lesions in some species, must be ruled out. Isolation of *E. coli* which do not produce LT, ST, and VT will confirm involvement of purely att-eff bacteria.

The second major virulence attribute of some EPEC is the production of potent cytotoxins. Toxins, produced by EPEC, which are capable of killing Vero cells *in vitro* have been termed **verotoxins** or **verocytotoxins (VT),** and the organisms which secrete them are **verotoxigenic *E. coli* (VTEC).** Several VT have been identified, at least one of which is nearly identical to a toxin produced by *Shigella dysenteriae*, **shigatoxin (SDT),** and they are sometimes referred to as **shigalike toxins (SLT).** The genetic information coding for these cytotoxins is carried by temperate bacteriophages. Two verotoxins, **VT1** and **VT2,** have been recognized in human *E. coli*. Production of VT1 (nearly identical with shigatoxin) is greatest in iron-depleted environments. Verotoxin 2 does not cross-react serologically with shigatoxin, and production is not iron regulated.

Verotoxins comprise an active A subunit, and several binding B subunits, which attach to glycolipid receptors on the cell surface. The A subunit is internalized in the cell, where it interferes with protein synthesis by inactivation of the 60 S ribosomal subunit. Both types of VT act similarly, but VT2 is less potent than VT1. *In vivo*, VT has an adverse effect on enterocytes in the intestine, but endothelial cells in small vessels are particularly prone to the cytotoxic effect of VT. Very young animals may lack the glycolipid VT receptor on small intestinal enterocytes, which may explain the relatively greater involvement of the colon in disease mediated by VTEC.

Although many *E. coli* produce VT in small amounts, VTEC do so in large quantities. Verotoxin-secreting AEEC have been implicated in diarrhea in calves; VTEC (serotype O6) of unknown adhesion are considered facultative pathogens causing diarrhea in cats. Non-AEEC VTEC cause edema disease and postweaning *E. coli* enteritis in swine, discussed in the next section.

In calves younger than 4 weeks (generally older than 3 days, and most commonly in the second week of life), strains of *E. coli* which may possess FY = Att25 are found occasionally. They adhere by an attaching-effacing mechanism, and secrete VT1. They composed less than 1–4% of isolates from calves younger than 1 month which died of *E. coli*-related disease in surveys in the United States and United Kingdom, but in some areas they are a significant cause of morbidity and mortality. Serotypes O5, O26, and O111 are involved, and since the characteristic syndrome produced is one of erosive fibrinohemorrhagic enterocolitis, these isolates may be characterized as **enterohemorrhagic *E. coli* (EHEC).** Although all EHEC are verotoxigenic, not all VTEC are EHEC.

In humans, serotypes O26 and O157 especially are implicated in hemorrhagic colitis and are considered EHEC; 0111 is considered enteropathogenic. Serotypes 026 and 0111 are primarily of human origin and are probably accidental in calves, where they lack the EAF normally found on human class I EPEC. Serotype O157 is more commonly isolated from bovine sources (feces, meat, milk), and in addition to causing hemorrhagic colitis in humans, has been implicated in hemolytic–uremic syndrome, also mediated by VT. Lesions have been produced by experimental O157 infection in pigs and calves, but spontaneous disease in animals due to this serotype has yet to be recognized.

The syndrome induced by EHEC in calves is one of diarrhea, with the development of dysentery, marked by bright red blood in feces, in some cases. Fever is not characteristic, and animals may remain bright until the effects of dehydration supervene. Death may occur within several days of onset of illness, but animals will recover within 7–10 days in some cases.

At necropsy, the gross lesions are usually confined to the spiral colon and rectum, though the distal small intestine and cecum are occasionally involved with a mild fi-

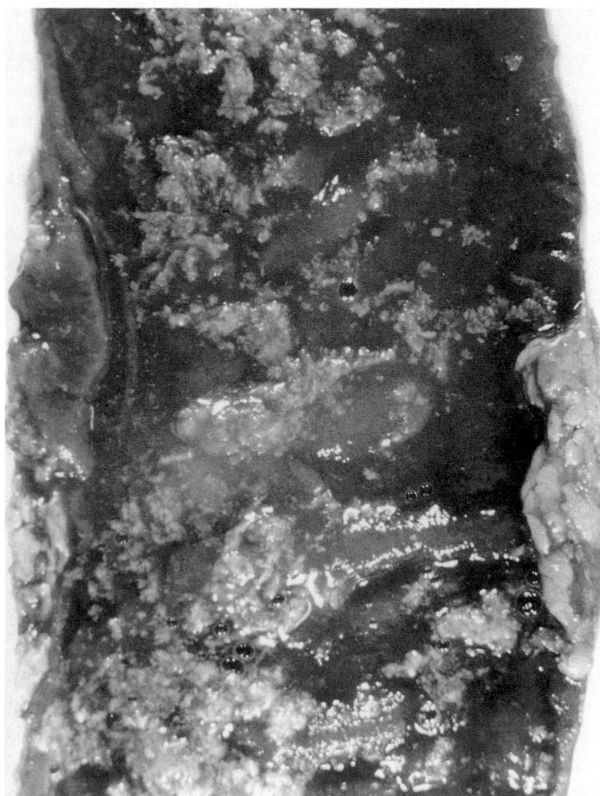

Fig. 1.121 Fibrinohemorrhagic enteritis. Ileum. Calf. Enterohemorrhagic *E. coli* infection. (Courtesy of M. Schoonderwoerd and R. Clarke.)

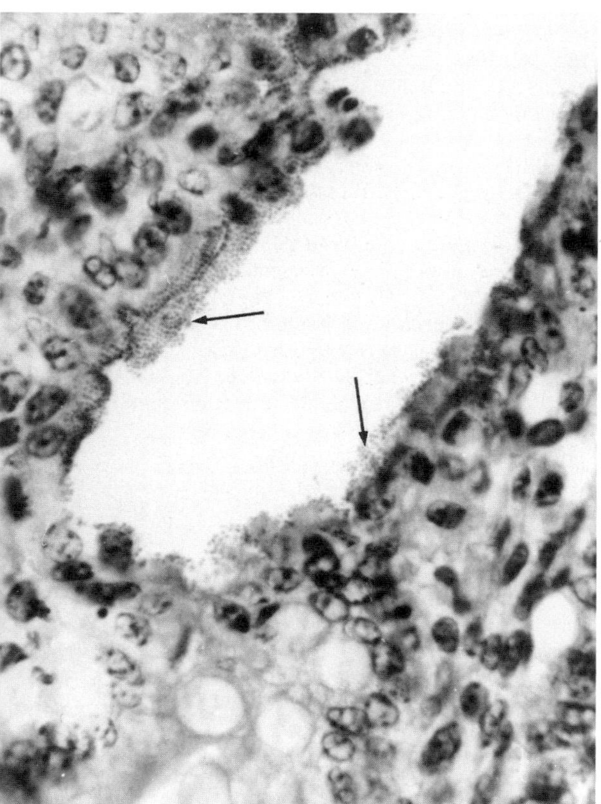

Fig. 1.122 Colon. Calf. Enterohemorrhagic *E. coli* infection. Adherent bacteria (arrows) on surface of enterocytes. (Courtesy of M. Schoonderwoerd and R. Clarke.)

brinous or fibrinohemorrhagic enteritis (Fig. 1.121). In the colon, changes vary from mild patchy congestion of the mucosa to marked mucosal reddening, with adherent mucus, necrotic debris, and blood; the colonic contents are fluid and frequently blood-tinged. There may be congestion of the margins of mucosal folds in the rectum, or an overt fibrinohemorrhagic proctitis. Mesenteric lymph nodes are often enlarged, especially along the ileum, and occasionally there may be lesions (arthritis, serositis) suggesting septicemia.

Microscopically, in affected small intestine, the profile of villi is ragged or markedly scalloped, and they are blunted, moderately atrophic, or fused. Epithelial cells on villi in small bowel, and on the colonic surface, where lesions are most severe, are short, rounded up, and in some cases exfoliating singly or in small clumps, causing focal microerosions. Cells in some areas may be markedly attenuated. The microvillous border is indistinct, and covered by a heavy layer of prominent Gram-negative coccobacilli (Fig. 1.122). Lesions in large bowel may extend down into glands, which may be dilated, lined by flattened epithelium, and filled with sloughed epithelium and leukocytes. In the small intestine, foci of bacterial adherence may be patchy, on the sides of the upper third of villi, with extensive surrounding areas of normal epithelium. Crypts in areas of atrophic small intestine may be elongate, with numerous mitotic figures. In severely affected bowel, the mucosa and submucosa are congested, edematous, and occasional microvascular thrombi may be present. Sloughed enterocytes, erythrocytes, neutrophils, fibrin, and bacteria are in the lumen.

EHEC occur frequently in association with other agents causing neonatal diarrhea in calves, especially *Cryptosporidium,* rotavirus, and coronavirus. Appropriate laboratory investigation should be undertaken to rule out viral agents. The EHEC are differentiated from AEEC by production of a more severe clinical syndrome, with blood, which is probably mediated by local cytotoxic effects of VT on enterocytes and vascular endothelium. Determination of O serotype and demonstration of VT production by the organism in culture confirm the etiology. In section, they are differentiated from ETEC and *Cryptosporidium* as described for AEEC.

Bibliography

Abaas, S. *et al.* Cytotoxin activity of Vero cells among *Escherichia coli* strains associated with diarrhea in cats. *Am J Vet Res* **50:** 1294–1296, 1989.

Batt, R. M. *et al.* Ultrastructural damage to equine small intestinal epithelium induced by enteropathogenic *Escherichia coli. Equine Vet J* **21:** 373–375, 1989.

Broes, A. *et al.* Natural infection with an attaching and effacing *Escherichia coli* in a diarrheic puppy. *Can J Vet Res* **52:** 280–282, 1988.

Cantey, J. R., and Blake, R. K. Diarrhea due to *Escherichia coli* in the rabbit: A novel mechanism. *J Infect Dis* **135:** 454–462, 1977.

Chanter, N. *et al.* Dysentery in calves caused by an atypical strain of *Escherichia coli* (S102-9). *Vet Microbiol* **12:** 241–253, 1986.

Hall, G. A. *et al.* Dysentery caused by *Escherichia coli* (S102-9) in calves: Natural and experimental disease. *Vet Pathol* **22:** 156–163, 1985.

Hall, G. A., Chanter, N., and Bland, A. P. Comparison in gnotobiotic pigs of lesions caused by verotoxigenic and nonverotoxigenic *Escherichia coli. Vet Pathol* **25:** 205–210, 1988.

Helie, P. *et al.* Experimental infection of newborn pigs with an attaching and effacing *Escherichia coli* O45:K"E65" strain. *Infect Immun* **59:** 814–821, 1991.

Janke, B. H. *et al.* Attaching and effacing *Escherichia coli* infections in calves, pigs, lambs, and dogs. *J Vet Diagn Invest* **1:** 6–11, 1989.

Janke, B. H. *et al.* Attaching and effacing *Escherichia coli* infection as a cause of diarrhea in young calves. *J Am Vet Med Assoc* **196:** 897–901, 1990.

Karmali, M. A. Infection by verocytotoxin-producing *Escherichia coli. Clin Microbiol Rev* **2:** 15–38, 1989.

Law, D. Virulence factors of enteropathogenic *Escherichia coli. J Mol Microbiol* **26:** 1–10. 1988.

Mainil, J. G. *et al.* Shigalike toxin production and attaching effacing activity of *Escherichia coli* associated with calf diarrhea. *Am J Vet Res* **48:** 743–748, 1987.

Moon, H. W. *et al.* Attaching and effacing activities of rabbit and human enteropathogenic *Escherichia coli* in pig and rabbit intestines. *Infect Immun* **41:** 1340–1351, 1983.

Morris, J. A., Chanter, N., and Sherwood, D. Occurrence and properties of FY(Att25)$^+$ *Escherichia coli* associated with diarrhoea in calves. *Vet Rec* **121:** 189–191, 1987.

Moxley, R. A., and Francis, D. H. Natural and experimental infection with an attaching and effacing strain of *Escherichia coli* in calves. *Infect Immun* **53:** 339–346, 1986.

Okerman, L. Enteric infections caused by nonenterotoxigenic *Escherichia coli* in animals: Occurrence and pathogenicity mechanisms. A review. *Vet Microbiol* **14:** 33–46, 1987.

Pearson, G. R. *et al.* Natural infection with an attaching and effacing *Escherichia coli* in the small and large intestines of a calf with diarrhoea. *Vet Rec* **124:** 297–299, 1989.

Peeters, J. E., Charlier, G. J., and Raeymaekers, R. Scanning and transmission electron microscopy of attaching effacing *Escherichia coli* in weanling rabbits. *Vet Pathol* **22:** 54–59, 1985.

Pospischil, A. *et al.* Attaching and effacing bacteria in the intestines of calves and cats with diarrhea. *Vet Pathol* **24:** 330–334, 1987.

Rothbaum, R. *et al.* A clinicopathologic study of enterocyte-adherent *Escherichia coli:* A cause of protracted diarrhea in infants. *Gastroenterology* **83:** 441–454, 1982.

Schoonderwoerd, M. *et al.* Colitis in calves: Natural and experimental infection with a verotoxin-producing strain of *Escherichia coli* O111:NM. *Can J Vet Res* **52:** 484–487, 1988.

Tzipori, S., Gibson, R., and Montanaro, J. Nature and distribution of mucosal lesions associated with enteropathogenic and enterohemorrhagic *Escherichia coli* in piglets and the role of plasmid-mediated factors. *Infect Immun* **57:** 1142–1150, 1989.

Wray, C., McLaren, I., and Pearson, G. R. Occurrence of "attaching and effacing" lesions in the small intestine of calves experimentally infected with bovine isolates of verocytotoxic *E. coli. Vet Rec* **125:** 365–368, 1989.

c. EDEMA DISEASE AND POSTWEANING *ESCHERICHIA COLI* ENTERITIS **Edema disease** is a distinct syndrome in pigs characterized by sudden death, or the development of nervous signs, associated with enteric colonization by certain serotypes of usually hemolytic *E. coli*. The disease occurs most commonly in pigs within a few weeks after weaning, or after other change in feeding or management. It often occurs in association with outbreaks of postweaning *E. coli* enteritis. Rare reports exist of edema disease in suckling and mature animals. The disease may be sporadic or occur as an outbreak, usually affecting the best animals in a group, and mortality often approaches 100% of affected animals. Edema disease and postweaning *E. coli* enteritis have apparently declined in prevalence in many parts of North America, perhaps with the use of concentrate rations based largely on soybeans and corn, rather than other grains.

A soluble factor (**edema disease principle (EDP)** or *E. coli* neurotoxin) released in the gut by some serotypes of *E. coli* (mainly O138, O139, O141) has been implicated as the cause of edema disease. This is a verotoxin **[SLT II variant (SLT IIv)],** produced by the O serotypes of *E. coli* implicated in the etiology of the disease, and the lesions of edema disease are reproduced in pigs inoculated intravenously with pure SLT IIv. The genetic code for SLT IIv is 94% homologous with that of VT2, but is not phage mediated.

The factors predisposing to enteric colonization and adhesion by these strains are unknown. The serogroups involved seem to be normal members of the gut flora of weaned pigs. Weaning, changes in ration, or accompanying alterations in the enteric microenvironment may favor proliferation of these strains of *E. coli*. They stick to the microvillus border of enterocytes on villi in the small intestine, presumably by the medium of some sort of adhesin. They do not use an attaching–effacing mechanism, nor do they possess recognized pilus adhesins. The presence of a space around adherent bacilli in electron micrographs may imply the presence of unstained pili or a capsule.

Some strains of *E. coli* which cause edema disease also produce secretory enterotoxin. Diarrhea is not a usual concomitant of edema disease in individual animals, and SLT IIv has a low capacity to cause secretion in intestinal loops in comparison with ST and SLT I. However, some other animals in the group may develop typical postweaning *E. coli* enteritis, described subsequently. Significant gross or microscopic lesions in the intestinal mucosa do not occur in edema disease, which appears to be a classical enterotoxemia, the active principle being absorbed from the gut and acting at a distant site. However, the means by which the toxin enters the circulation is unknown.

Experimentally, the target of SLT IIv, like other verotoxins, is vascular endothelium, particularly of small arteries and arterioles in the gastric and colonic submucosa and brain. The organ tropism speculatively may be attributed to the differential distribution of the SLT IIv receptor, globotetraosylceramide, on endothelium. Vascular lesions at these sites are sometimes seen in animals dying acutely, and showing typical postmortem lesions of edema. They are more consistently encountered in survivors, or in pigs with a subacute clinical course in which nervous signs are prominent, but in which gross edema at necropsy is not. The angiopathy, in its early stages in experimental intoxication, is recognized by swelling of endothelial cells and intramural and perivascular hemorrhage. Pyknosis and karyorrhexis of smooth muscle nuclei, often accompanied by fibrinoid degeneration or hyalin change in the tunica media, may be seen in subacute spontaneous cases. Proliferative mesenchymal elements are found in the tunica media and tunica adventitia in more advanced cases. However, inflammation is not at any stage a prominent component of the angiopathy, nor of the associated edema in most sites, and thrombosis of vessels is rarely encountered. Edema is probably due to vessel damage during the early stages of the angiopathy. The lesions are distinct from those which might be expected with endotoxemia.

Swine with edema disease may die without premonitory signs. Others may have anorexia, or more characteristically, show nervous signs, usually of less than a day's duration. An unsteady staggering gait, knuckling, ataxia, prostration and tremors, convulsions, and paddling occur. A hoarse squeal, the hoarseness attributed to laryngeal edema and dyspnea, may also be noted clinically.

At necropsy, lesions in acute deaths may be subtle or absent. Typically, edema is variably present in one or more sites. However, it may be mild and must be carefully sought, especially by slipping the suspected area over subjacent tissue. Subcutaneous edema may be present in the frontal area and over the snout, in the eyelids, and in the submandibular, ventral abdominal, and inguinal areas. Internally, there may be some hydropericardium, and serous pleural and peritoneal effusion, perhaps accompanied by mild or moderate pulmonary edema. More commonly, the serous surfaces merely appear glistening and wet. Edema of the mesocolon, of the submucosa of the cardiac glandular area of the stomach over the greater curvature, and of mesenteric lymph nodes is most consistently found. The gastric submucosal edema should be sought by carefully cutting through the muscularis to the submucosa. The edema fluid is clear, and slightly gelatinous (Fig. 1.123). It is rarely blood-tinged, and overt hemorrhage is usually not present in uncomplicated edema disease. The stomach is often full of feed, but the small intestine is relatively empty, and the mucosa is grossly normal. The colon may contain somewhat inspissated feces.

In swine dying after a more prolonged clinical course, gross edema often is not present, though enlargement of mesenteric lymph nodes is present in a large proportion of cases. A few pigs may show usually bilateral symmetrical foci of yellowish malacia in the brain stem at various levels from basal ganglia to medulla.

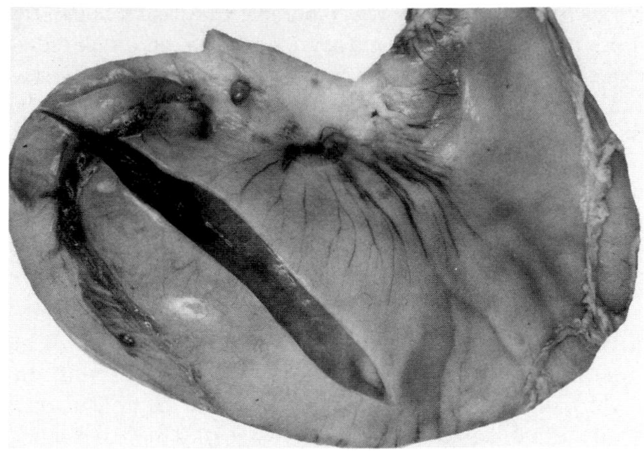

Fig. 1.123 Edema of stomach wall. Edema disease. Pig.

Edema in the sites of predilection mentioned is the main microscopic lesion in swine dying acutely. It generally is devoid of much protein and contains few erythrocytes and inflammatory cells. A proportion of animals will also have meningeal edema and distended Virchow–Robin spaces in the brain. Vascular lesions may not be well developed

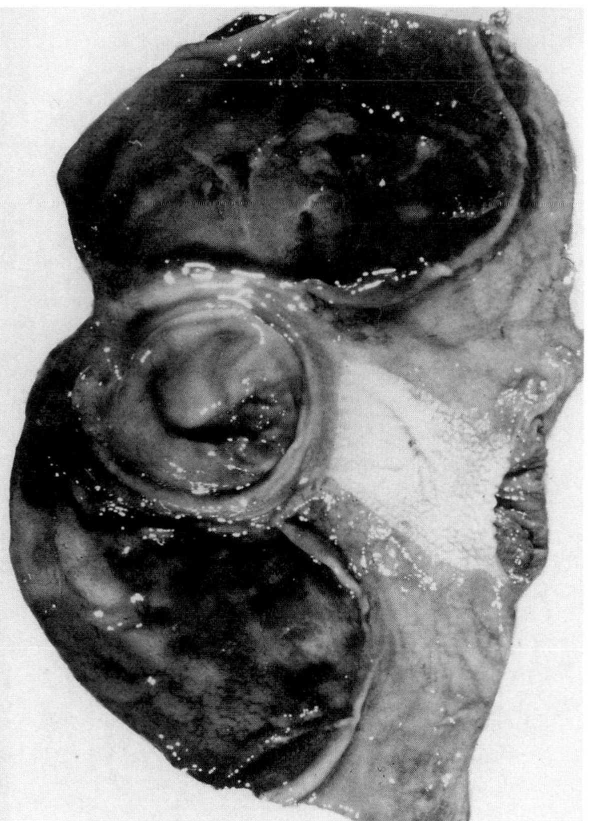

Fig. 1.124 Postweaning colibacillosis. Pig. Deep red areas of venous infarction in the gastric mucosa.

in pigs dying suddenly. When present they usually consist of edema, hemorrhage, myocyte necrosis, and hyalin degeneration in the tunica media. Angiopathy is more consistently found in cases of longer standing. Affected vessels may be found in any tissue in the carcass. Brain edema and focal encephalomalacia in the brain stem are associated with the presence of lesions in cerebral vessels; necrosis may be a sequel to edema and ischemia. Cerebrospinal angiopathy of swine is probably a manifestation of edema disease.

A diagnosis of edema disease is based on nervous signs or sudden death in growing pigs, in association with typical gross and microscopic lesions, when they are present. In acute cases, heavy growth of hemolytic *E. coli* of one of the three common serotypes associated with edema disease is usual on culture of the small and large bowel. In animals with more chronic signs, these strains may have been superseded by others as the dominant *E. coli* populating the intestine. Tests for production of SLT IIv by bacteria cultured from affected animals, or for its presence in gut content, may become routine as techniques for *in vitro* assay are refined.

Edema disease must be differentiated from enteritis and endotoxemia due to *E. coli* in postweaning pigs; from mulberry heart disease in animals dying suddenly; and from salt poisoning, *Salmonella* meningoencephalitis, and other infectious encephalitides, in animals with nervous signs.

Postweaning *E. coli* enteritis (coliform enteritis of weaned pigs) typically occurs during the first week or two following weaning, or after some other change in feed or management. It is usually associated with hemolytic *E. coli* of the same serotypes primarily implicated in edema disease, as well as serotype O149. The two diseases often occur in the same population of pigs, though usually affecting different animals. Typically, postweaning colibacillosis is a disease of high morbidity and variable mortality, with loss of condition in pigs suffering prolonged illness. Diarrhea is usually yellow and fluid, and stains the perineum. Deaths which occur may or may not follow a prior episode of diarrhea, and often appear to be related to endotoxemia.

In fatal cases, there may be bluish-red discoloration of the skin and evidence of dehydration. Deep red gastric venous infarcts are present in almost all cases (Fig. 1.124). The small intestine is flaccid. The mucosa may be normal in color and the content, creamy. In other animals the mucosa of the distal small intestine will be congested and the contents, watery and perhaps blood-tinged or brown with flecks of yellow mucus (Fig. 1.125). Cecal and colonic lesions are usually mild, but there may be some congestion and fibrinous exudate in the proximal large bowel. Mesenteric lymph nodes may be somewhat enlarged, congested, and juicy. Other organs are usually unremarkable grossly.

The pathogenesis of postweaning *E. coli* enteritis is poorly understood, and the microscopic pathology is not

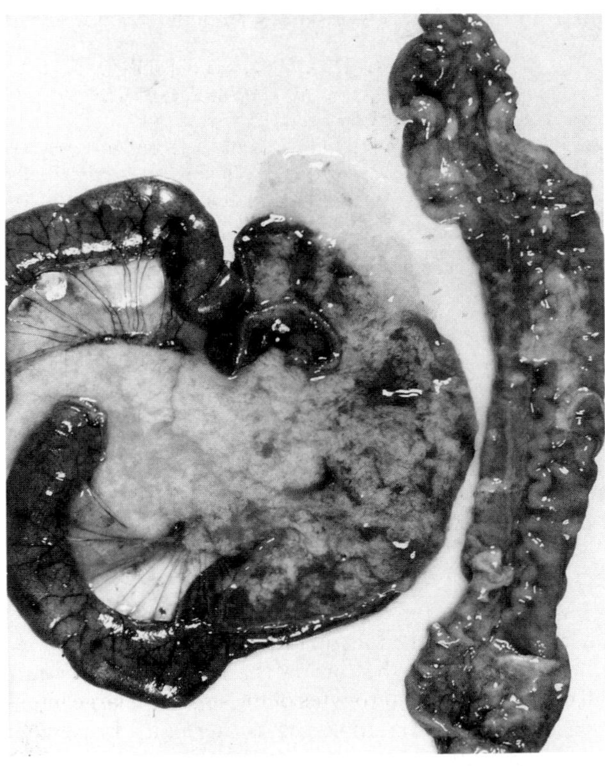

Fig. 1.125 Postweaning colibacillosis. Pig. Acute catarrhal enteritis. Congested, flaccid small intestine.

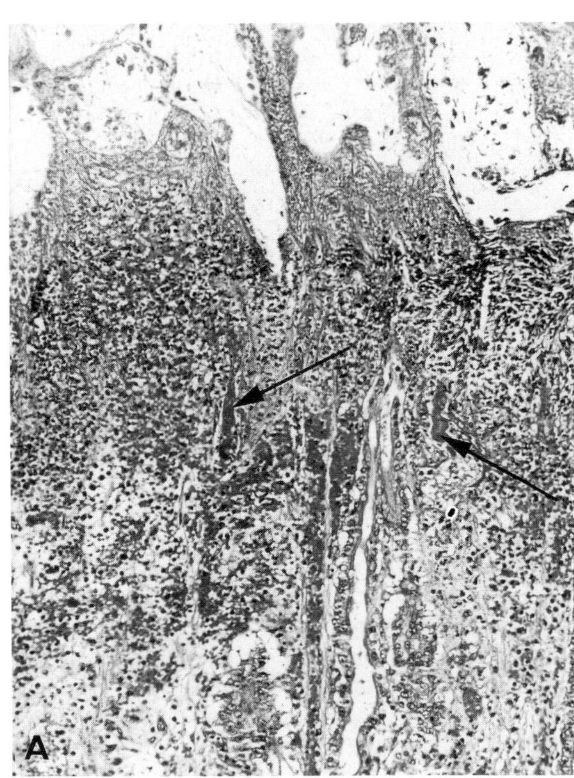

Fig. 1.126A Postweaning colibacillosis in a pig. Thrombosis of venules (arrows) and necrosis of the superficial gastric mucosa in venous infarction.

well described. In swine with diarrhea, *E. coli* may be attached to the surface of villi by means not clearly related to known adhesins, though K88 pili may be present, mainly on O149 strains. Atrophy of villi does not seem to be evident, and diarrhea is presumed to be mediated by enterotoxins (STb, alone or in combination with STa and LT) secreted by *E. coli* of the serotypes involved. The contribution of verotoxin to diarrhea is unclear, but since SLT IIv is much less enterotoxic than ST, this may be minimal. Furthermore, VT is secreted by only a minority of implicated isolates. Mortality in animals with prolonged diarrhea and few gross intestinal or extraintestinal lesions may be ascribed to dehydration. In animals dying of more acute disease, there is local microvascular thrombosis in sections of congested mucosa (Fig. 1.126A,B), and the gross and microscopic lesions in other organs, especially those related to gastric mucosal and submucosal thrombosis and venous infarction, are suggestive of endotoxemia. Hemolytic *E. coli* of the implicated strains are consistently isolated in virtually pure culture from the lower small intestine and colon. However, they are present in the spleen and liver in only a few cases, suggesting terminal bacteremia.

The factors predisposing to the massive colonization of hemolytic *E. coli* are unclear. Loss of lactogenic immunity, a favorable environment for proliferation of bacterial strains with specific nutrient requirements, and promotion of epithelial colonization by the effects of antecedent rotavirus infection, have been variously implicated.

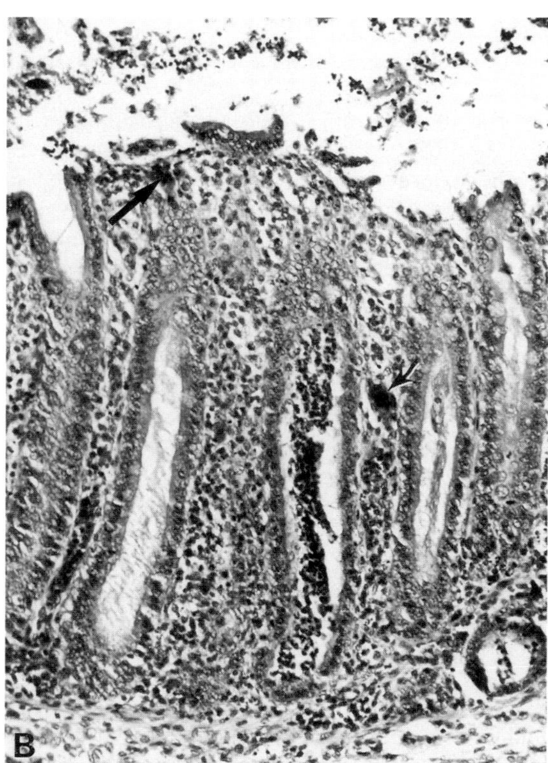

Fig. 1.126B Postweaning colibacillosis. Pig. Erosion and effusion from colonic surface, and accumulation of neutrophils in glands, associated with thrombosis of some venules in the lamina propria (arrows).

A diagnosis of postweaning colibacillosis is suggested by the gross lesions in animals dying acutely or subacutely, and it is confirmed by culture and serotyping of associated strains of *E. coli*. The fatal disease must be differentiated from edema disease, proliferative hemorrhagic enteropathy, salmonellosis, and swine dysentery. Postweaning diarrhea due to uncomplicated rotavirus infection, transmissible gastroenteritis, or associated with classical enterotoxigenic K88$^+$ *E. coli* and attaching–effacing O45:K"E65" *E. coli,* is usually nonfatal.

Bibliography

Bertschinger, H. U., and Pohlenz, J. Bacterial colonization and morphology of the intestine in porcine *Escherichia coli* enterotoxemia (edema disease). *Vet Pathol* **20:** 99–110, 1983.

Gannon, V. P. J, and Gyles, C. L. Characteristics of the shiga-like toxin produced by *Escherichia coli* associated with porcine edema disease. *Vet Microbiol* **24:** 89–100, 1990.

Gannon, V. P. J., Gyles, C. L., and Wilcock, B. P. Effects of *Escherichia coli* shiga-like toxins (verotoxins) in pigs. *Can J Vet Res* **53:** 306–312, 1989.

Hampson, D. J., and Fu, Z. F. Preweaning supplementary feed and porcine post-weaning diarrhoea. *Res Vet Sci* **44:** 309–314, 1988.

Hoblet, K. H. *et al.* Study of porcine postweaning diarrhea involving K88$^{(-)}$ hemolytic *Escherichia coli. Am J Vet Res* **47:** 1910–1912, 1986.

Lecce, J. G. *et al.* Rotavirus and hemolytic enteropathogenic *Escherichia coli* in weanling diarrhea of pigs. *J Clin Microbiol* **16:** 715–723, 1982.

MacLeod, D. L., Gyles, C. L., and Wilcock, B. P. Reproduction of edema disease of swine with purified shiga-like toxin-II variant. *Vet Pathol* **28:** 66–73, 1991.

Methiyapunc, S., Pohlenz, J. F. L., and Bertschinger, H. U. Ultrastructure of the intestinal mucosa in pigs experimentally inoculated with an edema disease-producing strain of *Escherichia coli* (O139:K12:H1). *Vet Pathol* **21:** 516–520, 1984.

Moon, H. W., Schneider, R. A., and Moseley, S. L. Comparative prevalences of four enterotoxin genes among *Escherichia coli* isolated from swine. *Am J Vet Res* **47:** 210–212, 1986.

Nagy, B., Casey, T. A., and Moon, H. W. Phenotype and genotype of *Escherichia coli* isolated from pigs with postweaning diarrhea in Hungary. *J Clin Microbiol* **28:** 651–653, 1990.

Richards, W. P. C., and Fraser, C. M. Coliform enteritis of weaned pigs. A description of the disease and its association with hemolytic *Escherichia coli. Cornell Vet* **51:** 245–257, 1961.

Sarmiento, J. I., Casey, T. A., and Moon, H. W. Postweaning diarrhea in swine: Experimental model of enterotoxigenic *Escherichia coli* infection. *Am J Vet Res* **49:** 1154–1159, 1988.

d. ENTEROINVASIVE *ESCHERICHIA COLI* Strains of *E. coli* are recognized, infecting humans and certain other species, which have the capacity to invade or to be internalized by surface enterocytes of the small and large intestine, in which they multiply. In this sense they resemble *Shigella* in primates, and *Salmonella*. The enteroinvasiveness of *Shigella* and some strains of *E. coli* appears to be correlated with the presence of a high-molecular-weight plasmid coding for outer membrane proteins (OMP) involved in invasion. Multiplication of the organism within epithelial cells results in local erosion and ulceration, associated with acute inflammation in the mucosa. Although in shigellosis, septicemia does not usually occur, bacteria may be present in inflamed mesenteric lymph nodes or liver in some enteroinvasive *E. coli* infections in laboratory animals.

Among domestic animals, enteroinvasive colibacillosis has been confirmed experimentally only in neonatal swine, using a strain of O101 *E. coli*. Spontaneous enteritis which appears to be due to enteroinvasive *E. coli* is encountered rarely in piglets up to weaning and in calves younger than 2 weeks. Diarrhea in experimentally infected piglets is described as gray-yellow, watery, and containing small clots. The gross findings may not be remarkable, or the intestine may appear congested in comparison with that in most diarrheic piglets. In spontaneous cases suspected of being due to enteroinvasive *E. coli,* the gastric fundus may be congested also, and this correlates with the presence of venous infarction visible microscopically. Experimental enteroinvasive colibacillosis in piglets causes villus atrophy comparable in severity to that induced by the common viruses of neonates. Enterocytes appear cuboidal or flattened, and some are seen lysing. The lamina propria is edematous; capillaries are congested and infiltrated by neutrophils and other inflammatory cells. In spontaneous cases thrombi may be evident in proprial capillaries and submucosal lymphatics. Neutrophils and tissue fluid effuse into the lumen between villi through epithelial discontinuities. Similar microthrombosis, proprial inflammation, enterocyte destruction, and effusion may be found in the cecum and colon. Intracellular organisms of O serogroup 101 were demonstrated by immunoperoxidase staining in the experimental study, but are not generally recognized in spontaneous cases suspected to be due to enteroinvasive *E. coli.* Edema and neutrophil accumulation in sinusoids of mesenteric lymph nodes are present. Experimental enteroinvasive colibacillosis in piglets has been associated with malabsorption and protein loss into the gut, presumably due to villus atrophy and effusive enteritis, respectively.

In calves, lesions suspected to be due to enteroinvasive *E. coli* grossly resemble mild salmonellosis. The mucosa of the lower small intestine, cecum, and spiral colon is congested, and may be covered by a fine fibrinous exudate. The content is fluid and may appear blood-tinged. Mesenteric lymph nodes are enlarged and wet. The microscopic lesions resemble those described in pigs, and must be differentiated from those due to AEEC or VTEC, and coronavirus.

Bibliography

Hornich, M. *et al.* Malabsorption in newborn piglets with diarrhoeic *Escherichia coli* infection and transmissible gastroenteritis. *Zbl VetMed (B)* **24:** 75–86, 1977.

Okerman, L. Enteric infections caused by non-enterotoxigenic *Escherichia coli* in animals: Occurrence and pathogenicity mechanisms. A review. *Vet Microbiol* **14:** 33–46, 1987.

e. Septicemic Colibacillosis Generalized systemic infection with *E. coli* occurs commonly in calves, and less commonly or sporadically among young animals of the other domestic species. Predisposition to infection is a prerequisite for *E. coli* septicemia. This usually results from reduced transfer or absorption of maternal colostral immunoglobulin, or from intercurrent disease or debilitation. But certain strains of *E. coli,* especially O78:K80, O86:K61, O26:K60, and O2:K1 in calves and lambs, and O115:K"V165" in pigs and calves, are particularly associated with septicemia, and may possess characteristics which enhance their ability to invade and proliferate systemically in compromised animals.

Among factors conferring virulence on these strains are plasmids coding for colicin V (Col V), and for the production of a specific toxin and surface antigen (Vir). Col V plasmids carry genes coding for aerobactin, a bacterial hydroxamate siderophore permitting survival in low-iron environments; factors resisting effects of serum such as complement activation; and hydrophobic properties which impede phagocytosis. The Vir plasmid, which is less commonly carried, codes for a pilus, and causes production of a toxin which is lethal in chicks, and which presumably is active in other species. Plasmids with genes for surface antigen 31A in *E. coli* pathogenic for calves also code for aerobactin. Hemolysin seems to promote virulence of some invasive strains of *E. coli* in experimental situations.

The portal of entry of *E. coli* causing septicemia is unclear and probably varies somewhat. The navel in the neonate, the upper respiratory tract and possibly the tonsil, and the intestine are likely sites. The nasopharyngeal route appears to be particularly important in ruminants. Enteritis is not a necessary, or even common, concomitant of colisepticemia in animals. Invasive strains given to animals with adequate levels of immunoglobulin are usually limited to colonization of the intestine, and local carriage to the mesenteric lymph nodes. Nevertheless, a capacity to colonize the gut, perhaps mediated by fimbriae, may be the first requirement for virulence in the potentially septicemic serotype O115 in pigs.

Colisepticemia is most commonly a disease of neonates, and may vary from peracute septicemia and endotoxemia resulting in sudden death, to subacute or chronic disease in which signs relate to bacterial localization, especially in the meninges, joints, and eyes.

The lesions associated with colisepticemia in young animals of any species, especially calves, lambs, and foals, may vary from subtle to obvious. Mortality in hypogammaglobulinemic neonates may occur acutely with little in the way of abnormal gross findings. These may be limited to mildly congested or blue-red, slightly rubbery lungs, and a firm spleen, perhaps with evidence of omphalitis. Microscopic changes in the lungs include thickening of alveolar septa by mononuclear cells and neutrophils, and effusion of lightly fibrinous exudate and a few neutrophils into alveoli. There may be a corona of neutrophils around white pulp in the spleen, and neutrophils may be present in abnormal numbers in circulation in many organs, including lung and hepatic sinusoids. Kupffer's cells also may be prominent in sinusoids in the liver. Fibrin thrombi may be evident in pulmonary capillaries, glomeruli, and hepatic sinusoids. Some calves will develop acute interstitial nephritis with foci of neutrophil accumulation, which with time evolve into white-spotted kidney, in surviving animals.

More severe acute cases will show evidence of serosal hemorrhage, including petechiae or ecchymoses on the epicardium and endocardium and perhaps parietal and visceral pleura. There may be slight serosanguinous pericardial fluid. The lungs may be deep red-blue, rubbery, and fail to collapse. Interlobular septa may be slightly separated by edema, and froth or fluid may be present in the major airways. Meningeal vessels may be congested, and the meninges, wet. The abomasum or stomach may have focal superficial ulcers, or more extensive deep red areas of venous infarction. There may be evidence of diarrhea and dehydration, with congestion of the small intestine. Microscopic lesions resemble those previously described, with more severe congestion, thrombosis, and edema in lungs, and perhaps other tissues. In cases not examined for some time after death, clumps of small bacilli may be seen in vessels throughout the body. The vascular permeability, thrombosis, and hemorrhage reflect endotoxemia and its sequelae.

Subacute cases may develop localized infection, often multiple, on serous surfaces and in the joints and meninges. Fibrinous peritonitis, pleuritis and pericarditis, fibrinopurulent arthritis, and meningitis are commonly found, alone or in variable combinations. Affected animals may have a history of lameness ascribable to arthritis, nervous signs due to meningitis, or general debilitation. Microscopic examination reveals the lesions already described in animals with active systemic disease, with the addition of extensive congestion and edema of inflamed serous surfaces, associated with an acute fibrinous inflammatory exudate.

In lambs, congestion and edema of the mucosa of turbinates and sinuses, perhaps with mucopurulent to hemorrhagic sinusitis, have been described. Fibrinous polyserositis and arthritis are sporadic manifestations of *E. coli* septicemia in swine, and must be differentiated from the more significant *Haemophilus, Mycoplasma,* and streptococcal infections causing these lesions. Colisepticemia is a sporadic cause of mortality in litters of young puppies.

Diagnosis of colisepticemia is based on the isolation of *E. coli* in large numbers from more than one parenchymatous organ or other internal site, other than mesenteric lymph node (preferably liver, spleen, lung, or kidney), or from a site of serosal localization, in conjunction with compatible gross and/or microscopic lesions.

Watery mouth, a syndrome characterized by salivation, depression, loss of appetite, and abomasal and abdominal distension, is associated with *E. coli* infection/bacteremia in lambs younger than 3 days in Great Britain. At necropsy, affected lambs are in poor condition. They may have unclotted milk and mucinous fluid in the distended abomasum; there is gas in the abomasum and intestine, and meconium retention is common. It is hypothesized that *E. coli* colonize the bowel, and in some manner cause loss of motility and functional obstruction. Fluid and gas accumulate in the abomasum. Bacteremia/septicemia is terminal.

Bibliography

Askaa, J., Jacobsen, K. B., and Sorensen, M. Neonatal infections in puppies caused by *Escherichia coli* serogroups O4 and O25. *Nord Vet Med* **30:** 486–488, 1978.

Besser, T. E., and Gay, C. C. Septicemic colibacillosis and failure of passive transfer of colostral immunoglobulin in calves. *Vet Clin North Am: Food Anim Pract* **1:** 445–459, 1985.

Cordy, D. R. Pathomorphology and pathogenesis of bacterial meningoventriculitis of neonatal ungulates. *Vet Pathol* **21:** 587–591, 1984.

Dassouli-Mrani-Belkebir, A. *et al.* Characters of *Escherichia coli* O78 isolated from septicaemic animals. *Vet Microbiol* **17:** 345–356, 1988.

Espinasse, J. *et al.* A new diarrhoeic syndrome with ataxia in young Charolais calves: Clinical and microbiological studies. *Vet Rec* **128:** 422–425, 1991.

Fairbrother, J. M. *et al.* Pathogenicity of *Escherichia coli* O15:K"V165" strains isolated from pigs with diarrhea. *Am J Vet Res* **50:** 1029–1036, 1989.

Linklater, K. A. Watery mouth in lambs. *Vet Annual* **29:** 88–92, 1989.

Lopez-Alvarez, J., and Gyles, C. L. Occurrence of the vir plasmid among animal and human strains of invasive *Escherichia coli. Am J Vet Res* **41:** 769–774, 1980.

Mason, R. W., and Corbould, A. Colisepticemia of lambs. *Aust Vet J* **57:** 458–460, 1981.

Said, A. M. O. *et al.* Virulence factors and markers in *Escherichia coli* from calves with bacteremia. *Am J Vet Res* **49:** 1657–1660, 1988.

Smith, H. W. Transmissible pathogenic characteristics of invasive strains of *Escherichia coli. J Am Vet Med Assoc* **173:** 601–607, 1978.

Wilkie, I. W. Polyserositis and meningitis associated with *Escherichia coli* infection of piglets. *Can Vet J* **22:** 171–173, 1981.

2. *Salmonellosis*

The genus *Salmonella* is named for Salmon, who first described infection with *S. choleraesuis* in detail, although diseases in humans caused by *Salmonella* spp. had been described earlier. It is proposed that *Salmonella* has a single species, *S. enterica,* with several subspecies, and many (~2200) antigenically distinct serovars (serotypes), which are based on the somatic or O antigens, and H or flagellar antigens. In conventional terminology, the serovars are treated as species. They are usually designated on the basis of the locality in which the specific type was first isolated or identified, or their host preference and the clinical syndrome they may produce. Most serovars may be potentially pathogenic, but the virulence of many is undefined. However, salmonellosis in domestic animals is usually caused by a few types that are somewhat host specific, like *S. abortus-ovis* (sheep), *S. choleraesuis* (swine), and a few which are not host specific, like *S. typhimurium*. Salmonellosis is one of the most serious zoonotic diseases. Phage typing or restriction endonuclease analysis of plasmids is desirable when there is evidence of transmission from animals to humans, or when epidemiologic tracing is necessary.

Probably salmonellosis in animals should be regarded as many diseases, because of the variety of susceptible animal species, the variety of serovars which are well-known pathogens, and the poorly defined circumstances in which the two interact to produce the disease. However, some general features of salmonellosis may be noted here.

Stressors are often implicated in salmonellosis, and disease is usually more common and severe in young animals. The more common stress factors which have been associated with salmonellosis in most species of domestic animals include transportation, starvation, changes in the ration, overcrowding, age, pregnancy, parturition, exertion, anesthesia, surgery, intercurrent disease, and oral treatment with antibiotics and anthelmintics.

There are many examples of enhancement of susceptibility to salmonellosis by intercurrent disease. The best-known association is that between the virus of hog cholera and *S. choleraesuis,* an association so close as to have caused early pathologists to disregard the bacterium as a primary pathogen. Salmonellosis sometimes complicates viral diseases of carnivores and has also been observed in cattle infected with foot-and-mouth disease and bovine virus diarrhea.

There is clearly an age susceptibility to clinical disease and somewhat also to infection. Adult animals are less likely to suffer generalized or septicemic infections than are the young. When adults become infected they are more likely to cast it off or become symptomless carriers for indefinite periods. There is no sound explanation of why young animals are more susceptible than adults. The containment of many young animals in limited areas is conducive to high degrees of contamination of the local environment and to rapid spread of the infection. The concentration of animals is also of importance in adults, particularly horses and sheep. In these species outbreaks are more common when the animals are closely confined. Often coupled with close confinement are the rigors attending it, especially during long travel with irregular and inadequate feeding and watering. Less tangible environmental effects are suggested by the seasonal occurrence of salmonellosis in pigs and horses; however, seasonal changes in management may predispose to disease.

The disease in adult cattle is usually sporadic, and there are often predisposing conditions such as parturient paresis, ketosis, mastitis, and parasitic infestations. The stress of anesthesia and surgery may account in part for the serious outbreaks of salmonellosis which occur in hospitalized animals at veterinary schools.

The main route of transmission is undoubtedly by ingestion. Most of the basic information on the pathogenesis has been obtained through experimental infection in laboratory animals and *in vitro* models. Although the data obtained are valuable, they may not be completely applicable to domestic animals. Susceptibility to particular serovars varies among and within species. Some strains of *S. muenster* which cause a subclinical infection in mice are highly fatal for calves.

The clinical and pathologic syndromes of salmonellosis may vary from a localized enterocolitis to a septicemia. Certain serovars tend to be associated mainly with enterocolitis, e.g., *S. typhimurium* in most species except mice, in which it causes a typhoidlike illness. Other serovars, especially those with a high degree of host specificity, like *S. typhi* (humans), *S. dublin* (cattle), and *S. choleraesuis* (swine) tend to cause septicemia. There may be overlap between the two forms of disease, and if the animal survives, a carrier state usually follows.

The pathogenesis of salmonellosis may be divided into several stages: entry of the bacteria into the host and attainment of the primary site of infection, usually the enterocyte; attachment to the surface (colonization); and invasion of the enterocytes. In those cases in which bacteremia follows, the organisms must be able to survive and replicate in macrophages and disseminate to other sites, e.g., liver, lung, joints, meninges, or placenta and fetus. The course and outcome of *Salmonella* infection is affected by chromosomal and extrachromosomal (plasmid-, bacteriophage-, transposon-mediated) virulence determinants in the organism, and the response of the host to these factors. Chromosomal genes tend to code for virulence factors involved in attachment and invasion of *Salmonella,* whereas the ability to survive in macrophages after invasion is enhanced in some serovars by specific plasmids.

For infection to take place, *Salmonella* must be present in sufficient numbers; generally a minimal infective oral dose of 10^7–10^9 organisms is needed to infect large domestic animals. After ingestion, the *Salmonella* must overcome nonspecific resistance factors, including bactericidal actions of salivary enzymes, and the acid pH of gastric juices. Mucus and lysozymes in the glycocalyx, peristalsis, and constant sloughing of enterocytes may interfere with attachment. Those organisms that survive the nonspecific resistance factors may colonize and invade the enterocytes. *Salmonella* have been demonstrated in the Peyer's patches as early as 6 hr postinoculation.

The ability to attach, invade, and penetrate enterocytes is crucial to virulence, and the first step in the development of salmonellosis. Considerable research has focused on the large number of genes involved, and their coordinate regulation of expression, in this complex process. The genome of *S. typhimurium* is about 4800 kb long, which amounts to approximately 3000 genes; of these <1000 have been mapped. Many of the virulence factors involved in the various stages of the pathogenesis of salmonellosis have not been fully defined. A number of known virulence factors contribute to the pathogenesis of salmonellosis, including motility, pili or fimbriae, lipopolysaccharides, and enterotoxins.

Motility, associated with the presence of flagella, is characteristic of many *Salmonella* serovars. Bacterial motility is generally not considered to be an important virulence determinant; however, motility may enhance the movement of bacteria through the glycocalyx and facilitate the attachment to specific receptor sites on enterocytes.

Fimbriae (pilar adhesins) are present on salmonellae, and they may play a role in colonization of the gut. Adherence of *Salmonella* to intestinal epithelial cells apparently takes place in two stages. The first stage is reversible, since the organisms can be washed off easily. Weak ionic and non-ionic interactions between bacterial and host-cell membrane surfaces are thought to be the binding forces responsible for this attachment. The second stage of adherence is irreversible; it occurs after a lag period, and it is characterized by degeneration of the microvilli on the epithelial cells and the formation of membrane-bound vacuoles (endosomes) containing *Salmonella*. This process is referred to as receptor-mediated endocytosis. Both stages of adherence are likely to be enhanced by mannose-sensitive (type 1), or less commonly, mannose-resistant (type 3) fimbriae, which bind to specific surface receptors on epithelial cells. Type 1 fimbriae apparently make the bacterial cell wall more hydrophobic and attract it to the negatively charged intestinal epithelial cells. *Salmonella* have 200–300 pili or fimbriae, but the role of these pilar adhesins in the pathogenesis of salmonellosis remains controversial, since some investigators have failed to demonstrate any difference in adherence between fimbriated and nonfimbriated strains of *Salmonella*. Some strains of *S. typhimurium* possess a nonfimbrial, mannose-resistant, hemagglutinating adhesin, which promotes adherence to mammalian cells *in vitro*. In chicks, colonization of *Salmonella* occurs more readily in the absence of the normal enteric microflora, which may be related to decreased competition for specific receptor sites on enterocytes.

The **lipopolysaccharide** (LPS) moiety of *Salmonella* with smooth cell walls consists of an O-specific side chain, a core portion, and a lipid A portion. Most *Salmonella* isolated from animals have smooth cell walls, and this feature influences virulence in several ways. These strains are more invasive, and are more successful at avoiding phagocytosis and lysis by phagolysosomes after invasion. Lipopolysaccharides reduce the susceptibility of the organisms to the host's cationic proteins; they stimulate local prostaglandin synthesis and prevent the activation and deposition of complement on the bacterial surface. The main function of LPS may be to facilitate survival in the intestinal tract and eventual entry into deeper tissues. The involvement of LPS in invasion apparently varies with *Salmonella* species, since some strains of *S. typhimurium* do not require intact LPS to invade epithelial cells *in vitro*. On the other hand, more host-specific *Salmonella* species such as *S. typhi* and *S. choleraesuis* require intact LPS or O side chains. The lipid A portion of LPS is responsible for the endotoxin-mediated effects of *Salmonella* infection that are seen in the systemic form of the disease. Septicemia (endotoxemia) typically causes fever, leukopenia, hemoconcentration, lactic acidosis, coagulopathies, hypotension, and death. Apparently, LPS usually is a chromosome-mediated characteristic, but the cell wall also may be affected by genes carried in plasmids and bacteriophages.

Invasion of the enterocytes, especially those in the ileum, occurs within 12 hr of oral infection. The ultrastructural changes of *Salmonella* infection in the intestine were first described in experimental infections of guinea pigs. Large numbers of organisms are present in the lumen, on the surface of the brush border, and in enterocytes. There is an increase in the number of neutrophils in the gut lumen and within intercellular spaces, and some of these contain bacteria. Degeneration of microvilli, characterized by loss of filamentous cores, is associated with close adherence of bacteria. Other degenerative changes consist of elongation, swelling, budding, and fusion of microvilli, and loss of the terminal web.

The organisms usually appear to invade the cells through the brush border; however, they may also enter the mucosa through the intercellular junctional complex. The bacteria are located in the cytoplasm within membrane-bound vacuoles, which may also contain remnants of microvilli and cytoplasmic debris. Most *Salmonella* organisms remain intact, multiply, and produce enterotoxins during their transcellular migration in endosomes. Many bacteria are often present in a single enterocyte during the early stages of infection, but cellular damage is mild and transient. The *Salmonella*-receptor complex dissociates as a result of the acidification of the endosomal content, allowing the receptor site to return to the apical plasma membrane and repeat the processes of endocytosis. After 24 hr, most of the bacteria are located within membrane-bound vacuoles in macrophages in the lamina propria. Many organisms are evident in the lumina of crypts, but invasion of cryptal epithelial cells evidently does not take place.

Although the early changes associated with *Salmonella* infection in enterocytes in other host species have similarities to those in the guinea pig, there are some notable differences. Ligated intestinal loops of pigs infected with *S. typhimurium* and *S. choleraesuis* did not have degenerative changes in the microvilli, bacteria were not seen to penetrate the apical membrane, there were fewer intracellular organisms, and most were not membrane bound. Both serovars caused destruction of villi, resulting in marked villus atrophy. The early inflammatory reaction was mainly neutrophilic, but few of these were seen to phagocytize bacteria. Interestingly, increased bactericidal activity has been reported in pigs orally infected with *S. typhimurium*.

In contrast to the findings in pigs, marked ultrastructural changes are seen in epithelial cells of isolated colon segments in ponies inoculated with *S. typhimurium* and with culture lysates of this organism. These changes consist of separation of epithelial cells, swelling of the endoplasmic reticulum, increased electron-dense bodies, and some degeneration of microvilli. The latter is seen only in lysate-inoculated segments. Many apical phagolysosomes occur in epithelial cells of segments inoculated with viable organisms. In addition, there is moderate submucosal edema and a neutrophilic reaction in the lumen, lamina propria, and submucosa. Similar, but milder, changes occur in colon segments inoculated with cholera toxin.

Toxins may mediate the secretion of electrolyte and fluid by some invasive strains of *Salmonella*. The significance of heat-labile or heat-stable **enterotoxins,** the effects of which are described under enterotoxigenic *E. coli,* is not so clearly defined for enteric salmonellosis. Cyclic AMP may play a role in secretion of fluids into the gut lumen, but the mechanism involved is poorly understood. *Salmonella* infection stimulates adenylate cyclase activity in the rabbit ileum, but the level of stimulation is considerably less than that produced by cholera toxins. Fluid secretion occurs in the presence or absence of gross lesions in the mucosa. A polymorphonuclear inflammatory reaction is evident just prior to the onset of fluid secretion, but at the height of fluid exsorption, the mucosa is relatively normal. Enterocolitis associated with salmonellosis may result in increased synthesis and secretion of prostaglandins, which in turn stimulate mucosal adenylate cyclase activity, causing abnormalities in fluid, sodium, and chloride transport.

Fluid accumulation (probably enterotoxin mediated) and mucosal lesions have been observed in ligated loops of small intestine in pigs and calves inoculated with *S. typhimurium,* and also in pigs with *S. choleraesuis*. Oral infection of pigs with *S. heidelberg* produces a syndrome similar to that seen with enterotoxigenic diarrheal diseases. It is characterized by fluid exsorption in the small intestine and colon, but the typical necrotizing and ulcerative mucosal lesions seen with *S. typhimurium* and *S. choleraesuis* are absent. Fluid accumulation has also been demonstrated in isolated colon segments of ponies inoculated with *S. typhimurium* culture lysates. Similar fluid exsorption occurred in colon segments inoculated with cholera toxin.

As a result of the fluid exsorption, which occurs mainly in the lower small intestine, a large volume of fluid reaches the colon. Diarrhea is, at least in part, due to the inability of the damaged colon to absorb this fluid.

A **cytotoxin** or verotoxin similar to the shiga neurotoxin produced by *Shigella dysenteriae* has been associated with some serovars of *Salmonella*. Cytolytic activity is probably due to inhibition of protein synthesis. This activity is located on the bacterial outer membrane and has been demonstrated in lysates of *Salmonella,* but not in intact organisms. This toxin apparently chelates cations, such as Ca^{2+} and Mg^{2+} ions, resulting in ultrastructural changes within the cell membrane, permitting selective leakage of molecules. The degeneration and necrosis of enterocytes in salmonellosis may be associated in part with such a cytotoxin.

Vascular degeneration and thrombosis of mucosal vessels are common features of *Salmonella* enteritis. The vascular lesions may be due to action of large amounts of **endotoxins** absorbed through the damaged mucosa, or released locally. The effect of cytotoxin on the endothelial cells also may be involved in the pathogenesis of these lesions.

Invading *Salmonella* in some species enter the mucosa through M cells in the Peyer's patches, and host specificity of some *Salmonella* serovars may be associated in part with specific receptor sites on these cells. When bacteria invade through M cells, smaller numbers of *Salmonella* may enter through enterocytes in other areas of the small intestine. However, the M cell is not the main site of attachment in some hosts, for instance, in *S. typhimurium* infections of calves and pigs.

In salmonellosis characterized by enterocolitis, the organisms usually do not disseminate beyond the mucosa and the mesenteric lymph nodes, and the ensuing inflammation remains confined to the intestine.

The outcome of an infection with *Salmonella* is determined by the genetic virulence determinants of the invading organism and the ensuing humoral and cell-mediated immune response of the host. *Salmonella* are considered to be facultative intracellular pathogens, and invading strains must have the genetic information to survive and replicate within macrophages in order to cause a bacteremia or septicemia. The virulence of several serovars commonly associated with infections in animals, including *S. typhimurium, S. dublin,* and *S. choleraesuis,* is enhanced by serovar-specific plasmids which provide these serovars with increased ability to survive in macrophages. Mutant strains that lack the plasmids have reduced virulence. Such plasmids were found in $>60\%$ of *Salmonella* of animal origin in New York State. Whether plasmids enhance resistance of *Salmonella* to humoral immunity remains a moot point. After invasion, flagellar antigens appear to contribute to the ability of the organism to survive in macrophages, through an unknown mechanism. Macrophages actively phagocytize bacteria coated with complement. Bacterial LPS prevents this process and thus interferes with phagocytosis of *Salmonella*. Phagocytosis of *Salmonella* is also repressed by porins, hydrophobic bacterial cell-surface proteins that function as transmembrane diffusion channels. A virulence (Vi) antigen, the mode of action of which is unknown, is found in certain invasive strains of *Salmonella*. However, when this antigen is missing, the strain is less virulent.

Salmonella taken up by resident macrophages elicit a major immune response in the host. There is considerable controversy about the roles played by cell-mediated and humoral immunity in the pathogenesis of salmonellosis. *Salmonella* infection results in the release of lymphokines by specifically stimulated T lymphocytes; they activate macrophages which phagocytize the organisms.

Once the *Salmonella* organisms have crossed the mucosa, they may enter the bloodstream via the lymphatics, perhaps carried in macrophages, and cause septicemia or transient bacteremia, or they may remain indefinitely in the gut-associated lymphoid tissues and mesenteric lymph nodes. Increased susceptibility to salmonellosis in animals with intercurrent disease, or subjected to stress, may be related to relaxation of cell-mediated immunity to the organism. Septicemia may be of variable duration and severity but, as a rule, it is rapidly fatal in young animals. If, however, there is transient bacteremia, the organisms are removed by the fixed macrophages, especially of the spleen, liver, and bone marrow. They may continue to proliferate in such extravascular locations and cause another bacteremic phase, which may be fatal as a septicemia or result in secondary localization.

The carrier state is important in the epidemiology of the disease. Whether *Salmonella* can maintain themselves in the intestine is not clear; to some extent, at least, the fecal flora is likely to depend on intermittent seeding from the bile, or from macrophages in the lamina propria and gut-associated lymphoid tissue. The duration of the carrier state may be prolonged, or animals may rid themselves of the infection, probably by means of cell-mediated immunity. The carrier state is an unstable one, for it appears that if the carrier is subjected to some stress or debilitating disease, it may succumb to disease; this often seems to occur in adult cattle. The carrier animal is a potential threat to any other animal it contacts, either directly, or through the medium of its excreta, or by-products such as bone or meat meal.

Bibliography

Chang, E. B. *Salmonella* bacterial adherence and penetration of mucosal cells: Inducing role of the epithelium. *Gastroenterology* **97:**1055–1056, 1989.

Clarke, R. C., and Gyles, C. L. Virulence of wild and mutant strains of *Salmonella typhimurium* in ligated intestinal segments of calves, pigs, and rabbits. *Am J Vet Res* **48:** 504–510, 1987.

Clarke, R. C. *et al.* Plasmids of *Salmonella muenster* and their relation to virulence. *Can J Vet Res* **51:** 436–439, 1987.

D'Aoust, J.-Y. Pathogenicity of foodborne *Salmonella. Int J Food Microbiol* **12:** 17–40, 1991.

Dunlap, N. E. *et al.* A "safe-site" for *Salmonella typhimurium* is within splenic cells during the early phase of infection in mice. *Microb Pathogen* **10:** 297–310, 1991.

Finlay, B. B., and Falkow, S. *Salmonella* as an intracellular parasite. *Mol Microbiol* **3:** 1833–1841, 1989.

Finlay, B. B., Heffron, F., and Falkow, S. Epithelial cell surfaces induce *Salmonella* proteins required for bacterial adherence and invasion. *Science* **243:** 940–943, 1989.

Galan, J. E., and Curtiss, R., III. Expression of *Salmonella typhimurium* genes required for invasion is regulated by changes in DNA supercoiling. *Infect Immun* **58:** 1879–1885, 1990.

Gevaert, D., Haesebrouck, F., and Devriese, L. Kiem-gastheer interacties bij *Salmonella* infecties: een overzicht over virulentiefactoren en immuniteit. *Vlaams Diergeneeskd Tijdschr* **59:** 43–48, 1990.

Giannella, R. A. Importance of the intestinal inflammatory reaction in *Salmonella*-mediated intestinal secretion. *Infect Immun* **23:** 140–145, 1979.

Hsu, H. S. Pathogenesis and immunity in murine salmonellosis. *Microbiol Rev* **53:** 390–409, 1989.

Iglewski, B. H., and Clark, V. L. (eds.). "Molecular Basis of Bacterial Pathogenesis." San Diego, California, Academic Press, 1990.

Kawahara, K. *et al.* Identification and mapping of mba regions of the *Salmonella choleraesuis* virulence plasmid pKDSC50 responsible for mouse bacteremia. *Microb Pathogen* **8:** 13–21, 1990.

Le Minor, L., and Popoff, M. Y. Designation of *Salmonella enterica* sp. nov., nom. rev., as the type and only species of the genus *Salmonella. Int J Syst Bacteriol* **37:** 465–468, 1987.

McDonough, P. L. *et al.* Virulence determinants of *Salmonella typhimurium* from animal sources. *Am J Vet Res* **50:** 662–670, 1989.

Murray, M. J. Salmonella: Virulence factors and enteric salmonellosis. *J Am Vet Med Assoc* **189:** 145–147, 1986.

Murray, M. J. *et al.* Comparative effects of cholera toxin, *Salmonella typhimurium* culture lysate, and viable *Salmonella typhimurium* in isolated colon segments in ponies. *Am J Vet Res* **50:** 22–28, 1989.

Nnalue, N. A., and Lindberg, A. A. *Salmonella choleraesuis* strains deficient in O antigen remain fully virulent for mice by parenteral inoculation but are avirulent by oral administration. *Infect Immun* **58:** 2493–2501, 1990.

Ou, J. T., and Baron, L. S. Strain differences in expression of virulence by the 90-kilobase pair virulence plasmid of *Salmonella* serovar Typhimurium. *Microb Pathogen* **10:** 247–251, 1991.

Reed, W. M., Olander, H. J., and Thacker, H. L. Studies on the pathogenesis of *Salmonella heidelberg* infection in weanling pigs. *Am J Vet Res* **46:** 2300–2310, 1985.

Smith, G. S., Lumsden, J. H., and Wilcock, B. P. Neutrophil bactericidal capability in experimentally induced salmonellosis in pigs. *Am J Vet Res* **42:** 1332–1334, 1981.

Takeuchi, A. Electron microscope studies of experimental *Salmonella* infection. I. Penetration into the intestinal epithelium by *Salmonella typhimurium*. *Am J Pathol* **50:** 109–136, 1967.

Wallis, T. S. *et al.* The nature and role of mucosal damage in relation to *Salmonella typhimurium*-induced fluid secretion in the rabbit ileum. *J Med Microbiol* **22:** 39–49, 1986.

a. Salmonellosis in Swine Many serovars of *Salmonella* have been isolated from swine, and with poultry and cattle, they form an important reservoir of the organism. The bacteria are carried in the lamina propria of the intestine, but also in the regional lymph nodes of the alimentary tract, so that carrier animals may not excrete the organism in the feces.

Salmonellosis occurs in feeder pigs, usually 2–4 months of age. It is very uncommon in sucklings and adult swine.

Three syndromes are associated with *Salmonella* infections in swine. Septicemic salmonellosis is usually associated with the host-adapted *S. choleraesuis* var. *kunzendorf,* although enteric lesions may be present with this serovar. Sporadic infections with *S. dublin* have also been associated with septicemia in nursing pigs. *Salmonella typhimurium* most commonly causes acute or chronic enterocolitis, including a necrotizing proctitis which may lead to rectal stricture. *Salmonella typhisuis* infection is characterized by ulcerative enterocolitis, as well as caseous tonsillitis and lymphadenitis.

Detailed consideration of these three syndromes is warranted because salmonellosis is one of the most important diseases of swine.

Salmonella choleraesuis was once thought to be the cause of hog cholera because gross lesions of septicemic salmonellosis and acute hog cholera are similar. The latter disease is often complicated by *S. choleraesuis,* the bacterium being recovered from 10 to 50% of pigs with hog cholera. Other predisposing factors mentioned earlier generally also apply to salmonellosis in swine.

The major clinical manifestations of *S. choleraesuis* infection are septicemia and enteritis; they usually occur separately. Septicemia is more common. Oral inoculation of *S. choleraesuis* results initially in septicemia and acute enterocolitis, followed in some cases by large necrotic and ulcerative lesions (button ulcers) in the colonic mucosa. Enteritis is not necessarily chronic, or even clinically evident. Interstitial pneumonia and multifocal hepatic necrosis are the most consistent systemic lesions. Immunocytochemical techniques reveal the preferential location of *S.choleraesuis* in the colon and surface of ileal M cells in Peyer's patches. The invasive capability of this serovar is indicated by the presence of large numbers of organisms in proprial macrophages and regional lymph nodes.

Salmonellosis which is clinically septicemic is usually fatal. Death may occur quickly without observed illness, or after a course of a week or more. There is a high fever; characteristic but not pathognomonic blue discoloration of the skin, especially of the tail, snout, and ears (Fig. 1.127); posterior weakness; dyspnea which often leads to misdiagnosis of primary pneumonia; and sometimes terminal convulsions. Sows may abort during the septicemic phase of infection. Pigs recovered from this phase may have dry gangrene of the ears and tail, posterior paralysis, blindness, and diphtheritic enteritis. The chronic or enteric form may develop from the acute but is usually insidious from the onset. It is characterized by loose yellow feces containing flakes of fibrin, progressive emaciation and debility, and eventual death. Some recover but fail to thrive, often partly owing to chronic bronchopneumonia.

At autopsy there is a bluish or purplish discoloration of the skin, which may be very intense about the head and ears. There may be superficial necrosis of the ears. Typically there are petechial hemorrhages in many organs and tissues. The lymph nodes are almost invariably hemorrhagic. The visceral nodes are more frequently and obviously involved than the peripheral ones, with the exception of those of the throat, which are usually hemorrhagic. The mesenteric lymph nodes are greatly enlarged; they may be speckled with hemorrhages in the parenchyma or in the peripheral sinus.

There may be hemorrhages, petechial or as small discrete blebs, on the laryngeal mucosa (Fig. 1.128). The lungs do not collapse because there is frothy fluid in the respiratory passages. They may be pale blue or purple. Beneath the visceral pleura there are small dark foci of hemorrhage. The lungs are wet, and there is fluid in the interlobular tissue. The changes are best appreciated in the posterior lobes, because the anterior lobes are often the seat of acute lobular pneumonia. These pulmonary changes, attributable in part to endotoxin, account for the respiratory signs observed clinically. The pneumonia is interstitial because of endotoxemia and embolic organ-

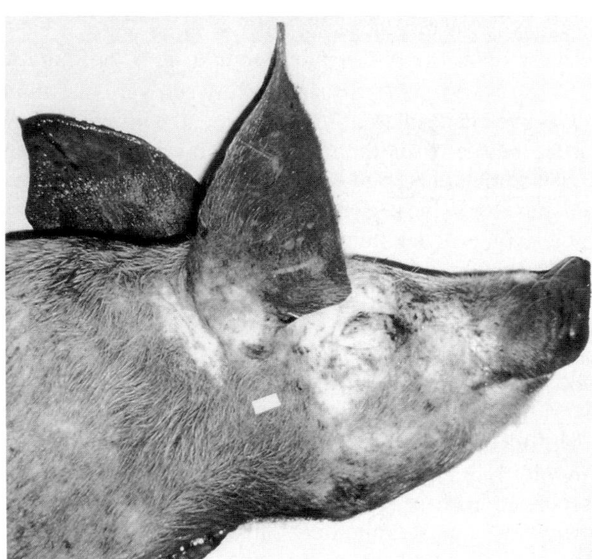

Fig. 1.127 Septicemic salmonellosis. Pig. Note blue-red congestion of skin of ears, snout, and neck due to microvascular thrombosis in endotoxemia.

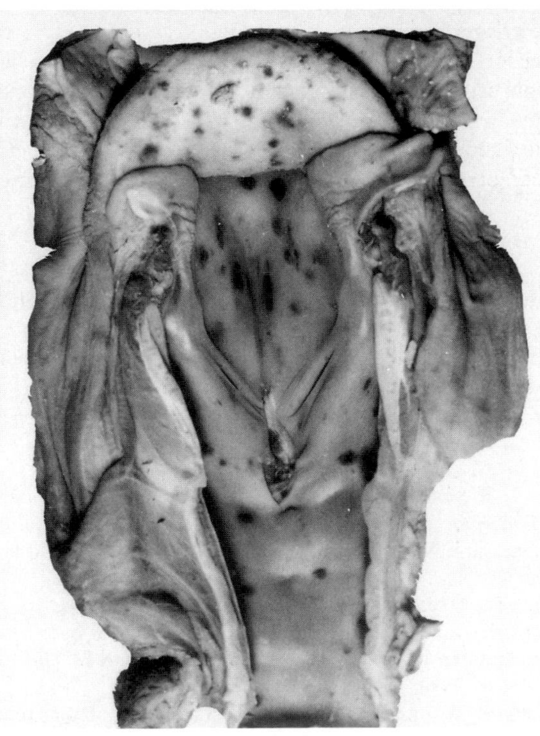

Fig. 1.128 Porcine salmonellosis. Laryngeal hemorrhages.

isms. The lobar anteroventral pneumonia may be due to ascending *Salmonella* alveolitis and bronchiolitis. Occasionally, the injury to the alveolar septa by *Salmonella* results in extensive fibrinous pneumonia of the posterior lobes. The cardiac serosae often bear petechiae, and in some more virulent infections, there is fibrinohemorrhagic pericarditis with scant fluid exudation.

The spleen in enlarged, deep blue, firm with sharp edges; little blood oozes from the cut surface. There may be petechiae on the capsule, but the marginal infarcts of hog cholera are not present. The enlargement of the spleen and absence of infarcts distinguish salmonellosis from hog cholera. Other causes of splenomegaly, such as erysipelas, other septicemias, and African swine fever, must be differentiated.

The liver is usually congested, and focal hemorrhages may be visible in the capsule. In some cases the hemorrhages are very large, involving up to half of the central area in a lobule. They may be scattered at random throughout the liver or grouped, often at the edge of a lobe. In some, there are tiny yellow foci of necrosis, referred to as paratyphoid nodules (Fig. 1.129).

Pinpoint hemorrhages are consistently present in the renal cortex. There may be only a few in each kidney, or they may be so numerous as to cause the turkey-egg appearance. The kidneys may be of normal color, or the cortices may be pale, and the medulla, intensely congested as in other septicemias. In some, there are petechiae in the pelvic and ureteral epithelium. In almost all cases hemorrhages are present beneath the epithelium of the bladder.

The stomach shows the intense red-black color of the severe congestion and venous infarction common to endotoxemia in pigs. If the animal survives a week or more, the superficial necrotic layer of the affected gastric mucosa sloughs. There may be no lesions in the intestine. There may be a catarrhal enteritis or, more frequently, the enteritis is hemorrhagic, increasing in severity lower in the tract and terminating in a hemorrhagic ileitis. The mucosae of the colon and cecum may be normal, but if the course is prolonged, there is hyperemia, fibrinohemorrhagic inflammation, or button ulcers (Fig. 1.130).

Petechial hemorrhages may occur in the meninges and brain, but there is no sign of gross inflammation. Localization sometimes occurs in synovial membranes, producing polysynovitis and sometimes polyarthritis. It is more usual to have an increase in the volume of fluid with red velvety hypertrophy of the synovial villi. The gross features described are usually not all present in any one case.

The histologic changes which occur in internal organs in acute disease are mainly associated with endothelial damage due to endotoxin, and focal localization of bacteria. The discoloration of the skin is initially due to intense dilation, congestion, and thrombosis of capillaries and venules in the dermal papilla. There is activation and necrosis of the endothelial cells in affected vessels. The renal lesions vary but affect principally the glomeruli. In some there is diffuse glomerulitis, and this is associated with mild nephrosis and hyaline casts. In others, the glomerulitis is exudative and hemorrhagic, and in these, a great many capillary loops contain hyaline thrombi. The hemorrhages seen grossly come from the glomeruli and from the wide venules of the outer cortex, although some are from intertubular capillaries. Embolic bacterial colonies are occasionally seen in the glomerular and intertubular capillaries. Fibrin thrombi may also be found in the afferent arterioles and interlobular arteries. Endotoxemia causes the gross and microscopic lesions seen in most organs.

The pulmonary lesions are also characterized by thrombosis and vasculitis and a largely mononuclear cellular response in alveolar septa. There is a flooding of the alveoli by edema fluid and moderate numbers of alveolar macrophages. This is the usual histologic picture; the extremes are an acute fibrinous inflammation or a few scattered parenchymal hemorrhages.

In the liver, the paratyphoid nodules may be found in

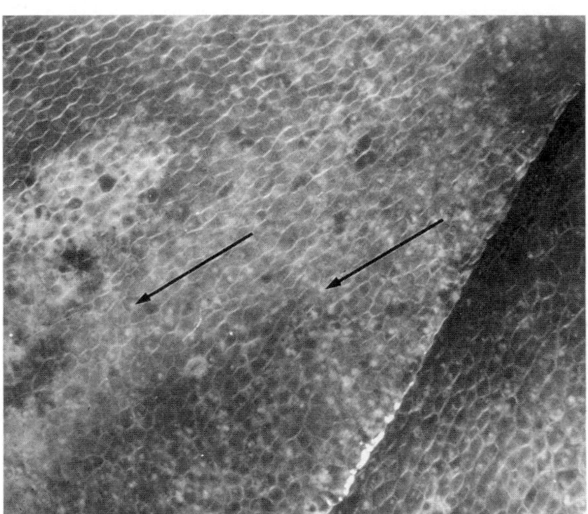

Fig. 1.129 Porcine salmonellosis. Paratyphoid nodules (arrows) in liver. *Salmonella* septicemia.

all transitional stages from foci of nonspecific necrosis to reactive granulomas. Typically there are few neutrophils, and whether the nodules are necrotic or reactive depends on their duration. The initial change is focal coagulation necrosis. About the margins the macrophages accumulate and form small histiocytic granulomas, which expand and displace the surrounding parenchymal cords.

In the spleen there are some scattered hemorrhages, but the overall histologic impression is of increased histiocytes with a scattering of neutrophils. The follicles are small and rather inactive. Very small foci of necrosis, containing many bacteria, may be sparse or relatively numerous, and these develop a reactive macrophage response and form the typical paratyphoid nodules.

Meningoencephalomyelitis occurs in a proportion of cases of septicemic salmonellosis. The lesion is fundamentally a vasculitis. There may be petechiae in the meninges but, microscopically, there is an infiltration of large mononuclear cells in the pia–arachnoid and concentrated about the veins. There is also sludging of these cells and polymorphs, including eosinophils, in the veins. Similar lesions may occur at any level in the brain. In some cases the walls of many veins are necrotic, and there may be a mononuclear cell reaction in the walls and surrounding neuropil. Only a few neutrophils and eosinophils form part of the inflammatory cell reaction in these areas. The parenchymal lesions consist of a disseminated focal granulomatous encephalitis. Areas of malacia may be associated with the granulomas. Microabscesses form in those few cases in which bacterial emboli are detectable. Glial nodules are typical of the healed phase. These lesions occur in the spinal cord as well.

Salmonella typhimurium infection in swine produces a syndrome which differs from that of *S. choleraesuis* in a number of ways. Clinically, the disease occurs in feeder pigs and is characterized by fever, inanition, and yellow watery diarrhea, which may contain blood and mucus, especially in the later stages. The diarrhea may be chronic and intermittent. There is a high morbidity but low mortality. Most pigs recover but may remain carriers for variable periods, and some may develop rectal stricture. The organism persists in tonsils, lower intestinal tract, and submandibular and ileocolic lymph nodes.

The pathogenesis and morphology of the enteric lesions differ from those described for *S. choleraesuis* enteritis. The lesions with *S. typhimurium* infection are mainly confined to the colon, cecum, and rectum, usually with minor involvement of the distal small intestine. There is an acute enterocolitis with formation of a pseudodiphtheritic membrane on the mucosal surface. Button ulcers are not associated with this or other nonhost-adapted serovars. Immunocytologic techniques do not reveal any predilection for specific sites in the intestine. It may be demonstrated in the mesenteric lymph nodes 24 hr postinfection, and these may be enlarged. Systemic dissemination and septicemia are rare.

Rectal stricture is thought to be a sequel in most cases to ulcerative proctitis of ischemic origin, caused by *S. typhimurium*. It is characterized clinically by marked progressive distension of the abdomen, loss of appetite, emaciation, and soft feces. At autopsy, there is marked dilation of the colon, which is caused by narrowing of the rectum, 1–10 cm anterior to the anus (Fig. 1.131). The stricture is usually <1.0 cm in diameter and varies in length from 0.5 to 20 cm. There is marked fibrous thickening of the rectal wall, which may contain microabscesses. The dilation of the colon, anterior to the stricture, may consist of a well-demarcated widened area several centimeters long and wide. The colonic mucosa in this area is usually ulcerated and may be covered by fibrinous exudate. In some cases, there is more gradual dilation of the entire colon, with ulceration of the mucosa just anterior to the stricture. The mucosa is always excessively corrugated; this is mainly the result of marked thickening of the internal muscularis. Anastomoses of the small intestine and/or colon to the dilated portion of the descending colon may occur. Localized chronic peritonitis is often associated with the dilated segments of the colon.

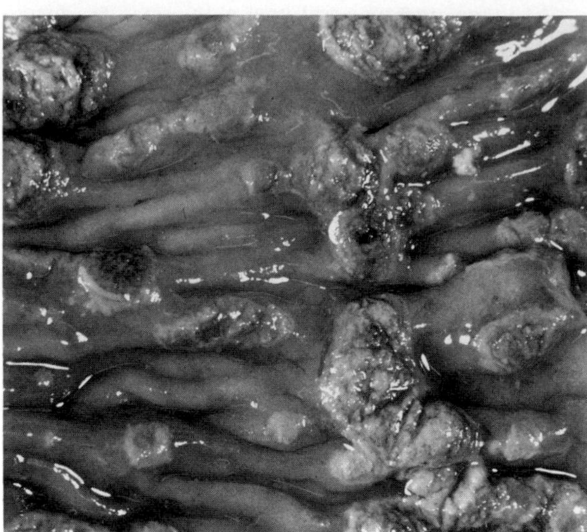

Fig. 1.130 Porcine salmonellosis. Bottom ulcers in colon.

Microscopically, the strictures are the result of marked fibrosis of the gut wall, with almost complete obliteration of the normal structures. The mucosa is generally completely absent. The luminal surface is covered by debris, fibrin, and neutrophils. A few veins in the wall contain well-organized thrombi. The colonic lesions are those of a mild to severe necrotizing ulcerative colitis described earlier.

The stricture is located in an area of rectum which has a relatively poor blood supply, namely the junction of the circulatory fields of the caudal mesenteric and pudendal arteries. Ulcerative proctitis is consistently found in swine with typhlocolitis due to *S. typhimurium* infection. Granulation of such lesions probably leads to cicatrization and stricture. The location, the persistent nature of this lesion in some pigs, and its limited capacity to heal are probably related to the restricted blood supply of the affected area.

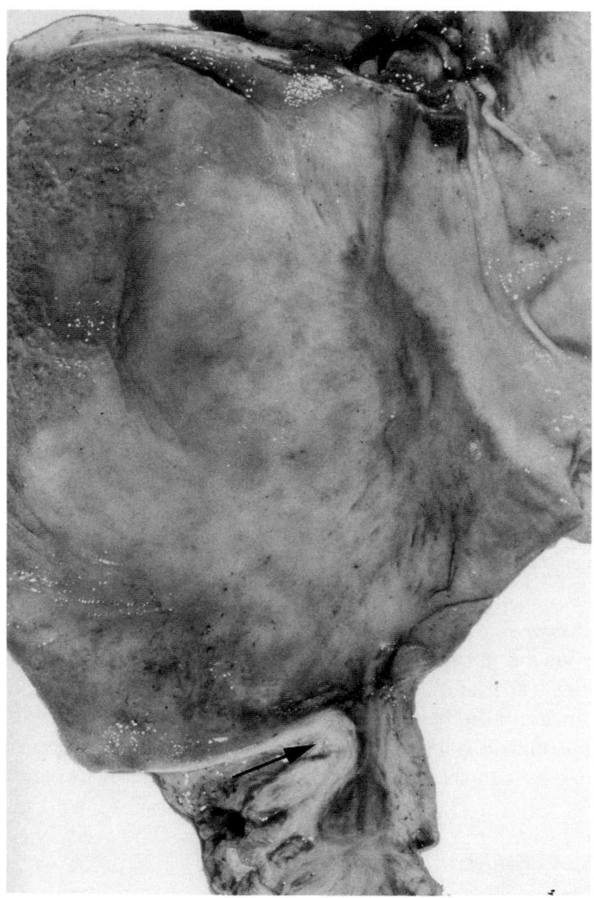

Fig. 1.131 Porcine salmonellosis. Rectal stricture. Opened colon is massively dilated anterior to stricture in rectum (arrow).

The lesions in the colon and cecum, with greater collateral blood supply, heal more rapidly, usually without further complications. At the time of autopsy, *S. typhimurium* may not be isolated because of loss of the carrier state. Alternatively, rectal stricture may result from ischemia due to noninfectious causes, such as rectal prolapse.

Salmonella typhisuis infection is an uncommon condition in pigs. The disease, called paratyphoid in Europe, is now known to cause disease in pigs in the Americas and Asia. It is a progressive disease of 2 to 4-month-old pigs, clinically characterized by intermittent diarrhea, emaciation, and frequently, massive enlargement of the neck region, the latter associated with caseous palatine tonsillitis, cervical lymphadenitis, and parotid sialoadenitis. There is also circular or buttonlike to confluent ulceration of the mucosa of the ileum, cecum, colon, and rectum. Other less frequent findings are caseous lymphadenitis of the mesenteric lymph nodes, interstitial pneumonia, hepatitis, and pericarditis.

The differential diagnosis of septicemic salmonellosis includes other septicemias which occur in feeder swine, such as peracute erysipelas, *Haemophilus,* and streptococcal infections. It is important to differentiate *S. choleraesuis* infection from hog cholera and African swine fever.

The enteric forms of salmonellosis must be differentiated from other enteritides in weaned swine, particularly postweaning *E. coli* enteritis, swine dysentery, and intestinal adenomatosis. Isolation of *S. choleraesuis* and *S. typhimurium* from animals with typical lesions confirms a diagnosis with those agents, which are usually easy to recover. The host-adapted *S. typhisuis* is a very fastidious organism that requires special procedures for isolation.

Bibliography

Arbuckle, A. B. R. Villous atrophy in pigs orally infected with *Salmonella choleraesuis*. *Res Vet Sci* **18:** 322–324, 1975.

Barnes, D. M., and Bergeland, M. E. *Salmonella typhisuis* infection in Minnesota swine. *J Am Vet Med Assoc* **152:** 1766–1770, 1968.

Buckley, H. G., and Donnelly, W. J. C. *Salmonella dublin* infection in piglets. *Ir Vet J* **24:** 74–78, 1970.

Ehrensperger, F. *et al.* Megacolon in fattening pigs. *Schweiz Arch Tierheilk* **120:** 477–483, 1978.

Fenwick, B. W., and Olander, H. J. Experimental infection of weanling pigs with *Salmonella typhisuis*: Effect of feeding low concentrations of chlortetracycline, penicillin, and sulfamethazine. *Am J Vet Res* **48:** 1568–1573, 1987.

Lawson, G. H. K., and Dow, C. Experimental infection of pigs with smooth and rough strains of *Salmonella choleraesuis. J Comp Pathol* **75:** 83–88, 1965.

Nordstoga, K., and Fjolstad, M. Porcine salmonellosis. III. Production of fibrinous colitis by intravenous injections of a mixture of viable cells of *Salmonella choleraesuis* and disintegrated cells of the same agent, or hemolytic *Escherichia coli. Acta Vet Scand* **11:** 380–389, 1970.

Olson, L. D. Anastomoses of intestinal tract as a sequela to rectal stricture in swine. *Can J Comp Med* **43:** 102–105, 1979.

Pospischil, A., Wood, R. L., and Anderson, T. D. Peroxidase–antiperoxidase and immunogold labeling of *Salmonella typhimurium* and *Salmonella choleraesuis* var. *kunzendorf* in tissues of experimentally infected swine. *Am J Vet Res* **51:** 619–624, 1990.

Reed, W. M., Olander, H. J., and Thacker, H. L. Studies on the pathogenesis of *Salmonella typhimurium* and *Salmonella choleraesuis* var. *kunzendorf* infection in weanling pigs. *Am J Vet Res* **47:** 75–83, 1986.

Schwartz, K. J. Salmonellosis in swine. *Compend Cont Ed Pract Vet* **13:** 139–146, 1991.

Wilcock, B. P. Experimental *Klebsiella* and *Salmonella* infection in neonatal swine. *Can J Comp Med* **43:** 200–206, 1979.

Wilcock, B. P., and Olander, H. J. Neurologic disease in naturally occurring *Salmonella choleraesuis* infection in pigs. *Vet Pathol* **14:** 113–120, 1977.

Wilcock, B. P., and Olander, H. J. The pathogenesis of porcine rectal stricture. II. Experimental salmonellosis and ischemic proctitis. *Vet Pathol* **14:** 43–55, 1977.

Wood, R. L., Pospischil, A., and Rose, R. Distribution of persistent *Salmonella typhimurium* infection in internal organs of swine. *Am J Vet Res* **50:** 1015–1021, 1989.

b. Salmonellosis in Horses The most common serovar in horses in most areas is *S. typhimurium,* and its prevalence is increasing. Other serovars are usually associated with sporadic cases of disease. Many horses are *Salmonella* carriers, and when they are stressed, diarrhea follows.

Treatment with antibiotics, especially orally, increases the risk of salmonellosis. Resistance to certain antibiotics is associated with the presence of resistance (R) plasmids that may be transferred to other bacteria, of the same or different species, by conjugation or transduction. Antibiotic-resistant *Salmonella* may not respond to treatment, and antimicrobial therapy may increase the potential for infection and disease, because of the suppression of the normal flora. Antibiotic resistant strains have been associated with outbreaks of salmonellosis at veterinary teaching hospitals. An antibiotic-resistant strain of *S. agona* appears to be emerging in horses in the United States of America.

Salmonellosis in horses may be manifested clinically as peracute (usually septicemic), acute, and chronic forms, and as an asymptomatic carrier state.

The septicemic form occurs most commonly in foals 1–6 months of age. These animals are usually with their dams at pasture, and predisposing factors are unclear. The infection in foals tends to be fatal. Affected animals are lethargic and develop severe diarrhea, often with characteristic green color, which may contain casts and blood. They are febrile and waste rapidly, to die in 2–3 days. Some survive for a week or more, and these may develop signs of pneumonia, osteitis, polyarthritis, and meningoencephalitis.

The primarily enteric forms of the disease are more likely to occur in older horses. Most of the predisposing factors mentioned earlier apply to horses. Salmonellosis is an occupational hazard of horses, since most are exposed to long periods of transport, and to exertion due to overwork or excessive training.

Clinically, the acute disease is characterized by diarrhea and fever for a period of 1–2 weeks, followed by recovery or death. The chronic form persists for weeks or months. Affected horses pass soft, unformed manure, which resembles cow feces. They lose their appetite, with subsequent progressive loss of weight and condition. In later stages, they become dehydrated and emaciated. The carrier state is somewhat controversial. Some investigators were unable to confirm long-term carriers in horses; others were able to recover *Salmonella* from feces of recovered animals for months. Reinfection may complicate attempts to determine whether an animal is a carrier.

The gross lesions are those of enteritis and/or septicemia; the former are most consistently found at autopsy. As a rule, the longer the course, the lower in the intestine does one find the most severe lesions.

Acute septicemic cases show small hemorrhages on the serous membranes, especially the pericardium and peritoneum, and enlargement of the spleen. In others, petechiae are present on the valvular endocardium, bladder mucosa, renal and adrenal cortices, and meninges, but none of these is consistent. The splenic enlargement is most

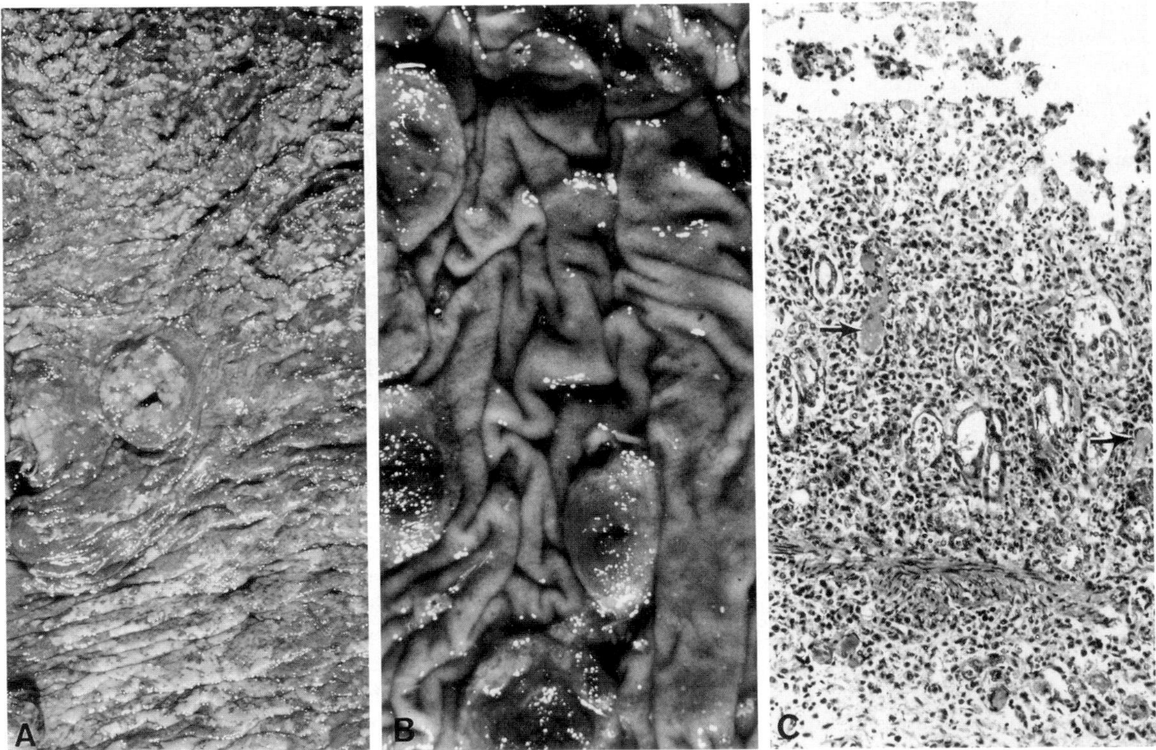

Fig. 1.132 Equine salmonellosis. (A) Focal and coalescent ulceration and diphtheresis involving ileocecal valve and mucosa. (B) Nodular ulcerative lesions in colon. Chronic salmonellosis. (C) Superficial necrosis and effusion from colonic mucosa. Foal. *S. typhimurium*. Several thrombosed vessels are in the propria (arrows).

marked in peracute cases, and the organ is dark and pulpy. The visceral lymph nodes are always enlarged, juicy, and often hemorrhagic. Marked pulmonary congestion and edema, renal cortical pallor, and medullary congestion may occur.

The main lesions are in the stomach and intestines. In **peracute or septicemic cases,** there is intense hyperemia of the gastric mucosa, probably venous infarction, with some edema and scattered hemorrhage. The small intestine may be congested with a mucous or hemorrhagic exudate. In **acute cases,** there is diffuse and intense fibrinohemorrhagic inflammation of the cecum and colon overshadowing any lesions in the upper intestine, and leading rapidly to superficial necrosis of the mucosa and a grayish-red pseudomembrane (Fig. 1.132A). In **chronic salmonellosis,** enteric lesions may be few or subtle. Some animals have extensive or patchy fibrinous or ulcerative lesions of the cecum and colon. In others raised circumscribed lesions about 2–3 cm in diameter may be evident, with a gelatinous submucosa and ulcerated mucosa. Some such lesions are more fibrinous, and resemble button ulcers (Fig. 1.132B).

Histologic alterations of significance are usually limited to the intestine. However, in septicemic animals, lesions typical of endotoxemia are present in lung, liver, kidney, spleen, and adrenal. There may be acute ileocecocolic lymphadenitis, and inflammation in sites of localization, such as growth plates in long bones, and the meninges. Depending on the duration of the enteritis, hemorrhage, necrosis, or diphtheresis may predominate, but the infiltrating leukocytes are largely mononuclear. The superficial coagulation necrosis of the mucosa may extend over large areas. A layer of fibrinocellular exudate may cover the necrotic mucosa. Fibrin thrombi are frequently present in the capillaries of the lamina propria (Fig. 1.132C). There is usually marked congestion of submucosal vessels, which is accompanied by considerable edema. Horses with acute enterocolitis, including cases of salmonellosis, may develop pulmonary aspergillosis, possibly due to invasion of the damaged intestinal mucosa by *Aspergillus* spp.

Bibliography

Begg, A. P. *et al.* Some aspects of the epidemiology of equine salmonellosis. *Aust Vet J* **65:** 221–223, 1988.

Carter, M. E., Dewes, H. G., and Griffiths, O. V. Salmonellosis in foals. *N Z Vet J* **3:** 78–83, 1979.

Carter, J. D. *et al.* Salmonellosis in hospitalized horses: Seasonality and case fatality rates. *J Am Vet Med Assoc* **188:** 163–167, 1986.

Cook, W. R. Diarrhea in the horse associated with stress and tetracycline therapy. *Vet Rec* **93:** 15–17, 1973.

Donahue, J. M. Emergence of antibiotic-resistant *Salmonella agona* in horses in Kentucky. *J Am Vet Med Assoc* **188:** 592–594, 1986.

Eugster, A. K., Whitford, H. W., and Mehr, L. E. Concurrent rotavirus and *Salmonella* infections in foals. *J Am Vet Med Assoc* **173:** 857–858, 1978.

Henninger, R. W. Proximal enteritis in a quarter horse stallion. *Compend Cont Ed Pract Vet* **8:** S53–S58, 1986.

Hird, E. W. *et al.* Risk factors for salmonellosis in hospitalized horses. *J Am Vet Med Assoc* **188:** 173–177, 1986.

Ikeda, J. S., and Hirsh, D. C. Common plasmid encoding resistance to ampicillin, chloramphenicol, gentamicin, and trimethoprim-sulfadiazine in two serotypes of *Salmonella* isolated during an outbreak of equine salmonellosis. *Am J Vet Res* **46:** 769–773, 1985.

McCain, C. S., and Powell, K. C. Asymptomatic salmonellosis in healthy adult horses. *J Vet Diagn Invest* **2:** 236–237, 1990.

Owen, R. ap R., Fullerton, J., and Barnum, D. A. Effects of transportation, surgery, and antibiotic therapy in ponies infected with *Salmonella*. *Am J Vet Res* **44:** 46–50, 1983.

Palmer, J. E., Benson, C. E., Whitlock, R. H. *Salmonella* shed by horses with colic. *J Am Vet Med Assoc* **187:** 256–257, 1985.

Puotunen-Reinert, A., and Huskamp, B. Acute postoperative diarrhoea in colic horses. *J S Afr Vet Assoc* **57:** 5–11, 1986.

Roberts, M. C., and O'Boyle, D. A. The prevalence and epizootiology of salmonellosis among groups of horses in southeast Queensland. *Aust Vet J* **57:** 27–35, 1981.

Slocombe, R. F., and Slauson, D. O. Invasive pulmonary aspergillosis of horses: An association with acute enteritis. *Vet Pathol* **25:** 277–281, 1988.

Smith, B. P. *et al.* Equine salmonellosis: Experimental production of four syndromes. *Am J Vet Res* **40:** 1072–1077, 1979.

Traub-Dargatz, J. L., Salman, M. D., and Jones, R. L. Epidemiologic study of salmonellae shedding in the feces of horses and potential risk factors for development of the infection in hospitalized horses. *J Am Vet Med Assoc* **196:** 1617–1622, 1990.

Wenkoff, M. S. *Salmonella typhimurium* septicemia in foals. *Can Vet J* **14:** 284–287, 1973.

c. Salmonellosis in Cattle There are differences between the disease in young and adult cattle. The serovars usually incriminated are *S. typhimurium* and *S. dublin,* the latter having often in the past been classified as *S. enteritidis*. These serovars are of worldwide distribution. Formerly *S. dublin* in North America was found mainly in the states west of the Rocky Mountains; however, it is now commonly isolated in areas east of this mountain range. Wherever it is found, it tends to show some specific adaptation to cattle and to occur in epizootics, whereas the other infections are more often sporadic. Whatever the serovar, the manifestations of infection in individual animals are similar, except that bacteremia and dissemination of infection are more common with *S. dublin* than with other serovars.

It is unusual to find salmonellosis in calves younger than a week, in contrast to colibacillosis, which usually affects very young animals. **In calves,** salmonellosis is a febrile disease typified by dejection, dehydration, and usually diarrhea. Diarrhea is not always present, but when it is, the feces are yellow or grayish, and have a very unpleasant odor. In older calves, there may be blood and mucus in the feces. In less acute cases there may be delayed evidence of localization in the lung and synovial structures. Morbidity and mortality may be considerable, especially in calves which are confined, such as in vealer operations. Experimental infections in calves indicate that survival is related inversely to the numbers of *Salmonella* in the inoculum, and directly to the age of the calves.

The general appearance at autopsy of a calf with salmonellosis may resemble one with septicemic colibacillosis. However, enlargement of mesenteric lymph nodes and gross enteric lesions are generally observed in salmonellosis. There is moderately severe gastrointestinal inflammation, acute swelling and hemorrhage of the visceral lymph nodes, and some petechiation of serous membranes. The enteritis may be catarrhal, but sometimes it is hemorrhagic, or more commonly causes exudation of yellowish fibrin (Figs. 1.133, 1.134). The mucosa overlying the lymphoid tissues may become necrotic and slough. In animals with fibrinous enteritis, the bowel wall is somewhat turgid, and the serosa may have a ground-glass appearance. There is often a diffuse, but perhaps mild, fibrinous peritonitis.

The intestinal lesions are usually most severe in the ileum, especially during the early stages of the disease. With time the jejunum and colon become involved, but the duodenum remains relatively normal. The regional distribution of the lesions may, in part, be related to differences in the level of bacterial colonization of the mucosa.

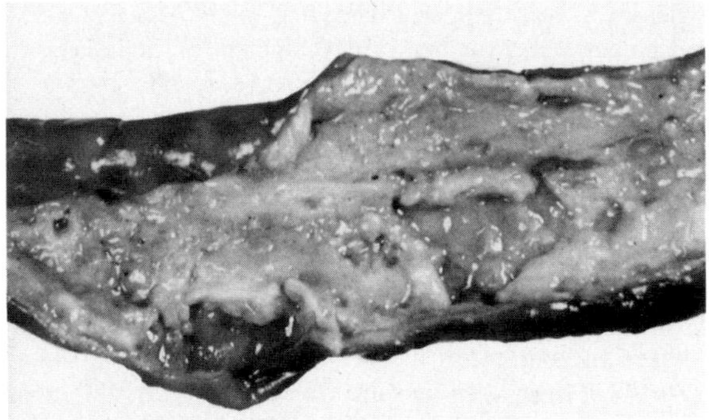

Fig. 1.133 Diphtheritic enteritis. Calf. Salmonellosis.

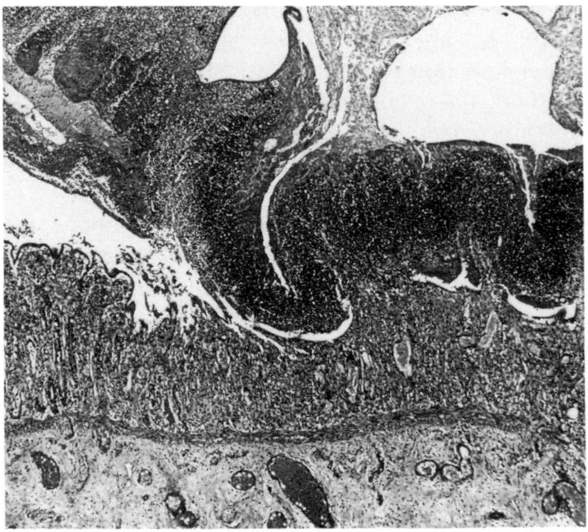

Fig. 1.134 Bovine salmonellosis. Diphtheritic membrane on the surface of the ileum. Exudate arises from eroded mucosa in which crypts of Lieberkühn are sparse or absent.

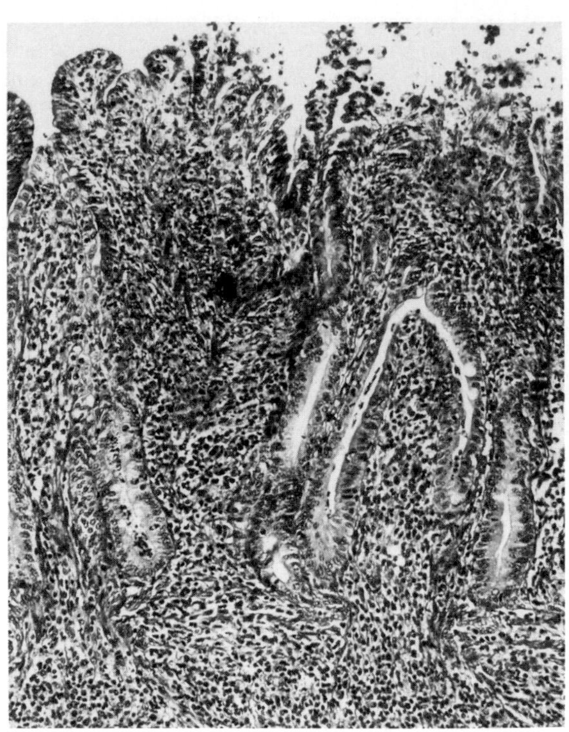

Fig. 1.135 Bovine salmonellosis. Atrophy of villi, exfoliation of surface epithelium, and effusion of neutrophils in ileum 12 hr after inoculation with *S. typhimurium*. (Courtesy of R. Clarke and C. L. Gyles.)

Twelve hours after oral infection of calves with *S. typhimurium*, the numbers of bacteria are generally lower in the abomasum and duodenum than in the lower intestinal tract, whereas they are relatively constant from the jejunum through to the rectum.

The early microscopic lesions in the small intestine consist of a thin layer of fibrinocellular exudate on the surface of short and blunt villi (Figs. 1.135). This is followed by extensive necrosis and ulceration of the mucosa, with fibrin and neutrophils exuding from the ulcerated areas into the lumen (Figs. 1.136, 1.137). The lamina propria may be moderately infiltrated by mononuclear inflammatory cells. Fibrin thrombi are often evident in proprial capillaries. There is also marked submucosal edema, and the centers of lymphoid follicles in the Peyer's patches are necrotic. The mucosal damage is usually too extensive to be explained solely on the basis of ischemia due to microvascular thrombosis. Similar erosion, ulceration, and fibrinous effusion occur in the proximal large bowel.

Scanning electron microscopy of small intestine shows large numbers of bacteria on a tattered mucosal surface. Clusters of enterocytes slough off short and blunt villi (Fig. 1.138). Strands of fibrin emerge from the mucosal defects and cover the mucosa. Ultrastructurally, the lesions are similar to those previously described for guinea pigs, except that there is more damage to epithelium in calves experimentally infected with *S. typhimurium*.

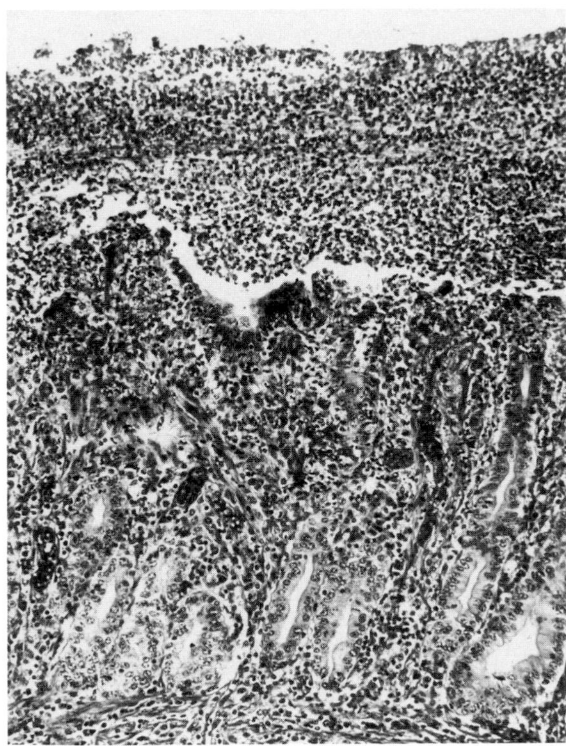

Fig. 1.136 Bovine salmonellosis. Atrophy of villi, erosion, and effusion of neutrophils and fibrin into lumen. Some thrombosis of proprial vessels 36 hr after inoculation with *S. typhimurium*. (Courtesy of R. Clarke and C. L. Gyles.)

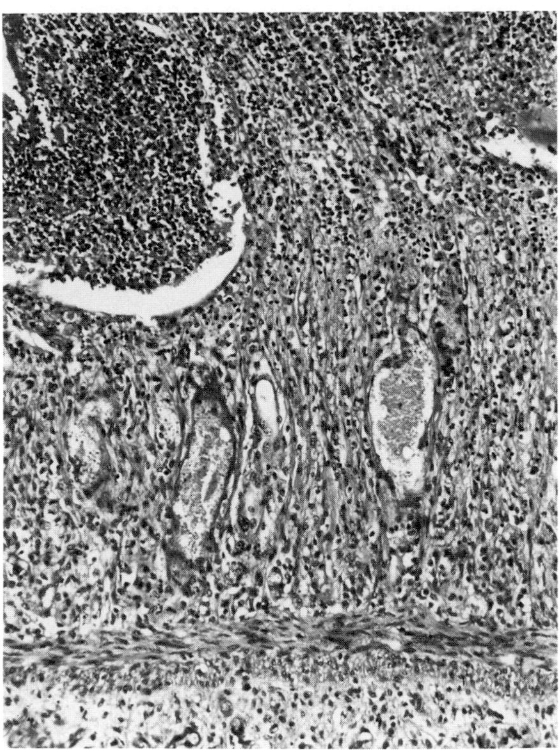

Fig. 1.137 Bovine salmonellosis. Eroded ileal mucosa, largely devoid of crypts of Lieberkühn. Fibrin and neutrophils in lumen.

Characteristic changes usually occur in the liver and spleen, but may be absent in peracute septicemic cases. There is often fibrinous cholecystitis. In acute cases, the spleen is enlarged and pulpy as a result of congestion, but this is soon replaced by acute splenitis, present as miliary, tiny foci of necrosis or as reactive nodules. The liver is often pale and beset with many minute paratyphoid nodules, which may require microscopy for detection. In the spleen, macrophage reaction is sometimes diffuse. Paratyphoid granulomas may also be found microscopically in the kidney, lymph nodes, and bone marrow. These probably represent a cell-mediated immune response to embolic bacteria. In those animals that survive the acute phase of the disease, the inflammatory changes in lymphoid tissues progress to an immunologic response, characterized by a diffuse reaction of medium-sized and large lymphocytes in the follicles, and plasma cells in the sinusoids. There may be marked cortical atrophy of the thymus. In calves with acute septicemia, pulmonary congestion and edema are visible at necropsy, with interstitial thickening of pulmonary alveolar septa by mononuclear cells in tissue section. There may be thrombosis of septal capillaries, and some effusion of edema fluid and macrophages into alveolar spaces.

In subacute salmonellosis in calves, there may be anterior bronchopneumonia, usually with adhesions and small abscesses. Purulent exudate is in synovial cavities, and the organism is recoverable in pure culture from such affected joints and tendon sheaths. It may be mixed with *Actinomyces pyogenes* and *Pasteurella* in the lungs. Mixed infections of *Salmonella* with other diarrheagenic agents, including bovine coronavirus, rotavirus, bovine virus diarrhea, and cryptosporidia have been reported.

Salmonellosis in adult cattle may occur in outbreaks as it does in calves, but more often it is sporadic, and it may cause chronic diarrhea and loss of condition. The source of infection is usually the carrier animal. Other sources, such as feed containing protein of animal origin, or bone meal, should be considered when the disease is caused by an uncommon serovar. Abortions are most common with *S. dublin*, but may occur with any serovar. In some herds this may be the only clinical evidence of infection, although other animals often excrete the offending serovar in the feces. The carrier state of *S. dublin* infection in adult cattle may persist for years, sometimes for life, in contrast to infections with other serovars, which rarely persist for more than 18 months. Dairy cows may persistently shed salmonella, especially *S. dublin,* in milk and cause infections in humans who drink raw milk; *S. dublin* in humans is often fatal. The morbid changes in adult cattle correspond to those in calves except that there is more pleural hemorrhage, and the enteritis may be more hemorrhagic and fibrinous. The histologic changes in the liver and other organs are the same as those seen in calves.

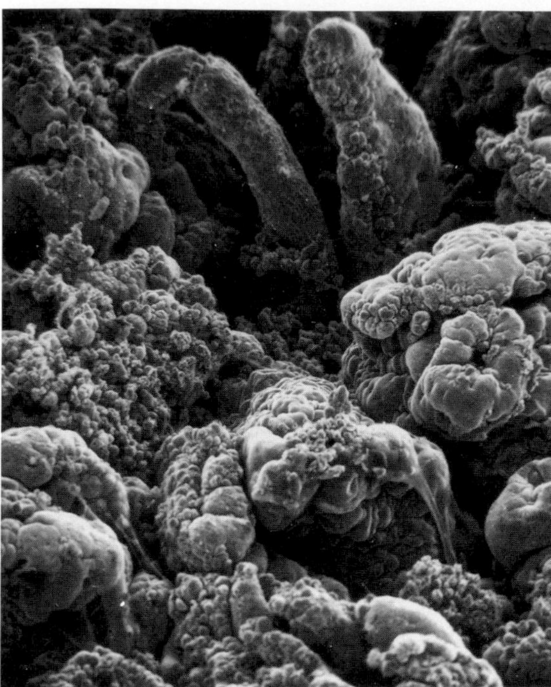

Fig. 1.138 Bovine salmonellosis. Scanning electron micrograph. Ileum. Calf 12 hr postinoculation with *S. typhimurium*. Villi are atrophic, and rounded cells are exfoliated from surface. (Courtesy of R. Clarke and C. L. Gyles.)

Bibliography

Bulgin, M. S. *Salmonella dublin*: What veterinarians should know. *J Am Vet Med Assoc* **182:** 116–118, 1983.

Clegg, F. G. *et al.* Outbreaks of *Salmonella newport* infection in dairy herds and their relationship to management and contamination of the environment. *Vet Rec* **112:** 580–584, 1983.

Donovan, G. A. *Salmonella dublin* infection in calves at a north Florida dairy farm. *Compend Cont Ed Pract Vet* **6:** S587–S590, 1984.

Hall, G. A., Jones, P. W., and Aitken, M. M. The pathogenesis of experimental intraruminal infections of cows with *Salmonella dublin*. *J Comp Pathol* **88:** 409–417, 1978.

Hall, G. A. *et al.* Pathology of calves with diarrhoea in southern Britain. *Res Vet Sci* **45:** 240–250, 1988.

Rings, D. M. Salmonellosis in calves. *Vet Clin North Am: Food Anim Pract* **1:** 529–539, 1985.

Smith, B. P. *et al.* Bovine salmonellosis: Experimental production and characterization of the disease in calves, using oral challenge with *Salmonella typhimurium*. *Am J Vet Res* **40:** 1510–1513, 1979.

Tablante, N. L., Jr., and Lane, V. M. Wild mice as potential reservoirs of *Salmonella dublin* in a closed dairy herd. *Can Vet J* **30:** 590–592, 1989.

Teuscher, E., Couture, Y., and Matovelo, J. A. Observations on the pathology of experimental salmonellosis (*S. typhimurium*) in calves, with special consideration of the haematopoietic organs (thymus, mesenteric lymph nodes, spleen, and bone marrow). *Schweitz Arch Tierheilk* **130:** 195–210, 1988.

Wray, C., and Sojka, W. J. Experimental *Salmonella typhimurium* infection in calves. *Res Vet Sci* **25:** 139–143, 1978.

Wray, C., and Roeder, P. L. Effect of bovine virus diarrhoea–mucosal disease virus infection on *Salmonella* infection in calves. *Res Vet Sci* **42:** 213–218, 1987.

Wray, C. *et al.* A three-year study of *Salmonella dublin* infection in a closed dairy herd. *Vet Rec* **124:** 532–535, 1989.

d. Salmonellosis in Sheep As well as abortion caused by *S. abortus-ovis,* abortion and neonatal death may follow infection of pregnant ewes by any species of *Salmonella*. Whereas the prevalence of *S. abortus-ovis* in Great Britain seems to be waning, *S. montevideo,* on the other hand, has been associated with abortions in several flocks in the British Isles. Salmonellosis is not a common disease in sheep, but outbreaks are always severe and may cause very heavy losses. Predisposing influences are necessary, and these are usually provided by circumstances which enforce congregation. Deprivation of food and water for 2–3 days may be sufficient and, coupled with fatigue, is the usual predisposing factor when sheep are transported or confined in holding yards. Deaths usually continue for a week to 10 days after debilitating circumstances have been remedied.

The serovars usually found in sheep are *S. typhimurium, S. arizonae,* and *S. enteritidis*. *Salmonella dublin* is increasing in prevalence in Great Britain and the midwestern states of the United States. Experimental inoculation of sheep with *S. arizonae* produces infection but rarely disease. Under natural conditions, this host-adapted organism is frequently considered to be a secondary infection to some other disease, or an incidental finding in apparently healthy animals. Most serovars produce the same sort of disease, which closely resembles that seen in cattle both clinically and at autopsy. The major findings are fibrinohemorrhagic enteritis and septicemia.

Bibliography

Brown, D. D., Ross, J. G., and Smith, A. F. G. Experimental infections of sheep with *Salmonella typhimurium*. *Res Vet Sci* **21:** 335–340, 1976.

Hannam, D. A. R., Wray, C., and Harbourne, J. F. Experimental *Salmonella arizonae* infection of sheep. *Br Vet J* **142:** 458–466, 1986.

Hunter, A. G. *et al.* An outbreak of *S. typhimurium* in sheep and its consequences. *Vet Rec* **98:** 126–130, 1976.

Linklater, K. A. Abortion in sheep associated with *Salmonella montevideo* infection. *Vet Rec* **112:** 372–374, 1983.

Meinershagen, W. A., Waldhalm, D. G., and Frank, F. W. *Salmonella dublin* as a cause of diarrhea and abortion in ewes. *Am J Vet Res* **31:** 1769–1771, 1970.

Pritchard, J. *Salmonella arizonae* in sheep. *Can Vet J* **31:** 42, 1990.

e. Salmonellosis in Carnivores *Salmonella* may often be recovered from apparently healthy dogs and cats. However, primary disease rarely occurs. In these species, too, nosocomial infections are sometimes associated with hospitalization and antibiotic therapy. In dogs, salmonellosis may be secondary to canine distemper. It can cause bronchopneumonia, acute hemorrhagic gastroenter-

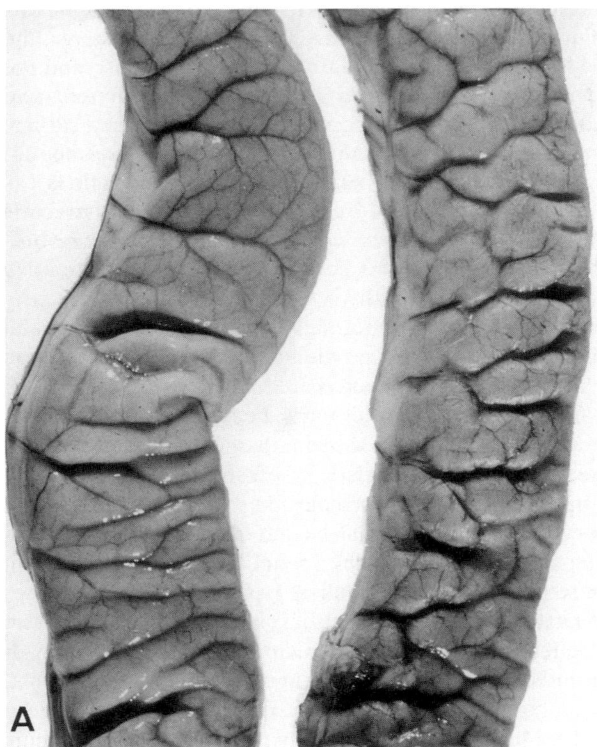

Fig. 1.141A Porcine intestinal adenomatosis complex. Exaggerated reticular pattern of folds on serosal aspect of the ileum.

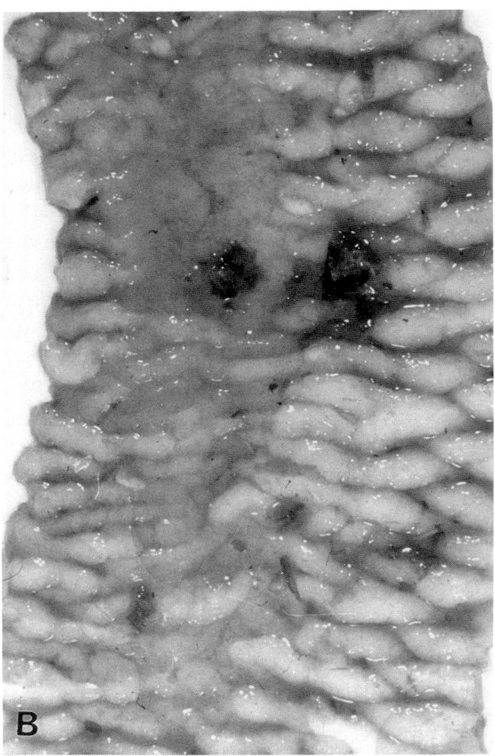

Fig. 1.141B Porcine intestinal adenomatosis complex. Raised nodular or ridgelike areas of thickened mucosa in the ileum, resulting from hypertrophy of glands.

ileum and proximal large intestine. The cerebriform pattern of serosal folding is evident in such cases (Fig. 1.142). Necrotic enteritis may be a sequel to other enterocolitides in swine, but adenomatosis is probably the most common primary lesion.

Microscopically, coagulation necrosis of the mucosa may be focal and superficial, with local effusion of neutrophils and fibrin into the lumen, and an acute inflammatory infiltrate at the margin of the necrotic tissue. Frequently, necrosis extends to involve most of the thickness of the mucosa, sometimes penetrating to the submucosa. A few islands of viable adenomatous crypts or glands may be left deep among the necrotic debris. Tissue in the upper ileum at the proximal margin of the zone of mucosal necrosis should be examined for adenomatosis, since in severe cases of necrotic enteritis, no remnants of abnormal mucosa may persist elsewhere. Masses of bacteria, presumably fecal anaerobes, are found superficially in the necrotic tissue. With time, granulation tissue develops in ulcerated areas.

Regional ileitis is the term applied to contracted tubular distal ileum, which may have an ulcerated mucosa, perhaps with a few raised foci of surviving proliferative mucosa. Granulation of ulcerated gut may result in progressive stricture of the lumen. More characteristically there is hypertrophy of the external muscle layer. Idiopathic ileal muscular hypertrophy also occurs in swine, apparently independent of antecedent adenomatosis. Granulomatous regional ileitis and mesenteric lymphadenitis in swine, nontuberculous and distinct from adenomatosis, has been described from Finland.

Proliferative hemorrhagic enteropathy is the fourth syndrome in the intestinal adenomatosis complex. It is a dis-

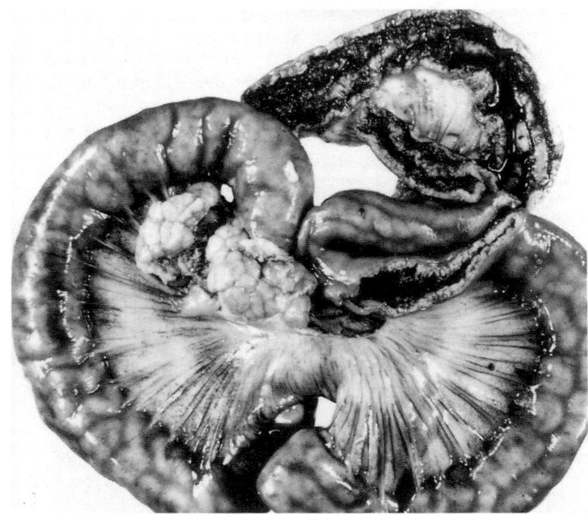

Fig. 1.142 Porcine intestinal adenomatosis complex. Necrotic enteritis. Thick ileal wall, enlarged lymph nodes, and opaque mesentery.

tinctive clinical entity, characterized by acute or subacute intestinal hemorrhage and anemia. Animals may exsanguinate so quickly as to die without passing blood. Others pass dark tarry feces for several days. This syndrome is more common in young adults, rather than growing pigs. It is usually sporadic, or of relatively low morbidity, but as many as half the clinically recognized cases may die.

Animals dead of proliferative hemorrhagic enteropathy are pale. The typical cerebriform pattern is evident on the external surface of the distal ileum, which is thickened and turgid (Fig. 1.143A). Fluid blood, or a loose or firm fibrin and blood clot may be present in the ileum (Fig. 1.143B), and the contents of the cecum and colon may contain dark bloody digesta and feces. The mucosa of the affected ileum usually resembles that in uncomplicated adenomatosis, and overt points of hemorrhage or ulceration are rarely discernible grossly. Rather the animals appear to suffer widespread diapedesis from the mucosa.

In tissue sections from animals dead with the hemorrhagic syndrome, there is extensive erosion and necrosis of adenomatous epithelium in the superficial mucosa (Fig. 1.144). An acute inflammatory infiltrate is present in the upper lamina propria, small vessels are thrombosed, and heavy effusion of neutrophils onto the mucosal surface and into lumina of glands is evident. Fibrin and hemorrhage emanating from superficial mucosal vessels are in the intestinal lumen. More extensive coagulation necrosis of the mucosa is associated occasionally with the hemorrhagic syndrome. It has been suggested that proliferative hemorrhagic enteropathy is the result of a hypersensitivity reaction to release of normally occult intracellular bacterial antigen from its intracellular location, by degeneration or phagocytosis of infected epithelium.

The diagnosis of proliferative hemorrhagic enteropathy at autopsy is based on the presence in the distal ileum of gross lesions characteristic of adenomatosis, in association with massive hemorrhage from the lower small intestine. The condition must be differentiated from hemorrhagic ulceration of the pars esophagea, and from mesenteric torsion, as well as from less common causes of gastrointestinal bleeding in swine. Less hemorrhagic manifestations of the adenomatosis complex must be differentiated from acute or chronic salmonellosis, postweaning *E. coli* enteritis, and from acute swine dysentery.

The diagnosis of the intestinal adenomatosis complex is confirmed by finding intracellular *Campylobacter*-like

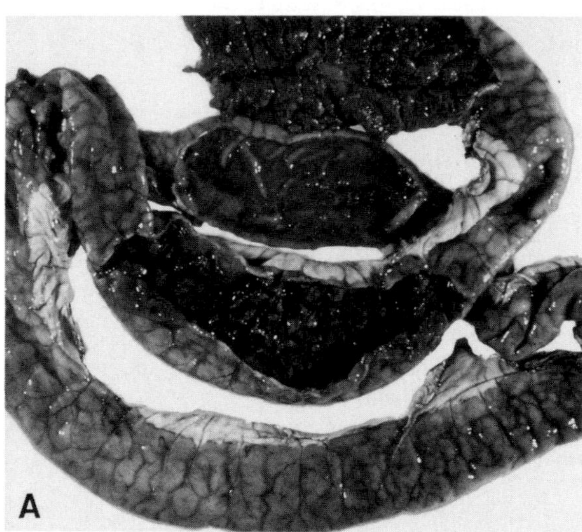

Fig. 1.143A Porcine intestinal adenomatosis complex. Folded necrotic mucosa, and fibrinohemorrhagic exudate in terminal ileum.

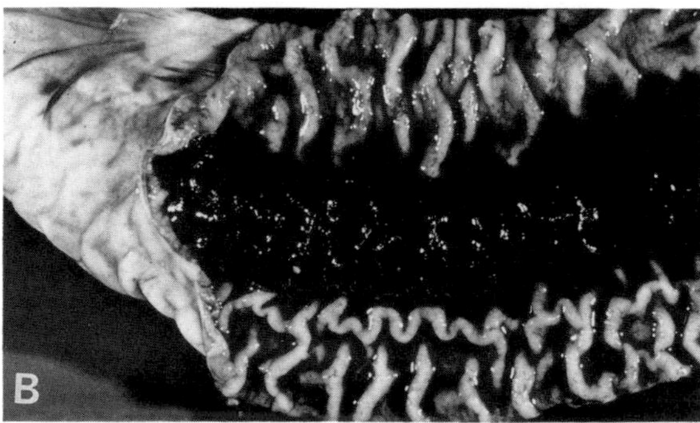

Fig. 1.143B Porcine intestinal adenomatosis complex. Proliferative hemorrhagic enteropathy. Hemorrhage and blood clot in terminal ileum. Nodular folded mucosa.

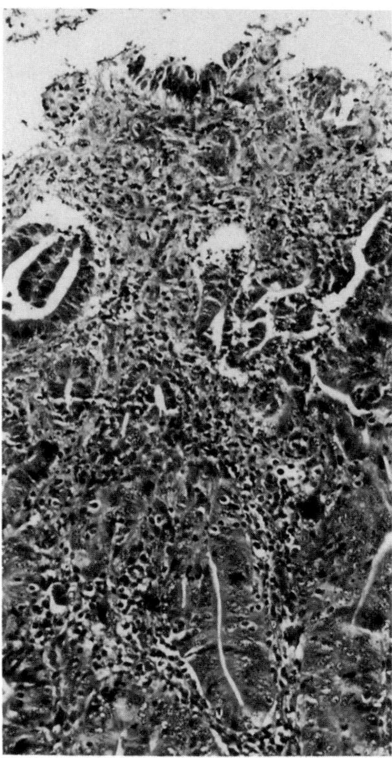

Fig. 1.144 Porcine intestinal adenomatosis complex. Proliferative hemorrhagic enteropathy. Superficial necrosis of mucosa associated with thrombosis of small vessels, hemorrhage, and effusion of fibrin and neutrophils.

organisms. They may be seen in smears of mucosal scrapings stained by the modified Koster's acid-fast method or with specific immunofluorescent techniques. Their intracellular location and association with typical adenomatous lesions is demonstrated in silver-stained tissue sections. Culture is not possible, and isolation of other *Campylobacter* species is of no etiologic significance.

Bibliography

Eriksen, K., Landsverk, T., and Bodahl, E. G. Cell differentiation in intestinal adenomatosis of pigs studied by histochemistry of laminin and enzymes of epithelial and subepithelial tissue. *Res Vet Sci* **49:** 1–7, 1990.

Gebhart, C. J. *et al.* Cloned DNA probes specific for the intracellular *Campylobacter*-like organism of porcine proliferative enteritis. *J Clin Microbiol* **29:** 1011–1015, 1991.

Jonsson, L. and Martinsson, K. Regional ileitis in pigs. Morphological and pathogenetical aspects. *Acta Vet Scand* **17:** 223–232, 1976.

Landsverk, T., and Nordstoga, K. Intestinal adenomatosis in pigs. A pathomorphological investigation. *Nord Vet Med* **33:** 77–80, 1981.

Lawson, G. H. K. *et al.* Proliferative haemorrhagic enteropathy. *Res Vet Sci* **27:** 46–51, 1979.

Lomax, L. G., and Glock, R. D. Naturally occurring porcine proliferative enteritis: Pathologic and bacteriologic findings. *Am J Vet Res* **43:** 1608–1614, 1982.

Lomax, L. G. *et al.* Porcine proliferative enteritis: Experimentally induced disease in cesarean-derived colostrum-deprived pigs. *Am J Vet Res* **43:** 1622–1630, 1982.

Love, D. N., and Love, R. J. Pathology of proliferative haemorrhagic enteropathy in pigs. *Vet Pathol* **16:** 41–48, 1979.

McOrist, S., and Lawson, G. H. K. Reproduction of proliferative enteritis in gnotobiotic pigs. *Res Vet Sci* **46:** 27–33, 1989.

McOrist, S. *et al.* Early lesions of proliferative enteritis in pigs and hamsters. *Vet Pathol* **26:** 260–264, 1989.

Roberts, L. *et al.* Porcine intestinal adenomatosis and its detection in a closed pig herd. *Vet Rec* **104:** 366–368, 1979.

Rowland, A. C., and Rowntree, P. G. M. A haemorrhagic bowel syndrome associated with intestinal adenomatosis in the pig. *Vet Rec* **91:** 235–241, 1972.

Schultheiss, P. C., Kurtz, H. J., and Glassman, D. Retrospective study of *Campylobacter* species isolated from porcine diagnostic case material. *J Vet Diagn Invest* **1:** 181–182, 1989.

Ward, G., and Winkelman, N. L. Recognizing the three forms of proliferative enteritis in swine. *Vet Med* **85:** 197–203, 1990.

Yates, W. D. G. *et al.* Proliferative hemorrhagic enteropathy in swine: An outbreak and review of the literature. *Can Vet J* **20:** 261–268, 1979.

b. INTESTINAL ADENOMATOSIS IN OTHER SPECIES Lesions resembling those described in the intestinal adenomatosis complex of swine, and associated with intracellular *Campylobacter*-like organisms, have been described in many species. They include ileal hyperplasia or proliferative ileitis, the cause of "wet tail" in hamsters; proliferative ileitis in puppies; intestinal adenomatosis in a foal; duodenal hyperplasia in guinea pigs; enterotyphlocolitis in rabbits; intestinal adenomatosis affecting the cecum and colon in blue foxes; proliferative colitis in ferrets; and adenocarcinomas of the colon in rats. Typically, the disease causes diarrhea and loss of body condition, and in blue foxes, rectal prolapse is common.

Though the disease can be transmitted to hamsters from swine, using intestinal homogenates, it is not known whether the agents seen in adenomatosis of the various species are related or the same. Adenomatous epithelium is occasionally seen in mesenteric lymph nodes in swine. In rats, in which the lesion behaves like a well-differentiated adenocarcinoma, intracytoplasmic *Campylobacter*-like organisms are in epithelium metastatic to the regional lymph nodes.

Though often cited as an example of this class of lesion, terminal ileitis or regional enteritis in lambs is not associated with intracellular *Campylobacter*-like organisms, and is discussed elsewhere in this chapter, with Border disease. Similarly, though grouped by some with adenomatosislike lesions, enteritis in rusa deer associated with *C. hyointestinalis,* to be discussed, is not characterized by intracellular bacteria.

Bibliography

Collins, J. E., and Libal, M. C. Proliferative enteritis in two pups. *J Am Vet Med Assoc* **183:** 886–889, 1983.

Duhamel, G. E., and Wheeldon, E. B. Intestinal adenomatosis in a foal. *Vet Pathol* **19:** 447–450, 1982.

Elwell, M. R., Chapman, A. L., and Frenkel, J. K. Duodenal hyperplasia in a guinea pig. *Vet Pathol* **18:** 136–139, 1981.

Eriksen, K., and Landsverk, T. Electron microscopy of intestinal adenomatosis in the blue fox, *Alopex lagopus*. *J Comp Pathol* **102:** 279–290, 1990.

Eriksen, K., Landsverk, T., and Bratberg, B. Morphology and immunoperoxidase studies of intestinal adenomatosis in the blue fox, *Alopex lagopus*. *J Comp Pathol* **102:** 265–278, 1990.

Fox, J. G. *et al.* Proliferative colitis in ferrets. *Am J Vet Res* **43:** 858–864, 1982.

Schoeb, T. R., and Fox, J. G. Enterocecocolitis associated with intraepithelial *Campylobacter*-like bacteria in rabbits (*Oryctolagus cuniculus*). *Vet Pathol* **27:** 73–80, 1990.

Stills, H. F., and Hook, R. R., Jr. Experimental production of proliferative ileitis in Syrian hamsters (*Mesocricetus auratus*) by using an ileal homogenate free of *Campylobacter jejuni*. *Infect Immun* **57:** 191–195, 1989.

Vandenberghe, J. *et al.* Spontaneous adenocarcinoma of the ascending colon in Wistar rats: The intracytoplasmic presence of a *Campylobacter*-like bacterium. *J Comp Pathol* **95:** 45–55, 1985.

c. ENTERITIS ASSOCIATED WITH *CAMPYLOBACTER* SPP. ***Campylobacter jejuni*** and ***C. coli*** are common causes of diarrhea in humans. *Campylobacter* enteritis and salmonellosis vie for supremacy in this regard in many areas. *Campylobacter jejuni* and *C. coli* also cause enteritis in animals.

Virulence resides in part in the production of secretory enterotoxin, and *C. jejuni* is more commonly enterotoxigenic than *C. coli;* cytotoxins have also been reported. *Campylobacter jejuni* colonizes the surface mucus layer and adheres to the mucosa, by mechanisms which are as yet unclear, and it often attains the systemic circulation, though it is not found within epithelium. Like salmonellosis, *Campylobacter* infection may be zoonotic. Many human infections are acquired by drinking raw milk, or from other animal foodstuffs, especially poultry products. Chickens are common asymptomatic shedders of *C. jejuni*. Some human cases have been associated with diarrhea in family pets, particularly puppies.

Campylobacter jejuni has been associated with diarrhea characterized by the presence of blood and mucus in some dogs, despite the fact that it often can be isolated from a high proportion of asymptomatic animals. It also has been isolated from dogs with parvoviral enteritis and other viral infections; it is not known whether concurrent infection with these agents is synergistic. The role of *Campylobacter* as a significant primary pathogen in dogs is not proven. Mild enteritis and colitis have been described in naturally infected dogs, although in experimentally infected gnotobiotic and conventional dogs, lesions are limited to mild mucosal colitis. Erosive colitis has been associated with *C. jejuni* infection in mink, and was reproduced experimentally. *Campylobacter jejuni* is isolated commonly from cats, but usually not in assocation with diarrhea.

A catalase-negative thermophilic organism, termed *Campylobacter upsaliensis,* has been isolated from the feces of dogs with and without diarrhea, and from normal cats. A similar agent has been associated with chronic diarrhea in dogs. *Campylobacter*-like organisms were on the surface of the biopsied intestinal mucosa in one such case, which had atrophic villi and dilation and hypertrophy of intestinal crypts.

Campylobacter jejuni, and *C. fetus* subsp. *fetus* have been isolated from the feces of normal cattle and from diarrheic calves, cattle, and sheep, many of them suffering from disease due to other agents. *Campylobacter hyointestinalis* has also been circumstantially associated with diarrhea in calves, and in rusa deer with an ileotyphlocolitis and vibrios in mucus on the mucosal surface. Experimental inoculation of *C. jejuni, C. coli,* and *C. hyointestinalis* into calves and lambs may result in passage of mucoid feces, and the production of mild enterocolitis in animals examined microscopically. A few crypt abscesses, goblet cell discharge, and focal acute inflammatory infiltrates are evident; organisms are in mucus on the surface, mainly in the large intestine. Signs of experimental infection are mild, and further work is needed to prove the significance of these *Campylobacter* species in ruminants. For many years *C. (Vibrio) coli* was proposed as the cause of winter dysentery in cattle; coronavirus is now implicated in the etiology of that condition.

Campylobacter jejuni also has been isolated from the feces of a number of scouring foals, but the significance of the infection is unclear.

Campylobacter coli is the species commonly isolated from the intestine of swine. As *Vibrio coli* it was long associated with swine dysentery, but did not induce enteritis in experimentally inoculated gnotobiotic pigs. More recent reports of diarrhea in conventional swine inoculated orally with *C. coli* need confirmation. Though experimental infections with *C. jejuni* in neonatal gnotobiotic pigs produce a mild mucosal colitis, similar to that in experimentally infected dogs, there is little evidence that this agent is a significant cause of spontaneous disease in swine.

Weaner colitis in sheep is a diarrhea of high morbidity and low mortality, reported from southeastern Australia, and associated with an unidentified *Campylobacter* species, not *C. jejuni.* Chronic diarrhea in weaned sheep, usually ~ 6 months old, must be differentiated from gastrointestinal parasitism. At necropsy, there is abnormally fluid colonic content, but mucosal lesions are not seen; chronically affected animals may have edema and loss of body condition suggestive of enteric protein loss. Microscopically, there is erosive typhlocolitis. Goblet cells are depleted in number, and multifocal erosion, or occasionally, ulceration, of the mucosa is evident. The lamina propria is infiltrated by a predominantly neutrophilic reaction, which in severe cases may extend to the submucosa. Scattered glands are distended by neutrophils and necrotic debris. Consistently, a layer of bacteria is present covering surface epithelial cells and in crypts. Though visible in routine sections, they are seen best with silver stains. Under the electron microscope, these bacteria adhere to the cell between microvilli, by one pole of the organism, but they do not invade. The disease has been reproduced by inoculation of the thermophilic catalase-negative *Campylobacter*-like organism, which is isolated from spontaneous cases on modified mycoplasma agar base medium.

Bibliography

Boosinger, T. R., and Powe, T. A. *Campylobacter jejuni* infections in gnotobiotic pigs. *Am J Vet Res* **49:** 456–458, 1988.

Davies, A. P., Gebhart, C. J., and Meric, S. A. *Campylobacter*-associated chronic diarrhea in a dog. *J Am Vet Med Assoc* **184:** 469–471, 1984.

Diker, K. S., Diker, S., and Özlem, M. B. Bovine diarrhea associated with *Campylobacter hyointestinalis. J Vet Med (B)* **37:** 158–160, 1990.

Dillon, A. R., Boosinger, T. R., and Blevins, W. T. *Campylobacter* enteritis in dogs and cats. *Compend Cont Ed Pract Vet* **9:** 1176–1183, 1987.

Fox, J. G. *et al.* "*Campylobacter upsaliensis*" isolated from cats as identified by DNA relatedness and biochemical features. *J Clin Microbiol* **27:** 2376–2378, 1989.

Gardner, D. E., and Young, G. W. *Campylobacter* in foals. *N Z Vet J* **35:** 116–117, 1987.

Hill, B. D., Thomas, R. J., and Mackenzie, A. R. *Campylobacter hyointestinalis*-associated enteritis in Moluccan rusa deer (*Cervus timorensis* subsp. *moluccensis*). *J Comp Pathol* **97:** 687–693, 1987.

Jopp, A., and Orr, M. B. Enteropathy and nephropathy associated with "winter scour" in hoggets. *N Z Vet J* **28:** 195, 1980.

Junttila, J. *et al. Campylobacter*-associated epidemic in cats. *Compan Anim Pract* **1(7):** 16–18, 1987.

Macartney, L. *et al.* Experimental infection of dogs with *Campylobacter jejuni. Vet Rec* **122:** 245–249, 1988.

Malik, R., and Love, D. N. The isolation of *Campylobacter*

jejuni/coli from pound dogs and canine patients in a veterinary hospital. *Aust Vet Practit* **19:** 16–18, 1989.

McOrist, S., Stephens, L. R., and Skilbeck, N. Experimental reproduction of ovine weaner colitis with a *Campylobacter*-like organism. *Aust Vet J* **64:** 29–31, 1987.

Olubunmi, P. A., and Taylor, D. J. Production of enteritis in pigs by the oral inoculation of pure cultures of *Campylobacter coli*. *Vet Rec* **111:** 197–202, 1982.

Shane, S. M., and Montrose, M. S. The occurrence and significance of *Campylobacter jejuni* in man and animals. *Vet Res Commun* **9:** 167–198, 1985.

Stansfield, D. G., Hunt, B., and Kemble, P. R. *Campylobacter* gastroenteritis in fattening lambs. *Vet Rec* **118:** 210–211, 1986.

Stephens, L. R. *et al.* Colitis in sheep due to a *Campylobacter*-like bacterium. *Aust Vet J* **61:** 183–187, 1984.

Terzolo, H. R. *et al.* Enteric *Campylobacter* infection in gnotobiotic calves and lambs. *Res Vet Sci* **43:** 72–77, 1987.

Walker, R. I. *et al.* Pathophysiology of *Campylobacter* enteritis. *Microbiol Rev* **50:** 81–94, 1986.

Warner, D. P., and Bryner, J. H. *Campylobacter jejuni* and *Campylobacter coli* inoculation of neonatal calves. *Am J Vet Res* **45:** 1822–1824, 1984.

5. *Swine Dysentery*

Swine dysentery is a highly infectious disease, mainly of weaned pigs, which is characterized by diarrhea, with mucus, blood, or fibrin in the feces. It probably occurs wherever swine are raised. As long ago as 1924, swine dysentery was known to be experimentally transmissible by dosing young pigs with colonic contents from affected pigs. For many years *Campylobacter (Vibrio) coli* was thought to cause swine dysentery, but *Serpula (Treponema) hyodysenteriae* is now known to be the cause. It is a Gram-negative, anaerobic but oxygen-tolerant spirochete, 6–9 μm long and 0.4 μm in diameter. It produces strong beta hemolysis on blood agar plates. The organism is motile, moving in serpentine fashion; it is loosely coiled and has seven to nine axial filaments which extend like flagella at each end of the cell.

Swine dysentery can be reproduced by feeding pure cultures of *S. hyodysenteriae* to specific pathogen-free and conventionally reared swine. Experimental reproduction of the disease in gnotobiotic pigs requires the presence of anaerobic bacteria indigenous to the normal colon, along with *S. hyodysenteriae*. There is apparently a synergistic action between the spirochete and the other anaerobes, mainly *Bacteroides* and *Fusobacterium*. These probably provide a suitable microenvironment and substrates essential for the *Serpula* to proliferate.

Another spirochete, classified as *Serpula (Treponema) innocens,* but perhaps a complex of species, also occurs in the large bowel of pigs. It is nonhemolytic or only weakly so, and differs in some biochemical reactions from *S. hyodysenteriae*. Its role in spontaneous disease is controversial. Though *S. innocens* is found in normal pigs, it also has been associated with diarrhea that resembles a mild form of swine dysentery, and in the United Kingdom is termed grower scour, or nonspecific colitis. At least some strains of *S. innocens* seem mildly pathogenic for swine.

The pathogenesis of swine dysentery is still incompletely understood. *Serpula hyodysenteriae* colonizes the mucus on the mucosal surface, in the lumen of colonic glands, and mucus in goblet cells. Lesions, including necrosis of surface epithelium, are associated with the presence of large numbers of spirochetes and other anaerobic bacteria on the mucosa. Attachment of spirochetes to host cells has not been observed *in vivo,* and invasion is not essential for epithelial necrosis to occur. When spirochetes invade surface epithelial cells, they appear to do so through lateral membranes, and do not attach to and penetrate the luminal membrane. *Serpula* usually do not invade beyond the epithelial cells. Liberation of toxins by *S. hyodysenteriae,* and possibly other anaerobes, may result in necrosis of superficial epithelium, perhaps directly, or as a result of local microvascular compromise.

The result is mucosal colitis, characterized by superficial erosion, with hyperplasia of cells in colonic glands, and hypersecretion of mucus. Thrombosis of capillaries and venules in the superficial areas of the colonic mucosa and the gastric fundic mucosa (venous infarction) is probably due to absorption, through the damaged mucosa, of endotoxins released by Gram-negative bacteria.

The diarrhea in swine dysentery is due to malabsorption of fluids and electrolytes in the colon. This presumably results from damage to the superficial colonic epithelium. The normal colon of the pig has a tremendous absorptive capacity. Interference with colonic absorption results in severe diarrhea and dehydration. Active fluid secretion by the colon, associated with bacterial enterotoxins, does not occur in swine dysentery. Fluid and electrolyte transport are normal in the small intestine. Prostaglandins released during inflammation do not appear to be implicated in the development of diarrhea.

There is usually an introduction of pigs, presumably carriers, into a herd prior to an outbreak. Once established in a herd, the infection tends to remain enzootic, and although treatment can effect a rapid clinical amelioration, it may not be curative, and relapses at greater or lesser intervals can occur. Apparently infection is not followed by a substantial immunity, although individual carrier pigs are resistant to further challenge with *S. hyodysenteriae* after recovery from disease. The morbidity may reach 90% and mortality, 30%. Many of the factors predisposing to salmonellosis also apply to swine dysentery.

The disease occurs in pigs of all ages older than ~2–3 weeks old, but particularly in pigs 8–14 weeks of age. Once initiated, it spreads rapidly by pen contact. The disease is initially febrile, but with the onset of diarrhea, fever tends to subside. The initial diarrheic feces are thin, semisolid, and without blood or mucus; it is usually only after 1–2 days of diarrhea that blood and mucus appear in the feces. Some pigs die peracutely without showing diarrhea, and many which show diarrhea do not have dysentery, but pass feces which contain much mucus.

Pigs which die of swine dysentery are usually gaunt with a contracted abdomen; the eyes are sunken; and there may be bluish discoloration of the abdominal skin.

Associated lesions may include pericardial serous effusion, and intense congestion of the gastric mucosa due to venous infarction. The intestinal lesions, especially in young pigs dying acutely, and those that have been treated, can be easily overlooked because the mucosal colitis may be mild, patchy, and often more catarrhal than fibrinous.

In typical cases, dehydration gives a semiopaque ground-glass appearance to the serosa, and the wall of the cecum and colon is thickened. The colonic content in these cases is usually scant, and porridgelike dirty gray to reddish brown and greasy in appearance. The mucosa, with patchy foci of light fibrin exudation, has the velvety thickening of catarrhal secretion (Fig. 1.145A). The most severe lesions approach those of salmonellosis in the extent and severity of fibrin effusion. The production of mucus in swine dysentery becomes copious in many chronic cases because of remarkable goblet-cell hyperplasia.

The earliest microscopic lesions are characterized by discrete areas of necrosis and erosion in the superficial mucosa. Thin layers of fibrinocellular exudate cover the eroded areas. In more advanced cases, the areas of necrosis become more diffuse but remain superficial, and exudation is more copious (Fig. 1.145B). There may be minor bleeding from small vessels in eroded mucosa. Fibrin thrombi are evident in the capillaries and venules of the superficial lamina propria. There is usually some edema of the lamina propria, submucosa, and serosa. There is initially expulsion of mucus from the basilar portions of the crypts (Fig. 1.146A). In concert with the increased turnover of epithelial cells associated with the superficial necrosis, there is hyperplasia of cells deeper in the glands. The crypts are elongated, lined by proliferative basophilic epithelial cells which have large nuclei, and few differentiated goblets (Fig. 1.146B). Often, crypts subsequently become dilated and contain necrotic debris. Others have marked goblet cell hyperplasia, and copious mucus production.

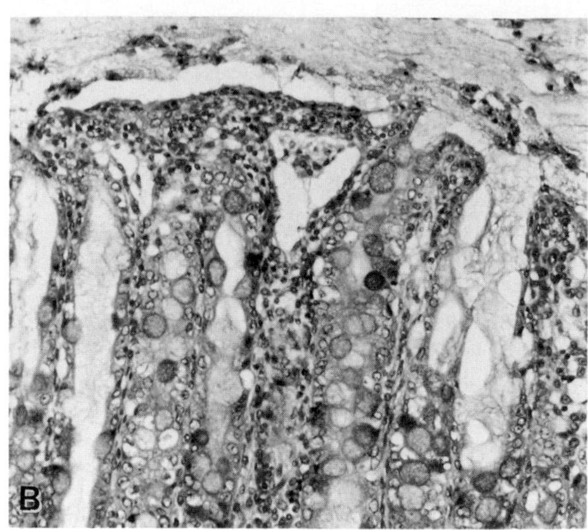

Fig. 1.145B Swine dysentery. Flattened and exfoliating epithelium on mucosal surface, and edema of superficial lamina propria. Mucus in glands and on surface, mixed with neutrophils and exfoliated epithelium.

Large numbers of spirochetes are easily demonstrated using Warthin–Starry or similar silver stains, mainly in the areas of superficial erosion and in the lumen of crypts.

Ultrastructurally, large numbers of spirochetes are on the surface and within the cytoplasm of epithelial cells. Fewer organisms are present in the intercellular spaces between superficial epithelial cells, in the lumen of crypts,

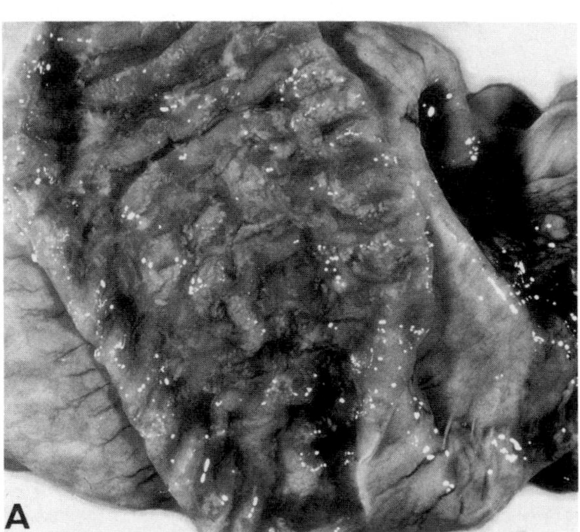

Fig. 1.145A Swine dysentery. Patchy fibrinocatarrhal exudate on the colonic mucosa.

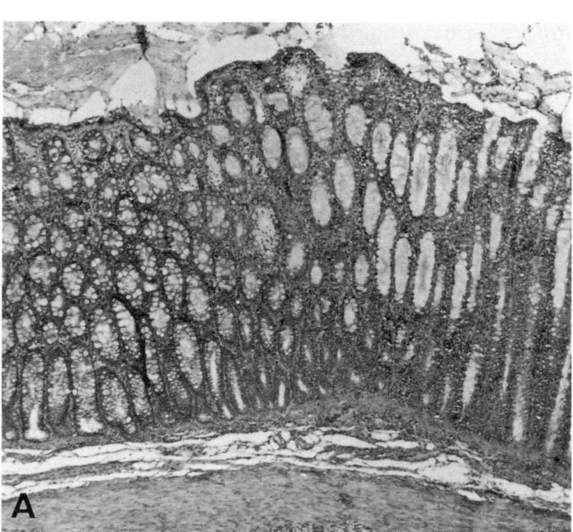

Fig. 1.146A Swine dysentery. Hyperplastic glands with few goblet cells adjacent to mucosa with normal density of goblet cells. Copious mucus on surface.

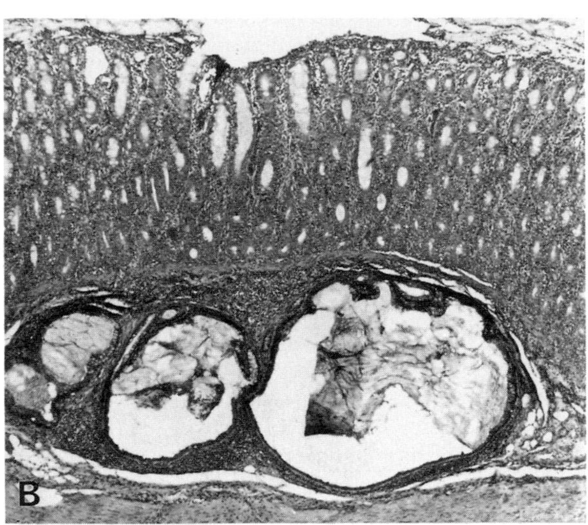

Fig. 1.146B Swine dysentery. Hyperplastic glandular lining virtually devoid of goblet cells; colitis cystica profunda or herniation of mucous glands into submucosal lymphoid tissue.

and occasionally in the lamina propria. Degenerative changes in the epithelial cells are characterized by loss of microvilli, clumping of nuclear chromatin, and swelling of the mitochondria and the rough endoplasmic reticulum.

Bibliography

Ferguson, H. W., Neill, S. D., and Pearson, G. R. Dysentery in pigs associated with cystic enlargement of submucosal glands in the large intestine. *Can J Comp Med* **44:** 109–114, 1980.

Harris, D. L. *et al.* Swine dysentery: Studies of gnotobiotic pigs inoculated with *Treponema hyodysenteriae, Bacteroides vulgatus,* and *Fusobacterium necrophorum. J Am Vet Med Assoc* **172:** 468–471, 1978.

Joens, L. A. *et al.* Location of *Treponema hyodysenteriae* and synergistic anaerobic bacteria in colonic lesions of gnotobiotic pigs. *Vet Microbiol* **6:** 69–77, 1981.

Kennedy, M. J. *et al.* Association of *Treponema hyodysenteriae* with porcine intestinal mucosa. *J Gen Microbiol* **134:** 1565–1576, 1988.

Kinyon, J. M., Harris, D. L., and Glock, R. D. Enteropathogenicity of various isolates of *Treponema hyodysenteriae. Infect Immunol* **15:** 638–646, 1977.

Schmall, L. M., Argenzio, R. A., and Whipp, S. C. Pathophysiologic features of swine dysentery: Cyclic nucleotide-independent production of diarrhea. *Am J Vet Res* **44:** 1309–1316, 1983.

Spearman, J. G., Nayar, G., and Sheridan, M. Colitis associated with *Treponema innocens* in pigs. *Can Vet J* **29:** 747, 1988.

Stanton, T. B. *et al.* Reclassification of *Treponema hyodysenteriae* and *Treponema innocens* in a new genus, *Serpula* gen. nov., as *Serpula hyodysenteriae* comb. nov. and *Serpula innocens* comb. nov. *Int J Syst Bacteriol* **41:** 50–58, 1991.

Teige, J., Jr. *et al.* Swine dysentery: A scanning electron microscopic investigation. *Acta Vet Scand* **22:** 218–225, 1981.

Wilcock, B. P., and Olander, H. J. Studies on the pathogenesis of swine dysentery. *Vet Pathol* **16:** 450–465, 1979.

6. *Diseases Associated with Enteric Clostridial Infections*

Most of the important enteric clostridial diseases occur in herbivores and are caused by one or the other of the five toxigenic types of *Clostridium perfringens.* Hemorrhagic enteritis in dogs is associated with an untyped *C. perfringens,* and *C. difficile* is implicated in necrotizing enteritis in foals and dogs. Occasionally other members of the genus are associated with diseases of the alimentary tract. *Clostridium chauvoei* may affect the tongue and the smooth muscle of the lower alimentary tract, causing a blackleglike myositis. *Clostridium botulinum* causes toxicoinfectious botulism in horses, and by ingestion of toxin, botulism in cattle. Braxy, abomasitis caused by *C. septicum,* is discussed with gastritis.

There are five types of *C. perfringens,* designated A–E, which are differentiated on the basis of their production of the four major antigenic lethal exotoxins. A strain formerly classified as type F is now regarded as a subtype of type C. The major exotoxins are alpha, beta, epsilon, and iota; the relationships between the five types and the four toxins are listed.

Toxin	Alpha	Beta	Epsilon	Iota
Type A	+ +	−	−	−
B	+	+ +	+	−
C	+	+ +	−	−
D	+	−	+ +	−
E	+	−	−	+ +

+ +, significant toxin, +, small amount, −, none detected

Eight minor toxins are produced by *C. perfringens,* and some of these may be useful in identification of types and in division of types A, B, and C into varieties.

The **alpha toxin** is a lecithinase which acts on cell membranes, producing hemolysis or necrosis of cells. The nature of the **beta toxin** is not clear. It is common to those strains (B and C) which cause enteritis, is necrotizing, trypsin labile, and appears to have a paralyzing effect on the intestine. The **epsilon toxin** is produced as an inactive prototoxin that is activated by enzymic digestion. In culture, the appropriate enzymes (the minor toxins kappa and lambda) may be produced by the organism. In the intestine, trypsin is an effective activator. The prototoxin is produced only during periods of growth. The **iota toxin** also is elaborated as a prototoxin and activated by proteolytic enzymes either in culture (lambda toxin) or in the intestine; it increases capillary permeability. **Kappa toxin** is a collagenase and **lambda,** a nonspecific proteinase. Other minor toxins include mu, a hyaluronidase, and delta, a hemolysin. The enterotoxin produced by certain strains is subsequently discussed.

There is not always a clear distinction between the different types of *C. perfringens.* Some strains lose their ability to produce one or more of their toxins when stored or cultured, and this complicates the identifications of isolates and the assessment of their significance in disease outbreaks.

Clostridial diseases of the intestine often are called enterotoxemias. Disease produced by *Clostridium perfringens* type D, whose epsilon exotoxin is elaborated in the intestine but exerts its important effects on distant organs such as brain and kidney, is an enterotoxemia. The hemolytic disease attributed to type A is also an enterotoxemia, but in general, the other types produce local intestinal lesions. The production of an **enterotoxin,** distinct from the classical exotoxins, by some types of *C. perfringens,* is potentially confusing. This enterotoxin is elaborated only by sporulating cells and is released on lysis of the cells. It is, almost exclusively, a product of type A strains but is identified occasionally from type C and very rarely from type D strains. The enterotoxin is not involved in the pathogenesis of enterotoxemia (pulpy-kidney disease) caused by the latter strains. It is significant in food poisoning by type A strains in humans, where it has also been associated with antibiotic treatment-related diarrhea, infantile diarrhea, and sudden infant death syndrome.

Bibliography

McDonel, J. L. Toxins of *Clostridium perfringens* types A, B, C, D, and E. *In* "Pharmacology of Bacterial Toxins," F. Dorner and J. Drews (eds.), pp. 477–517. Oxford, Pergamon Press, 1986.

a. *Clostridium perfringens* Type A *Clostridium perfringens* type A is the most common of the five types and is the only one associated with the microflora of both soil and intestinal tract. Its major toxin is the alpha toxin, and it also produces the enterotoxin.

This is one of several clostridia that produce gas gangrene in humans and animals. The production of gas gangrene in wound and puerperal infections probably is a composite effect of the major and minor toxins elaborated by the organism. The necrotizing and hemolytic activity of the alpha toxin is assisted by the collagenase and hyaluronidase which disrupt connective tissues and permit the infection to spread. Other wound contaminants, not necessarily clostridial, also can be important in lesion development.

The significance of type A strains in enteric diseases other than food poisoning in humans and necrotic enteritis of chickens is not clear. Their postulated causative association with equine colitis X is discussed elsewhere. There is a single case report of a fatal infection with *C. perfringens* type A in a neonatal foal with hemorrhagic diarrhea, severe abdominal pain, depression, and dehydration. Macroscopic lesions in this foal consisted of excessive serosanguineous fluid in the peritoneal cavity, and extensive subserosal hemorrhages on the intestine. The small intestine was distended with gas and foul-smelling bloody fluid, which extended into the large intestine. The mucosa of the small intestine was dark purple. Microscopic lesions were confined to the gut, mainly the small intestine, and were characterized by diffuse and marked necrosis and desquamation of the villous mucosa. The remnants of the necrotic villi were covered by large numbers of Gram-positive rods, consistent with clostridia. There was also marked hyperemia and hemorrhage of the lamina propria, submucosa, and subserosa without a significant leukocytic reaction. Intravenous inoculation of *C. perfringens* type A in ponies resulted in acute colic and hemorrhagic gastroenterocolitis.

Clostridium perfringens type A has been associated with white scours in suckling pigs and diarrhea in feeder pigs. The pigs had a necrotizing enterocolitis, villus atrophy, and serositis. A similar syndrome was reproduced with oral inoculation of viable *C. perfringens* type A into gnotobiotic colostrum-deprived and weaner pigs. Type A has been suspected of causing disease in cattle, but proof is often lacking. Calves inoculated intraruminally with *C. perfringens* type A developed anorexia, depression, bloat, and diarrhea, and some of these calves died. Lesions included variable degrees of abomasitis and abomasal ulcers.

A very rare disease of calves and lambs characterized by acute intravascular hemolysis is also associated with type A infections. Affected animals may be found dead or moribund, and jaundice and hemoglobinuria may be evident clinically. At autopsy icterus, anemia, and other changes of severe, acute, intravascular hemolysis are prominent. Severe diarrhea may occur in calves, but enteric lesions are likely to be obscured by rapid autolysis. This hemolytic disease must be distinguished from other causes of acute intravascular hemolysis such as leptospirosis, bacillary hemoglobinuria caused by *Clostridium novyi* type D (*haemolyticum*), and chronic copper poisoning. Presumably the hemolytic effect of the exotoxin is responsible for the intravascular hemolysis. Given that type A strains are commonly found in the intestines of ruminants, and that alpha toxin given intravenously is destroyed rapidly, it is apparent that there must be complex pathogenetic requirements for the development of this disease. The pathogenesis may be somewhat analogous to that of enterotoxemia caused by type D, which is discussed subsequently.

Bibliography

Dart, A. J. *et al.* Enterotoxaemia in a foal due to *Clostridium perfringens* type A. *Aust Vet J* **65:** 330–331, 1988.

Jestin, A., Popoff, M. R., and Mahé, S. Epizootiologic investigations of a diarrheic syndrome in fattening pigs. *Am J Vet Res* **46:** 2149–2151, 1985.

McGowan, B., Moulton, J. E., and Rood, S. E. Lamb losses associated with *Clostridium perfringens* Type A. *J Am Vet Med Assoc* **133:** 219–221, 1958.

Niilo, L., and Cho, H. J. Clinical and antibody responses to *Clostridium perfringens* type A enterotoxin in experimental sheep and calves. *Can J Comp Med* **49:** 145–148, 1985.

Ochoa, R., and Kern, S. R. The effects of *Clostridium perfringens* type A enterotoxin in Shetland ponies—Clinical, morphologic, and clinicopathologic changes. *Vet Pathol* **17:** 738–747, 1980.

Olubunmi, P. A., and Taylor, D. J. *Clostridium perfringens* type A in enteric diseases of pig. *Trop Vet* **3:** 28–33, 1985.

Popoff, M. R., and Jestin, A. Enteropathogenicity of purified *Clostridium perfringens* enterotoxin in the pig. *Am J Vet Res* **46:** 2147–2148, 1985.

Roeder, B. L. *et al.* Experimental induction of abdominal tympany, abomasitis, and abomasal ulceration by intraruminal inoculation of *Clostridium perfringens* type A in neonatal calves. *Am J Vet Res* **49:** 201–207, 1988.

Rose, A. L., and Edgar, G. Enterotoxaemic jaundice of cattle and sheep. A preliminary report on the aetiology of the disease. *Aust Vet J* **12:** 212–220, 1936.

b. *CLOSTRIDIUM PERFRINGENS* TYPE B *Clostridium perfringens* type B is reported from Europe, South Africa, and the Middle East but not from North America and Australasia. It causes lamb dysentery, usually in lambs younger than ~10 to 14 days, dysentery in calves of approximately the same age, and dysentery in foals within the first few days of life.

In lambs, death may occur without premonitory signs, but there is usually abdominal pain, especially when animals are forced to rise, and passage of semifluid dark feces mixed or coated with blood. The abdomen is often tympanitic. A more chronic form in older lambs, which among other diseases is known as "pine" in England, is characterized by unthriftiness and depression, reluctance to suckle, and a peculiar stretching when the animal rises; such cases are reputed to respond well to specific antiserum. Proof of the nature of their illness is lacking, although epidemiologically it does appear to be a chronic form of this disease.

Typical lesions are usually present, although in exceptional peracute cases, they may be indistinct. The first impression on opening the abdominal cavity is that there is mesenteric torsion, a not uncommon accident in young lambs. The characteristic lesion is an extensive hemorrhagic enteritis. Discrete and then confluent ulcerations develop if the course is long enough. In peracute cases, there may be only a few small patches of necrosis. The peritoneal cavity often contains a small amount of serous or bloodstained fluid.

In cases with more severe and deeply penetrating mucosal ulcerations, there may be an overlying peritonitis with red fibrin strands on the local mesentery and intestinal adhesions. The ulcers are usually visible through the serosa as purplish areas, and they may be limited to the small intestine or also involve the large intestine. On the mucosal surface, they are irregular but well defined by a sharp margin and rim of intense hyperemia, and they contain a yellow necrotic deposit; they may coalesce to form extensive areas of necrosis. Usually the intestinal contents are bloodstained and may appear to be composed of pure blood, but in lambs which live for 3–4 days, there may be little or no hemorrhage evident. In acute cases, the abomasal mucosa may be intensely congested. The mesenteric lymph nodes are edematous or intensely congested. Histologically the wall of the intestine is suffused with blood, and the areas of necrosis extend deep into the mucous membrane and may penetrate the muscularis mucosa to the muscle layers and peritoneum. In the necrotic tissue, there are large numbers of typical bacilli, but few inflammatory cells.

The lesions present in other organs are those of severe toxemia. The liver is usually pale and friable, but may be congested. The spleen is normal or slightly enlarged and pulpy. The kidneys may be enlarged, edematous, pale, and soft from toxic degeneration. The pericardial sac contains abundant clear gelatinous fluid, the myocardium is pale and soft, and hemorrhages beneath the serous membranes of the heart are almost constant. The lungs are often slightly congested and very edematous.

In areas in which this disease occurs, the diagnosis can be made with reasonable certainty on the basis of the history and the presence of the typical macroscopic lesions. Confirmation depends on finding large numbers of clostridia in the necrotic tissue of the ulcers and on the detection of toxins in the intestinal contents of fresh cadavers. The organism may be isolated only from the intestine of fresh cadavers.

The disease in calves caused by type B *C. perfringens* closely resembles that in lambs, usually affecting sucklings younger than 10 days, with a course of 2–4 days, characterized by prostration and dysentery. Older calves to 10 weeks sometimes are affected. It appears that calves are more likely to recover, albeit slowly, than are lambs. The intestinal lesion is an acute hemorrhagic enteritis with extensive mucosal necrosis and patchy diphtheritic membrane formations, especially in the ileum.

In foals also there is hemorrhagic enteritis with severe diarrhea. Suckling foals of 2 days to, rarely, some weeks of age are affected. The course of the illness is from 1 to 2 days. The intestine is intensely hyperemic with a number of dark foci to 1 cm in diameter, which may develop into ulcerations. The contents of the intestine are bloodstained. Microscopically, there is marked necrosis of the mucosa, with large numbers of clostridia in the lesion. The disease is apparently rare in foals, but should be differentiated bacteriologically from infection with other clostridia, with *Actinobacillus equuli,* and from salmonellosis, which more typically involves the large bowel.

Bibliography

Dalling, T. Lamb dysentery. *J Comp Pathol* **39:** 148–163, 1926.

Stubbings, D. P. *Clostridium perfringens* enterotoxaemia in two young horses. *Vet Rec* **127:** 431, 1990.

c. *CLOSTRIDIUM PERFRINGENS* TYPE C *Clostridium perfringens* type C has a worldwide distribution and causes disease in adult sheep and goats, feeder cattle, and neonatal lambs, calves, foals, and pigs. Type C also causes necrotizing enteritis in humans. The prevalence of disease varies widely among countries, and among regions and species within countries. There are five antigenic subtypes within type C, all of which possibly affect young animals.

In adult sheep *C. perfringens* type C causes "struck,"

a disease of pastured animals, which has a mortality rate of 5–15% in some areas. The disease in adult goats probably is similar in most respects to that in sheep. Death usually occurs suddenly with terminal convulsive episodes, but some animals, with infections not so peracute, stand in a straining position, which probably indicates acute abdominal pain. In adult sheep, diarrhea or convulsions do not occur.

At necropsy, the peritoneal cavity contains as much as 3 liters of clear, pale yellow fluid, which clots on exposure to air and which becomes stained with hemoglobin if necropsy is delayed. The peritoneal vessels, especially of the omentum, small intestine, and urinary bladder, are intensely congested, and multiple subperitoneal hemorrhages may be present. The small intestine is intensely hyperemic, either in patches or along most of its length, and in the zones of hyperemia, there may be ulcers that may attain several centimeters in size. Ulcers usually are present, mostly in the jejunum, and are surrounded by a zone of hyperemia with deep red base, although in some, the necrotic material is dark green and adherent. The large intestine is normal. The primary intestinal lesion is superficial mucosal necrosis, which advances more deeply, with a peripheral leukocytic reaction, congestion, and hemorrhage. The organisms are limited to the necrotic tissue.

Lesions in other organs are those of severe toxemia and include copious pleural and pericardial transudate of gelatinous fluid and hemorrhages beneath the serous membranes of the heart. There is congestion and sometimes gross hemorrhage of the zona reticularis of the adrenal.

The causative organism may become bacteremic, and this accounts for the very different appearance when autopsy is delayed for some hours. In such instances, there is extensive bloodstained gelatinous fluid in the intermuscular septa and subcutis, and fluid in the serous cavities is stained. The muscles are soft, stained pink to black with blood, and emphysematous. Because of this change, struck may be confused with blackleg if postmortem examination is delayed.

The disease in feedlot cattle is similar to struck. Animals are found either dead or moribund, and congestion and hemorrhage of the gastrointestinal tract are prominent. The jejunal and ileal content is bloody with fibrin clots and necrotic debris. Excessive straw-colored pleural and pericardial fluid and petechiation of epicardium and endocardium are present. Autolysis and postmortem bloat occur rapidly, and differentiation from ruminal tympany and other clostridial diseases is necessary.

The diseases caused by type C in lambs, calves, pigs, and foals are very similar and will be discussed together. Affected animals usually are young sucklings, which contract the disease within the first few days of life, often within the first 12 hr if they have been confined. Foals and most clinically affected lambs die, but in calves and pigs, subacute disease may occur in which there is diarrhea and unthriftiness.

Often affected animals are found dead. Sick lambs may shiver, show abdominal pain, abdominal distension, dysentery, and prostration and die in 12 hr or less. Sick calves show abdominal pain, some show diarrhea of sudden onset, and death is preceded by spasmodic convulsions.

Similar lesions occur at autopsy in all species, but may be less severe in lambs. In lambs, the intestinal changes vary from a catarrh to an acute hemorrhagic enteritis with mucosal necrosis which, like lamb dysentery, suggests strangulation. The most prominent changes occur in the jejunum and ileum, the lumen of which may contain free blood, which forms a clotted cast in fresh cadavers. Sometimes there is merely acute hyperemia of a segment of jejunum with edema of the wall, a scant creamy intestinal content, and a few small ulcerations of the mucosa. The peritoneal cavity contains a small quantity of serous bloodstained fluid, and the local mesentery and peritoneum are often mildly inflamed, hyperemic, and bear red strands of fibrin. The mesenteric nodes are enlarged, wet, and congested. There is usually an excess of pericardial fluid and pulmonary interstitial edema. Ecchymoses on the serous membranes are nearly constant, and in a few cadavers all tissues, but especially the meninges and brain, are liberally sprinkled with small hemorrhages. These are sites of bacterial embolism, due to a massive terminal bacteremia by *C. perfringens*.

Other lesions are those of toxemia, and the histologic changes are the same as those of lamb dysentery. There is no reliable distinction between the two diseases except for the geographic distribution and the results of toxin analyses, which must be performed on both the intestinal contents and the cultured organism, since only the beta toxin may be detectable in the intestinal contents.

Clostridium perfringens type C causes hemorrhagic enteritis of suckling piglets in many parts of the world. Rarely, epizootics occur in 2 to 4-week-old pigs and in weaned pigs. The disease occurs as epizootics in affected herds and regions, and may then remain enzootic. Susceptibility varies, but whole litters are often affected, usually within the first week of life and often within the first 24 hr; the clinical course is about 1 day. Poor hygienic conditions, overcrowding, and antibiotic treatment are thought to be predisposing factors in some outbreaks. Affected animals pass bloodstained feces in the terminal stages, and there is marked hyperemia of the anus just prior to death. The predominant lesions occur in the small intestine, especially the jejunum, but the cecum and spiral colon often are involved, and occasionally lesions are confined to the large intestine. Lesions are similar in all areas, and in acute cases consist of intestinal and mesenteric hyperemia, extensive necrosis of the intestinal mucosa, and bloodstaining of the contents (Fig. 1.147). There may be emphysema of the intestinal wall, which becomes fragile. Mesenteric lymph nodes are red, and sanguineous peritoneal and pleural fluid is present. Fibrinous intestinal adhesions may develop.

Microscopically, the necrotic process extends deeply and sometimes penetrates the muscularis mucosae. Numerous typical bacilli inhabit the necrotic tissue and line up along the margin of involved villi. Older pigs may not

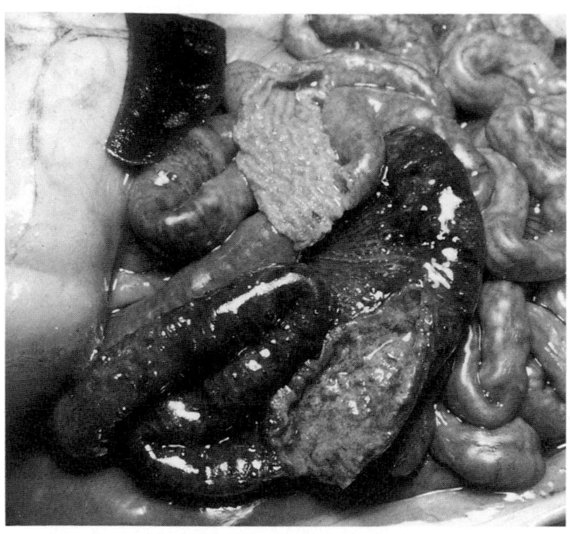

Fig. 1.147 Necrotizing enteritis. Piglet. *Clostridium perfringens* type C. (Courtesy of M. Bergeland.)

show intestinal hemorrhage but do have mucosal necrosis, and peritoneal and pericardial effusion.

Infection is acquired from the sow's feces, and lesions begin in the jejunum with adhesion of bacteria to, and necrosis of, epithelium on the villus tips. The cells slough, and extension of the necrotizing process then is nonselective and involves all the structures of the villi as it extends toward the crypt. The disease is not reproducible with toxins of *C. perfringens* type C, but requires viable organisms with the ability to attach to the enterocytes.

The disease due to type C in foals has been reported from the United States of America, Canada, and Australia. It usually occurs in foals <4 days of age. Typical clinical signs include weakness, yellow to brown watery diarrhea or dysentery, colic, and dehydration. Affected foals usually die in <24 hr. Macroscopic lesions are those of an acute hemorrhagic necrotizing enteritis usually in the distal two thirds of the small intestine, although in some cases, most of the small and large intestine may be affected. The microscopic lesions are similar to those described previously in the other species. In foals the lesions must be differentiated from those seen with other clostridia.

Bibliography

Arbuckle, J. B. R. The attachment of *Clostridium welchii (C. perfringens)* type C to intestinal villi of pigs. *J Pathol* **106:** 65–72, 1972.

Drolet, R., Higgins, R., and Cécyre, A. Necrohemorrhagic enterocolitis caused by *Clostridium perfringens* type C in a foal. *Can Vet J* **31:** 449–450, 1990.

Greig, A. An outbreak of *C. welchii* type C enterotoxaemia in young lambs in South West Scotland. *Vet Rec* **96:** 179, 1975.

Lauerman, L. H., Jensen, R., and Pierson, R. E. *Clostridium perfringens* Type C enterotoxemia in feedlot cattle and sheep. *Am Assoc Vet Lab Diagnost 20th Annu Proc* 363–364, 1977.

McEwen, A. D., and Roberts, R. S. Struck: Enteritis and peritonitis of sheep caused by a bacterial toxin derived from the alimentary canal. *J Comp Pathol* **44:** 26–49, 1931.

Niilo, L. Toxigenic characteristics of *Clostridium perfringens* Type C in enterotoxemia of domestic animals. *Can J Vet Res* **51:** 224–228, 1987.

Niilo, L., Harries, W. N., and Jones, G. A. *Clostridium perfringens* Type C in hemorrhagic enterotoxemia of neonatal calves in Alberta. *Can Vet J* **15:** 224–226, 1974.

Sims, L. D. *et al.* Haemorrhagic necrotizing enteritis in foals associated with *Clostridium perfringens. Aust Vet J* **62:** 194–196, 1985.

Weibel, W., Häni, H., and Zimmermann, W. Ein Ausbruch von *Clostridium perfringens*-Enteritis bei Saugferkeln in der Schweiz. *Schweiz Arch Tierheilk* **125:** 553–556, 1983.

d. *Clostridium perfringens* Type D Enterotoxemia (pulpy kidney disease, braxylike disease, overeating disease) caused by the toxins of *C. perfringens* type D is an important disease of sheep and goats with a worldwide distribution. It occurs occasionally in calves. There is a single case report of possible type D enterotoxemia in a filly. Focal symmetric encephalomalacia of sheep is caused by the epsilon toxin of type D.

In most lambs and calves with type D enterotoxemia, the course is peracute, and the animal is found dead. Lambs and calves may die in a few minutes in convulsions, and calves often bawl as from severe pain. Animals which survive longer may show excessive salivation, rapid breathing, hyperesthesia, straining, opisthotonus, and terminal coma or convulsions. In adult sheep, in which the clinical course may be several days, diarrhea with the passage of dark semifluid feces is common. In sheep, subacute cases may occur and be followed by recovery. In some such cases, neurologic signs may develop. These include blindness, ataxia, head pressing, and posterior paresis, and the lesions of focal symmetric encephalomalacia are present in the brains of such cases. On other occasions these lesions are not preceded by signs of enterotoxemia. In goats, signs of enterotoxemia similar to those in sheep and lambs may be seen, but chronic enterotoxemia characterized by abdominal distension and pain, depression, and dark green diarrhea may persist for several days to weeks. Nervous signs do not occur.

In lambs dead of acute enterotoxemia, the carcass usually is well nourished. In those with a course of 1–2 days, often there is evidence of a dark scour about the rump. Putrefactive changes occur rapidly. In some rapidly fatal cases, there are no lesions. Often there is excessive straw-colored pericardial fluid, which clots on exposure to air; congestion and edema of the lungs, which may be severe enough to produce froth in all the respiratory passages; and hemorrhage beneath the endocardium of the left ventricle. There may be hemorrhages beneath other serous membranes (Fig. 1.148) such as the epicardium, and blotchy hemorrhages beneath the parietal peritoneum are characteristic. Sometimes the liver is congested and the spleen, enlarged and pulpy. There is no gastrointestinal inflammation visible at necropsy. Short lengths of the small intestine are distended with gas, and are hyperemic.

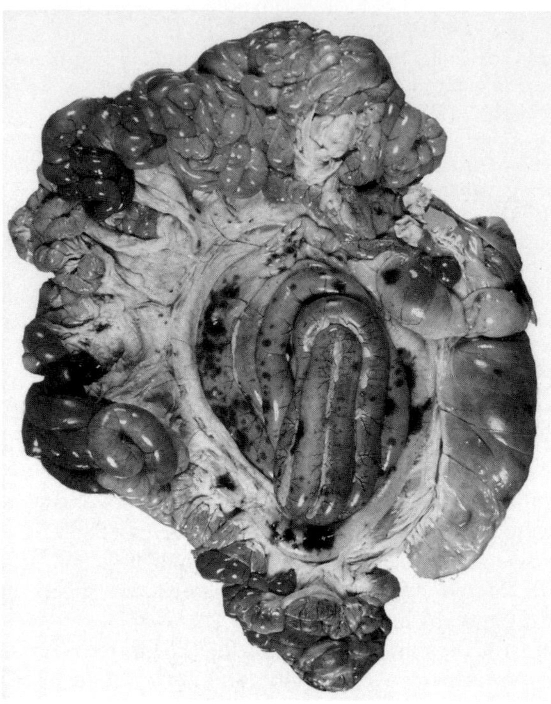

Fig. 1.148 *Clostridium perfringens* type D enterotoxemia. Peritoneal hemorrhages. Sheep.

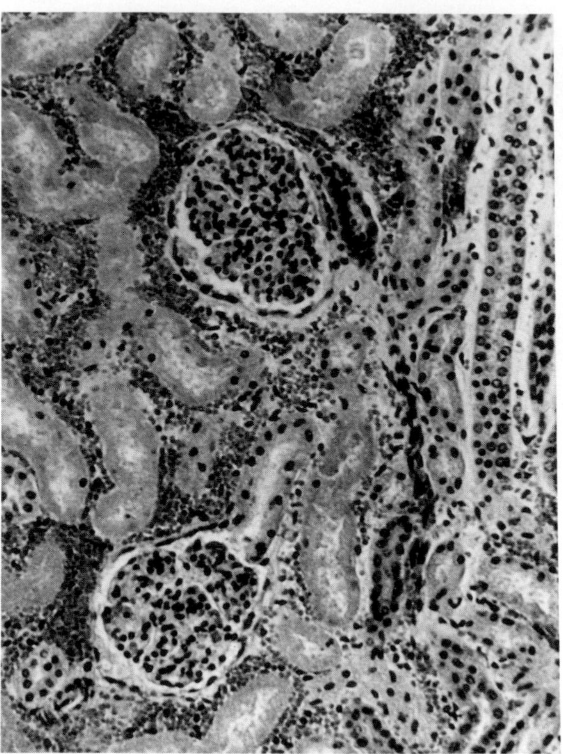

Fig. 1.149 *Clostridium perfringens* type D enterotoxemia. Nephrosis and intertubular hemorrhage. Sheep.

The intestinal content is creamy in animals that die rapidly, but in those that live for some hours, the contents, especially of the lower intestine, are more fluid and dark green.

In experimental cases and natural cases examined immediately after death, there are no specific renal lesions. The kidneys often are congested, and autolysis leads within a few hours to the intertubular hemorrhages which are characteristic of the disease (Fig. 1.149). Similarly, autolysis that is unusually rapid is responsible for the pulpy kidney of enterotoxemia. Both of these lesions can be useful diagnostic aids.

In adult sheep, the lesions are the same as those in lambs, but are more consistent and more advanced, with the exception of renal autolysis, which occurs less rapidly, and less commonly progresses to the stage of pulpiness.

Brain lesions occur in lambs with subacute enterotoxemia, and these are sufficiently consistent to be of diagnostic significance. They develop in two patterns; each is bilaterally symmetric. The commonest pattern involves the basal ganglia, internal capsule, dorsolateral thalamus, and substantia nigra; there are some minor variations of the pattern, but the lesions always are of the same type (Fig. 1.150). The second pattern affects the white matter of the frontal gyri, sparing only the communicating U fibers. The lesion begins with edema and the leakage of plasma and then red cells from the venules and capillaries in the affected areas. The altered permeability of the vessels is diffuse throughout the brain, sparing only heavily myelinated tracts, such as the optic tracts and corpus callosum. This is well demonstrated by vital staining with trypan blue. The least change visible by light microscopy is the accumulation of protein droplets around small venules. Electron microscopically, severe damage to vascular endothelium is apparent, and there is swelling of protoplasmic astrocytes. The foot processes around blood vessels and the processes around neurons are most severely swollen. Edema and hemorrhage lead to malacia in the affected areas.

Lesions in calves dying of enterotoxemia caused by *C. perfringens* type D closely resemble those in lambs. Affected calves are usually 1–3 months of age. Splenic swelling is more common in calves than in lambs, and rapid autolysis of the kidney is not a prominent finding. However, subcapsular congestion and hemorrhage occur (Fig. 1.151) and sometimes a blackish clot of blood to 1.0 cm thick forms a rather even cast around the kidney.

The histologic changes in enterotoxemia include, in addition to the brain lesions described, mild degeneration and necrosis of the epithelium of the proximal convoluted tubules with edema, congestion, and interstitial hemorrhage in the renal cortex, and congestion of the medulla (these are autolytic changes but are useful diagnostically); superficial desquamation in the intestine with congestion, and numerous typical bacilli in the contents; congestion and hemorrhage of the spleen with disruption of reticulum; subepicardial hemorrhage and degeneration in the Purkinje network; and proteinaceous edema fluid in the lungs. All of these changes are secondary to endothelial damage

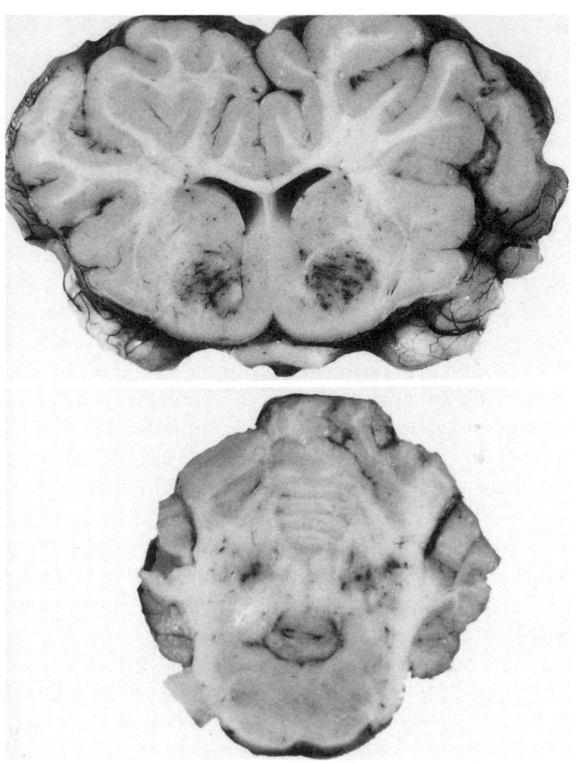

Fig. 1.150 *Clostridium perfringens* type D enterotoxemia. Focal symmetric encephalomalacia. Sheep. Hemorrhages and softening in internal capsules and cerebellar white matter.

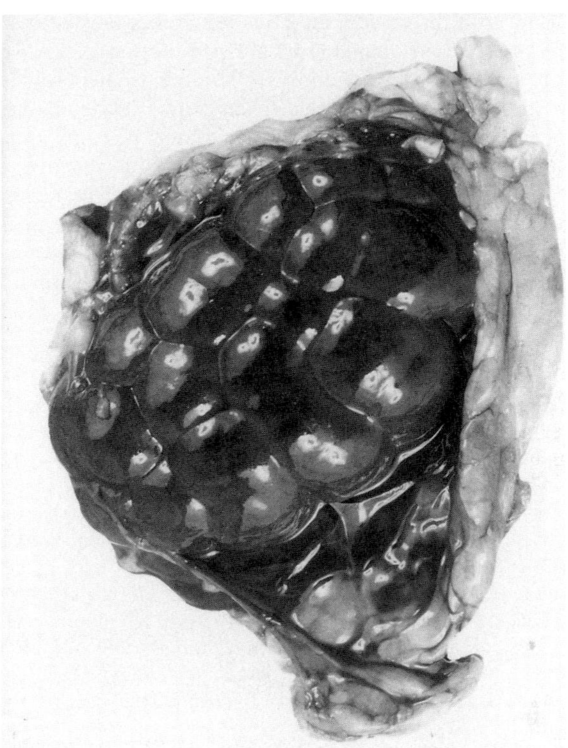

Fig. 1.151 *Clostridium perfringens* type D enterotoxemia. Renal cortical hemorrhage. Calf.

produced by the epsilon toxin. The nature of the clinical syndrome, including the severity and extent of the nervous disorder, probably depends on the amount and rate of absorption of this toxin.

Type D enterotoxemia may be seen in both adult goats and kids. Four forms of the disease are recognized in goats: peracute, acute, chronic, and subclinical. The peracute disease is similar to that seen in lambs. The acute form is characterized by diarrhea and abdominal discomfort. Affected animals either recover or die within 2–4 days after the onset of clinical signs. The chronic form of the disease may last for a few days or weeks. Weight loss and diarrhea are its main clinical features. The principal macroscopic lesions in the acute and chronic disease are mild to severe hyperemia of the mucosa, especially of the distal small intestine, cecum, and spiral colon. The affected areas may be covered by a thin layer of fibrin. The intestinal contents are olive green to red and mucoid. The mesenteric lymph nodes are enlarged and edematous. Hydropericardium, pulmonary edema, and pulpy kidneys may be seen, but are inconsistent.

In natural cases, the microscopic lesions in the small intestine vary from a mild pleocellular leukocytic reaction in the lamina propria to a mild fibrinous enteritis. In the latter, the tips of the villi are necrotic, eroded, and covered by fibrinocellular exudate. Villus atrophy may follow. The leukocytic reaction in the lamina propria extends into the edematous submucosa. The proprial and submucosal vessels are congested. Essentially similar lesions occur in the large intestine, bearing in mind the anatomic differences. There is lymphocytolysis in the centers of the lymphoid follicles of the mesenteric lymph nodes. Lesions in the lungs and kidneys may be similar to, but are less consistent than, those seen in lambs. Cerebral edema may be present, but focal symmetric encephalomalacia has not been reported in goats with enterotoxemia.

Experimental intraduodenal inoculation of whole cultures of *C. perfringens* type D in kids results mainly in a colitis of the spiral colon. The reasons for the different manifestations of enterotoxemia in sheep and goats are unknown. It is thought to be due to a caprine-specific effect of the epsilon toxin on the intestinal mucosa. The possibility that other toxins (entero- or cytotoxin) affect the enteric mucosa must be considered. Type D enterotoxemia in goats must be differentiated from gastrointestinal nematodiasis, grain overload, and salmonellosis.

Hemoconcentration and hyperglycemia occur in enterotoxemia. Hemoconcentration is secondary to loss of fluid into tissues and cavities through injured vascular endothelium. The increase in blood glucose is probably due to rapid mobilization of hepatic glycogen, possibly stimulated by hepatocyte-bound epsilon toxin. Other mechanisms have been proposed, including the release of catecholamines due to the central stimulation of the sympathetic division of the autonomic nervous system, resulting from brain edema. The catecholamines activate adenylate cyclase, enhancing the production of cAMP, which stimulates glycogenolysis leading to hyperglycemia. The blood glucose may reach very high levels and spills into the urine, providing very good circumstantial evidence for diagnosis of the disease. The absence of glucosuria after some hours postmortem is of no significance, as early postmortem growth of bacteria in the urine destroys the glucose. Glucosuria may occur in calves and presumably in goats but does not occur in starved animals with depleted glycogen stores.

Bibliography

Blackwell, T. E. *et al.* Differences in signs and lesions in sheep and goats with enterotoxemia induced by intraduodenal infusion of *Clostridium perfringens* type D. *Am J Vet Res* **52:** 1147–1152, 1991.

Buxton, D., Linklater, K. A., and Dyson, D. A. Pulpy kidney disease and its diagnosis by histological examination. *Vet Rec* **102:** 241, 1978.

Gardner, D. E. Pathology of *Clostridium welchii* type D enterotoxaemia. II. Structural and ultrastructural alterations in the tissues of lambs and mice. *J Comp Pathol* **83:** 509–524, 1973.

Gardner, D. E. Pathology of *Clostridium welchii* type D enterotoxaemia. III. Basis of the hyperglycaemic response. *J Comp Pathol* **83:** 525–529, 1973.

Hartley, W. J. A focal encephalomalacia of lambs. *N Z Vet J* **4:** 129–135, 1956.

Oxer, D. T. Enterotoxaemia in goats. *Aust Vet J* **32:** 62–66, 1956.

Stubbings, D. P. *Clostridium perfringens* enterotoxaemia in two young horses. *Vet Rec* **127:** 431, 1990.

von Rotz, A., Corboz, L., and Waldvogel, A. *Clostridium perfringens* Type D-Enterotoxämie der Ziege in der Schweiz. Pathologisch-anatomische und bakteriologische Untersuchungen. *Schweiz Arch Tierheilk* **126:** 359–364, 1984.

e. *Clostridium perfringens* Type E *Clostridium perfringens* type E causes intestinal disease in calves and rabbits. Calves die acutely and have a congested ulcerated abomasum, and hemorrhagic enteritis, which occurs segmentally along the small intestine. Mesenteric nodes are enlarged and red, and pericardial effusion and serosal hemorrhages may be present.

Bibliography

Hart, B., and Hooper, P. T. Enterotoxaemia of calves due to *Clostridium welchii* Type E. *Aust Vet J* **43:** 360–363, 1967.

f. Other Clostridial Diseases An acute hemorrhagic necrotizing enteritis has been associated with *C. difficile* in neonatal foals. Clinically these foals have diarrhea, colic, weakness, and dehydration. They die within 24 hr after onset of clinical signs. The lesions are similar to those described under *C. perfringens* type C infection, from which they must be differentiated. *Clostridium difficile* and its cytotoxin have also been demonstrated in feces of nonfatal cases of diarrhea in foals, but the significance of this finding is unclear since other enteropathogens may have been involved. *Clostridium difficile,* and possibly other clostridia are thought to be associated with some cases of colitis X, described elsewhere.

Clostridium difficile and its cytotoxin have been demonstrated in feces of dogs with chronic diarrhea. Descriptions of lesions are not available, since all dogs responded to treatment with metronidazole. The organism is frequently shed in feces of normal dogs, which makes the significance of its presence difficult to interpret, until Koch's postulates have been fulfilled. This organism causes a pseudomembranous colitis in humans, often, but not necessarily, with a history of antibiotic treatment. The pathogenesis and diagnosis of the disease caused by this organism are briefly discussed in the next section.

Hemorrhagic canine gastroenteritis (canine gastrointestinal hemorrhage syndrome) occurs sporadically. It is associated with *Clostridium perfringens.* Usually a peracute, hemorrhagic gastroenteritis develops, and the specific *C. perfringens* type is not identified; recurrent diarrhea associated with a type A strain is also recorded. Dogs with the peracute disease often are found dead lying in a pool of bloody excreta. Sometimes hemorrhagic diarrhea is noted prior to death. Autopsy reveals hemorrhagic enteritis and colitis, and sometimes hemorrhage gastritis is present (Fig. 1.152). Colonic lesions tend to be more severe. Microscopically there is hemorrhagic necrosis of the gastrointestinal mucosa, which extends from the luminal surface into the mucosa. Numerous clostridia may line the necrotic intestinal structures or be distributed through the detritus, but they do not invade the intact tissue (Fig. 1.153). Multiple serotypes of clostridia have been associated with hospital-acquired, usually nonfatal, cases of diarrhea in dogs. *Clostridium perfringens* enterotoxin has been demonstrated twice as frequently in hospitalized

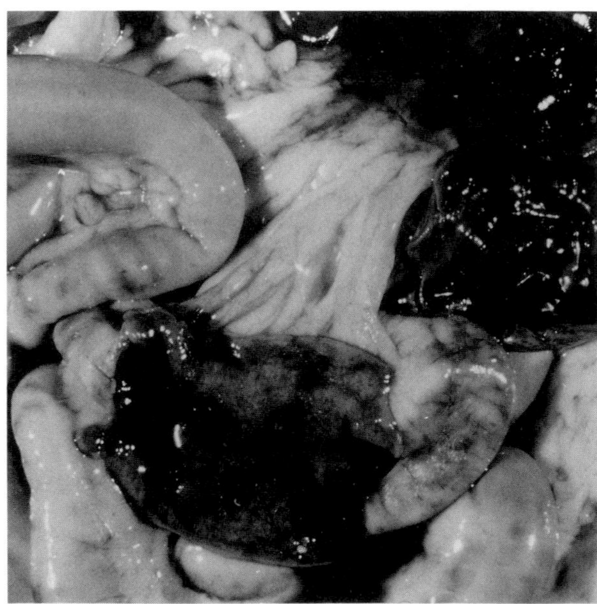

Fig. 1.152 Hemorrhagic enteritis in a dog with canine gastrointestinal hemorrhage syndrome, associated with untyped *C. perfringens.*

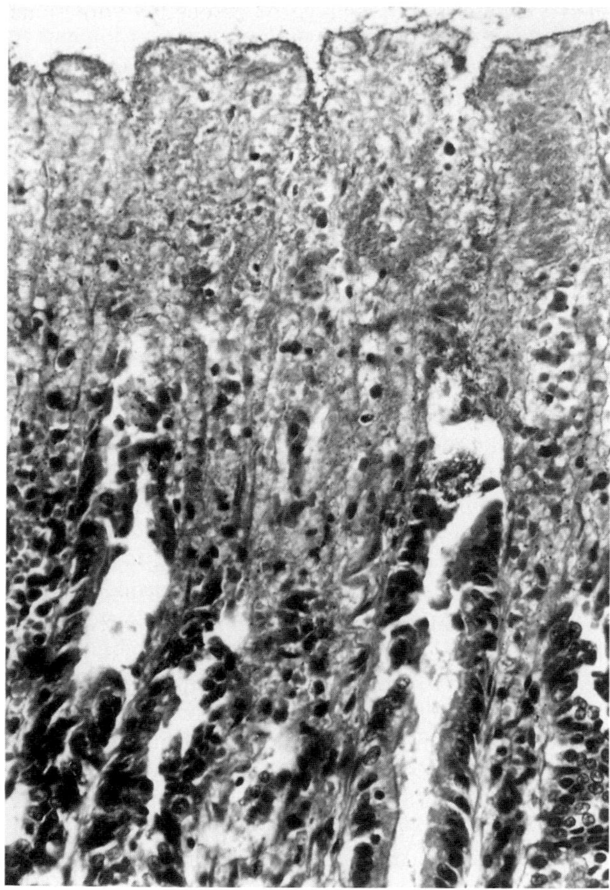

Fig. 1.153 Coagulation necrosis and hemorrhage in the superficial mucosa. Colon. Canine gastrointestinal hemorrhage syndrome. The mucosal surface is highlighted by a dark rim of clostridia.

dogs with diarrhea compared to controls without diarrhea. Feces vary from watery, to mucoid, to bloody in a few of the affected dogs. Diarrhea lasts for several days. The lesions in a fatal case were similar to those previously described in dogs with hemorrhagic enteritis and colitis, except they were mainly located in the ileum. The acute cases must be differentiated from canine parvoviral enteritis, shock gut, and warfarin toxicity or other coagulopathy.

Bibliography

Berry, A. P., and Levett, P. N. Chronic diarrhoea in dogs associated with *Clostridium difficile* infection. *Vet Rec* **118:** 102–103, 1986.

Burrows, C. F. Canine hemorrhagic gastroenteritis. *J Am Anim Hosp Assoc* **13:** 451–458, 1977.

Carman, R. J., and Lewis, J. C. M. Recurrent diarrhoea in a dog associated with *Clostridium perfringens* type A. *Vet Rec* **112:** 342–343, 1983.

Jones, R. L., Adney, W. S., and Shideler, R. K. Isolation of *Clostridium difficile* and detection of cytotoxin in the feces of diarrheic foals in the absence of antimicrobial treatment. *J Clin Microbiol* **25:** 1225–1227, 1987.

Jones, R. L. *et al.* Hemorrhagic necrotizing enterocolitis associated with *Clostridium difficile* infection in four foals. *J Am Vet Med Assoc* **193:** 76–79, 1988.

Kruth, S. A. *et al.* Nosocomial diarrhea associated with enterotoxigenic *Clostridium perfringens* infection in dogs. *J Am Vet Med Assoc* **195:** 331–334, 1989.

Prescott, J. F. *et al.* Haemorrhagic gastroenteritis in the dog associated with *Clostridium welchii*. *Vet Rec* **103:** 116–117, 1978.

Prescott, J. F. *et al.* A method for reproducing fatal idiopathic colitis (colitis X) in ponies and isolation of a clostridium as a possible agent. *Equine Vet J* **20:** 417–420, 1988.

g. The Pathogenesis and Diagnosis of Clostridial Enteric Infections The pathogenesis of some of the enteric clostridial diseases is extraordinarily circuitous. More is known of the pathogenesis of enterotoxemia caused by *C. perfringens* type D than of the others, and this can be exemplary: disease due to types A and E may develop in the same way, but types B and C usually affect the newborn and probably have a more simple pathogenesis. In all of the diseases the organisms multiply rapidly in the intestine, and disease results from the activity of the bacterial exotoxins.

Many animals harbor the specific clostridial organisms in their alimentary canal at least transiently, but in small and harmless numbers. Under certain circumstances they grow profusely and produce toxins in overwhelming concentration.

Enterotoxemia of pastured lambs occurs mainly in the spring when pastures are abundant and lush, and usually the best lambs are affected. It is possible that intestinal hypomotility may be a primary factor, which allows clostridia to proliferate in the small intestine instead of being carried by peristalsis to the colon. Whether it is the level of nutrients or other factors in ingested pasture which predispose to the development of enterotoxemia is unclear. Pulpy kidney is not solely a disease of green lush pastures; it also occurs on pastures of little but coarse fibrous grass, and in sheep fed pelleted feeds. In these circumstances the relationship to diet is obscure.

Lambs fed large amounts of grain or concentrate are highly susceptible, thus the synonym overeating disease. The manner in which overeating leads to clostridial enterotoxemia is complex. Cultures of *C. perfringens* type D given orally are largely destroyed in the rumen and abomasum. The few organisms which reach the intestine proliferate rapidly and produce toxin, but when the numbers are no longer reinforced by escapees from the stomach, they are rapidly cleared from the intestine by peristalsis. If the cultures are administered into the duodenum, the concentrations of organisms and toxin in the intestine become much larger than those after oral dosing, but not large enough to cause anything but diarrhea. The disease can be reproduced successfully if the diet of the sheep is suddenly changed to grain or concentrate before administering the culture.

The critical factor is almost certainly the presence of starch in the small intestine, providing a suitable substrate for these saccharolytic bacteria, and they proliferate to immense numbers—perhaps more than 1×10^9 organisms per gm of intestinal contents—and produce correspondingly large amounts of toxin. When the rumen is provided suddenly with excessive quantities of food, or food of a different type, there is a delay before the ruminal flora can adapt. In this period, undigested or partially digested food may escape into the intestine, and if starch is there, as it is with overeating on grain, *C. perfringens* type D is likely to take advantage of it. The epsilon prototoxin is activated by digestive enzymes, especially the combination of trypsin and chymotrypsin.

The concentration of toxin must be maintained at high levels for several hours if it is to cause intoxication, rather than just diarrhea. The outcome depends not only on the concentration of toxin in the intestine, but also on the length of time it is maintained, the size of the sheep, and whether there is circulating antitoxin. Some sheep possess epsilon antitoxin, attesting to previous nonfatal intoxication, and they are highly resistant to the disease. Even with high intestinal concentrations of toxin, only small amounts reach the bloodstream. A high concentration of epsilon toxin facilitates its own absorption from the intestine, probably in part by increasing the permeability of the mucosa. Necrosis of epithelium and moderate atrophy of villi are evident in some animals with type D enterotoxemia, and it is reasonable to assume that epithelial damage precedes the facilitated absorption.

Probably the disease develops in the same way in the calf as in the sheep. The virtual confinement of the disease to calves which are overfed suggests that this is the case. The acute disease in goats probably has a similar pathogenesis, but the chronic disease, with lesions confined to the intestine, appears to be caused by local effects of type D toxins. This form of the disease has not been investigated in detail.

The epsilon toxin binds to receptors on the endothelial cells, especially in the brain and renal tubular epithelial cells, resulting in changes described earlier.

The pathogenesis of enterotoxemia produced by type A bacteria is obscure. In lambs it occurs under circumstances similar to those of type D enterotoxemia. Nothing is known of the permeability of the ruminant intestine to alpha toxin, but the syndrome described in both lambs and calves is consistent with the action of a hemolytic toxin in the circulation.

The contribution of enterotoxin from type A strains to enteric diseases of animals probably is minimal. A brief description of the mechanisms involved in the pathogenesis of the diarrhea seems warranted, since type A strains are a possible cause of diarrhea in animals. The type A enterotoxin is heat labile, and it is trypsin activated. It stimulates fluid and electrolyte loss and mucosal damage in the ileum and to a lesser extent in the jejunum of rabbits, and it is cytotoxic to tissue cultures. The cellular basis for enterotoxin activity appears to be associated with a single class of protein receptor on the enterocytes. Ultrastructurally, the enterotoxin produces blebs in the brush-border membranes. Physiologic activities of the enterotoxin include changes in permeability in plasma membranes for ions, amino acids, and nucleotides. Degeneration and necrosis of enterocytes are thought to be due to the influx of Ca^{2+} ions. The effect on the mucosa further increases mucosal permeability, resulting in more loss of fluids and electrolytes.

The diseases in young animals caused by *C. perfringens* type B and type C are principally diseases of the intestine, and this suggests that the pathogenesis is more direct. This is particularly true of type C hemorrhagic enteritis in pigs.

Cultures of type B or type C given orally produce disease much more consistently than do type D. Types B and C possess the beta toxin, which is probably responsible for the severe intestinal lesion. However, the earlier literature must be interpreted with caution, since beta toxin has been purified only relatively recently, and in earlier studies, toxin may have been contaminated with alpha and other toxins. It is possible that types B and C need not attain the high concentration in the intestine that type D must to initiate illness. Both bacteria and toxins are required to induce disease. Beta toxin is trypsin labile, and circumstances such as low enzyme levels in young animals, very high levels of toxin, or trypsin inhibitors could be important. Sows' colostrum contains a trypsin inhibitor. It is not known whether colostrum in other species possesses this factor. Although both lamb dysentery and hemorrhagic enterotoxemia occur in pastured animals, they are most serious in confined animals. Under these circumstances disease spreads rapidly among the susceptible age group, as would be expected of any virulent infection.

Often the most vigorous and presumably the best nourished lambs and calves succumb, and on occasion there may be a nutritional predisposition to these diseases. Pig bel, a necrotizing jejunitis of humans in New Guinea that probably is caused by the beta toxin, has been causally related to consumption of heat-stable trypsin inhibitors in sweet potatoes. Naturally occurring protease inhibitors in soybeans appear to have a similar effect in guinea pigs. Intraduodenal inoculation of *C. perfringens* type C in combination with soybean flour produces acute fatal hemorrhagic enterotoxemia in lambs.

"Struck" in adult sheep caused by type C is prevalent when the grass is short in late winter or early spring. It is also a disease of the best-conditioned sheep, but the place of nutritional factors in its pathogenesis, and in the pathogenesis of disease caused by type C in feedlot cattle, has not been examined.

Clostridium difficile produces two toxins. Toxin A, an enterotoxin, causes mucosal lesions followed by fluid accumulation in several species of laboratory animals. Toxin B, a cytotoxin, may act synergistically with toxin A. It is cytotoxic for a variety of tissue culture cell lines *in vitro,* but the significance of this in the pathogenesis of diarrhea remains unclear. This toxin is highly fatal when given parenterally.

The diagnosis of outbreaks of enteric diseases caused by clostridia may be difficult. A history of sudden deaths in appropriate environmental circumstances, age groups, etc., should provoke a suspicion. Gross lesions in one or more reasonably fresh carcasses are often characteristic enough to provide a working diagnosis. Glucosuria may be demonstrable in type D enterotoxemia, but its absence does not preclude the disease. Confirmation of type D enterotoxemia can be based on microscopic brain lesions in sheep, but in this and other suspected clostridial diseases, bacteriologic proof should be sought. The organisms should be isolated and typed, and toxin should be sought by mouse inoculation and protection with specific antitoxin. Examinations should be made as soon after death as is possible. Very autolyzed carcasses generally are unsuitable, as the toxin is rapidly destroyed postmortem, and the intestinal flora very quickly becomes mixed.

The contents of the small intestine should be examined for toxin; in adult sheep which have shown diarrhea, it is well to examine the contents of cecum and colon if toxin is not found in the small intestine. If storage is necessary prior to animal inoculation, gut content should be frozen. There is no critical concentration of toxin which is diagnostic for pulpy kidney disease or other enteric clostridial diseases. The presence of toxin in conjunction with typical lesions is considered significant. The absence of demonstrable toxin does not preclude a presumptive diagnosis if other characteristic findings are evident. Negative results on a toxin analysis made more than 4 hr after death do not eliminate clostridial disease as the cause of death. Gram-stained smears should be made from various levels of the intestine or from discrete mucosal lesions. The smears usually reveal large numbers of bacilli with the morphology of *C. perfringens*. In pulpy kidney disease, and the other clostridial enteritides, the bacteria are present in smears in pure, or virtually pure, population.

Clostridium difficile is slow growing and often becomes contaminated on nonselective anaerobic media. Selective agar plates (cycloserine–cefoxitin–fructose agar) improve the chances of recovering this organism. Some strains are nontoxigenic; cytotoxin must be demonstrated in gut contents or feces by *in vitro* neutralization and mouse neutralization tests.

Bibliography

Al-Mashat, R. R., and Taylor, D. J. Production of diarrhoea and enteric lesions in calves by the oral inoculation of pure cultures of *Clostridium sordellii*. *Vet Rec* **112:** 141–146, 1983.

Bullen, J. J., and Batty, I. Experimental enterotoxaemia of sheep: The effect on the permeability of the intestine and the stimulation of antitoxin production in immune animals. *J Pathol Bacteriol* **73:** 511–518, 1957.

Buxton, D., and Morgan, K. T. Studies of lesions produced in the brains of colostrum deprived lambs by *Clostridium welchii* (*C. perfringens*) type D toxin. *J Comp Pathol* **86:** 435–447, 1976.

Finnie, J. W. Histopathological changes in the brain of mice given *Clostridium perfringens* type D epsilon toxin. *J Comp Pathol* **94:** 363–370, 1984.

Fleming, S. Enterotoxemia in neonatal calves. *Vet Clin North Am: Food Anim Pract* **1:** 509–514, 1985.

Lyerly, D. M. *et al.* Effects of *Clostridium difficile* toxins given intragastrically to animals. *Infect Immun* **47:** 349–352, 1985.

McClane, B. A., Hanna, P.C., and Wnek, A.P. *Clostridium perfringens* enterotoxin. *Microb Pathogen* **4:** 317–323, 1988.

McDonel, J. L. *Clostridium perfringens* toxins (type A, B, C, D, E). *Pharmacol Ther* **10:** 617–655, 1980.

Moon, H. W., and Dillman, R. C. Comments on clostridia and enteric disease in swine. *J Am Vet Med Assoc* **160:** 572–573, 1972.

Niilo, L. Experimental production of hemorrhagic enterotoxemia by *Clostridium perfringens* type C in maturing lambs. *Can J Vet Res* **50:** 32–35, 1986.

Niilo, L. *Clostridium perfringens*. *In* "Pathogenesis of Bacterial Infections in Animals," C. L. Gyles and C. O. Thoen (eds.), pp. 80–86. Ames, Iowa, Iowa State University Press, 1986.

Niilo, L. *Clostridium perfringens* type C enterotoxemia. *Can Vet J* **29:** 658–664, 1988.

Sterne, M. Clostridial infections. *Br Vet J* **137:** 443–454, 1981.

7. Mycobacterial Enteritis: Paratuberculosis (Johne's Disease)

Various *Mycobacterium* spp. can cause enteric lesions in animals. They may occur in typical tuberculosis due to *M. bovis* (see The Respiratory System, Chapter 6 of this volume). *Mycobacterium intracellulare* has been isolated from granulomas in mesenteric lymph nodes of pigs in various countries. Typical *Mycobacterium avium* is an environmental organism that causes tuberculosis in birds. It occasionally produces systemic disease in mammals, which usually seem to be immunocompromised. There may be an enteric component to disseminated infections, and *M. avium* has also been associated with granulomatous enteritis and ulcerative colitis in horses, discussed previously in this chapter. *Mycobacterium avium silvaticum,* the wood pigeon mycobacterium, causes tuberculosis in birds, and may cause paratuberculosislike disease in mammals. All of these infections are of minor importance in domestic animals compared to paratuberculosis, or Johne's disease, in ruminants.

Johne's disease is caused by *Mycobacterium avium paratuberculosis* infection in ruminants. The etiologic agent of Johne's disease has been reduced to subspecific status within *M. avium* on the basis of the high (>90%) DNA homology among typical paratuberculosis strains and type strains of *M. avium avium*. The Johne's disease agent, which in culture is slow growing, and dependent on mycobactin as a source of iron, may be a host-adapted antigen-deficient rough variant of *M. avium*. However, it does possess an unique suite of cultural and biochemical traits, and genetic characteristics, which differentiates it from *M. avium avium* and *M. a. silvaticum*.

Infections by *M. a. paratuberculosis* also can be produced in pigs, horses, and asses, and spontaneous disease is reported, rarely, in Equidae. Typical clinical signs may occur, but gross lesions in these species are modest or absent, and histologic lesions often are mild. The infection can be transmitted to mice, hamsters, guinea pigs, rabbits, and macaques. It also has been implicated in some cases of Crohn's disease in humans.

Strains of *M. a. paratuberculosis* may differ in cultural characteristics and in pathogenicity for the various species of ruminants. Strains that produce an intensely orange pigment in tissues and in cultures sometimes are isolated from sheep, and occasionally from cattle, in Great Britain and the Faeroe Islands. It is assumed that all strains are capable of infecting cattle, sheep, and goats. However, a Norwegian strain from goats seems to have low virulence in experimentally inoculated calves, though bovine strains are pathogenic for goats, and sheep strains are virulent in cattle. Channel Island breeds and beef shorthorn cattle appear to be unusually susceptible. Whether this is genuinely breed related, or due to factors such as dissemination by trade within the breed, or high prevalence within herds, which increase the opportunity for infection, is unclear.

The epidemiology and pathogenesis of Johne's disease are best understood in **cattle**, and are assumed to be similar in sheep and goats. Exposure is mainly by ingestion of organisms shed in the feces of an infected animal. Young animals are more susceptible than old to experimental infection. Adults may become infected, but are less likely to develop the disease, and often recover from the infection. The critical age for susceptibility to an infection which will ultimately produce clinical disease is ~6 months. This age-dependent resistance is reflected in the ability of the macrophages of resistant animals to restrict intracellular growth of bacteria, but not to lyse them.

Bacteria taken up through the mucosa replicate within macrophages. They are initially found in Peyer's patches. Although the major lesions of Johne's disease usually are confined to the ileum, large intestine, and draining lymph nodes, the infection is generalized. In both clinical and subclinical cases, the organism can be cultured from a variety of parenchymatous organs and widely distributed lymph nodes, and it has also been found in the gonads of both sexes. In fulminating infections, there is a bacteremia, in blood or in infected phagocytes.

Organisms may be excreted in milk, semen, and urine, and intrauterine infections occur, even when the dam is clinically normal. Bovine fetuses may be infected as early as the first trimester of gestation. A prevalence of 26% has been reported for intrauterine infection when the dam is culture positive, suggesting that *in utero* infection may be epidemiologically significant, but this is debated. Excretion of the organism in milk may also contribute to infection of offspring. The organism has not been demonstrated in the milk of ewes, but congenital and uterine infection do occur.

The incubation period of Johne's disease is protracted and irregular. Some carriers, in which bacteria persist in the mucosa and draining lymph nodes, may be infected for life without showing signs. The relationship between immune events and stages of the disease is speculative. Cell-mediated immunity clearly plays a role in the development of mucosal lesions and the onset of clinical disease. Exacerbations of clinical disease often are associated with parturition, a low nutritional plane, heavy milk yield, and intercurrent disease.

The pathogenesis of Johne's disease is related to the granulomatous immunoinflammatory response in the lamina propria in the small intestine, and the associated villus atrophy that develops. Malabsorption in the ileum, and filtration secretion from inflamed mucosa, overloads the capacity of the colon to resorb electrolyte and fluid; the function of the colon itself may be compromised by mycobacterial infection. There is malabsorption of amino acids, and enteric loss of plasma proteins, causing negative nitrogen balance and a decline in body condition. Hypoproteinemia, when it develops, will further promote filtration secretion.

Clinically affected animals are usually 2 years of age or older. The typical manifestation of Johne's disease is profuse diarrhea passed effortlessly. Clinical signs may be intermittent, with long intervening periods of remission. Emaciation is progressive and ultimately fatal, but the appetite is often retained, and animals remain bright, until the terminal stages.

There is little correlation between the severity of the clinical syndrome and the severity of the lesions. Many animals allowed to die have gross and microscopic lesions so slight that they would be easily missed unless specifically sought; on the other hand, severe lesions can be found in animals which appear relatively healthy.

Advanced cases of Johne's disease are emaciated, with marked loss of muscle mass and serous atrophy of fat depots, intermandibular edema, and fluid effusion in the body cavities. Plaques of intimal fibrosis and mineralization may be evident in the thoracic aorta. Specific gross lesions occur in the intestine and regional lymph nodes. The mesenteric nodes, particularly the ileocecal, are always enlarged, sometimes remarkably so, pale, and edematous, especially in the medulla. Lymphangitis is common, and the lymphatic vessels often can be traced as thickened cords from the intestinal serosa through the mesentery to the mesenteric nodes (Fig. 1.154). Often lymphangitis is the only recognizable gross change, and is specific enough to justify a presumptive diagnosis of Johne's disease at necropsy. The intestinal serosa often has a slight granular and diffusely opaque appearance because of subserosal edema and cellularity.

Mucosal lesions may occur from the duodenum to the rectum; they may be segmental or continuous. They are usually best developed in the lower ileum (Fig. 1.155), and in the upper large intestine. The ileocecal valve is frequently described as enlarged, and this area is considered by some to be the earliest and most consistently affected, but abnormalities in this vicinity may not be notable.

The classical intestinal change is diffuse thickening of the mucosa, which is folded into transverse rugae. When well developed, the mucosal folds cannot be smoothed out by stretching. This lesion is due to accumulations of chronic inflammatory cells and edema in the mucosa and submucosa. The crests of the folds are often slightly reddened by congestion or multiple petechial hemorrhages, and the mucosal surface is velvety, but there is usually no

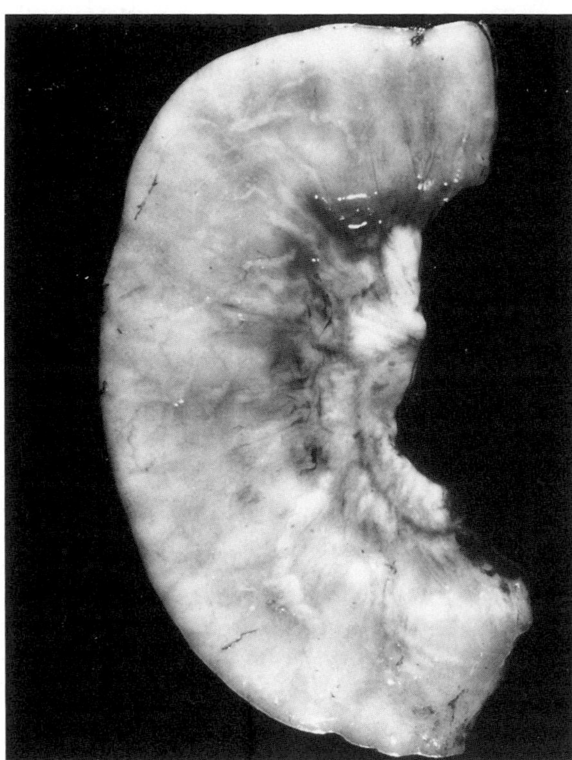

Fig. 1.154 Johne's disease. Serosal edema and lymphangitis (arrow). Sheep.

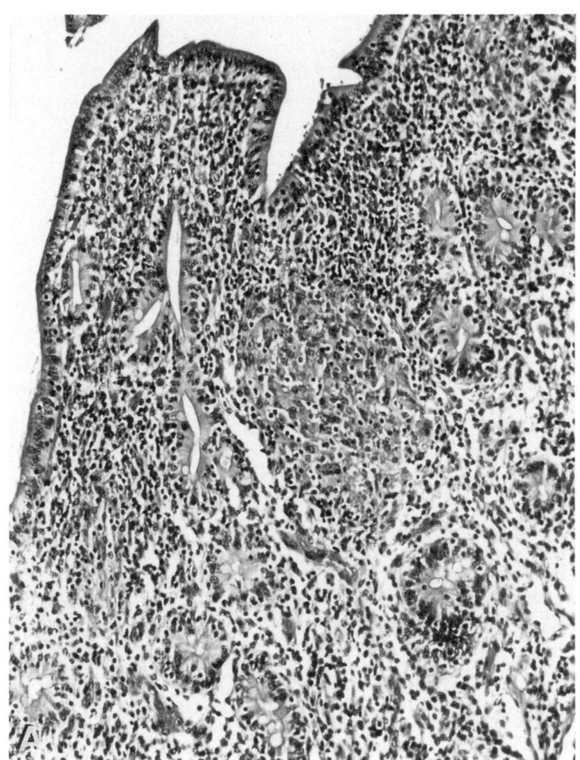

Fig. 1.156A Johne's disease. Aggregate of macrophages in hypercellular lamina propria.

excess mucus. The minimal recognizable gross change is a very slight fleshy or velvety thickening of the mucosa, which must be sought in suspect cases.

When gross lesions are well developed, the characteristic microscopic change, granulomatous transmural enteritis, is obvious. But in cattle in which gross changes are minimal or absent, the microscopic abnormalities are more subtle. In these the lamina propria is diffusely infiltrated with lymphocytes and plasma cells, and a large number of eosinophils. There may be very few macrophages (Fig. 1.156A), and the most characteristic change is an infiltrate of lymphocytes and plasma cells in the submucosa, and associated with the submucosal and mesenteric lymphatics.

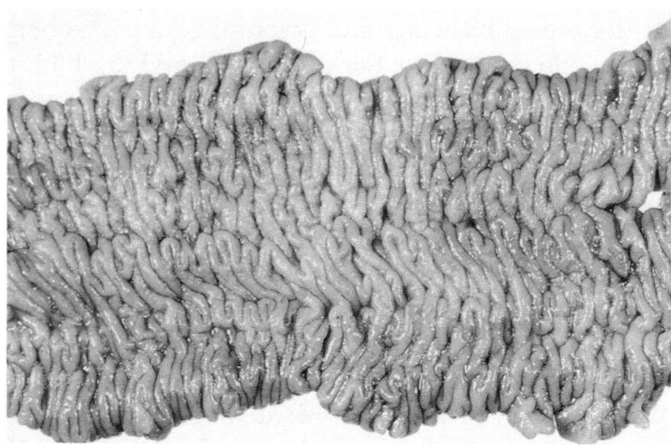

Fig. 1.155 Johne's disease. Thickened mucosal folds. Jejunum. Cow.

In more clear-cut cases, villi are moderately to markedly atrophic, and macrophages are focally or diffusely distributed, in the villi, or deeper in the lamina propria, as part of an increased chronic inflammatory cell infiltrate. Giant cells may be present. The inflammatory infiltrate may abnormally separate and displace crypts, which are elongate, with hyperplastic epithelium. Crypts may be distended with mucus and exfoliated cells, probably because of compression and obstruction of their mouths by edema and inflammatory cells (Fig. 1.156B). Masses of epithelioid macrophages may accumulate in the submucosa. Foci of necrosis may occur within these aggregates of macrophages (Fig. 1.157), but in cattle, caseation and mineralization are extremely rare.

Lymphangitis is one of the most consistent changes. Initially the lymphatics are surrounded by lymphocytes and plasma cells, and many contain plugs of epithelioid cells in the lumen. Granulomas may form in the wall and project into the lumen. These nodules may undergo some central necrosis.

Granulomatous lymphadenitis occurs in mesenteric lymph nodes in advanced cases. In the early stages, there is histiocytosis of the subcapsular sinus. Ultimately, nodular or diffuse infiltrates of epithelioid macrophages and

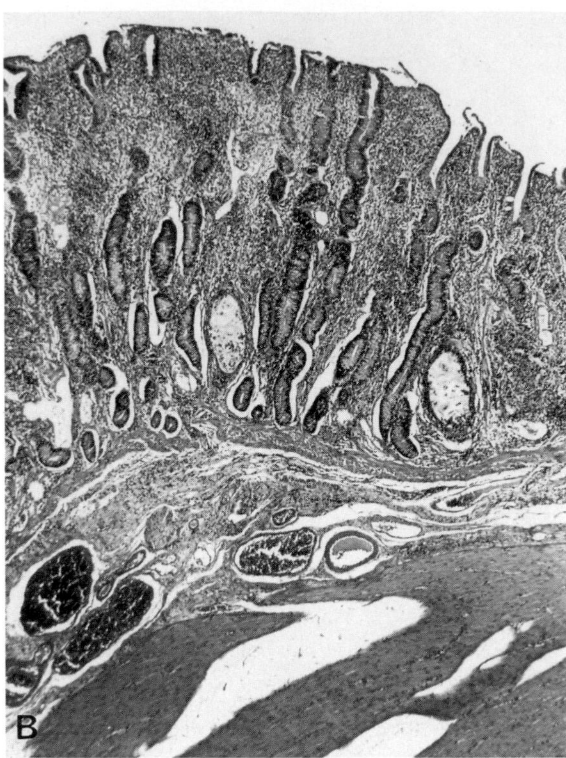

Fig. 1.156B Johne's disease. Blunt atrophic ileal villi, and hyperplastic and occasionally cystic, crypts. Edema of lamina propria, submucosa, and muscularis. Note heavy inflammatory infiltrate in lamina propria. Cow.

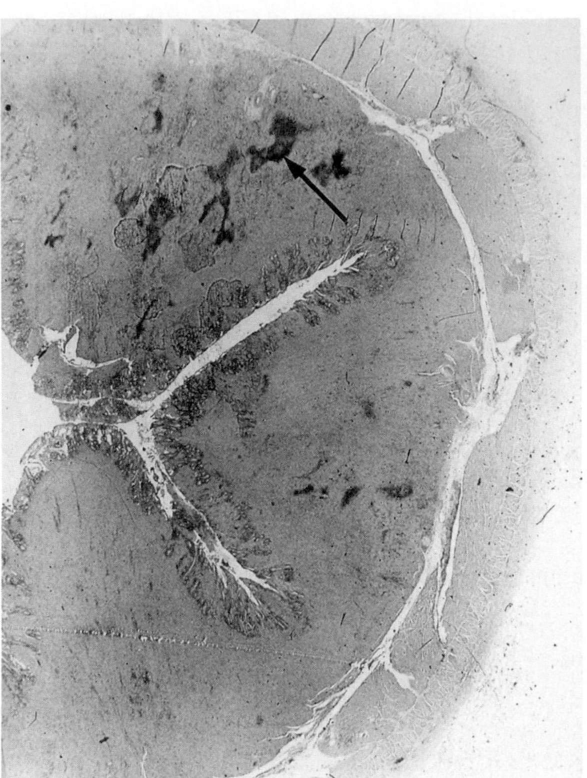

Fig. 1.157 Johne's disease. Hemisection of ileum showing diffuse infiltration of cells and small areas of necrosis (arrow).

giant cells may replace much of the cortex, and infiltrate the medullary sinusoids.

Of the other organs and tissues from which the bacilli may be isolated in cattle, lesions have been described only in the liver, hepatic lymph nodes, and very rarely, the kidney and lungs. These are characteristically focal granulomas. They are most common in the liver, where foci of epithelioid cells and lymphocytes are found in the triads and scattered throughout the parenchyma. These lesions usually contain demonstrable bacilli, if macrophages are evident.

In **sheep and goats,** Johne's disease also occurs only in adults and is characterized by chronic wasting; there may be breaks in the wool in sheep, and submandibular edema due to hypoproteinemia. The feces are often normal; they may be soft and unpelleted, but overt diarrhea is unusual, except intermittently in the terminal stages, perhaps because of the innately greater efficiency of electrolyte and fluid absorption in the colon of these species. In **farmed deer,** Johne's disease is clinically similar, but there are reports of disease in animals younger than a year old.

In sheep, goats, and deer, enteric gross lesions are often mild, with little obvious thickening, and no transverse ridges; they are easily missed at necropsy. In sheep and goats, the bowel occasionally is quite remarkably thickened, and the lymphatics may be knotted as well as corded, the knots being focal granulomatous accumulations of epithelioid cells and lymphocytes. Goats, and some sheep, develop foci of tuberclelike caseation, often with calcification, in the mucosa, the submucosa, on the peritoneal surface of the bowel, and in the lymphatics. Some are recognizable grossly as whitish foci in the mucosa or lymphatics, 1–4 mm in diameter, and there is modest surrounding fibrosis. Tubercles in the lymph nodes of goats and deer may mineralize (Fig. 1.158), and be large enough to replace much of the node. In sheep infected with the pigmented strain of the organism, the mucosa and lymph nodes may be orange. Scattered lymph nodes elsewhere in the body, and liver, lung, spleen, and other organs may contain focal granulomatous lesions in sheep and goats. Some may mineralize. Lesions resembling those of lepromatous leprosy, with axonal degeneration in the sciatic nerves and brachial plexus, have been reported in goats. Amyloidosis of renal glomeruli, and occasionally other tissues, is also reported in goats.

In all species, the organism is usually readily demonstrable in macrophages and giant cells in the lesions when appropriately stained by acid-fast techniques. However, in some clinical cases, an extensive search may have to be made for individual macrophages bearing a few acid-fast bacilli. When there are few organisms, they may best be demonstrated by fluorescent or immunoperoxidase staining. The pigmented strains of the organism are invariably present in large numbers in sheep. But in tubercles

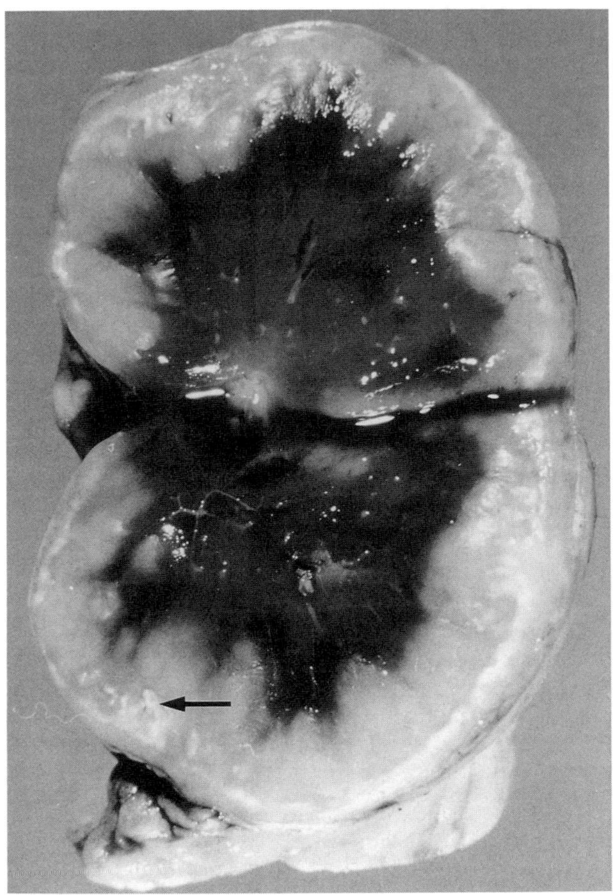

Fig. 1.158 Ileocecal lymph node. Goat. Paratuberculosis. Hyperplasia of lymphocytes in the cortex. White foci of mineralized caseous exudate in cortex (arrow).

in sheep and goats, the organisms may be too few to be demonstrated except by culture.

Johne's disease in sheep, and especially in goats and deer, may resemble tuberculosis, on account of the caseation and mineralization of enteric lesions or mesenteric lymph nodes. In cattle, there is almost never any caseation or calcification; this, the diffuseness of the lesion, and the absence of ulceration and reactive fibrosis, distinguish Johne's disease from intestinal tuberculosis.

However, it is not possible to conclusively separate infection with *M. a. paratuberculosis* from other mycobacterial infections in mammals solely on the basis of gross or microscopic lesions. Isolation of the organism is required. The ileocecal lymph node, and affected segments of gut, are candidate sites for culture to confirm a diagnosis. Isolation may be difficult to accomplish, especially from sheep.

Bibliography

Allen, W. M., Berrett, S., and Patterson, D. S. P. A biochemical study of experimental Johne's disease. I. Plasma protein leakage into the intestine of sheep. *J Comp Pathol* **84:** 381–384, 1974.

Angus, K. W. Intestinal lesions resembling paratuberculosis in a wild rabbit (*Oryctolagus cuniculus*). *J Comp Pathol* **103:** 101–105, 1990.

Buergelt, C. D. *et al.* Pathological evaluation of paratuberculosis in naturally infected cattle. *Vet Pathol* **15:** 196–207, 1978.

Camphausen, R. T., Jones, R. L., and Brennan, P. J. Antigenic relationship between *Mycobacterium paratuberculosis* and *Mycobacterium avium*. *Am J Vet Res* **49:** 1307–1310, 1988.

Carrigan, M. J., and Seaman, J. T. The pathology of Johne's disease in sheep. *Aust Vet J* **67:** 47–50, 1990.

Chiodini, R. J., Van Kruiningen, H. J., and Merkal, R. S. Ruminant paratuberculosis (Johne's disease): The current status and future prospects. *Cornell Vet* **74:** 218–262, 1984.

Cimprich, R. E. Equine granulomatous enteritis. *Vet Pathol* **11:** 535–547, 1974.

Dierckins, M. S., Sherman, D. M., and Gendron-Fitzpatrick, A. Probable paratuberculosis in a Sicilian ass. *J Am Vet Med Assoc* **196:** 459–461, 1990.

Fodstad, F. H., and Gunnarsson, E. Postmortem examination in the diagnosis of Johne's disease in goats. *Acta Vet Scand* **20:** 157–167, 1979.

Gezon, H. M. *et al.* Identification and control of paratuberculosis in a large goat herd. *Am J Vet Res* **49:** 1817–1823, 1988.

Hamilton, H. L. *et al.* Intestinal multiplication of *Mycobacterium paratuberculosis* in athymic nude gnotobiotic mice. *Infect Immun* **57:** 225–230, 1989.

Hines, S. A. *et al.* Disseminated *Mycobacterium paratuberculosis* infection in a cow. *J Am Vet Med Assoc* **190:** 681–683, 1987.

Larsen, A. B., Moon, H. W., and Merkal, R. J. Susceptibility of swine to *Mycobacterium paratuberculosis*. *Am J Vet Res* **32:** 589–595, 1971.

Lepper, A. W. D., and Wilks, C. R. Intracellular iron storage and the pathogenesis of paratuberculosis. Comparative studies with other mycobacterial, parasitic, or infectious conditions of veterinary importance. *J Comp Pathol* **98:** 31–53, 1988.

Mair, T. S. *et al.* Generalised avian tuberculosis in a horse. *Equine Vet J* **18:** 226–230, 1986.

Mokresh, A. H., and Butler, D. G. Granulomatous enteritis following oral inoculation of newborn rabbits with *Mycobacterium paratuberculosis* of bovine origin. *Can J Vet Res* **54:** 313–319, 1990.

Morin, M. Johne's disease (paratuberculosis) in goats: A report of eight cases in Quebec. *Can Vet J* **23:** 55–58, 1982.

Patterson, D. S. P., and Barrett, S. Malabsorption in Johne's disease in cattle: An *in vitro* study of L-histidine uptake by isolated intestinal tissue preparations. *J Med Microbiol* **2:** 327–334, 1969.

Pemberton, D. H. Diagnosis of Johne's disease in cattle using mesenteric lymph node biopsy: Accuracy in clinical suspects. *Aust Vet J* **55:** 217–219, 1979.

Riemann, H. *et al.* Paratuberculosis in cattle and free-living exotic deer. *J Am Vet Med Assoc* **174:** 841–843, 1979.

Saitanu, K., and Holmgaard, P. An epizootic of *Mycobacterium intracellulare,* serotype 8 infection in swine. *Nord Vet Med* **29:** 221–226, 1977.

Saxegaard, F. Experimental infection of calves with an apparently specific goat-pathogenic strain of *Mycobacterium paratuberculosis*. *J Comp Pathol* **102:** 149–156, 1990.

Seitz, S. E. *et al.* Bovine fetal infection with *Mycobacterium paratuberculosis*. *J Am Vet Med Assoc* **194:** 1423–1426, 1989.

Shackelford, C. C., and Reed, W. M. Disseminated *Mycobacterium avium* infection in a dog. *J Vet Diagn Invest* **1:** 273–275, 1989.

Thorel, M.-F., Krichevsky, M., and Lévy-Frébault, V. Numerical taxonomy of mycobactin-dependent mycobacteria, emended description of *Mycobacterium avium,* and description of *Mycobacterium avium* subsp. *avium* subsp. nov., *Mycobacterium avium* subsp. *paratuberculosis* subsp. nov., and *Mycobacterium avium* subsp. *silvaticum* subsp. nov. *Int J Syst Bacteriol* **40:** 254–260, 1990.

Van Kruiningen, H. J., Ruiz, B., and Gumprecht, L. Experimental disease in young chickens induced by a *Mycobacterium paratuberculosis* isolate from a patient with Crohn's disease. *Can J Vet Res* **55:** 199–202, 1991.

Williams, E. S., Snyder, S. P., and Martin, K. L. Pathology of spontaneous and experimental infection of North American wild ruminants with *Mycobacterium paratuberculosis. Vet Pathol* **20:** 274–291, 1983.

8. Enterocolitis of Foals Caused by Rhodococcus equi

Rhodococcus (Corynebacterium) equi, is an opportunistic intracellular pathogen. Thought formerly to be primarily a soil-associated organism, it is now also believed to be part of the normal intestinal flora of horses. It usually is associated with suppurative bronchopneumonia of foals. About half the pneumonic foals also have ulcerative colitis, and in some foals, intestinal lesions alone occur.

The development of intestinal lesions appears to be dose related, in that reproduction of the disease requires repeated oral infection. In natural disease, continual exposure to bacteria in swallowed respiratory exudate probably is an important source of infection in those animals with pneumonia.

Gross lesions may occur throughout the small and large intestines, but usually are most severe over Peyer's patches in small intestine, and in the cecum, large colon, and related lymph nodes (Fig. 1.159A). Mucosal lesions consist of irregular ulcers to 1–2 cm in diameter, often covered by purulent or necrotic debris (Fig. 1.159B). Edema of the wall of the gut may be severe. Lymph nodes often are massively enlarged by edema and by caseous or purulent foci, which may obliterate the structure of the node. Occasionally, massively enlarged abscessed lymph nodes are found without evidence of concurrent enteritis.

Microscopically, infection seems to occur by penetration of the specialized epithelium over Peyer's patches or intestinal lymphoid follicles. An initial neutrophilic response occurs, and erosions of the epithelium develop subsequently. Macrophages and neutrophils accumulate in the lamina propria. The macrophages contain aggregates of *R. equi* but do not destroy them. Later, necrosis of lymphoid follicles occurs, and deep ulcers develop, which contain masses of neutrophils, macrophages, and multinuclear giant cells. Pyogranulomatous lymphangitis

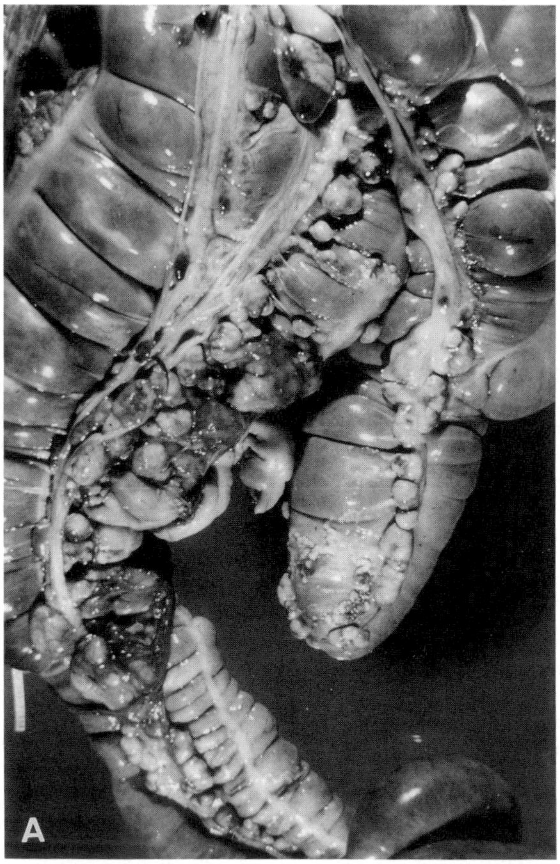

Fig. 1.159A *Rhodococcus equi* infection. Foal. Enlarged suppurative cecal and colic lymph nodes.

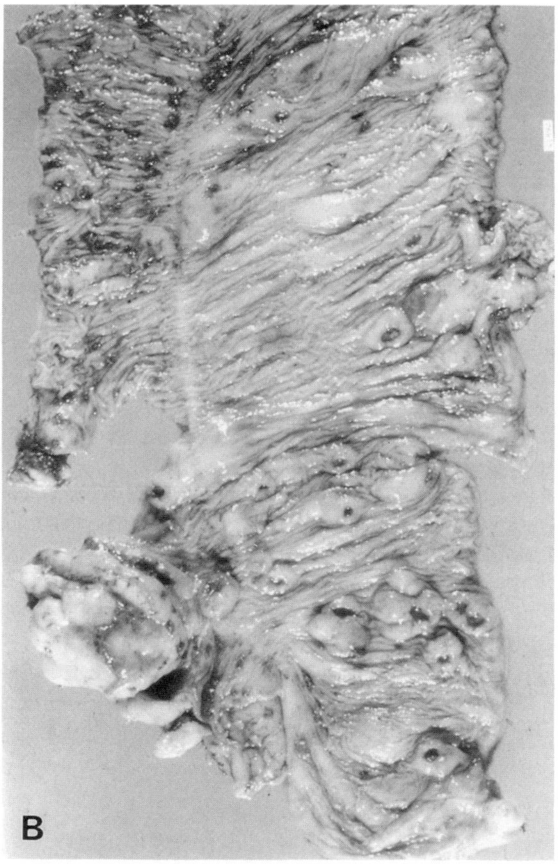

Fig. 1.159B *Rhodococcus equi* infection. Foal. Craterous ulcerated lesions on colonic mucosa.

and mesenteric lymphadenitis characterize the chronic enteric disease.

Bibliography

Barton, M. D., and Hughes, K. L. *Corynebacterium equi:* A review. *Vet Bull* **50:** 65–80, 1980.

Cimprich, R. E., and Rooney, J. R. *Corynebacterium equi* enteritis in foals. *Vet Pathol* **14:** 95–102, 1977.

Ellenberger, M. A., and Genetzky, R. M. *Rhodococcus equi* infections: Literature review. *Compend Cont Ed Pract Vet* **8:** S414–S424, 1986.

Johnson, J. A., Prescott, J. F., and Markham, R. J. F. The pathology of experimental *Corynebacterium equi* infection in foals following intragastric challenge. *Vet Pathol* **20:** 450–459, 1983.

Zink, M. C., Yager, J. A., and Smart, N. L. *Corynebacterium equi* infections in horses, 1958–1984: A review of 131 cases. *Can Vet J* **27:** 213–217, 1986.

9. Enterococcus durans *Enteritis*

Enterococcus (Streptococcus) durans is a small Gram-positive coccus, found in the environment and the gut of various species, which has been associated occasionally with diarrhea in suckling pigs, puppies, foals, and suckling rats.

These bacteria adhere to the microvillous surface of enterocytes by fine filamentous pili. In tissue section, they form a layer of small cocci crowded on the surface of epithelial cells over the entire villus, at any level of the small intestine. There is minimal associated mucosal damage or inflammation, and the organisms isolated from foals do not produce secretory enterotoxins. Malabsorption associated with reduced brush-border enzyme activity may explain diarrhea. Although in spontaneous cases in piglets, *E. durans* is frequently associated with other pathogens, the organism isolated from foals produced diarrhea when inoculated alone into gnotobiotic pigs.

Bibliography

Collins, J. E. *et al. Enterococcus (Streptococcus) durans* adherence in the small intestine of a diarrheic pup. *Vet Pathol* **25:** 396–398, 1988.

Hoover, D. *et al.* Streptococcal enteropathy in infant rats. *Lab Anim Sci* **35:** 635–641, 1985.

Jergens, A. E. *et al.* Adherent Gram-positive cocci on the intestinal villi of two dogs with gastrointestinal disease. *J Am Vet Med Assoc* **198:** 1950–1952, 1991.

Tzipori, S. *et al. Streptococcus durans:* An unexpected enteropathogen of foals. *J Infect Dis* **150:** 589–593, 1984.

10. Bacteroides fragilis-*Associated Diarrhea*

Bacteroides fragilis is a non-spore-forming obligate anaerobe, which is part of the normal enteric flora. Some strains secrete an enterotoxin and have been associated with diarrhea in piglets, calves, lambs, foals, and humans. Enterotoxigenic strains or cell-free culture filtrates cause secretion in ligated lamb or calf intestinal loops, and bacterial inocula cause diarrhea when administered orally to gnotobiotic piglets. The syndrome produced is one of undifferentiated neonatal diarrhea, with accumulation of fluid content in a flaccid small and large intestine, and no other remarkable gross lesions.

Microscopic lesions are most consistent in the large intestine of experimentally inoculated animals. Bacteria do not adhere to the surface. Surface enterocytes round up and exfoliate, whereas crypt epithelium becomes hyperplastic. Similar exfoliation of enterocytes sometimes occurs on the tips and sides of villi in the ileum. Mild to moderately severe acute inflammatory cell infiltrates may be evident in the lamina propria of affected bowel, and effusing through the damaged epithelial surface into the lumen. Ultrastructurally, affected cells lose their intercellular interdigitations; microvilli are shortened or absent; and the terminal web is disrupted. Exfoliative epithelial lesions have also been described in the colon of a spontaneous case of *B. fragilis* enteritis in a piglet.

Bibliography

Collins, J. E. *et al.* Exfoliating colitis associated with enterotoxigenic *Bacteroides fragilis* in a piglet. *J Vet Diagn Invest* **1:** 349–351, 1989.

Myers, L. L., Shoop, D. S., and Byars, T. D. Diarrhea associated with enterotoxigenic *Bacteroides fragilis* in foals. *Am J Vet Res* **48:** 1565–1567, 1987.

Myers, L. L., Collins, J. E., and Shoop, D. S. Ultrastructural lesions of enterotoxigenic *Bacteroides fragilis* in rabbits. *Vet Pathol* **28:** 336–338, 1991.

11. Enteritis Due to Chlamydia psittaci

Chlamydia are obligate intracellular parasites. *Chlamydia psittaci* infects animals and humans. *Chlamydia psittaci* is divisible into two types; type 1 is associated with abortion, pneumonia, or enteric disease, and type 2, with polyarthritis, encephalitis, or conjunctivitis. The nonenteric diseases are discussed in appropriate chapters elsewhere in these volumes.

The intestinal tract is the natural habitat for *Chlamydia*. Most infections probably are inapparent, but the intestine may be an important portal of entry in the development of systemic infections leading to hepatitis, arthritis, encephalitis, pneumonia, and abortion in ruminants. Enteritis may accompany or presage these diseases, and occasionally *Chlamydia* causes severe enteric disease in calves.

Following oral infection, *Chlamydia* infects mainly the enterocytes on the tips of ileal villi. These cells are in the G_1 phase of the cell cycle; cells in this phase are required by *Chlamydia* as a site for multiplication. Chlamydiae also infect other cells including goblet cells, enterochromaffin cells, and macrophages. Macrophages may transport chlamydiae systemically prior to destruction by the organisms they carry.

Chlamydia adsorbs to the brush border of enterocytes and enters the cell by pinocytosis. Following multiplication of organisms in the supranuclear region, the cells degenerate. Chlamydiae are released into the gut lumen, and into the lamina propria, where they infect endothelial cells of lacteals, are released, and become systemic.

Gastrointestinal disease caused by *Chlamydia* usually

is a problem of calves younger than 10 days, but may affect older calves, and may produce recurrent diarrhea. Watery diarrhea, dehydration, and death are often accompanied by lesions, though not necessarily signs, of hepatitis, interstitial pneumonia, and arthritis. Gross lesions may occur in the abomasum and throughout the intestinal tract but are most consistent and severe in the terminal ileum. Mucosal edema, congestion, and petechiae, sometimes with ulceration, are usually observed. Serosal hemorrhages and focal peritonitis may occur. Histologically, chlamydial inclusions may be demonstrable with Giemsa or Macchiavello's stain in vacuoles in the supranuclear region of the enterocytes. Central lacteals and capillaries are dilated, and neutrophils and monocytes infiltrate the lamina propria. Occasionally, granulomatous inflammation occurs in the intestinal submucosa and extends into the mesentery and to the serosa, to produce the peritonitis observed grossly. Crypts in the small and large intestine may be dilated, lined by flattened epithelium, and contain inflammatory exudate.

Chlamydia has also been recognized in the cecocolic mucosa of swine, complicating experimental infections with *Salmonella typhimurium,* but it seems not to be a primary pathogen in that species.

Bibliography

Doughri, A. M., Young, S., and Storz, J. Pathologic changes in intestinal chlamydial infection of newborn calves. *Am J Vet Res* **35:** 939–944, 1974.

Ehret, W. J. *et al.* Chlamydiosis in a beef herd. *J S Afr Vet Assoc* **46:** 171–179, 1975.

Pospischil, A., and Wood, R. L. Intestinal *Chlamydia* in pigs. *Vet Pathol* **24:** 568–570, 1987.

Reggiardo, C. *et al.* Diagnostic features of chlamydia infection in dairy calves. *J Vet Diagn Invest* **1:** 305–308, 1989.

Shewen, P. E. Chlamydial infection in animals: A review. *Can Vet J* **21:** 2–11, 1980.

12. Equine Monocytic Ehrlichiosis

This condition, also called Potomac horse fever and equine ehrlichial colitis, first defined clinically in 1979, is characterized by fever, leukopenia, depression, loss of appetite, and diarrhea. It is caused by *Ehrlichia risticii,* a member of the Rickettsiales, which are obligate intracellular bacterial pathogens. *Ehrlichia* spp. replicate within the phagosome of the host cell, in contrast to most other rickettsiae, which are free within the cytoplasm. Equine monocytic ehrlichiosis was first described in the Potomac river valley, and is associated with other river valleys in the northeastern United States. The condition is not commonly diagnosed as a cause of death elsewhere, though antibody has been reported from horses in many parts of North America, and in Europe. It is distinct from equine ehrlichiosis, which is found predominantly in California. That condition is caused by *Ehrlichia equi,* which usually infects granulocytes; *E. risticii* infects mainly monocytes.

The disease may be highly variable. Many infected animals seem not to get sick. Others develop severe colic, subcutaneous edema, laminitis, and shock: as many as 30% of those which do become ill will die if not treated. Potomac horse fever typically occurs in the summer. Though rickettsiae are usually vector borne, this has not been demonstrated for *E. risticii;* oral transmission is possible experimentally, but the epidemiology is not that of a contagious disease.

The incubation period in experimental infections is about 9–14 days, and diarrhea begins 1–3 days after the onset of fever. Diarrhea may be mild, with cow-pat feces, or progress to become profuse and watery, with dehydration ensuing. Not all experimentally infected animals develop disease.

At necropsy of spontaneous cases, small vesicles are reported in the oral cavity, and epicardial hemorrhages and pulmonary congestion and hemorrhage, compatible with endotoxemia, are described. These are not reported in experimental cases, nor is laminitis. The lesions of the gastrointestinal tract are the most significant, in both spontaneous and experimental cases. In some animals there may be focal or more extensive erosions in the gastric mucosa, perhaps with some overlying fibrinous exudate. Lesions in the small intestine are generally limited to segmental areas of mucosal congestion or hyperemia, with occasional focal ulcers or hemorrhage, and are much less consistent and severe than those in the cecum and colon. The content of the large bowel is abnormally fluid, and may have a brown or red-brown color, and foul odor. In the cecum and colon, there may be patches of hyperemia 5–10 cm in diameter, aggregates of small ulcers a few millimeters in diameter, and petechial hemorrhages. Sometimes the mucosa of the entire cecum is widely hyperemic. Ulcers and petechial hemorrhage are more severe and consistent in the right dorsal colon. The small colon is usually unaffected grossly.

Microscopic lesions are most consistent in the large intestine; similar changes may be evident in small bowel. In areas of gross hyperemia there is marked congestion and superficial hemorrhage in the mucosa. Associated with these lesions are superficial epithelial necrosis, erosion, and fibrin effusion. The mucosal surface is denuded, or perhaps covered by a fibrinocellular exudate, and epithelium in the upper half of crypts is attenuated. Deeper parts of crypts are dilated and may contain necrotic epithelium and inflammatory cells. An abnormally intense mixed inflammatory cell population is in the lamina propria, and sometimes, the submucosa. Lymphoid tissue in the gut, mesenteric lymph nodes, and spleen is moderately involuted, compatible with the effects of the stress of systemic illness.

Organisms are not evident in hematoxylin and eosin-stained tissue. They are visible, in colon, and less consistently, in cecum, small colon, and small intestine, with modified Steiner silver stain. They appear as small clusters of 10–15 fine brown dots, less than 1 μm in diameter, in the apical cytoplasm of epithelial cells deep in crypts, or as more numerous, smaller black structures distributed in the cytoplasm of macrophages in the periglandular lamina propria, or in a few glandular epithelial cells. Mast cell granules also take this stain, but are larger, and very heavily stained. Spirochetes in glands also stain, but are extracellular, and have distinct morphology. Immunoperoxidase procedures conclusively demonstrate the organisms in tissue sections. Ultrastructurally, small dense elementary bodies may be found, alone or in small clusters in vacuoles in the cytoplasm of macrophages, mast cells, and crypt epithelium, or as the morula – aggregates of larger, more open organisms in the same locations.

Bibliography

Breider, M. A., Callahan, G., and Corstvet, R. E. Detection of *Ehrlichia risticii* using an avidin–biotin–immunoperoxidase staining system. *J Vet Diagn Invest* **1:** 215–218, 1989.

Cordes, D. O. *et al.* Enterocolitis caused by *Ehrlichia* sp. in the horse (Potomac horse fever). *Vet Pathol* **23:** 471–477, 1986.

Dutta, S. K. *et al.* Disease features in horses with induced equine monocytic ehrlichiosis (Potomac horse fever). *Am J Vet Res* **49:** 1747–1751, 1988.

Holland, C. J. Biologic and pathogenic properties of *Ehrlichia risticii:* The etiologic agent of equine monocytic ehrlichiosis. *In* "Ehrlichiosis," J.C. Williams and I. Kakoma (eds.), pp. 68–77. Dordrecht, Holland, Kluwer, 1990.

McDade, J. E. Ehrlichiosis—A disease of animals and humans. *J Infect Dis* **161:** 609–617, 1990.

Perry, B. D. Potomac horse fever. *Vet Ann* **28:** 108–113, 1988.

Rikihisa, Y., Perry, B. D., and Cordes, D. O. Ultrastructural study of erhlichial organisms in the large colons of ponies infected with Potomac horse fever. *Infect Immun* **49:** 505–512, 1985.

Steele, K. E., Rikihisa, Y., and Walton, A. M. Ehrlichia of Potomac horse fever identified with a silver stain. *Vet Pathol* **23:** 531–533, 1986.

Whitlock, R.H. *et al.* Potomac horse fever: Clinical characteristics and diagnostic features. *Proc Am Assoc Vet Lab Diagnost* **27:** 103–124, 1984.

C. Mycotic Diseases of the Gastrointestinal Tract

1. Intestinal Phycomycosis and Aspergillosis

Mycotic invasion of the wall of the gastrointestinal tract is a common sequel to many diseases and lesions affecting the mucosa, and it may be the precursor to systemic infection. It is generally agreed that one or more of heavy fungal challenge, disruption of the normal flora, a primary local lesion, or lowered host resistance, is required for establishment of mycotic disease in the gut. Spores probably are carried across the mucosa by macrophages in the normal course of events, and only if phagocyte function is compromised, permitting germination, will they establish in the deeper tissues or become disseminated. Neutrophil function seems important in prevention of establishment of mycoses, whereas T cell-mediated macrophage activity is involved in resolution of lesions.

Organisms associated with alimentary tract mycoses are *Aspergillus;* zygomycetes of the family Mucoraceae, including the genera *Absidia, Mucor,* and *Rhizopus;* the oomycete *Pythium;* and entomophthoracetes such as *Basidiobolus* and *Conidiobolus*. *Candida* spp. may also invade the wall of the alimentary canal; that is subsequently considered separately. Enteric manifestations of histoplasmosis are also discussed.

Aspergillus has relatively uniform narrow (3–6 μm) hyphae with relatively numerous septa; it typically displays acute angled dichotomous branching. Mucoraceous fungi are characterized in their invasive mycelial form by broad (6–25 μm), coarse, irregular hyphae, with infrequent septation and random branching, sometimes surrounded by an eosinophilic sleeve in tissue sections. *Pythium* spp. have relatively narrow (to 9–10 μm), thick-walled hyphae, with almost parallel walls and occasional septa; they branch at about right angles. In entomophthoramycosis, hyphae may vary from 5 to 25 μm in diameter, with thin, irregularly parallel walls, infrequent septa, and rare random branching. They are characteristically surrounded by a wide sheath or sleeve of eosinophilic material in tissue section.

Lesions occur anywhere in the gastrointestinal tract, including the forestomachs of ruminants, and in the mesenteric lymph nodes. Clinical signs may be related specifically to the location of lesions (vomition, bloody diarrhea), or be nonspecific (malaise, weight loss), or be absent. Three types of lesion are produced: hemorrhagic and infarctive, caseating, and granulomatous.

Mucoraceous fungi and *Aspergillus* typically cause hemorrhagic and infarctive lesions. This is illustrated by the mycotic rumenitis following grain overload or neonatal infectious bovine rhinotracheitis (IBR) infection in ruminants. They frequently complicate Peyer's patch necrosis in cattle with mucosal disease, and are seen along the margins of the abomasal folds in calves with bacterial septicemia, or in neonatal infectious bovine rhinotracheitis (IBR) infection. Mucoraceous fungi are found at any level of the gastrointestinal tract; *Aspergillus* tends to be most common in the abomasum. These fungi have a propensity to invade mucosal and submucosal veins, producing thrombosis and venous infarction. Characteristically there is full-thickness necrosis of the gut wall, which grossly is edematous and red-black due to venous stasis and hemorrhage. Often there is a relatively mild inflammatory response to the fungi. Spread to the liver and more distant organs via the portal and systemic circulations is not uncommon.

Mycotic ileitis and colitis in cats occasionally may be a sequel to panleukopenia. Intestinal lesions caused by the fungi (often *Aspergillus*) may be hemorrhagic and necrotizing with a prominent cellular response, but sometimes are small, localized, and difficult to find. In the latter cases, lesions of panleukopenia in the intestine, and multifocal mycotic emboli in the lung suggest the pathogenesis. The lung appears to be the favored site of dissemination in cats. Mycotic enteritis with dissemination is a rare sequel to canine parvovirus enteritis.

The gastrointestinal tract is probably a common portal of entry for many sporadic, disseminated zygomycoses, and aspergillosis, in animals. The presence of fungal hyphae in mesenteric lymph node granulomas of many clinically normal cattle indicates that, contrary to general impressions, invasion by these agents across the intestinal mucosa does not lead invariably to systemic disease. Fungi may produce a localized granulomatous lesion in specialized lymphoid tissue of the Peyer's patch or may be carried to the regional lymph node, while the mucosal lesion, if any, heals. In the lymph nodes a granulomatous response, with giant cells which contain hyphal fragments, often develops; asteroid bodies may form around *Aspergillus* spp. Usually the granulomatous lesions produce little or moderate enlargement of lymph nodes, but sometimes a massive, caseating lymphadenitis results, with adhesions to adjacent structures.

Entomophthoromycosis involving the gastrointestinal tract has been reported in a few dogs. Ulcerative stomatitis, gastritis, and enteritis is reported, with induration of involved tissues by a granulomatous inflammatory reaction containing the typical hyphae. In horses, entomophthoromycosis due to *Conidiobolus* may involve the lips and pharynx, as well as the nostrils and nasal mucosa.

Pythiosis (oomycosis), due to *Pythium* spp., occurs in tropical and subtropical areas, where it is best recognized as a cause of cutaneous lesions in horses (see The Skin and Appendages, Volume 1, Chapter 5). However, it causes enteric disease in dogs, and less commonly, horses, and perhaps cats. There is segmental thickening and ulceration of the stomach and small intestine, with transmural granulomatous inflammation, sometimes extending to involve the pancreas, or causing granulomatous peritonitis, with adhesions of the omentum. Obstruction may occur. Lymphovascular channels on the intestinal serosa are thickened, and the mesenteric lymph nodes are greatly enlarged and frequently embedded in a granulomatous mass. Small, firm or caseous yellow foci may be embedded in the firm fibrotic reactive tissue. Segments of bowel may be infarcted. Granulomatous inflammation is evident in the mucosa, and especially the submucosa; it extends along lymphatics transmurally. Granulomas, with a local mixed inflammatory infiltrate, often including eosinophils, may have liquefactive or caseous necrotic centers. Characteristic hyphae are difficult to see with hematoxylin and eosin; they are best exposed, in the areas of necrosis or centers of granulomas, by silver stains. Similar lesions are reported in horses with intestinal obstruction.

Definitive diagnosis of mycotic lesions requires culture, which may be difficult, and identification of the isolate, which is frequently a specialist activity. If possible, granulomatous lesions of the gut should always be cultured for fungi as well as bacteria, in order to increase the frequency of specific diagnosis. Mycotic lymphadenitis must be differentiated from a mycobacterial, actinomycotic, or nocardial lesion. A presumptive diagnosis may be based on morphologic characteristics of organisms in tissue sections. Immunochemical procedures using specific antibody may add to the confidence of a morphologic diagnosis.

Bibliography

Allison, N., and Gillis, J. P. Enteric pythiosis in a horse. *J Am Vet Med Assoc* **196:** 462–464, 1990.

Angus, K. W., Gilmour, N. J. L., and Dawson, C. O. Alimentary mycotic lesions in cattle: A histological and cultural study. *J Med Microbiol* **6:** 207–213, 1973.

Connole, M. D. Review of animal mycoses in Australia. *Mycopathologia* **111:** 133–164, 1990.

Cordes, D. O., and Shortridge, E. H. Systemic phycomycosis and aspergillosis of cattle. *N Z Vet J* **16:** 65–80, 1968.

Jensen, H. E., Schønheyder, H., and Jørgensen, J. B. Intestinal and pulmonary mycotic lymphadenitis in cattle. *J Comp Pathol* **102:** 345–355, 1990.

Miller, R. I. Gastrointestinal phycomycosis in 63 dogs. *J Am Vet Med Assoc* **186:** 473–478, 1985

Munro, R. *et al.* Systemic mycosis in Scottish red deer (*Cervus elaphus*). *J Comp Pathol* **95:** 281–289, 1985.

Pavletic, M. M., Miller, R. I., and Turnwald, G. H. Intestinal infarction associated with canine phycomycosis. *J Am Anim Hosp Assoc* **19:** 913–919, 1983.

Reed, W. M. *et al.* Gastrointestinal zygomycosis in suckling pigs. *J Am Vet Med Assoc* **191:** 549–550, 1987.

Slocombe, R. F., and Slauson, D. O. Invasive pulmonary aspergillosis of horses: An association with acute enteritis. *Vet Pathol* **25:** 277–281, 1988.

Smith, J. M. B. "Opportunistic Mycoses of Man and Other Animals." Kew, U. K., C.A.B. International Mycological Institute, 1989.

Taylor, R. L., and Kintner, L.D. Phycomycosis of feedlot cattle. *J Am Vet Med Assoc* **174:** 371–372, 1979.

2. *Candidiasis*

Candida spp. are normal inhabitants of the alimentary tract of animals, existing as budding yeasts in association with mucosal surfaces. When there are changes in the mucosae, particularly squamous mucosae, or in the mucosal flora, the yeasts may become invasive; branching, filamentous pseudohyphae and hyphae largely replace the yeast forms. Only a few of the almost 200 *Candida* species cause candidiasis; in animals, the most important are *Candida albicans* and *C. tropicalis*.

Changes in the mucosal flora usually result from antibiotic therapy, which reduces the numbers of anaerobic bacteria and allows proliferation of *Candida* spp. Environmental and social stress, and treatment with anticancer and antiinflammatory agents may also predispose to candidiasis.

Candida spp., especially *C. albicans*, are capable of adhesion to epithelium, and this is important in virulence. Hypha formation is favored by carbohydrates such as sucrose, or polysaccharides which are less readily fermentable than glucose. Glucose is necessary for keratinolysis by the fungus. An endotoxin released during reproduction and death of *Candida* organisms may cause local damage, permit deeper penetration into squamous epithelium, and perhaps promote systemic dissemination.

Candida spp. occasionally are opportunistic invaders of mucosal lesions anywhere in the alimentary tract, but other fungi are more likely to take advantage of this kind of lesion, particularly in older animals. Candidiasis is mainly a disease of keratinized epithelium in young animals, especially pigs, calves, and foals. Accumulation of keratin due to anorexia probably contributes to the extensiveness of lesions in all species by increasing the substrate available to the fungus. Systemic dissemination is by embolization from primary sites of gastrointestinal colonization and local invasion. Foci of necrosis with a mainly neutrophilic infiltrate, and containing masses of proliferating organisms, are found in organs such as the spleen, liver, kidney, and heart.

In pigs *Candida* spp. often invade the parakeratotic material that accumulates on the gastric squamous mucosa. Apparently these infections are innocuous. Thrush is candidiasis of the oral cavity; it is seen occasionally in young pigs, especially those raised on artificial diets, or in pigs with intercurrent disease. Lesions may be confined to the tongue, hard palate, or pharynx, but often involve the esophagus and gastric squamous mucosa as well. Rarely the glandular stomach is involved. Grossly the lesions are yellow-white, smooth, or wrinkled plaques more or less covering the mucosa. Histologically, the epithelium is spongy and contains yeasts and abundant hyphae and pockets of neutrophils and bacteria beneath the cornified layer. Congestion of vessels and a few inflammatory cells are present in the mucosal propria. Desquamation of the epithelium may produce small ulcers.

In calves, candidiasis occurs following prolonged antibiotic therapy and in association with rumen putrefaction. Lesions are seen most often in the ventral sac of the rumen but may involve the omasum and reticulum and occasionally the abomasum. Grossly the lesions resemble those of thrush in pigs, but the keratin layer tends to be thicker, less diffuse, and light gray. In the omasum the leaves may be stuck together by the mass of fungus-riddled keratin. Disseminated candidiasis occurs more often in calves than in pigs, probably because of the relatively prolonged survival of calves with alimentary lesions. Candidiasis in calves must be differentiated from alimentary herpesvirus infections.

Gastroesophageal candidiasis in foals involves the squamous epithelium and is associated with ulceration adjacent to the margo plicatus. Colic and anorexia are seen, and are probably related to the development of the ulcers, which may perforate, causing peritonitis.

In tissues, the presence of oval or round blastospores about 3–6 μm in diameter, which may be budding, mixed with pseudohyphae comprising chains of elongate yeastlike cells, or with tubular septate hyphae, permits a provisional identification of *Candida* spp. Silver or PAS stain enhances the organisms in section.

Bibliography

Gilardi, G. L. Nutrition of systemic and subcutaneous pathogenic fungi. *Bacteriol Rev* **29:** 406–424, 1965.

Gross, T. L., and Mayhew, I. G. Gastroesophageal ulceration and candidiasis in foals. *J Am Vet Med Assoc* **182:** 1370–1373, 1983.

Jubb, T. F. Systemic candidiasis in a Suffolk ram. *Aust Vet J* **65:** 333–335, 1988.

McClure, J. J., Addison, J. D., and Miller, R. I. Immunodeficiency manifested by oral candidiasis and bacterial septicemia in foals. *J Am Vet Med Assoc* **186:** 1195–1197, 1985.

Osborne, A. D., McCrae, M. R., and Manners, M. J. Moniliasis in artificially reared pigs and its treatment with Nystatin. *Vet Rec* **72:** 237–241, 1960.

Smith, J. M. B. "Opportunistic Mycoses of Man and Other Animals." Kew, U. K., C.A.B. International Mycological Institute, 1989.

3. Intestinal Histoplasmosis

Histoplasma capsulatum is a soil organism of worldwide distribution. The disease, histoplasmosis, is endemic in certain areas, such as the Mississippi and Ohio river valleys of the United States of America, and in parts of southern Ontario and the Ottawa–St. Lawrence river valleys in Canada. There are sporadic cases elsewhere. It is important in humans and dogs, and occurs occasionally in other species. Infection generally occurs via inhalation of spores, and if lesions occur, usually they are confined to the lungs. Dissemination, with hepatic, splenic, and sometimes gastrointestinal lesions, develops in some dogs. It is associated with a heavy exposure, youth, and perhaps some degree of host immunoincompetence. Infec-

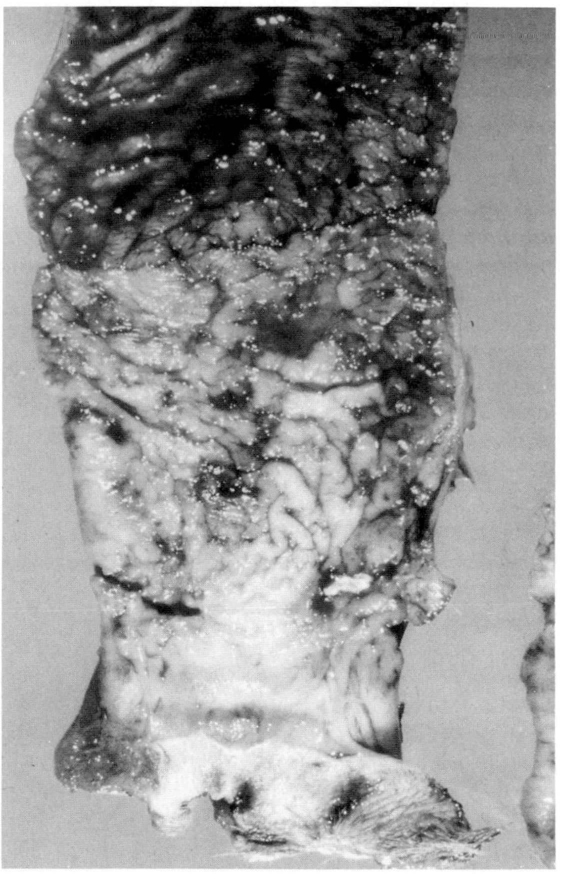

Fig. 1.160 Ulcerative colitis. Dog. Histoplasmosis.

tion also can be produced by ingestion, and the rare examples of disease confined to the gastrointestinal tract may develop in this manner. Intestinal infection by ingestion of infected sputum also is possible.

Disseminated histoplasmosis is a disease predominantly of young dogs that usually present with weight loss, generalized lymphadenopathy, and often diarrhea with blood, and tenesmus. Intestinal histoplasmosis is reported as part of disseminated disease in cats, and as an isolated lesion in a horse.

At postmortem there may be hemorrhagic enteritis involving small and large intestine, or granulomatous thickening of the mucosa and intestinal wall with ulceration (Fig. 1.160), or no apparent lesions. Mesenteric lymph nodes often are markedly enlarged. Histologically, lesions, characteristically transmural granulomatous inflammation, may occur in stomach, and small or large intestine. The nonulcerated areas of the mucosa contain focal to diffuse infiltrations of macrophages laden with *H. capsulatum* organisms within cytoplasmic vacuoles. The mucosa may be grossly thickened by the infiltrate, causing necrosis and ulceration. The cellular reaction may extend through the muscularis to the serosa. Macrophages filled with organisms are particularly prominent in the lymphoid tissue of the gut and the mesenteric nodes. Periodic acid–Schiff stain highlights the organisms in tissues. Microscopic diagnosis of gastrointestinal histoplasmosis is not difficult, but grossly the disease must be distinguished from intestinal lymphoma, and in the colon, from colitis of other types. Histoplasmosis is discussed in detail with The Hematopoietic System (Volume 3, Chapter 2).

Bibliography

Berry, C. L. The development of the granuloma of histoplasmosis. *J Pathol* **97:** 1–10, 1969.

Clinkenbeard, K. D. *et al.* Canine-disseminated histoplasmosis. *Compend Cont Ed Pract Vet* **11:** 1347–1360, 1989.

Dade, A. W., Lickfeldt, W. E., and McAllister, H. A. Granulomatous colitis in a horse with histoplasmosis. *Vet Med Small Anim Clin* **68:** 279–281, 1973.

Mahaffey, E. *et al.* Disseminated histoplasmosis in three cats. *J Am Anim Hosp Assoc* **13:** 46–51, 1977.

D. Protothecal Enterocolitis

Prototheca spp. are colorless algae closely related to *Chlorella*. They are ubiquitous in raw and treated sewage and in water, and are found in feces, plant sap, and slime flux of trees. Two species, *P. zopfii* and *P. wickerhamii*, cause disease in animals; infections with both may occur in the same animal.

Lesions caused by *Prototheca* spp. include cutaneous infections of cats and humans, mastitis in cows, and disseminated infections in dogs. The intestine and the eye are the most commonly involved sites in protothecosis of dogs.

Factors predisposing to the development of intestinal protothecosis are poorly understood. Skin infections are thought to result from traumatic inoculation, and it is possible that in the alimentary tract *Prototheca* is an opportunistic invader of existing mucosal lesions. The chronicity of the disease and the mild host response are not consistent with a virulent infection. In dogs, collies seem over-represented among the cases reported, suggesting breed-related susceptibility or immune compromise.

Chronic, intractable, bloody diarrhea or passage of bloodstained feces, is a frequent presenting sign, with progressive weight loss. Hemorrhagic and ulcerative colitis is a prominent enteric lesion, but changes may develop also in the small intestine. Mesenteric lymph nodes may be enlarged.

The mild host response to infection is characteristic of protothecosis; usually only a few lymphocytes and monocytes are present. In early lesions the extracellular organisms are scattered in the lamina propria, but later they fill the lamina propria and often are packed in cords in the connective tissue of the submucosa. Lacteals are distended, whereas lymphatics and the sinuses of draining lymph nodes are filled with organisms.

Prototheca in sections resemble somewhat cryptococcal organisms. They range from 5-μm spheres to 9- $\times$ 2-μm ovoids, with a refractile capsule, and are positive with PAS and silver stains. The presence of endosporulation with formation of 2–20 sporangiospores within a single sporangium characterizes *Prototheca* spp. and *Chlorella* spp. *Chlorella* contain PAS-positive cytoplasmic starch granules that are PAS negative following diastase digestion; *Prototheca* do not contain these granules. Differentiation of the genera by a fluorescent antibody test using formalin-fixed material is also possible.

Bibliography

Chandler, F. W., Kaplan, W., and Callaway, C. S. Differentiation between *Prototheca* and morphologically similar green algae in tissue. *Arch Pathol Lab Med* **102:** 353–356, 1978.

Migaki, G. *et al.* Canine protothecosis: Review of the literature and report of an additional case. *J Am Vet Med Assoc* **181:** 794–797, 1982.

Pore, R. S. *et al. Prototheca* ecology. *Mycopathologia* **81:** 49–62, 1983.

Sudman, M. S., and Kaplan, W. Antigenic relationships between *Chlorella* and *Prototheca* spp. *Sabouraudia* **12:** 364–370, 1974.

Thomas, J. B., and Preston, N. Generalized protothecosis in a collie dog. *Aust Vet J* **67:** 25–27, 1990.

E. Gastrointestinal Helminthosis

The diagnosis of disease due to gastrointestinal helminths must be made with knowledge of their pathogenic potential and the mechanisms by which it is expressed. Parasites are much more common than the diseases they cause, and helminthiasis, the state of infection, must be differentiated clearly from helminthosis, the state of disease.

Gastrointestinal helminths fall into five categories, according to pathogenesis of disease.

The first group resides free in the lumen of the intestine,

competing with the host for nutrients in the gut content. They are generally of low pathogenicity, except for rare massive infections, and are not likely to be lethal, except by obstruction. Some of these worms, in sufficient numbers, may cause subclinical disease such as inefficient growth, or clinical disease in the form of ill thrift; others are essentially nonpathogenic. The ascarids, small strongyles (cyathostomes) of horses, and tapeworms such as *Moniezia* and *Taenia* spp. fall into this group, as may *Physaloptera,* in the stomach of carnivores.

A second group of helminths, all nematodes, primarily cause blood loss. These worms feed on the mucosa, causing bleeding, or they actively suck blood. Anemia, hypoproteinemia, and their sequelae cause production loss, clinical disease, and death. *Haemonchus* in the abomasum, the hookworms of carnivores and ruminants in the intestine, the large strongyles of horses, and *Oesophagostomum radiatum* in cattle are the main examples.

The third group, composed of nematodes and some flukes, causes mainly protein-losing gastroenteropathy, usually associated with inappetence and diarrhea. In the abomasum, *Ostertagia* and *Trichostrongylus axei* cause mucous metaplasia and hyperplasia of gastric glands, achlorhydria, and diarrhea. In the small intestine, *Cooperia, Nematodirus, Strongyloides, Trichostrongylus,* and larval paramphistomes in sheep and cattle cause villus atrophy. This may cause malabsorption of nutrients, electrolytes, and water, but probably more important is the associated loss of endogenous protein into the gut.

The villus atrophy which occurs in these infections may be largely immune mediated. Crypts become hypertrophic, and cells on the mucosal surface in animals with subtotal or total villus atrophy are often attenuated. There may be filtration secretion from chronically inflamed mucosa, or transient leaks of tissue fluid and inflammatory cells between epithelial cells. Microerosion of the mucosa occurs in severe cases. Physical damage to the mucosa due to feeding activity of the nematodes is unlikely; however, in fluke infestations, this may be superimposed. Disease due to these agents is marked by diarrhea and by weight loss, which is probably mainly the result of the interaction of inappetence and enteric protein loss.

Trichuris spp. reside partly in tunnels in the epithelium on the mucosal surface of the cecum and colon. Mucosal typhlocolitis results, which may be in part related to the immunoinflammatory response to the worms. In heavy infestations, erosion results in loss of absorptive function, and effusion of tissue fluids, or, in severe cases, hemorrhagic exudate. More subtle alteration in colonic function, perhaps again immune mediated, is caused by *Oesophagostomum columbianum* in sheep. Mucus hypersecretion and diarrhea occur.

The fourth group causes physical trauma to the intestinal wall by burrowing into or inciting inflammatory foci in the submucosa or deeper layers. In the stomach, various species of spirurids embed in the mucosa, or establish in cystic spaces in the submucosa. In the intestine, acanthocephala cause local ulceration by their thorny hold-fast organ; larval stages of equine cyathostomes, and *Oesophagostomum* spp. become encapsulated in the submucosa. Protein loss may occur from ulcerated areas, or when larvae emerge from the submucosa. The potential exists for perforation of the stomach or bowel, or for complications due to sepsis of submucosal nodules. Adhesion of inflamed serosal surfaces associated with nodules or perforations may impair motility.

Finally, some intestinal helminths, among them a few in the previously mentioned categories, have effects at sites distant from the gut. This is usually the result of migrating larval stages of the worm, either in definitive or intermediate hosts. Larval *Habronema,* ascarids, hookworms, and equine strongyles may cause lesions in a variety of extraintestinal sites in the definitive host. Larval ascarids and taeniid metacestodes may cause lesions or signs due to migration in nonenteric locations in accidental or intermediate hosts.

A diagnosis of helminthosis should be reserved for cases in which, ideally, three criteria are met: (1) the helminth is present, in numbers consistent with disease; (2) the lesions (if any) typically caused by the agent, are identified; and (3) there is a syndrome compatible with the pathogenic mechanisms known to be associated with the worm. Only a presumptive diagnosis can be made if the syndrome, and preferably lesions, are present, but worms are not. This is appropriate only if treatment is very recent, and the condition of the animal such that it would have been virtually moribund prior to therapy, since response to treatment is usually rapid.

In many cases, it may be necessary and reasonable to base the diagnosis on only the presence of an adequate number of worms, associated with an appropriate syndrome, since autolysis may preclude critical examination of intestinal tissues. This is also appropriate for the establishment of a rapid presumptive diagnosis at autopsy. However, quantitation of the worm burden is highly desirable. To this end, appropriate samples of gastric and intestinal content and mucosa should be collected, and estimates made of the number of worms they contain, using standard parasitologic techniques. Many species of nematodes are difficult to see, and impossible to enumerate with the naked eye. Others, such as the hookworms, though usually visible, may be so sparsely distributed that they are overlooked or dismissed. An accurate estimate of the number might reveal sufficient to ascribe significance to the burden.

It is not acceptable to diagnose helminthosis only on the basis of the presence of worms, without evidence of an appropriate disease state. Nor is it an acceptable diagnosis when a syndrome such as wasting and diarrhea, or anemia, is recognized without identifying the presence of worms or their characteristic lesions.

Bibliography

Arundel, J. H. "Parasitic Diseases of the Horse." Veterinary Review No. 28, Sydney, N.S.W., Australia, University of Sydney Postgraduate Foundation in Veterinary Science, 1985.

Bremner, K. C. The pathophysiology of parasitic gastroenteritis of cattle. *In* "Biology and Control of Endoparasites," L. E. A. Symons, A. D. Donald, and J. K. Dineen (eds.), pp. 277–289. Sydney, Australia, Academic Press, 1982.

Castro, G. A. Immunophysiology of enteric parasitism. *Parasitol Today* **5:** 11–19, 1989.

Chitwood, M., and Lichtenfels, J. R. Identification of parasitic metazoa in tissue sections. *Exp Parasitol* **32:** 407–519, 1972.

Dargie, J. D. The pathophysiological effects of gastrointestinal and liver parasites in sheep. *In* "Digestive Physiology and Metabolism in Ruminants," Y. Ruckebusch and P. Thivend (eds.), pp. 349–371. Lancaster, U.K., MTD Press, 1980.

Drudge, J. H., and Lyons, E. T. Pathology of infections with internal parasites in horses. *The Blue Book* **27:** 267–275, 1977.

Holmes, P. H. Pathophysiology of nematode infections. *Int J Parasitol* **17:** 443–451, 1987.

Holmes, P. H. Pathophysiology of parasitic infections. *Parasitology* **94:** S29–S51, 1987.

Jordan, H. E., and Stair, E. L. Documenting clinical gastrointestinal parasitism: Worm-burdens—A valuable tool. *Proc Am Assoc Vet Lab Diagnost* **26:** 241–248, 1983.

Kassai, T. *et al.* Standardized nomenclature of animal parasitic diseases (SNOAPAD). *Vet Parasitol* **29:** 299–326, 1988.

Levine, N. D. "Nematode Parasites of Domestic Animals and of Man." 2nd Ed. Minneapolis, Minnesota, Burgess, 1980.

Lichtenfels, J. R. Helminths of domestic equids. *Proc Helm Soc Wash* **42** Special Issue, 1975.

Poynter, D. Some tissue reactions to the nematode parasites of animals. *Adv Parasitol* **4:** 321–383, 1966.

Russell, D. A., and Castro, G. A. Physiology of the gastrointestinal tract in the parasitized host. *In* "Physiology of the Gastrointestinal Tract," L.R. Johnson (ed.), pp. 1749–1779. New York, Raven Press, 1987.

Slocombe, J. O. D. Pathogenesis of helminths in equines. *Vet Parasitol* **18:** 139–153, 1985.

Steel, J. W., and Symons, L. E. A. Nitrogen metabolism in nematodosis of sheep in relation to productivity. *In* "Biology and Control of Endoparasites," L. E. A. Symons, A. D. Donald, and J. K. Dineen (eds.), pp. 235–256. Sydney, Australia, Academic Press, 1982.

Sykes, A. R. Nutritional and physiological aspects of helminthiasis in sheep. *In* "Biology and Control of Endoparasites," L. E. A. Symons, A. D. Donald, and J. K. Dineen (eds.), pp. 217–234. Sydney, Australia, Academic Press, 1982.

Symons, L. E. A. "Pathophysiology of Endoparasitic Infection." Sydney, Australia, Academic Press, 1989.

Titchen, D. A., and Reid, A. M. Putative roles of peptides in the genesis and control of parasitic diseases. *In* "Aspects of Digestive Physiology of Ruminants," A. Dobson and M. J. Dobson (eds.), pp. 217–237. Ithaca, New York, Comstock, 1988.

Zajak, A. M. The role of gastrointestinal immunity in parasitic infections of small animals. *Sem Vet Med Surg (Small Anim)* **2:** 274–281, 1987.

1. Parasitic Diseases of the Abomasum and Stomach

a. OSTERTAGIOSIS A complex of related genera and species of trichostrongylid nematodes, including *Ostertagia,* parasitize the abomasum of ruminants. The nomenclature of these worms is in a state of flux; for the sake of simplicity, the disease that they cause will be termed ostertagiosis. Ostertagiosis is probably the most important parasitism in grazing sheep and cattle in temperate climatic zones throughout the world. It causes subclinical loss in production, and clinical disease characterized by diarrhea, wasting, and in many cases, death. *Ostertagia ostertagi* and the associated *O. lyrata* infect cattle. Sheep and goats are infected by *Teladorsagia* (*Ostertagia*) *circumcincta,* and by the associated *T. trifurcata.* Some cross-infection by these genera occurs between sheep and cattle, but is of minor significance. Other species of *Ostertagia* and related genera, including *Teladorsagia, Marshallagia, Spiculopteragia,* and *Camelostrongylus* infect wild ruminants, including farmed deer; some may also parasitize the abomasum of cattle, sheep, and goats. Their behavior in general resembles that of the *Ostertagia* and *Teladorsagia.*

The life cycle is direct. Third-stage larvae exsheath in the rumen and enter glands in the abomasum where they undergo two molts. Normally, early fifth-stage larvae emerge to mature on the mucosal surface, beginning between the eighth and twelfth day after infection in *T. circumcincta* infections in sheep, and about 17–21 days after *O. ostertagi* infection in cattle. However, a proportion of larvae ingested may persist in glands in a hypobiotic state at the early fourth stage, only to resume development and emerge at a future time, perhaps many months hence. The prepatent period is about 3 weeks.

During the course of larval development, the normal architecture of the gastric mucosa is altered by interstitial inflammation, and mucous metaplasia and hyperplasia of the epithelium lining glands. In sheep infected with *T. circumcincta,* mucous metaplasia and hyperplasia occurs in infected and surrounding glands early in infection, reaching a peak about the time of emergence of larvae onto the mucosal surface. In cattle with *O. ostertagi* only glands infected with larvae undergo significant mucous change until about the time larvae leave the glands for the surface of the mucosa. Mucous change then becomes more widespread, involving uninfected glands in the vicinity of those which contained larvae.

In both species, affected glands are lined by mucous neck cells which proliferate, displacing parietal cells. Glands elongate, and the affected areas of mucosa thicken (Fig. 1.61A,B). In developing lesions the gland lining is cuboidal or low columnar, and mitotic figures are frequent. In infected glands the lining in many cases is flattened adjacent to worms (Fig. 1.161C), but is composed of tall columnar mucous cells elsewhere in the gland. The undifferentiated mucous cells lining uninfected glands also eventually differentiate into tall columnar mucous cells. If infection is not heavy, lesions are limited to a radius of a few millimeters around infected or previously infected glands. These form raised nodular pale areas in the mucosa, often with a slightly depressed center. Confluence of these lesions in heavily infected animals leads to the development of widespread areas of irregularly thickened mucosa with a convoluted surface pattern, likened to Morocco leather. With time, severely affected mucosa may be composed almost totally of somewhat dilated, elongate glands lined by columnar mucous cells. With loss of the

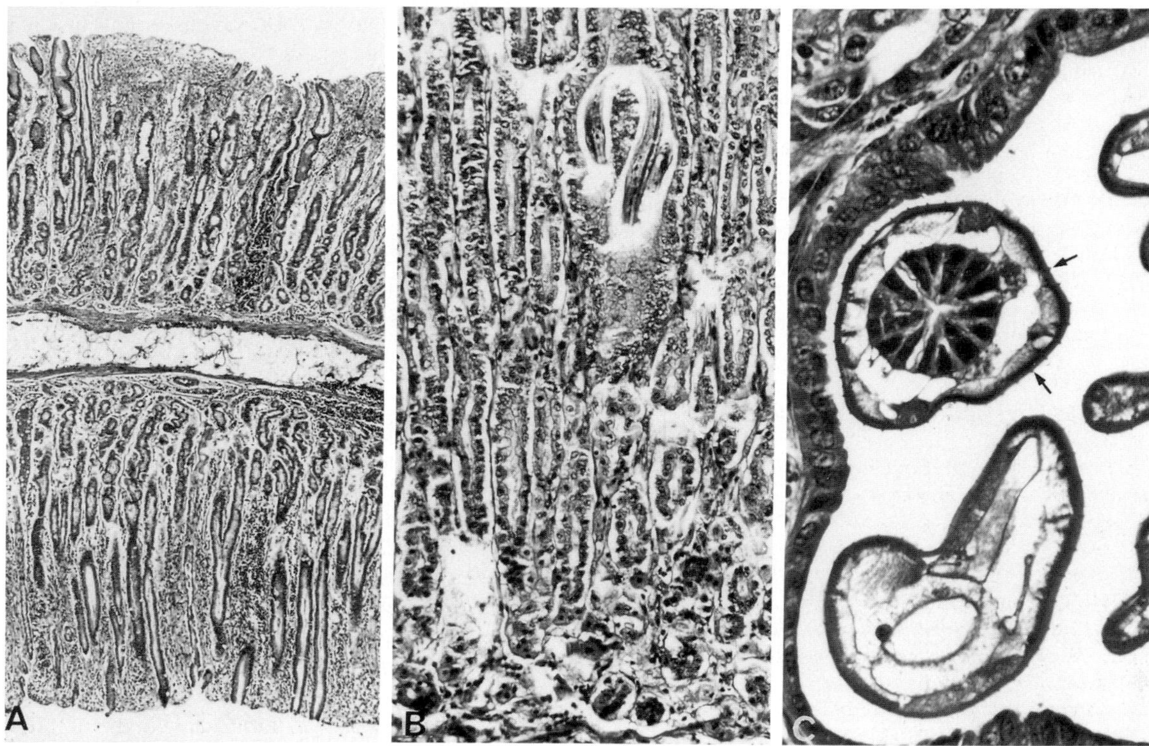

Fig. 1.161 Ostertagiosis. Abomasum. Ox. (A) Mucous metaplasia and hyperplasia thickening fundic mucosa on abomasal fold. Moderate inflammatory infiltrate in propria between glands. (B) Mucous metaplasia and hyperplasia deep in fundic mucosa. Larva in section in gland. (C) *Ostertagia* in dilated gland lined by cuboidal mucous neck cells. Longitudinal cuticular ridges are visible as fine projections on the nematode (arrows).

worm burden, through treatment or natural attrition, the mucosa gradually returns to normal.

Mucous metaplasia and hyperplasia is accompanied by a mixed population of inflammatory cells in the lamina propria. The epithelial lesion itself may be immune mediated. Infiltrates of lymphocytes are present between glands deep in infected mucosa within a few days after infection of sheep with *Teladorsagia,* and lymphoid follicles with germinal centers evolve in these sites. Lymphocytes, plasma cells, eosinophils, and a few neutrophils are present between glands in the infected abomasum, and *Ostertagia* seem to secrete an eosinophil chemotactic factor. There may be edema of the lamina propria associated with permeability of proprial vessels, which in experimental *Camelostrongylus* infection occurs as early as 4 days after infection. Globule leukocytes are common in the lining of infected glands. A few eosinophils, neutrophils, and effete epithelial cells may be seen in the lumen of glands.

Mucosal lesions lead to achlorhydria, elevation of plasma pepsinogen levels, and loss of plasma protein. Widespread replacement of parietal cells by mucous neck cells results in progressive and massive decline in hydrogen ion secretion. In severe cases the abomasal content has a pH of up to 7 or more, and a high sodium ion concentration. The pathogenic significance of associated failure to hydrolyze protein in the abomasum, and of increased numbers of bacteria in content, is unclear. Mucous metaplasia and achlorhydria in ovine ostertagiosis occur in the face of substantially increased gastrin secretion, which is not stimulated simply by failure of antral acidification. The permeability of the mucosa is also increased, which is reflected in back-diffusion of pepsinogen from the lumen of glands to the propria, and ultimately to the circulation. Intercellular junctions between poorly differentiated mucous neck cells are permeable also to plasma protein in tissue fluids, emanating from the leaky small vessels in the inflamed lamina propria. Significant loss of protein occurs into the lumen of the abomasum.

The cardinal signs of ostertagiosis in sheep and cattle are loss of appetite, diarrhea, and wasting. The cause of reduced appetite is unclear, but the elevated serum gastrin levels which occur in ostertagiosis may have a central effect on satiety, or peripheral effects on gastrointestinal motility, which would depress feed consumption. Diarrhea is associated with marked elevation in abomasal pH, but the mechanisms by which it occurs are also obscure. Plasma protein loss into the gastrointestinal tract, in combination with reduced feed intake, seems largely responsible for the weight loss and hypoproteinemia which occur in clinical ostertagiosis, and for loss in productive efficiency which occurs in subclinical disease.

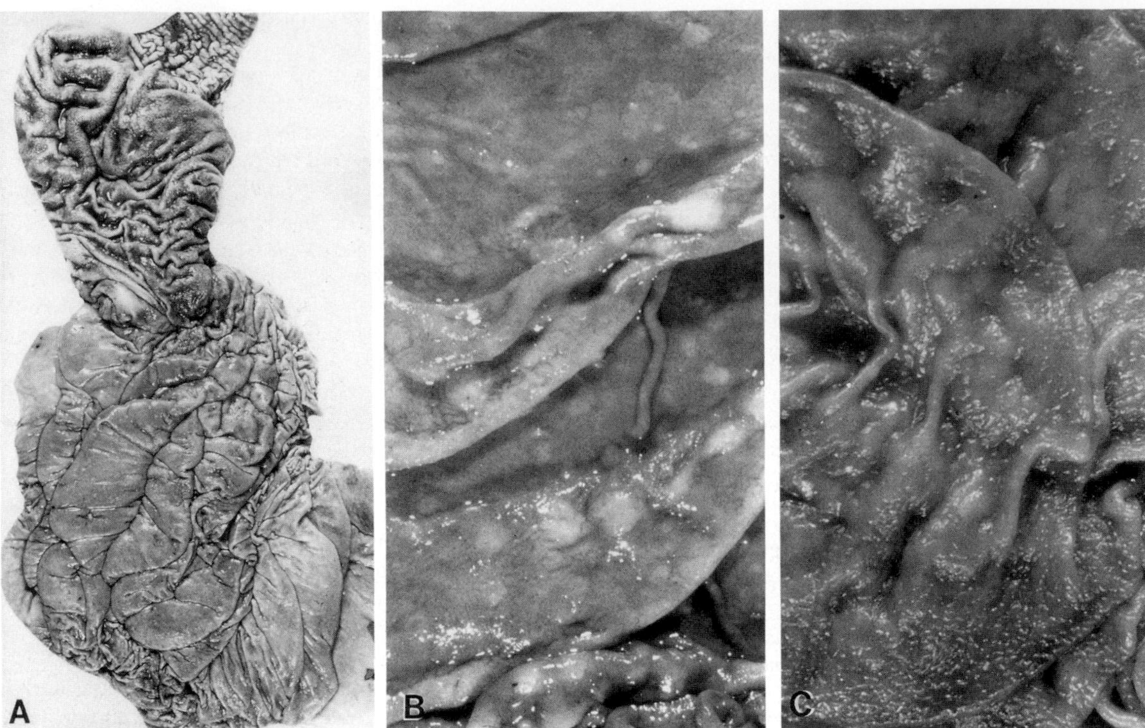

Fig. 1.162 Ostertagiosis. Abomasum. (A) Acute edematous gastritis. Ox. (B) Individual nodules and some confluent lesions. Sheep. (C) Confluent thickening of hyperplastic glandular mucosa. Sheep.

Clinical ostertagiosis occurs under two sets of circumstances. The first, type I disease, is seen in lambs or calves at pasture during or shortly after a period of high availability of infective larvae. It is due to the direct development, from ingested larvae, of large numbers of adult worms, over a relatively short period. In contrast, type II disease is due to the synchronous maturation and emergence of large numbers of hypobiotic larvae from the mucosa, and it occurs when intake of larvae is likely to be low or nonexistent. It may occur in yearlings during the winter in the northern hemisphere, or during the dry summer period in Mediterranean climates. Heifers about the time of parturition may succumb, and this syndrome is also occasionally seen in animals experiencing environmental stress of any type.

Types I and II ostertagiosis do not differ fundamentally in the signs or lesions they present. Animals will have a history of depression, inappetence and diarrhea, and weight loss consistent with the severity and duration of the other signs. There may be edema of subcutaneous tissues and mesenteries, and accumulation of fluid in the body cavities. The carcass may be wasted, and the liver is often atrophic, and the gallbladder dilated, as a result of inanition. The content of the abomasum is fluid. It may be slightly foul smelling, in contrast to the normal sharply acidic odor of abomasal content. The rugae often have substantial submucosal edema (Fig. 1.162A). The mucosa will have widespread individual or confluent thickened, pale mucosal nodules (Fig. 1.162B,C), or will show diffuse thickening and corrugation over much of the gastric lining. Both fundic and pyloric areas are involved. The mucosa may be reddened and perhaps focally eroded, with a superficial light fibrinous exudate in occasional cases.

The diagnosis is indicated at autopsy by an abnormally elevated abomasal pH (>4.5), in association with typical gross lesions on the mucosa. The adult worms are brown and threadlike, as long as 1.5 cm, but very difficult to see on the mucosa with the unaided eye. Abomasal contents and washings should be quantitatively examined for the presence of emergent or adult *Ostertagia* and other nematodes. The mucosa, or a known portion of it, should be digested to permit recovery and quantitation of preemergent stages. Significant worm burdens in sheep are in the range of 10,000–50,000 or more. In cattle more than 40,000–50,000 adult worms may be present, and in outbreaks of Type II disease hundreds of thousands of hypobiotic larvae are often detected in the abomasal mucosa. Typically, there is widespread mucous metaplasia and hyperplasia in dilated glands in sections of abomasum. *Ostertagia* are recognized in sections, on the mucosal surface or in glands, by the presence of prominent longitudinal cuticular ridges, which project from the surface of worms cut transversely. In some cases, the worm burden may have been lost through attrition or recent treatment, and the diagnosis must be presumptive, based on the characteristic mucosal lesions.

Bibliography

Al Saqur, I. *et al.* Observations on the infectivity and pathogenicity of three isolates of *Ostertagia* spp. sensu lato in calves. *Res Vet Sci* **32:** 106–112, 1982.

Anderson, N. Aspects of the biology of *Ostertagia ostertagi* in relation to the genesis of ostertagiasis. *Vet Parasitol* **27:** 13–21, 1988.

Anderson, N. *et al.* Experimental *Ostertagia ostertagi* infections in calves: Results of single infections with five graded dose levels of larvae. *Am J Vet Res* **27:** 1259–1265, 1966.

Anderson, N., Hansky, J., and Titchen, D. A. Effects of plasma pepsinogen, gastrin, and pancreatic polypeptide of *Ostertagia* spp. transferred directly into the abomasum of sheep. *Int J Parasitol* **15:** 159–165, 1985.

Anderson, N., Reynolds, G. W., and Titchen, D. A. Changes in gastrointestinal mucosal mass and mucosal and serum gastrin in sheep experimentally infected with *Ostertagia circumcincta*. *Int J Parasitol* **18:** 325–331, 1988.

Armour, J., and Ogbourne, C. P. "Bovine Ostertagiasis: A Review and Annotated Bibliography. Commonwealth Institute of Parasitology Misc. Publ. No. 7, 1982 St. Albans, U.K.

Connan, R. M. Type II ostertagiosis in farmed red deer. *Vet Rec* **128:** 233–235, 1991.

Coop, R. L. *et al.* Effect of *Ostertagia ostertagi* on lamb performance and cross resistance to *O. circumcincta*. *Res Vet Sci* **39:** 200–206, 1985.

Entrocasso, C. *et al.* The sequential development of type I and type II ostertagiasis in young cattle with special reference to biochemical and serological changes. *Vet Parasitol* **21:** 173–188, 1986.

Fox, M. T. *et al. Ostertagia ostertagi* infection in the calf: effects of a trickle challenge on appetite, digestibility, rate of passage of digesta, and liveweight gain. *Res Vet Sci* **47:** 294–298, 1989.

Hilton, R. J., Barker, I. K., and Rickard, M. D. Distribution and pathogenicity during development of *Camelostrongylus mentulatus* in the abomasum of sheep. *Vet Parasitol* **4:** 231–242, 1978.

Klesius, P. H. *et al.* Visualization of eosinophil chemotactic factor in abomasal tissue of cattle by immunoperoxidase staining during *Ostertagia ostertagi* infection. *Vet Parasitol* **31:** 49–56, 1989.

Lichtenfels, J. R., Pilitt, P. A., and Lancaster, M. B. Systematics of the nematodes that cause ostertagiasis in cattle, sheep, and goats in North America. *Vet Parasitol* **27:** 3–12, 1988.

Snider, T. G. *et al.* Sequential histopathologic changes of type I, pre-type II and type II ostertagiasis in cattle. *Vet Parasitol* **27:** 169–179, 1988.

Sykes, A. R., Coop, R. L., and Angus, K. W. The influence of chronic *Ostertagia* infection on the skeleton of growing sheep. *J Comp Pathol* **87:** 521–529, 1977.

b. HEMONCHOSIS Hemonchosis is a common and severe disease in some parts of the world. *Haemonchus* species require a period of minimal warmth and moisture for larval development on pasture. As a result, they tend to be most important in tropical or temperate climates with hot wet summers. *Haemonchus contortus* infects mainly sheep and goats, whereas *H. placei* occurs mainly in cattle. Though *H. contortus* and *H. placei* will infect the heterologous host, the host–parasite relationship appears to be less well adapted, and the species do appear to be genetically distinct. *Mecistocirrus digitatus* causes disease very similar to hemonchosis in cattle and sheep in Southeast Asia and Central America.

By exploitation of hypobiosis or retardation of larvae, populations of *H. contortus* are able to persist in the abomasum of the host through periods of climatic adversity, such as excessive cold or dryness. Disease can be expected in animals, especially females, experiencing the synchronous spring rise or periparturient development and maturation of previously hypobiotic larvae, and in young animals heavily stocked at pasture during periods of optimal larval development and availability. Resistance to reinfection occurs much more reliably in calves infected with *H. placei* than in sheep infected with *H. contortus*.

Haemonchus, commonly called the large stomach worm, or barber's pole worm, is ~2 cm long. Females give the species its common name by their red color, against which the white ovaries and uterus stand out. The male is a little shorter and a uniform deep red. These worms are equipped with a buccal tooth or lancet, and fourth-stage and adult worms suck blood. Ingested third-stage larvae enter glands in the abomasum, where they molt to the fourth stage and persist as hypobiotic larvae, or from which they emerge as late fourth-stage larvae to continue development in the lumen. The prepatent period for *H. contortus* in sheep is ~15 days, and for *H. placei* in cattle is ~26–28 days.

Hemonchosis may present as peracute or acute disease, resulting from the maturation or intake of large numbers of larvae. It may cause more insidious chronic disease, if worm burdens are lower. The pathogenicity of *Haemonchus* infection, whatever its manifestation, is the result of bloodsucking activity, which causes anemia and hypoproteinemia. Large numbers of *Haemonchus* administered to sheep do cause changes resembling those occurring in ostertagiosis, including achlorhydria, increased plasma pepsinogen and serum gastrin, with some mucosal inflammation, and architectural alterations in the abomasal glands. However, these appear to be experimental phenomena, and do not contribute significantly to the spontaneous disease.

Individual *Haemonchus* worms in sheep cause the loss of about 0.05 ml of blood per day. On the order of a tenth to a quarter of the erythrocyte volume may be lost per day by heavily infected lambs; the plasma loss is concomitant and may be several hundreds of milliliters. The potential for the rapid onset of profound anemia and hypoproteinemia in heavily infected animals is obvious. Such animals succumb quickly, some even before the maturation of the worm burden. Less heavily infected animals may be able to withstand the anemia and hypoproteinemia for a time. They compensate by expanding erythropoiesis twofold to threefold, and increasing hepatic synthesis of plasma protein. However, they are unable to compensate adequately for the enteric iron loss, despite intestinal reabsorption of a proportion of the excess, and they ultimately succumb some weeks later to iron-loss anemia, when iron reserves are depleted. Low-level infections may contribute to subclinical loss of production or ill thrift through chronic enteric protein and iron loss. Low-protein rations compound the effect of infection.

The clinical syndrome may vary somewhat. Some animals are found dead, without the owner's observing illness. Others lack exercise tolerance, fall when driven, or are reluctant to stand or move, so weak are they from anemia. Edema of dependent portions, especially the submandibular area or head in grazing animals is often observed. In primary hemonchosis, there is no diarrhea; diarrhea may occur if intercurrent infection with large numbers of other gastrointestinal helminths occurs.

The postmortem appearance of animals with hemonchosis is dominated by the extreme pallor of anemia, apparent on the conjunctiva and throughout the internal tissues. The liver is pale and friable. There is usually edema of subcutaneous tissues and mesenteries, with hydrothorax, hydropericardium, and ascites, reflecting the severe hypoproteinemia. In animals with more chronic disease, perhaps complicated by a low plane of nutrition, there may be depletion of fat depots and atrophy of muscle mass. The abomasal content is usually fluid, and dark red-brown, because of the presence of blood (Fig. 1.163). The abomasal rugae may be edematous because of hypoproteinemia, and focal areas of hemorrhage are evident over the surface. In animals which are not decomposing, the worms will be evident to the naked eye: if alive, writhing on the mucosal surface; if dead, less obvious and free in the content.

In clinically affected sheep and goats, usually about 1000–12,000 worms are found. The severity of the disease is a function of the number of worms on one hand, and to some extent, the size of the animal on the other. In lambs, 2000–3000 worms is a heavy burden, whereas in adult sheep and goats, 8000–10,000 are associated with fatal infection. Burdens of fewer than 500–1000 *Haemonchus* are unlikely to cause death in animals on a good plane of nutrition, but may contribute to inefficiency in production, or cause ill thrift, and perhaps mortality, if the quality of feed declines.

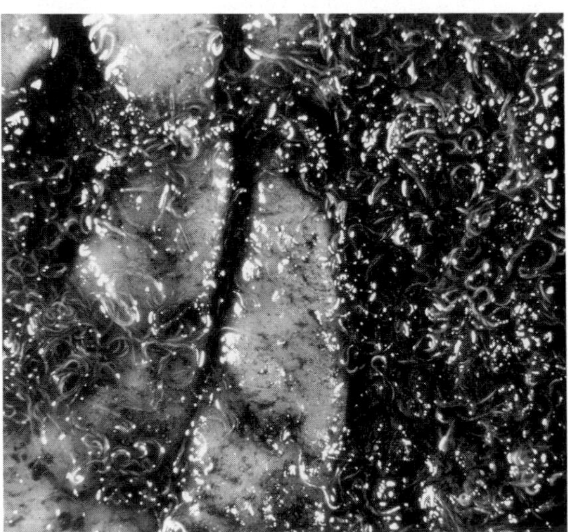

Fig. 1.163 *Haemonchus contortus* in acid-hematin-tinged abomasal content. Sheep.

A high egg count is usually found on fecal flotation, since *Haemonchus* is a prolific egg layer. However, in peracute prepatent infections, no eggs will be present. In recently treated animals, no worms may be present, and the diagnosis may have to be presumptive. On the other hand, treated animals returned to contaminated pasture may succumb to reinfection within 2–3 weeks.

Bibliography

Abbott, E. M., Parkins, J. J., and Holmes, P. H. Studies on the pathophysiology of chronic ovine haemonchosis in Merino and Scottish blackface lambs. *Parasitology* **89:** 585–596, 1984.

Abbott, E. M., Parkins, J. J., and Holmes, P. H. Influence of dietary protein on the pathophysiology of haemonchosis in lambs given continuous infections. *Res Vet Sci* **45:** 41–49, 1988.

Bremner, K. C. The parasitic life cycle of *Haemonchus placei* (Place) Ransom (Nematoda: Trichostrongylidae). *Aust J Zool* **4:** 146–151, 1956.

Dargie, J. M., and Allonby, E. W. Pathophysiology of single and challenge infection of *Haemonchus contortus* in Merino sheep: Studies on red cell kinetics and the "self-cure" phenomenon. *Int J Parasitol* **5:** 147–157, 1975.

Euzeby, J., amd Graber, M. *Mecistocirrus digitatus* Von Linstow 1906, parasite du bétail de la Guadeloupe. *Bull Soc Pathol Exot Luxemb* **67:** 84–94, 1974.

Fernando, S. T. The life cycle of *Mecistocirrus digitatus,* a trichostrongylid parasite of ruminants. *J Parasitol* **51:** 156–163, 1965.

Jennings, F. W. The anaemias of parasitic infections. *In* "Pathophysiology of Parasitic Infection," E. J. L. Soulsby, (ed.), pp. 41–67. New York, Academic Press, 1976.

Le Jambre, L. F. Hybridization studies of *Haemonchus contortus* (Rudolphi, 1893) and *H. placei* (Place, 1893) (Nematoda: Trichostrongylidae). *Int J Parasitol* **9:** 455–463, 1979.

Nicholls, C. D. *et al.* Hypergastrinaemia of sheep infected with *Haemonchus contortus. Res Vet Sci* **45:** 124–126, 1988.

O'Sullivan, B. M., and Donald, A. Responses to infection with *Haemonchus contortus* and *Trichostrongylus colubriformis* in ewes of different reproductive status. *Int J Parasitol* **3:** 521–530, 1973.

Roberts, F. H. S. Reactions of calves to infestation with the stomach worm *Haemonchus placei* (Place, 1893) Ransom 1911. *Aust J Agric Res* **8:** 740–767, 1957.

Rowe, J. B. *et al.* The effect of haemonchosis and blood loss into the abomasum on digestion in sheep. *Br J Nutr* **59:** 125–139, 1988.

Salman, S. K., and Duncan, J. L. The abomasal histology of worm-free sheep given primary and challenge infections of *Haemonchus contortus. Vet Parasitol* **16:** 43–54, 1984.

C. *TRICHOSTRONGYLUS AXEI* INFECTION *Trichostrongylus axei* infects the abomasum of cattle, sheep, and goats, and the stomach of horses. It has a direct life cycle, third stage infective larvae entering tunnels in the epithelium of the foveolae and neck of gastric glands in both fundic and pyloric areas. The worms live throughout their life partly embedded in intraepithelial tunnels at about this level of the mucosa. They molt to the fourth stage about a week after being ingested and to the fifth stage by ~2 weeks after infection. The prepatent period is ~3 weeks in calves and sheep and about 25 days in horses.

Infections with *T. axei* are usually part of a mixed gastrointestinal helminthosis. However, in all hosts, this species alone is capable of inducing disease, if present in sufficient numbers. After a period of several weeks, mucous metaplasia and hyperplasia are seen in glands in infected areas of the mucosa. Mucous neck cells replace parietal and peptic cells, and the glands increase markedly in depth and appear slightly dilated. This change is associated with an infiltrate of eosinophils and lymphocytes, especially in the superficial lamina propria. In severely affected animals, flattening of surface epithelium with desquamation, or erosion of the mucosa, develops, accompanied by effusion of neutrophils, eosinophils, and tissue fluid. The inflammatory reaction in the propria is most intense in the vicinity of erosions, and no specific reaction is associated with worms in epithelial tunnels. Fibroplasia may occur in the superficial propria in eroded areas.

In light infestations there may be no changes visible in the abomasum other than congestion of the mucosa. The gross lesions present in heavy *T. axei* infections reflect the hypertrophy of glands, and superficial erosion. Circular or irregular raised white plaques of thickened infected mucosa stand out against the background of more normal tissue. The surface of the mucosa generally is covered by a heavy layer of mucus. Erosions or shallow ulcers may be present, especially on the tips of abomasal folds. In severe infections the entire mucosa appears edematous and congested.

Infection in horses is uncommon and is related usually to sharing pasture with sheep or cattle. In chronically infected horses, white raised plaques (Fig. 1.164) or nodular areas of mucosa are present, covered by tenacious mucus and surrounded by a zone of congestion. Mucosal lesions may be confluent in heavily infected animals, and erosions and superficial ulceration may be encountered. Infection may extend into the proximal duodenum, where polypoid masses of hypertrophic glandular mucosa are occasionally observed. Plasma pepsinogen levels may be elevated.

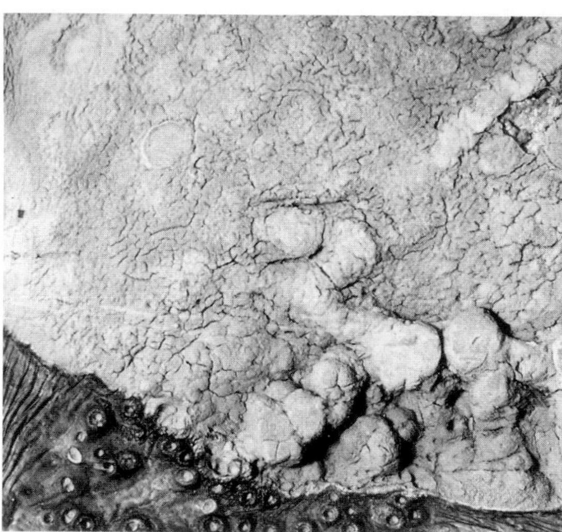

Fig. 1.164 Hypertrophic gastritis. Gastric mucosa. Horse. Trichostrongylosis. (Courtesy of N. O. Christensen and the *Skandinavisk veterinartidskrift*.)

Achlorhydria develops in heavily infected sheep and cattle, associated with diarrhea, particularly in the latter species. Dehydration may prove severe in scouring calves. Plasma pepsinogen and gastrin levels increase, and hypoproteinemia and wasting occur. This suggests that the mucous metaplasia in the glands is associated with increased permeability and that plasma protein loss occurs into the gastrointestinal tract.

Though *T. axei* is not common as a primary cause of disease in any species, it should be sought at autopsy of animals with signs of wasting and perhaps diarrhea. The typical gross lesions in the stomach are distinctive in horses. In ruminants, they must be differentiated from those due to *Ostertagia,* with which animals may be intercurrently infected. The worms are very fine, and gastric washes or digestion are required to recover them quantitatively. The distinctive intraepithelial location of *T. axei* in section differentiates it from other nematodes inhabiting the abomasum of ruminants and the stomach of horses.

Bibliography

Herd, R. P. Serum pepsinogen concentrations of ponies naturally infected with *Trichostrongylus axei. Equine Vet J* **18:** 490–491, 1986.

Leland, S. E. *et al.* Studies on *Trichostrongylus axei* (Cobbold, 1879). VII. Some quantitative and pathologic aspects of natural and experimental infections in the horse. *Am J Vet Res* **22:** 128–138, 1961.

Purcell, D. A., Ross, J. G., and Todd, J. R. The pathology of *Trichostrongylus axei* infection in calves and sheep. *In* "Pathology of Parasitic Diseases," S. M. Gaafar (ed.), pp. 295–302. Lafayette, Indiana, Purdue, 1971.

Ross, J. G., Purcell, D. A., and Todd, J. R. Investigations of *Trichostrongylus axei* infections in calves: Observations using abomasal and intestinal cannulae. *Br Vet J* **125:** 149–158, 1970.

Snider, T. G. *et al.* High concentration of serum gastrin immunoreactivity and abomasal mucosal hyperplasia in calves infected with *Ostertagia ostertagi* and/or *Trichostrongylus axei. Am J Vet Res* **49:** 2101–2104, 1988.

d. Gastric Parasitism in Horses The commonest parasites of the equine stomach are larvae of the bot flies of the genus ***Gasterophilus.*** Though they are not helminths, it is convenient to consider them here. There are six species of the genus, the common ones being *G. intestinalis, G. nasalis,* and *G. haemorrhoidalis,* and the uncommon ones being *G. pecorum, G. nigricornis,* and *G. inermis.* The ova are deposited on the ends of the coat hairs in the face, intermandibular region, or on the lower body and legs. The eggs hatch spontaneously, or when stimulated by licking. The first-stage larvae penetrate the oral mucosa, molt, emerge, and migrate down the alimentary canal.

Gasterophilus intestinalis usually wander about in tunnels in the superficial mucosa of the cheeks, tongue, or gums for 3–4 weeks before moving to periodontal pockets containing purulent exudate in the gingival sulcus on the lingual aspect of molars, especially in the upper arcade. Here they molt before moving on to the base of the tongue, and to the stomach. This is the most common species, and in the stomach it attaches itself to the squamous mucosa of the cardia to complete its subsequent molts. *Gasterophilus nasalis* first invade the gums, where they may be associated with pockets of purulent exudate in the interdental spaces, then pass to the stomach and settle on the pyloric mucosa and in the first ampulla of the duodenum. Members of any of these species may occasionally be found attached to the pharynx and esophagus but, except for *G. pecorum,* which congregates in the pharynx and causes pharyngitis, these preliminary migrations are uneventful for the host. In the summer following the deposition of the ova, the larvae leave the stomach and pass out in the feces to pupate. Those of *G. pecorum* and *G. haemorrhoidalis* may attach themselves for a short while to the wall of the rectum.

It is generally assumed that the larvae of *Gasterophilus* have little effect on their host. They may, however, produce obvious gastric lesions. Infestations by bots usually involve scores or occasionally hundreds, scattered, or more commonly grouped together in rosettelike colonies on the pars esophagea (Fig. 1.165), especially on the cranial aspect of the stomach. The larvae fasten themselves to the mucosa by the chitinous oral hooks, and they bore into the mucosa. They apparently subsist on blood, exudate, and detritus, producing focal erosions and ulcerations at the point of contact. These defects in the cardia are surrounded by a narrow rim of hyperplastic squamous epithelium. Usually the number of epithelial defects exceeds the number of larvae, suggesting that they move about on the mucosa.

Severe infestations produce a dense pock-marked appearance of the pars esophagea, with chronic inflammatory thickening. Ulcers may occur in the glandular mucosa and rarely, a large proportion of the affected pyloric mucosa may be lost. Healing occurs when the larvae migrate on, but may be complicated by secondary bacterial infection. Histologically, the ulcers penetrate the submucosa, which is chronically inflamed. The deep layers of eroded epithelium and the epithelial margins of ulcers in the squamous mucosa become hyperplastic and develop rete pegs. Other exceptional untoward sequelae include subserosal abscessation, perforation with hemorrhage or peritonitis, and inflammatory stricture of the pylorus. There seems to be no relationship between bot infestations and the development of gastric ulcers in the pars esophagea.

The **spirurid nematodes** *Draschia megastoma, Habronema majus,* and *H. muscae* are also parasitic in the stomach of horses. The adult worms are 1–2 cm in length. The latter two species lie on the mucosal surface and are probably insignificant except possibly for a few erosions and mild gastritis. *Draschia megastoma* burrows into the submucosa to produce large tumorlike nodules (Fig. 1.166).

Habronema majus mainly uses *Stomoxys calcitrans* as its intermediate host and the other two species use various muscid flies. The *Habronema* larvae in the feces are swallowed by maggots of the appropriate intermediate host and persist through pupation and maturation of the fly. They leave the host fly via the proboscis when it seeks moisture, for instance, on the lips. Horses may also be infected when they swallow parasitized flies. Larvae deposited on or in cutaneous wounds, or in the eye, invade the skin or conjunctiva and provoke an intense local reaction, which becomes granulomatous and densely infiltrated with eosinophils (see The Skin and Appendages, Volume 1, Chapter 5). Occasionally *Draschia* and *Habro-*

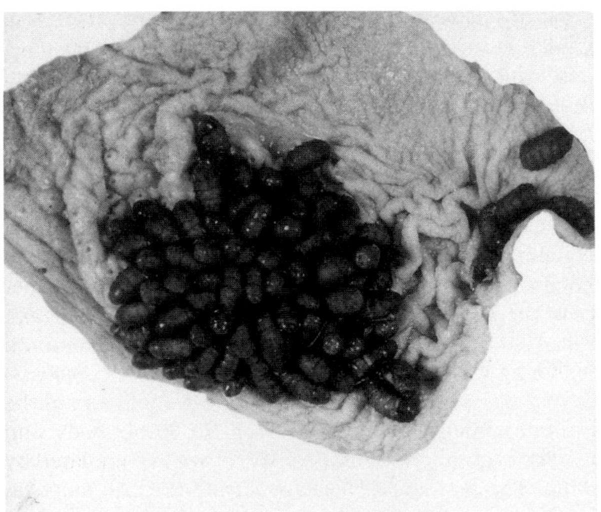

Fig. 1.165 *Gasterophilus* larvae on gastric mucosa. Horse.

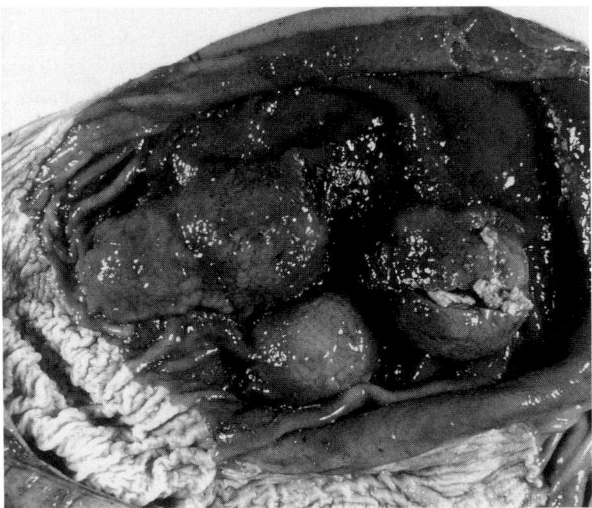

Fig. 1.166 Nodules containing *Draschia megastoma* in the submucosa of glandular mucosa, near margo plicatus. Purulent content in sectioned nodule.

nema larvae may be found in the brain, or in the lungs, where they may become encapsulated and mineralize.

The only one of concern in the stomach is *Draschia megastoma,* which burrows into the submucosa of the fundus, usually within a few centimeters of the margo plicatus. Within the submucosa, the worms provoke a surrounding granulomatous reaction, which contains them in a central core of necrotic and cellular detritus. Eosinophils are present in large numbers. The granulomas cause the overlying mucosa to bulge into the gastric lumen, forming protrusions as large as ~5 cm in diameter, with a small fistulous opening to the lumen. The nodules generally produce no clinical disturbance, though they have been considered to lead rarely to abscessation, adhesions of the stomach to the spleen, or perforation when infected with pyogenic bacteria.

Bibliography

Cogley, T. P. Effects of migrating *Gasterophilus intestinalis* larvae (Diptera: Gasterophilidae) in the mouth of the horse. *Vet Parasitol* **31:** 317–331, 1989.

Lyons, E. T. *et al.* Parasites in lungs of dead equids in Kentucky: Emphasis on *Dictyocaulis arnfieldi. Am J Vet Res* **46:** 924–927, 1985.

Price, R. E., and Stromberg, P. C. Seasonal occurrence and distribution of *Gasterophilus intestinalis* and *Gasterophilus nasalis* in the stomachs of equids in Texas. *Am J Vet Res* **48:** 1225–1232, 1987.

Principato, M. Classification of the main macroscopic lesions produced by larvae of *Gasterophilus* spp. (Diptera: Gasterophilidae) in free-ranging horses in Umbria. *Cornell Vet* **78:** 43–52, 1988.

Sweeney, H. J. The prevalence and pathogenicity of *Gasterophilus intestinalis* larvae in horses in Ireland. *Irish Vet J* **43:** 67–73, 1990.

Waddell, A. H. The pathogenicity of *Gasterophilus intestinalis* larvae in the stomach of the horse. *Aust Vet J* **48:** 332–335, 1972.

e. Gastric Parasitism in Swine Gastric parasitism is not of great clinical or pathologic importance in swine and is rare in pigs reared in modern total confinement systems. *Ascaris suum,* normally inhabiting the small intestine, may migrate or reflux to the stomach after death. *Hyostrongylus rubidus* is probably the most significant parasite of the stomach of swine; it and the various spirurids are more common in pigs allowed to forage. *Ollulanus tricuspis* is reported in pigs. It is more commonly encountered in cats, and is discussed with gastric parasitism in dogs and cats.

Hyostrongylus rubidus is a trichostongylid nematode with a typical life cycle. Third-stage larvae enter glands in the stomach, especially in the fundic region, where they develop and molt twice. Preadult and adult worms emerge onto the gastric mucosa ~18–20 days after ingestion. The lesions produced by *Hyostrongylus* resemble those caused by *Ostertagia* in ruminants. During the course of larval development, there is mucous metaplasia and hyperplasia of the lining of infected and neighboring glands, and dilation of infected glands. The lamina propria in infected mucosa is edematous and infiltrated by lymphocytes, plasma cells, and eosinophils, and lymphoid follicles develop deep in the mucosa. Neutrophils and eosinophils may transmigrate the epithelium into dilated glands, the lining of which may become quite attenuated. Effusion of neutrophils and fibrin may occur through transient gaps, or more extensive erosions, in the surface of the mucosa. Larval nematodes are found in the gastric glands in sections, whereas adults are mainly on the surface of the mucosa.

During the course of development of the worms, the mucous metaplasia and hyperplasia cause the formation of pale nodules in the vicinity of infected glands (Fig. 1.167A). In heavy infections these may become confluent, causing the development of an irregularly thickened convoluted mucosa (Fig. 1.167B), most notable in the fundic area and along the lesser curvature. Adult worms are fine, red, and threadlike in the gastric mucus; they are difficult to see with the naked eye. Mucosal nodularity is most apparent during larval development, and perhaps persists around glands containing inhibited larvae. In established heavy infections the mucosa is not so thickened. It is pinkish brown, corrugated, and covered with excess mucus. There may be focal or diffusely eroded areas with pale fibrin evident on the surface, and occasionally ulceration of the glandular mucosa has been associated with hyostrongylosis.

Experimental infections of moderate degree do not produce obvious clinical signs or loss of production. However, loss of plasma protein has been documented in heavy *Hyostrongylus* infections. Inappetence, diarrhea, and reduced weight gains and feed efficiency also occur in these circumstances. In the field, hyostrongylosis is associated mainly with the thin-sow syndrome. It seems probable that hyostrongylosis may interact with nutritional and metabolic factors in contributing to this syndrome. Hyostrongylosis is confirmed by total worm count on the gastric mucosa and digests, in association with compatible gross and microscopic lesions in the stomach.

Spirurid nematodes parasitizing the porcine stomach include *Physocephalus sexalatus, Ascarops strongylina, A. dentata,* and *Simondsia paradoxa. Physocephalus* and *Ascarops* utilize dung beetles as intermediate hosts; the intermediate host of *Simondsia* is not known. *Ascarops* and *Physocephalus* are common in many parts of the world, in swine with access to grazing. Large numbers of worms are required to cause ill thrift. Worms in affected pigs may be free in the lumen or partly embedded in the mucosa, which may be congested and edematous, or eroded and ulcerated with a fibrinous exudate on the surface. There may be chronic interstitial inflammation and fibrosis in the mucosa. *Simondsia* is found in swine in Europe and Asia. The posterior portion of the female worm is globular, and is embedded in palpable nodules as large as 6–8 mm in diameter in the gastric mucosa. *Gnathostoma hispidum* may cause lesions in the liver, and submucosal nodules in the gastric wall of pigs, similar to those produced by *G. spinigerum* in carnivores.

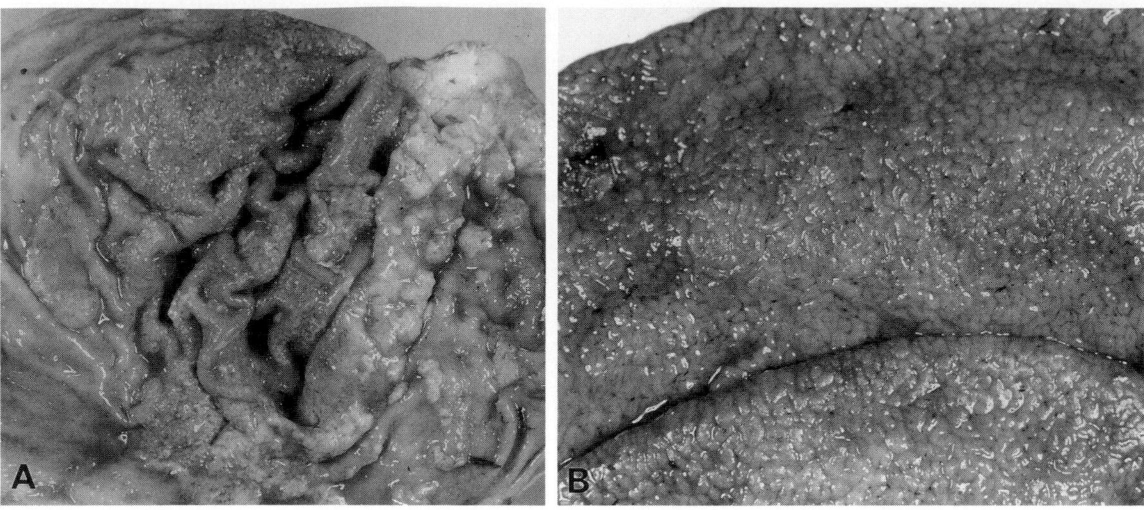

Fig. 1.167 Hyostrongylosis. Pig. (A) Hypertrophic, catarrhal gastritis. (B) Abnormally rugose mucosa.

Bibliography

Castelino, J. B., Herbert, I. V., and Lean, I. J. The live-weight gain of growing pigs experimentally infected with massive doses of *Hyostrongylus rubidus* (Nematoda) larvae. *Br Vet J* **126:** 579–582, 1970.

Dey-Hazra, A. *et al.* Gastrointestinal loss of plasma proteins in *Hyostrongylus*-infected pigs. *Z Parasitenkd* **38:** 14–20, 1972.

Kendall, S. B., and Small, A. J. *Hyostrongylus rubidus* in sows at pasture. *Vet Rec* **5:** 388–390, 1974.

Stewart, T. B., Hale, O. M., and Marti, O. G. Experimental infections with *Hyostrongylus rubidus* and the effects on performance of growing pigs. *Vet Parasitol* **17:** 219–227, 1984/85.

Stockdale, P. H. G. Pathogenesis of *Hyostrongylus rubidus* in growing pigs. *Br Vet J* **130:** 366–373, 1974.

Stockdale, P. H. G. *et al.* Hyostrongylosis in Ontario. *Can Vet J* **14:** 265–268, 1973.

Titchener, R. N., Herbert, I. V., and Probert, A. J. Plasma protein loss in growing pigs during the prepatent and early patent periods of infection with high doses of *Hyostrongylus rubidus* larvae. *J Comp Pathol* **84:** 399–406, 1974.

Varma, S. *et al.* Pathology of *Ascarops strongylina, Physocephalus sexalatus* and *Simondsia paradoxa,* the stomach worms of swine. *Arch Vet* **13:** 41–46, 1978.

f. Gastric Parasitism in Dogs and Cats Parasites are uncommonly encountered in the stomach of dogs and cats at autopsy, and most are incidental findings, or postmortem migrants from the intestine.

Gnathostoma spinigerum occurs in the stomach of dogs and cats, and of a variety of nondomestic carnivores. It is more common in areas with warm climates. The life cycle of this spirurid nematode involves *Cyclops* as an aquatic invertebrate intermediate host, and a variety of fish, amphibia, or reptiles as second intermediate hosts. Third-stage larvae may also persist in the tissues of mammalian transport hosts. The life cycle dictates that infected animals have the opportunity to forage and scavenge. Ingested third-stage larvae may migrate in the liver, leaving tracks of necrotic debris, which eventually heal by fibrosis. In heavy infections, lesions associated with larval migration may be found elsewhere in the abdominal and pleural cavities, and in the skin. Adults are found in groups of as many as 10 in nodules in the gastric submucosa. Nodules are are as large as ~5 cm in diameter, and open into the gastric lumen. Portions of nematodes may protrude through this opening. The worms lie in a pool of blood-tinged purulent exudate in the lumen of the nodule, the wall of which is composed of granulation tissue and reactive fibrous stroma. A mixed inflammatory infiltrate is in the wall of the nodules, and focal granulomas may center on nematode ova trapped in the connective tissue. Infection with *Gnathostoma* has been considered significant. Illness and death may be associated with disturbance of motility, chronic vomition, and occasional rupture of verminous nodules onto the gastric serosa, leading to peritonitis.

A number of species of ***Physaloptera,*** including *P. praeputialis* (cat), *P. rara* (dogs and wild Canidae and Felidae), and *P. canis* (dog) are found in the stomach of dogs and cats. These nematodes utilize arthropod intermediate hosts and probably some vertebrate transport hosts. The adult worms, which may be mistaken for small ascarids, are found in the stomach, where they may be free in the lumen. More commonly they are attached as individuals or in small clusters to the gastric mucosa. Ulcers may be formed, and the anterior end of the worm may be embedded in the submucosa. Hyaline PAS-positive material surrounds the anterior end of some worms, perhaps anchoring them in the tissue. These nematodes are not highly pathogenic, though heavy burdens may have the potential to cause significant gastric damage and protein loss into the lumen. They have been associated with chronic vomition.

Cylicospirura felineus and members of the genus ***Cyathospirura*** may be found in the stomach of domestic and wild felids. *Cylicospirura* are usually found in the submucosal nodules, similar to those formed by *Gnathostoma,* whereas *Cyathospirura* is usually found free in the lumen, or sometimes associated with *Cylicospirura* in gastric nodules. The pathogenicity of these species is poorly defined, but is likely to be low.

Ollulanus tricuspis is a small trichostrongyle, ~1 mm long, which inhabits the stomach of cats and swine. It is viviparous, and third-stage larvae developing in the uterus of the female are transmitted in vomitus. As a result, infection is usually not detected by usual fecal examination, and infection with this species may go unnoticed. In some parts of the world it is common, particularly in cat colonies and cats which roam. Clinical signs and gross lesions due to *O. tricuspis* are uncommon. Vomition, anorexia, and weight loss are the signs most frequently associated with infection.

The worms lie beneath the mucus on the surface of the stomach, or partly in gastric glands. Infection is associated with increased numbers of lymphoid follicles deep in the gastric mucosa, increased interstitial connective tissue in the mucosa, and numerous globule leukocytes in the gastric epithelium. Heavy infection results in mucous metaplasia and hyperplasia of gastric glands, causing the surface of the stomach to be thrown into thickened convoluted folds, grossly resembling idiopathic hypertrophic gastritis of dogs. Gastric glands are often separated by the heavy reactive fibrous stroma in the mucosa. In gastric biopsies, this suite of microscopic changes in the mucosa should be recognized as characteristic of *Ollulanus* infection, even if worms are not present. *Ollulanus* are characterized in section by the numerous longitudinal cuticular ridges (synlophe) recognized as projections on the surface of sectioned worms. In cats which have been vomiting, there may be associated reflux esophagitis.

Capillaria putorii has also been reported from the stomach of cats. It is probably an uncommonly recognized inhabitant of the intestine, which may be found in the stomach because of intestinal reflux at or after death. It is probably of little significance in either site.

Ascarids, hookworms, and tapeworms normally found in the small intestine may also be found, as postmortem artefacts, in the stomach.

Bibliography

Beveridge, I., Presidente, P. J. A., and Arundel, J. H. *Gnathostoma spinigerum* infection in a feral cat from New South Wales. *Aust Vet J* **54:** 46, 1978.

Burrows, C. F. Infection with the stomach worm *Physaloptera* as a cause of chronic vomiting in the dog. *J Am Anim Hosp Assoc* **19:** 947–950, 1983.

Coman, B. J., Jones, E. H., and Driesen, M. A. Helminth parasites and arthropods of feral cats. *Aust Vet J* **57:** 324–327, 1981.

Greve, J. H., and Kung, F. Y. *Capillaria putorii* in domestic cats in Iowa. *J Am Vet Med Assoc* **182:** 511–513, 1983.

Hargis, A. M. *et al.* Chronic fibrosing gastritis associated with *Ollulanus tricuspis* in a cat. *Vet Pathol* **19:** 320–323, 1982.

Hargis, A. M., Prieur, D. J., and Blanchard, J. L. Prevalence, lesions, and differential diagnosis of *Ollulanus tricuspis* infection in cats. *Vet Pathol* **20:** 71–79, 1983.

Hasslinger, M. A. *Ollulanus tricuspis,* the stomach worm of the cat. *Feline Pract* **14:** 22–35, 1984.

Kirkpatrick, C. E. *et al.* Gastric gnathostomosis in a cat. *J Am Vet Med Assoc* **190:** 1437–1439, 1987.

Nayak, B. C., and Rao, A. T. Pathology of gastric lesions in *Gnathostoma spinigerum* infection in a dog. *Ind Vet J* **49:** 750–753, 1972.

Wilson, R. B., and Presnell, J. C. Chronic gastritis due to *Ollulanus tricuspis* infection in a cat. *J Am Anim Hosp Assoc* **26:** 137–139, 1990.

2. *Intestinal Helminth Infections*

a. *STRONGYLOIDES* INFECTION *Strongyloides* spp. parasitize all species of domestic animals considered here. Ruminants are infected by *S. papillosus;* horses, by *S. westeri;* swine, mainly by *S. ransomi;* dogs, by *S. stercoralis;* and cats, by *S. felis, S. planiceps* (*S. catti*), and *S. stercoralis* in the small intestine, and by *S. tumefaciens* in the colon. The parasitic worms are parthenogenetic females, which produce larvae capable of direct infection of the host, or of developing into a free-living generation of males and females. The offspring of the free-living generation then adopt a parasitic existence.

Infection by third-stage larvae takes place by skin penetration, or to a lesser extent by ingestion and probably subsequent penetration of the gastrointestinal mucosa. Larvae attain the bloodstream, and in young animals, break out into pulmonary alveoli. They migrate to the large airways, whence they are carried up the mucociliary escalator to be swallowed, and establish in the small intestine. Alternatively, in species other than *S. stercoralis* and *S. felis,* prenatal, or much more important, transmammary, infection occurs. Infective early fourth-stage larvae are mobilized from muscle or adipose tissue in the periparturient female. They may cross the placenta shortly before birth, or are shed in the milk for several weeks after parturition. No somatic migration is required prior to establishment of these larvae in the gut of the new host.

The suckling young may develop patent infections within 1–2 weeks of birth. The prepatent period is short, and development of free-living larvae or the free-living generation is rapid. If sanitation is poor, and large numbers of larvae derived from parasitic or free-living generations of the worm are in the substrate, infection through the skin may be considerable. Dermatitis of contact surfaces may be associated with skin penetration. Heavy intestinal infections may be a significant cause of morbidity and mortality in neonatal or suckling animals under appropriate epizootiologic circumstances.

Typically infecting the anterior small intestine of all species, *Strongyloides* larvae establish in tunnels in the epithelium about the base of villi or in upper crypts, and they persist in that location (Fig. 1.168). Adult worms are small, only 2–6 mm long, depending on species. In sufficient numbers, they cause the development of villus atrophy, associated with a mixed, but mainly mononuclear inflammatory cell infiltrate into the lamina propria. Cryptal epithelium is hyperplastic. Villi are stumpy, or there is

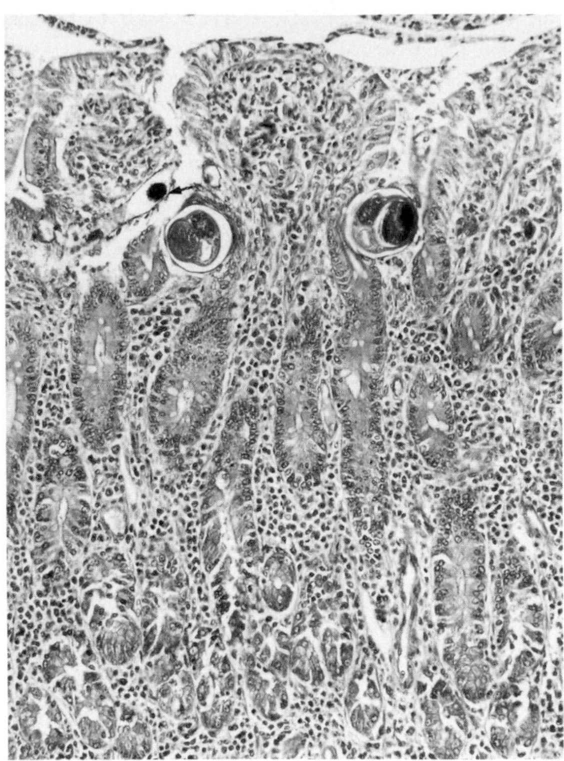

Fig. 1.168 *Strongyloides westeri* in tunnels at base of a moderately atrophic villus. Intestine of foal with diarrhea. An ovum is in a tunnel on an adjacent villus (arrow).

subtotal villus atrophy. Surface epithelium is usually low columnar to cuboidal, with an indistinct brush border; it may be squamous, or in some cases, eroded. In such circumstances, focal effusion of neutrophils and tissue fluid into the lumen is seen. The nematodes are usually found in tunnels in the surface epithelium, not beneath the basal lamina. In animals with severe atrophy, they may be in crypts of Lieberkühn. Embryonated or larvating ova may be retained in epithelial tunnels, and help to distinguish this nematode in tissue section from *Trichostrongylus,* in hosts in which both species occur.

Strongyloides ransomi is responsible for diarrhea in suckling piglets in some parts of the world. Minor local hemorrhage occurs as larvae migrate through the lungs, and thickening of alveolar septa is reported, associated with scattered aggregates of lymphocytes and plasma cells. In the duodenum, villus atrophy is associated with local malabsorption of amino acids, and with protein loss into the gut. In heavy infections, amino acid malabsorption is not compensated for by increased absorption in more distal intestine. Diarrhea occurs, presumably the result of malabsorption. Debilitation is the product of anorexia, protein loss into the gut, and nutrient malabsorption. Plasma gastrin levels are elevated in this infection, but the pathogenetic significance of this is obscure. This disease must be considered in enzootic areas, and differentiated from the other causes of undifferentiated diarrhea in suckling piglets >6–10 days of age. Specific gross lesions other than those associated with diarrhea may be absent. Moderate to severe clinical disease in 3 month old pigs is associated with 20,000–70,000 worms, most in the anterior 30–40% of the small intestine. Worms are evident in mucosal scrapings at autopsy.

Strongyloides westeri commonly infects foals. It is associated with diarrhea, occasionally fatal, in some animals younger than 4–5 months. It is claimed that skin lesions by larval penetration may permit entry of *Rhodococcus equi,* which causes lymphadenitis. Millions of larvae are necessary to cause fatal infections experimentally. The gross findings at necropsy do not indicate the cause, which may be suggested by finding worms in gut scrapings and confirmed by their association with atrophic villi in tissue section (Fig. 1.168).

Strongyloides papillosus may cause diarrhea and, in occasional overwhelming infections, death, in suckling ruminants, or young animals being artificially reared. The lesions, and presumably the pathogenesis of *S. papillosus* infection, are typical of the genus.

Strongyloides stercoralis infections are most commonly fatal in puppies younger than 2–3 months, often from kennel environments. Affected dogs are wasted and dehydrated with evidence of diarrhea, perhaps blood tinged, but the intestine may only be congested or unremarkable at autopsy. Severe villus atrophy and heavy mononuclear interstitial infiltates are evident in the duodenum of affected dogs. Occasionally larvae may be present in granulomas in the lamina propria and submucosa. This suggests the possibility of autoinfection, or colonic penetration and systemic migration by filariform larvae originating in the gut. This occurs in *S. stercoralis* infections in humans and primates, and experimentally, in immunosuppressed dogs. Focal interstitial pneumonia may be associated with pulmonary migration.

Strongyloides felis may cause mild focal granulomatous or eosinophilic interstitial pneumonia in response to lung migration of larvae. In some cases there is local adenomatous hyperplasia of the crypts of Lieberkühn in the vicinity of worms in the small intestine, but no more general lesions. Diarrhea is uncommon.

Strongyloides tumefaciens in cats has been associated rarely with chronic diarrhea. It differs from the other species discussed, in being associated with the formation in the colon of submucosal nodules of proliferative glands, in which the worms are found. It is uncertain whether this is a specific lesion induced by infection, or merely herniation of infected colonic glands into space left by involution of a submucosal lymphoid follicle.

Bibliography

Dey-Hazra, A., Enigk, K., and Kohn, H. P. Intestinal absorption of palmitate and 2-aminoisobutyric acid in piglets infected with *Strongyloides ransomi. Res Vet Sci* **22:** 353–356, 1977.

Dey-Hazra, A. *et al.* Protein synthesis changes in the liver of piglets infected with *Strongyloides ransomi. Vet Parasitol* **5:** 339–351, 1979.

Enigk, K., and Dey-Hazra, A. Intestinal plasma and blood loss in piglets infected with *Strongyloides ransomi*. *Vet Parasitol* **1:** 69–75, 1975.

Enigk, K., Dey-Hazra, A., and Batke, J. Zur Klinischen Bedeuteing und Behandlung des galktogen erworbenen *Strongyloides*. Befalls der Fohlen. *Dtsch Tierärztl Wochenschr* **81:** 605–607, 1974.

Etherington, W. G., and Prescott, J. F. *Corynebacterium equi* cellulitis associated with *Strongyloides* penetration in a foal. *J Am Vet Med Assoc* **177:** 1025–1027, 1980.

Garcia, F. T. *et al.* Intestinal function and morphology in strongyloidiasis. *Am J Trop Med Hyg* **26:** 859–865, 1977.

Giese, W., Dey-Hazra, A., and Enigk, K. Enteric loss of plasma proteins in *Strongyloides* infection of pigs. *Int J Parasitol* **3:** 631–639, 1973.

Greer, G. J., Bello, T. R., and Amborski, G. F. Experimental infection of *Strongyloides westeri* in parasite-free ponies. *J Parasitol* **60:** 466–472, 1974.

Harmeyer, J. *et al.* Messung der intestinalen Resorptionsstorung durch *Strongyloides*-Befall bei Ferkeln. *Z Parasitenkd* **41:** 47–60, 1973.

Lyons, E. T., Drudge, J. H., and Tolliver, S. C. On the life cycle of *Strongyloides westeri* in the equine. *J Parasitol* **59:** 780–787, 1973.

Malone, J. B. *et al. Strongyloides tumefaciens* in cats. *J Am Vet Med Assoc* **171:** 278–280, 1977.

Moncol, D. J. Supplement to the life history of *Strongyloides ransomi* Schwartz and Alicata, 1930 (Nematoda: Strongyloididae) of pigs. *Proc Helminth Soc Wash* **42:** 86–92, 1975.

Nwaorgu, O. C., and Connan, R. M. The importance of arrested larvae in the maintenance of patent infections of *Strongyloides papillosus* in rabbits and sheep. *Vet Parasitol* **7:** 339–346, 1980.

Schad, G. A., Hellman, M. E., and Muncey, D. W. *Strongyloides stercoralis:* Hyperinfection in immunosuppressed dogs. *Exp Parasitol* **57:** 287–296, 1984.

Speare, R., and Tinsley, D. J. *Strongyloides felis:* An "old" worm rediscovered in Australian cats. *Aust Vet Practit* **16:** 10–18, 1986.

Stewart, T. B., Stone, W. M., and Marti, O. G. *Strongyloides ransomi:* Prenatal and transmammary infection of pigs of sequential litters from dams experimentally exposed as weanlings. *Am J Vet Res* **37:** 541–544, 1976.

Stone, W. M., and Smith, F. W. Infection of mammalian hosts by milk-borne nematode larvae: A review. *Exp Parasitol* **34:** 306–312, 1973.

Turner, J. H., and Shalkop, W. T. Larval migration and accompanying pathological changes in experimental ovine strongyloidiasis. *J Parasitol* **44:** 28–38, 1958.

b. INTESTINAL TRICHOSTRONGYLOSIS Members of the genus *Trichostrongylus* parasitize the anterior small intestine of ruminants the world over. They cause significant subclinical inefficiency in production, or clinical disease characterized by diarrhea, ill thrift, and, in some cases, death. The most important species infecting sheep and goats are *T. colubriformis, T. vitrinus,* and *T. rugatus;* others include *T. longispicularis, T. falculatus, T. capricola,* and *T. probolurus. Trichostrongylus colubriformis* and *T. longispicularis* also parasitize cattle. Though some *T. axei* may be found in the duodenum of cattle and sheep, this species is primarily parasitic in the abomasum.

Trichostrongylosis is most important in zones with a cool climate at some time of the year, but without extreme winters. It is an extremely important problem in many sheep-grazing areas of New Zealand, Australia, South Africa, South America, and the United Kingdom. Though gastrointestinal helminthosis is usually a mixed infection, *Trichostrongylus* often dominates, and appears to be a significant pathogen in its own right.

The life cycle is direct. Ingested third-stage larvae exsheath in the acid abomasal environment and establish preferentially in the proximal 5–6 m of the small intestine in sheep. A small proportion of the population settles in the abomasal antral mucosa near the pylorus. The larvae in the intestine enter tunnels above the basal lamina, between enterocytes, mainly at the base of villi (Fig. 1.169A), and they persist throughout their life at least partially embedded in the epithelium. Usually, infecting larvae all develop, over ~2 weeks, into adult worms, with a prepatent period of ~16–18 days. Hypobiosis appears to be relatively uncommon among members of the genus *Trichostrongylus,* and the circumstances by which it is stimulated are unclear. When it occurs, larvae are retarded in development at the parasitic third stage.

Experimental infections of all *Trichostrongylus* species studied indicate that the lesions and pathogenesis of disease caused by them are similar, though *T. vitrinus* seems more pathogenic than *T. colubriformis* and *T. rugatus.*

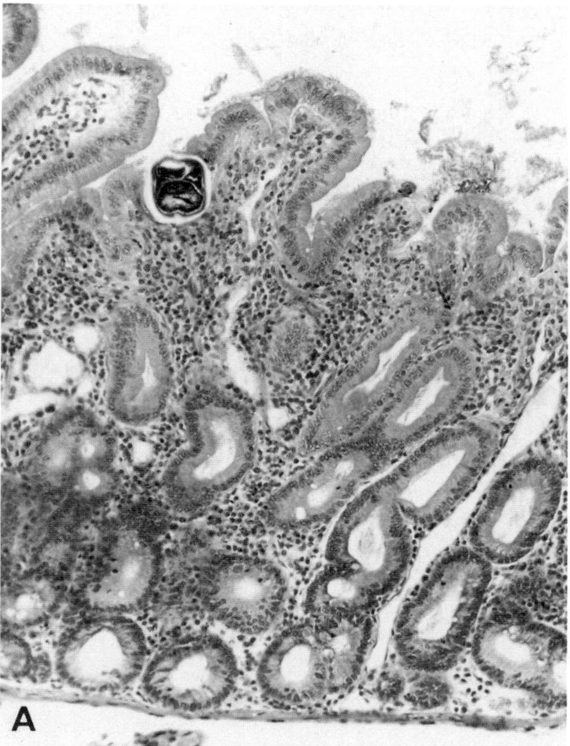

Fig. 1.169A Subtotal villus atrophy. *Trichostrongylus colubriformis,* intestine, sheep. Exfoliation of enterocytes, focal effusion of tissue fluid, dilated crypts, and mononuclear cells in lamina propria.

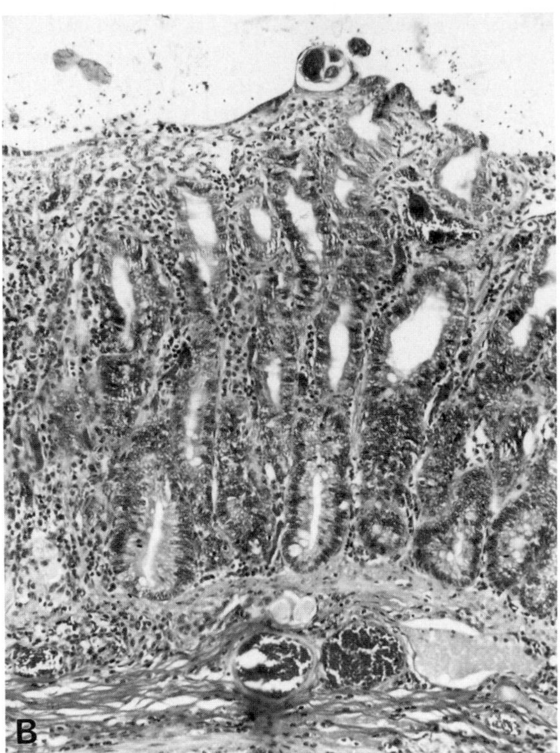

Fig. 1.169B Severe villus atrophy in intestinal trichostrongylosis. Sheep. Surface epithelium is attenuated or eroded, and crypts are hyperplastic. Nematode in tunnel in surface epithelium.

Villus atrophy occurs in areas of intestine populated heavily by the worms, and the severity of the lesion within individual animals is correlated with the local density of the worms. The mechanism by which the atrophy occurs has not been investigated. However, in experimental infections, hyperplasia of cryptal epithelium seems to precede the onset of villus atrophy. It may be that the lesion is induced by cell-mediated immune mechanisms, which stimulate proliferation by the epithelial proliferative compartment, and interfere with differentiation of cells emerging from crypts. In the rabbit model, there is a fourfold increase in the rate of cell production, and a twofold increase in the rate of cell movement along villi in the infected gut.

The established lesion is characterized microscopically by villus atrophy, which may vary considerably in severity, in association with elongate, dilated, often straight, crypts, containing many mitotic cells (Figs. 1.169A,B). Goblet cells may be numerous in some infected animals. In animals with subtotal villus atrophy, the surface epithelium may vary from tall, columnar, relatively normal-appearing cells, to more domed or cuboidal epithelium lacking a well-defined brush border. Ultrastructurally, such epithelium appears poorly differentiated, containing numerous polyribosomes in the cytoplasm, and with stumpy, sparse, and irregularly oriented microvilli. The levels of brush-border enzymes, notably alkaline phosphatase, peptidases, and maltase, are diminished in affected areas of intestine. In animals with subtotal villus atrophy, exfoliating rounded enterocytes are seen, as are focal and probably transient leaks of neutrophils and tissue fluids through the epithelial surface. In animals with more severe atrophy, the surface epithelium is flattened between the openings of crypts, and erosions of the mucosa may be evident, from which inflammatory cells and tissue fluid effuse.

The lamina propria in the affected area of intestine is populated by a moderately heavy mixed inflammatory cell population. Lymphocytes and plasma cells are prominent between crypts, with an admixture of eosinophils. Globule leukocytes may be present in the epithelium of crypts and occasionally villi, but this is often not marked in severely affected mucosa. In the superficial lamina propria, neutrophils often accumulate beneath the epithelium, and in areas of erosion or previous erosion, there may be a thin transversely oriented layer of connective tissue. Inflammatory cells do not seem to be specifically attracted to worms in tunnels in the surface epithelium. Abnormal permeability of the endothelium of capillaries and venules in heavily infected mucosa has been demonstrated, and edema of the lamina propria may be evident in these areas.

The disease is marked clinically by depression, inappetence, which may be mild or profound, and by diarrhea and wasting. The cause of the inappetence is unclear. It is suggested that it may be related to abnormalities in levels of some gastrointestinal hormones; it can be associated with concurrent gastrointestinal hypomotility, and gastric hyposecretion of acid with atrophy of fundic parietal cell mass. The pathogenesis of the diarrhea is also uncertain. It too is associated with the period when inappetence and gastric dysfunction occur. Though local malabsorption of nutrients, and presumably electrolytes and water, occurs in the duodenum, it seems unlikely that the absorptive capacity of the remaining small intestine and large bowel would be overwhelmed.

Weight loss or reduced productive efficiency is not related to nutrient malabsorption, since net absorption of nutrients over the length of the small intestine does not seem to be severely affected. Rather, the interaction of reduced feed consumption with increased loss of endogenous nitrogen into the gut seems to be responsible. There is considerable effusion of plasma protein into the intestine of infected animals, and this, coupled with exfoliation of epithelium, which appears to be turning over at an increased rate, is the source of protein loss. In trichostrongylosis, compensation for increased catabolism of plasma protein and mucosal epithelial protein is at the expense of anabolic processes elsewhere in the body. Wool and muscle growth are hindered in subclinical disease. In severely affected animals, breaks in the wool, muscle wasting, reduced skeletal growth, and osteoporosis are related to reduced deposition, or catabolism, of somatic and cutaneous protein, associated probably with functional hyperadrenocorticism. In addition, reduced mineralization of bone may be compounded by reduced intestinal absorption of phosphorus, and by loss of endogenous calcium, probably complexed with plasma albumin. The pathogenesis of trichostrongylosis in calves and goats is similar to that in sheep.

Animals succumbing to trichostrongylosis are usually cachectic and dehydrated. Dark green scoured feces will be on the skin or wool of the escutcheon or breech. There may be serous atrophy of internal fat depots, and marked atrophy of skeletal muscle. The subcutis is tacky. There may be edema of the mesentery and perhaps serous effusion into the body cavities, associated with hypoproteinemia, if dehydration is not severe. Mesenteric lymph nodes are enlarged and juicy. The content of the abomasum is abnormally fluid, and it may be greater than pH 4. The intestines are flaccid, and the small bowel contains thin, fluid, green content, which in the duodenum may appear somewhat mucoid. The large intestine may contain similar fluid or pasty green feces. These are usually foul smelling, probably due to products of bacterial action on protein.

The mucosa of the duodenum in the freshly killed animal may be glistening and pink, but in spontaneous mortalities with superimposed postmortem change, it will be unremarkable. Examination of the duodenal mucosa of freshly dead animals using a hand lens or dissecting microscope will reveal patchy or diffuse atrophy of villi, and fine white or translucent threadlike worms, ~5–8 mm long, entwined on the mucosal surface. The proximal third of the small intestine (~5–7 m) contains the bulk of the population of *Trichostrongylus*. A worm count on the small bowel usually reveals 15,000–80,000 *Trichostrongylus* in severe clinical infections. Subclinical or mild disease may be associated with fewer worms. The diagnosis is based on recovery of substantial populations of *Trichostrongylus* spp. in association with the clinicopathologic syndrome and villus atrophy. Mixed infections with other genera are common.

Bibliography

Barker, I. K. Intestinal pathology associated with *Trichostrongylus colubriformis* infection in sheep: Histology. *Parasitology* **70:** 165–171, 1975.

Barker, I. K. Intestinal pathology associated with *Trichostrongylus colubriformis* infection in sheep: Vascular permeability, and ultrastructure of the mucosa. *Parasitology* **70:** 173–180, 1975.

Barker, I. K., and Titchen, D. A. Gastric dysfunction in sheep infected with *Trichostrongylus colubriformis*, a nematode inhabiting the small intestine. *Int J Parasitol* **12:** 345–356, 1982.

Beveridge, I. *et al.* Comparison of the effects of infection with *Trichostrongylus colubriformis, T. vitrinus,* and *T. rugatus* in Merino lambs. *Vet Parasitol* **32:** 229–245, 1989.

Bown, M. D., Poppi, D. P., and Sykes, A. R. The effects of a concurrent infection of *Trichostrongylus colubriformis* and *Ostertagia circumcincta* on calcium, phosphorus, and magnesium transactions along the digestive tract of lambs. *J Comp Pathol* **101:** 11–20, 1989.

Coop, R. L., and Angus, K. W. The effect of continuous doses of *Trichostrongylus colubriformis* larvae on the intestinal mucosa of sheep and liver vitamin A concentration. *Parasitology* **70:** 1–9, 1975.

Coop, R. L., Angus, K. W., and Sykes, A. R. Chronic infection with *Trichostrongylus vitrinus* in sheep. Pathological changes in the small intestine. *Res Vet Sci* **26:** 363–371, 1979.

Gregory, P. C. *et al.* The influence of a chronic subclinical infection of *Trichostrongylus colubriformis* on gastrointestinal motility and digesta flow in sheep. *Parasitology* **91:** 381–396, 1985.

Hennessey, D., and Pritchard, R. K. Functioning of the thyroid gland in sheep infected with *Trichostrongylus colubriformis*. *Res Vet Sci* **30:** 87–92, 1981.

Horak, I. G., Clark, R., and Gray, R. S. The pathological physiology of helminth infestations. III. *Trichostrongylus colubriformis*. *Onderstepoort J Vet Res* **35:** 195–224, 1968.

Hoste, H. *Trichostrongylus colubriformis:* Epithelial cell kinetics in the small intestine of infected rabbits. *Exp Parasitol* **68:** 99–104, 1989.

Hoste, H., and Mariana, J. Cl. *Trichostrongylus colubriformis:* Epithelial cell migration in the proximal and distal small intestine of infected rabbits. *Exp Parasitol* **68:** 347–353, 1989.

Jones, D. G. Intestinal enzyme activity in lambs chronically infected with *Trichostrongylus colubriformis:* Effect of anthelmintic treatment. *Vet Parasitol* **12:** 79–89, 1983.

Kimambo, A. E. *et al.* Effect of prolonged subclinical infection with *Trichostrongylus colubriformis* on the performance and nitrogen metabolism of growing lambs. *Vet Parasitol* **28:** 191–203, 1988.

Roseby, F. B. Effect of *Trichostrongylus colubriformis* (Nematoda) on the nutrition and metabolism of sheep. III. Digesta flow and fermentation. *Aust J Agric Res* **28:** 155–164, 1977.

Shayo, M. E., and Benz, G. W. Histopathologic and histochemic changes in the small intestine of calves infected with *Trichostrongylus colubriformis*. *Vet Parasitol* **5:** 353–364, 1979.

Steel, J. W., Symons, L. E. A., and Jones, W. O. Effects of level of larval intake on the productivity and physiological and metabolic responses of lambs infected with *Trichostrongylus colubriformis*. *Aust J Agric Res* **31:** 821–838, 1980.

Sykes, A. R., Coop, R. L., and Angus, K. W. Experimental production of osteoporosis in growing lambs by continuous dosing with *Trichostrongylus colubriformis* larvae. *J Comp Pathol* **85:** 549–559, 1975.

Symons, L. E. A., and Hennessy, D. R. Cholecystokinin and anorexia in sheep infected by the intestinal nematode *Trichostrongylus colubriformis*. *Int J Parasitol* **11:** 55–58, 1981.

Taylor, S. M., and Pearson, G. R. *Trichostrongylus vitrinus* in sheep. II. The location of nematodes and associated pathological changes in the small intestine during clinical infection. *J Comp Pathol* **89:** 405–412, 1979.

Waller, P. J., Donald, A. D., and Dobson, R. J. Arrested development of intestinal *Trichostrongylus* spp. in grazing sheep and seasonal changes in the relative abundance of *T. colubriformis* and *T. vitrinus*. *Res Vet Sci* **30:** 213–216, 1981.

Wilson, W. D., and Field, A. C. Absorption and secretion of calcium and phosphorus in the alimentary tract of lambs infected with daily doses of *Trichostrongylus colubriformis* or *Ostertagia circumcincta* larvae. *J Comp Pathol* **93:** 61–71, 1983.

c. *Nematodirus* and *Cooperia* Infection ***Nematodirus*** species infect the anterior third of the small intestine of ruminants. The most important species are *N. helvetianus,* which infects cattle; *N. spathiger, N. filicollis,* and *N. abnormalis,* which infect sheep, goats, and cattle; and *N. battus,* a parasite mainly of sheep, which will cause disease in calves.

The life cycle is direct. However, hatching of infective larvae of *N. battus* and *N. filicollis* from the egg is delayed. Eggs of *N. battus* deposited on the ground in one year hatch the next spring, following a period of conditioning by cold over winter. The epizootiologic pattern is that of infection of a susceptible lamb crop during one year by larvae produced by the previous year's lambs. Under these conditions, with many infective larvae, parasitic enteritis dominated by *Nematodirus* may occur. The larvae of *N. spathiger* and *N. helvetinus* are not delayed in hatching, and their epizootiologic pattern resembles that of *Trichostrongylus* spp. in grazing animals. They often form part of a mixed population of worms in parasitic gastroenteritis in grazing lambs and calves. The disease may occur in yarded calves as well as animals at pasture.

Third-stage larvae enter the deeper layers of the mucosa, perhaps entering crypts. Larvae emerge at the fourth or fifth stage to take up residence coiled among the villi, with their posterior ends protruding toward the lumen. They normally do not penetrate the epithelium.

The presence of large numbers of some *Nematodirus* species is associated with the development of villus atrophy, which is usually moderate in comparison with that induced by *Strongyloides* or *Trichostrongylus*. The villi are compressed by the pressure of entwined nematodes, and the impression of the longitudinal cuticular ridges or synlophe is present on the surface of enterocytes adjacent to the worms. Local erosions may occur at such sites. Villi are stumpy, bifurcate, perhaps fused, or ridgelike surface alterations may replace the normal villous structures. Crypts may appear elongate and dilated.

Surface enterocytes may be domed, with loss of the prominent brush border, and irregular nuclear polarity. Ultrastructurally such cells appear poorly differentiated and have irregular, deformed microvilli. Biochemical studies reveal reduction in levels of mucosal alkaline phosphatase and disaccharidases, which correlate with the severity of diarrhea in affected sheep. If villus atrophy is severe, the ability of the worms to maintain their position may be compromised. They may enter crypts with their anterior end, move to more normal mucosa lower in the small bowel, or perhaps be lost from the gut.

The pathogenesis of the villus atrophy has not been determined, but it may be related to the development of an immune response to the nematodes in the lumen. A moderate mixed inflammatory response with substantial numbers of lymphocytes, plasma cells, and eosinophils is evident in the lamina propria. The presence of such an infiltrate, and moderate shortening of villi associated with poorly differentiated surface enterocytes, is consistent with the postulated induction of villus atrophy by cell-mediated immune activity in the lamina propria.

Lambs and calves with nematodirosis develop severe dark green diarrhea, which stains the escutcheon or the breech of lambs. Affected animals may become inappetent, scour and waste for several weeks before recovering, or they may die acutely. Disease is presumably mainly related to malabsorption and loss of appetite. Protein loss into the gut apparently has not been investigated. At necropsy, other than the changes associated with dehydration and cachexia, findings are limited to fluid mucoid content in the upper small intestine, and soft or fluid feces in the colon. The mucosa of the duodenum is usually unremarkable or perhaps hyperemic with excess mucus on the surface. Worm counts will reveal tangled cottony masses of elongate, lightly coiled nematodes in heavy *Nematodirus* infections. Clinical disease is associated with populations of ~10,000–50,000 or more *Nematodirus*.

Cooperia infect the upper small intestine of ruminants. The important species include *C. curticei* mainly in sheep and goats; and *C. pectinata, C. punctata,* and *C. oncophora,* mainly in cattle. Though both sheep and cattle may suffer from mixed burdens of helminths containing or dominated by populations of *Cooperia,* this species seems to be more significant in cattle, especially in cool temperate regions.

Cooperia has a typical trichostrongylid life cycle, but larvae do have the capacity to undergo hypobiosis to carry the population through periods of regular climatic adversity. The normal prepatent period is ~16–20 days. Like *Nematodirus, Cooperia* do not tunnel in the epithelium, but rather brace or coil themselves among villi to maintain their place in the intestine. In sections, the compression of epithelium adjacent to the worms, and the impressions left on enterocytes by the longitudinal cuticular ridges are apparent. In light infections the worms are concentrated in the anterior third of the small intestine. Heavier infections, perhaps because they are associated with villus atrophy and therefore loss of the substrate against which to brace, are more evenly distributed down the intestine.

Heavy burdens of *Cooperia* in calves, >70,000–80,000 nematodes, may be associated with inappetence, reduced weight gain, or weight loss and diarrhea, with protein-losing enteropathy in experimental infections. The associated atrophy of villi is concomitant with reductions in the brush-border enzymes. The syndrome is typical of intestinal helminthosis, and the diagnosis is confirmed by finding large numbers of the fine, coiled *Cooperia* in the small intestine.

Bibliography

Ahluwalia, J. S., and Charleston, W. A. G. Studies on the pathogenicity of *Cooperia curticei* for sheep. *N Z Vet J* **23:** 197–199, 1975.

Alicata, J. E., and Lynd, F. T. Growth rate and signs of infection in calves experimentally infected with *Cooperia punctata*. *Am J Vet Res* **22:** 704–707, 1961.

Armour, J. *et al.* Pathophysiological and parasitological studies on *Cooperia oncophora* infections in calves. *Res Vet Sci* **42:** 373–381, 1987.

Armour, J. *et al.* Clinical nematodiriasis in calves due to *Nematodirus battus* infection. *Vet Rec* **123:** 230–231, 1988.

Benz, G. W., and Ernst, J. V. Alkaline phosphatase activities in intestinal mucosa from calves infected with *Cooperia punctata* and *Eimeria bovis*. *Am J Vet Res* **37:** 896–899, 1976.

Beveridge, I., Martin, R. R., and Pullman, A. L. Development of the parasitic stages of *Nematodirus abnormalis* in experimentally infected sheep and associated pathology. *Proc Helminthol Soc Wash* **52:** 119–131, 1985.

Borgsteede, F. H. M., and Hendriks, J. Experimental infections with *Cooperia oncophora* (Railliet, 1918) in calves. Results of single infections with two graded dose levels of larvae. *Parasitology* **78:** 331–342, 1979.

Catchpole, J., and Harris, T. J. Interaction between coccidia and *Nematodirus battus* in lambs on pasture. *Vet Rec* **124:** 603–605, 1989.

Coop, R. L., Angus, K. W., and Mapes, C. J. The effect of large doses of *Nematodirus battus* on the histology and biochemistry of the small intestine of lambs. *Int J Parasitol* **3:** 349–361, 1973.

Coop, R. L., Sykes, A. R., and Angus, K. W. The pathogenicity of daily intakes of *Cooperia oncophora* larvae in growing calves. *Vet Parasitol* **5:** 261–269, 1979.

Mapes, C. J., Coop, R. L. and Angus, K. W. The fate of large infective doses of *Nematodirus battus* in young lambs. *Int J Parasitol* **3:** 339–347, 1973.

Martin, J., and Lee, D. L. *Nematodirus battus:* Scanning electron microscope studies of the duodenal mucosa of infected lambs. *Parasitology* **81:** 573–578, 1980.

Randall, R. W., and Gibbs, H. C. Effects of clinical and subclinical gastrointestinal helminthiasis on digestion and energy metabolism in calves. *Am J Vet Res* **42:** 1730–1734, 1981.

Samizadeh-Yazd, A., and Todd, A. C. Observations on the pathogenic effects of *Nematodirus helvetianus* in dairy calves. *Am J Vet Res* **40:** 48–51, 1979.

d. Hookworm Infection Members of the ancylostomatidae infect dogs, cats, ruminants, and swine. Hookworms of the genus *Globocephalus* appear to be of little significance in swine. In dogs, *Ancylostoma caninum, A. braziliense,* and *A. ceylanicum* occur. The former is most common in tropical, subtropical, and warm temperate zones of Africa, Australia, Asia, and North America, where adequate humidity for larval development occurs. *Ancylostoma braziliense* occurs in dogs and cats in the tropics and subtropics, whereas *A. ceylanicum* is found in both species in Sri Lanka and Southeast Asia. *Uncinaria stenocephala* occurs in dogs in cool temperate regions of Europe and North America. *Ancylostoma tubaeformae* occurs only in the cat.

Ancylostoma spp. are capable of infecting the host by four routes: (1) orally, with direct development to adult worms in the intestine; (2) by skin penetration, resulting in movement through the bloodstream to the lungs, and thence via the trachea to the pharynx and gut; (3) by the lactogenic transmission of third-stage larvae mobilized from dormancy in the skeletal muscle of parturient bitches; and (4) in occasional instances, by prenatal transplacental transmission of mobilized larvae. The latter route of transmission does not apparently occur in *A. braziliense* infection. Some larvae of *A. caninum* may become arrested at the third stage in the intestine, to resume development at a later time.

Ancylostoma spp. all usually inhabit the small intestine, where they move about the surface, several times a day attaching to feed, then moving on. They penetrate deeply into the mucosa, sometimes to, or through, the muscularis mucosae, taking a plug of tissue into the large buccal capsule. Tissue is lacerated by prominent teeth, and anticoagulant is released, permitting persistent blood flow. Bloodsucking activity begins when larvae enter the adult stage, in *A. caninum* ~8 days after infection. Blood loss is maximal while worms are attaining maturity between 12 and 16 days after infection, and then again during the peak period of egg production after ~3.5 weeks of infection. The prepatent period for *A. caninum* is ~15 days.

Ancylostomosis is the result of persistent blood loss, resulting in anemia and hypoproteinemia. There is considerable variation in the bloodsucking activity, and therefore the pathogenicity, of the members of the genus. *Ancylostoma caninum* consumes in the range of 0.01–0.2 ml of blood per worm per day. The amount of blood lost per worm is least in heavier infections. Pups several months old with populations of the order of 300–400 worms may lose 10–30% of their blood volume per day, depending on body weight. *Ancylostoma ceylanicum* also causes anemia, but *A. braziliense* seems to cause insignificant blood loss. *Ancylostoma tubaeformae* in cats is a significant bloodsucker. Experimentally, about 200 worms may cause anemia, weight loss, and mortality in 1.5-kg cats.

The anemia in ancylostomosis is at first normochromic and normocytic. If adequate iron reserves and hematopoietic capacity are mustered, the animal may be able to equilibrate the rate of red cell production with the increased rate of loss, stabilizing the mass of the reduced circulating red cell population. Small size, poor iron reserves, and the low level of iron in bitch's milk make suckling pups with ancylostomosis susceptible to rapid development of the microcytic hypochromic anemia characteristic of iron deficiency.

Acute fatal ancylostomosis occurs most commonly in pups only 2–3 weeks of age, infected via the bitch's milk. Heavy infections acquired by this route may result in death from anemia and hypoproteinemia within a few days of the initiation of bloodsucking activity, and before eggs are present in the feces. Anemia may also lead to mortality of pups after a course of longer duration. Percutaneous infection results in disease in older dogs held in runs or kennels under conditions of moisture and temperature conducive to larval development on the ground. Dermatitis due to larval penetration may be observed between the toes or on ventral contact surfaces of the body. Ancylostomosis in older dogs is usually typified by anemia, lack of exercise tolerance, weakness, and emaciation. Feces may be diarrheic, dark red or black, and are often mucoid. Though diarrhea may occur, and there is some evidence for mild malabsorption and subtle atrophy of the intestinal mucosa, the major effect of ancylostomosis is due to increased loss of erythrocytes, iron, and plasma protein.

Animals dying of ancylostomosis are characteristically extremely pale. There is often glistening edema of subcutaneous tissues and mesenteries, and serous effusion into body cavities, attributable to hypoproteinemia. In chronic infections, cachexia may be evident. If recent exposure to heavy percutaneous infection has occurred, there may be dermatitis, and numerous focal hemorrhages scattered in the pulmonary parenchyma, reflecting disruption of vessels by larvae breaking out into alveoli. The liver has the blotchy pallor of anemia. The intestinal content throughout the entire length is mucoid and deep red, from the erythrocytes voided into it by the worms (Fig. 1.170). The latter are visible, ~1–1.5 cm long, translucent, gray or red, depending on when they last consumed blood, dispersed over the mucosa, sometimes into the large intestine. They are often attached to the mucosa, and pinpoint red sites of recent feeding activity may be scattered over the intestinal surface. Relatively few *A. caninum* are required to cause death. In a young pup as few as 20–50 worms may be present in fatal infections, and they may be sufficiently sparsely scattered as to be overlooked, if not sought. In older animals with chronic or more acute fatal disease, 300–400, or less commonly, several thousands of worms, may be present.

Uncinaria stenocephala infects mainly by the oral route; percutaneous infection is not efficient, though dermatitis may result; and prenatal and lactogenic transmission appear not to occur. This species sucks little blood and is much less pathogenic than is *A. caninum*. However, heavy infections with this species, arising usually in contaminated communal kennel environments, may cause clinical disease and occasional mortality in pups. Nonspecific lethargy, inappetence, and ill thrift are signs of infection, perhaps with diarrhea; anemia does not occur. Disease is associated with burdens of more than ~1000 worms. Worms, each ~5–10 mm long, may be particularly distributed in the distal half of the small bowel, and sometimes are found in the colon in heavy infections. They are often embedded in the mucosa in freshly dead animals. The intestinal mucosa appears thickened, with scattered focal hemorrhages at sites of attachment.

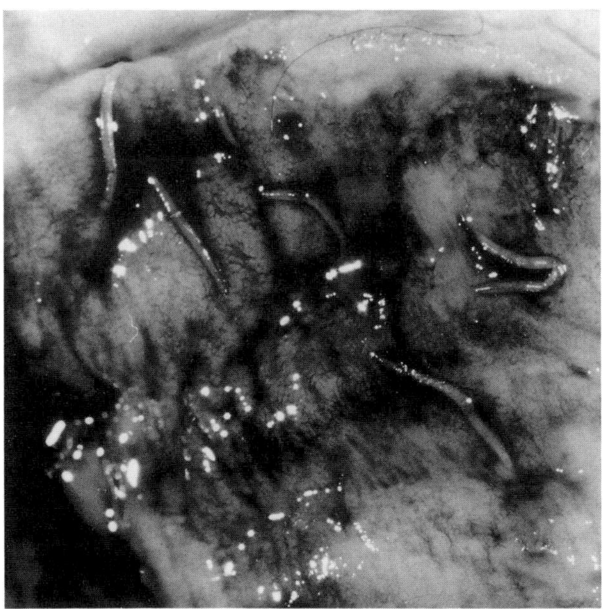

Fig. 1.170 Robust *Ancylostoma caninum* nematodes attached to mucosa. Small intestine. Pup died from exsanguination by hookworms. Gut content is bloody.

The presence of large numbers of worms is associated with moderate atrophy and thickening of villi. The surface epithelium is irregular. Focal aggregates of mononuclear cells and some neutrophils are in the vicinity of the anterior end of worms embedded deep in the mucosa, a plug of tissue within their buccal cavity. Disease due to *U. stenocephala* may be related to villus atrophy, with protein loss into the gut, and perhaps malabsorption. Hypoproteinemia may be evident, but anemia does not occur. A similar syndrome may be associated with heavy infections of *A. braziliense,* in which hypoproteinemia also occurs.

The **hookworms of ruminants** include the following: in cattle, *Bunostomum phlebotomum* and in India and Indonesia, *Agriostomum vryburgi;* in sheep, *Bunostomum trigonocephalum* and, in India and Southeast Asia, Africa, and South America, *Gaigeria pachyscelis*. The life cycle of these nematodes is typical of hookworms. *Bunostomum* third-stage larvae infect by the oral or percutaneous routes, whereas *Gaigeria* infect only across the skin. Eggs and larval stages on the ground are extremely susceptible to desiccation, and hookworm disease in ruminants is most common in tropical or subtropical areas during wet seasons. However, stabled animals in cooler temperate areas may suffer disease resulting from larvae invading the skin from contaminated bedding. Following skin penetration, the usual pattern is seen, with migration of larvae to the lungs where they molt to the fourth stage, and subsequently pass up the trachea to the digestive tract. Larvae taken in by ingestion spend some time in the deep mucosa of the intestine before emerging to mature in the lumen of the small intestine. The prepatent period of *Bunostomum* is long, ~7–8 weeks. *Gaigeria* larvae migrate via the lungs, and worms begin to lay eggs ~10 weeks after infection.

Both *Bunostomum* and *Gaigeria* cause hemorrhagic anemia and hypoproteinemia, especially in animals younger than a year. These species often occur with mixed gastrointestinal helminth burdens, and their effects are at least additive to those of the other worms. They may be primary pathogens. Several hundred *Bunostomum* may cause signs in lambs and a few hundred to a few thousand are found in clinical or fatal infections in calves. As few as 20–30 *Gaigeria* will cause anemia and hypoproteinemia in lambs and kids, though several times that number may be more usual in fatal cases. The size of the animal, the status of its iron reserves, and the plane of nutrition, especially the level of protein, are likely to influence the pathogenicity of these species.

At autopsy, the lesions expected in anemia and hypoproteinemia are evident. *Bunostomum* are found often in the lower half of the small intestine, whereas *Gaigeria* tends to be concentrated high in the duodenum. Blood and bite marks may be evident on the mucosa in the infected areas of intestine, but hemorrhage may be occult. The relatively low numbers of worms associated with disease, and their peculiar distribution, dictate that the entire gut be examined and flushed, and a careful search be made for these species in suspect cases. Hemonchosis may occur concurrently, or should be eliminated as a diagnosis, as should fasciolosis, and in cattle, *Oesophagostomum radiatum* infection.

Bibliography

Ansari, M. Z., Singh, K. S., and Iyer, P. K. R. A note on histological studies on the experimental infection of *Gaigeria pachyscelis* Railliet and Henry, 1910, in natural and laboratory animals. *Indian J Anim Sci* **49:** 491–493, 1979.

Areekul, S., Tipayamontri, U., and Ukoskit, K. Experimental infection of *Ancylostoma braziliense* in dogs and cats in Thailand. II. Blood loss. *S E Asian J Trop Med Publ Health* **5:** 230–235, 1974.

Baker, K. P., and Grimes, T. D. Cutaneous lesions in dogs associated with hookworm infestation. *Vet Rec* **87:** 376–379, 1970.

Buelke, D. L. Hookworm dermatitis. *J Am Vet Med Assoc* **158:** 735–739, 1971.

Carroll, S. M., and Grove, D. I. Response of dogs to challenge with *Ancylostoma ceylanicum* during the tenure of a primary hookworm infection. *Trans R Soc Trop Med Hyg* **80:** 406–411, 1986.

Carroll, S. M. *et al.* Transmission electron microscopical studies of the site of attachment of *Ancylostoma ceylanicum* to the small bowel mucosa of the dog. *J Helminthol* **58:** 313–320, 1984.

Gibbs, H. C. On the gross and microscopic lesions produced by the adults and larvae of *Dochmoides stenocephala* (Railliet, 1884) in the dog. *Can J Comp Med* **22:** 382–385, 1958.

Hart, R. J., and Wagner, A. M. The pathological physiology of *Gaigeria pachyscelis* infection. *Onderstepoort J Vet Res* **38:** 111–116, 1971.

Jacobs, D. E. The epidemiology of hookworm infection of dogs in the UK. *Vet Ann* **18:** 220–224, 1978.

Kalkofen, U. P. Intestinal trauma resulting from feeding activities of *Ancylostoma caninum*. *Am J Trop Med Hyg* **23:** 1046–1053, 1974.

Kalkofen, U. P. Hookworms of dogs and cats. *Vet Clin North Am: Small Anim Pract* **17:** 1341–1354, 1987.

Lee, K. T., Little, M. D., and Beaver, P. C. Intracellular (muscle-fiber) habitat of *Ancylostoma caninum* in some mammalian hosts. *J Parasitol* **61:** 589–598, 1975.

Migasena, S., Gilles, H. M., and Maegraith, B. G. Studies in *Ancylostoma caninum* infection in dogs. II. Anatomical changes in the gastrointestinal tract. *Ann Trop Med Parasitol* **66:** 203–207, 1972.

Miller, T. A. Blood loss during hookworm infection, determined by erythrocyte labeling with radioactive ^{51}Chromium. II. Pathogenesis of *Ancylostoma braziliense* infection in dogs and cats. *J Parasitol* **52:** 856–865, 1966.

Nascimento, A. A. *et al.* Estudos clínico e anátomo-patholôgico em ovinos (*Ovis aries*) e em caprinos (*Capra hircus*) infestados experimentalmente com *Gaigeria pachyscelis* Railliet and Henry, 1910 (Nematoda: Ancylostomatoidea). *Ars Vet* **4:** 113–124, 1988.

Onwuliri, C. O. E., Nwosu, A. B. C., and Anya, A. O. Experimental *Ancylostoma tubaeforme* infection of cats: Changes in blood values and worm burden in relation to single infections of varying size. *Z Parasitenkd* **64:** 149–155, 1981.

Pacenovsky, J., and Brezanska, M. Penetration of *Bunostomum phlebotomum* larvae into the body of cattle. *Vet Med Praha* **13:** 277–383, 1968.

Pearson, G. R. *et al.* Uncinariasis in kennelled foxhounds. *Vet Rec* **110:** 328–331, 1982.

Schad, G. A., and Page, M. R. *Ancylostoma caninum:* Adult worm removal, corticosteroid treatment, and resumed development of arrested larvae in dogs. *Exp Parasitol* **54:** 303–309, 1982.

Smith, B. L., and Elliot, D. C. Canine pedal dermatitis due to percutaneous *Uncinaria stenocephala* infection. *N Z Vet J* **17:** 235–239, 1969.

Soulsby, E. J. L., Venn, J. A. J., and Green, K. N. Hookworm disease in British cattle. *Vet Rec* **67:** 1124–1125, 1955.

Spellman, G. G., Jr., and Nossel, H. L. Anticoagulant activity of dog hookworm. *Am J Physiol* **220:** 922–927, 1971.

Stoye, M. Untersuchungen uber die Moglichkeit pranataler und galaktogener Infektionen mit *Ancylostoma caninum* Ercolani 1859 (Ancylostomidae) beim Hund. *Zentralbl Veterinaermed (B)* **20:** 1–39, 1973.

Walker, M. J., and Jacobs, D. E. Pathophysiology of *Uncinaria stenocephala* infections of dogs. *Vet Ann* **25:** 263–271, 1985.

Williams, J. C. *et al.* Experimental and natural infection of calves with *Bunostomum phlebotomum*. *Vet Parasitol* **13:** 225–237, 1983.

e. *TRICHURIS* INFECTION *Trichuris* species, the whipworms, are so called because of their long, thin anterior end and shorter, stouter posterior portion. They inhabit the cecum, and occasionally the colon, of all the domestic animals considered here, except the horse. The host–parasite relationships include the following: in dogs, *T. vulpis;* in cats, *T. campanula* and *T. serrata;* in swine, *T. suis;* in sheep and goats, *T. ovis, T. globulosa, T. skrjabini;* in cattle, *T. discolor* and less commonly *T. ovis* and *T. globulosa*.

The life cycle is direct. Larvated ova are resistant to climatic insult, and persist in contaminated environments for several years. Ingestion of larvated eggs leads to release of third-stage larvae, which enter the mucosa of the anterior small intestine for as long as 7–10 days, before returning to the lumen and passing on to the cecum where they establish their adult existence. The prepatent period varies from ~6–7 weeks in the case of *T. suis* to 11–12 weeks for *T. vulpis*. In rare instances, disease may occur during the prepatent period, in which case, ova will not be in the feces.

In all species the anterior end of the worm is embedded at least partially in tunnels within the surface epithelium (Fig. 1.171), but not normally breaching the basal lamina. Light infections apparently cause little morphologic alteration in the mucosa and no disease. Although *Trichuris* ingest blood, disease associated with them is not usually related to this activity. Moderate infection of *T. vulpis* in dogs is associated with a mild mucosal colitis. There is a moderate mixed inflammatory infiltrate in the lamina propria between glands. Superficial vessels are congested, and scattered neutrophils may be present in the lamina propria beneath the surface epithelium. There is focal loss of goblet cells on the surface. These are replaced by low columnar or cuboidal cells, some of which may be exfoliat-

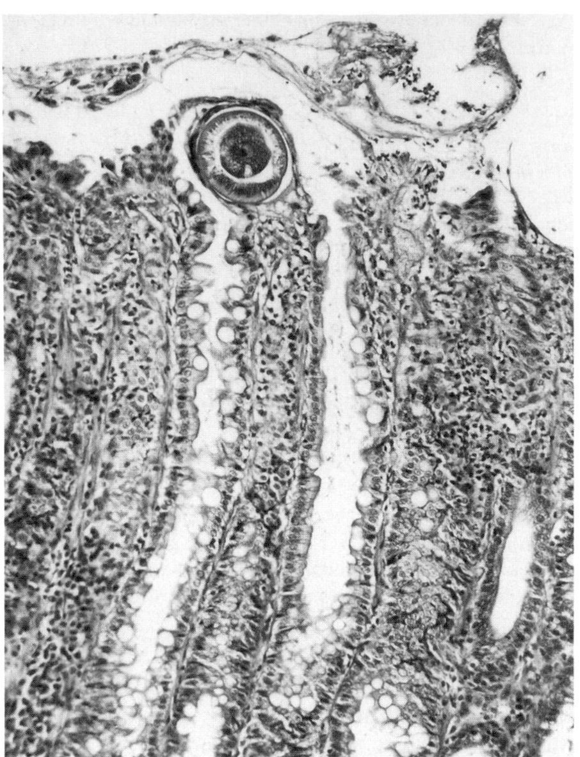

Fig. 1.171 Mild erosive colitis. Dog. *Trichuris vulpis*. Anterior end of nematode is in tunnel in surface epithelium. There is exfoliation of epithelium, and effusion of neutrophils and fibrin from the surface.

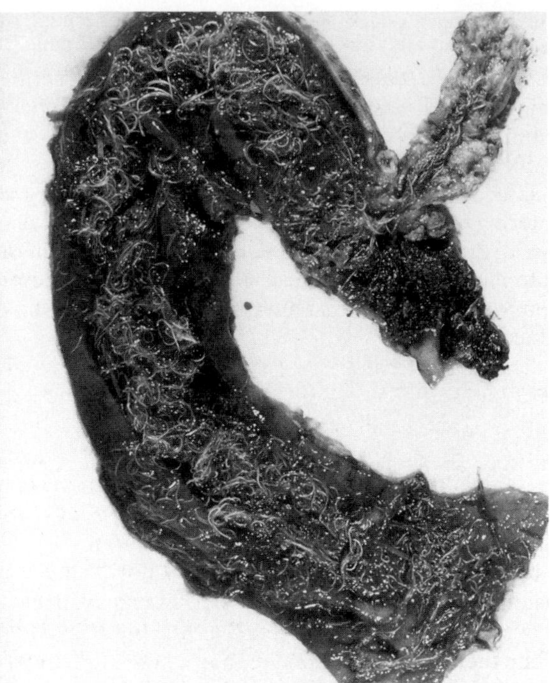

Fig. 1.172 *Trichuris vulpis* typhocolitis. Dog.

ing. Focal erosion may also be evident, and effusion of a few neutrophils and tissue fluid is evident through leaks or erosions on the surface. Goblet cells may be sparser than normal in glands in affected areas, which often appear longer than usual, and are lined by hyperplastic epithelium.

Heavy infection with *Trichuris* is associated with severe and often hemorrhagic typhlitis or typhlocolitis in all species. In the **dog,** large populations of worms overflow their normal habitat and infect the mucosa of the ascending, and often more distal, colon, sometimes extending to the rectum. The signs are chronic diarrhea or dysentery, perhaps with some weight loss. The blood and foul odor of the feces is related to hemorrhage and effusion of tissue fluid from the eroded mucosal surface. The mucosa is thickened, red, and edematous. The colonic content is fluid or porridgelike, and brown, tinged pink or red. Masses of tangled worms are visible on the mucosa (Fig. 1.172). Microscopically the mucosa is widely eroded, or mildly ulcerated, and effusion of inflammatory exudate and blood is evident. Glandular epithelium is hyperplastic. Occasionally, *T. vulpis* infection may be associated with local or regional transmural lesions, with granulomatous foci and fibroplasia in deeper layers of the mucosa. Sometimes ova or worms are in these aberrant locations. Other transmural lesions may be the result of bacteria entering through mucosa damaged by *Trichuris*. *Balantidium* infection has been reported as a rare complication of *Trichuris* infection in dogs with access to swine yards.

Trichuris suis infection in **swine,** if heavy enough, may cause mucohemorrhagic typhlocolitis, which is associated with anorexia, diarrhea or dysentery, dehydration, ill thrift, and in some cases, death. The disease is most common in animals exposed to dirt yards contaminated with infective *Trichuris* ova. The lesion is one of mucosal colitis, resembling that described in the dog. There is thickening of the mucosa with mucus hypersecretion from hypertrophic glands, coupled with erosion of, and effusion from, the mucosal surface. Lesions are more severe in swine with conventional gut flora, than in those reared germ free, or free of known enteric pathogens. Some contribution of the normal anaerobe flora to the development of lesions more severe than mild catarrhal colitis is apparent.

The large bowel in swine with *Trichuris* is thickened and congested, possibly with focal hemorrhages. The surface is glistening with mucus, perhaps with some fibrin exudation. The gross appearance may resemble that found in swine dysentery, and the microscopic lesions are similar. However, closer examination will reveal the presence of the nematodes over the mucosa. Usually the thicker posterior end of the worms is noted. They may resemble at first glance *Oesophagostomum,* and only on more careful observation is the elongate threadlike anterior end seen.

The signs of the disease appear to be referable to loss of colonic absorptive function, and probably partly because of effusion of protein into the lumen. Though erythrocyte loss does occur, it is a minor component of the pathogenesis.

Trichurosis in **sheep** and **cattle** resembles that described in swine. The disease usually occurs in animals concentrated in areas contaminated by ova; hence, it may occur in stabled or yarded cattle. Outbreaks in sheep may be associated with hand feeding or congregation of animals at watering points. Affected animals develop chronic diarrhea with brown feces or dysentery, and loss of condition. At autopsy the lesions are those of cachexia and hypoproteinemia, associated with a mucohemorrhagic typhlitis or typhlocolitis.

A diagnosis of trichurosis in all species is usually readily made at autopsy. The worms have a characteristic morphology and are usually easily seen on the inflamed mucosal surface. In section, the thin anterior end of the nematodes, embedded in tunnels in the surface epithelium, contains the stichosome esophagus typical of members of the Trichuroidea, and a single bacillary band. The ova may be seen in the body of worms, in the gut lumen, or occasionally in tissue. They are barrel-shaped, have a thick wall, and plugs at both poles of the egg. *Capillaria* spp. and their ova may be similar in tissue section, but are not expected in the cecum and colon.

Bibliography

Batte, E. G. *et al.* Pathophysiology of swine trichuriasis. *Am J Vet Res* **38:** 1075–1079, 1977.

Beck, J., and Beverley-Burton, M. The pathology of *Trichuris, Capillaria* and *Trichinella* infections. *Helminthol Abstracts* **37:** 1–26, 1968.

Beer, R. J. S. Studies on the biology of the life-cycle of *Trichuris suis* Schrank 1788. *Parasitology* **67:** 253–262, 1973.

Beer, R. J. S., and Lean, I. J. Clinical trichuriasis produced experimentally in growing pigs. Part 1: Pathology of infection. *Vet Rec* **93:** 189–195, 1973.

Beveridge, I., and Green, P. E. Species of *Trichuris* in domestic ruminants in Australia. *Aust Vet J* **57:** 141–142, 1981.

Ewing, S. A., and Bull, R. W. Severe chronic canine diarrhea associated with *Balantidium–Trichuris* infection. *J Am Vet Med Assoc* **149:** 519–520, 1966.

Frechette, J. L. *et al.* Infection des jeunes bovins par *Trichuris discolor. Can Vet J* **14:** 243–246, 1973.

Hall, G. A., Rutter, J. M., and Beer, R. J. S. A comparative study of the histopathology of the large intestine of conventionally reared, specific pathogen-free and gnotobiotic pigs infected with *Trichuris suis. J Comp Pathol* **86:** 285–292, 1976.

Hendrix, C. M., Blagburn, B. L., and Lindsay, D. S. Whipworms and intestinal threadworms. *Vet Clin North Am: Small Anim Pract* **17:** 1355–1375, 1987.

Malik, R. *et al.* Severe whipworm infection in the dog. *J Small Anim Pract* **31:** 185–188, 1990.

Perdrizet, J. A., and King, J. M. Whipworm (*Trichuris discolor*) infection in dairy replacement heifers. *J Am Vet Med Assoc* **188:** 1063–1064, 1986.

Ruben, R. Studies on the common whipworm of the dog, *T. vulpis. Cornell Vet* **44:** 36–39, 1954.

Rutter, J. M., and Beer, R. J. S. Synergism between *Trichuris suis* and the microbial flora of the large intestine causing dysentery in pigs. *Infect Immunol* **11:** 395–404, 1975.

Widmer, W. R., and Van Kruiningen, H. J. *Trichuris*-induced transmural ileocolitis in a dog—an entity mimicking regional enteritis. *J Am Anim Hosp Assoc* **10:** 581–585, 1974.

f. *Oesophagostomum* and *Chabertia* Infection Members of the genus *Oesophagostomum* infect sheep, cattle, and swine. They form inflammatory nodules in the wall of the intestine, incited by histotropic larval stages. Ill thrift, diarrhea and, in cattle, anemia are induced by adult populations in the lumen of the colon.

In **sheep,** two species, *O. columbianum* and *O. venulosum,* are probably most significant; the former is considerably more pathogenic and is particularly important in warm temperate to tropical areas. Third-stage *O. columbianum* penetrate deeply into the lamina propria, or sometimes to the submucosa, mainly in the small intestine, where they normally spend ~1 week. They molt, emerge, and mature in the colon. However, a proportion of fourth-stage larvae enters a second histotropic phase in nodules in the colonic submucosa. Adult worms in the colon may be pathogenic for lambs. Burdens of only a few hundred *O. columbianum* are associated with anorexia, mucoid feces or diarrhea, and ill thrift. The effects of infection may be exacerbated by intercurrent malnutrition.

At autopsy of animals with clinical oesophagostomosis, the carcass is emaciated, the mesenteric lymph nodes are enlarged, and the colonic mucosa is thickened, congested, and covered by a layer of mucus in which the worms are scattered. There is hyperplasia of goblet cells, and the lamina propria contains a heavy mixed inflammatory infiltrate with eosinophils and many immune-active cells. Globule leukocytes are in the epithelium of glands. Nodules caused by histotropic fourth-stage larvae, mainly in the large intestine, are ~0.5–1 cm in diameter and are composed of a central caseous or mineralized core surrounded by a thin, fibrous encapsulating stroma. Microscopically, the nematode (or its remnants) is present among a mass of necrotic debris in which eosinophils are prominent. Giant cells and macrophages may surround the necrotic material. Similar nodules may be found in liver, lungs, mesentery, and mesenteric lymph nodes. Those in the deeper layers of the gut project from the serosal surface, hence the name pimply gut. They may cause adhesion to adjacent loops of gut or to other organs, and rarely may incite intussusception or peritonitis. However, in most cases, nodules are incidental findings at autopsy. They are probably the response to histotropic fourth-stage larvae in hosts sensitized by third-stage larvae, or by prior infection. The nodules caused by the histotropic third stage consist of small concentrations of suppurative exudate which resolve as minor foci of granulomatous inflammation after the evacuation of the larvae.

Oesophagostomum venulosum is a much less significant parasite. It seldom causes significant nodule formation; when it does, the nodules are small and mainly in the cecum and colon. Adult worm burdens are usually not considered particularly pathogenic.

In **cattle,** two species, *O. radiatum* and *O. venulosum* occur, the former being the significant parasite. The life cycle is similar to that of *O. columbianum*. The disease caused by *O. radiatum* is characterized by loss of appetite, reduced productive efficiency, anemia, hypoproteinemia, and diarrhea. Anemia results from hemorrhage at sites of larval emergence, and from mucosal erosions and discontinuities in the gland lining, associated with maturing and adult populations of worms. Blood loss is exacerbated by impaired coagulation, probably the result of consumption of clotting factors, the initiating mechanism for which is unclear. Considerable exudation of tissue fluids and plasma protein from colonic lesions, in addition to that due to hemorrhage, contributes to the hypoproteinemia and gastrointestinal protein loss. Reduced growth, or loss in condition, is mainly the product of the interaction between protein effusion into the gut and inappetence. Diarrhea presumably results in part from loss of colonic absorptive capacity.

Oesophagostomosis may be fatal in calves. Animals may be pale from anemia, and edematous from hypoproteinemia. Cases of some duration will be cachectic. Colonic lymph nodes are enlarged. The mucosa of the colon is grossly thickened and folded by edema and increased mixed inflammatory cell infiltrates, including many immune active cells, in the lamina propria. Colonic submucosal lymphoid follicles are large and active. Effusion of tissue fluid and blood cells may be evident through small leaks between cells, or from erosions in glands or on the surface. Pathogenic worm burdens in calves are in the range of ~1000–10,000 *O. radiatum*. Although repeated exposure to infective larvae may result in the accumulation of large numbers of fourth-stage worms in nodules, formation of nodules has little pathogenic significance in cattle.

In **swine,** *O. dentatum, O. quadrispinulatum,* and several other species occur in the large intestine; the two mentioned are most widespread. The life cycle is typical of the genus. Third-stage larvae enter the wall of the cecum and colon, where they encyst and molt to the fourth stage, emerging ~1 week later to mature in the lumen. The larvae initially lie about the level of the base of the mucosa. They incite a reaction which causes local loss of the muscularis mucosae, so that the nodule formed involves both mucosa and submucosa, and the larvae ultimately reside in the submucosa. The nodules are grossly ~1–20 mm in diameter, umbilicate, and may contain yellow or black cheesy exudate in the center. An eosinophilic cyst wall surrounds the third-stage larva. Nearby lymphatics may undergo thrombosis. Once the larvae molt and begin to move to the lumen, an intense influx of eosinophils and neutrophils occurs into the nodules, and a focus of necrotic debris and fibrin lies over the evacuated nodule. Mucosal and submucosal edema causes thickening of the wall of the large bowel, and contraction of the cecum. Gross and microscopic lesions resolve over the ensuing weeks as most larvae leave the mucosa.

Oesophagostomosis in swine is a mild, usually subclinical disease. Occasional diarrhea, depression in weight gain, and inefficiency of feed conversion may occur, especially during the period of emergence of larvae and maturation of worms in the lumen of the large intestine. Burdens of ~3000–20,000 adult worms are associated with subclinical disease experimentally. The nematodes are ~1–2 cm long, white, and are present in mucus on the surface of the gut, or in luminal content. Occasionally, infection with *Oesophagostomum,* particularly mucosal damage precipitated by larval encystment, may predispose to necrotic enteritis in association with anaerobic flora and perhaps *Balantidium*. Massive repeated challenge will cause severe typhlocolitis, but this seems to be purely an experimental phenomenon. Mortality should rarely, if ever, be ascribed to oesophagostomosis in pigs.

Chabertia ovina, a robust worm ~1–2 cm long, inhabits the colon of sheep, goats, and cattle. It is particularly a problem in cooler climatic zones, mainly in sheep. The life cycle resembles that of *Oesophagostomum,* third-stage larvae encysting in the wall of the small intestine, then emerging to mature in the cecum and colon. Disease in sheep is associated with the presence of mature worms in the colon. Feces are soft, mucoid, and perhaps blood flecked, and ill thrift may occur. The adults penetrate to the muscularis mucosae and take a plug of mucosa into the buccal capsule; minor hemorrhage may be related to physical trauma to the mucosa. More significant is loss of plasma protein from the mucosa, associated with numerous focal sites of trauma, and with widespread areas of mononuclear infiltration in the mucosa and submucosa. There is also hyperplasia of goblet cells. Grossly the lesions are characterized by edema of all layers of the wall of infected parts of the colon, and enlargement of colonic lymph nodes. Worms are generally concentrated in the proximal portion of the spiral colon, and the area they inhabit may have numerous hemorrhagic foci corresponding to sites of former attachment. Pathogenic burdens may be as few as 150 worms, and the species must be sought in its usual site of predilection or be missed.

Bibliography

Bawden, R. J. Relationships between *Oesophagostomum columbianum* infection and the nutritional status of sheep. III. Serum and tissue protein changes. *Aust J Agric Res* **20:** 965–970, 1969.

Bremner, K. C., and Fridemanis, R. *Oesophagostomum radiatum* in calves: Intestinal hemorrhage associated with larval emergence. *Exp Parasitol* **36:** 24–429, 1974.

Bremner, K. C., and Fridemanis, R. A defibrination syndrome in calves caused by histotropic larvae of *Oesophagostomum radiatum*. *J Comp Pathol* **85:** 83–390, 1975.

Clark, R. G., Mason, P. C., and Fennessy, P. F. Nodular lesions in the absence of *Oesophagostomum columbianum*. *N Z Vet J* **26:** 33, 1978.

Dash, K. M. The life cycle of *Oesophagostomum columbianum* (Curtice, 1890) in sheep. *Int J Parasitol* **3:** 843–851, 1973.

Dobson, C. Changes in the protein content of the serum and intestinal mucus of sheep with reference to the histology of the gut and immunological response to *Oesophagostomum columbianum* infections. *Parasitology* **57:** 201–219, 1967.

Elek, P., and Durie, P. H. The histopathology of the reactions of calves to experimental infection with the nodular worm *Oesophagostomum columbianum* (Rudolphi, 1803). II. Reaction of the susceptible host to infection with a single dose of larvae. *Aust J Agric Res* **18:** 549–559, 1967.

Hale, O. M. *et al.* Influence of an experimental infection of nodular worms (*Oesophagostomum* spp.) on performance of pigs. *J Anim Sci* **52:** 316–322, 1981.

Herd, R. P. The pathogenic importance of *Chabertia ovina* (Fabricius, 1788) in experimentally infected sheep. *Int J Parasitol* **1:** 251–263, 1971.

McCracken, R. M., and Ross, J. G. The histopathology of *Oesophagostomum dentatum* infections in pigs. *J Comp Pathol* **80:** 619–623, 1970.

Poelvoorde, J., and Berghen, P. Experimental infection of pigs with *Oesophagostomum dentatum:* Pathogenesis and parasitology of repeated mass infection. *Res Vet Sci* **31:** 10–13, 1981.

Shelton, G. C., and Griffiths, H. J. *Oesophagostomum columbianum:* Experimental infections in lambs. Effects of different types of exposure on the intestinal lesions. *Pathol Vet* **4:** 413–434, 1967.

Stewart, M. *et al.* The energy and nitrogen metabolism and performance of pigs infected with *Oesophagostomum dentatum. Anim Prod* **36:** 137–142, 1983.

Stewart, T. B., and Gasbarre, L. C. The veterinary importance of nodular worms (*Oesophagostomum* spp.). *Parasitol Today* **5:** 209–213, 1989.

Stockdale, P. H. G. Necrotic enteritis of pigs caused by infection with *Oesophagostomum* spp. *Br Vet J* **126:** 526–530, 1970.

g. EQUINE STRONGYLOSIS Members of the Strongylidae are common nematode parasites of the cecum and colon in horses, usually present as mixed infections. The subfamily Strongylinae are the large strongyles, including the important genus *Strongylus* and the less significant genera *Triodontophorus, Oesophagodontus,* and *Craterostomum.* Members of this group are plug feeders or bloodsuckers, and *Strongylus* spp. undergo extensive extraintestinal migrations. The subfamily Cyathostominae, or small strongyles, includes eight genera of nematodes, among several of which the species of the superseded genus *Trichonema* have now been dispersed. Adults of this group feed mainly on intestinal contents, and are of little pathogenic significance. However, emergence of histotropic larval stages from the gut wall may cause disease.

i. *Large Strongyles* ***Strongylus vulgaris*** is common, and is the most significant nematode parasitic in horses. Larval forms cause endoarteritis in the mesenteric circulation, resulting in colic and thromboembolic infarction of the large bowel, whereas the adults cause anemia and ill thrift. Infective third-stage larvae, ingested from pasture, penetrate the mucosa of the small and large intestine, and molt to the fourth stage. They enter the lumina of small arterioles, up which they migrate, on or under the intima, to reach the cranial mesenteric artery within 3 weeks. Three or four months later, after molting in that location to the fifth stage, the immature adults return down the mesenteric arteries to the wall of the cecum or colon, where they encapsulate in the subserosa, forming nodules ~5–8 mm in diameter. Returning larvae in nodules are surrounded by necrotic debris, neutrophils, some eosinophils and macrophages, and the adjacent arteriole may be thrombosed. They eventually break into the lumen of the large bowel, especially cecum and right ventral colon, where they mature in another 1–2 months, ~6–7 months after infection. Some larvae may become trapped and encapsulated in arterioles in the mesentery on their way back to the gut, and remain there to eventually die.

Endoarteritis associated with migration and establishment of larvae in the cranial mesenteric artery and its branches is discussed with The Cardiovascular System (Volume 3, Chapter 1), as are the consequences of aberrant migration in the aorta and other arteries. Syndromes associated with aberrant migration include cerebrospinal nematodiasis and iliac thrombosis. Lesions of the cranial mesenteric artery and of the cecal and colic arteries may lead to colic as a result of reduced perfusion or thromboembolism, or perhaps due to impingement on autonomic ganglia in the vicinity of the arterial root at the aorta. Though many older horses are infected with adult worms, or have arterial lesions, the complications of colic and infarction caused by this parasite are most common in young horses. An acute syndrome, characterized by pyrexia, anorexia, depression, and weight loss, diarrhea, or constipation, colic and infarction of intestine occurs in foals infected with large numbers of larvae, but not often in animals previously exposed to infection.

Strongylus edentatus is also common and has a life cycle characterized by extensive larval migration. Third-stage larvae enter the intestinal wall and pass in the portal system to the liver where they incite inflammatory foci. Here they molt to the fourth stage and, ~30 days after infection, begin migrating through the hepatic parenchyma. The foci of inflammatory reaction in the liver are probably related to antigens released by migrating and trapped larvae. They consist of a core of necrotic eosinophils, with a surrounding fibrous capsule, a mixture of neutrophils, eosinophils, and mononuclear cells, or recent necrotic foci or tracks infiltrated by neutrophils and a few eosinophils.

By 8–10 weeks after infection, larvae are migrating from the liver via the hepatic ligaments. Hemorrhagic tracks may be produced in the hepatic parenchyma. Parenchymal scars and tags of fibrous tissue on the hepatic capsule, especially the diaphragmatic surface (Fig. 1.173), commonly found at autopsy, are the legacy of migrating *S. edentatus.* Those migrating in the hepatorenal ligament enter the retroperitoneal tissue of the flank where they may be encountered, often associated with local hemorrhage. Larvae in aberrant locations in the omentum, hepatic ligaments, and diaphragm may become encapsulated in eosinophilic granulomas and destroyed. Omental adhesions may also be a sequel to aberrant larval migration. In the flank, larvae persist for several months, molting to the fifth stage before returning from the right flank via the cecal ligament to the cecum and origin of the colon. Here they form nodules and edematous or hemorrhagic plaques in the wall of the gut, eventually perforating to the lumen where they mature and begin to lay eggs ~10–12 months

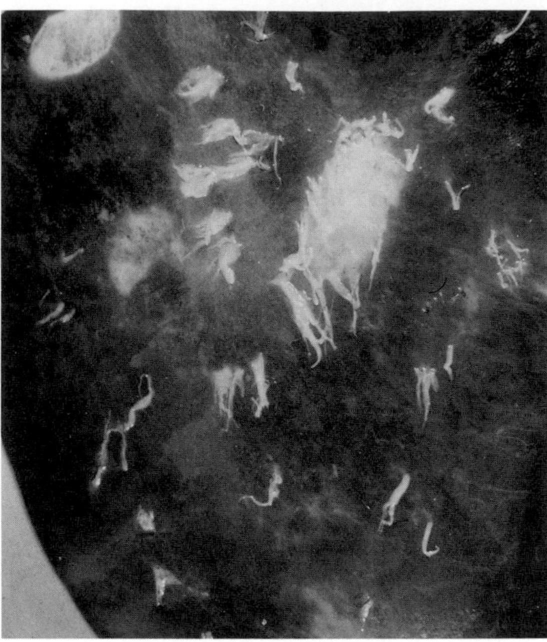

Fig. 1.173 Fibrous tags and capsular scars, associated with migration of larval *Strongylus edentatus*, on the diaphragmatic surface of a horse liver.

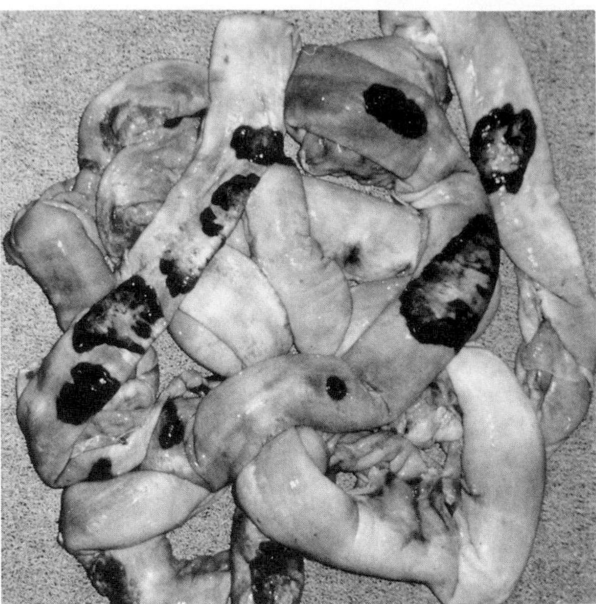

Fig. 1.174 Hemomelasma ilei, large subserosal plaques of resolving hemorrhage on the small intestine of a horse, associated with damage caused by migrating larvae of large strongyles.

after infection. Lesions associated with the larval migration of *S. edentatus* are usually incidental findings at autopsy.

Strongylus equinus is less prevalent and abundant than the other two members of the genus. Exsheathed third-stage larvae penetrate to the deeper layers of the wall of the ileum, cecum, and colon, molt to the fourth stage and produce hemorrhagic subserosal nodules, before moving to the liver through the peritoneal cavity. They migrate in the hepatic parenchyma for 6–7 weeks, then leave the liver, probably via the hepatic ligaments, to the pancreas and peritoneal cavity, where they molt to the fifth stage ~4 months after infection. They regain the lumen of the cecum and especially right ventral colon, by an unknown route, probably by direct penetration from the peritoneal cavity or pancreas. Larval *S. equinus* may wander retroperitoneally in the flanks, perirenal fat, omentum, and to the diaphragm, and occasionally, the lungs. Eggs appear in the feces of the horse ~8–9 months after infection. Larval migration by this species causes lesions in the bowel wall and hepatic parenchyma similar to those produced by *S. edentatus*.

Hemomelasma ilei is the term applied to slightly elevated subserosal hemorrhagic plaques, 1–2 cm × 3–4 cm in size, found usually along the antimesenteric border of the distal small intestine, or rarely on the large bowel (Fig. 1.174). They are associated with trauma by migrating larvae of *S. edentatus* in particular, but may be caused by larvae of any of the *Strongylus* spp. These lesions are composed of edema, hemorrhage, and a mixed population of leukocytes, with macrophages ingesting erythrocytes prominent in evolving lesions. Occasionally a fragment of nematode or cuticle, or a migratory track, may be found in section. With time these lesions resolve to yellow, brown, or tan fibrotic plaques, as red cells engulfed by macrophages are destroyed and the products of hemoglobin breakdown are reduced to iron and bile pigments, and removed from the site, which scars. The presence of haemomelasma ilei is sometimes associated with clinical, but nonfatal, colic. However, the lesion is not uncommon as an incidental finding and probably is a rare cause of clinical signs.

The other genera in the Strongylinae, *Triodontophorus, Oesophagodontus,* and *Craterostomum,* have life cycles which probably involve local migration of developing larvae into the deeper layers of the mucosa or the submucosa in the large intestine. Here they form small nodules before emerging to mature in the lumen of the cecum and colon. Larval members of these genera may contribute to the syndrome associated with emergence of larval cyathostomes, described subsequently.

Adults of all species in the Strongylinae are plug feeders and bloodsuckers. In sufficient numbers they may cause ill thrift and anemia, as the result of active hematophagia and blood loss from recent sites of feeding activity. Increased albumin catabolism causing accelerated turnover of the plasma pool, and reduced red cell survival, have been demonstrated in horses infested with relatively low numbers (<100) of *S. vulgaris*. *Triodontophorus tenuicollis,* the most important species of that genus, tends to attach to the mucosa in clusters, usually in the right dorsal colon, causing local congestion and ulceration. *Triodontophorus* may be associated with significant blood loss.

ii. ***Cyathostomes*** The small strongyles, or cyathostomes, are essentially nonpathogenic as adults, despite the fact that tens or many hundreds of thousands may be in the content of the large bowel, and that they may browse on the mucosal surface to some extent. The larval stages migrate into the deep mucosa or submucosa of the large bowel (mainly cecum and ventral colon) to molt and develop, before emerging to the lumen to molt again and mature. In the mucosa they are surrounded by a fibrous capsule, and there may be a moderate mixed inflammatory reaction containing eosinophils in the mucosa and adjacent submucosa. A similar but more intense reaction is seen around larvae in the submucosa. Emergence of larvae causes rupture of the muscularis mucosae and intense local eosinophilia and edema, followed by infiltration of neutrophils and macrophages. The third- or fourth-stage larvae may undergo hypobiosis or retarded development, persisting in the mucosa, only to mature sporadically, or perhaps more synchronously, as the adult population in the lumen turns over or is lost. Adults are found predominantly in the dorsal and ventral colon; only a small minority are in the cecum.

Mucosal nodules are up to only a few millimeters in diameter, slightly raised red or blackish, and may be umbilicate. Incision reveals a small translucent gray or red larval nematode. In heavy infections the mucosa of the cecum and colon may be diffusely pocked by such nodules.

Disease attributable to larval cyathostomes usually occurs in heavily infected horses at the time of turnover of the adult population. It is due to emergence of large numbers of hypobiotic larvae over a short period, somewhat analogous to type II ostertagiosis in cattle. This occurs in the late winter, spring, and early summer in northern temperate climates. It is a disease of horses older than a year. Little resistance is apparent to repeated infection. Animals develop a syndrome characterized by diarrhea, ill thrift or cachexia, and hypoalbuminemia, perhaps with passage of immature cyathostomes in the feces. In animals dying or killed at this time, numerous nodules, containing immature cyathostomes or recently ruptured, are present in the mucosa of the cecum and colon. The mucosa and submucosa are edematous, and the mucosa, congested. If mucosal damage is severe there may be a fibrinous exudate on the eroded or ulcerated surface. Many recently emerged fourth-stage or early fifth-stage larvae may be in the luminal content. The cecal and colic lymph nodes may be enlarged and wet, and the mesentery of the large bowel, edematous. Diarrhea and wasting are presumably due to reduced absorptive function, and loss of protein is associated with the damage to the colonic mucosa caused by emerging larvae.

Bibliography

Drudge, J. H., and Lyons, E. T. Large strongyles: Recent advances. *Vet Clin North Am: Equine Pract* **2:** 263–280, 1986.

Enigk, K. Further investigations on the biology of *Strongylus vulgaris* (Nematoda) in the host animal. *Cornell Vet* **63:** 247–263, 1973.

Harmon, B. G., Ruoff, W. W., and Huey, R. Cyathostome colitis and typhlitis in a filly. *Compend Cont Ed Pract Vet* **8:** S301–S306, 1986.

McCraw, B. M., and Slocombe, J. O. D. *Strongylus edentatus:* Development and lesions from ten weeks postinfection to patency. *Can J Comp Med* **42:** 340–356, 1978.

McCraw, B. M., and Slocombe, J. O. D. *Strongylus equinus:* Development and pathological effects in the equine host. *Can J Comp Med* **49:** 372–383, 1985.

Morgan, S. J. *et al.* Histology and morphometry of *Strongylus vulgaris*-mediated equine mesenteric arteritis. *J Comp Pathol* **104:** 89–99, 1991.

Ogbourne, C. P. Pathogenesis of cyathostome (*Trichonema*) infections of the horse. A review. Commonwealth Institute of Helminthology, No. 5, 1978 St. Albans, U.K.

Ogbourne, C. P., and Duncan, J. L. *Strongylus vulgaris* in the horse: Its biology and veterinary importance. 2nd Ed. Commonwealth Institute of Helminthology No. 9, 1985 St. Albans, U.K.

Reinemeyer, C. R. Small strongyles: Recent advances. *Vet Clin North Am: Equine Pract* **2:** 281–312, 1986.

h. Ascarid Infection Members of the Ascarididae are common and important parasites of swine, horses, dogs, cats, water buffalo, and to a lesser extent, cattle. They do not occur normally in sheep and goats. Their importance is related to incidental and sometimes significant lesions caused by larvae during migration in the tissues of definitive and accidental hosts, and to the effects of adult worms in the small intestine of the definitive host.

Ascaris suum is a large parasite, females measuring as long as 40 cm, usually found in the upper half of the small intestine of swine. The life cycle is direct. Infective larvae, present in the resistant egg, are released in the intestine and penetrate the mucosa to be carried in the portal blood to the liver. They then pass to the lungs in the blood, and break out of capillaries into alveoli. Third-stage larvae may be found in liver and lung 3–5 days after infection. Larvae move up the respiratory tree to the pharynx, where they are swallowed, arriving in the intestine about a week after infection. Worms mature in the intestine, and begin to lay eggs ~2 months after infection. Small doses of eggs more commonly give rise to patent infections than do large doses. This probably results from excessive loss of migrating larvae due to resistance incited by the antigenic mass of the heavier infections.

Larval migration induces lesions in the liver and lungs (Fig. 1.175A,B). Infections heavy enough to cause clinical signs are rare in swine reared under conditions of good hygiene and husbandry. However, respiratory signs characterized by dyspnea (commonly termed thumps) may occur in piglets if large numbers of larvae migrate through the lungs. Gross lesions in pigs, associated with pulmonary migration of ascarids, are limited largely to numerous focal hemorrhages scattered over and through the pulmonary parenchyma. There may be some edema, congestion, and failure of the lung to collapse due to bronchiolar constriction and alveolar emphysema.

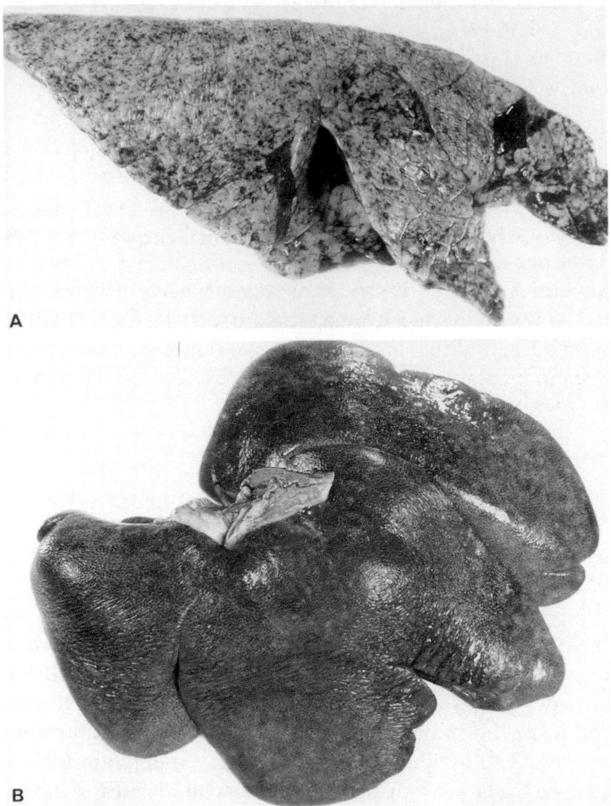

Fig. 1.175 (A) Multifocal parenchymal hemorrhages caused by migrating larval *Ascaris suum*. Lung. Pig. (B) Interstitial hepatitis caused by larvae of *Ascaris suum*. Pig.

Microscopically there is an eosinophilic bronchiolitis. Bronchioles are surrounded by macrophages and eosinophils, and the bronchiolar mucosa is thrown into small folds, the epithelium frequently disorganized or perhaps eroded. The bronchiolar wall is infiltrated by eosinophils, which are also present, with necrotic debris, in the lumen. The architecture of small airways may be obscured or obliterated by the reaction, the outlines of some bronchioles recognizable only by the persistent smooth muscle of the wall. Interstitial infiltrates of eosinophils and macrophages are most dense about bronchioles, but diffuse out into surrounding parenchyma, thickening alveolar septa, and diminishing the size of alveoli. Small branches of the pulmonary artery are also cuffed by eosinophils, lymphocytes, and macrophages, and eosinophils may be seen transmigrating the wall of vessels.

Larvae are usually readily found in section. They may be present in alveoli, alveolar ducts, bronchioles, or bronchi, perhaps surrounded by eosinophils. In more chronic cases, larvae in tissue are in eosinophilic granulomas. The worms may be dead in cases of some standing, and are recognized only as an eosinophilic remnant or some bits of cuticle. Like all larval ascarids of mammals, *A. suum* in the lungs have lateral alae visible in section.

Lesions in the liver due to migrating *A. suum*, though not causing clinical disease, do result in considerable economic loss from condemnation at meat inspection. At first exposure to larvae, the lesions are related to mechanical damage caused by the worms, subsequent repair, and hypersensitivity reactions to excretory and secretory products of the larvae. Initially, hemorrhagic tracks are present near portal areas and throughout lobules. They are visible through the capsule as pinpoint red areas, perhaps slightly depressed and surrounded by a narrow pale zone. Erythrocytes, and within a few days, neutrophils and eosinophils, fill the space left in the parenchyma by the larva. These lesions collapse and heal by fibrosis, causing scarring which involves most intensely the adjacent portal tracts. However, fibrosis extends diffusely through more distant tracts, emphasizing lobular outlines. There is a heavy eosinophil infiltrate in fibrotic septa, which becomes most obvious beginning ~10–14 days after infection. In sensitized pigs, fewer larval tracks and hemorrhages occur, but a heavy infiltrate of eosinophils is found in portal tracts within a few days of infection, followed several weeks later by the formation of lymphocyte aggregates and follicles. Granulomatous foci containing giant cells, macrophages, and eosinophils may center on the remnants of larvae trapped and destroyed in the liver.

The inflammatory infiltrates in livers of animals exposed to larval ascarids may become severe and diffuse, and this is reflected in the gross appearance of the liver, which has extensive milk spots, and prominent definition of lobules. The liver is firm, and heavy scars may become confluent, obliterating some lobules, and extending out to exaggerate interlobular septa throughout the liver. Where pigs are raised intensively, it is now rare to encounter extreme fibrosis of the liver associated with ascarid migration.

The pathogenicity of adult ascarids in the intestine is poorly defined. Heavy infections may obstruct the gut, being visible as ropelike masses throughout the intestinal wall. Ascarids may occasionally pass to the stomach and be vomited or migrate up the pancreatic or bile ducts. Sometimes biliary obstruction and icterus, or purulent cholangitis, may ensue. Rarely, intestinal perforation occurs. Relatively subtle morphologic changes are induced in the intestine by *Ascaris* infection in swine. These include substantial hypertrophy of the muscularis externa, and elongation of the crypts of Lieberkühn, though height of villi may not be significantly reduced. Hypertrophy and exhaustion of the goblet cell population, and increased proprial infiltrates of eosinophils and mast cells are also observed in infected intestine. The presence of ~80–100 worms in 3-month-old swine fed low protein rations may depress feed intake and the efficiency of feed conversion. *Ascaris lumbricoides* in humans interferes with carbohydrate, fat, and protein absorption, and *A. suum* probably has a similar influence. The effects of infection seem to be most apparent in animals on diets marginal in energy, and in quantity and quality of protein.

Ascaris suum also infects animals other than swine. In sheep, and occasionally cattle, immature ascarids may be found in the intestine. Dyspnea and coughing associated with eosinophilic pneumonia, and focal eosinophilic hepatitis, may occur in lambs exposed to *A. suis;* mortality may occur, rarely. Liver lesions in lambs are usually too small to be significant at meat inspection.

In calves exposed to yards contaminated by pig feces containing *Ascaris* eggs, severe acute interstitial pneumonia may occur. Respiratory signs of dyspnea, tachypnea, coughing, and increased expiratory effort are usually first seen ~7–10 days after exposure, when large numbers of larvae are present in the lungs. Deaths may ensue over the following few days, and the lungs are moderately consolidated, light pink to deep red, with alveolar and interstitial emphysema and interlobular edema. Microscopically, there is thickening of alveolar septa, and effusion of fibrin, proteinaceous edema fluid, and macrophages into alveoli. Hemorrhage into alveoli may also occur. Larvae are present in alveoli and bronchioles and provoke acute bronchiolitis. Neutrophils are found around larvae in bronchioles; eosinophils may be present but are not prominent in animals dying acutely. In addition to being usually readily observed in tissue sections, larvae may be recovered from the airways by washing with saline, or from minced lung in saline or digestion fluid, by use of a Baermann apparatus. Tens of thousands to millions of larvae may be present in the lungs of fatal cases.

Bibliography

Andersen, S. *et al.* Experimental *Ascaris suum* infection in piglets. *Acta Pathol Microbiol Scand* **81:** 650–656, 1973.

Bernardo, T. M., Dohoo, I. R., and Donald, A. Effect of ascariasis and respiratory diseases on growth rates in swine. *Can J Vet Res* **54:** 278–284, 1990.

Bindseil, E. The tissue reaction to migrating larvae of *Ascaris suum*. *In* "Parasitic Zoonoses. Clinical and Experimental Studies," E. J. L. Soulsby, (ed.), pp. 313–318. New York, Academic Press, 1974.

Brown, D., Hinton, M., and Wright, A. I. Parasitic liver damage in lambs with particular reference to the migrating larvae of *Ascaris suum*. *Vet Rec* **115:** 300–303, 1984.

Clark, E. G., Von Dewitz, A., and Acompanado, G. Spurious *Ascaris suum* infection in lambs. *Can Vet J* **30:** 903, 1989.

Copeman, D. B. Immunopathological response of pigs in ascariasis. *In* "Pathology of Parasitic Diseases," S. M. Gaafar (ed.), pp. 135–145. Lafayette, Indiana, Purdue Univ. Studies, 1971.

McCraw, B. M., and Greenway, J. A. *Ascaris suum* infection in calves. III. Pathology. *Can J Comp Med* **34:** 247–255, 1970.

Nesheim, M. C. Nutritional aspects of *Ascaris suum* and *A. lumbricoides* infections. *In* "Ascariasis and Its Public Health Significance," D. W. T. Crompton, M. C. Nesheim, and Z. S. Pawlowski (eds.), pp. 147–160. London, Taylor and Francis, 1985.

Stephenson, L. S. *et al. Ascaris suum:* Nutrient absorption, growth, and intestinal pathology in young pigs experimentally infected with 15-day-old larvae. *Exp Parasitol* **49:** 15–25, 1980.

Urban, J. F., Jr., Romanowski, R.D., and Steele, N.C. Influence of helminth parasite exposure and strategic application of anthelmintics on the development of immunity and growth of swine. *J Anim Sci* **67:** 1668–1677, 1989.

Yang, S., Gaafar, S. M., and Bottoms, G. D. Effects of multiple-dose infections with *Ascaris suum* on blood gastrointestinal hormone levels in pigs. *Vet Parasitol* **37:** 31–44, 1990.

Parascaris equorum is the ascarid of horses. It is widespread and common in young horses; it may contribute to ill thrift and occasionally causes death by obstruction. *Parascaris equorum* is a large nematode, females being as long as half a meter. The life cycle resembles that of *A. suum*. Similarly, hepatic and pulmonary lesions are associated with larval migration, and coughing may occur at the time larvae are in the lungs, if infections are heavy. The prepatent period is ~10–15 weeks. The lesions in the lungs of foals with migrating *Parascaris* larvae, ~2 weeks after infection, are like those described in swine with *Ascaris*. Animals with resolving pulmonary lesions develop subpleural nodular accumulations of lymphocytes as large as 1 cm in diameter, and there may be lymphocytic cuffing of pulmonary vessels.

It is possible to establish heavy infections of *P. equorum* in the intestines of foals a few months old, but not in yearlings, where larvae appear to be killed during hepatopulmonary migration. However, in heavily infected foals, many worms are lost from the intestine prior to patency, suggesting the possibility of an effect of crowding on the population of growing worms. A heavy burden of ascarids in the intestine may reduce weight gains in growing foals. Inappetence occurs, but increased plasma protein catabolism or loss into the gut does not. Reduced weight gain and hypoalbuminemia may be due to decreased protein intake. Ascarid infection may reduce rate of intestinal transit. Heavy burdens can be associated with obstruction, intussusception or, rarely, perforation of the intestine.

Bibliography

Austin, S. M. *et al. Parascaris equorum* infections in horses. *Compend Cont Ed Pract Vet* **12:** 1110–1118, 1990.

Clayton, H. M. Ascarids: Recent advances. *Vet Clin North Am: Equine Pract* **2:** 313–328, 1986.

Clayton, H. M., Duncan, J. L., and Dargie, J. D. Pathophysiological changes associated with *Parascaris equorum* infection in the foal. *Equine Vet J* **12:** 23–25, 1980.

DiPietro, J. A., Boero, M., and Ely, R. W. Abdominal abscess associated with *Parascaris equorum* infection in a foal. *J Am Vet Med Assoc* **182:** 991–992, 1983.

Nicholls, J. M. *et al.* A pathological study of the lungs of foals infected experimentally with *Parascaris equorum*. *J Comp Pathol* **88:** 261–274, 1978.

Srihakim, S., and Swerczek, T. W. Pathologic changes and pathogenesis of *Parascaris equorum* infection in parasite-free pony foals. *Am J Vet Res* **39:** 1155–1160, 1978.

The **ascarids of small animals** are *Toxascaris leonina,* infecting both cats, and dogs, and *Toxocara canis* and *Toxocara cati* infecting the dog and cat, respectively. All occur in the small intestine, mainly in young animals. *Toxascaris leonina* has a life cycle which may be direct, but can involve a paratenic host. In the definitive host, larvae ingested in infective ova enter the wall of the gut, where they remain for several weeks, molting to the fourth stage and emerging to the intestinal lumen to molt again and mature. The prepatent period is ~10–11 weeks. In the paratenic host, such as the mouse, third stage larvae are found encapsulated in granulomas in many tissues but mainly the wall of the intestine, where they may be visible as pale foci 1–2 mm in diameter. They are infective to the definitive host if the paratenic host is eaten.

Toxocara canis has a complex life cycle. Puppies may be infected by ingestion of larvated ova, in which case larvae follow the pathway of hepatopulmonary movement in the bloodstream, and tracheal migration to the pharynx and gut, though some reach other tissues in the circulation. In older dogs most larvae ingested in eggs are disseminated in the circulation to various tissues, where they encyst, rather than undergoing development and a tracheal migration. In the pregnant bitch, these larvae are mobilized, crossing the placenta to infect the fetus after day 42 of gestation. In the fetus, they remain in the liver, passing to the lungs after birth. Transmammary transmission of mobilized second-stage larvae also occurs, infecting the neonate via the colostrum. In addition, paratenic hosts may be infected by ingestion of larvated eggs. In a wide variety of species, infective larvae are disseminated hematogenously to many organs, where they settle, mainly in muscle. In some abnormal hosts, including humans, a syndrome termed visceral larva migrans is described, characterized by eosinophilia, general malaise, and perhaps signs related to granulomatous reactions to larvae in the eye, liver, lungs, and brain. Larvae in paratenic hosts eaten by young dogs undergo tracheal migration before maturing in the gut.

Toxocara cati may infect cats directly from the larvated egg, via paratenic hosts, or, in kittens, by the transmammary route from the postparturient queen. Prenatal infection apparently does not occur. Larvae hatching from eggs migrate via the liver, lungs, and trachea, whereas those taken in from milk or prey do not. Following tracheal migration or ingestion in milk or prey, larvae enter the gastric wall, whereas fourth-stage larvae are found in the gastric contents, and the wall and lumen of the small intestine. *Toxocara cati* may also be a cause of visceral larva migrans in humans.

Focal hemorrhages may be found in the lungs of puppies with migrating *T. canis* larvae. Larval *T. canis* are occasionally found in or associated with eosinophilic granulomas in the tissues of pups and older dogs, though a clinical syndrome comparable to visceral larva migrans occurs only very rarely, if at all, in the dog. Inflammatory foci are most commonly seen grossly in the kidney, as white elevated spots 1–2 mm in diameter in the cortex beneath the capsule. They may be encountered in section in any organ, and are composed of a small focus of macrophages, lymphocytes, and plasma cells, with a few eosinophils, and possibly containing a larva. Larvae may be destroyed in such foci, which heal by scarring. Considering the large numbers of larvae which must move through the tissues of dogs, and in many cases be sequestered there, relatively few are encountered incidentally, free or encapsulated in granulomas. Granulomas incited by *T. canis* larvae may be found in the eye on ophthalmoscopic examination, and retinitis, post-inflammatory retinopathy, and blindness associated with *T. canis* larvae confirm that ocular larva migrans is a significant entity in dogs. There are rare reports of encapsulated *T. canis* larvae associated with eosinophilic gastroenteritis in German shepherd dogs, and a somewhat similar syndrome has been produced experimentally by superinfection with large numbers of *T. canis*. Occult lesions similar to those occurring in dogs may be found in the tissues of cats infected with *T. canis*, though ocular larva migrans has not been found.

Toxocara cati developing in the mucosa of the stomach and intestine may provoke a mild granulomatous response composed of lymphocytes and a few macrophages about the coiled larva. Larvae free of such a response are also found in the mucosa and submucosa.

Heavy infections of ascarids in puppies and kittens, usually those reared in unhygienic communal environments, may result in ill thrift. The most significant effects are those caused in the stomach and intestine by maturing *T. canis* in young puppies infected prenatally. The animals may develop weakness, lethargy, and vomition, which is occasionally fatal. At autopsy the animal appears poorly grown for its age, pot-bellied, and cachectic, and masses of maturing worms are present in the intestine (Fig. 1.176)

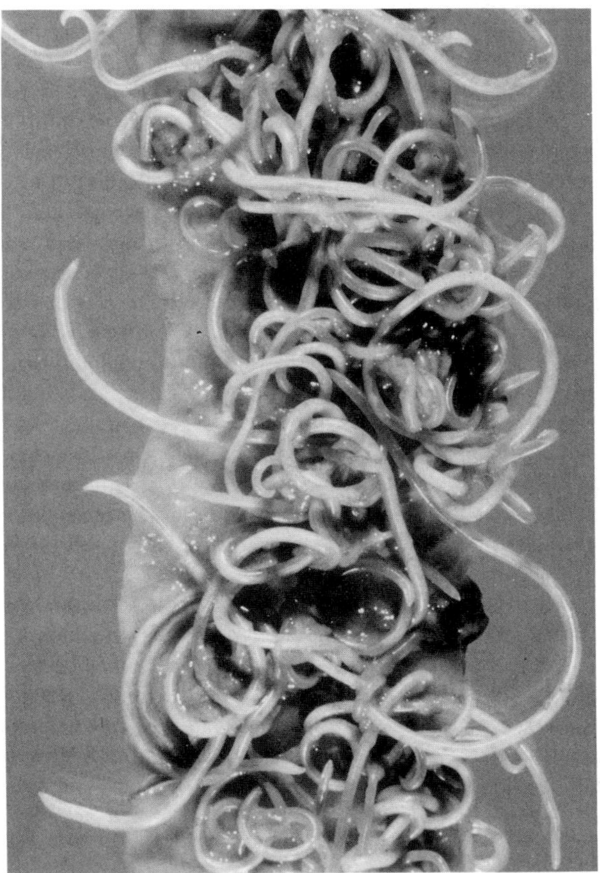

Fig. 1.176 Tangled mass of *Toxocara canis* in the small intestine of a pup.

and perhaps stomach. Sometimes as much as 20% of the body weight of young puppies may be accounted for by the worm burden. *Toxocara cati* may be associated with clinical disease but usually not death, in kittens to several months of age. Medial hypertrophy of the pulmonary artery in cats has been associated with *T. cati* and *T. canis* infection; whether it is causal is unclear. Disease is rarely attributed to *T. leonina*.

Mature *T. cati* are as long as ~10 cm; *T. canis* are as long as ~18 cm. In freshly dead animals they are often coiled like a spiraled spring. They may maintain their place in the intestine by bracing against the gut wall in this way. The mechanism by which adults of these ascarids in the intestinal lumen impair growth has not been investigated. Ascarids occasionally enter the bile or pancreatic ducts, and many perforate those structures or the intestine.

Bibliography

Fitzgerald, P. R., and Mansfield, M.E. Visceral larva migrans (*Toxocara canis*) in calves. *Am J Vet Res* **31:** 561–566, 1970.

Greve, J. H. Somatic migration of *Toxocara canis* in ascarid-naive dogs. *In* "Pathology of Parasitic Diseases," S. M. Gaafar (ed.), pp. 147–159. Lafayette, Indiana,Purdue Univ. Studies, 1971.

Hayden, D. W., and Van Kruiningen, H. J. Experimentally induced canine toxocariasis: Laboratory examinations and pathologic changes, with emphasis on the gastrointestinal tract. *Am J Vet Res* **36:** 1605–1614, 1975.

Johnson, B. W. *et al.* Retinitis and intraocular larval migration in a group of Border collies. *J Am Anim Hosp Assoc* **25:** 623–629, 1989.

Parsons, J. C. Ascarid infections of cats and dogs. *Vet Clin North Am: Small Anim Pract* **17:** 1307–1339, 1987.

Parsons, J. C., Bowman, D. D., and Grieve, R. B. Pathological and haematological responses of cats experimentally infected with *Toxocara cati* larvae. *Int J Parasitol* **19:** 479–488, 1989.

Toxocara (*Neoascaris*) *vitulorum* infects the small intestine of young calves of domestic cattle, mainly in the tropics and subtropics, and it is especially significant in water buffalo.

The life cycle involves transmammary transmission of third-stage larvae mobilized from the tissues of the dam within a few days of parturition. The larvae attain the liver of the calf and undergo a tracheal migration. Patency occurs within ~1 month of birth, but worms are expelled within a short time, and by ~ 2–3 months of age, none is present.

Signs of infection include foul-smelling diarrhea and ill thrift. Immature and mature worms both contribute to the signs. Heavily infected calves may die in an emaciated state, with burdens of as many as 400–500 worms as much as 30 cm long in the intestine. Occasionally, migration up the bile duct, or perforation of the gut may occur.

Bibliography

Roberts, J. A. The life cycle of *Toxocara vitulorum* in Asian buffalo (*Bubalus bubalis*). *Int J Parasitol* **20:** 833–840, 1990.

Srivastava, A. K., and Sharma, D. N. Studies on the occurrence, clinical features and pathomorphological aspects of ascariasis in buffalo calves. *Vet Res J* **4:** 160–162, 1978.

Warren, E. G. Observations on the migration and development of *Toxocara vitulorum* in natural and experimental hosts. *Int J Parasitol* **1:** 85–99, 1971.

i. *PROBSTMAYRIA* AND *OXYURIS* INFECTIONS *Probstmayria vivipara,* the small pinworm of horses, is viviparous, and as a result, massive proliferation of the population can occur endogenously. The worms are minute, ~3 mm long, and may be present in the millions on the mucosa and in the content of the cecum and right ventral colon. Despite the large number which may be present, they do not appear to be pathogenic.

Oxyuris equi, the large pinworm of horses, also is relatively innocuous. The fourth-stage larvae in the dorsal colon do have a large buccal capsule and feed on plugs of mucosa; in massive numbers they may be of significance. The adults probably live in the content. The male is ~1 cm long, but the female may be 4–15 cm, with a narrow tail composing as much as 75% of the body length. They lay eggs in the perianal area, and their main significance is the resulting irritation.

Bibliography

Smith, H. J. *Probstmayria vivipara* pinworms in ponies. *Can J Comp Med* **43:** 341–342, 1979.

j. CESTODE INFECTION Adult tapeworms inhabit the gastrointestinal tract, or the ducts of the liver and pancreas, where they are generally of minor significance. They are flattened, segmented colonies of sequentially maturing hermaphroditic reproductive units, or proglottids, forming an elongate strobila a few millimeters to many meters long. The Eucestoda are attached to the host by a specialized hold-fast organ, or scolex, which usually has four suckers, and perhaps a rostellum, sometimes armed with hooks. The Cotyloda may have elongate muscular grooves (bothridia) on the scolex. Cestodes lack an alimentary tract and absorb nutrients through the specialized absorptive surface or tegument of the proglottids. Any effects they have on the host are related to competition for nutrients in the lumen of the intestine, or result from tissue damage caused by scolices of species which embed themselves deeply in the mucosa or submucosa.

Carnivores may be infected by tapeworms which use certain prey species as intermediate hosts. Metacestodes, or larvae, of members of the Taeniidae use as intermediate hosts some species of domestic animals and, accidentally, humans. They may cause disease, result in economic loss due to condemnation of tissues or organs at meat inspection, or have zoonotic significance.

Adult cestodes in tissue section are flattened, with internal organs in a loose parenchymatous matrix, often containing calcareous corpuscles in the outer region, and lacking tubular digestive structures. They are segmented, and the scolex may be encountered at the anterior end, attached to the intestine.

Bibliography

Schmidt, G. D. "Handbook of Tapeworm Identification." Boca Raton, Florida, CRC Press, 1986.

Wardle, R. A., McLeod, J. A., and Radinovsky, S. "Advances in the Zoology of Tapeworms, 1950–1970." Minneapolis, Minnesota, University of Minnesota Press, 1974.

i. *Ruminants* In ruminants the more common and widely distributed intestinal tapeworms are *Moniezia expansa, M. benedini,* and *Thysaniezia (Helictometra) giardi. Stilesia globipunctata* is found in the small intestine of sheep and goats in Europe, Asia, and Africa, whereas *S. hepatica* occurs in the bile ducts of ruminants in Africa and Asia. *Thysanosoma actinioides* occurs in the small intestine, and pancreatic and bile ducts of ruminants in North and South America. *Avitellina* spp. occur in the small intestine of sheep and other ruminants in parts of Europe and Asia. The intermediate hosts of these tapeworms are oribatid mites or psocids (book lice).

Heavy infestations of the small intestine by *Moniezia, Thysaniezia,* and *Avitellina* are associated by some with diarrhea and ill thrift in young lambs and calves. However, the evidence suggests that *Moniezia* is harmless; no effect on production or clinical signs can confidently be assigned to it. Concomitant gastrointestinal nematode parasitism may well be present and significant.

The scolex of *Stilesia globipunctata* may be embedded in mucosal nodules 6–10 mm in diameter in the upper small intestine, with the threadlike strobila streaming into the lumen. There is a chronic inflammatory reaction around the scolex, which is deep in the mucosa, plugs of tissue being grasped by the suckers. Glands in the vicinity are hyperplastic, causing the nodules. The presence of as many as a hundred of these nodules has been associated with wasting, edema, and diarrhea.

Stilesia hepatica and *Thysanosoma actinioides* may cause mild fibrosis and ectasia of the bile ducts. Worms are often concentrated in the segmented saclike dilations in the duct. These worms cause economic loss through condemnation of infected livers at meat inspection, and in areas where infection is common, this cost may be very significant.

Bibliography

Allen, R. W. The biology of *Thysanosoma actinioides* (Cestoda: Anoplocephalidae) a parasite of domestic and wild ruminants. *Bull Agric Exp Stn New Mexico State Univ* **69:** 1973.

Amjadi, A. R. Studies on histopathology of *Stilesia globipunctata* infections in Iran. *Vet Rec* **88:** 486–488, 1971.

Bergstrom, R. C. How serious are *Moniezia* infections in cattle and sheep? *Vet Med* **80:** 72–75, 1985.

Boisvenue, R. J., and Hendrix, J. C. Studies on the location of adult fringed tapeworms, *Thysanosoma actinioides,* in feeder lambs. *Proc Helminthol Soc Wash* **54:** 204–206, 1987.

Elliott, D. C. Tapeworm (*Moniezia expansa*) and its effect on sheep production: The evidence reviewed. *N Z Vet J* **34:** 61–65, 1986.

ii. *Horses* The cestodes found in horses are *Anoplocephala perfoliata,* which colonizes the proximal cecum, especially at the ileocecal junction, and *A. magna* and *Paranoplocephala mamillana* in the small intestine and occasionally the stomach. The latter worm is small, less than 5 cm in length, and is rarely associated with disease or lesions. *Anoplocephala magna* tends to live in the lower small intestine, where it can attain a length of 80 cm, and a width of 2.5 cm. All use oribatid mites as intermediate hosts. Heavy infections have been associated with erosive or ulcerative enteritis, and rarely with intestinal perforation.

Anoplocephala perfoliata is more commonly associated with lesions, and occasionally with mortality. In areas of concentrated mucosal attachment by clusters of as many as several hundred of this stumpy species, especially at the ileocecal orifice, erosion and ulceration of the mucosa are observed. The depressed surface is often covered by a fibrinous exudate, perhaps with some hemorrhage, or there may be a local verrucous granulating mass projecting into the lumen. Chronic lesions of this sort may be associated with unthriftiness. Partial obstruction of the ileocecal orifice may occur rarely, but no clear relationship is established between infection with *A. perfoliata* and the development of ileal muscular hypertrophy. Ileocecal and cecocecal intussusception, and occasionally, perforation of the intestine, have also been associated with infection by this tapeworm.

Bibliography

Bain, S. A., and Kelly, J. D. Prevalence and pathogenicity of *Anoplocephala perfoliata* in a horse population in South Auckland. *N Z Vet J* **25:** 27–28, 1977.

Barclay, W. P., Phillips, T. N., and Foerner, J. J. Intussusception associated with *Anoplocephala perfoliata* infection in five horses. *J Am Vet Med Assoc* **180:** 752–753, 1982.

Beroza, G. A. *et al.* Cecal perforation and peritonitis associated with *Anoplocephala perfoliata* infection in three horses. *J Am Vet Med Assoc* **183:** 804–806, 1983.

Lyons, E. T. *et al.* Prevalence of *Anoplocephala perfoliata* and lesions of *Draschia megastoma* in thoroughbreds in Kentucky at necropsy. *Am J Vet Res* **45:** 996–999, 1984.

Owen, Rh., Jagger, D. W., and Quan-Taylor, R. Caecal intussusceptions in horses and the significance of *Anoplocephala perfoliata. Vet Rec* **124:** 34–37, 1989.

iii. *Carnivores* Dogs may be parasitized by *Diphyllobothrium* spp., as may be humans, cats, swine, and many other fish-eating mammals. The adults can be large, attaining lengths of 12–15 m in humans, though those in animals tend to be shorter. The worm is ~2 cm across, and marked centrally by the uterus containing dark eggs, which are operculate. Intermediate stages occur in copepods and fish. The adult worm matures in the intestine of piscivorous mammals. Macrocytic hypochromic anemia associated with vitamin B_{12} deficiency, probably induced by competitive absorption from the gut by the worm, is reported in some humans with diphyllobothriosis. Infection by *Diphyllobothrium* spp. is rarely, if ever, associated with clinical disease in animals.

Spirometra species are, like *Diphyllobothrium,* members of the class Cotyloda, and their life cycle is similar. The taxonomy of the genus is difficult, but among recognized species are *S. mansonoides,* infecting dogs, cats, and raccoons in North and South America, *S. mansoni* in dogs and cats in East Asia and South America, and *S. erinacei,* found in cats and dogs in Australia and the Far East. Prospective hosts must have the opportunity for predation, since they are infected by the plerocercoid or sparganum found in the body cavity of the second intermediate host, usually an amphibian or reptile, or in another transport host.

Spargana can also occur in carnivores, swine, or even humans, if the procercoid in the first intermediate host, the *Cyclops,* is ingested, usually while drinking. Spargana are white, ribbonlike, but otherwise structureless worms up to several centimeters long. They may be found, free or encysted in a thin, noninflammatory fibrous capsule, in the peritoneal cavity and intermuscular or subcutaneous tissue. A chronic inflammatory reaction may occur about dead spargana. The adult worms are nonpathogenic. Plerocercoids are of significance in humans, where they migrate mainly in the subcutaneous tissues.

Mesocestoides spp. occasionally infect dogs, as well as other mammals and some birds, in North America, Europe, Asia, and Africa. These members of the Eucestoda have a life cycle involving an insect or mite, and a vertebrate as second intermediate host. In the latter, infective tetrathyridia, ~1–2 cm long, flat, narrow, and bearing an invaginated scolex with four suckers, are found in the body cavities, liver, and lung. Tetrathyridia have the capacity for asexual multiplication, resulting in massive infections of intermediate hosts such as amphibia and reptiles, as well as dogs, cats, and other mammals. In the intestine of definitive hosts, *Mesocestoides* adults also may replicate asexually, and heavy infections may occur as a result of this, or from the consumption of large numbers of tetrathyridia in an intermediate host. Animals infected with intestinal *Mesocestoides* may develop diarrhea. Tetrathyridia replicating in the intestine of the dog also may penetrate the gut wall, and proliferate in the peritoneal cavity.

Tetrathyridia in the abdominal cavity of dogs and cats may cause peritoneal effusion (parasitic ascites), perhaps with the development of pyogranulomatous peritonitis and adhesions. Tetrathyridia 1–2 mm in diameter are scattered in the thick creamy exudate, along with similar size white bodies, composed of necrotic parasite and host cellular debris. There may be villous mesothelial proliferation and fibrous adhesions, with a mixed interstitial inflammatory infiltrate. Metacestodes with an unarmed scolex may be evident in sections. Mild infections may be discovered incidentally at necropsy. *Mesocestoides* infection of the abdominal cavity must be differentiated from peritoneal infections by cysticerci of several *Taenia* spp., which occur very rarely in carnivores.

Dipylidium caninum occurs in the dog, cat, fox, and occasionally, children. It is ubiquitous. The narrow worms, to 0.5 m long, have distinctive cucumber-seedlike segments, and are often encountered incidentally in the small intestine at autopsy. They are of no pathologic significance. Cysticercoids develop in fleas and perhaps in the dog louse *Trichodectes canis*. Infection in the normal definitive hosts, or in accidental ones such as humans, is by ingestion of fleas containing cysticercoids.

Bibliography

Boreham, R. E., and Boreham, P. F. L. *Dipyllidium caninum:* Life cycle, epizootiology, and control. *Compend Cont Ed Pract Vet* **12:** 667–675, 1990.

Kirkpatrick, C. E. *et al.* Use of praziquantel for treatment of *Diphyllobothrium* sp. infection in a dog. *J Am Vet Med Assoc* **190:** 557–558, 1987.

Mueller, J. F. The biology of *Spirometra. J Parasitol* **60:** 3–14, 1974.

Stern, A. *et al.* Canine *Mesocestoides* infections. *Compend Cont Ed Pract Vet* **9:** 223–231, 1987.

Williams, J. F., Lindsay, M., and Engelkirk, P. Peritoneal cestodiasis in a dog. *J Am Vet Med Assoc* **186:** 1103–1105, 1985.

k. TAENIID TAPEWORMS Taeniid cestodes are the most important tapeworms in domestic animals, not because of the effects of the adult worm in the carnivorous definitive host, but rather because of the metacestodes, or larval forms, in intermediate hosts. Single oncospheres hatch from the egg in the upper small intestine, penetrate the epithelium, and are carried in the portal blood to the liver. Some species of metacestodes migrate in the liver, eventually to enter the peritoneal cavity. Others persist to develop in the liver, whereas still others pass on to the heart, lungs, and systemic circulation, establishing in muscle or a variety of other sites and tissues. Metacestodes may be found occasionally in organs other than the site of predilection.

Taeniid metacestodes assume four basic forms. The **cysticercus** is a fluid-filled, thin-walled, but muscular cyst, into which the scolex and neck of a single larval tapeworm are invaginated. The **strobilicercus** is a modification of this theme; late in larval development the scolex evaginates and is connected to the terminal bladder by a segmented strobila, so that it resembles a tapeworm, several centimeters long. The **coenurus** is a single or loculated fluid-filled cyst, in which up to several hundred nodular invaginated scolices are present in clusters on the inner wall. Each scolex is capable of developing into a single adult cestode in the intestine of the definitive host. The **hydatid cyst** is a uni- or multilocular structure, on the inner germinal membrane of which brood capsules develop. Within the brood capsules, invaginated protoscolices form. Brood capsules may float free in the cyst fluid, where they are termed hydatid sand. Internal daughter cysts can develop. Release of brood capsules or protoscolices into tissues, as a result of rupture of the hydatid cyst, may lead to development of new cysts. The alveolar hydatid cyst proliferates by budding externally.

Taenia taeniaeformis infects the intestine of domestic cats and some wild felids, and the strobilicercus, *Cysticercus fasciolaris,* is found in the liver of small rodents. The adults are as long as 60 cm, have no neck, and posterior segments are somewhat bell shaped, so that this species is readily differentiated from the other cestodes found in the feline small intestine. Usually, only a few worms are present in the cat, and they are of no consequence.

Taenia pisiformis is common in the small intestine in dogs and some wild canids, which prey on rabbits and hares. *Cysticercus pisiformis* migrates in the liver of the intermediate host, causing hemorrhagic tracks, which are infiltrated by a mixed inflammatory reaction, and ultimately heal by scarring. The pea-size cysticerci encyst in a thin, noninflammatory fibrous capsule on the mesentery or omentum, or on the ligaments of the bladder. Occasionally, cysticerci persist beneath the hepatic capsule. Burdens of 20–30 worms, sometimes more, may be present in the intestine of the dog.

Taenia hydatigena infects the dog, and the metacestode, *Cysticercus tenuicollis,* the long-necked bladder worm, or false hydatid, is found in the peritoneal cavity of sheep, cattle, and swine, and occasionally other species. Immature cysticerci in the liver migrate through the parenchyma for several weeks as they develop, before emerging to encyst on the peritoneum anywhere in the abdominal cavity. The immature cysticerci are less than a centimeter long, ovoid, and translucent. They cause tortuous hemorrhagic tracks similar to those produced by immature liver flukes, and if large numbers are present, they may cause a syndrome of depression and icterus identical to acute fascioliasis.

Heavily infected livers, with 4000–5000 actively migrating cysticerci, are mottled due to the subcapsular and parenchymal hemorrhagic foci and tracks. Cysticerci to 6–8 mm long may be present beneath or breaching the capsule by about 3 weeks after infection. In severe cases hemorrhage into the abdominal cavity may occur, but this is uncommon. Hepatic necrosis due to migrating cysticerci may predispose to germination of clostridial spores, and the development of black disease or bacillary hemoglobinuria, though these are more often complications of fascioliasis.

Cysterci trapped in the liver may persist in a fibrous capsule, or be destroyed in a cystic eosinophilic granuloma, which may mineralize; this is common on the diaphragmatic surface where the falciform ligment is attached. Usually, the intensity of infection is low, and a few, but occasionally scores of cysticerci, delicate, translucent, fluctuant, fluid-filled cysts to 5 cm or more in diameter, are contained in individual thin, noninflammatory fibrous capsules scattered on the peritoneal serosa. A single invaginated scolex on a long neck is present in each cysticercus. When a cyst degenerates, it is destroyed by a granulomatous reaction, and the fibrotic mass may mineralize.

Hepatic migration by *C. tenuicollis* may, at any stage, cause condemnation of lamb and pig liver at meat inspection.

Taenia ovis infects the intestine of the dog, whereas the metacestode, *Cysticercus ovis,* is in the muscle of sheep, where it causes cysticercosis, or sheep measles. Cysticercosis of muscle caused by *C. ovis,* by *C. bovis* in cattle, and by *C. cellulosae* in swine and other species, including dogs, is considered with Muscles and Tendons (Volume 1, Chapter 2). The adult stages of the latter two cysticerci, *T. saginata* and *T. solium,* respectively, occur in the small intestine of humans.

Taenia multiceps occurs in the intestine of dogs and wild canids, but the metacestode, *Coenurus cerebralis,* develops in the brain and spinal cord of sheep and other ungulates, and rarely, in humans. In the goat, coenuri may also occur in other organs, beneath the skin, and intramuscularly. The migration of small metacestodes in the central nervous system may cause tortuous red or yellowish gray tracks in the brain due to traumatic hemorrhage and malacia, and nervous signs or death may occur at this stage. More commonly, signs of central nervous disease, termed "sturdy" or "gid," do not develop until coenuri, to 4–5 cm in diameter, have developed more fully, 4–8 months after infection. Cysts may be present at any level and depth in the brain and spinal cord, and projecting into the cerebral ventricles, but they are most common near the surface of the parietal cortex in the cerebrum. They cause increased intracranial pressure, hydrocephalus, necrosis of adjacent brain, and sometimes lysis, perhaps extending to perforation, of the overlying cranial bone. Coenuri developing in the spinal cord may cause paresis or paralysis.

Taenia serialis infects dogs and foxes throughout the world. The larval coenurus is found in the subcutaneous and intermuscular connective tissue of lagomorphs. Usually, large numbers of tapeworms are found incidentally in the intestine of infected dogs, presumably because of the development of many worms from the numerous scolices in one or more coenuri. Several cases of cerebral coenurosis in cats, from Australia and North America, have been ascribed to the metacestode of *T. serialis*.

Cysticerci and coenuri are recognized in tissue sections as generally cystic structures with an eosinophilic outer layer or tegument, which may appear fibrillar or almost ciliate on the outermost surface. Beneath the tegumental cells a less cellular area, which may contain calcareous corpuscles, gives way to a weblike, lightly cellular matrix, and the central open fluid-filled portion of the cyst. No internal organs are seen. Muscular inverted scolices, with suckers, and (in all but *C. bovis*) hooks on the rostellum, may be encountered in favorable sections, extending into the center of the metacestode. Size and shape of hooks may assist in a specific diagnosis, if they are fully developed. Immature migrating metacestodes lack organized scolices. Other sources should be consulted for details on the taxonomy and specific identification of adult and larval taeniid tapeworms.

Echinococcus spp. tapeworms occur in the small intestine of a number of species of carnivores, predominantly canids. In enzootic areas the distinctive metacestodes, or hydatid cysts, are commonly found in normal or accidental intermediate hosts. Humans may become infected accidentally with the metacestode, and echinococcosis or hydatidosis is a significant public health problem where carnivores shedding *Echinococcus* eggs come in close contact with humans.

The taxonomy of the genus is complex. There appear to be four species, of which at least some have strains or biotypes that may be recognized on the basis of biochemical, morphologic, or genetic characteristics, biological behavior, and ecology. These strains seem to be based on adaptations to prey–predator relationships among definitive and intermediate hosts, which are relatively isolated geographically and ecologically. Since *Echinococcus* species may be self-fertilizing, they have a high potential for forming double recessives. The large number of genetically identical worms that may result from asexual reproduction by the cystic metacestode developing from a single oncosphere gives the genus a high capacity for establishment of mutant populations. These adaptive advantages may predispose to the development of strains.

The species are *Echinococcus granulosus, E. multilocularis, E. oligarthus,* and *E. vogeli*. The latter two involve sylvatic cycles in Central and South America, with felids and canids as definitive hosts, respectively, and rodents as intermediate hosts in which polycystic hydatidosis occurs; *E. vogeli* may infect humans. The other two species may use domestic animals as definitive hosts, and will be considered further here.

Echinococcus granulosus uses the dog and some other canids as the definitive host. The most widespread strain uses a sheep–dog cycle, and has been disseminated wherever there is pastoral husbandry of sheep. It is significant as a potential zoonosis in many parts of Eurasia and the Mediterranean region, some parts of the United Kingdom, North America, South America, continental Australia, and Africa. Eradication has been accomplished, or virtually so, in Iceland, New Zealand, and Tasmania. Other dog strains affecting domestic animals include those in horses, cattle, camels, pigs, water buffalo, goats, and humans. Sylvatic cycles include these: in Eurasia and North America, cervid–wolf; in Argentina, hare–fox; in Sri Lanka, deer–jackal; in Australia, macropod–dingo. Typically, cysts which develop in the intermediate host to which the strain is adapted are fertile, and a high proportion contain brood capsules and protoscolices. Oncospheres infecting other hosts either may not establish, or, more commonly, develop into sterile cysts which do not produce protoscolices. Thus, knowledge of the local cycles of *E. granulosus* may permit interpretation and prediction of the patterns of fertility and sterility of cysts found in the various potential intermediate hosts.

In the small intestine of the definitive host, protoscolices evaginate and establish between villi and in the crypts of Lieberkühn. The scolex distends the crypt, and the epithelium is gripped by the suckers and occasionally eroded, but there is little or no inflammatory response. The worms which develop are short, usually less than 6–7 mm long. They commonly have only 3–5 proglottids, the caudal gravid one making up almost half the length of the worm. Burdens of *E. granulosus* are often heavy, no doubt due to the large numbers of protoscolices ingested at a meal containing one or more hydatid cysts. The heavily infected intestine is carpeted by the tiny white blunt projections, partially obscured between the villi; the worms may resemble lymphangiectasia. Enteric signs are not normally encountered in dogs with intestinal hydatid tapeworms.

Penetration of oncospheres released from eggs in the intestine of the intermediate host takes them into the subepithelial capillaries, or perhaps the lacteal. The majority probably migrate via the liver, some carrying on to the lungs and general circulation. However, those gaining the lacteal may bypass the liver, entering the vena cava with the lymph, and either are filtered out in the pulmonary circulation or are disseminated. Hydatid cysts occur most commonly in the liver and lung, with some strain and host species variation in the relative prevalence in these organs. In sheep they may be more common in lungs, whereas in cattle and horses, the liver is the usual site of establishment. Less commonly in domestic animals, the brain, heart, bone, and subcutaneous tissue may be sites of development of hydatid cysts. A single cyst, or up to several hundreds, may be present, displacing tissue in infected organs. Disease is rarely attributed to hydatidosis in animals, even in those heavily infected. However, strategic location of one or more cysts may lead to heart failure, bloat, or central nervous signs. Condemnation of infected organs at meat inspection causes economic loss.

Hydatid cysts are usually spherical, turgid, and fluid filled. They usually measure 5–10 cm in diameter in domestic animals; rarely, cysts in animals may be larger, but in humans, hydatid cysts can become huge. On the other hand, some fertile cysts in equine livers may be as small as 2–3 mm across. The lining of fertile cysts is studded with small granular brood capsules, which contain protoscolices, and hydatid sand, composed of free brood capsules and protoscolices, is in the fluid. The lining of sterile cysts is smooth. Though the potential exists for development of internal daughter cysts, and rare exogenous budding by herniated cysts, most hydatid cysts in domestic animals are unilocular. However, they may be irregular or distorted in shape because of the variable resistance of parenchyma and portal tracts or bronchi and by the profiles of bone or other resistant tissues.

Microscopically, immature hydatid cysts are surrounded by an infiltrate of mixed inflammatory cells including giant cells and eosinophils. As they develop, a layer of granulation tissue, which may contain round cells and eosinophils, invests the cyst, and this evolves so that the inner portion of the fibrous capsule is composed of mature collagenous connective tissue, which is relatively acellular. Within this, and in close apposition, is the acellular lamellar hyaline outer layer of the hydatid cyst wall, which, with time, may become hundreds of micrometers thick. This layer is composed of a polysaccharide–protein complex, and is PAS positive. The cyst is lined by the thin syncytial germinal layer from which the brood capsules form on fine pedicles. If the cyst is ruptured and protoscolices are released into tissue, secondary cysts may form from them.

Hydatid cysts may degenerate. The inner structures collapse, and the mass becomes caseous and may mineralize. Degenerate hydatid cysts may resemble tuberculous lesions or metastatic squamous cell carcinoma, but for the fact that they can often be shelled out of the fibrous capsule. In section, among necrotic debris, macrophages, and giant cells, remnants of the lamellar outer membrane, and perhaps the rostellar hooklets of degenerate protoscolices may be recognized, to confirm the origin of the lesion.

Echinococcus multilocularis has a holarctic distribution, the adults occurring mainly in foxes, and the metacestodes in small rodents, especially voles and lemmings. Dogs and cats may also become infected with the worms in enzootic areas. Though the parasite is principally arctic, the cycle is found in the northern prairie area of North America as far south as Iowa and Illinois, and in parts of central and western Europe. The mature cestodes in the intestine are similar to, but smaller than, *E. granulosus*. In the intermediate host, the metacestode infects mainly the liver, forming a cystic structure with internal brood capsules and protoscolices, but it is capable of external budding. As a result, racemose proliferative masses of metacestodes infiltrate infected livers. They may metastasize via the bloodstream to the lungs or bone, or implant in the peritoneal cavity. The inflammatory reaction to alveolar hydatids comprises macrophages, perhaps giant cells, lymphocytes, and plasma cells in an encapsulating fibrous stroma. The metacestodes are rarely found in domestic animals, but may infect humans who ingest eggs shed by infected carnivores.

Bibliography

Arundel, J. H. A review of cysticercoses of sheep and cattle in Australia. *Aust Vet J* **48:** 140–155, 1972.

Bryan, R. T., and Schantz, P. M. Echinococcosis (hydatid disease). *J Am Vet Med Assoc* **195:** 1214–1217, 1989.

Bundza, A., Finley, G. G., and Easton, K. L. An outbreak of cysticercosis in feedlot cattle. *Can Vet J* **29:** 993–996, 1988.

Cranley, J. C. Problems in the postmortem diagnosis of equine hydatidosis. *Ann Trop Med Parasitol* **78:** 199–203, 1984.

de Aluja, A. S. and Vargas, G. The histopathology of porcine cysticercosis. *Vet Parasitol* **28:** 65–77, 1988.

Doherty, M. L. *et al.* Outbreak of acute coenuriasis in adult sheep in Ireland. *Vet Rec* **125:** 185, 1989.

Eckert, J., and Thompson, R. C. A. *Echinococcus* strains in Europe: A review. *Trop Med Parasitol* **39:** 1–8, 1988.

Edwards, G. T. Small fertile hydatid cysts in British horses. *Vet Rec* **108:** 460–461, 1981.

Edwards, G. T., and Herbert, I. V. The course of *Taenia hydatigena* infections in growing pigs and lambs: Clinical signs and postmortem examination. *Br Vet J* **136:** 256–264, 1980.

Jepson, P. G. H., and Hinton, M. N. An enquiry into the causes of liver damage in lambs. *Vet Rec* **118:** 584–587, 1986.

Kingston, N. *et al.* Cerebral coenuriasis in domestic cats in Wyoming and Alaska. *Proc Helminthol Soc Wash* **51:** 309–314, 1984.

Lymbery, A. J. *et al.* Biochemical and molecular identification of species of *Taenia*. *Aust Vet J* **66:** 227, 1989.

Okolo, M. I. O. Observations on *Cysticercus cellulosae* in the flesh of rural dogs. *Int J Zoonoses* **13:** 286–289, 1986.

Slocombe, R. F. *et al.* Cerebral coenuriasis in a domestic cat. *Aust Vet J* **66:** 92–93, 1989.

Sweatman, G. K., and Henshall, T. C. The comparative biology and morphology of *Taenia ovis* and *Taenia krabbei*, with observations on the development of *T. ovis* in domestic sheep. *Can J Zool* **40:** 1287–1311, 1962.

Sweatman, G. K., and Plummer, P. J. G. The biology and pathology of the tapeworm *Taenia hydatigena* in domestic and wild hosts. *Can J Zool* **35:** 94–109, 1957.

Thompson, R. C. A. (ed.). "The Biology of *Echinococcus* and Hydatid Disease." London, George Allen and Unwin, 1986.

Thompson, R. C. A., and Allsopp, C. E. (eds.). "Hydatidosis: Veterinary Perspectives and Annotated Bibliography." Wallingford, UK, C.A.B. International, 1988.

Trees, A. J. *et al.* *Taenia hydatigena:* A cause of persistent liver condemnations in lambs. *Vet Rec* **116:** 512–516, 1985.

Verster, A. A taxonomic revision of the genus *Taenia* Linnaeus, 1758 s. str. *Onderstepoort J Vet Res* **37:** 3–58, 1969.

I. Intestinal Fluke Infection Trematode infections of the intestine of domestic animals are, on the whole, uncommon. Dogs and cats in many parts of the world may be infected with *Alaria* spp., the second intermediate hosts for which are frogs or other amphibia. *Heterophyes heterophyes, Metagonimus yokagawi,* and *Echinochasmus perfoliatus* may infect dogs and cats fed fish which contain metacercariae. The former two occur in the Mediterranean area and the Far East; the latter in Eurasia. *Cryptocotyle* spp., most commonly parasitic in piscivorous birds, may also be found in dogs, cats, and mink fed infected marine fish.

Enteritis is attributed to *Alaria, Echinochasmus,* and *Cryptocotyle*. The flukes attach to the mucosa by suckers, and perhaps cause their effects by local irritation, erosion, and ulceration, which large numbers of them may induce. The production of excessive intestinal mucus and hemorrhagic enteritis have been associated with intestinal fluke infection in small animals. The flukes involved are small, less than 4–5 mm long, and must be sought carefully at autopsy.

Nanophyetus salmincola occurs in the small intestine of dogs, cats, and humans, and in various fish-eating wild mammals and birds in the northwestern United States of America, Vancouver Island, Canada, and Eastern Siberia. Its distribution is determined by that of the snails which are the first intermediate hosts. The second intermediate hosts are fish, especially members of the Salmonidae. The adult flukes inhabit the small intestine where they penetrate and attach to the mucosa. Large numbers may cause mucoid or hemorrhagic enteritis.

Nanophyetus salmincola transmits the agents of Elokomin fluke fever and salmon poisoning disease to animals consuming raw salmon infected with metacercaria. Elokomin fluke fever is caused by a rickettsial agent and affects a wide range of carnivores, whereas salmon poisoning disease is caused by the closely related *Neorickettsia helminthoeca,* possibly in combination with the agent of Elokomin fluke fever. *Neorickettsia helminthoeca* causes disease only in Canidae. Both diseases are reported only in North America.

Salmon poisoning disease has an incubation period of about 5–7 days, and is characterized clinically by pyrexia, anorexia, depression, weakness, and weight loss. There may be serous nasal discharge and mucopurulent conjunctivitis. Diarrhea with tenesmus develops; feces are scant yellowish and mucoid or watery, often with some blood. The condition usually is fatal; only 5–10% of infected dogs recover. They are immune to reinfection. The disease must be differentiated from canine distemper and canine parvovirus infection.

At autopsy, lesions are most consistently found in the lymphoid tissues. There is generalized enlargement of lymph nodes, especially in the abdominal cavity. Involved nodes are edematous, and on cut surface they have a yellowish hue with prominent cortical follicles. Enlarged tonsils are everted from their fossae. The thymus is often increased in size in young dogs, and the spleen may be swollen and congested. Prominent splenic lymphoid tissue is reported in foxes but is not obvious in dogs. Intestinal lymphoid tissue is prominent. Peyer's patches and other intestinal lymphoid aggregates are elevated above the mucosal surface, and there may be petechial hemorrhages on the mucosa. Lymphoid tissue near the ileocecocolic valve may ulcerate and bleed. Ileocolic intussusception occurs in many cases. The liver of foxes becomes friable, and may rupture, causing hemorrhage into the peritoneal cavity. Focal hemorrhages may be seen in the mucosa of the bladder, and subpleural hemorrhages to 2 cm in diameter usually occur.

The microscopic changes in lymph nodes include depletion of lymphocytes, focal necrosis with neutrophilic infiltrates, and an increase in the number of histiocytes in the cortex and medulla. Similar changes may occur in the thymus, and splenic follicles may undergo necrosis. Elementary bodies of the *Neorickettsia* may be demonstrated in the cytoplasm of macrophages in lymphoid tissue, and in other visceral organs, by use of Giemsa or Macchiavello's stains. In the small intestine the flukes may be present embedded deep in the mucosa, though usually little reaction to them is present.

Lesions of the central nervous system occur in most cases. Leptomeninges may be somewhat opaque, but the lesions are best recognized microscopically. They are composed of macrophage accumulations in the leptomeninges and Virchow–Robin spaces, and focal gliosis in the parenchyma. Meningeal reaction is perhaps most consistent over the cerebellum, and consists of mild or moderate perivascular or more diffuse accumulations of histiocytes. Similar cells may cuff small and medium-sized vessels throughout the parenchyma. Focal gliosis is relatively sparsely distributed but seems most common in the brain stem. Elementary bodies are also demonstrable in macrophages in the central nervous system, and the diagnosis is usually made on the basis of this finding in macrophages in lymphoid tissue and/or brain. The organisms can be isolated and grown on primary canine monocyte cultures and in several other cell-culture systems, but this is not a routine procedure.

Paramphistome infections in ruminants may cause significant intestinal disease. The adults, of the genera *Paramphistomum, Cotylophoron, Calicophoron, Ceylonocotyle, Gastrothylax, Fischoederius,* and *Carmyerius,* occur in the forestomachs of ruminants in various areas around the world. Infection is most common in warm temperate to tropical areas. In the rumen, the reddish pear-shaped adult flukes, with their characteristic anterior and posterior suckers, are considered innocuous, though some papillae may become atrophic and slough.

When ingested, metacercariae encysted on herbage give rise to immature flukes which inhabit the duodenum, where massive infections may cause severe enteritis. In cattle, water buffalo, and American bison, the species incriminated in disease include *P. cervi, P. microbothrium, P. explanatum, Calicophoron calicophorum,* and various species of *Cotylophoron, Gastrothylax,* and *Fischoederius.* In sheep and goats, *P. microbothrium, P. ichikawai, P. cervi, P. explanatum, G. crumenifer, Cotylophoron cotylophorum,* and *F. cobboldi* have been associated with disease. The species involved vary with the host and geographic area.

After ~3–5 weeks in the small intestine, the worms normally migrate forward, through the abomasum, to establish and mature in the reticulorumen. However, if massive infection occurs, growth in the small intestine is retarded, and flukes may persist for months in the duodenum, prolonging the course of disease.

Calves and lambs with intestinal paramphistomosis are depressed and inappetent. Fetid diarrhea usually develops within several weeks of infection, and may contain immature flukes. Soiling of the perineum and escutcheon, and tenesmus, may be severe. Hypoproteinemia is reflected in submandibular edema in some animals, and anemia is reported to occur occasionally. Sheep may die within 5–10 days, and cattle and water buffalo, after a course of 2–3 weeks of disease. Morbidity and mortality can be substantial, and survivors may suffer considerable loss in condition.

The carcass may be in good or cachectic condition, depending on the duration of the disease, and there may be edema of subcutaneous tissues, abomasal folds, and mesentery, and fluid in the body cavities, due to hypoproteinemia. The gallbladder is frequently distended with bile, associated with inappetence. The mesenteric lymph nodes are enlarged and edematous. The anterior small intestine appears congested externally, and immature paramphistomes, deeply penetrating the intestinal wall, may be visible through the serosa. Occasionally, they will perforate the gut and be found free in the abdominal cavity. The mucosal surface of the duodenum is edematous, thickened, corrugated, and covered with mucus. Many immature pink or brown paramphistomes, a few millimeters long, are scattered over the surface and embedded in the mucosa. Some are free in clusters in the lumen, and the digesta, which is thin and mucoid, may appear somewhat blood-tinged. Most larval paramphistomes are in the first 3 m of small intestine. In advanced infections, some may be present migrating forward on the abomasal mucosa, or already in the forestomachs.

In section, small larval paramphistomes are found deep in the lamina propria, occasionally in the submucosa, and sometimes in Brunner's glands. Larger immature forms are attached to the surface of the mucosa by a plug of tissue taken into the acetabulum. There is atrophy of villi, elongation of crypts, and possibly erosion or ulceration of the mucosa in heavily infected areas. A mixed inflammatory infiltrate is in the lamina propria but, often, little specific reaction is present to flukes in tissue. The lesions are somewhat reminiscent of those in severe trichostrongylosis, but for the difference in appearance of the offending helminths. Protein loss into the gut, coupled with loss of appetite, seems to be the most important pathophysiologic consequence. The pathogenesis of the diarrhea is unclear.

The other fluke occurring in the intestine of ruminants is *Skjrabinotrema ovis,* associated with catarrhal enteritis in sheep in Eurasia.

In **swine,** the paramphistomes *Gastrodiscoides* and *Gastrodiscus* may be found in the colon, where they are of little significance. *Fasciolopsis buski* and *Artyfechinostomum malayanum* may infect the small intestine of swine, as well as humans. They are of little importance in pigs other than as reservoirs for human infection.

In **horses** in Africa and India, the paramphistomes *Gastrodiscus aegyptiacus* and *Pseudodiscus colinsi* occur in the large bowel. Larvae of the former species have been associated with severe colitis in horses, but they are generally nonpathogenic.

Intestinal schistosomiasis, due mainly to *Schistosoma* spp. in ruminants, and *Heterobilharzia* in dogs, may cause protein-losing enteropathy, associated perhaps with granulomatous enteritis in response to deposition of ova in mucosal venules (see The Cardiovascular System, Volume 3, Chapter 1).

Flukes in tissue section are generally somewhat flattened or globose, with a loose mesenchymal parenchyma in which the internal structures are suspended. The cuticle is eosinophilic, and may be spiny. Muscular oral and acetabular suckers, and pharynx may be encountered in sections. Ceca are usually present, and elements of the male and female reproductive systems in these typically hermaphroditic adult worms (excepting the schistosomes) may be seen. The uterus may contain ova with a tan-yellow or brown shell, perhaps with an operculum, and ova are often seen in the intestinal lumen or in tissue. The developing miracidium may be present in ova. Schistosomes are recognized by their intravascular location and sexual dimorphism, the leaf-like male perhaps enveloping the slender cylindrical female within the gynocophoric canal, in section.

Bibliography

Azzie, M. A. J. Pathological infection of thoroughbred horses with *Gastrodiscus aegyptiacus. J S Afr Vet Med Assoc* **46:** 77–78, 1975.

Booth, A. J., Stogdale, L., and Grigor, J. A. Salmon-poisoning disease in dogs on southern Vancouver Island. *Can Vet J* **25:** 2–6, 1984.

Boray, J. C. The pathogenesis of ovine intestinal paramphistomosis due to *Paramphistomum ichikawai. In* "Pathology of Parasitic Diseases," S.M. Gaafar (ed.), pp. 209–216. Lafayette, Indiana, Purdue University Studies, 1971.

Dargie, J. D. The impact on production and mechanisms of pathogenesis of trematode infections in cattle and sheep. *Int J Parasitol* **17:** 453–463, 1987.

Dinnik, J. A., and Dinnik, N. N. The life cycle of *Paramphistomum microbothrium* Fischoeder, 1901 (Trematoda, Paramphistomidae). *Parasitology* **44:** 285–299, 1954.

Durie, P. H. The paramphistomes (Trematoda) of Australian ruminants. II. The life history of *Ceylonocotyl streptocoelium* (Fischoeder) Nasmark and of *Paramphistomum ichikawai* Fukui. *Aust J Zool* **1:** 193–222, 1953.

Durie, P. H. The paramphistomes (Trematoda) of Australian ruminants. 3. The life history of *Calicophoron calicophorum* (Fischoeder) Nasmark. *Aust J Zool* **4:** 152–157, 1956.

Eduardo, S. L. *Artyfechinostomum malayanum* (Leiper, 1911) Mendheim, 1943 (Tremtoda: Echinostomatidae) from pigs in the Philippines. *Phil J Vet Med* **26:** 25–27, 1989.

Farrell, R. K., Leader, R. W., and Johnston, S. D. Differentiation of salmon-poisoning disease and Elokomin fluke fever: Studies with the black bear (*Ursus americanus*). *Am J Vet Res* **34:** 919–922, 1973.

Fernandes, B. J. *et al.* Systemic infection with *Alaria americana* (Trematoda). *Can Med Assoc J* **115:** 1111–1114, 1976.

Hayden, D. W. Alariasis in a dog. *J Am Vet Med Assoc* **155:** 889–891, 1969.

Herd, R. P., and Hull, B.L. *Paramphistomum microbothrioides* in American bison and domestic beef cattle. *J Am Vet Med Assoc* **179:** 1019–1020, 1981.

Hibler, S. C., Hoskins, J. D., and Greene, C. E. Rickettsial infections in dogs. Part III. Salmon disease complex and haemobartonellosis. *Compend Cont Ed Pract Vet* **8:** 251–256, 1986.

Horak, I. G. Host–parasite relationships of *Paramphistomum microbothrium* Fischoeder, 1901, in experimentally infected ruminants with particular reference to sheep. *Onderstepoort J Vet Res* **34:** 451–540, 1967.

Horak, I. G. Paramphistomiasis of domestic ruminants. *Adv Parasitol* **9:** 33–72, 1971.

Knapp, S. E., and Milleman, R. E. Salmon-poisoning disease. *In* "Infectious Diseases of Wild mammals," 2nd Ed., J. W. Davis, L. H. Karstad, and D. O. Trainer (eds.), pp. 376–387. Ames, Iowa, Iowa State University Press, 1981.

Lawrence, J. A. Bovine schistosomiasis in southern Africa. *Helminthol Abstr* **47:** 261–270, 1978.

Vercruysse, J. *et al.* Pathology of *Schistosoma curassoni* infection in sheep. *Parasitology* **91:** 291–300, 1985.

m. ACANTHOCEPHALAN INFECTIONS The Acanthocephala are a phylum of parasitic animals which have an elongate saclike body, no internal alimentary canal, and use as the hold-fast a spiny protrusible proboscis. The life cycle typically involves obligate development in an intermediate host, usually an arthropod, and perhaps the utilization of a paratenic host to facilitate transmission. The acanthocephala of concern in domestic animals are in the genera *Macracanthorhynchus* and *Oncicola*.

Macracanthorhynchus hirudinaceus is the thorny-headed worm of swine, infecting the small intestine. The life cycle involves dung beetles or other Scarabaeidae, and foraging or rooting swine are prone to infection. Males are ~10 cm long, and the females to 30–40 cm long, slightly pink, curved, and tapering posteriorly. The proboscis has about six rows of hooks, and is used to penetrate deeply into the intestinal wall. It incites a local granulomatous nodule called a strawberry mark, with a purulent focus about the embedded proboscis. The proboscis may penetrate the muscularis, and the nodules around the proboscis, ~1 cm in diameter, may be visible on the serosal surface of the gut as gray or yellow suppurative foci, surrounded by a halo of hyperemic tissue. They occasionally perforate, causing peritonitis. As the parasites move about in the gut, abandoned sites of attachment granulate, forming a firm fibrous nodule, which may persist for some time in the wall of the gut. Severely infected pigs may suffer ill thrift and perhaps anemia, probably related partly to the potential for plasma protein loss and hemorrhage from numerous focal ulcerative lesions. *Macracanthorhynchus catalinum* and *M. ingens* are smaller but similar thorny-headed worms which inhabit the intestine of a variety of wild carnivores, and occasionally the dog.

Oncicola canis occurs in the small intestine of wild carnivores, and occasionally the dog and cat. Intermediate hosts are presumably arthropods, with insectivorous vertebrates acting as paratenic hosts. As many as several hundred worms, 0.5–1.5 cm long and dark gray, may infest the small intestine; usually infections are light. The proboscis is embedded to the subserosal level, and a focal nodular lesion develops about it. Associated disease, or complications such as perforation, are apparently rare.

Bibliography

Nelson, M. J., and Nickol, B. B. Survival of *Macracanthorhynchus ingens* in swine and histopathology of infection in swine and raccoons. *J Parasitol* **72:** 306–314, 1986.

Zao, B., Taraschewski, H., and Mehlhorn, H. Licht- und elektronmicroscopische Untersuchungen zur Histopathogenität von *Macracanthorhynchus hirudinaceus* (Archiacanthocephala) in experimentell infizierten Hausschweinen. *Parasitol Res* **76:** 355–359, 1990.

F. Protozoal Infections

1. Coccidiosis

The coccidia are members of the protozoan phylum Apicomplexa, intracellular parasites characterized at some stage of the life cycle by a typical apical complex of organelles at one end of the organism. Members of the suborder Eimeriorina, which we shall consider together under coccidiosis, all have a similar basic life cycle. It begins with infection of a cell, usually in the intestinal mucosa, by a sporozoite released from a sporocyst in the lumen of the gut. One or more cycles of asexual division, termed schizogony or merogony, follow, and the merozoites produced infect other cells, forming another generation of meronts, or transforming to sexual stages, termed gamonts. Gamonts subsequently develop into nonmotile female macrogametes, and motile male forms or microgametes. A nonmotile zygote produced by union of micro- and macrogametes forms an oocyst. Sporogony, production of sporocysts containing infectious sporozoites within the oocyst, may occur in the host, or more commonly, after the resistant oocysts are passed in feces.

Members of the genus *Eimeria* are homoxenous, sexual and asexual development taking place in a single host. *Isospora* spp. may be homoxenous, or optionally heteroxenous (*Cystoisospora*), in which case asexual stages occur in an intermediate host. The members of the genera *Toxoplasma, Sarcocystis, Hammondia, Besnoitia, Frenkelia,* and *Caryospora* are all heteroxenous. The heteroxenous genera exploit natural prey–predator relationships. In general, sexual development takes place in the intestinal mucosa of a predator, whereas at least one generation of asexual replication, often several, occurs in the tissues of one or more species of prey.

In the domestic animals we are considering, asexual and sexual development of *Eimeria* spp. is limited normally to the intestinal mucosa, and may involve stages within the lamina propria or epithelium. In the definitive host, asexual and sexual development of the *Isospora* spp. parasitic in domestic animals is also usually limited to the intestinal mucosa. In the heteroxenous *Isospora* spp., *Toxoplasma, Sarcocystis, Hammondia, Besnoitia, Frenkelia,* and in *Neospora,* asexual stages in the intermediate hosts may be found in a variety of tissues, and in *Caryospora,* sexual stages also occur in the tissues of the prey species. Depending on the parasite and the stage of development, the range of tissues infected may be wide or narrow. As examples, *Toxoplasma* and *Neospora* may infect phagocytic and parenchymal cells in many organs in the intermediate host; *Sarcocystis* spp. typically infect endothelium and finally myocytes; and *Caryospora* have been implicated in dermal coccidiosis in immunosuppressed dogs (see The Skin and Appendages, Volume 1, Chapter 5).

The endogenous stages of coccidia are all intracellular, except, temporarily, the merozoite and microgamete. Mature developmental stages are usually readily recognized; immature forms may not be easily identifiable. Trophozoites, small, undifferentiated, rounded, basophilic forms with a single nucleus, usually within a parasitophorous vacuole in the host cell, are found at three stages of the life cycle. They occur following invasion by the infective sporozoite, prior to merogony; following invasion by a merozoite, prior to a subsequent generation of merogony; and following invasion by a merozoite, prior to differentiation into a recognizable gamont. Developing meronts are multinucleate. Merogony usually involves endopolygeny, multiple fission, or apparent budding of merozoites from the periphery of the meront or from infoldings of it. A single residual body, surrounded by slightly curved, fusiform or banana-shaped uninucleate merozoites, or many spherical clusters of merozoites with a central residuum, may be present. A second form of replication, termed endodyogony, occurs in meronts of many of the heteroxenous coccidia. Two daughter organisms develop within a mother organism, which is destroyed when they are released. The location of a meront, and the number of merozoites it contains, vary with the species and the generation of merogony. A very few, or as many as tens or hundreds of thousands of merozoites may be released from a single meront.

Microgamonts mature in two steps. The first involves enlargement of the gamont and proliferation of nuclei. During the second phase the microgametes differentiate about the periphery of the gamont, which may become deeply folded or fissured by invaginations. Immature microgametocytes during these stages may resemble developing schizonts. However, fully differentiated microgametes differ from merozoites in being small, densely basophilic, comma-shaped, with 2–3 flagella. They may be present in swirling masses, perhaps with some residual bodies, in mature microgametocytes. Macrogametes, the female stage, have a large nucleus with a prominent nucleolus, and with time they usually enlarge to contain refractile eosinophilic plastic granules or wall-forming bodies, which give rise to the layers of the oocyst wall. Mature macrogametes typically have prominent wall-forming bodies, contain clear or PAS positive amylopectin granules, and a large nucleus and nucleolus.

Fertilization by the microgamete leads to development of the zygote, and subsequent formation of the oocyst wall. The oocyst wall comprises one to two clear or eosinophilic refractile membranes in most species of coccidia, but the outer wall of some species can be very thick and densely amphophilic. The contained sporont is spherical, with nucleus and nucleolus, and amylopectin granules in the cytoplasm. Sporulation usually occurs outside the host, but in *Sarcocystis* and *Frenkelia,* it occurs in the tissue of the definitive host; in *Caryospora,* sporulated oocysts develop in tissues of the prey host. Sporozoites are enclosed within sporocysts, which in turn are contained by the oocyst wall. Oocysts of most coccidia, or sporocysts of *Sarcocystis* and *Frenkelia,* are passed in the feces.

Coccidia of domestic animals are relatively host, organ, and tissue specific. Asexual stages of *Toxoplasma* and *Neospora* are the obvious exception to this generalization. Species of *Eimeria* and *Isospora* rarely occur in more than one genus of host. Similar coccidia occurring in related genera of hosts, when tested, usually prove incapable of cross-infection. The coccidia of sheep and goats exemplify this, and our concepts of the species infecting these hosts have been modified considerably as a result. The epizootiologic connotations of high host specificity are obvious. Within a host, infections are commonly organ or site and tissue specific, so that a given life-cycle stage of a species of coccidium typically infects a certain type of cell at a particular level of the intestine, or other target site. Asexual and sexual stages may have different site and tissue specificities. The location of the endogenous stages, and their morphology, may give a strong indication of the species of coccidium infecting the animal.

The economic cost of coccidiosis in the food animal species is considerable, in terms of mortality, morbidity, subclinical disease, and the cost of prevention and treatment. It is even more so in chickens. In dogs and cats, coccidiosis is a minor problem, and in horses, coccidia probably do not cause disease. The development of coccidiosis is a function of the innate virulence of the organism, the size and viability of the inoculum, and the susceptibility of the host. Some species of coccidia are much more commonly associated with disease than are others.

Virulence reflects a number of factors. Among these are the location and type of cell infected by various stages of the organism, the function of infected cells, and the degree of host reaction stimulated by infection. The biotic potential of the organism within the host (i.e., the degree of asexual replication) coupled with the size of inoculum, determines to some extent the number of cells infected by subsequent asexual and sexual generations of the coccidium. Provided that the later generations are pathogenic, a high biotic potential increases the virulence of the organism.

The effects of infection on the host cell are several, and vary somewhat with the infecting species. Infected cells may be functionally compromised. They may hypertrophy; nuclei may enlarge, or a considerable amount of cytoplasm may be displaced; and the outer membrane of infected cells may be modified highly, perhaps to facilitate metabolic exchange. The intercellular relationships may be affected. The rate of movement of infected epithelial cells up villi is altered in some cases, and epithelial cells infected by some species seem more resistant to autolysis. At least in chickens, and perhaps in mammals, epithelial cells infected by coccidia may migrate into the lamina propria. The release of merozoites and oocysts is cytolytic, and if this is synchronous and widespread, as may occur in heavy infections, considerable loss of function may be expected. This may result in villus atrophy if many surface epithelial cells are lost, as in piglets infected by *Isospora suis*. On the other hand, massive coccidial infection and cytolysis in the intestinal crypts and glands may have a radiomimetic effect; erosion and ulceration of the colon is a sequel to severe cryptal damage in bovine coccidiosis.

Immunoinflammatory reactions may be incited by coccidial infection. In experimental systems, resistance to coccidial infection is thymus dependent, and is largely mediated by T cell-promoted intracellular killing. It seems to be directed mainly against asexual stages in the life cycle. Villus atrophy in coccidiosis may also be related to cell-mediated immune reactions. In chickens infected with *Eimeria acervulina,* atrophy of villi is preceded by a hyperproliferative state in the crypts of Lieberkühn, characteristic of atrophy associated with cell-mediated immunity.

In *E. neischultzi*-infected rats, the development of villus atrophy is also associated with competent cell-mediated immune mechanisms. Villus atrophy associated with chronic coccidiosis in sheep and goats perhaps has a similar pathogenesis.

In mammals, acute inflammatory reactions in intestinal coccidiosis are most commonly associated with heavy infection and destruction of cells by the sexual stages and oocysts, rather than in response to asexual stages. This contrasts with *E. necatrix* infection in chickens, where acute hemorrhage occurs around schizonts in the lamina propria. In toxoplasmosis and neosporosis, necrosis and focal acute or chronic inflammatory reactions may be incited by actively replicating asexual stages in many organs. A syndrome characterized by hemorrhage occurs in some species infected with asexual stages of *Sarcocystis,* about the time that merogony occurs in vascular endothelium. This may be mediated in part by endothelial damage and by activation and consumption of clotting factors.

The effects of intestinal coccidiosis in mammals vary with the host–parasite system. They mainly relate to malabsorption induced by villus atrophy, or to anemia, hypoproteinemia, and dehydration due to exudative enteritis and colitis caused by epithelial erosion and ulceration. A neurotoxin has been associated with the development of nervous disorders in cattle with coccidiosis. Many species of coccidia appear to have little pathogenic effect under normal circumstances. This may reflect relative insulation from host defense mechanisms due to their largely intraepithelial location, or it may be associated with a relatively low biotic potential. However, even some species of coccidia developing in cells in the lamina propria, in large numbers, seem innocuous.

Coccidiosis is typically a disease of intensively managed animals. It is especially important in naive young animals exposed to a high level of infection. This is predisposed for by high contamination rates associated with crowding, yarding, or high stocking rates on pasture. A damp substrate promotes oocyst sporulation and survival, and practices such as feeding on the ground, or the natural propensity of young animals to nibble or perhaps indulge in coprophagy, may promote infection. Although infections may not proceed to patency, chronic ingestion of oocysts may cause an intestinal immune response, villus atrophy, and perhaps ill thrift, in some situations. Immune reactions may only halt development of, but not kill, endogenous asexual stages. Epizootiologic evidence suggests that under some circumstances, there may be relaxation of resistance and resumption of development of the organisms, ultimately expressed in disease. This seems the likely explanation for outbreaks of bovine coccidiosis occurring during midwinter in freezing climates, or in postparturient stabled dairy cattle.

Coccidiosis caused by members of the genera *Eimeria* and *Isospora* in the various species will be considered further here. Cryptosporidiosis and the heteroxenous organisms, including *Toxoplasma, Neospora,* and *Sarcocystis,* will be considered subsequently.

Bibliography

Ball, S. J., Pittilo, R. M., and Long, P. L. Intestinal and extraintestinal life cycles of eimeriid coccidia. *Adv Parasitol* **28:** 1–54, 1989.

Gardiner, C. H., Fayer, R., and Dubey, J. P. "An Atlas of Protozoan Parasites in Animal Tissues." U.S. Dept. of Agriculture, Agriculture Handbook No. 651, 1988.

Kirkpatrick, C. E., and Dubey, J. P. Enteric coccidial infections. *Isospora, Sarcocystis, Cryptosporidium, Besnoitia,* and *Hammondia. Vet Clin North Am: Small Anim Pract* **17:** 1405–1420, 1987.

Levine, N. D. "Veterinary Protozoology." Ames, Iowa, Iowa State University Press, 1985.

Levine, N. D. "The Protozoan Phylum Apicomplexa." Boca Raton, Florida, CRC Press, 1988.

Levine, N. D., and Ivens, V. "The Coccidian Parasites (Protozoa, Apicomplexa) of Carnivores." Illinois Biological Monographs, No 51. Urbana, Illinois, University of Illinois Press, 1981.

Levine, N. D., and Ivens, V. "The Coccidian Parasites (Protozoa, Apicomplexa) of Artyodactyla." Illinois Biological Monographs, No 55. Urbana, Illinois, University of Illinois Press, 1986.

Long, P. L. (ed.). "Coccidiosis of Man and Domestic Animals." Boca Raton, Florida, CRC Press, 1990.

a. COCCIDIOSIS IN CATTLE Over a dozen species of *Eimeria* parasitize cattle; of these, *Eimeria zuernii* and *E. bovis* are potentially highly pathogenic, whereas several others, notably *E. ellipsoidalis* and *E. auburnensis,* may cause diarrhea, but probably not death. Coccidial infection is common, and it usually comprises several species.

Disease occurs mainly in calves or weaned feeder cattle younger than ~1 year, when one or both of the potentially pathogenic species produce heavy infection. It may occur in animals at pasture or on range, concentrated at waterholes, but is most common in animals in feedlots or yards where the level of sanitation is not high. The stress of shipping, cold weather, or intercurrent disease may be associated with outbreaks, which can occur in midwinter when oocyst transmission is expected to be poor. Bovine parvovirus infections have been associated with outbreaks of coccidiosis in a dry environment in northern Australia. Reactivation of latent schizonts in tissue may explain coccidiosis in stressed animals, or at a time when transmission is unlikely. Recrudescence of infection has been demonstrated in glucocorticoid-treated calves infected with *E. zuernii,* but not with *E. bovis.*

Coccidiosis is characterized by diarrhea, which may progress to dysentery with mucus, and tenesmus, perhaps causing rectal prolapse. Animals dehydrate, become hyponatremic and perhaps anemic. Morbidity may be high, but mortality is usually low. The duration of severe disease is ~3–10 days, after which most cases recover, since infection is essentially self-limiting. Some animals develop concurrent nervous signs, including tremors, nystagmus, opisthotonus, and convulsions, and many of these die within a few days.

The signs in bovine coccidiosis due to *E. zuernii* and *E.*

bovis occur when the epithelium in the glands of the cecum and colon is infected by second-generation schizonts and gametocytes. In heavily infected animals, disease, and perhaps death, can occur before many oocysts are passed in the feces. The life cycles of both agents are similar, two schizogonous generations preceding gametogony. The first-generation schizont of ***E. bovis*** infects hypertrophic endothelial cells in lacteals on the upper part of villi in the lower small intestine, several meters proximal to the ileocecal valve. These schizonts may be large, to ~300 μm in diameter, and are visible to the naked eye as pinpoint white nodular foci in the mucosa. They contain tens of thousands of merozoites, but are invested by only a narrow rim of mononuclear inflammatory cells, unless they degenerate, when a marked local mixed reaction develops, including neutrophils and macrophages. Merozoites released from these schizonts ~14–18 days after infection enter cells deep in cecal and colonic glands. In heavy infections, crypts of Lieberkühn in the terminal ileum may also be infected. Here they produce small second generation schizonts, which in turn release merozoites, infecting other cells in the gland. Gametogony may begin as early as 15 days after infection, and oocyst production peaks ~19–21 days after infection.

The first-generation schizonts of ***E. zuernii*** may be about the same size as those of *E. bovis*. However, they are most common in the terminal meter of the ileum and are located in the lamina propria below the crypt–villus junction, often deep near the muscularis mucosae, rather than in the endothelium of the lacteal; hence, they are not so readily visible grossly as those of *E. bovis*. The second-generation schizonts and gamonts of *E. zuernii* also occur in glands of the cecum and colon, but not the terminal ileum. The merozoites tend to be somewhat longer (to 15 μm) and schizonts more numerous and of greater diameter (~14 μm) than those of *E. bovis*. The timing of the development of *E. zuernii* infection is similar to that of *E. bovis*. First-generation schizonts of *E. bovis* occasionally reach the mesenteric lymph node, where they may mature, with no significance.

Animals dying of coccidiosis have fecal staining of the hindquarters, and may be somewhat cachectic and anemic. The gross enteric lesions in severe cases are those of fibrinohemorrhagic typhlocolitis, which may extend to the rectum; if *E. bovis* is involved, the terminal ileum may be affected (Fig. 1.177), and perhaps a few schizonts will be visible in ileal villi. The contents of the large bowel are usually abnormally fluid, and may vary from brown to black to overtly bloody, possibly with flecks of mucus or fibrin. The mucosa is edematous, with exaggerated longitudinal and perhaps transverse folds, which may be congested in a tiger-stripe pattern, or more diffusely petechiated. Submucosal edema is also marked. Fibrin strands or a patchy diphtheritic membrane may be present on the mucosa (Fig. 1.178), and fibrin casts can form. In milder cases, lesions are limited to congestion and edema of the mucosa.

In animals dying at the peak of infection, virtually all cells lining cecal and colonic glands in many areas are infected by small schizonts, gamonts, or developing oocysts. Cells infected by *E. bovis* tend to dissociate and

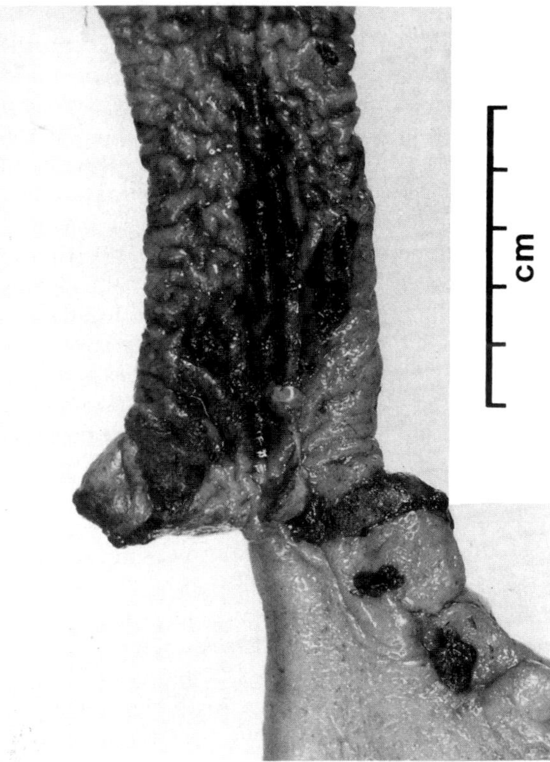

Fig. 1.177 Bovine coccidiosis. Acute enteritis. Mucosal thickening, large and minute ulcerations, and hemorrhages.

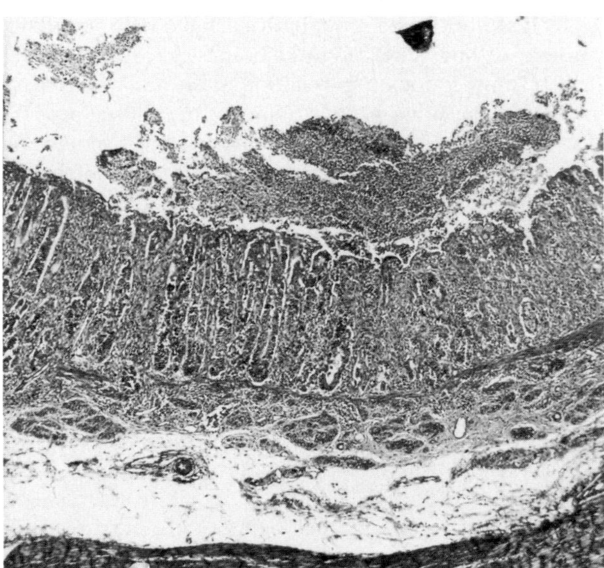

Fig. 1.178 Bovine coccidiosis. Damaged colonic glands and inflammatory exudate.

project into the lumen of the gland. Where infected epithelium remains more or less intact, the surface does not erode, and effusion or exudate is not apparent. However, as cells are disrupted and oocysts are released into the lumen of glands, the remaining glandular epithelium becomes extremely attenuated, or the gland collapses (Fig. 1.179A). Concurrently, the surface epithelium becomes squamous, or the mucosa is eroded, and effusion of fibrin, neutrophils, and hemorrhage occurs from dilated, congested superficial vessels. Oocysts released into the lumen of the colon may be seen in the exudate (Fig. 1.179B). At the same time, the mucosa begins to collapse, and the lamina propria is infiltrated by neutrophils, eosinophils, lymphocytes, macrophages, and plasma cells (Fig. 1.179C). Oocysts trapped in denuded glands in the collapsed mucosa may be surrounded by small giant cells.

If destruction is widespread, and the animal survives sufficiently long, the mucosa may ulcerate to the level of the muscularis mucosae, and begin to granulate. In areas where the lesion is patchy, glands which have been relatively spared may become lined with hyperplastic epithelium, making an attempt to regenerate the mucosa. Flattened epithelial cells spread from these glands across the denuded surface, beneath the diphtheritic exudate. A few crenated oocysts in small giant cells in the stromal remnants of the mucosa may be all the evidence of coccidiosis found in lesions in animals surviving for 7–10 days.

Malabsorption due to mucosal damage in the cecum and colon, and inflammatory effusion and hemorrhage, explain the enteric signs of coccidiosis. The nervous signs in bovine coccidiosis are not associated with recognized lesions in the brain; they have been related to a neurotoxin found in the blood of affected animals, which often are also copper deficient.

The gross lesions of coccidiosis in cattle must be differentiated from those in salmonellosis, bovine virus diarrhea, rinderpest, malignant catarrhal fever, and bovine adenovirus infection, all of which may cause typhlocolitis. Coccidiosis can often be simply confirmed at autopsy by finding large numbers of developing stages in mucosal scrapings. Oocysts of *E. bovis* are ovoid, smooth, and ~28 × 21 μm; those of *E. zuernii* are subspherical to ovoid, smooth and ~18 x 15 μm.

Although other coccidia are unlikely to be the primary cause of diarrhea or death in cattle, several have distinctive endogenous stages which may be recognized in tissue section. ***Eimeria auburnensis*** has a giant first-generation schizont, which may be confused with those of *E. bovis* and *E. zuernii*. However, they are present usually 6–12 m cranial to the ileocecal valve and form in the epithelium deep in crypts of Lieberkühn, though this may not be apparent because of plane of section, or following their migration into the lamina propria. Second-generation schizonts and gamonts of *E. auburnensis* develop in the

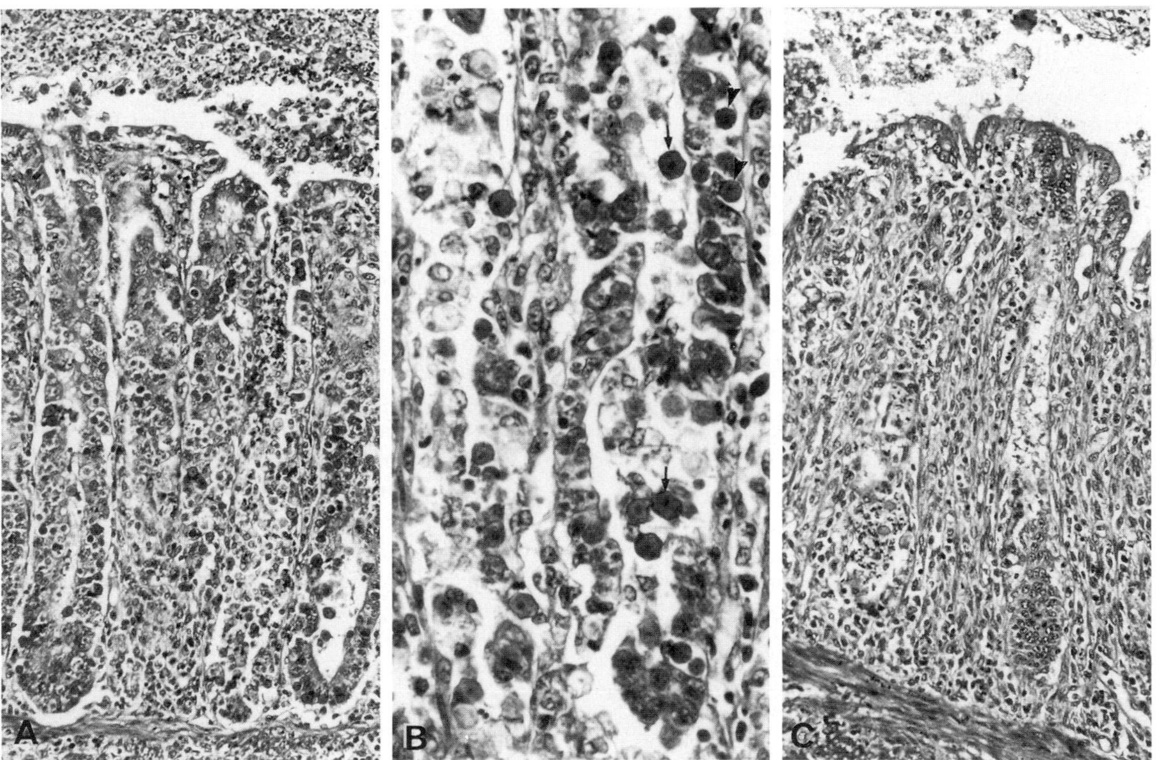

Fig. 1.179 Bovine coccidiosis. (A) Heavy infection and destruction of colonic glands by gamonts. Exudate covers mucosa. (B) Destruction of colonic glands by developing gamonts (arrowheads). Oocysts are in the lumen of some glands (arrows). (C) Destruction of colonic glands. Only a few glands remain in the mucosa.

lamina propria in the ileum, small schizonts, in villi, and gamonts in the deeper lamina propria. Microgametocytes may be several hundred μm across. Oocysts are ~38 × 23 μm.

The other bovine coccidium with gamonts apparently developing in the lamina propria is *E. bukidnonensis*. Oocysts of this species are large, ~48 × 35 μm and thick walled, with a micropyle, and have been found in the lamina propria. *Eimeria alabamensis* develops in vacuoles within the nucleus of epithelial cells in small intestine and, in heavy infections, the large bowel. Both schizonts and gamonts may be found together within the same nucleus. Gamonts of *Eimeria kosti* have been described in the epithelium deep in the abomasal glands. None of these organisms is particularly pathogenic.

Eimeria bareillyi is associated with clinical coccidiosis in water buffalo calves. The serosal vessels in the distal half of the small intestine are congested, and the lumen of the lower small bowel contains creamy or yellow fluid content in which some mucus, fibrin, or blood may be present. Focal to coalescent pale, raised plaques or polypoid masses may be present on the mucosa, or the surface may appear granular and necrotic, with petechial hemorrhages. The gross changes are caused by hypertrophy of crypts and villi, on which virtually every cell is infected with developing gamonts or oocysts. *Eimeria bareillyi* will not cross-transmit to domestic cattle, though *E. ellipsoidalis* and *E. zuernii* of bubaline origin will. *Eimeria zuernii* is pathogenic in water buffalo.

Bibliography

Bürger, H.-J. *Eimeria*-Infektionen beim Rind. *Berl Münch Tierärztl Wschr* **96:** 350–357, 1983.

Chobotar, B., and Hammond, D. M. Development of gametocytes and second asexual generation stages of *Eimeria auburnensis* in calves. *J Parasitol* **55:** 1218–1228, 1969.

Davis, L. R., and Bowman, G. W. Observations on the life cycle of *Eimeria bukidnonensis* Tubangui 1931, a coccidium of cattle. *J Protozool* **11** (Suppl.): 17, 1964.

Davis, L. R., Bowman, G. W., and Boughton, D. C. The endogenous development of *Eimeria alabamensis* Christensen 1941, an intranuclear coccidium of cattle. *J Protozool* **4:** 219–225, 1957.

Elibihari, S., and Hussein, M. F. *Eimeria kosti* sp. n., an abomasal coccidium from a cow. *Bull Anim Health Prod Afr* **22:** 105–107, 1974.

Friend, S. C. E., and Stockdale, P. H. G. Experimental *Eimeria bovis* infection in calves: A histopathological study. *Can J Comp Med* **44:** 129–140, 1980.

Isler, C. M., Bellamy, J. E. C., and Wobeser, G. A. Pathogenesis of neurological signs associated with bovine enteric coccidiosis: A prospective study and review. *Can J Vet Res* **51:** 261–270, 1987.

Jubb, T. F. Nervous disease associated with coccidiosis in young cattle. *Aust Vet J* **65:** 353–354, 1988.

Kennedy, M. J., and Kralka, R. A. A survey of *Eimeria* spp. in cattle in central Alberta. *Can Vet J* **28:** 124–125, 1987.

Lindsay, D. S., Dubey, J. P., and Fayer, R. Extraintestinal stages of *Eimeria bovis* in calves and attempts to induce relapse of clinical disease. *Vet Parasitol* **36:** 1–9, 1990.

Parker, R. J. *et al.* Coccidiosis associated with postweaning diarrhoea in beef calves in a dry tropical region. *Aust Vet J* **61:** 181–183, 1984.

Sanyal, P. K., and Ruprah, N. S. Endogenous stages and pathology in *Eimeria zurnii* coccidiosis in buffalo calves. *S L Vet J* **32:** 22–25, 1984.

Sanyal, P. K., Ruprah, N. S., and Chhabra, M. B. Attempted transmission of three species of *Eimeria* Schneider, 1875 of buffalo-calves to cow-calves. *Ind J Anim Sci* **55:** 301–304, 1985.

Shastri, U. V., and Krishnamurthi, R. A note on pathological lesions in clinical bubaline coccidiosis due to *Eimeria bareillyi*. *Ind J Anim Sci* **45:** 46–47, 1975.

Stockdale, P. H. G. The pathogenesis of the lesions produced by *Eimeria zuernii* in calves. *Can J Comp Med* **41:** 338–344, 1977.

Stockdale, P. H. G. *et al.* Some pathophysiological changes associated with infection of *Eimeria zuernii* in calves. *Can J Comp Med* **45:** 34–37, 1981.

b. Coccidiosis in Sheep and Goats Coccidial infection is universal in sheep and goats, and coccidiosis can be a significant problem in the young of both species. Consideration of the etiology of coccidiosis in these species is complicated by the morphologic similarity of the coccidia infecting sheep and goats. Assumptions on the potential for cross-infection of coccidia between sheep and goats, and of the species found in each host, have been revised as new taxonomic and biologic information has come to light.

At present, about a dozen species of coccidia are found in each of sheep and goats. Of these, three (*E. pallida, E. caprovina,* and *E. punctata*) may occur in both sheep and goats, though the validity of *E. punctata* as a species is questioned. Eight species pairs of *Eimeria* occur, in which the coccidia look and behave similarly in sheep and goats, but do not cross-infect. Listing the sheep-adapted species of each pair first, these are *E. ahsata–E. christenseni; E. ovinoidalis–E. ninakohlyakimovae; E. bakuensis (ovina)–E. arloingi; E. granulosa–E. jolchijevi; E. crandallis–E. hirci; E. faurei–E. apsheronica; E. parva–E. alijevi; E. intricata–E. kocharli.* Two species are unique to sheep, *E. weybridgensis* (formerly *E. arloingi* B), and *E. marsica;* in goats, one species, *E. caprina,* is unique. In addition, giant schizonts of an unknown coccidian, termed *Globidium gilruthi,* are seen incidentally as pinpoint white foci in the abomasum of sheep and goats. The taxonomic confusion has been carried over into descriptions of the natural or experimental disease, since many infections were of mixed species, resulted from inocula of poorly defined species of coccidia, or occurred under circumstances in which the oocysts associated were not described. However, although the taxonomic picture has changed, the syndromes associated with coccidiosis in sheep and goats have not.

Coccidiosis in these species is a disease of young animals. Under conditions of intensive pastoral husbandry or confinement, lambs and kids are exposed to oocysts of many species of coccidia within the first few days of life. A degree of protection against subsequent challenge with oocysts of a species of coccidium is conferred by previous infection with that species. Coccidiosis seems to occur mainly in susceptible animals, those with limited experience of infection, exposed to conditions in which infection pressure is relatively high; hence, the disease may occur in lambs and kids held in sheds or yards with the ewes or does. Under these circumstances, animals as young as 3 weeks may develop signs and perhaps die. Weaned lambs, presumably exposed to only light infections while at range, are also prone to coccidiosis when brought into feedlots. In young suckled animals and those in feedlots, exposed to large numbers of oocysts, signs may occur before oocysts are passed. Suckling lambs, ~5–8 weeks old, reared at pasture at relatively heavy stocking rates, may also develop signs, and occasionally die. Under these conditions, the disease needs to be differentiated from gastrointestinal helminthosis, which may be concurrent.

Outbreaks of coccidiosis in confined lambs and kids are usually acute and characterized by moderate morbidity and low mortality; there is green or yellow watery diarrhea, occasionally with blood or mucus. Yarded and grazing animals may also suffer weight loss, or subclinical ill thrift. Signs are usually associated with lesions in the lower small intestine, caused by *E. ahsata* and *E. bakuensis* in lambs, and their analogs in goats, *E. christenseni* and *E. arloingi,* or with typhlocolitis, caused by *E. ovinoidalis* in sheep, and *E. ninakohlyakimovae* in goats. Some pathogenicity is also ascribed to *E. faurei, E. intricata, E. parva,* and *E. crandallis* in sheep, and presumably to their analogs in goats. Infections may be mixed, and gross and microscopic lesions may reflect this.

Eimeria ovinoidalis in sheep and ***E. ninakohlyakimovae*** in goats presumably have similar endogenous development. In the sheep, giant schizonts to 300 μm in diameter develop in cells deep in the lamina propria, in the terminal ileum. They release merozoites, which enter epithelium in the glands of the cecum and colon, and perhaps distal ileum. Here small second-generation schizonts evolve, and other cells in glands in the same area subsequently become infected by the gametocytes.

These species are considered highly pathogenic, and *E. ovinoidalis* is often associated with disease in feedlot lambs. Lesions other than those related to diarrhea, dehydration, and hypoproteinemia are limited to the terminal ileum, and especially the cecum and proximal colon, and are associated with second-generation schizogony and gametogony. Affected areas of gut are edematous and thickened, and there may be focal or more diffuse congestion and hemorrhage in the mucosa. Heavily infected animals may have bloodstained feces. Occasionally, pinpoint white foci, the giant schizonts, may be seen in the mucosa of the ileum. In sections, schizonts and gamonts are in many or most cells lining glands in affected areas. Neutrophils and macrophages may accumulate in response to merozoites released from ruptured giant schizonts, but the most significant microscopic lesions are those in the cecum and colon, which resemble those in cattle due to *E. bovis* and *E. zuernii.* ***Eimeria caprina*** in goats also seems to have pathogenic potential. Like *E. ninakohlyakimovae,* it causes typhlocolitis; the small intestine is not involved.

Eimeria christenseni and *E. arloingi* in goats and their analogs, *E. ahsata* and *E. bakuensis* in sheep, are also associated with serious disease. They seem to have somewhat similar developmental cycles and lesions, though interpretation of the literature is clouded by confusion among these species. Many cases of coccidiosis in lambs attributed to *E. bakuensis* (as *E. arloingi*) may have in fact been due to *E. ahsata,* since the unsporulated oocysts, though of differing sizes, can be confused.

Eimeria christenseni has a developmental cycle which involves giant schizonts to nearly 300 μm across in the endothelium of the lacteal in villi in the middle small intestine. The more mature of these may detach and appear to lie free in the lacteal, dilating the villi. Second-generation schizogony and gametogony occur in epithelial cells lining the crypts and villi, mainly in the small intestine 4–6 m below the abomasum, but in heavy infections, also in terminal small bowel. Gamonts are usually below the host cell nucleus, though this is variable, and multiple infections of host cells are common. In heavy infections every cell in a number of contiguous crypt–villus units may be infected. Though there may be an acute local reaction around ruptured primary schizonts, clinical disease is associated with the subsequent stages of development, diarrhea occurring during the late prepatent and patent periods. Affected intestine may be congested and edematous. Numerous pale white or yellow foci from a few millimeters to a centimeter in diameter, often visible from the serosa, are present as slightly raised plaques on the mucosa of the small bowel. These foci are areas of intense infection of cryptal and villus epithelium by gamonts and developing oocysts, and have been dubbed oocyst patches. There may be some hemorrhage into the intestine, but the feces are rarely bloody.

Eimeria arloingi undergoes a development similar to that of *E. christenseni* (Fig. 1.180A,B) and causes similar gross and microscopic lesions in goats, with minor differences. First-generation schizonts are most numerous in the lacteals of villi in the lower jejunum, gamonts are mainly above the host cell nucleus, and the associated grossly visible plaques in the mucosa (Fig. 1.181A,B) may tend to be more distal in the small intestine, and occasionally involve the large bowel. *Eimeria ahsata* and *E. bakuensis* in sheep are similar.

Nodular polypoid structures, sometimes pedunculate, and about 0.3–1.5 cm in diameter, are encountered in the small intestinal mucosa of sheep and goats, usually as an incidental finding. These masses comprise hypertrophic crypt–villus units, in which virtually every epithelial cell is infected by mainly gametocytic stages of coccidia, which, in sheep, are probably *E. bakuensis* and *E. ahsahta.* Adjacent mucosa appears normal and is uninfected. The term pseudoadenomatous has been used to describe these polypoid lesions, and the oocyst patches or plaques previously discussed in coccidia-infected sheep and goats. The infected epithelial cells appear somewhat hypertro-

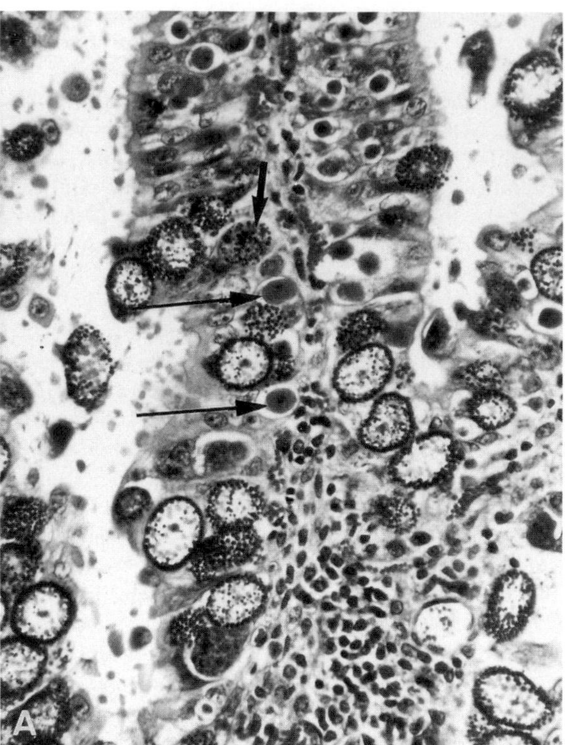

Fig. 1.180A Coccidiosis. *Eimeria arloingi*. Goat. Undifferentiated gamonts (long arrow), macrogametocytes (short arrow), and microgametocytes infect epithelial cells.

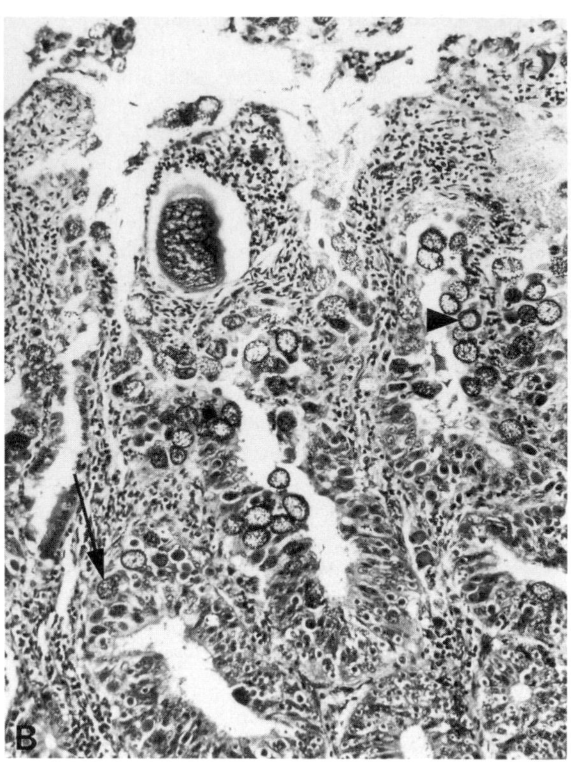

Fig. 1.180B Coccidiosis. *Eimeria arloingi*. Goat. Ileum. Large schizont in lacteal. Gamonts (arrow) and developing oocysts (arrowhead) in epithelium of crypts and villi.

phic, with eosinophilic cytoplasm and prominent brush borders. Often these coccidia-infected cells do not slough rapidly postmortem, in contrast to their uninfected fellows. This may aid a histologic diagnosis in otherwise autolytic gut in clinical cases.

Why masses of infected cells apparently persist in chronically infected animals without clinical disease is unclear. However, the plaques and polyps may be the result of mitogenic stimuli from progamonts, the immature stages in crypt epithelium, which appear to divide by binary fission in synchrony with the infected host cell. They would thus supply a continuous stream of infected cells, in which the coccidia mature as the cell moves up the villus. Occasionally, macrophages and giant cells are seen massing at the base of crypts in the centers of polyps, apparently destroying infected epithelium, perhaps as part of the immune response.

Coccidiosis may also cause ill thrift and diarrhea in suckling or weanling lambs 5–6 weeks old heavily stocked on pasture. In the United Kingdom, *E. crandallis,* which develops largely in the ileum, and *E. ovinoidalis* are associated mainly with this syndrome. *Eimeria weybridgensis (E. arloingi* B*),* which infects most of the length of the small intestine, may contribute also. The only gross lesion in affected lambs is congestion and thickening of the mucosa of the lower small intestine.

Under some circumstances, probably sudden exposure to large doses of oocysts, *E. crandallis,* at least, causes villus atrophy in infected areas of intestine. Giant first-generation schizonts develop in crypt cells, which after infection, migrate into the lamina propria. Masses of merozoites which disperse into the intestinal lumen from these schizonts infect enterocytes over wide areas. As the infection progresses, villi become stumpy or disappear, and in small bowel and cecum, crypts are straight, hypertrophic, and contain proliferative epithelium. Asexual or, more commonly, sexual stages of coccidia are present in epithelium on the surface of the mucosa. In hyperplastic crypts, epithelial cells are infected by progamonts, which seem to be dividing in synchrony with host cells. Masses of macrophages may invest and invade the base of infected crypts, and apoptosis of infected and uninfected cells may occur, resulting in attenuation of surviving crypt epithelium. In heavy infections, there also may be thickening of the cecal mucosa by hyperplastic coccidia-infected cells. Occasionally, areas of small intestine and cecum, in which there has been severe damage to crypts, may become eroded.

Such lesions, if widespread, may cause malabsorption or perhaps protein-losing enteropathy. It is unclear whether atrophy of villi is the result of excess loss of epithelium directly due to the effects of coccidial infection, or whether it is mediated by an immune response.

Eimeria apsheronica in the goat has minor pathogenic

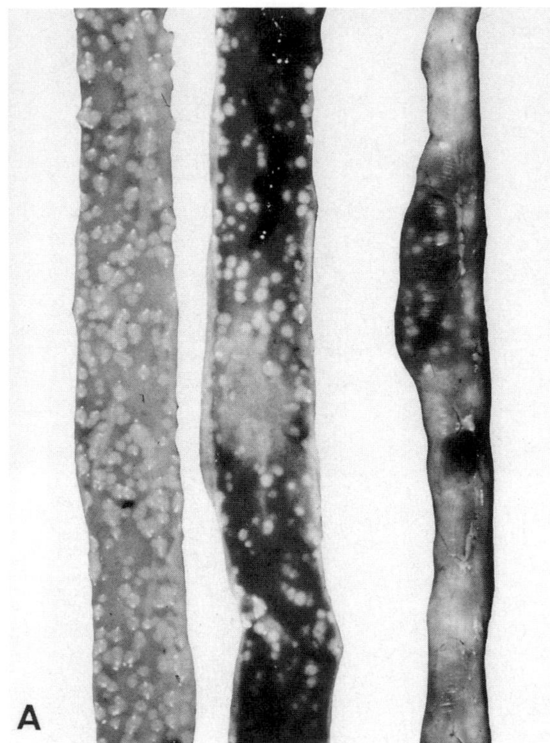

Fig. 1.181A Coccidiosis. Goat. White nodules on mucosa are visible from serosa (right). Hemorrhage in lumen, *Eimeria arloingi*. (Courtesy of P. A. Taylor.)

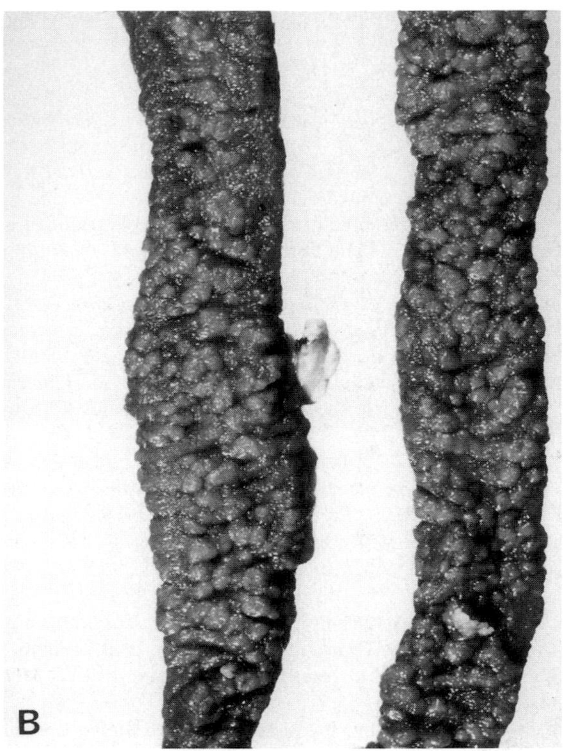

Fig. 1.181B Coccidiosis. Goat. Chronic coccidiosis showing mucosal hypertrophy.

potential. Giant schizonts develop in the lamina propria of villi throughout the small intestine and in the cecum; second-generation schizonts are in the epithelium on villi in the small intestine, and in the cecum, but not the colon. Gametocytes have the same distribution. Pale foci in the mucosa, where gametocytes are concentrated, and focal areas of erosion and hemorrhage may occur in heavily infected animals.

Large schizonts are often encountered incidentally in submucosal lymphatics, or in the subcortical or medullary sinusoids of mesenteric lymph nodes in sheep and goats. Sometimes they may be visible grossly in these locations as pinpoint white foci. Occasionally, coccidial gametocytes or oocysts may also develop in intestinal lymphoid aggregates and mesenteric lymph nodes, where they may provoke a mild granulomatous reaction. Stages in lymph nodes probably result from establishment of sporozoites or primary merozoites swept from the lacteal into the lymphatic drainage early in infection. Development in such sites is not uncommon, but aberrant, and likely to be a dead end. The species involved appear mainly to be those previously considered, with a giant primary schizont developing in the lacteal.

In coccidiosis, oocysts are usually numerous in feces, but this is neither constant in, nor necessarily indicative of, disease. Mucosal scrapings or tissue sections of mucosa containing large numbers of asexual and gametogenous coccidial forms, in association with diarrhea, and perhaps some hemorrhage into the intestine, support the diagnosis, in the absence of other syndromes such as gastrointestinal helminthosis.

Bibliography

Chapman, H. D. The effects of natural and artificially acquired infections of coccidia in lambs. *Res Vet Sci* **16:** 1–6, 1974.

Desser, S. S. Extraintestinal development of Eimeriid coccidia in pigs and chamois. *J Parasitol* **64:** 933–935, 1978.

Foreyt, W. J. Coccidiosis and cryptosporidiosis in sheep and goats. *Vet Clin North Am: Food Anim Pract* **6:** 655–669, 1990

Gregory, M. W., and Catchpole, J. Ovine coccidiosis: Pathology of *Eimeria ovinoidalis* infection. *Int J Parasitol* **17:** 1099–1111, 1987.

Gregory, M. W., and Catchpole, J. Ovine coccidiosis: Heavy infection in young lambs increases resistance without causing disease. *Vet Rec* **124:** 458–461, 1989.

Gregory, M. W., and Catchpole, J. Ovine coccidiosis: The pathology of *Eimeria crandallis* infection. *Int J Parasitol* **20:** 849–860, 1990.

Gregory, M. W. *et al.* Ovine coccidiosis: Observations on "oocyst patches" and polyps in naturally acquired infections. *Int J Parasitol* **17:** 1113–1124, 1987.

Hilali, M. Studies on globidial schizonts in the abomasum of Norwegian sheep. *Acta Vet Scand* **14:** 22–43, 1973.

Kanyari, P. W. N. *Eimeria apsheronica* in the goat: Endogenous development and host cellular response. *Int J Parasitol* **20:** 625–630, 1990.

Lima, J. D. Development of *Eimeria* species in mesenteric lymph nodes of goats. *J Parasitol* **65:** 976–978, 1979.

Lima, J.D. Prevalence of coccidia in domestic goats from Illinois, Indiana, Missouri, and Wisconsin. *Int Goat Sheep Res* **1:** 234–241, 1980.

Lima, J. D. Life cycle of *Eimeria christenseni* Levine, Ivens and Fritz, 1962 from the domestic goat, *Capra hircus* L. *J Protozool* **28:** 59–64, 1981.

Mason, P. Naturally acquired coccidia infection in lambs in Otago. *N Z Vet J* **25:** 30–33, 1977.

McDougald, L. R. Attempted cross-transmission of coccidia between sheep and goats and description of *Eimeria ovinoidalis* sp. n. *J Protozool* **26:** 109–113, 1979.

Norton, C. C. Coccidia of the domestic goat *Capra hircus,* with notes on *Eimeria ovinoidalis* and *E. bakuensis* (syn. *E. ovina*) from the sheep *Ovis aries. Parasitology* **92:** 279–289, 1986.

Norton, C. C., and Catchpole, J. The occurrence of *Eimeria marsica* in the domestic sheep in England and Wales. *Parasitology* **72:** 111–114, 1976.

Pout, D. D. Coccidiosis of lambs. III. The reaction of the small intestinal mucosa to experimental infections with *E. arloingi* "B" and *E. crandallis. Br Vet J* **130:** 45–53, 1974.

Prasad, R. S., Chabra, M. B., and Singh, R. P. Clinical coccidiosis in kids associated with *Eimeria christenseni. Ind Vet J* **58:** 330–332, 1981.

Savin, F., Dincer, S., and Milli, U. The life cycle and pathogenicity of *Eimeria arloingi* (Marotel, 1905) Martin, 1909, in Angora kids and an attempt at its transmission to lambs. *Zbl Vet Med (B)* **27:** 392–397, 1980.

Taylor, S. M. *et al.* Diarrhea in intensively reared lambs. *Vet Rec* **93:** 461–464, 1973.

Wacha, R. S., Hammond, D. M., and Miner, M. L. The development of the endogenous stages of *Eimeria ninakohlyakimovae* (Yakimoff and Rastegaieff, 1930) in domestic sheep. *Proc Helminthol Soc Wash* **38:** 167–180, 1971.

Yvore, P. *et al.* Experimental coccidiosis in the young goat: Parasitic development and lesions. *Int Goat Sheep Res* **1:** 163–167, 1980.

c. Coccidia in Horses The only coccidium of horses reported with any frequency is *Eimeria leuckarti,* which is found in horses and donkeys the world over. In one survey of foals in Germany, it was found in 100%. It may also occur in older animals. Its reputation for pathogenicity rests largely on the distinctive large gamonts being found by pathologists in the lamina propria of the small intestine in animals dead of obscure enteric disease. However, implication of *E. leuckarti* in the disease process is rarely, if ever, convincing, and it is encountered incidentally in the intestine of horses dead of other clearly defined conditions. Furthermore, heavy experimental inoculations, producing many gamonts in the gut and heavy oocyst passage, have failed to elicit clinical signs.

The stages present in the lamina propria of villi are giant microgametocytes and macrogametes, developing in markedly hypertrophic host cells, probably of mesenchymal origin (Fig. 1.182). The microgametocytes are as large as ~250 μm in diameter, and when mature they contain swirling masses of microgametes. Immature microgametocytes very much resemble some of the giant schizonts of other species of coccidia, and have frequently been referred to as such; this stimulated the application of the term *Globidium* to the organism. However, the only schizont containing merozoites that has been recognized in horses was very small (12.5 μm in diameter), and in the epithelium of the ileum. The macrogametes have distinctive large eosinophilic or Schiff-positive granules, which may be individual or confluent. The host cells are markedly hypertrophic with a fibrillar periphery, and the enlarged nucleus forms a crescent along one side of the parasitophorous vacuole. There is no inflammatory response to the gamonts, and only a mild reaction to degenerate stages in the lamina propria.

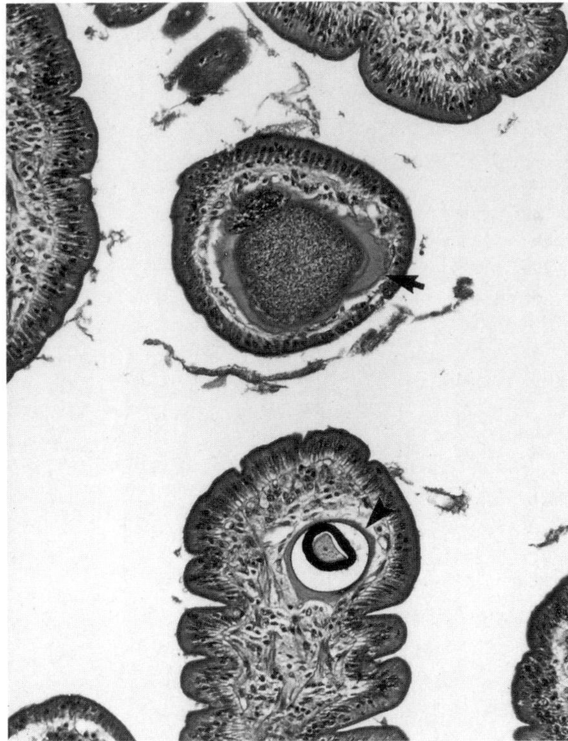

Fig. 1.182 Microgametocyte (arrow) and developing oocyst (arrowhead) of *Eimeria leuckarti* in lamina propria. Horse.

Bibliography

Barker, I. K., and Remmler, O. The endogenous development of *Eimeria leuckarti* in ponies. *J Parasitol* **58:** 112–122, 1972.

Bauer, C. Prevalence of *Eimeria leuckarti* (Flesch, 1883) and intensity of faecal oocyst output in a herd of horses during a summer grazing season. *Vet Parasitol* **30:** 11–15, 1988.

Bauer, C., and Bürger, H.-J. Zur Biologie von *Eimeria leuckarti* (Flesch, 1883) der Equiden. *Berl Münch Tierärztl Wschr* **97:** 367–372, 1984.

d. Coccidiosis in Swine At least 8–10 species of *Eimeria* are thought to occur in swine, along with a single species of *Isospora.* The latter, *I. suis,* is the most important; it causes porcine neonatal coccidiosis, a disease of piglets from ~5–6 days to ~2–3 weeks of age. This disease is recognized in the United States, Canada, the

United Kingdom, and western Europe; it also occurs in Australia, and probably wherever swine are reared intensively. The condition is most severe in herds where continuous farrowing and total confinement are practiced, and some laboratories report a prevalence of 10–50% among scouring baby pigs. Rapid sporulation (12 hr), and short prepatent period (5 days), promote rapid build-up of infection in a farrowing house.

Porcine neonatal coccidiosis has a high morbidity, and usually a low but variable mortality. It causes yellow watery diarrhea, dehydration, loss of condition and death, or at least a temporary check in growth. Some animals may runt severely. Illness usually begins at ~7–10 days of age. Piglets continue to nurse, but may vomit clotted milk. At autopsy, many piglets have the typical appearance of undifferentiated neonatal diarrhea, with no specific gross findings in the gastrointestinal tract other than fluid yellow content. However, the intestine in some animals with coccidiosis may look turgid, rather than flaccid, and in a minority of animals a fibrinous or fibrinonecrotic exudate is present in the lower portion of the small intestine. Occasionally, casts will form.

Isospora suis replicates in the epithelium on the distal third of villi (Fig. 1.183), mainly in the jejunum and ileum, though infected cells may be found in the duodenum and colon in a few animals. Piglets usually become infected within the first day or two of life, perhaps by coprophagy of the sow's feces. Merogony occurs in vacuoles in the cytoplasm, usually beneath the nucleus of the host cell. Infection of host cells is maximal 4–5 days after infection, and by 5 days, gametogony is evident. The onset of lesions and clinical signs corresponds with this period of heavy infection of cells, which undergo lysis. Villi may become markedly atrophic. The surface epithelium which remains is cuboidal to squamous, and infected epithelial cells may be seen degenerating or exfoliating (Fig. 1.184). Erosions may develop at the tips of villi (Fig. 1.185). In the remnant

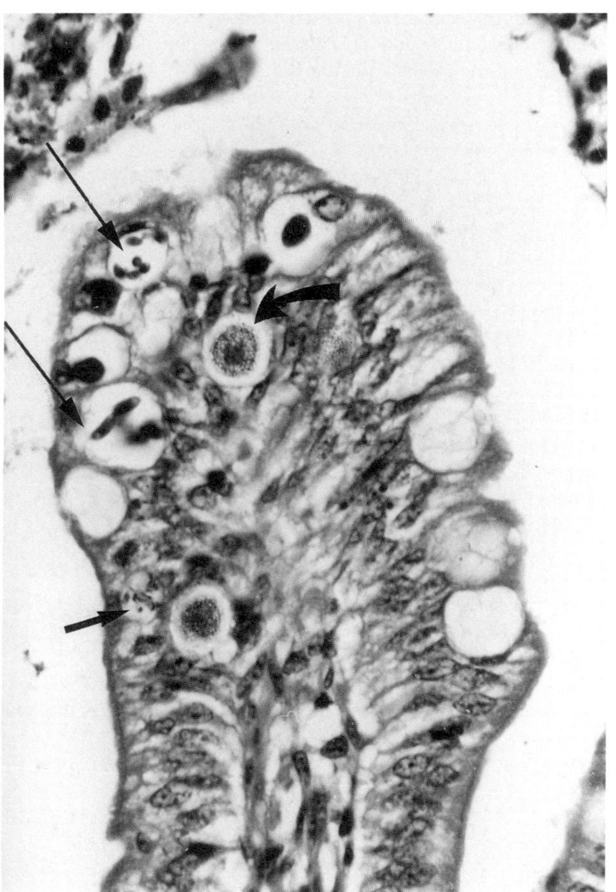

Fig. 1.183 Meronts containing merozoites (long arrows), developing oocysts (curved arrow), and a microgametocyte (arrow) in epithelial cells. Pig. *Isospora suis* infection.

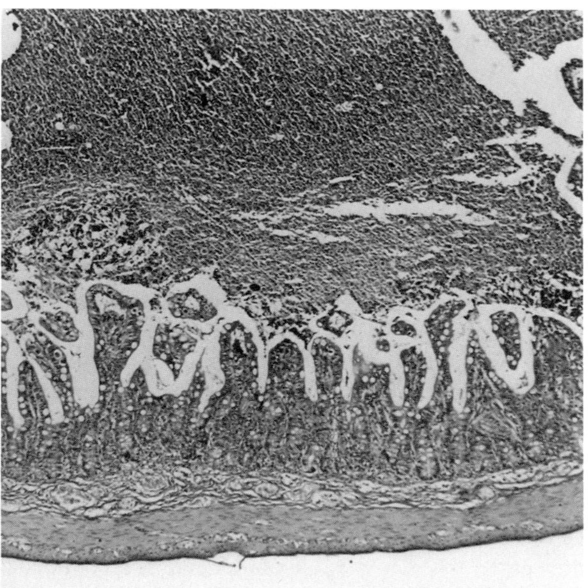

Fig. 1.184 Blunting and atrophy of villi. Pig. *Isospora suis* infection. Lumen contains massive numbers of exfoliated epithelial cells, inflammatory cells, and coccidial stages, which appear grossly as exudate.

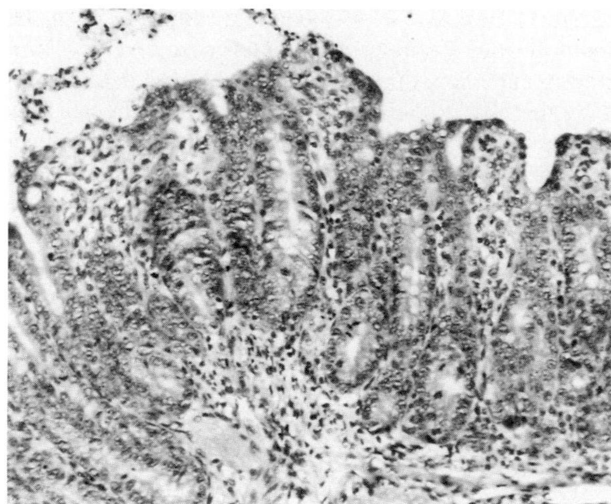

Fig. 1.185 *Isospora suis* infection. Surface epithelium is severely attenuated. There is erosion and effusion at tips of villi.

of the villus, neutrophil infiltration, a moderate increase in round cells, and an eosinophilic proteinaceous material, perhaps collagen, may be present in the lamina propria. Effusion of neutrophils and fibrin from the eroded tips of villi contributes to the fibrinonecrotic membrane seen in some animals, and ulceration can occur. Gram-positive cocci are often present in the exudate. In animals surviving for a few days, the cryptal epithelium may be markedly hyperplastic.

The severity of the lesions is a function of the size of the inoculum and the age of the pigs. Heavier inocula, within limits, produce more cellular damage and villus atrophy; fibrinonecrotic enteritis indicates ingestion of a large dose of oocysts. However, severe lesions may not be associated with heavy shedding of oocysts, since relatively few gamonts are able to develop in the reduced population of epithelial cells remaining on villi. The severity of lesions and signs is much greater in piglets a few days old in comparison with those 2 weeks of age. This relates partly to the lower rate of replication of epithelium in the crypts of young piglets, and therefore the development of more severe villus atrophy. The smaller size of young piglets also makes them more susceptible to the effects of malabsorption and diarrhea. Animals previously exposed to *I. suis* have relatively strong resistance to challenge.

A diagnosis of coccidiosis must be considered in scouring neonatal piglets, and is suggested strongly by the presence of fibrinonecrotic enteritis in the distal small bowel. Atrophy of villi may be recognized at autopsy using a hand lens or stereomicroscope, or in tissue section. Asexual or sexual stages may be found in smears of mucosal scrapings. The distinctive binucleate type I meronts and pairs of large (12–18 μm in smears, 8–13 μm in sections) type I merozoites may be found in jejunal mucosa in the early phase of diarrheal disease. Multinucleate type II meronts and numerous small type II merozoites are the predominant stage during the clinical phase of disease. In section these form clusters of 2–16 organisms like bunches of bananas, perhaps with a small residual body, in the parasitophorous vacuole in the enterocyte.

Macro- and microgamonts are present in moderate numbers by the fifth day of infection, and a few oocysts may also be seen. Microgametocytes are ~9–16 μm in diameter, and are multinucleate. Oocysts in tissue sections are oval, ~15 × 12 μm, whereas those in smears are ~18 × 16 μm. Coccidial stages may be difficult to find in animals which have been ill for several days. Oocysts may not be found in feces, either because the infection is not yet patent, the patent period has passed, or the lesions are very severe, reducing the number of oocysts produced.

Coccidiosis in older swine is due to several *Eimeria* species, and is uncommon. It typically occurs in animals with access to yards or pasture contaminated with oocysts. Weaners and growing pigs are affected. The species considered potentially pathogenic include *E. scabra, E. debliecki,* and *E. spinosa*. It is difficult to produce disease in experimentally inoculated pigs; *E. scabra* is probably the most pathogenic. Coccidiosis in swine due to *Eimeria* spp. is usually sporadic, or affects a few pigs in a group. Typically it causes diarrhea of a few days' duration, loss of appetite, and perhaps transient ill thrift, or in severe cases, emaciation. Occasionally animals die.

Lesions are usually limited to the lower small intestine, which may be congested or hemorrhagic, though overt blood is rarely found in the feces. Large numbers of schizonts, gamonts, and developing oocysts are in epithelial cells on villi and sometimes in crypts. Atrophy of villi, or erosion and local hemorrhage or inflammatory effusion may be evident, the lamina propria is edematous, and desquamated epithelium and oocysts are in the lumen of the gut. Rarely, heavily infected animals may have lesions in the large intestine. The species involved are diagnosed on the basis of the morphology of oocysts in feces or mucosal scrapings.

Coccidial gamonts and oocysts of a species resembling *E. debliecki* have been found infecting epithelium on the papilliform mucosa of cystic bile ducts in porcine liver. This is probably an aberrant site of development.

Bibliography

Ernst, J. V. Pathogenicity in pigs experimentally infected with *Eimeria spinosa*. *J Parasitol* **7:** 1254–1257, 1987.

Eustis, S. L., and Nelson. D. T. Lesions associated with coccidiosis in nursing piglets. *Vet Pathol* **18:** 21–28, 1981.

Harleman, J. H., and Meyer, R. C. Pathogenicity of *Isospora suis* in gnotobiotic and conventionalised piglets. *Vet Rec* **116:** 561–565, 1985.

Hill, J. E. *et al.* Coccidosis caused by *Eimeria scabra* in a finishing hog. *J Am Vet Med Assoc* **186:** 981–983, 1985.

Joyner, L. P. Coccidiosis in pigs. *Vet Ann* **22:** 140–144, 1982.

Koudela, B., Vítovec, J., and Štěrba, J. Concurrent infection of enterocytes with *Eimeria scabra* and other enteropathogens in swine. *Vet Parasitol* **35:** 71–77, 1990.

Lindsay, D. S. *et al.* Diagnosis of neonatal porcine coccidiosis caused by *Isospora suis*. *Vet Med Small Anim Clin* **78:** 89–95, 1983.

Lindsay, D. S., Blagburn, B. L., and Boosinger, T. R. Experimental *Eimeria debliecki* infections in nursing and weaned pigs. *Vet Parasitol* **25:** 39–45, 1987.

Lindsay, D. S., Current, W. L., and Taylor, J. R. Effects of experimentally induced *Isospora suis* infection on morbidity, mortality, and weight gains in nursing pigs. *Am J Vet Res* **46:** 1511–1512, 1985.

Matuschka, F.-R., and Heydorn, A. O. Die Entwicklung von *Isospora suis* Biester und Murray 1934 (Sporozoa: Coccidia: Eimeriidae) im Schwein. *Zool Beitr* **26:** 405–476, 1980.

Robinson, Y. *et al.* Experimental transmission of intestinal coccidiosis to piglets: Clinical, parasitological, and pathologic findings. *Can J Comp Med* **47:** 401–407, 1983.

Stuart, B. P., and Lindsay, D. S. Coccidiosis in swine. *Vet Clin North Am: Food Anim Pract* **2:** 455–468, 1986.

Stuart, B. P. *et al.* Coccidiosis in swine: Dose and age response to *Isospora suis*. *Can J Comp Med* **46:** 317–320, 1982.

Vetterling, J. M. Coccidia (Protozoa: Eimeriidae) of swine. *J Parasitol* **51:** 897–912, 1965.

Vítovec, J., Koudela, B., and Štěrba, J. Pathology and pathogenicity of *Eimeria scabra* (Henry, 1931) in experimentally infected pigs. *Folia Parasitol* **34:** 299–304, 1987.

e. Coccidiosis in Dogs and Cats Although several species of *Eimeria* have been reported from dogs and cats, their status as genuine parasites of these hosts is in doubt. The significant coccidia of dogs and cats are members of the genus *Isospora,* considered here, and of the genera *Toxoplasma, Sarcocystis, Hammondia, Besnoitia,* and *Neospora,* dealt with subsequently. *Caryospora* spp. may occasionally produce dermal coccidosis in immunosuppressed dogs.

Isospora spp. are characterized by oocysts which are passed unsporulated in feces, and which, when sporulated, have two sporocysts, each with four sporozoites. Some species are homoxenous; others are optionally heteroxenous. Following ingestion of sporulated oocysts of heteroxenous species, transport hosts, usually prey species such as mice and other small rodents, but sometimes other hosts, are infected by large sporozoitelike hypnozoites in phagocytic cells in lymph nodes and other tissues. These, when ingested by the predator, resume development in the intestine, and lead to asexual and sexual development in the definitive host. Heteroxenous passage is not obligatory, and sporulated oocysts are also directly infective to the definitive host.

Coccidiosis in the dog and cat is largely a clinical entity, and usually nonfatal. The lesions of coccidiosis in small animals are poorly defined, and care must be taken not to ascribe disease to these organisms simply on the basis of the presence of endogenous stages in the mucosa of animals dead of enteric disease. Rotavirus and coronavirus might be expected to produce similar signs; however, genuine cases of fatal coccidiosis do occur, though few are recorded in the literature. Affected animals are young, and usually from environments such as pet shops, animal shelters, or kennels where standards of sanitation may not be high. There is a history of diarrhea of several days' duration, and the animal is dehydrated. Other than mild hyperemia of the mucosa and excessively fluid content of the small intestine and colon, gross lesions in the gut may not be evident. Microscopically, there may be moderate atrophy of villi, with attenuation of surface enterocytes, and perhaps effusion of acute inflammatory exudate from the tips of some eroded villi. Asexual and sexual stages of coccidia will be evident in moderate to large numbers in the epithelium or lamina propria of villi. In some cases, the large bowel may be infected, with exfoliation of surface epithelium, and the accumulation of necrotic debris in some dilated glands.

In **dogs,** four species of *Isospora* are recognized. Meronts of *Isospora canis* develop in the subepithelial lamina propria of the villi in the distal small intestine and, to a lesser extent, in large bowel. Gamonts occur beneath and within the epithelium of the ileum and large intestine, and the oocyst is the largest among *Isospora* spp. of dogs, being ~38 × 30 μm. Endogenous stages of *I. burrowsi* occur in epithelial cells, and in the lamina propria of the tips of villi in the distal two thirds of the small intestine. *Isospora neorivolta* develops mainly in proprial cells beneath the epithelium in the tips of villi in the distal half of the small intestine, and rarely in the cecum and colon. Occasional stages may be in the epithelium. *Isospora ohioensis* develops exclusively in epithelial cells, mainly in the distal portions of villi along the length of the small bowel, especially in the ileum, and occasionally in the large bowel. It may be the most pathogenic species in dogs. The oocysts of *I. burrowsi, I. ohioensis* and *I. neorivolta* are similar. Original literature should be consulted for details which will permit differentiation of these species in tissue. *Isospora canis* and *I. ohioensis* are known to be heteroxenous. Meronts of an unknown coccidian, probably an *Isospora* sp., have been found in the intrahepatic bile ducts of a dog, associated with severe suppurative cholangiohepatitis.

In **cats,** two heteroxenous *Isospora* spp. occur. Meronts and gamonts of *I. felis* develop in epithelium of villi in the small intestine, and occasionally in epithelium in the large bowel. The oocyst is large, ~43 × 33 μm. *Isospora rivolta* also develops in epithelium on villi and in crypts and glands in the small and large intestine. Oocysts are ovoid, ~25 × 23 μm. Subepithelial schizonts and gamonts of an unknown coccidian, possibly an *Isospora* species, have been associated with fatal enteritis in a cat.

Bibliography

Dubey, J. P. Taxonomy of *Sarcocystis* and other coccidia of cats and dogs. *J Am Vet Med Assoc* **170:** 778–782, 1977.

Dubey, J. P. Pathogenicity of *Isospora ohioensis* infection in dogs. *J Am Vet Med Assoc* **173:** 192–197, 1978.

Kirkpatrick, C. E., and Dubey, J. P. Enteric coccidial infections. *Isospora, Sarcocystis, Cryptosporidium, Besnoitia,* and *Hammondia. Vet Clin North Am: Small Anim Pract* **17:** 1405–1420, 1987.

Levine, N. D., and Ivens, V. "The Coccidian Parasites (Protozoa, Apicomplexa) of Carnivores." Illinois Biological Monographs, No 51. Urbana, Illinois, University of Illinois Press, 1981.

Lipscombe, T. P. *et al.* Intrahepatic biliary coccidiosis in a dog. *Vet Pathol* **26:** 343–345, 1989.

McKenna, P. B., and Charleston, W. A. G. Coccidia (Protozoa:Sporozoasida) of cats and dogs. IV. Identity and prevalence in dogs. *N Z Vet J* **28:** 128–130, 1980.

Olson, M. E. Coccidiosis caused by *Isospora ohioensis*-like organisms in three dogs. *Can Vet J* **26:** 112–114, 1985.

Pospischil, A. *et al.* A fatal case of an unusual coccidiosis in a cat: Asexual and sexual development of parasites in macrophages. *Zbl Vet Med (B)* **31:** 141–150, 1984.

Trayser, C. V., and Todd, K. S. Life cycle of *Isospora burrowsi* n. sp. (Protozoa: Eimeriidae) from the dog *Canis familiaris. Am J Vet Res* **39:** 95–98, 1978.

2. *Heteroxenous Apicomplexan Protozoa*

Toxoplasma, Sarcocystis, Besnoitia, Hammondia, Frenkelia, and *Neospora* compose the group considered here. With the exception of *Neospora,* these heteroxenous members of the Apicomplexa are known to utilize carnivores as definitive hosts, and have one or more generations of merogony in the tissues of various species of prey. Merogonous stages of *Neospora* are recognized in dogs and herbivores; the definitive host and life cycle are not known. *Frenkelia,* as far as is known, utilizes only raptorial birds as definitive hosts, and small rodents as intermediate hosts. It will not be considered further.

a. TOXOPLASMOSIS *Toxoplasma gondii* uses members of the Felidae as definitive hosts. It is optionally heteroxenous; cats may be infected directly by ingestion of oocysts, but probably most commonly by ingestion of asexual stages in the tissues of prey species. These intermediate hosts are infected by oocysts shed in the feces of cats, or perhaps by a variety of other routes subsequently considered. Five stages of asexual development are recognized in the intestinal epithelium of cats infected with tissue cysts from intermediate hosts. The gametocytes also develop in epithelium on villi, especially in the ileum. In heavy infections, exfoliation of infected epithelium from villi is associated with the development of villus atrophy, and occasional spontaneous cases of diarrhea in kittens seem to be caused by *Toxoplasma*-induced atrophy of villi and malabsorption.

In intermediate hosts, and in cats, extraintestinal asexual development occurs in a variety of organs and tissues. Rapidly dividing forms (tachyzoites) may by endodyogeny proliferate in cells in many sites for an indefinite number of generations, and are the stage associated with acute toxoplasmosis in cats and other species. Eventually, tachyzoites induce the formation of a cyst wall in a host cell, and divide slowly, forming bradyzoites, which reside in quiescent tissue cysts.

Toxoplasma gondii is unique among the protozoa in its ability to parasitize a wide range of hosts and tissues. It is one of the most ubiquitous of organisms; experimentally, essentially all homeothermic animals can be infected, and natural infections occur in birds, nonhuman primates, rodents, insectivores, herbivores, and carnivores, including domestic species and humans. Serologic surveys indicate that infection is widespread in most species of domestic animals; however, except for abortions in sheep and goats, overt disease is sporadic and rare.

Transmission may occur by a number of different routes. The shedding of oocysts in the feces of cats and wild Felidae has been mentioned earlier. Transplacental infection occurs commonly in sheep and goats and sporadically in swine and humans. Carnivorous animals and humans may become infected by ingesting cysts containing bradyzoites in tissues of infected animals. Excretion of *T. gondii* in the semen of goats and rams has been observed experimentally, but venereal transmission is not considered to be significant. Tachyzoites have been demonstrated in milk from experimentally infected goats. However, the chance of the organisms being in the milk of spontaneously infected goats is very small, since apparently, large numbers of infecting oocysts are required for tachyzoites to be excreted in the milk.

Systemic toxoplasmosis occurs most commonly in young animals, especially immunologically immature neonates; in immunocompromised hosts; or in species such as marsupials and highly arboreal primates, which probably evolved in isolation from exposure to cats. In dogs, canine distemper, ehrlichiosis, and lymphosarcoma are commonly concomitant with toxoplasmosis. The infection in juveniles may be acquired pre- or postnatally. After ingestion, *Toxoplasma* organisms penetrate the intestinal mucosa. In cats the enterointestinal cycle and systemic infection occur almost simultaneously. In other animals the tachyzoites are the first stage of infection, after invasion of the lamina propria by sporozoites released from the oocyst, or by bradyzoites released from the tissue cyst digested from food in the intestine.

Dissemination of *Toxoplasma* occurs in lymphocytes, macrophages, granulocytes, and as free forms in plasma. From the intestine the organism may follow two routes. It may spread via the lymphocytes to the regional nodes and from there in the lymph to the bloodstream; or it may pass in the portal circulation to the liver and from there to the systemic circulation. Further dissemination occurs to a wide variety of organs. Tachyzoites actively invade or are phagocytosed by host cells and are surrounded in a parasitophorous vacuole. Tachyzoites proliferate, destroying the host cell, and cell to cell transmission may occur within infected organs.

Necrosis is common, and appears to be directly related to the rapid replication of tachyzoites. There is no evidence that *T. gondii* produces a toxin. The outcome of infection is determined by a number of factors, including the number and strain of *Toxoplasma* in the infecting dose, and the species, age, and immune status of the host. Lesions in visceral organs are usually evident within 1–2 weeks after oral infection. Variable numbers of tachyzoites are usually found in the vicinity of the necrotic areas.

Specific immunity develops within a few days after infection; the cell-mediated arm is most significant in toxoplasmosis. This reduces the severity of infection but usually does not terminate it. Immune animals develop a chronic or dormant form of *Toxoplasma* infection, which is characterized by the formation of cysts, containing bradyzoites. These are mainly located in the brain, skeletal muscle, and myocardium. The formation of cysts is accompanied by the disappearance of tachyzoites from the circulation and visceral organs. Cyst formation may take place as early as 1–2 weeks after infection, and they may persist for months, possibly years. Intracellular encystment protects the bradyzoites from both cellular and humoral immune mechanisms. Inflammation is usually not associated with cysts. When the level of resistance drops below a critical level, for example, because of treatment with immunosuppressive drugs, intercurrent disease, or other factors which depress immunity, a chronic infection may become reactivated. The cysts rupture and cause a severe inflammation, which is mainly hypersensitive in character. Apparently, released bradyzoites rarely survive to infect other cells.

The clinical signs of toxoplasmosis vary considerably, depending on the organs affected. The most consistent signs reported are fever, lethargy, anorexia, ocular and nasal discharges, and respiratory distress. Neurologic signs include incoordination, circling, tremors, opisthotonus, convulsions, and paresis. Paresis is often associated with radiculitis and myositis. In the dog, signs may coexist with those of canine distemper and are not sufficiently distinctive to allow ready differentiation. Immunosuppression by intercurrent distemper may activate latent *Toxoplasma* infection.

Systemic toxoplasmosis has been reported in most species of domestic animals. The hallmarks are interstitial pneumonitis, focal hepatic necrosis, lymphadenitis, myocarditis, and nonsuppurative meningoencephalitis. Pulmonary lesions are probably most consistently found, followed by central nervous system lesions. The lesions in the various organs are morphologically similar in most species, varying mainly in degree.

Macroscopic lesions in the lung vary from irregular gray foci of necrosis on the pleural surface to a hemorrhagic pneumonia with confluent involvement of the ventral portions. Careful examination of the liver usually reveals either areas of focal necrosis or irregular mottling, and edema of the gallbladder. The spleen is enlarged, as are lymph nodes, which are wet and often red. Pleural, pericardial, and peritoneal effusions occur irregularly. Pale areas may be evident in the myocardium and skeletal muscle. Occasionally, the pancreas is the most severely affected organ, in which case an acute hemorrhagic reaction may involve the entire organ. Yellow, small, superficial intestinal ulcers with a hyperemic border have been reported in piglets. Large, pale areas of necrosis may be present in the renal cortices, mainly in goats and kittens. Chronic granulomatous toxoplasmosis may involve the intestine in older cats and produce annular areas of thickening. The mucosa overlying the granulomas may be ulcerated.

Microscopically, the early pulmonary lesions are characterized by diffuse interstitial pneumonia; the alveolar septa are thickened by a predominantly mononuclear inflammatory cell reaction with a few neutrophils and eosinophils. Macrophages and fibrinous exudate fill the alveoli. Foci of necrosis involving the alveolar septa, bronchiolar epithelial cells, and blood vessels are scattered throughout the lobules. These lesions are soon followed by regenerative changes, which are characterized by hyperplasia and hypertrophy of alveolar lining cells, mainly type II pneumocytes: so-called epithelialization of alveoli. In some areas this may be so marked as to give the affected areas an adenomatous appearance. Tachyzoites are usually evident in alveolar macrophages and may also be found in bronchiolar epithelial cells and the walls of blood vessels.

In the liver, irregular foci of coagulation necrosis are scattered at random throughout the lobules. There is usually little evidence of inflammation associated with the necrotic areas. Variable numbers of tachyzoites may be present in hepatocytes and Kupffer's cells, usually at the periphery of the lesions. A moderate lymphocytic reaction may be found in periportal areas and around central veins in cats. In this species, tachyzoites have been observed also in bile duct epithelial cells. If the pancreas is involved, there is extensive peripancreatic fat necrosis, with areas of coagulation necrosis in parenchyma. Numerous tachyzoites are usually evident in both ductal and acinar cells.

Lesions in lymph nodes are often associated with infection in the corresponding organ. They are characterized by irregular areas of coagulation necrosis, mainly in the cortex. A moderate inflammatory reaction may be evident at the periphery of the necrotic areas. There may be necrosis and depletion of lymphocytes in the follicles. In more chronic cases, the changes are those of nonspecific hyperplasia of lymphoid cells in cortical and paracortical areas, with a large macrophage population in the medullary sinusoids. Tachyzoites may be seen in phagocytic cells in sinusoids. Similar lesions may occur in the spleen. Necrotic areas are mainly located in the red pulp in this organ.

In the heart and skeletal muscle, foci of necrosis and mononuclear cell inflammation may be part of toxoplasmosis. There is often some difficulty in distinguishing between tachyzoites and mineralization of mitochondria in myocytes but, at some distance from areas of acute reaction, inert cysts can usually be identified in healthy fibers.

Brain lesions may vary in appearance. In the most fulminating cases, cerebral lesions may be relatively inconspicuous. They consist of a nonsuppurative meningoencephalitis with multifocal areas of necrosis and often malacia. There is swelling of endothelial cells, necrosis of vessel walls, and vasculitis. There may be marked perivascular edema and hyperplasia of perithelial cells. Tachyzoites and occasionally cysts may be found in vessel walls, and in necrotic areas in both gray and white matter at all levels of the brain. If survival is prolonged, residual cerebral lesions consist of microglial nodules along with more extensive hyperplasia of perithelial cells and perivascular fibrosis, which tend to make the vessels very obvious. At this stage tachyzoites are rare, and cysts 30 μm in diameter with a wall of amorphous acidophilic material ~0.5 μm thick, located in areas away from the lesions, may be the only form seen. Spinal cord lesions resemble those seen in the brain.

The placental and fetal lesions associated with *Toxoplasma* infection and abortion are described with The Female Genital System (Volume 3, Chapter 4), and ocular lesions with The Eye and Ear (Volume 1, Chapter 4).

The finding of tachyzoites and/or cysts in association with areas of coagulation necrosis in one or more organs, is highly suggestive of toxoplasmosis. With the exception of the dormant cysts which may be found in brain, the accidental discovery of *Toxoplasma* in routine sections is rare. The inference from this is that, in spite of the ubiquity of the infection, when *Toxoplasma* is found in sections in association with lesions, it is probably significant. The encephalitic form of toxoplasmosis in pigs must be differentiated from pansystemic viral infections with brain lesions, such as pseudorabies, hog cholera, African swine fever, and viral encephalitides. These diseases are discussed elsewhere. In sheep and horses, lesions of the central nervous system due to *Toxoplasma*-like organisms must be differentiated from those due to *Sarcocystis,* which tend to be associated with vessels. The lung lesions in cats with toxoplasmosis resemble those of feline calicivirus infection (see The Respiratory System, Chapter 6 of this volume). In dogs, and fetal and neonatal ruminants, *Neospora caninum* infection must be differentiated, as discussed subsequently with that agent.

Serologic tests are of limited value in the diagnosis of disease associated with *T. gondii* infection. The fluorescent antibody or immunoperoxidase technique using specific antiserum may be applied to infected tissues for antigen recognition. Ultimately, probes to detect specific nucleic acid sequences may be effective diagnostic tools.

Bibliography

Buxton, D. Ovine toxoplasmosis: A review. *J R Soc Med* **83:** 509–511, 1990.

Dubey, J. P. Direct development of enteroepithelial stages of *Toxoplasma* in the intestines of cats fed cysts. *Am J Vet Res* **40:** 1634–1637, 1979.

Dubey, J. P. Toxoplasmosis in dogs. *Canine Pract* **12(6):** 7–21, 26–28, 1985.

Dubey, J. P. A review of toxoplasmosis in pigs. *Vet Parasitol* **19:** 181–223, 1986.

Dubey, J. P. A review of toxoplasmosis in cattle. *Vet Parasitol* **22:** 177–202, 1986.

Dubey, J. P. Toxoplasmosis in cats. *Feline Pract* **16(4):** 12–26, 44–45, 1986.

Dubey, J. P. Toxoplasmosis. *Vet Clin North Am: Small Anim Pract* **17:** 1389–1403, 1987.

Dubey, J. P., and Beattie, C. P. "Toxoplasmosis of Animals and Man." Boca Raton, Florida, CRC Press, 1988.

Dubey, J. P., and Johnstone, I. Fatal neonatal toxoplasmosis in cats. *J Am Anim Hosp Assoc* **18:** 461–467, 1982.

Dubey, J. P. *et al.* Caprine toxoplasmosis: Abortion, clinical signs, and distribution of *Toxoplasma* in tissues of goats fed *Toxoplasma gondii* oocysts. *Am J Vet Res* **41:** 1072–1076, 1980.

Dubey, J. P. *et al.* Fatal toxoplasmosis in dogs. *J Am Anim Hosp Assoc* **25:** 659–664, 1989.

Dubey, J. P. *et al.* Lesions in fetal pigs with transplacentally induced toxoplasmosis. *Vet Pathol* **27:** 411–418, 1990.

Dubey, J. P. *et al.* Acute primary toxoplasmic hepatitis in an adult cat shedding *Toxoplasma gondii* oocysts. *J Am Vet Med Assoc* **197:** 1616–1618, 1990.

Frenkel, J. K. Pathophysiology of toxoplasmosis. *Parasitol Today* **4:** 273–278, 1988.

Greig, A. Toxoplasmosis in sheep. *Vet Ann* **30:** 85–91, 1990.

Hutchinson, W. M. *et al.* The life cycle of the coccidian parasite, *Toxoplasma gondii,* in the domestic cat. *Trans R Soc Trop Med Hyg* **65:** 380–399, 1971.

Jolly, R. D. Toxoplasmosis in piglets. *N Z Vet J* **17:** 87–89, 1969.

Johnson, A. M. *Toxoplasma:* Biology, pathology, immunology, and treatment. *In* "Coccidiosis of Man and Domestic Animals," P. L. Long (ed.), pp. 121–153. Boca Raton, Florida, CRC Press, 1990.

Parker, G. A. *et al.* Pathogenesis of acute toxoplasmosis in specific-pathogen-free cats. *Vet Pathol* **18:** 786–803, 1981.

Smart, M. E. *et al.* Toxoplasmosis in a cat associated with cholangitis and progressive pancreatitis. *Can Vet J* **14:** 313–316, 1973.

b. NEOSPOROSIS *Neospora caninum,* which causes toxoplasmosis-like disease in dogs and neonatal ruminants, is known only from meronts in tissue; the definitive host and life cycle are yet to be discovered. *Neospora* has been associated with systemic and central nervous system disease in dogs, and with abortion and central nervous system disease in neonatal ruminants. Tachyzoites undergoing endodyogony, and cysts containing bradyzoites are found in the tissues of affected animals. The mode of transmission is not completely known. Transplacental transmission occurs in ruminants and dogs; some subclinically infected bitches have given birth to successive litters of pups which became affected within the first few months of life. Transmission may also occur by ingestion of infected tissue, as in toxoplasmosis.

Dogs of all ages may be affected, but disease seems most characteristic as encephalomyelitis, polyradiculoneuritis, and polymyositis in puppies older than ~5 weeks, and perhaps involving several animals in a litter. Ascending paralysis, muscle contraction causing hyperextension of the limbs, cervical weakness, and dysphagia may progress to death, or animals will stabilize with posterior paralysis. In adult dogs, there are signs of widespread involvement of the central nervous system, and disseminated disease may be evident, with polymyositis, myocarditis, and dermatitis associated with parasite infection. Though disease may be precipitated or exacerbated by glucocorticoid administration experimentally, *Neospora* is a primary pathogen, independent of immunosuppression.

In acute infections there may be hepatic enlargement with coalescing areas of pallor, related to widespread necrosis of hepatocytes; streaky pallor of muscles due to myonecrosis, mineralization, and nonsuppurative myositis; and pulmonary congestion and edema, due to subacute alveolitis. Tachyzoites are common in affected tissues.

Nonsuppurative encephalomyelitis is associated with the presence of tachyzoites and tissue cysts in neurons and neuropil; the degree of necrosis, gliosis, neovascularization, and demyelination presumably depends to some extent on the duration of the lesion. Retinitis is also reported in association with *Neospora,* as is pyogranulomatous ulcerative dermatitis in one dog.

In abortions in ruminants, *Neospora* may be associated with necrotizing placentitis, myositis, and nonsuppurative encephalomyelitis.

Tachyzoites are approximately ovoid, ~5–7 μm long, and are found in small groups or large clusters, free in the cytoplasm, or in parasitophorous vacuoles in many types of cells throughout the body. Tissue cysts are found only in the brain and spinal cord. They are spherical or slightly elongate, to ~110 μm in greatest dimension. The cyst wall is ~1–4 μm thick, usually greater than the width of the bradyzoites, which are slender (1.5 × 7 μm), slightly curved, with an obvious nucleus; they stain weakly PAS positive.

Neospora must be distinguished from *Toxoplasma* in all species, and from *Sarcocystis* in aborted fetuses. *Neospora* tachyzoites resemble those of *Toxoplasma* in tissue section. Ultrastructurally, *Neospora* tachyzoites have over 11 rhoptries, whereas there are few in *Toxoplasma*. *Toxoplasma* always is found in a membrane-bound vacuole in the cytoplasm; *Neospora* tachyzoites often are not within a parasitophorous vacuole. *Neospora* tissue cysts are relatively uncommonly encountered, especially in acute cases. They are distinguished from *Toxoplasma* by the thicker wall (thinner than 0.5 μm in *Toxoplasma*). The organisms in tissue are also distinguishable by immunohistochemistry using specific immune serum. *Sarcocystis* meronts divide by endopolygony in endothelium in domestic animals; they are not in a parasitophorous vacuole; and merozoites lack rhoptries. Sarcocysts in muscle cells are within a parasitophorous vacuole; they have a distinct wall; and they are usually subdivided internally by septa.

Bibliography

Anderson, M. L. *et al. Neospora*-like protozoan infection as a major cause of abortion in California dairy cattle. *J Am Vet Med Assoc* **198:** 241–244, 1991.

Dubey, J. P. *Neospora caninum:* A look at a new *Toxoplasma*-like parasite of dogs and other animals. *Compend Cont Ed Pract Vet* **12:** 653–663, 1990.

Dubey, J. P., and Lindsay, D. S. *Neospora caninum*-induced abortion in sheep. *J Vet Diagn Invest* **2:** 230–233, 1990.

Dubey, J. P. *et al.* Newly recognized fatal protozoan disease of dogs. *J Am Vet Med Assoc* **192:** 1269–1285, 1988.

Dubey, J. P., Hartley, W. J., and Lindsay, D. S. Congenital *Neospora caninum* infection in a calf with spinal cord anomaly. *J Am Vet Med Assoc* **197:** 1043–1044, 1990.

Dubey, J. P., Koestner, A., and Piper, R. C. Repeated transplacental transmission of *Neospora caninum* in dogs. *J Am Vet Med Assoc* **197:** 857–860, 1990.

Dubey, J. P. *et al.* Fatal congenital *Neospora caninum* infection in a lamb. *J Parasitol* **76:** 127–130, 1990.

c. *Hammondia* Infection *Hammondia* spp. are obligatorily heteroxenous organisms, with the cat (*H. hammondi*) and dog (*H. heydorni*) as definitive hosts. They are also known as *Toxoplasma hammondi* and *Isospora bahiensis,* respectively. *Toxoplasma*-like oocysts are shed in the feces of the definitive host and are infectious to intermediate hosts, mammals and birds (*H. hammondi*), and ruminants (*H. heydorni*). Here, bradyzoites develop in cysts in striated muscle, which are infective when ingested by the carnivore. Disease is not associated with infection of intermediate hosts; diarrhea may occur in heavily infected dogs.

Bibliography

Dubey, J. P., and Williams, D. S. F. *Hammondia heydorni* infection in sheep, goats, moose, dogs, and coyotes. *Parasitology* **81:** 123–127, 1980.

Frenkel, J. K., and Dubey, J. P. *Hammondia hammondi* gen. nov. sp. nov. from domestic cats, a new coccidian related to *Toxoplasma* and *Sarcocystis*. *Z Parasitenk* **45:** 3–12, 1975.

Nassar, A. M., Hilai, M., and Rommel, M. *Hammondia heydorni* infection in camels (*Camelus dromedarius*) and water buffaloes (*Bubalus bubalis*) in Egypt. *Z Parasitenkd* **69:** 693–694, 1983.

d. *Sarcocystis* Infection *Sarcocystis* spp. are obligatorily heteroxenous. Inconspicuous sexual stages occur in the epithelium at the tips of villi in the small intestine of carnivores, and oocysts sporulate in the subepithelial lamina propria, producing two sporocysts within a thin oocyst wall. Sporocysts containing four sporozoites are shed in feces. These are infective to intermediate hosts, in which several generations of merogony occur in vascular endothelium, and a final cyst containing merozoites (bradyzoites) is formed in myocytes and occasionally in other cells. Ingestion of tissue cysts containing bradyzoites initiates gametogony in the definitive host. There is apparently no resistance to the development of gamonts, and no disease is associated with them in the definitive host.

Many species of *Sarcocystis* are recognized, based on prey–predator cycles. Sporogony of a given species usually occurs in only one or a few genera of carnivores. The number of species capable of acting as intermediate hosts may be narrow or wide, depending on the species of *Sarcocystis*.

Sarcocystis cysts in ovine, and occasionally, bovine muscle may be grossly visible, causing losses at meat inspection. There is mounting evidence that *Sarcocystis* is involved in the etiology of eosinophilic myositis in cattle. *Sarcocystis* infection in cattle (*S. cruzi*), sheep (*S. tenella*), and swine (*S. miescheriana*), and, experimentally, in goats (*S. capracanis,*) may cause an acute fatal disease characterized by anemia and widespread hemorrhage, or chronic ill thrift. Cattle develop inappetence, weight loss, reduced milk yield, hyperexcitability, hair loss, and in some animals, nervous signs. Both syndromes are initiated during the endothelial phase of the infection. Abortion occurs during this phase in some species. Abortion associated with the acute disease is the result of the systemic illness, and the fetus usually is not infected. However, in cattle, some abortions, seen in otherwise clinically normal animals, are associated with meronts of *Sarcocystis* in the placenta and in vascular endothelium of the fetus, especially in the brain, and with nonsuppurative encephalitis. Encephalitis is occasionally associated with *Sarcocystis* infection in sheep, and in horses *Sarcocystis neurona* is the cause of protozoal myeloencephalitis. Details of these syndromes are discussed in the chapters on Muscle and Tendon (Volume 1, Chapter 2), The Female Genital System (Volume 3, Chapter 4) and The Nervous System (Volume 1, Chapter 3).

A *Sarcocystis*-like agent has also been implicated in mortality of Rottweiler dogs with hepatitis, encephalitis, and dermatitis. The origin and species involved are unknown.

Bibliography

Cawthorn, R. J., and Speer, C. A. *Sarcocystis:* Infection and disease of humans, livestock, wildlife, and other hosts. *In* "Coccidiosis of Man and Domestic Animals," P. L. Long (ed.), pp. 91–120. Boca Raton, Florida, CRC Press, 1990.

Dubey, J. P. Lesions in sheep inoculated with *Sarcocystis tenella* sporocysts from canine feces. *Vet Parasitol* **26:** 237–252, 1988.
Dubey, J. P., Hartley, W. J., and Badman, R. T. Fatal perinatal sarcocystosis in a lamb. *J Parasitol* **75:** 980–982, 1989.
Dubey, J. P., Speer, C. A., and Fayer, R. "Sarcocystosis of Animals and Man." Boca Raton, Florida, CRC Press, 1989.
Dubey, J. P. *et al.* Condemnation of beef because of *Sarcocystis hirsuta* infection. *J Am Vet Med Assoc* **196:** 1095–1096, 1990.
Dubey, J. P. *et al.* Acute sarcocystosislike disease in a dog. *J Am Vet Med Assoc* **198:** 439–443, 1991.
Dubey, J. P. *et al. Sarcocystis neurona* n. sp. (Protozoa: Apicomplexa), the etiologic agent of equine protozoal myeloencephalitis. *J Parasitol* **77:** 212–218, 1991.
Fayer, R., and Dubey, J. P. Bovine sarcocystosis. *Compend Cont Ed Pract Vet* **8:** F130–F142, 1986.
Hong, C. B. *et al.* Sarcocystosis in an aborted bovine fetus. *J Am Vet Med Assoc* **181:** 585–588, 1982.
O'Toole, D. *et al.* Experimental microcyst sarcocystis infection in lambs: Pathology. *Vet Rec* **119:** 525–531, 1986.

e. *Besnoitia* Infection *Besnoitia* spp. are also obligatorily heteroxenous. Some stages of merogony, and gametogony, occur in the intestine of the definitive host, cats, where they are not known to be pathogenic. Oocysts are shed unsporulated. When sporulated they are *Isospora*-like, and so-called large forms of *Isospora bigemina* are *Besnoitia* spp. Meronts in the intermediate host develop in mesenchymal cells, probably fibroblasts, which become massively hypertrophic, forming cysts containing many clusters of merozoites (bradyzoites) in the host cell cytoplasm. The definitive hosts are not known for many *Besnoitia* species. Among domestic animals cysts of *Besnoitia besnoiti* may assume some significance in the skin of cattle (see The Skin and Appendages, Volume 1, Chapter 4), and *Besnoitia* cysts have been reported in association with laryngeal polyps in a horse.

Bibliography

Frenkel, J. K. *Besnoitia wallacei* of cats and rodents: With a reclassification of other cyst-forming isosporoid coccidia. *J Parasitol* **63:** 611–628, 1977.
Ito, S., and Shimura, K. The comparison of *Isospora bigemina* large type of the cat and *Besnoitia wallacei. Jpn J Vet Sci* **48:** 433–435, 1986.
Lane, J. G., Lucke, V. M., and Wright, A. I. Parasitic laryngeal papillomatosis in a horse. *Vet Rec* **119:** 591–593, 1986.
Smith, D. D., and Frenkel, J. K. *Besnoitia darlingi* (Protozoa: Toxoplasmatinae): Cyclic transmission by cats. *J Parasitol* **63:** 1066–1071, 1977.

3. *Cryptosporidiosis*

Cryptosporidium is a small apicomplexan protozoan parasite, found on the surface of epithelium in the gastrointestinal (Fig. 1.186A,B) and respiratory tracts of mammals, birds, and reptiles. Respiratory infection is most significant in birds, and disease in mammals is generally enteric.

Two species are recognized in mammals: *C. muris,* described by Tyzzer from the stomach of the mouse; and *C. parvum,* smaller, and initially described in the mouse intestine. *Cryptosporidium parvum* seems to be transmissible freely among mammals, whereas *C. muris* is recognized in the abomasum of ruminants and probably in the stomach of cats. Distinct species infect birds (*C. meleagridis* and *C. baileyi*), reptiles (*C. serpentis*), and fish (*C. nasorum*). Oocysts from birds do not infect mammals. Cryptosporidiosis is a zoonosis; some human cases, including some among veterinary students, have been associated with exposure to infected animals.

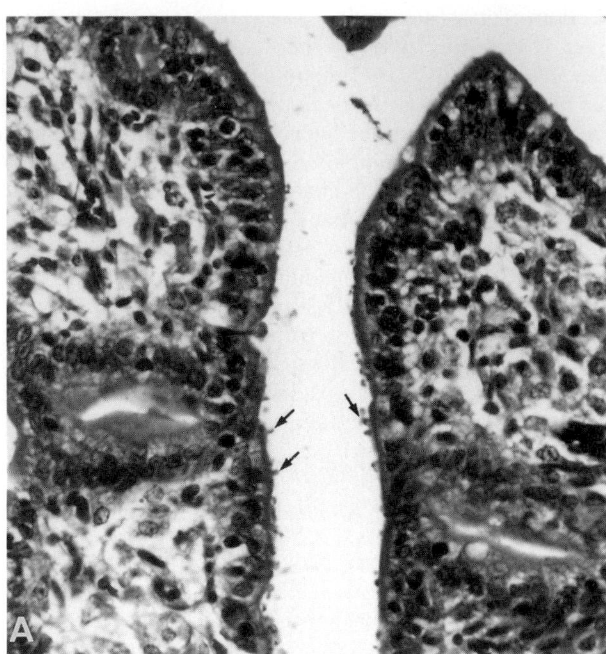

Fig. 1.186A Cryptosporidia, appearing as minute basophilic dots (arrows) on the brush border of enterocytes. Small intestine. Foal.

Cryptosporidium has a typical coccidian life cycle, with merogony, gametogony, and sporogony occurring in the brush border of infected epithelial cells; the prepatent period in calves is ~4 days. The organisms are within a vacuole formed by apposition of two unit membranes of the host cell, probably caused by inversion of a microvillus by the infecting sporozoite or merozoite. A specialized feeder organelle is usually present at the attachment zone in the base of the vacuole, between the infecting organism and the cytoplasm of the host cell. Developmental stages are small, in most cases ~2–6 μm in diameter. Undifferentiated meronts and gamonts are recognized as small basophilic trophozoites. Mature schizonts contain small falciform merozoites. Macrogamonts are ~5 μm in diameter, and contain small granules. Oocysts in tissue sections often are collapsed into a crescent shape. The various stages may be recognized in wax- or plastic-embedded sections under the light microscope but are best studied with the electron microscope. Oocysts may be demonstrated by fecal flotation, or in fecal smears stained with Giemsa, by a modified Ziehl–Neelsen technique, or with

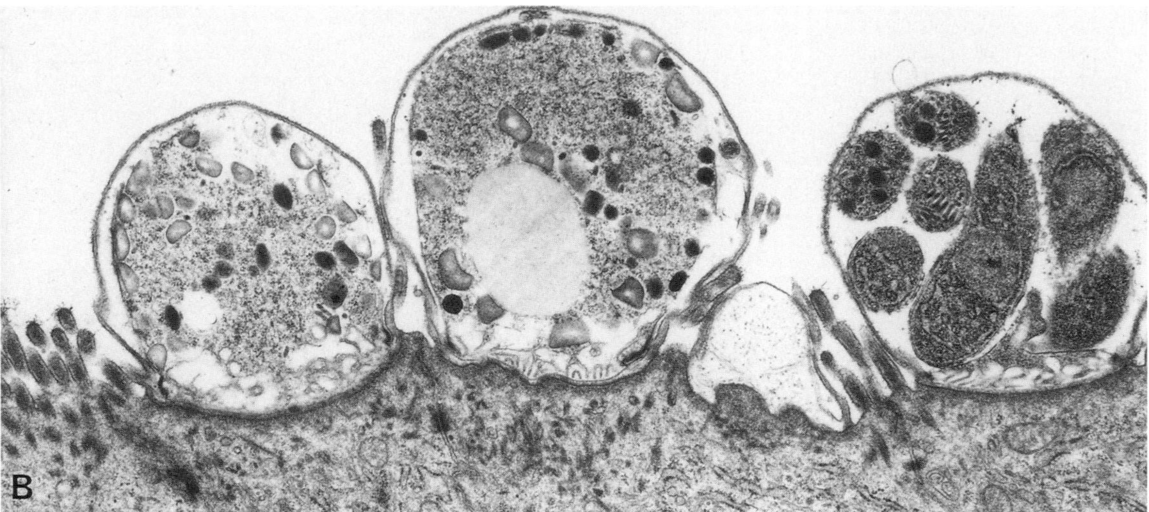

Fig. 1.186B Cryptosporidia attached to apex of enterocytes in small intestine. Two macrogametes and a schizont containing merozoites. (Courtesy of S. Tzipori.)

auramine O or fluorescein-labeled antibody and examined with ultraviolet light.

Two types of schizonts develop: type I produce up to eight merozoites, which recycle, producing either more type I schizonts, or a generation of type II schizonts; type II schizonts produce four merozoites, which become gametocytes. Oocysts sporulate within the host to contain four sporozoites. These also adopt two forms: thin-walled ones, which excyst within the gut, permitting autoinfection; and thick-walled ones, which are passed in the feces. The massive number of organisms found in clinically affected animals suggests that extensive recycling of merozoites from type I schizonts, and/or heavy autoinfection, takes place within the host.

The pathogenicity of cryptosporidia was not recognized until relatively recently, and how they cause disease is unknown. In some species, infection usually appears to be asymptomatic. Neonates seem particularly prone to cryptosporidiosis, and this is especially so among ruminants (calves, lambs, kids, red deer calves). Diarrhea, anorexia and depression in calves occurs usually between ~1 and 4 weeks of age, and in lambs about 5–14 days old. However, naive calves to 3 months of age are susceptible to infection and may develop diarrhea.

The prevalence of cryptosporidiosis in humans with acquired immunodeficiency syndrome (AIDS) implies that immunosuppression may be contributory to the development of disease. Heavy infections are also reported in Arabian foals with combined immunodeficiency, and cryptosporidiosis has occurred in cats with feline leukemia virus infection, and in dogs with canine distemper. In immunocompromised individuals, organisms may be present at any level of the gastrointestinal tract, from esophagus to colon. Liver, gall bladder, pancreas, and their ducts may also be involved, as may the respiratory tract. However, severe immunodeficiency does not appear to be a requirement for infection or disease in domestic animals. Cryptosporidia are incriminated sporadically as a cause of diarrhea in some animals, including pigs, in which they are usually considered incidental. Cryptosporidia frequently occur concurrent with enterotoxigenic *E. coli,* rotavirus, or coronavirus infection in neonatal ruminants. It is clear from experimental work that *Cryptosporidium* can be a primary pathogen, but the syndrome which it produces typically is not so severe as that generated by some other agents.

In all species, intestinal cryptosporidiosis is associated with villus atrophy of varying severity, characterized by blunting and some fusion of villi, and by hypertrophy of crypts of Lieberkühn (Fig. 1.187A,C). Surface epithelium is usually cuboidal, rounded, or low columnar, and sometimes exfoliating or forming irregular projections at tips of villi. Large numbers of cryptosporidia are usually visible in the microvillus border of cells on the villi (Fig. 1.187B), and not in crypts of Lieberkühn, although occasionally, the reverse is true. Organisms are most heavily distributed in the distal half of the small intestine, especially in ileum. However, they may occur in the cecum and colon, where they infect cells on the surface and occasionally in glands. In heavily infected large bowel, some attenuation of surface epithelium and dilation of crypts with necrotic debris may be evident. Mild proprial infiltrates of neutrophils and mixed mononuclear cells are present in both small and large intestine.

Diarrhea in cryptosporidiosis is due to malabsorption associated with villus atrophy; an immature population of epithelial cells on the surface; and perhaps to the occupation of a large proportion of the surface area of absorptive cells by the organisms. Mucosal lactase activity in infected calves is also significantly reduced. Hypersecretion by infected mucosa has not been demonstrated.

Cryptosporidiosis due to *C. parvum* is most significant

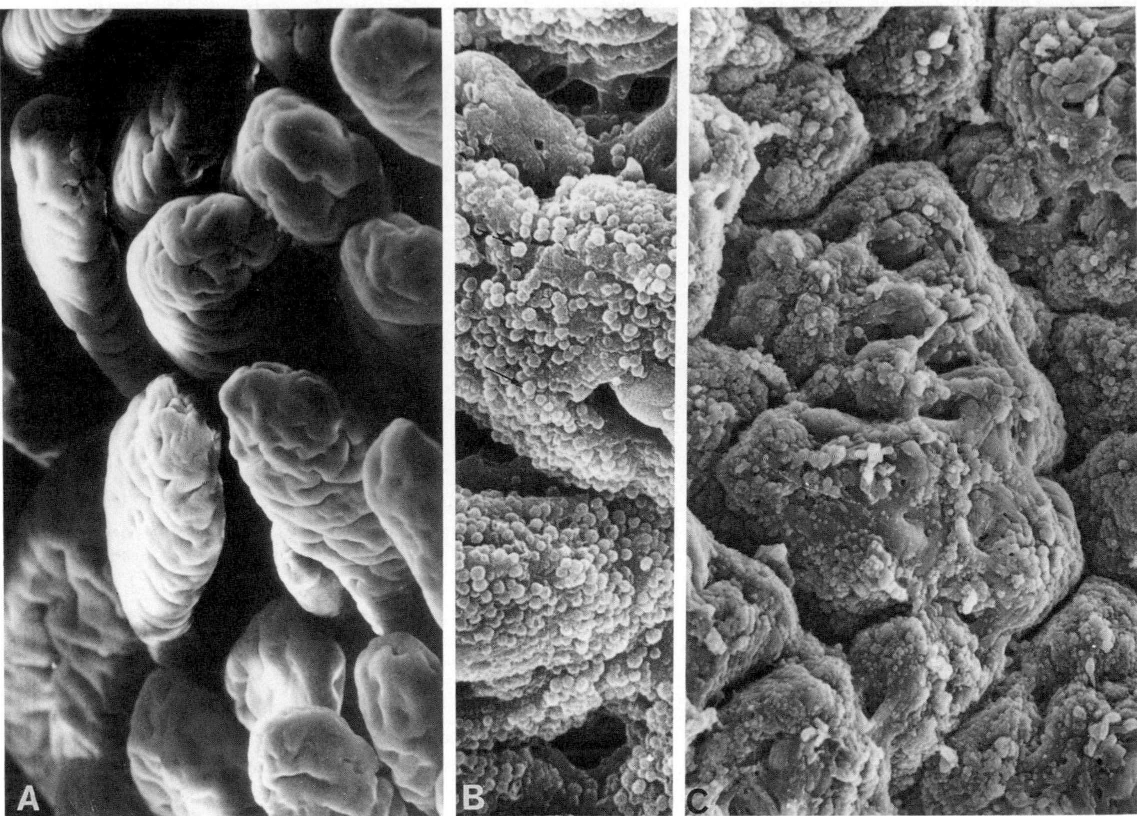

Fig. 1.187 Scanning electron micrographs. (A) Normal villi. (B) Detail of (C) showing cryptosporidia (arrows). (C) Villus atrophy associated with cryptosporidiosis. Cryptosporidia are visible as minute spheres on mucosal surface. (Courtesy of S. Tzipori.)

in calves, as a cause of undifferentiated neonatal diarrhea, in which it must be differentiated particularly from coronavirus and rotavirus infection. Frequently it is concurrent with other agents causing this syndrome; it tends to be most prevalent in animals ~2 weeks old. A similar situation occurs in lambs, though disease does not appear to be so common, or well recognized, in that species. It is a sporadic, or minor cause of sometimes fatal diarrhea in other species of ruminants, including goats, farmed red deer, and captive ungulates in zoos, usually occurring in neonates.

Though cryptosporidiosis can be induced experimentally in piglets, it is a rare cause of spontaneous disease in swine. It is only occasionally associated with disease of carnivores, and then often in probably immunocompromised animals. Though infection of foals is not uncommon, *Cryptosporidium* has been associated with disease mainly in animals with combined immunodeficiency, complicated by adenovirus infection. Disease has not occurred in successful experimental infections in foals, and the role of cryptosporidia in the etiology of neonatal diarrhea in foals is poorly defined.

The diagnosis is based on the presence of large numbers of cryptosporidia in sections of freshly fixed lower small intestine, preferably in association with villus atrophy. The organism must be differentiated from enterotoxigenic and enterocyte adherent-effacing *E. coli, Enterococcus durans,* and other agents attaching to the brush border of intestinal epithelium. Examination of smears of ileal mucosa stained with Giemsa may allow a rapid diagnosis, or permit a diagnosis on tissue from an animal dead for some hours.

Cryptosporidium muris in the abomasum of calves and older cattle is not associated with diarrhea, but plasma pepsinogen levels rise, and weight gains of some growing animals may be adversely affected. There is mucous metaplasia/hyperplasia in the fundic glands, which are dilated, with attenuation of the lining epithelium, on which cryptosporidia are numerous. Experimentally, *C. muris* will infect the stomach of cats. Rarely, cryptosporidia are seen in gastric biopsies from cats, sometimes associated with mild gastritis, but a causal relationship has not been established.

Bibliography

Anderson, B. C. Abomasal cryptosporidiosis in cattle. *Vet Pathol* **24:** 235–238, 1987.

Angus, K. W., and Blewett, D. A. (eds.). "Cryptosporidiosis." Proceedings of the First International Workshop. Edinburgh, Animal Diseases Research Association, 1989.

Argenzio, R. A. *et al.* Villous atrophy, crypt hyperplasia, cellular infiltration, and impaired glucose–Na absorption in enteric cryptosporidiosis of pigs. *Gastroenterology* **98:** 1129–1140, 1990.

Coleman, S. U. *et al.* Prevalence of *Cryptosporidium* sp. in equids in Louisiana. *Am J Vet Res* **50:** 575–577, 1989.

Current, W. L., and Blagburn, B. L. *Cryptosporidium:* Infections in man and domestic animals. *In* "Coccidiosis of Man and Domestic Animals," P.L. Long (ed.), pp. 155–185. Boca Raton, Florida, CRC Press, 1990.

Dubey, J. P., Speer, C. C., and Fayer, R. (eds.). "Cryptosporidiosis of Man and Animals." Boca Raton, Florida, CRC Press, 1990.

Goodwin, M. A., and Barsanti, J. A. Intractable diarrhea associated with intestinal cryptosporidiosis in a domestic cat also infected with feline leukemia virus. *J Am Anim Hosp Assoc* **26:** 365–368, 1990.

Green, C. E., Jacobs, G. J., and Prickett, D. Intestinal malabsorption and cryptosporidiosis in an adult dog. *J Am Vet Med Assoc* **197:** 365–367, 1990.

Harp, J. A., Woodmansee, D. B., and Moon, H. W. Resistance of calves to *Cryptosporidium parvum:* Effects of age and previous exposure. *Infect Immun* **58:** 2237–2240, 1990.

Heine, J. *et al.* Enteric lesions and diarrhea in gnotobiotic calves monoinfected with *Cryptosporidium* species. *J Infect Dis* **150:** 768–774, 1984.

Holland, R. E., Herdt, T. H., and Refsal, K. R. Pulmonary excretion of H_2 in calves with *Cryptosporidium*-induced malabsorption. *Dig Dis Sci* **34:** 1399–1404, 1989.

Mair, T. S. *et al.* Concurrent *Cryptosporidium* and coronavirus infections in an Arabian foal with combined immunodeficiency syndrome. *Vet Rec* **126:** 127–130, 1990.

Moore, D. A., and Zeman, D. H. Cryptosporidiosis in neonatal calves: 277 cases (1986–1987). *J Am Vet Med Assoc* **198:** 1969–1971, 1991.

Moore, J. A., Blagburn, B. L., and Lindsay, D. S. Cryptosporidiosis in animals including humans. *Compend Cont Ed Pract Vet* **10:** 275–287, 1988.

Pospischil, A. *et al.* Abomasal cryptosporidiosis in mountain gazelles. *Vet Rec* **121:** 379–380, 1987.

Reif, J. S. *et al.* Human cryptosporidiosis associated with an epizootic in calves. *Am J Publ Health* **79:** 1528–1530, 1989.

Sanford, S. E. Enteric cryptosporidial infection in pigs: 184 cases (1981–1985). *J Am Vet Med Assoc* **190:** 695–698, 1987.

Turnwald, G. H. *et al.* Cryptosporidiosis associated with immunosuppression attributable to distemper in a pup. *J Am Vet Med Assoc* **192:** 79–81, 1988.

Tzipori, S. Cryptosporidiosis in perspective. *Adv Parasitol* **27:** 63–129, 1988.

Tzipori, S. *et al.* Experimental cryptosporidiosis in calves: Clinical manifestations and pathological findings. *Vet Rec* **112:** 116–120, 1983.

4. Amoebiasis

Entamoeba histolytica is the cause of amoebiasis in humans, nonhuman primates, and, rarely, in other species including dogs and cattle; cats are susceptible to experimental infection. Infection in dogs is sporadic, probably acquired by exposure to cysts in feces from infected humans. Dogs tend not to pass encysted amoebae; hence, it has been suggested that they present little public health hazard, and are unlikely to support spread from dog to dog. However, under some circumstances, cysts may be shed, and fecal material containing motile trophozoites has been used to transmit infection orally to other dogs.

Amoebae usually are nonpathogenic inhabitants of the lumen of the large bowel, but sometimes they cause colitis. The diet and immune status of the host, and virulence attributes of various strains of the organism, seem to influence pathogenicity, but the precise host and parasite factors promoting invasion and necrosis are not known. Contact of amoebae with host cells, necessary for contact-dependent killing, is mediated by adhesins. Amoebae secrete several factors which alter membrane permeability, or are enterotoxic or cytotoxic, and pathogenic strains are erythrophagocytic. Amoebae attract and lyse neutrophils, which may exacerbate local tissue damage. They also release a factor which inhibits macrophage motility, and they generally suppress macrophage function.

Amoebiasis in dogs is associated with diarrheic or mucoid feces, perhaps with some blood, or with dysentery. Erosive mucosal colitis or ulcerative colitis occurs in dogs with amoebiasis, and disease seems more common or severe in animals with concomitant *Trichuris* or *Ancylostoma* infection.

Early lesions in human amoebiasis seem to be a diffuse acute mucosal colitis, with focal erosions or ulcerations. Amoebae, though scarce, may be found in mucus on the colonic surface, but are most numerous in the fibrinocellular exudate over erosions or superficial ulcers. Ulcers advance as an area of necrosis and predominantly neutrophilic infiltrate, causing loss of glands, and extending for the full depth of the mucosa. Established ulcerative amoebic colitis classically has a flask-shaped ulcer, the narrow neck through the mucosa, and the broad base in the submucosa. There amoebae, and necrosis, expand laterally, apparently less constrained by the architecture of the tissue. The ragged mucosal margin of the ulcer overhangs the excavation in the submucosa. The muscularis is rarely invaded. Amoebae may attain the deeper tissue via mucosal blood vessels or lymphatics. A mixed inflammatory reaction is present about the periphery of areas of necrosis.

Amoebae may be present, commonly in small clusters, in necrotic debris or in adjacent viable tissue, frequently not involved in an inflammatory reaction. Amoebae in tissue, often surrounded by a clear halo, may be spherical or irregular, with extended pseudopodia, and are ~6–50 μm in diameter. The nucleus has a central dense karyosome and peripheral chromatin clumps. The cytoplasm may appear foamy, can contain remnants of erythrocytes in phagolysosomes, and contains glycogen, which makes the cytoplasm PAS positive. The lesions of established amoebiasis in the colon of dogs resemble those in humans; the early lesions may as well.

Although dissemination of amoebae, with abscessation in other organs, especially liver, lung, and brain, is a relatively common complication in humans, it seems rare in dogs. One such case occurred in an animal with canine distemper.

Bibliography

Denis, M., and Chadee, K. Immunopathology of *Entamoeba histolytica* infections. *Parasitol Today* **4:** 247–252, 1988.

Jordan, H. E. Amebiasis (*Entamoeba histolytica*) in the dog. *Vet Med Small Anim Clin* **62:** 61–64, 1967.

Kretschmer, R. R. (ed.). "Amebiasis: Infection and Disease by *Entamoeba histolytica*." Boca Raton, Florida, CRC Press, 1990.

Ojcius, D. M., and Young, J. D.-E. A role for pore-forming proteins in the pathogenesis of parasites? *Parasitol Today* **6:** 163–165, 1990.

Perez-Tamayo, R. Pathology of amebiasis. *In* "Amebiasis," A. Martinez-Palomo (ed.), pp. 45–94. Amsterdam, Elsevier, 1986.

Pittman, F. E., El-Hashimi, W. K.,and Pittman, J. C. Studies of human amebiasis. II. Light- and electron-microscopic observations of colonic mucosa and exudate in acute amebic colitis. *Gastroenterology* **65:** 588–603, 1973.

Thorson, R. E., Seibold, H. R., and Bailey, W. S. Systemic amebiasis with distemper in a dog. *J Am Vet Med Assoc* **129:** 335–336, 1956.

Wittnich, C. *Entamoeba histolytica* infection in a German shepherd dog. *Can Vet J* **17:** 259–263, 1976.

5. Giardia *and Other Flagellates*

Giardia spp. are flagellate protozoa which inhabit the small intestine of a wide range of vertebrates. The taxonomy of the genus is difficult. It appears that three morphologically distinct groups exist, each with a relatively wide host range. *Giardia duodenalis* infection is common in humans, and is associated with disease in a few of them. *Giardia* from humans are infective for a wide range of mammals. There is circumstantial evidence that human giardiasis may be zoonotic in some cases, but this is the subject of debate. *Giardia duodenalis* occurs in dogs, cats, cattle, sheep, goats, and horses, and has been associated with disease, with varying degrees of credibility, in most of these hosts.

Giardia trophozoites are pyriform in outline, ~10–20 μm long by 5–15 μm wide and 2–4 μm thick, and convex on the dorsal surface. The concave ventral surface is modified by the presence of a disk, which functions in attachment. Nutrient absorption seems to occur through the dorsal surface. A pair of nuclei, two axonemes, two medial bodies, and four pairs of flagella are present. The organisms apply their ventral aspect to the microvillous surface of enterocytes (Fig. 1.188), usually between villi, in folds on the villous surface, or occasionally in crypts of Lieberkühn. *Giardia* have been demonstrated in the mucosa, but this is an unusual and probably aberrant location. Relatively resistant oval cysts are passed in the feces, and transmission is by the fecal–oral route.

The significance of *Giardia* as a pathogen in humans and other species has been controversial, since asymptomatic infection is the rule. There now is no doubt that under some circumstances *Giardia* may cause disease. How the host–parasite relationship is modified, and the pathogenesis of the disease, are still unclear.

In young dogs and cats, in which giardiosis is most important, though still uncommon, the main sign is intermittent or chronic diarrhea, which may persist for several months. The stool is soft, pale, mucoid, and greasy. Though appetite is not usually impaired, there may be a reduced growth rate or weight loss, suggesting malabsorption. A poor hair coat is attributed to deficiency of fat-soluble vitamins. Gastrointestinal dysfunction has not been extensively documented in animals. Some people with *Giardia* infection have malabsorption of *d*-xylose and vitamin B_{12}, with steatorrhea and hypocarotinemia. Excess fecal fat has been found in infected cats, but *d*-xylose malabsorption was not demonstrated in one dog with giardiosis.

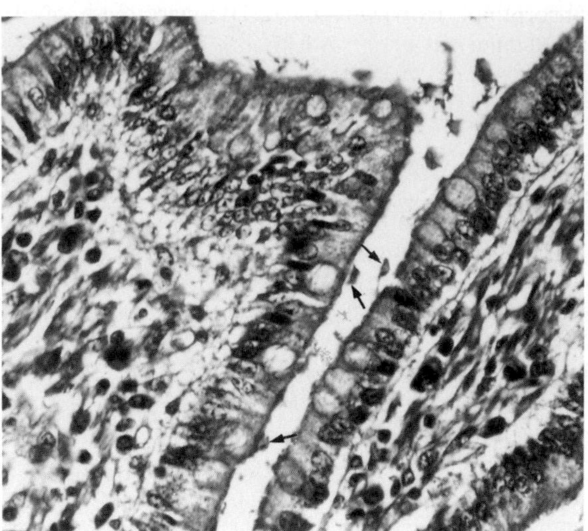

Fig. 1.188 *Giardia lamblia* (arrows) applied to brush border of enterocytes on villi. Dog.

Several mechanisms have been proposed to explain these findings. Although villus atrophy may occur in humans with giardiosis, this occurs mainly in a subgroup of patients with hypogammaglobulinemia. Marked histologic abnormality is not found in many cases of giardiosis in humans, and this seems also to be true for dogs and cats. In experimental murine giardiosis, infection is associated with hypertrophy of crypts and increased production of cells, combined with an increased rate of movement of enterocytes along villi. Intraepithelial lymphocytes are common in infected intestine, and altered epithelial kinetics may be related to cell-mediated immune reactions in the mucosa. Atrophy of villi has been associated with restoration of cell-mediated immune competence in *Giardia*-infected athymic mice, suggesting that immune phenomena may be involved in the pathogenesis of giardiosis.

Selective deficiencies in some brush border enzymes occur in humans with giardiosis. Possibly these are related to altered villus transit times, or to the direct effects of *Giardia* on microvilli, which may be deformed adjacent to adherent organisms, or diffusely shortened. *Giardia* may also inhibit the activity of pancreatic lipase, causing fat malabsorption. However, bacterial overgrowth of the small intestine may occur with *Giardia* infection, and associated bile salt deconjugation could explain steatorrhea in giardiosis. Possibly *Giardia* are capable of deconjugating bile salts.

Giardiosis is usually diagnosed clinically on the basis of typical cysts in fecal flotations, or trophozoites in intestinal aspirates or fecal smears, coupled with remission of clinical signs following therapy, and an inability to identify other potential causes of the signs. A diagnosis is sometimes based on findings in biopsies of small intestine, or at autopsy.

In dogs and cats, morphologic changes in the mucosa are not well defined. The mucosa may appear normal, but there may be equivocal blunting of villi, perhaps associated with a moderate infiltrate of mononuclear cells into the core of the villus, or a heavy population of intraepithelial lymphocytes. *Giardia* should be sought in animals with malabsorption syndromes. They lie between villi, and are usually evident as crescent shapes, applied by their concave surface to the brush border of epithelial cells. In favorable sections through the level of the nuclei, they may appear to have a pair of eyes. Trophozoites oriented along the plane of section may look as they do in smears, the paired nuclei giving the organism a facelike appearance. An abnormal number of bacteria, suggestive of overgrowth, may be present in the mucus and content in the vicinity, in symptomatic animals. A diagnosis of giardiosis should always be reserved for those cases in which no other explanation for the syndrome can be identified.

Giardiosis has been associated with mucosal colitis in dogs, but the association is not clearly causal.

Among animals other than dogs and cats, *Giardia* seems most convincingly to be associated with enteric signs in calves, which may pass soft mucoid feces, and have a reduced growth rate. However, the significance of infection in that and other species is very poorly defined. Experimental infection of calves has produced only equivocal diarrhea.

Trichomonas, or similar flagellates, are sometimes encountered in the feces of horses, dogs, cats, and cattle with diarrhea, but there is no established causal association between the organisms and disease.

Bibliography

Barlough, J. E. Canine giardiasis: A review. *J Small Anim Pract* **20:** 613–623, 1979.

Buret, A., Gall, D. G., and Olson, M. E. Effects of murine giardiasis on growth, intestinal morphology, and disaccharidase activity. *J Parasitol* **76:** 403–409, 1990.

Buret, A. *et al.* Zoonotic potential of giardiasis in domestic ruminants. *J Infect Dis* **162:** 231–237, 1990.

Buret, A. *et al.* Intestinal protozoa and epithelial kinetics, structure, and function. *Parasitol Today* **6:** 375–380, 1990.

Gasser, R. B. Is giardiasis a zoonosis? *Aust Vet J* **67:** 456, 1990.

Hartong, E. A., Gourley, W. K., and Arvanitakis, C. Giardiasis: Clinical spectrum and functional–structural abnormalities of the small intestinal mucosa. *Gastroenterology* **77:** 61–69, 1979.

Kirkpatrick, C. E. Feline giardiasis: A review. *J Small Anim Pract* **27:** 69–80, 1986.

Kirkpatrick, C. E. Giardiasis in large animals. *Compend Cont Ed Pract Vet* **11:** 80–86, 1989.

Meyer, E. A. (ed.). "Giardiasis." Amsterdam, Elsevier, 1990.

Oberhuber, G., and Stolte, M. Giardiasis: Analysis of histological changes in biopsy specimens of 80 patients. *J Clin Pathol* **43:** 641–643, 1990.

Taminelli, V. *et al.* Experimentelle Infektion von Kälbern und Schafen mit bovinen *Giardia*-isolaten. *Schweiz Arch Tierheilk* **131:** 551–564, 1989.

6. Balantidium

Balantidium is a large oval protozoan ~50–60 μm or more long, and ~25–45 μm wide, with a macronucleus and micronucleus, and covered by many cilia arrayed in rows. *Balantidium coli* occurs in the large bowel of swine, humans, and nonhuman primates. It is very common in pigs, and many infected humans live in close contact with swine. It has also been reported from several dogs with access to swine yards, as a complication of trichurosis.

Balantidium is normally present as a commensal in the lumen of the cecum and colon, but is capable of opportunistic invasion of tissues injured by other diseases. Its capacity to invade may be related to production of hyaluronidase. In swine, where the organisms are most commonly encountered by veterinary pathologists, *Balantidium* may be found at the leading edge of the necrotizing or ulcerative lesions of the large intestine which develop secondary to intestinal adenomatosis (Fig. 1.189), swine dysentery, or perhaps salmonellosis. Probably *Balantidium* are interacting with anaerobic colonic flora in perpetuating and advancing the necrotizing lesions which are themselves complications of the primary bacterial infection. *Balantidium* is recognized in tissue by large size, ovoid shape, the dense curved or kidney-shaped macronu-

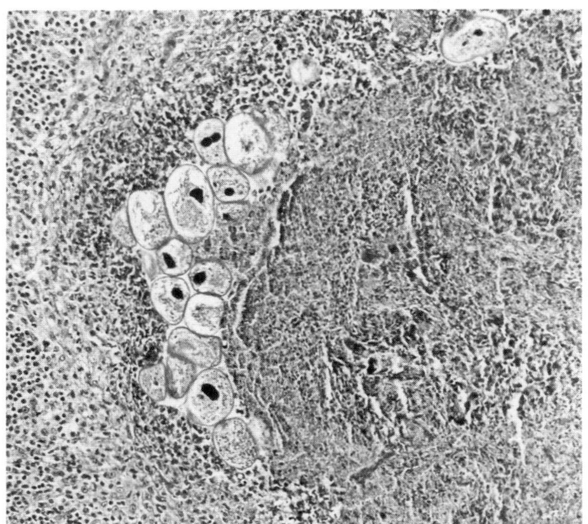

Fig. 1.189 *Balantidium coli* in ulcerated colon of pig with intestinal adenomatosis and necrotic enteritis.

cleus, and the presence of cilia (which may be accentuated by silver stains) in rows on the surface.

Bibliography

Arean, V. M., and Echevarria, R. Balantidiasis. *In* "Pathology of Protozoal and Helminthic Diseases," R. A. Marcial-Rojas (ed.), pp. 234–253. Baltimore, Maryland, Williams & Wilkins, 1971.

Ewing, S. A., and Bull, R. W. Severe chronic canine diarrhea associated with *Balantidium–Trichuris* infection. *J Am Vet Med Assoc* **149:** 519–520, 1966.

Acknowledgments

The authors wish to acknowledge the helpful criticism of portions of the manuscript by Suzanne Carman, Robert Clarke, Carlton Gyles, Philip Lautenslager, Michael Livesey, John Prescott, Jan Thorsen, and Bruce Wilkie. Jean Bagg and Carol Lee Ernst typed the manuscript, and Edward Eaton processed photographic illustrations. Janice Frame, Judy Henry, Adele Hulzebosch, Paul Innes, Gareth Jones, Martha Winhall, Patricia Weir, Pat Wallace, and Jo Boyle provided bibliographic or other assistance.

CHAPTER 2 The Liver and Biliary System

W. ROGER KELLY
University of Queensland, Australia

I. General Considerations

The liver is the major metabolic focus of the animal, and the dynamics of its synthetic, excretory, and catabolic processes are such that its content, at any instant, of various lipids, proteins, and carbohydrate, plus the host of other metabolites, is greatly exceeded by the daily throughput of these same compounds. So it is not surprising that minor perturbations of hepatic function will rapidly produce generalized changes in the gross and histologic appearance of the liver. Neither should it surprise that these changes, although obvious, may not signify important liver disease. Focal liver disease is also common as the result of the organ's acting as a catchment for the vast absorptive area of the gut, with all its resident microorganisms and parasites. These focal lesions may also be of little clinical significance, since the liver has vast reserves of function, and has a uniformity of structure at the subgross level which allows it to perform adequately after it has isolated even extensive focal lesions.

Liver lesions are common, yet seldom produce liver failure; their value in diagnosis is that often they indicate the presence and causes of disease in other organs and systems.

A. Hepatic Function

The metabolic functions of the liver seem almost infinite in variety and complexity. They are usually categorized broadly as synthetic, catabolic, detoxifying, secretory, and excretory, although there is always some overlap between categories. A detailed account of hepatic physiology is beyond the scope of this analysis, so discussion will be limited to disturbances of those functions more commonly encountered in liver disease.

The variety of synthetic functions is vast, but the liver's role in excretion of bile salts and synthesis of glucose, low-density lipoproteins, urea, and soluble plasma proteins (including soluble clotting factors) receives most attention in cases of disturbed liver function. Catabolic functions and capacity are likewise vast but, again, a relatively small proportion of these are considered by pathologists, the principal interest often being related to lipid and ketone metabolism.

Biotransformation and detoxification by the liver of substances absorbed from the bowel or synthesized in other organs is of much relevance to the study of hepatic disease, since it is now accepted that the manner and rate of these reactions may determine the nature, pattern, and severity of many examples of hepatotoxicity. The potency of these detoxification mechanisms may be profoundly altered by prior exposure to a wide range of naturally occurring compounds. As a general rule the liver is more important in detoxification of those compounds which are nonpolar: more water-soluble substances are more likely to be directly excreted by the kidneys.

The excretory function of the liver is intimately related to its detoxification functions, but the organ has the capacity to excrete various fairly simple substances, such as heavy metals, unchanged via the bile. If the difference between excretion and secretion is taken to be the production of waste versus useful compounds, then the liver tends to use similar pathways for both processes. The distinction becomes rather academic with consideration of the excretion/secretion of bile salts, since these products may be regarded as useful waste products because of their role in fat absorption from the gut. However, the processes of hepatic uptake, conjugation, intracytoplasmic transport, and canalicular discharge of bile salts are shared by a large number of other endogenous and exogenous compounds.

B. Hepatic Circulation

The hepatic artery, portal vein, and bile duct come together at the hilus of the liver and, within the liver, their radicles lie in a sheath of connective tissue in the portal triads, which is continuous with Glisson's capsule. The integrity of the liver depends on the integrity of these conduits, and it is also via these that most noxious influences are conveyed; the analysis of pathologic changes in the liver requires a recognition of these facts.

The shape of the liver depends on blood flow and biliary arrangements. The ratio of blood flow to parenchymal mass is the same in all parts of the liver, and a similar relationship is deduced for biliary volume. If blood flow or biliary drainage is impaired in part of the liver, the parenchyma of that part will atrophy; many alterations of gross form occur as responses to vascular or biliary disturbance. At the gross level there are also consistent differences in susceptibility to injury between lobes, some of which are attributable to differences in blood supply, biliary architecture, and anatomic location.

C. Functional Anatomy and Microcirculation

As stated earlier, the liver can respond uniformly across its various lobes to generalized metabolic insults, and this, coupled with the apparently monotonous uniformity of the normal parenchyma, can give the mistaken impression that the parenchyma is uniform in its susceptibility to injury. This apparent uniformity at the subgross level is belied, however, when intricate patterns of change appear in the organ after a wide range of generalized toxic, hypoxic, and infectious insults. Although normal hepatocytes show only minor morphologic differences, it is obvious in many damaged livers that the position of the hepatocyte relative to the various blood vessels and bile ducts is strongly correlated to its susceptibility to a whole range of noxious influences. It is therefore vital to develop some understanding of the relationship between the microcirculation and the parenchyma.

The traditional unit of liver structure is the hexagonal lobule, and it is still sometimes convenient to report pathologic changes in terms of the conventional lobule. However, descriptions in this chapter are based on Rappaport's concept of the hepatic acinus. This unit stresses the dependence of the liver on its afferent blood vessels and efferent bile ducts. The liver parenchyma is oriented to these conduits, and consists, in its smallest divisions, of acinar clumps of hepatic parenchyma, central to which are the portal triads, and which are supplied by the terminal portal venules. Thus the terminal portal triad lies at the center of the acinus and is surrounded by **periportal** hepatocytes (Rappaport's zone 1); this in turn is invested by the **midzone** (zone 2), and the hepatocytes of zone 3 will be referred to as **periacinar** (formerly centrilobular), and are usually (but not always) in close proximity to the hepatic venules (the central veins of the conventional lobule). A simple but useful analogy sees the microstructure of the liver as a rather compressed bunch of grapes. The spaces between the berries represent the terminal hepatic venules, whereas the ends of the stems of the bunch become the terminal portal triads. Each grape thus represents a microcirculatory and secretory unit or acinus (to use the terminology of a compound exocrine gland). To complete the analogy, the skins of the grapes are removed to depict the manner in which the sinusoids freely anastomose with one another across any border between adjacent acini.

The position of the hepatocyte in relation to the smallest portal triad determines some of its pathologic responses. The concept helps explain why, in certain planes of section, some hepatocytes may have periacinar reactions despite lying adjacent to larger portal triads. This acinar structure may not be readily apparent in sections of normal liver, but an acinar pattern will often be elegantly picked out during the course of a variety of acute and chronic liver diseases, ranging from acute hepatotoxicities to chronic fibrosis. In other words, whereas the normal liver has the form of a collection of lobules, in disease it behaves like an aggregation of acini.

Hepatocytes appear alike microscopically but are functionally heterogeneous. There are minor structural differences in the diameter of sinusoids and canaliculi and in the content of intracellular organelles. There are quite significant differences in the distribution of enzymes, and zonal variations in bile excretion.

Selection of the acinus as the descriptive unit should not imply a rigidity in its structure, blood supply, or biliary and lymphatic drainage. There is a vast potential for collateral circulation of blood, bile, and lymph through sinusoids, bile canaliculi, and spaces of Disse, respectively, so that, in disturbances of the steady state, adjacent acini may share the blood that flows through them and allow the passage of bile and lymph. If the steady state is permanently displaced, the parenchymal organization is rearranged to new afferent vascular arrangements.

The cells that line the sinusoids constitute an important component of the liver. Best known of these are the Kupffer cells, representatives of the monocyte–macrophage system, which possess potent phagocytic functions. These cells may not be so densely aggregated as their equivalents in spleen and lymph node, but their strategic location and large overall numbers make them an important component of the primary immunological defense system. By obscure mechanisms, microorganisms and other microscopic matter frequently get into the portal blood from the gut, and the Kupffer cells are responsible for ensuring that the hepatic venous blood is largely free from such particles. A consequence of this phagocytic activity is the frequent occurrence in otherwise normal livers of foci of inflammation and degeneration, the neighboring hepatocytes being injured indirectly.

The Kupffer cells are in the sinusoidal lumen, in contrast to the lipocytes, which are in the space of Disse, although how they are anchored there is not clear. Their numbers are greater in the periportal zone. The Kupffer cells can divide, but it is probable that their numbers are increased, or replenished after injury, mainly from monocytes of bone marrow origin. The Kupffer cells are extraordinarily efficient in removing microparticles and abnormal macromolecules from sinusoidal blood but only moderately so in the digestion of such materials. They are most prominent when they contain red cells, bile pigment, hemosiderin, or microbes. Lysosomal storage is also prominent in some of the metabolic storage diseases, which are considered collectively with the Nervous System (Volume 1, Chapter 3), in protoporphyria, and in hepatic phytotoxicosis involving storage of copper and iron.

The sinusoids are also lined by specialized endothelial cells with special transport functions, arranged as a highly fenestrated sheet, thus giving sinusoidal plasma direct access to the space of Disse. Thus the fluid in Disse's space between the endothelium and the cell membrane of the hepatocyte is equivalent to rather dilute plasma. A unique feature of the liver is the fact that hepatic lymph is derived directly from the content of Disse's space, which means that liver lymph is coagulable and contains all the other plasma proteins. This lymph normally flows in a retrograde direction to the portal triad and thence to the hilus of the liver, but when the volume of transudate is high, as in congested livers, alternative pathways for lymphatic drainage are recruited in the capsule and about hepatic veins.

The sinusoidal endothelium lacks a typical organized basement membrane, but the space of Disse contains extracellular matrix proteins, which may function as a low-density basement membrane with a regulatory role in exchanges between the plasma and hepatocyte. Examined in cell cultures, hepatocytes, lipocytes, and endothelial cells all contribute to the extracellular matrix in the space of Disse. The space of Disse may not be evident in biopsy specimens but becomes so as a result of shrinkage in postmortem tissues. It is the site of origin of almost all hepatic lymph which enters the lymphatics in the portal connective tissue.

The lipocytes, also known as Ito cells, are specialized for the storage of fat, vitamin A, and other lipid-soluble vitamins. Their distribution is quite dispersed, and they are difficult to identify in histologic sections unless they contain lipid vacuoles, which is often the case in cats and dogs. Lipocytes are capable of proliferation and of markedly increased synthesis of extracellular matrix, which may be abnormal in its protein, including collagen, content. The stimuli for lipocyte activation are not defined but, in general, are those which initiate parenchymal fibrosis. Platelet-derived growth factor appears to be an important mediator. In chronic disease, the delicate lining of the sinusoids may be so changed as to acquire the characteristics of capillaries as part of developing fibrosis or as a result of acquired exposure to pulsatile arterial blood flow.

D. Hematopoiesis

Hematopoiesis is a normal feature of the fetal liver, beginning very early in organogenesis when the liver assumes hematopoietic responsibility from the yolk sac, to become the main site until the bone marrow becomes productive at about midgestation. The activity is reduced in the late fetal period and normally ceases several weeks after birth but may continue in the presence of anemia. The hematopoiesis is largely erythropoiesis, and the focal clones of cells, which may be accompanied by megakaryocytes, are easily recognized. If granulopoiesis is also present, confusion can occur with inflammatory infiltrates, especially in neonates.

Hematopoiesis may resume in the liver in the myeloproliferative disorders, in chronic anemias such as those which result from immune hemolysis or marrow replacement, and in prolonged toxic/infective conditions such as pyometra in the bitch. These reactions, which are termed **myeloid metaplasia** or **extramedullary hematopoiesis,** are largely confined to the sinusoids and space of Disse. The predominant cell lineages reflect systemic demand and are governed by those rather than by hepatic factors.

E. Liver Regeneration

In spite of its high degree of differentiation, the liver retains to an almost embryonic degree the capacity to regenerate itself. The life span of hepatocytes is normally on the order of 30% of that of the animal itself. Replacement cells are normally derived from mitotic activity, which is largely confined to the periportal hepatocytes. However, patterns of regeneration are likely, in chronic liver disease, to reflect the embryologic origins of cells. There is good evidence that the extrahepatic and intrahepatic bile ducts have separate pathways of embryologic development. The intrahepatic ducts and canals of Hering arise by a process of transformation, which extends peripherally from the porta hepatis, from the embryonic plates of hepatocytes. It is not known why some embryonic hepatocytes develop into mature ones and why others differentiate as ducts, but it is suggested that the former is by induction by endothelial cells and the latter, by induction by ingrowing mesenchyme in the portal triads.

The full regenerative capacity of the tissue, however, is seen only after destruction of much of the parenchyma by noxious influences or its removal by surgery. The participation of hepatocellular regeneration in liver disease is discussed with Responses of the Liver to Injury (Section IV of this chapter).

F. Significance of the Hepatic Mass

There are four consequences of the large size of the liver which are sometimes overlooked. First, its mass, coupled with its relative fragility, has ballistic significance during episodes of abdominal violence.

Second, when there is widespread acute liver injury, a

large mass of damaged tissue has immediate and intimate access to a large volume of blood. This affects the homeostasis of the blood-clotting cycle, as well as releasing large amounts of hepatocellular debris into the general circulation: this will be considered further under Hemorrhage and Liver Failure (Section VII,D of this chapter).

Third, the hepatic sinusoidal bed holds a large quantity of blood, and this volume is subject to large variations according to different conditions. This means that the liver can play an important part in modifying splanchnic blood flow in such states as hypovolemic shock and anaphylaxis. In severe congestive heart failure, for example, the total body blood volume may increase by as much as 30%, and a large proportion of this increase is accommodated in the liver.

Fourth, the mass of the liver represents an important reserve of readily metabolizable nutrients to tide the animal over episodes of malnourishment, so variations in liver size must be considered in the light of recent nutritional history (see Hepatocellular Atrophy, Section IV,A of this chapter).

Bibliography

Arias, I. M. *et al.* "The Liver—Biology and Pathobiology" 2nd Ed. New York, Raven Press, 1988.

Evarts, R. P. *et al. In vivo* differentiation of rat liver oval cells into hepatocytes. *Cancer Res* **49:** 1541–1547, 1989.

Fausto, N., and Mead, J. E. Biology of disease. Regulation of liver growth: Protooncogenes and transforming growth factors. *Lab Invest* **60:** 4–13, 1989.

Friedman, S. L. *et al.* Hepatic lipocytes: The principal collagen-producing cells of normal rat liver. *Proc Natl Acad Sci USA* **82:** 8681–8685, 1985.

Jungermann, K., and Katz, N. Functional hepatocellular heterogeneity. *Hepatology* **2:** 385–395, 1982.

Kardon, R. H., and Kessell, R. G. Three-dimensional organization of the hepatic microcirculation in the rodent as observed in scanning electron micrographs of corrosion casts. *Gastroenterology* **79:** 72–81, 1980.

MacSween, R. N. M., Anthony, P. P., and Scheuer, P. J. (eds.). "Pathology of the Liver." Edinburgh, Scotland, Churchill Livingstone, 1987.

Phillips, M. J. *et al.* "The Normal Liver." New York, Raven Press, 1987.

Rappaport, A. M. Hepatic blood flow: Morphologic aspects and physiologic regulation. *Int Rev Physiol* **21:** 1–63, 1980.

Rozga, J., Jeppsson, B., and Bengmark, S. Hepatotrophic factors in liver growth and atrophy. *Br J Exp Pathol* **66:** 669–678, 1985.

Shah, K. D., and Gerber, M. A. Development of intrahepatic bile ducts in humans. *Arch Pathol Lab Med* **114:** 597–600, 1990.

Shiojiri, N. The origin of intrahepatic bile duct cells in the mouse. *J Embryol Exp Morphol* **79:** 25–39, 1984.

Starzl, T. E. *et al.* Portal hepatotrophic factors, diabetes mellitus and acute liver atrophy, hypertrophy, and regeneration. *Surg Gynecol Obstet* **141:** 843–858, 1975.

Van Eyken, P., Sciot, R., and Desmet, V. Intrahepatic bile duct development in the rat. *Lab Invest* **59:** 52–59, 1988.

Wisse, E., and Knook, D. L. (eds.). "Kupffer Cells and Other Liver Sinusoidal Cells." Amsterdam, Elsevier/North Holland Biomedical Press, 1977.

Zieve, L. *et al.* Hepatic regenerative enzyme activity after pericentral and periportal lobular toxic injury. *Toxicol Appl Pharmacol* **86:** 147–158, 1986.

II. Developmental Anomalies

Developmental anomalies occur, but most are not important. A variety of defects may accompany generalized malformations. As isolated defects, there may be absence or hypoplasia of one or more lobes, with corresponding hypertrophy of the others. Abnormal furrowing may produce additional lobes, and incisures of abnormal depth may isolate lobes. Accessory buttons of parenchyma may occur in the ligaments and in the thorax; these are frequently fibrotic and gray.

A. Cysts

Congenital cysts of the liver occur in all species. Their origins are diverse. **Intrahepatic congenital cysts** are probably derived from embryonic bile ducts. The embryogenesis of the bile ducts has not been clearly determined. The short intralobular portions of the ducts, the cholangioles, may have a common origin with the hepatic parenchyma from the distal portion of the hepatic anlage. The main bile ducts and the interlobular branches in the portal triad are probably derived from the proximal portion of the hepatic anlage. It also seems that many more embryonic cholangioles are formed than are actually necessary. Accordingly, cystic bile ducts may rise by failure of fusion of inter- and intralobular portions, or by failure of superfluous cholangioles to involute, or by establishment of the duct system with subsequent development of localized zones of atresia. The number, size, and degree of loculation of the cysts are quite variable. The walls are of connective tissue and are lined by a flattened or cuboidal epithelium. The content is clear and serous.

Serous cysts are occasionally found attached to the capsule on the diaphragmatic surface in calves, lambs, and foals. The cysts are usually small and multiple, but some are isolated and very large (Fig. 2.1A). Their origin is not

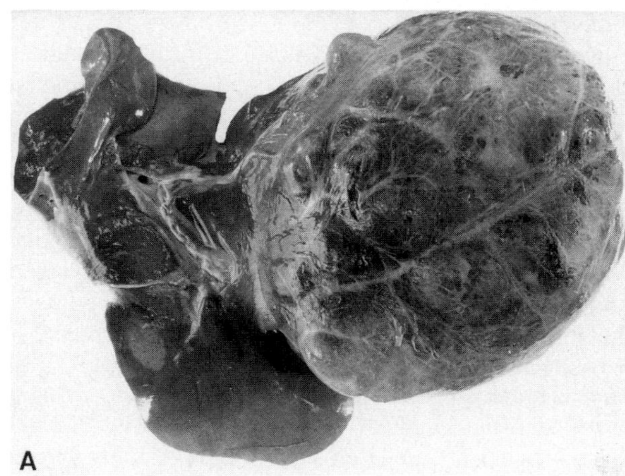

Fig. 2.1A Hepatic cyst. Sheep.

known, but it is variously postulated that they are serosal inclusion cysts, part of congenital polycystic biliary anomalies, or of endodermal origin. They do not contain bile. The incidence of these anomalies related to age suggests that a large proportion of them involute in the early postnatal period. To be distinguished are acquired cysts, parasitic cysts, and biliary cystadenomas.

One form of congenital hepatic cystic anomaly occurs in cats, piglets, and dogs, in which **multiple cysts** derived from **bile ducts** are found throughout the liver. The common bile duct is patent, communicates with the duodenum, yet is itself dilated. There are also polycystic renal anomalies in these animals, which may die of renal insufficiency; jaundice is not usually seen. The livers are often enlarged enough to cause abdominal distension and are riddled with large, softly fluctuant, irregular cysts that intercommunicate and whose content appears to be normal bile. An inherited basis for the disease has been proposed but not proven for dogs, and there is even less evidence for it in pigs, although the anomaly may appear in littermates.

B. Biliary Atresia

Anomalies of the extrahepatic biliary system include absence of gallbladder, and absence or **atresia** of one or more ducts. In carnivores, bile duct atresia may lead not only to jaundice, but also to vitamin D-deficiency rickets, due to inability to absorb fat-soluble vitamins.

An interesting occurrence of congenital atresia and other anomalies of the biliary tract has been reported in lambs and calves in Australia (Fig. 2.1B). Several hundred lambs and nine calves died in the outbreak as a result of chronic liver failure and icterus: epidemiologic features suggested that a plant toxin ingested by the dams during pregnancy was the cause of dysplasia and atresia of the cystic ducts. Affected animals had, for the most part, small, fibrotic gallbladders and firm livers, in which there was pronounced portal fibrosis and bile ductular hyperplasia, together with severe canalicular cholestasis. There was also renal tubular damage and bile staining. Many of the intrahepatic and renal changes were likely to have been secondary to the effects of chronic cholestasis, and the condition was held to be a primary dysgenesis of extrahepatic bile ducts. The significance of this condition is that it underscores the difficulty in differentiating heritable developmental conditions from those caused by *in utero* insults.

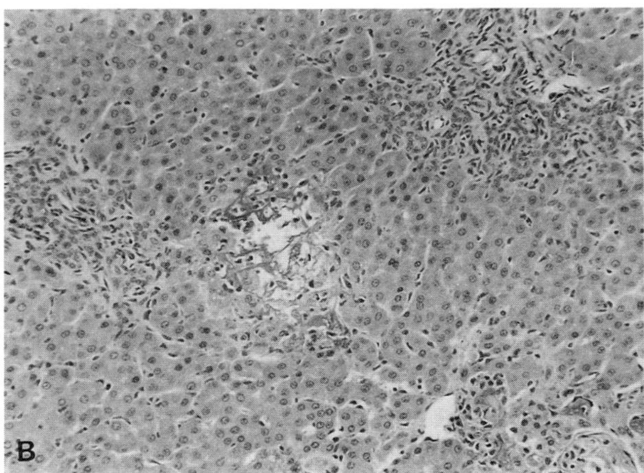

Fig. 2.1B Bile ductular proliferation and focal bile lake (center). Acquired congenital bile duct atresia. (Courtesy of P. A. W. Harper.)

C. Congenital Vascular Shunts

These include abnormal anastomotic connections between the hepatic artery and the portal vein, and the portosystemic shunts, which are between the portal vein and other systemic veins. Acquired shunts are discussed with Vascular Factors in Liver Injury (Section IX of this chapter).

Hepatic arterioportal fistulae are reported in dogs only. The number of cases reported is small but, because shunting between the portal and other veins is expected as a consequence of increased portal pressure, it is possible that some cases of portosystemic shunts include overlooked arteriovenous shunts. Demonstrable arterioportal shunts may be confined to one or more lobes, with many ramifying branches derived from dilated tortuous principals. Affected lobes may be enlarged, although the overall liver mass is reduced. Multiple shunts are present between the portal vein and the vena cava, using preexisting venous pathways. Ascites is present, an unusual finding in vein-to-vein shunts. Possibly as a reflection of high pulsatile pressure, bosses of proliferated smooth muscle project into the lumina of portal, hepatic, and sublobular veins, which may also show adventitial fibrosis.

Vein-to-vein portosystemic shunts occur mainly in dogs and cats; the patterns of abnormality are the same in both species and include, as major types, persistent sinus venosus, atresia of portal vein with multiple collateral connections to adjacent veins, direct shunting to the caudal vena cava or azygous vein, and connection to the caudal vena cava, which itself shunts to the azygous vein. Large breeds of dogs typically have large intrahepatic shunts, usually persistent ductus venosus, but sometimes other large intrahepatic communications. Small breeds of dogs, and cats, have mainly single large extrahepatic shunts between the portal vein and vena cava or azygous vein.

Congenital portosystemic shunts are seen in cats but are more frequent in dogs, which are mostly presented as adolescents with failure to thrive or with the nervous signs of hepatic encephalopathy (see Liver Failure, Section VII of this chapter). Often there is a clinical history of depression, convulsions and other nervous signs which are exacerbated on a high-protein diet, and which may be alleviated by dietary control. Because there is no cause of portal hypertension, there is usually no ascites in these animals.

The liver that has been bypassed by a congenital shunt

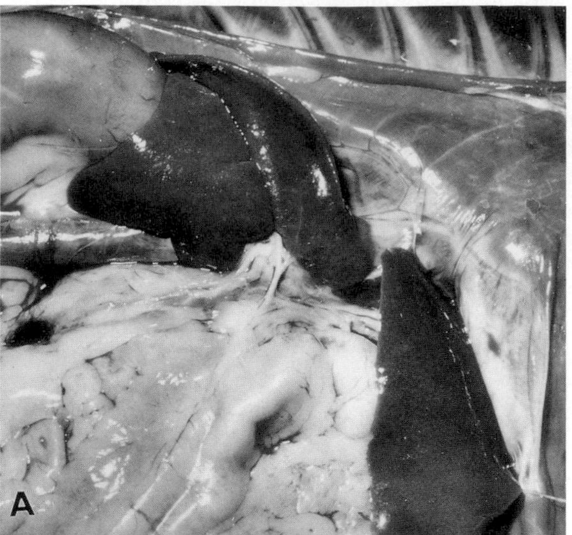

Fig. 2.2A Small liver in a pup with congenital portocaval shunt (persistent sinus venosus).

is very small (Fig. 2.2A) because it has been deprived of primary perfusion by portal hepatotrophic factors such as insulin, glucagon, and amino acids. With portosystemic shunting, these factors are diverted around the liver and are diluted in the total blood volume, so that they are present in much lower concentration in the blood which eventually reaches the liver. These livers may be smooth surfaced and normal in color and texture, but histologically, the hepatocytes are very small. Portal veins in the

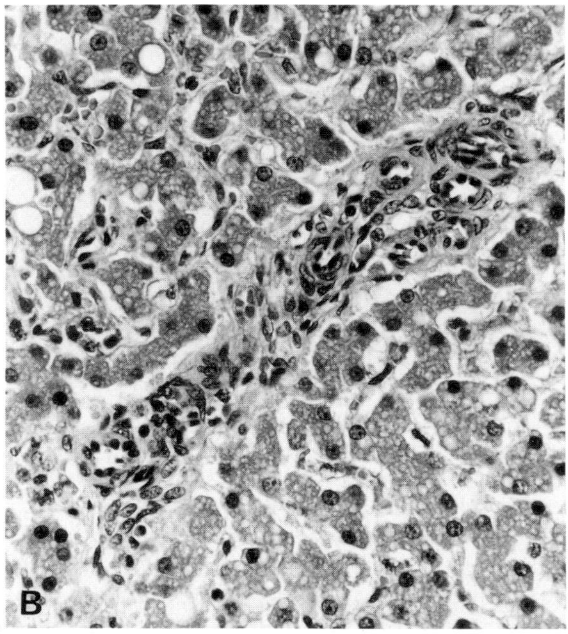

Fig. 2.2B Histology of (A). Portal triad. The portal venule is indiscernible, there are several hepatic arterioles, and hepatocytes are atrophic.

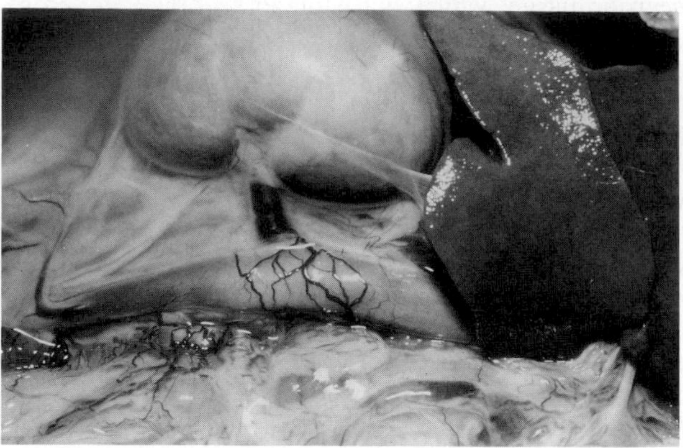

Fig. 2.3 Acquired portosystemic shunts (from mesentery to right renal vein) in chronic liver disease. The shunts are thin-walled and plexiform.

smaller triads are small or absent, and the hepatic arterioles are often prominent and multiple (Fig. 2.2B). Congenital portosystemic shunts should be easy to distinguish from shunts **acquired** due to chronic portal hypertension (see Vascular Factors in Liver Injury, Section IX of this chapter), in that the latter will be multiple, thin walled, and tortuous (Fig. 2.3).

Bibliography

Harper, P., *et al.* Congenital biliary atresia and jaundice in lambs and calves. *Aust Vet J* **67:** 18–23, 1990.

McKenna, S. C., and Carpenter, J. L. Polycystic disease of the kidney and liver in the Cairn terrier. *Vet Pathol* **17:** 436–442, 1980.

Van Den Ingh, T. S. G. A. M., and Rothuizen, J. Congenital cystic disease of the liver in seven dogs. *J Comp Pathol* **95:** 405–414, 1985.

Van Eyken, P., Sciot, R., and Desmet, V. Intrahepatic bile duct development in the rat. *Lab Invest* **59:** 52–59, 1988.

Webster, W. R., and Summers, P. M. Congenital polycystic kidney and liver syndrome in piglets. *Aust Vet J* **54:** 451, 1978.

III. Displacement, Torsion and Rupture

The lie of the liver should be observed as soon as the abdomen is opened. Most **displacements** are caudal, so that the margins of the liver come to be much behind the costal arch. Caudal displacements are the result of enlargement of the organ or caudal displacement of the diaphragm, the latter due to pleural effusion or other space-occupying lesion in the thorax. Congenital or acquired displacements in ventral and diaphragmatic hernias are common. Usually only one lobe goes into the thorax with other viscera; its blood supply may not be embarrassed, but usually it is severely congested and may rupture, or, given time, it will become indurated.

Torsion of individual lobes, usually the left lateral, occurs in swine and dogs, and the resultant infarction causes death through shock or hemorrhage. The lobe may contain clostridial spores, which are likely to germinate in the necrotic tissue, which will undergo putrefaction and be dry and crepitant compared to that of the other lobes.

Rupture of the liver occurs commonly as the result of trauma, because the organ is fragile relative to its mass. It is quite common for fatal liver rupture to be produced by the sudden accelerations and pressures of road accidents, without significant evidence of trauma to other parts of the body. This testifies to the relative fragility of the organ, which, although protected to some degree by its location, nevertheless offers little resistance to blunt trauma, particularly in the neonate. Large tears may develop in the liver capsule and hepatic parenchyma after trauma. In some cases of hepatic rupture, anastomosing linear patterns of fine, capsular fissures form that are quite shallow, but from which severe hemorrhage may issue until clotting seals them shortly before death, obscuring their significance (Fig. 2.4). Liver rupture is often clinically occult, since quite large ruptures may not disturb liver function much unless severe enough to cause rapid exsanguination, or unless the biliary tract is involved. Moderate blood loss from capsular ruptures is followed first by rapid coagulation, then fibrinolysis of most of the free clot. The liquid blood is then rapidly returned to the circulation by transdiaphragmatic lymphatic absorption, and, a day or so after the trauma, all that is seen is a delicate tracery of capsular tears which have been sealed by residual thrombus, with a little associated pale necrotic parenchyma. Rupture of major bile ducts leads to yellow-stained bile peritonitis, which may remain sterile and become chronic, or may be infected by enterohepatic circulation of bacteria such as clostridia. Rapid death ensues in the latter instance.

Diffuse hepatic disease with enlargement, in which the substance is friable and the capsule taut, provides a predisposition to rupture, which may occur spontaneously. Predisposing lesions include acute hepatitis, amyloidosis, severe congestion, fatty degeneration, and secondary neoplasms. Usually there is very little hemorrhage from spontaneous ruptures, which suggests that they occur in the terminal stages of the illness. Parasites that penetrate the capsule cause numerous small ruptures but seldom lead to significant hemorrhage. Fatal ruptures occur in foals during parturition, sometimes concurrent with costal fractures, and in the smaller species subject to energetic resuscitation.

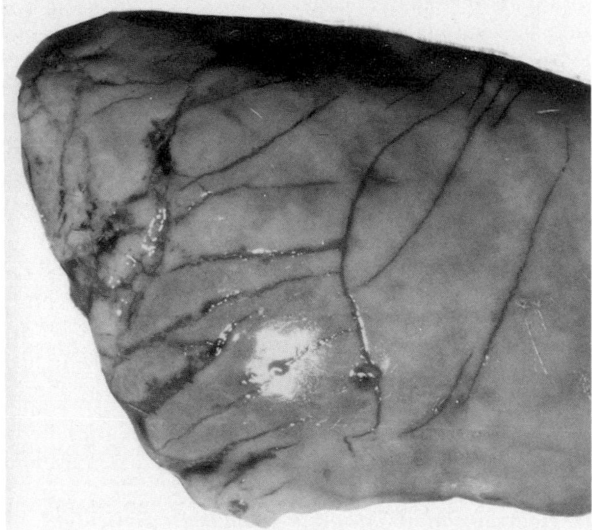

Fig. 2.4 Multiple linear capsular tears. Traumatic liver rupture. Dog.

IV. Hepatocellular Degenerations

Cells with a specialized range of metabolic function, such as muscle fibers or osteoblasts, as a rule have only a limited repertoire of reaction to injury. It is therefore not surprising that hepatocytes, with their diverse metabolic capacity, should exhibit a rather wider range of changes in response to various insults. It is not easy to establish with the light microscope whether or not these changes are reversible, as much depends on the nature of the insult and the relative speed of onset of its effects on the cell.

A. Hepatocellular Atrophy

The large mass of the liver allows a considerable reserve to be available for catabolism in starvation. Since the organ has large reserve function, great reduction in total hepatic mass can occur in catabolic states without much evidence of impaired hepatic function. Hepatocytes are not lost in this situation; they are simply reduced in volume. This is the basis of atrophy in severe malnutrition of slow onset and long duration, as seen, for example, in old grazing herbivores with poor teeth, and in marasmatic diseases. In such cases the liver is dark and small, and the capsule may appear too large for the organ, showing fine wrinkles on handling. These livers may even appear to be firmer than normal, due to condensation of normal stroma. Microscopic sections give an impression of greatly increased numbers of hepatocytes; these are small, with scant cytoplasm (Fig. 2.5). Portal triads and hepatic venules are closer together than normal due to the small size of the acini.

Atrophy of part of the liver may be a response to pressure or to impairment of blood or bile flow. Local pressure atrophy occurs adjacent to space-occupying lesions in the liver or as a result of chronic pressures from neighboring organs, such as distended rumen in the ox or colon in the horse. Chronic diffuse diseases of the biliary tract, such as sporidesmin poisoning and fascioliasis, are likely to cause atrophy of the left lobe in ruminants, probably as a result of the greater difficulty in maintaining adequate biliary drainage from this lobe, whose bile ducts are longer than those of the right in these species. The atrophy of biliary obstruction is complicated by some degree of inflammation and fibrosis superimposed on it. Hepatotrophic factors are components of the portal blood and are essential for the maintenance of normal hepatic mass.

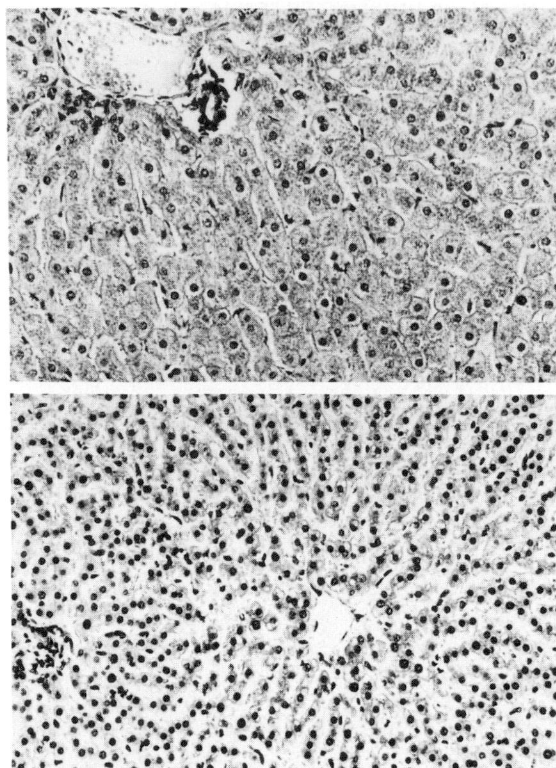

Fig. 2.5 Normal (top) and atrophic liver (bottom) at same magnification. Starvation. Sheep.

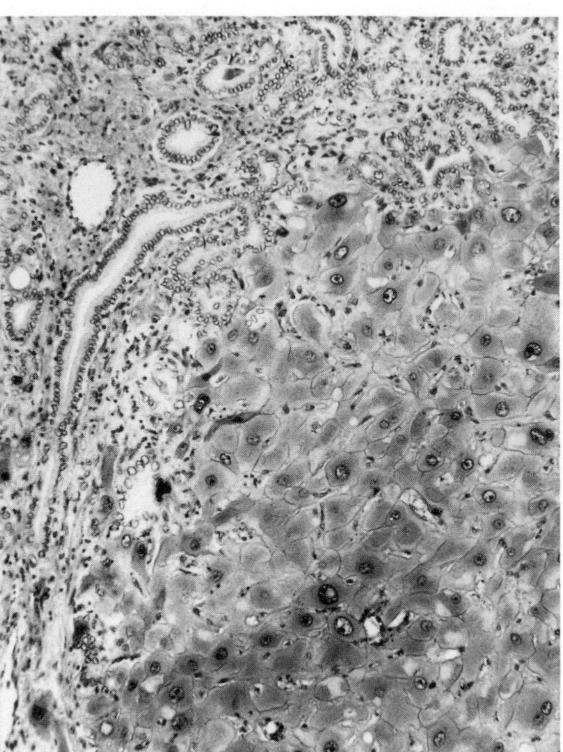

Fig. 2.6 Megalocytosis and bile duct proliferation in *Crotalaria* poisoning. Horse.

Thus atrophy of part or all of the liver occurs when portal blood is diverted or obstructed. The histologic features of this atrophy are similar to those of starvation atrophy.

B. Megalocytosis

The term **megalocytosis** was used first in the description of the changes of liver cell cytoplasm and nucleus that occur in pyrrolizidine alkaloid poisoning (Fig. 2.6). This form of megalocytosis has some specific features and is described under Chronic Hepatotoxicities (Section XI,D of this chapter). Very similar hepatocyte enlargement can be produced by other alkylating agents which have in common the capacity to replace hydrogen ions with alkyl radicals; the effect on DNA is to cause breaks and cross-links in the molecule, thus interfering with RNA transcription. Mycotoxins such as aflatoxin may produce megalocytosis which is histologically indistinguishable from that caused by the pyrrolizidine alkaloids. Hepatocellular mitosis is preceded by enlargement of the cells, and some degree of nuclear enlargement will be seen in any process that induces hepatocellular proliferation. Increased amounts of nuclear chromatin are present in prophase nuclei, which must be distinguished from those of megalocytosis. Mitoses may be rare even when expected, as in rapid regeneration following zonal necrosis, but may be frequent in other conditions, such as copper poisoning and lupinosis. Nuclei are normally diploid and uniform, but they may become tetraploid or even octoploid in cells that have large nuclei but which are otherwise normal.

C. Cytosegresomes

Cytosegresome formation (Councilman bodies, acidophilic bodies) produces spherical, refractile, eosinophilic structures seen in liver cells that have been sublethally injured by a variety of insults, ranging from hypoxia through a variety of intoxications to malnutrition, specific deficiencies, and some viral infections. They may be formed when masses of cytoplasmic organelles are gathered and condensed, and are sequestered from remaining cytoplasm by membranes that fuse with lysosomes (autolysosomes). They may also be derived from other hepatocytes that have undergone the form of shrinkage necrosis known as **apoptosis** (see Patterns of Hepatic Necrosis, Section V of this chapter) and whose condensed fragments are taken up by remaining hepatocytes (Fig. 2.7). These bodies can either be digested by lysosomal hydrolases (sometimes incompletely, to leave dense residual bodies) or extruded from the cytoplasm (exocytosis), to be taken up by Kupffer cells. Undigested remnants of these bodies may be observed at the light-microscopic level as lipofuscin granules.

D. Aggregation of Smooth Endoplasmic Reticulum

The volume of hepatocyte cytoplasm occupied by smooth endoplasmic reticulum varies with the location of

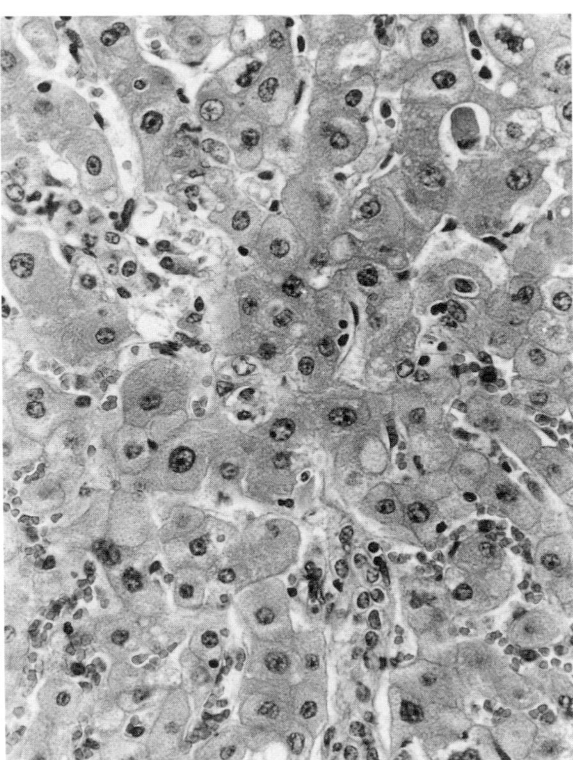

Fig. 2.7 *Lantana* poisoning. Ox. Hepatocellular swelling, hydropic (feathery) degeneration, and apoptosis.

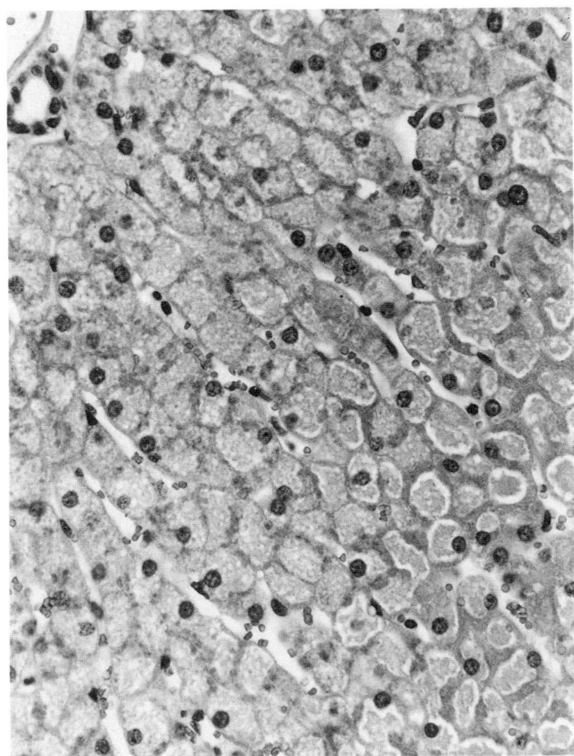

Fig. 2.8 Aggregation of smooth endoplasmic reticulum in hepatocyte cytoplasm in sublethal *Cestrum parqui* poisoning. Sheep. The reaction is most severe in the periacinar zone.

the cell within the acinus; periacinar hepatocytes usually have the largest amount. Hypertrophy of smooth endoplasmic reticulum is readily induced over a few days by exposure to a wide spectrum of compounds that are, before excretion, degraded in the liver by mixed-function oxidases; phenobarbitone is perhaps the best known of these inducing agents. The phenomenon of microsomal enzyme induction has considerable significance in the reaction of the liver to many hepatotoxins and will be dealt with further under Toxic Liver Disease (Section XI of this chapter).

In some intoxications the smooth endoplasmic reticulum forms granular aggregates in the cytoplasm within a few hours of exposure to the toxin. Although the bulk of the organelle seems to have increased, this reaction probably represents clumping of the normally dispersed reticulum, the functions of which are more likely to be depressed than enhanced in these circumstances.

The aggregated smooth endoplasmic reticulum forms a large, semidiscrete, eosinophilic mass, which tends to be separated from the rest of the cell content, and which displaces the nucleus and other organelles to the periphery (Fig. 2.8). In cells that survive, the deranged smooth endoplasmic reticulum may eventually be sequestered as a cytosegresome.

E. Intranuclear Inclusions

Besides the various nuclear inclusions associated with some virus infections, there are three types of inclusions that may be found in hepatocyte nuclei. The most common of these is the spherical, apparently hollow globule within the body of the nucleus (Fig. 2.9). These are membrane bound and are the result of cytoplasmic invagination into the nucleus, and ultrastructurally may be shown to contain such cytoplasmic components as glycogen and mitochondria. These inclusions are seen infrequently in otherwise normal livers but are more likely to occur in any chronically injured liver. They are particularly common in chronic pyrrolizidine alkaloid poisoning.

Another sort of intranuclear inclusion is the eosinophilic blocklike structure in which a regular crystal lattice can be seen with the electron microscope, and which is also present in nuclei of renal proximal tubular epithelium, probably with greater frequency. Their precise structure and significance are obscure; there is no heavy-metal component, as was once suspected. These inclusions are sometimes large enough to distort the nucleus. They are more likely to be found in old animals, particularly dogs, and should be distinguished from the acid-fast, noncrystalline intranuclear inclusions of lead poisoning. **Lead inclusions** are again more frequently seen in the renal tubular epithelium; they consist of lead–protein complex, have a characteristic furry appearance in electron micrographs, and are very electron dense.

Large eosinophilic intranuclear inclusions may be very frequent in the hepatocytes of individual **koalas**; there is

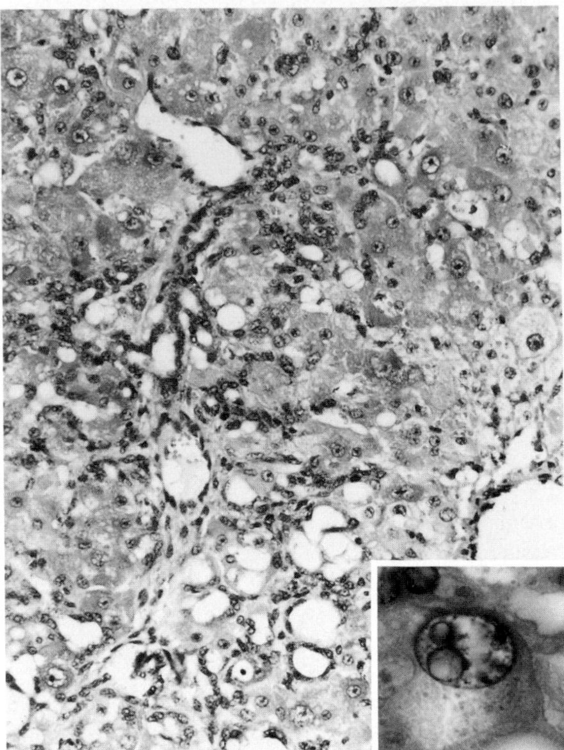

Fig. 2.9 Subacute aflatoxin poisoning. Calf. Bile ductule proliferation, megalocytosis, and nuclear vesiculation. (Inset) Intranuclear inclusions formed by invagination of cytoplasm into nucleus, seen in many subacute and chronic intoxications. (Courtesy of R. A. MacKenzie.)

no evidence of associated liver damage, and ultrastructural and other studies have not indicated their nature. The liver of this species is also remarkable for the density of lysosomal lipofuscinlike pigment in nearly all hepatocytes; this is presumably related in some way to their diet.

F. Hepatocellular Fusion

This is a rare phenomenon that may be found unexpectedly in cats; it has been produced in this species by experimental dioxin poisoning. The hepatocytes have a syncytial appearance due to fusion, then disappearance of adjacent cell membranes. In protoporphyria of Limousin cattle, small clusters of hepatocytes contain 4–10 or more closely packed nuclei, but it is not clear whether this represents fusion or multiple nuclear division. Syncytial cells characterize giant-cell hepatitis.

G. Pigmentation

Congenital melanosis occurs in calves and occasionally in lambs and swine. The deposits may be numerous and vary in size from flecks to irregular, bluish-black areas 2 cm or more in diameter. The melanin is confined to the capsule and the stroma. These deposits are sharply defined in young animals, but become more diffuse and fade with age.

The most striking example of **acquired melanosis** is the massive accumulation of melanin in hepatocytes of mature sheep and, less frequently, cattle after prolonged grazing on extensive unimproved pastures in inland eastern Australia, the Falkland Islands, and Scandinavia. The color of the affected livers ranges from a dull gray to uniform black, and there is usually a prominent acinar pattern. In severe cases there is also dusky pigmentation of the hepatic lymph nodes, lungs, and renal cortex. Histologically, the pigment is present as granules in lysosomes in hepatocytes and macrophages of the liver, the proximal tubular epithelium of the kidneys, and in alveolar and interstitial macrophages in the lung. There is no evidence of liver dysfunction, even in the blackest livers. The source of this pigment is not known, but the epidemiologic features of its occurrence indicate that it is derived from a component of the diet that after biotransformation, polymerization, and condensation, leaves an insoluble residue. This residue is sequestered within lysosomes without interfering further with hepatocellular function. Another possibility is that some dietary component is capable of inhibiting the catabolic sequence normally responsible for complete degradation of melanin precursors. The pigment first appears in periportal and midzonal hepatocytes (Fig. 2.10), which are probably the only cells to produce it. Release of pigment to other tissues may be through exocytosis or

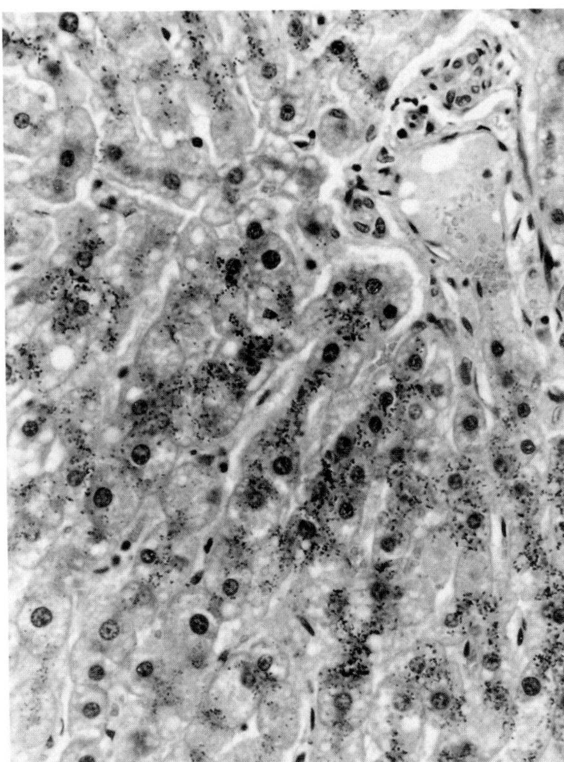

Fig. 2.10 Lysosomal pigment in periportal hepatocytes. Environmental melanosis. Sheep.

after normal necrobiosis. This environmental melanosis was originally characterized as a lipofuscin, with which class of residual lipid-based polymers it shares many histochemical reactions.

The chemical relationship between some melanins, **lipofuscin,** and **ceroid** can be difficult to determine, and the latter two pigments tend to be distinguished more by their origins and associations than by their structures. Ceroid is associated with peroxidation of fat deposits, and lipofuscin is the term given to small, golden, granular deposits derived from the lipid component of membranous organelles. Lipofuscin accumulates in hepatocellular lysosomes and indicates senility or some other cause of reduced membrane repair; the pigment is more obvious in cells near the periphery of the acinus and in atrophied cells. It is particularly common in the liver of old cats.

Lipofuscinlike pigment also accumulates in hepatocellular lysosomes of animals with deficiencies of enzymes involved with bile salt conjugation and transport, such as mutant Corriedale sheep, in which the liver becomes quite black.

Hemosiderin deposits are seldom sufficient to give gross discoloration, but if so, the color is dark brown. The pigment is detected microscopically as yellowish or brown crystals chiefly in the Kupffer cells, although small amounts may be found in hepatic cells. The ferric iron component of this pigment can be demonstrated by staining with Prussian blue; otherwise, it can easily be confused with lipofuscin.

In congenital **protoporphyria** of Limousin cattle, a dark golden brown pigment is present in portal areas, in Kupffer cells, sinusoidal endothelial, cells and heavily concentrated in the cytoplasm of hepatocytes, mainly in large secondary lysosomes as a lipofuscinlike material.

Diffuse hemosiderosis occurs quite commonly in all species, and its presence is suggestive of excess hemolytic activity relative to the rate of reutilization of iron. Thus it is seen in the hemolytic anemias, the anemia of copper deficiency, and in cachexia. It may be seen in the periacinar zones in severe chronic passive congestion of the liver. Localized hemosiderosis occurs in areas of hemorrhage. As well as being present in Kupffer cells, the pigment may be encrusted on the connective tissues. The pigment is normally present in the early neonatal period, when fetal hemoglobin is being replaced by mature hemoglobin.

Hemosiderosis should be distinguished from **hematin,** which is produced by the action of formic acid on hemoglobin following a prolonged postmortem interval, and is usually regarded as a histologic artefact. Hematin is also an iron-containing pigment, but the iron is in the reduced ferrous state and does not stain with ferricyanide. It takes the form of crystalline brown deposits, mainly within the blood vessels, and is darker than hemosiderin and occurs in irregular clumps, often extracellularly. Hematin may, however, be found in Kupffer cells and macrophages in small amounts.

Bile pigmentation may impart on olive-green color to the liver in diffuse obstructive biliary disease or intrahepatic cholestasis. Histologically, conjugated bile pigments may distend bile canaliculi, which then stand out microscopically as greenish-yellow stellate lakes between the hepatocytes (Fig. 2.11). In this case, the identity of the pigment is obvious, but when it is present in granular form in hepatocyte or Kupffer cell cytoplasm, it may easily be confused with hemosiderin and hematin. Death of individual hepatocytes releases the canalicular plugs into the space of Disse and the sinusoid.

The term **feathery degeneration** is applied to a type of hydropic change that occurs in hepatocytes in which there has been prolonged cholestasis. The cells are swollen and vacuolated and crisscrossed by a fine protoplasmic network that is brown with bile pigments.

Hemochromatosis, with some resemblance to the secondary form of the disease in humans, is rare in animals, but has been observed in cattle exposed to high levels of iron in pasture and water, and in sheep. The liver is enlarged and brownish with a diffuse fine nodularity, and the hepatic and adjacent lymph nodes are also darkened. Large amounts of iron are present in the hepatic parenchyma, the biliary epithelium, and the cortex of lymph nodes, and lesser amounts are present in the broad fibrous septa. The iron is stored predominantly in lysosomes. Brown discoloration of bone marrow resembles the osseous pigmentation of porphyria. The pathogenesis of nutritional siderosis is unknown.

Liver failure with fibrosis sometimes occurs in long-

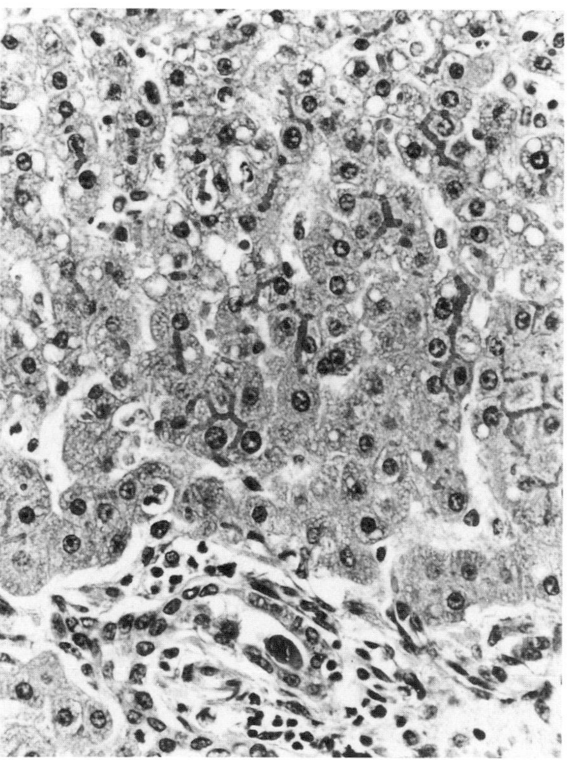

Fig. 2.11 Bile lakes in canaliculi and bile duct. Hemolytic disease (babesiosis). Ox.

term survivors in basenji and beagle dogs with the chronic hemolytic anemia of pyruvate kinase deficiency, and in poodles with familial nonspherocytic hemolytic anemia.

Brown crystalline deposits of 2,8-dihydroxyadenine have recently been described in hepatocytes and in other tissues in slaughtered cattle with no evidence of other disease. These accumulations were strongly birefringent under polarized light, and were seen in the cytoplasm of hepatocytes and macrophages of hepatic lymph nodes and as extracellular deposits in portal stroma and renal tubular lumina. Grossly, the portal stroma stood out as a greenish network. Affected lymph nodes were enlarged, and the medullary sinusoids were distended with greenish pasty material. The crystals were identified as 2,8-dihydroxyadenine by a panel of crystallographic methods and mass spectrometry, and it was suggested that a deficiency of adenine phosphoribosyltransferase might be responsible; however, this has not been confirmed.

Pigments of parasitic origin are particularly associated with flukes. Heavy deposits of black **iron–porphyrin** compound are formed about the cysts and migratory pathways of *Fascioloides magna*. Lesser amounts of similar pigment are deposited about bile ducts infested by *Fasciola hepatica* (see Helminthic Infections of Liver and Bile Ducts, Section X,D of this chapter). The presence of this pigment in the hilar nodes should suggest otherwise inapparent infestations by flukes. In schistosomiasis, the liver may be grayish in color owing to the accumulation of black pigment in Kupffer cells.

H. Hydropic Degeneration and Cloudy Swelling

These terms have been used for many years to describe cytoplasmic changes in cells prepared by conventional histologic techniques. It now seems agreed that cloudy swelling describes mitochondrial changes and dilatations of the cytoplasmic cytocavitary network that are nonspecific for types of injury or disease, being reflections of ischemic, toxic, and many other types of insult. These changes are also present in the early stages of autolysis. The mitochondrial changes include swelling, coagulation, and calcification.

Hydropic degeneration is a common change in hepatocytes in a number of diseases, ranging from mild intoxication to hypoxia, and is even seen in well-nourished animals that have recently fasted; in these, it probably represents fluid in the cytosol left after glycogen has been metabolized either pre- or postmortem. Insults such as hypoxia, damage by a wide range of toxins, and overload by bile pigment can all produce hydropic degeneration, so there is little specificity to the change. Any of the membranous compartments of the cytoplasm can be involved; thus hypoxia may produce lysosomal and mitochondrial vacuolation, whereas toxins that bind to endoplasmic reticulum may cause that organelle to take up large volumes of water.

Probably the most severe example of hepatocellular hydropic change is seen with glycogen accumulation in dogs with hyperadrenocorticoidism due either to functional adrenal cortical or pituitary tumors, or to treatment with glucocorticoids (Fig. 2.12A,B). The liver is enlarged, pale tan and, in long standing cases, may have scattered fatty hyperplastic nodules. The cytoplasm of the cells contains spaces with poorly demarcated edges; the cells

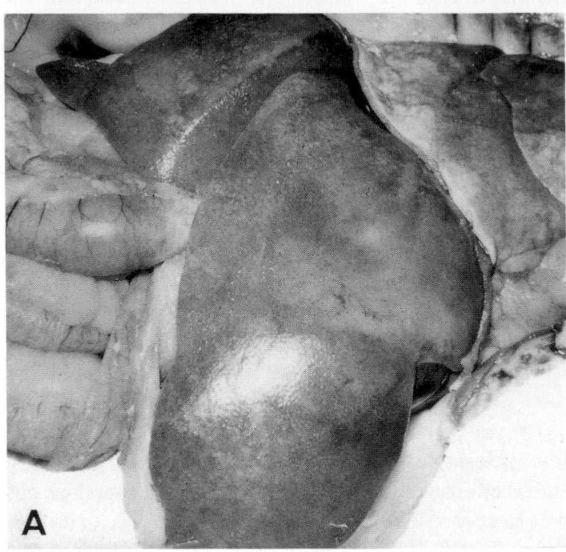

Fig. 2.12A Extreme hepatomegaly due to steroid hepatopathy (functional adrenocortical adenoma). For histology, see Fig. 2.12B.

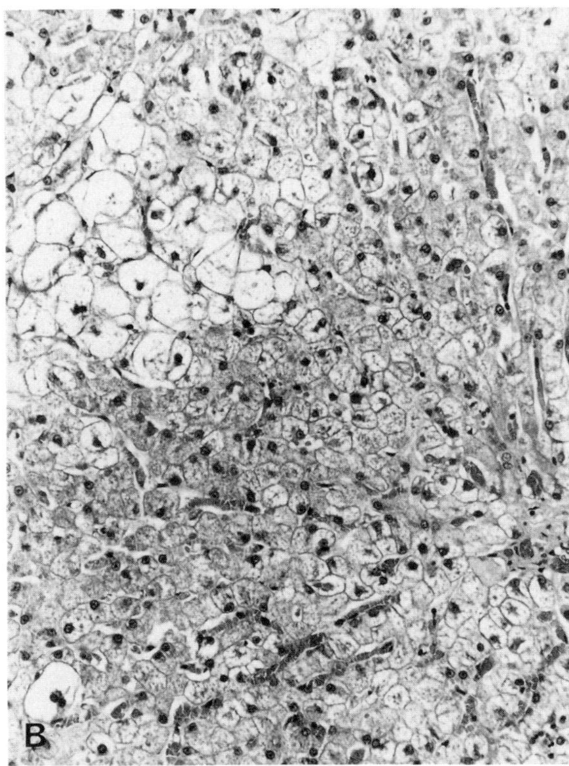

Fig. 2.12B Severe hydropic degeneration. Dog. Hypercorticoidism. Functional adrenocortical adenoma. Same liver as 2.12A.

are swollen, and the nucleus, although normal in appearance, is often displaced from its central position. Careful examination usually serves to distinguish the cytoplasmic spaces from those seen in fat infiltration, which should be spherical and have sharp borders. The amount of glycogen remaining in affected cells is very variable and can be assessed histologically only by use of stains such as periodic acid–Schiff (PAS). It will largely be a function of the original glycogen concentration and the postmortem interval.

It is sometimes impossible to distinguish hydropic from fatty change in routine sections, and special stains must be used; both changes may be present in the same cell. The severe hydropic change of hyperadrenocorticoidism seems to be completely reversible, and hydropic change due to other causes is usually regarded as such, but the change may be the earliest sign of impending hepatocyte necrosis.

Bibliography

Badylak, S. F., and Van Fleet, J. F. Tissue γ-glutamyl transpeptidase activity and hepatic ultrastructural alterations in dogs with experimentally induced glucocorticoid hepatopathy. *Am J Vet Res* **43:** 649–655, 1982.

Car, B. D., and Anderson, W. I. Giant cell hepatopathy in three aborted midterm equine fetuses. *Vet Pathol* **25:** 389–390, 1988.

Carlson, J. Endoplasmic reticulum storage disease. *Histopathology* **16:** 309–312, 1990.

Cornelius, C. E., Arias, I., and Osburn, B. I. Hepatic pigmentation with photophotosensitivity: A syndrome in Corriedale sheep resembling Dubin–Johnson syndrome in man. *J Am Vet Med Assoc* **146:** 709–713, 1965.

De Saram, W, Gallagher, C. H., and Goodrich, B. S. Melanosis of sheep liver. I. Chemistry of the pigment. *Aust Vet J* **45:** 105–108, 1969.

Hartley, W. J., Mullins, J., and Lawson, B. M. Nutritional siderosis in the bovine. *N Z Vet J* **7:** 99–105, 1959.

Lindmark, B. *et al.* Hepatocyte inclusions of 1-antichymotrypsin in a patient with partial deficiency of 1-antichymotrypsin and chronic liver disease. *Histopathology* **16:** 221–225, 1990.

McCaskey, P. C. *et al.* Accumulation of 2,8 dihydroxyadenine in bovine liver, kidneys, and lymph nodes. *Vet Pathol* **28:** 99–109, 1991.

Nordstoga, K. Hepatic lipofuscinosis in healthy Norwegian sheep. *Acta Vet Scand* **31:** 73–78, 1990.

Ossent, P., Stockli, R. M., and Pospischil, A. Emperipolesis of lymphoid neoplastic cells in feline hepatocytes. *Vet Pathol* **26:** 279–280, 1989.

Prasse, K. W. *et al.* Pyruvate kinase deficiency anemia with terminal myelofibrosis and osteosclerosis in a beagle. *J Am Vet Med Assoc* **166:** 1170–1175, 1975.

Randolf, J. F. *et al.* Familial nonspherocytic hemolytic anemia in poodles. *Am J Vet Res* **47:** 687–695, 1986.

Rogers, W. A., and Ruebner, B. H. Retrospective study of probable glucocorticoid-induced hepatopathy in dogs. *J Am Vet Med Assoc* **170:** 603–606, 1977.

Schleger, A. V. Histopathology of melanotic sheep liver. I. Histology and nonenzymic histochemistry. *Aust Vet J* **46:** 48–54, 1970.

Schleger, A. V. Histopathology of melanotic sheep liver. II. Enzymic histochemistry. *Aust Vet J* **46:** 55–61, 1970.

Searle, J. *et al.* The significance of cell death by apoptosis in hepatobiliary disease. *J Gastroenterol Hepatol* **2:** 77–96, 1987.

Stein, R. J., Richter, W. R, and Brynjolfsson, G. Ultrastructural pharmacopathology I. Comparative morphology of the livers of the normal street dog and pure bred beagle (intranuclear crystalline inclusions). *Exp Mol Pathol* **5:** 195–224, 1966.

Thompson, S. W., Sparanto, B. M., and Diener, R. M. Vacuoles in the hepatocytes of cortisone-treated dogs. *Am J Pathol* **63:** 135–148, 1971.

Thornburg, L. P., and Moody, G. M. Hepatic amyloidosis in a dog. *J Am Anim Hosp Assoc* **17:** 721–723, 1981.

Troyer, D. L. *et al.* Gross, microscopic, and ultrastructural lesions of protoporphyria in Limousin calves. *J Vet Med (A)* **38:** 300–305, 1991.

Weiden, P. L. *et al.* Long-term survival and reversal of iron overload after marrow transplantation in dogs with congenital hemolytic anemia. *Blood* **57:** 66–70, 1981.

Wilkie, I. W. *et al.* Giant-cell hepatitis in four aborted foals. A possible leptospiral abortion. *Can Vet J* **29:** 1003–1004, 1988.

I. Fatty Liver

Fatty liver is the term used to describe livers that contain more visible lipid in hepatocytes than one expects to see in that organ. This definition can include those examples of hepatocellular lipid accumulation that are more or less physiologic, such as seen in late pregnancy or heavy lactation in ruminants. In these animals, nutritional stress may lead to clinical ketosis, but clinically normal animals may have very fatty livers, and there is little diagnostic significance in mild degrees of fatty change.

The liver plays a vital role in the lipid economy of the body. Tissues such as skeletal muscle can directly utilize fatty acids that have been mobilized from the fat depots, but a far greater proportion of fatty acids from this source are taken up by the liver and transformed into triglyceride or are used directly by the liver, which derives most of its energy from the oxidation of fatty acids. The bulk of hepatocellular triglyceride is destined for the synthesis of low-density lipoproteins, which are secreted into the plasma and are more readily utilized by most tissues than are the fatty acids. Some of the lipid absorbed from the gut is presented directly to the liver as relatively water-soluble, short-chain fatty acids after transfer to portal blood. Long-chain fatty acids, however, after absorption as triglyceride in the form of chylomicra and transfer to the systemic circulation *via* the thoracic duct, are cleaved by endothelial lipase into free fatty acid, which may be either transported to the liver as albumin complexes, or incorporated directly into adipocyte triglyceride.

The synthesis and transport of lipoprotein within the hepatocyte are processes requiring a small but indispensable energy input. Thus any disturbance of protein and phospholipid synthesis or adenosine triphosphate (ATP) synthesis has the potential to inhibit lipoprotein synthesis or secretion. Triglyceride synthesis from incoming fatty acid, being less dependent on ATP synthesis and energy expenditure, may continue; the result is the accumulation of excess triglyceride in the hepatocyte cytoplasm.

The assembly of lipoprotein takes place in the cisternae of the granular endoplasmic reticulum, and any damage to the membranes of this structure or to the Golgi is likely to inhibit the rate of lipoprotein synthesis. This sort of disturbance seems to be the basis of the fatty liver in toxic liver injury. Excessive intake or mobilization of triglyceride may cause fatty acids to be presented to the liver in excess of its capacity to utilize them.

Small droplets of fat, usually in a periportal and juxtasinusoidal position, can normally be found in the liver. In lipidosis, the amount is increased, most of the increment occurring in the more peripheral portion of the acini. The amount of fat present in the earlier stages of degeneration is usually much more than can be appreciated microscopically. The fat accumulates in small globules in the cytoplasm, and these show little tendency to fuse. The nucleus is not displaced but may be distorted. Fatty change that is the result of acute cell injury, such as may be produced by toxins and acute anoxia, may not develop past the stage of forming small globules, its course being either to restitution or to death of the cell. Such livers may be of normal or reduced size but are not enlarged. They are yellowish, especially adjacent to the hepatic venules, but the color may not be readily evident, except in those areas ischemic from pressure of an adjacent viscus. The consistency is softer than normal. On the cut surface the architectural markings are obscure, although if there is some necrosis, the hepatic venules may be prominent and surrounded by a yellow halo.

In the more severe and long-standing degrees of hepatic lipidosis, most of the parenchymal cells are involved. Probably as a result of fusion of globules, each cell usually contains one large globule, which alters the contour of the cell and displaces the nucleus (Fig. 2.13). The sinusoids are compressed and appear anemic, and the tissue at low magnification resembles adipose tissue. Fat is also present in the epithelium of the bile ducts. Fatty change of this degree requires some time to develop and, therefore, implies a relatively mild cellular injury such as might result from nutritional and metabolic imbalances rather than from toxic or anoxic insult. With these severe degrees of degeneration, the liver is moderately or greatly enlarged, of a uniform light yellow color, and doughy. The edges are rounded, and the surface is smooth. The cut surface is uniform, greasy, and without acinar pattern unless there is also some congestion or zonal necrosis, in which case the cut surface is finely mottled red and yellow (Fig. 2.14). The least equivocal evidence of severe fatty change is the ability of the liver to float in water or fixative.

Severe fatty liver may not necessarily produce severe hepatic dysfunction, and the liver can return to normal structure and function once the metabolic defect has been corrected, especially if the duration of the lipid accumulation has not been long. There is, however, a range of chronic hepatic changes often seen in livers that have presumably been fatty for a long time. The assumption is usually made that these changes, which include fibrosis, pigment accumulation, and nodular hyperplasia, are directly related to the long-term presence of excess lipid in the hepatocytes or sinusoidal fat-storage cells. Fatty livers are very vulnerable to a wide range of toxic and nutritional insults, and the necrogenic effects of these are likely to be more potent initiators of fibrosis and remodeling than the long-term presence of the fat *per se*. Nevertheless, some chronic changes can be ascribed to long-term presence of lipid. These are most commonly seen in the livers of old dogs and include fatty cysts, ceroid accumulation and, rarely, calcifying focal fibrous reactions to accumulations of cholesterol.

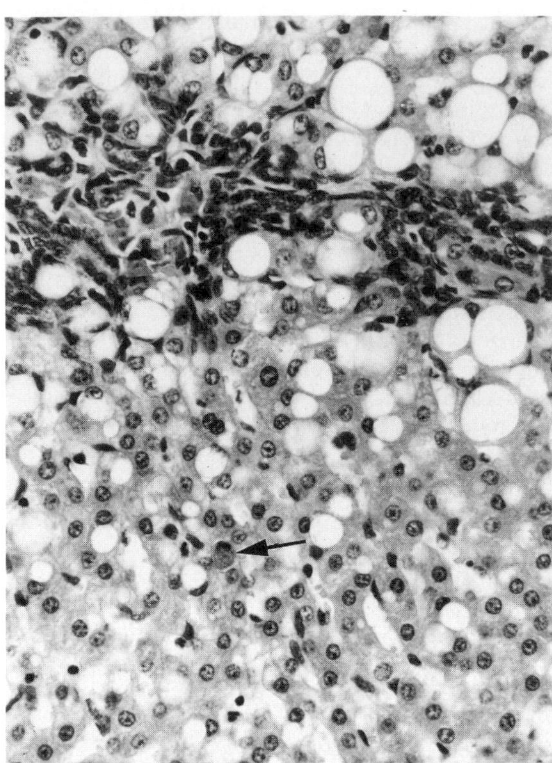

Fig. 2.13 Fatty change and cholangiolar proliferation. Ovine white liver disease. Ceroid in sinusoidal macrophage (arrow). (Courtesy of S. McOrist.)

When lipid accumulates rapidly and in large amounts, there is a tendency for groups of the fat-laden cells to rupture or fuse and eventually form a multinucleate rim about a foamy mass of lipid. This epithelial structure is known as a **fatty cyst,** as is the next stage, which occurs when released lipid is picked up by macrophages, which form foamy aggregations in sinusoids, the stroma of portal triads, and in hepatic venules (Fig. 2.15). These mesenchymal cells have only limited capacity for complete lysosomal digestion of neutral triglyceride; the result is progressive lipoperoxidation of the less saturated fatty acids, followed by polymerization of the reactive residues. These form complex and variable compounds, known collectively as **ceroid,** which are only slightly soluble in lipid solvents and are PAS positive, variably acid-fast, and autofluorescent. In histologic sections this pigment ap-

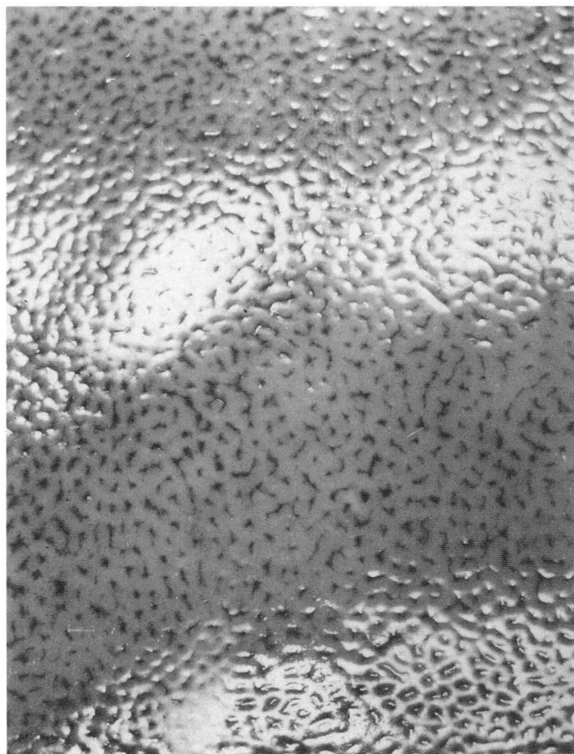

Fig. 2.14 Severe fatty liver with periacinar necrosis. Acute anemia in a fat goat.

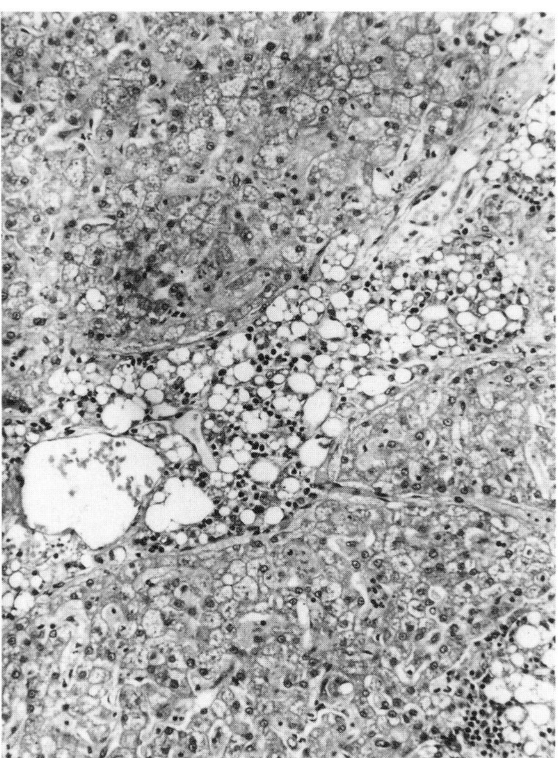

Fig. 2.15 Accumulations of lipid-filled macrophages (fatty cysts) in hepatic stroma. Dog.

pears as colorless or yellow irregular fragments associated with the lipid globules in macrophages and, to a lesser extent, hepatocytes. Considerable amounts of lipid and ceroid may find their way into the lymphatics in the hepatic stroma and into the portal lymph nodes, which become slightly enlarged, yellow-green, and rather oily on section. Most of the hepatocellular lipid may disappear from these livers, leaving the fatty cysts, and the result is a liver of relatively normal color, perhaps with a slightly nodular surface, with the stroma outlined by a delicate tracery of yellow ceroid deposit. It is difficult to distinguish these livers from those developing more pronounced remodeling, nodular regeneration, and regional atrophy, which are described with nodular regeneration under Idiopathic Chronic Liver Disease of Dogs (Section VI,F of this chapter).

Occasionally in the liver of old dogs there can be found sharply defined, fibrous, stony, hard masses, usually close to the surface, sometimes as much as 3–4 cm in diameter (Fig. 2.16). These masses are usually sufficiently mineralized to show up distinctly on clinical radiographs. The mineral appears to be deposited on a matrix of degenerate collagen, laid down about perivascular foci of foamy macrophages and accumulations of cholesterol. The fibrous tissue may be laid down in response to the continued presence of fat, ceroid, or cholesterol, but no reason is apparent for the strictly localized distribution of the reaction. There are no recognizable hepatocytes in these lesions.

Physiologic fatty liver occurs in late pregnancy and heavy lactation, particularly in ruminants. Obvious fat infiltration is also seen in neonates, especially in those species whose milk is relatively rich in fat. These livers are fatty enough to be pale to the naked eye.

Fasting an animal with reasonable fat reserves rapidly depletes hepatocellular stores of glycogen and *de novo* lipogenesis ceases. There follows a heavy demand on adipose tissue fat stores, since the liver, dependent primarily on fatty acid oxidation for its own considerable energy needs, must also provide a large amount of lipoprotein for export to other tissues. Under these circumstances, it appears that the synthesis and transport of low-density lipoprotein acts as a bottleneck in the movement of lipid through the hepatocyte. Triglyceride accumulates in the cytoplasm, particularly if starvation reduces the availability of protein and cofactors such as choline, which are essential to the synthetic process.

Ketosis of **ruminants** typically is associated with fatty liver. It is rather unrealistic to try to separate discussion of starvation from that of ruminant ketosis, especially from the morphologic point of view, as the differences are really quantitative. In biochemical terms, the difference seems to be related to the added stimulus for fatty acid oxidation caused by the drain of heavy pregnancy or lactation and the enormous potential for ketogenesis. In ewes freshly dead of pregnancy toxemia, one may see indistinct patches of white discoloration of abdominal fat, which

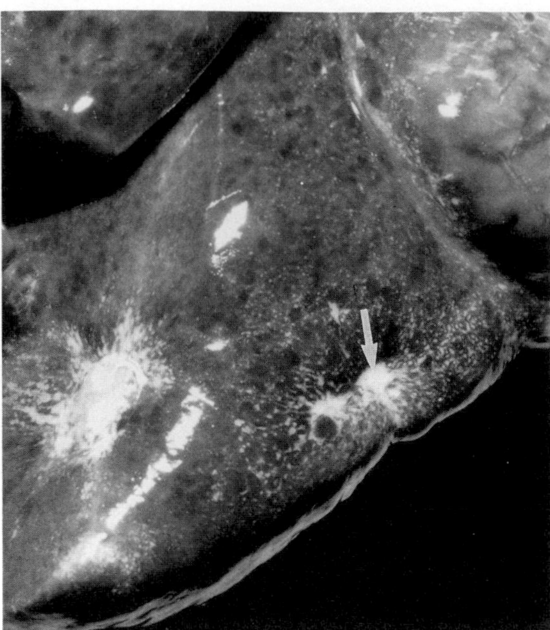

Fig. 2.16 Focal hepatic calcification (arrow). There is a hepatoma at upper right. Old dog.

may reflect accelerated lipolysis. These patches tend to be obscured by postmortem solidification of the fat. The fatty infiltration of hepatocytes in these animals is often most severe in the periportal zone, whereas the distribution of lipid in ketosis of cattle is predominantly periacinar.

Fatty liver of **diabetes** occurs when insulin is deficient or inactive due to lack of functioning receptors. There is greatly accelerated lipolysis from adipose tissue. The liver is thus presented with a large load of fatty acid, the mitochondrial oxidation of which is hindered by the shortage of ATP occasioned by reduced glucose availability. Lipoprotein synthesis is also reduced, partly because of the ATP limitation and partly as a result of reduced uptake by the liver of branched-chain amino acids. Insulin deficiency alone will produce fatty liver, but most cases in carnivores are associated with exocrine pancreatic insufficiency as well. This further reduces the availability of amino acids because of protein malabsorption. All these factors may combine to produce very fatty livers in chronic uncontrolled diabetes mellitus. The periacinar hepatocytes usually show the greatest degree of fatty infiltration, but the change is often diffuse and extreme, and the plasma may also be milky with triglyceride.

Lipoprotein synthesis and transport are dependent on oxidative metabolism, and **hypoxia** of hepatocytes leads to triglyceride accumulation. The two most common causes of hepatocellular hypoxia are anemia and reduced sinusoidal perfusion in passive venous congestion. The hepatocytes most severely affected are those in the periacinar zone (Fig. 2.17).

Local hypoxia is probably the basis for another example of fatty liver. Small, sharply demarcated patches of intense

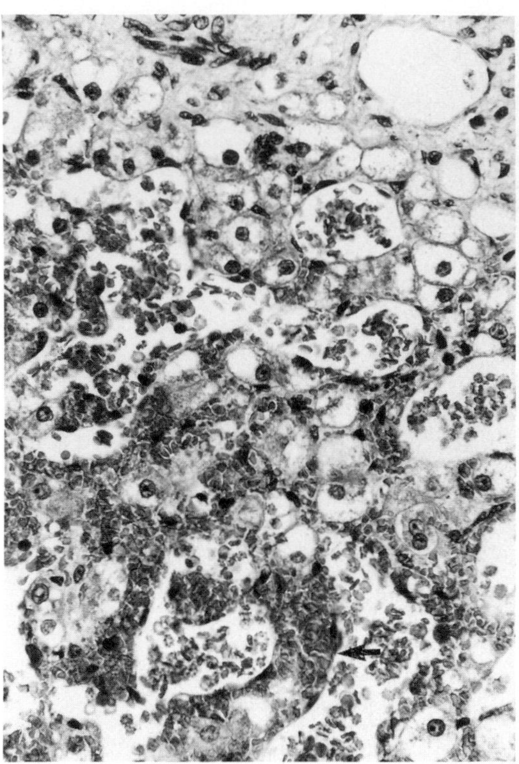

Fig. 2.17 Atrophy and loss of periacinar hepatocytes (arrow). They are replaced by erythrocytes within the remaining reticulin framework. Passive congestion. Dog.

fatty infiltration are often seen in bovine livers at or adjacent to sites of **capsular fibrous adhesions** (Fig. 2.18). These patches are neither swollen nor shrunken, extend usually less than a centimeter into the parenchyma, and are of the same consistency as normal liver. The acinar structure of these lesions is undisturbed, but the hepatocytes therein show pronounced lipidosis, presumably related to interference with local perfusion caused by tensions transmitted to the parenchyma by the adhesion.

Fatty liver due to **intoxication** is common. There are several stages of the cycle of hepatic lipid metabolism that can be affected selectively by various toxins to produce fatty liver. For example, it is possible experimentally to cause triglyceride accumulation by interfering with mitochondrial fatty acid oxidation with sublethal doses of cyanide, or by inhibiting apolipoprotein synthesis by administration of orotic acid. Most toxins that cause fatty liver in naturally occurring situations, however, also produce a greater or lesser degree of hepatocellular necrosis. Fatty liver occurring as a manifestation of toxic liver disease will be further discussed in that section, but the generalization may be made here that most important veterinary hepatic intoxications cause widespread membrane damage and/or disturbance of protein synthesis. These cause lipid accumulation in the hepatocyte by interfering with lipoprotein synthesis and export, as well as with fatty acid oxidation.

Whereas fatty liver in domestic animals is more fre-

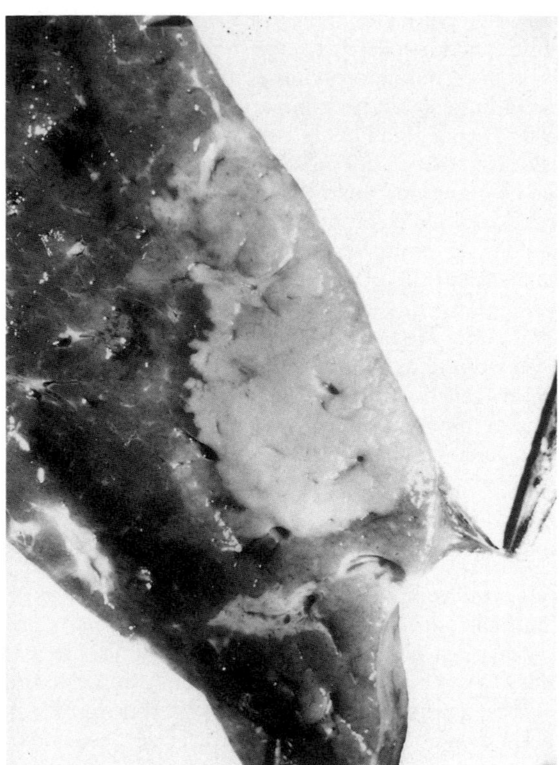

Fig. 2.18 Subcapsular focal fatty change associated with capsular adhesion. Ox.

quently associated with generalized interferences with energy metabolism, there are some specific nutritional **deficiencies** that will produce fatty liver; they have usually been defined under experimental conditions and have no valid naturally occurring equivalent. Choline deficiency, for example, in the absence of other suitable methyl donors, soon produces fatty liver as a result of reduced synthesis of lecithin and consequent impairment of triglyceride binding and transport. It is unlikely, however, that choline deficiency uncomplicated by other forms of malnutrition would occur in domestic animals; the same may be said of essential fatty acid deficiency, which also produces fatty liver in experimental animals.

One naturally occurring example of fatty liver that appears to be at least partly due to a specific deficiency is **ovine white-liver disease,** first described in lambs in New Zealand and now known to occur in southern Australia and Europe, and in goats. This is a syndrome of ill thrift, anorexia, mild normocytic normochromic anemia with, occasionally, photosensitization and icterus. The condition is associated with low liver cobalt levels and low plasma concentrations of vitamin B_{12}. Lambs younger than 1 year are more commonly affected than ewes, and pastures are likely to be adequate at the times of peak incidence in late spring and early summer; these epidemiologic features clearly indicate a different pathogenesis from that of pregnancy toxemia (ovine ketosis). The disease has been shown to be cobalt- and vitamin B_{12}-responsive, and there is clearly a degree of overlap between this condition and the more conventional forms of cobalt deficiency. Nevertheless, the liver pathology is sufficiently distinctive to allow classification as a separate entity.

In the early stages, the liver changes consist of vacuolar triglyceride accumulations in hepatocytes, usually most severe in the periacinar zones. In addition, ceroid pigment is present in all cases, early in hepatocytes and later also in sinusoidal cells and stromal macrophages. The fatty change may be very severe in the early stage, the liver being grossly swollen. A moderate degree of bile ductular proliferation is also a consistent feature (Fig. 2.13), and the epithelium of the smaller ductules in the triads is dysplastic. Spongy degeneration of cerebral white matter, typical of the hyperammonemia of hepatic failure, is present in some cases.

The disease can be produced in cobalt-deficient sheep fed diets high in propionate precursors, which may help explain the explosive nature of outbreaks on lush pasture. A role for mycotoxins has been suggested. Whatever the factor in its initiation, the metabolic disturbances of starvation are invoked by the severe inappetence, and these will no doubt confuse attempts to define the condition biochemically.

Equine hyperlipemia is almost exclusively a disease of ponies, and among these, the Shetland breed predominates. The disease is usually fatal after about a week. Pregnant or lactating mares are most likely to develop the disease, particularly if they are excessively fat and have recently suffered reduced feed intake due to onset of parturition or conditions such as laminitis or parasitism or other causes of stress. The clinical course is marked by somnolence, complete anorexia, and colic, progressing to mania in some cases, although most simply become progressively more depressed. Some ponies develop ventral subcutaneous edema, and most develop moderate diarrhea. All show marked increase in plasma triglyceride concentration, the lipid being predominantly very low density lipoprotein, but all other lipid fractions are elevated, and the concentration is sufficient to impart a striking milkiness to the serum and blood. Metabolic acidosis is a consistent feature in animals that die, and they also develop signs of disseminated intravascular coagulation.

The liver at necropsy is severely fatty and may have ruptured; the lipidosis also extends to heart and skeletal muscle, kidney, and adrenal cortex. The hepatic lipidosis is remarkable only by its severity; there may be some focal hepatocellular necrosis,and there is consistent prolongation of sulfobromophthalein retention times and elevation of serum alkaline phosphatase levels. Evidence of disseminated intravascular coagulation is seen as serosal hemorrhages and microscopic thrombi in various organs, and even gross infarction of myocardium and kidney. Small lipid emboli may be detected in frozen sections of lung, myocardium, and brain in these animals; their relationship to the microthrombosis is uncertain.

The pathogenesis of this disease is obscure. Since the excess lipid in liver and blood is in the form of triglyceride, the implication is that the liver is capable of esterifying fatty acid mobilized from depot fat. The triglyceride thus formed is presumably then exported to the plasma as low-density lipoprotein until the plasma transport mechanisms are saturated, at which stage fatty buildup in the hepatocyte begins. Another possibility is that there is an inability on the part of all tissues other than the liver to utilize fatty acids or low-density lipoproteins at the normal rate, while triglyceride synthesis from fatty acids continues in the liver.

It has been proposed that an underlying cause of pony hyperlipemia is a comparative resistance to insulin in susceptible animals, and that this is compounded in stressful episodes by increased levels of circulating cortisol. Various steroid hormones including glucocorticoids can interfere with insulin action, and hyperlipemic ponies often have elevated plasma insulin levels, which suggests reduced function of insulin receptors. However, plasma ketones are much less consistently elevated, which suggests that there is not much evidence of the increased ketogenesis which one might expect to follow impaired insulin utilization.

Fatty liver syndrome in **cats** has some features in common with hyperlipemia of ponies in that both occur in overfat, nutritionally stressed animals; there is hypertriglyceridemia, and the mortality rate is high. In the feline condition, however, there is no sex predilection, jaundice is frequently observed, and there may be severe periacinar hepatocellular necrosis, at least in the later stages. The liver has severe fatty accumulation in all hepatocytes; bile pigment accumulation, when seen, is mostly present in Kupffer cells and can be confused with polymerized lipid residues.

As with horses, the pathogenesis of this disease is obscure. Since the excess lipid in liver and blood is in the form of triglyceride, the implication is that the liver is capable of esterifying fatty acid mobilized from depot fat. The triglyceride thus formed is presumably then exported to the plasma as low-density lipoprotein until the plasma transport mechanisms are saturated, at which stage fatty buildup in the hepatocyte begins. Another possibility is that there is an inability on the part of all tissues other than the liver to utilize fatty acids or low-density lipoproteins at the normal rate, while triglyceride synthesis from fatty acids continues in the liver.

J. Lysosomal Storage Diseases

In common with other tissues in animals with heritable deficiency of specific lysosomal enzymes, liver cells may accumulate to a pathological degree the substrate normally catabolized by the missing enzyme. Such storage is, however, less obvious in the liver than in other tissues such as those of the central nervous system. One reason for this may be that hydropic and fatty changes in hepatocytes are so common that they do not attract the attention they receive in other tissues. Another is that there are likely to be more alternative catabolic and excretory pathways available to hepatocytes than to cells with more limited metabolic functions. This is suggested by the fact that in animals with ceroid- lipofuscinosis, the lysosomal storage is minimal in hepatocytes compared to that in the brain. Moreover, hepatic failure is rarely if ever recorded in these diseases, which are mostly manifested clinically by nervous dysfunction. Nevertheless, lysosomal storage of sugars, glycogen and cerebrosides, and other orphan substrates does occur in hepatocytes and Kupffer cells in individuals with the corresponding inborn errors of metabolism. Affected cells show variably severe vacuolar degeneration of either the fatty or hydropic types, or ill-defined expansions of the cytoplasm: Kupffer cells and bile-duct epithelium may be more severely affected than hepatocytes. Liver involvement in storage disease is probably best seen in some forms of glycogenosis, particularly in humans, in which species hepatomogaly may be observed.

K. Amyloidosis

Amyloid infiltration of the liver occurs in cattle, horses, dogs, and cats. In the carnivores the amyloidosis is primary, or at least not obviously secondary; in cattle it is secondary to some chronic tissue-destructive process; and in horses it occurs chiefly in those used for the production of hyperimmune serum. In cats there is an association with hypervitaminosis A. In each species it is part of generalized amyloidosis. The amyloid is deposited between the sinusoidal lining and the hepatocytes (Fig. 2.19)

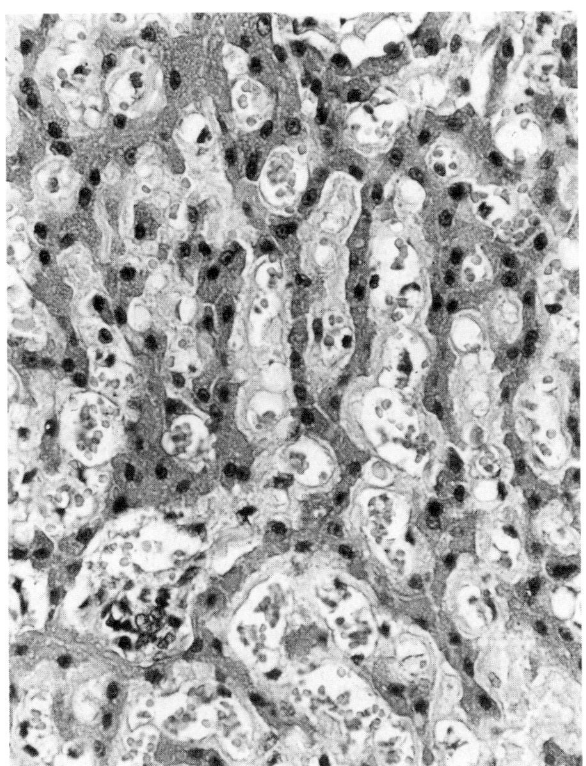

Fig. 2.19 Amyloid in the space of Disse compressing the hepatocellular plates. Cat.

and is sometimes found in the walls of the afferent vessels. The surrounded hepatocellular cords atrophy. Affected livers are enlarged, with rounded edges, pale and soft in horses, firm in cattle. The amyloid is deposited first in the parenchyma about the portal tracts and appears grayish and waxy. The liver is predisposed to rupture. Horses may develop icterus and other signs of hepatic failure, but cattle die first of the primary disease or from the uremia resulting from concurrent renal amyloidosis.

Bibliography

Black, H. *et al.* White liver disease in goats. *N Z Vet J* **36:** 15–17, 1988.

Bogin, E. *et al.* Biochemical changes associated with the fatty liver syndrome in cows. *J Comp Pathol* **98:** 337–347, 1988.

Caple, I. W. *et al.* Starvation ketosis in pregnant beef cows. *Aust Vet J* **53:** 289–291, 1977.

Collins, R. A., and Reid, I. M. A correlated biochemical and stereological study of periparturient fatty liver in the dairy cow. *Res Vet Sci* **28:** 373–376, 1980.

Haagsman, H. P., and Van Golde, L. M. G. Regulation of hepatic triacylglycerol synthesis and secretion. *Vet Res Commun* **8:** 157–171, 1984.

Henderson, G. D, Read, L. C., and Snoswell, A. M. Studies of liver lipids in normal, alloxan-diabetic and pregnancy-toxemic sheep. *Biochim Biophys Acta* **710:** 236–241, 1982.

Jeffcott, L. B, and Field, J. R. Current concepts of hyperlipaemia in horses and ponies. *Vet Rec* **116:** 461–466, 1985.

Katoh, N., and Kimura, K. Decreased protein kinase C activity in fatty liver from cattle. *Am J Vet Res* **50:** 1489–1492, 1989.

Lombardi, C. Considerations of the pathogenesis of fatty liver. *Lab Invest* **15:** 1–20, 1966.

Morris, M. D., Silversmit, D. B., and Hintz, H. F. Hyperlipoproteinemia in fasting ponies. *J Lipid Res* **13:** 383–389, 1972.

Reid, I. M. *et al.* The pathology of postparturient fatty liver in high-yielding dairy cows. *Invest Cell Pathol* **3:** 237–249, 1980.

Richards, R. B., and Harrison, M. R. White liver disease in lambs. *Aust Vet J* **57:** 565–568, 1981.

Sutherland, R. J., Cordes, D. O., and Carthew, G. C. Ovine white liver disease—an hepatic dysfunction associated with vitamin B_{12} deficiency. *N Z Vet J* **27:** 227–232, 1979.

Thornburg, L. P., Simpson, S., and Digilio, K. Fatty liver syndrome in cats. *J Am Anim Hosp Assoc* **18:** 397–400, 1982.

Ulvund, M. J. Ovine white liver disease (OWLD). Pathology. *Acta Vet Scand* **31:** 309–324, 1990.

V. Patterns of Hepatic Necrosis

Hepatocytes may be killed by toxic insult, activity of microorganisms or inflammatory cells, or by nutritional deficiencies and severe metabolic disturbances including hypoxia. Whatever the origin of the insult, the generation and propagation of free radicals is important in the mediation of many types of necrotizing liver injury.

Free radicals are particularly noxious for lipoprotein membranes. The membranes are composed of precise repeating lipoprotein subunits, which can be rapidly degraded by the action of these ions or reactive molecules, particularly as they tend to initiate self-propagating chain reactions. The hepatocyte, with its massive complement of membranous organelles, is therefore highly vulnerable to free radical damage unless protected by free radical scavengers such as reduced glutathione and vitamin E.

The later stages of hepatocellular degeneration, which eventually lead to the irreversible state of necrosis, are similar to those producing necrosis in other tissue, and reference to reviews of the subject in general pathology texts should be made for details of the ionic fluxes, disruption of cell and organelle membranes, and interference with energy metabolism that occur in the dying cell. Here, the various morphologic patterns of hepatic necrosis are described.

A. *Single-Cell Necrosis*

Necrobiosis is the term applied to the death of single effete cells in any tissue; it occurs more often in the liver than in many other organs, but the process is never obvious. The manner in which the cell disappears may not always be the same, but usually it is in the form of shrinkage necrosis known as apoptosis.

Apoptosis has become the accepted designation for the process whereby single cells are removed with minimal disturbance of the tissue of which they are a part. This process may in some situations be regarded as physiologic, as in the various remodelings that occur in the embryo or in cyclic changes in the reproductive tract. In others, it may be part of pathologic processes, such as rapidly growing malignancy or atrophy of accessory sex tissue following castration.

Apoptosis begins with sudden condensation of the cytoplasm and nucleus of a cell that is alive and still metabolically active; the process of apoptosis may in its earlier stages be energy dependent. Within a short interval, the cytoplasm is shredded away as membrane-bound fragments containing normal organelles (including fragments of nucleus) embedded in an electron-dense matrix. These fragments are rapidly engulfed by neighboring cells and by macrophages and, if they contain no nuclear chromatin, may be recognized under the light microscope as acidophilic or Councilman bodies. Larger fragments containing nuclear remnants are recognized as pyknotic fragments. The important distinctions from true necrosis are that at no stage do the apoptotic cells burst and release their content to the extracellular environment, and the apoptotic fragments are taken up, not only by Kupffer cells, but also by adjacent hepatocytes (Fig. 2.7). This dismantling of the cells occurs in such a fashion that there is little or no disturbance of local tissue form or function; there is none of the hemorrhage, scarring, or tissue defect that is produced by conventional necrosis. The process seems to have been evolved as a tidy means of deleting cells, whether they be surplus to requirement or damaged in certain ways. The process is quite inconspicuous, occurs rapidly, and tends to be overlooked unless its incidence is very high; this is perhaps why its nature and significance went unrecognized for so long. Nevertheless, once appreciated, apoptosis is seen in a wide variety of liver diseases, ranging from toxicities to immunologically mediated inflammations.

B. Coagulative Necrosis

This term may be applied to groups or zones of intact but dead hepatocytes which have shrunken slightly, stain intensely with eosin, and may have visible but distorted nuclei (Fig. 2.20). These cells may also be dehydrated but, in contrast to the metabolically driven self-dehydration of apoptosis, in coagulative necrosis, the removal of water is not an active process; the affected cells do not undergo spontaneous fragmentation and, when removed, they are taken up by macrophages, not by local surviving hepatocytes. It seems that coagulative necrosis, which is often seen in acute hepatotoxicity, is the result of sudden and catastrophic denaturation of cytosolic protein, which imparts a rather dense, rigid texture to the dead cells, somewhat preserving their shape.

C. Lytic Necrosis

In some circumstances, destruction of hepatocytes involves rapid swelling and disintegration of the cells, usually in groups. This pattern is also seen in some intoxications, often in the marginal zone between areas of coagulative necrosis and surviving hepatocytes. This suggests that, if the injury is not too rapidly fatal, there is time for failing sodium pumps to allow the cell to overhydrate and burst. Lytic necrosis may also be associated with foci of inflammation (Fig. 2.21A,B). The lysis in this situation is likely to be due to the activity of neutrophil leukocytes and macrophages and their hydrolytic enzymes.

D. Piecemeal Necrosis

Models of immune-mediated hepatocyte necrosis have emerged from studies of human viral hepatitis and some forms of drug-induced chronic hepatitis. The pattern of necrosis is sometimes referred to as piecemeal necrosis. The mechanisms may involve either direct damage to hepatocytes by the uptake of antigen–antibody complexes, or cooperation between macrophages and T lymphocytes. These may cause cell-mediated destruction of hepatocytes that have taken up these complexes or, perhaps, native antigen or virus. Whatever the agency, the mode of cell removal in this sort of injury often takes the form of apoptosis, which may be directly triggered by the immunologically competent cells. Whether these models are valid for any spontaneous liver disease in domestic animals remains to be proven. This type of liver injury is discussed further under chronic active hepatitis (in Section X,A,1 of this chapter), in which inflammation characteristically disrupts the limiting plate, giving an irregular appearance to the periportal zone.

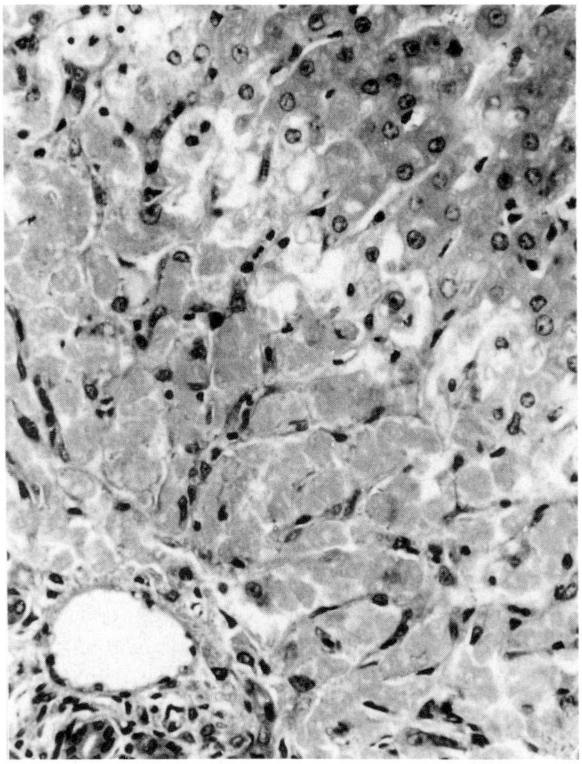

Fig. 2.20 Periportal necrosis in ngaione poisoning. Sheep. (Courtesy of A. A. Seawright.)

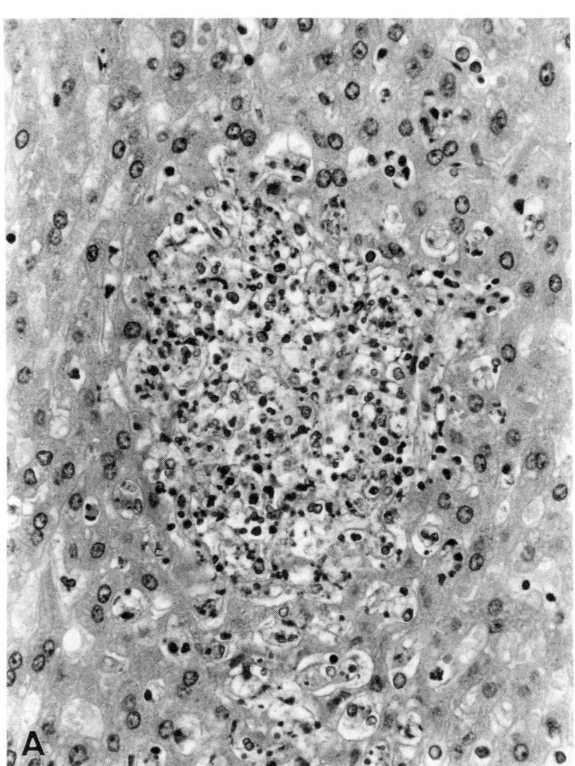

Fig. 2.21A Focal inflammation and lytic necrosis in salmonellosis.

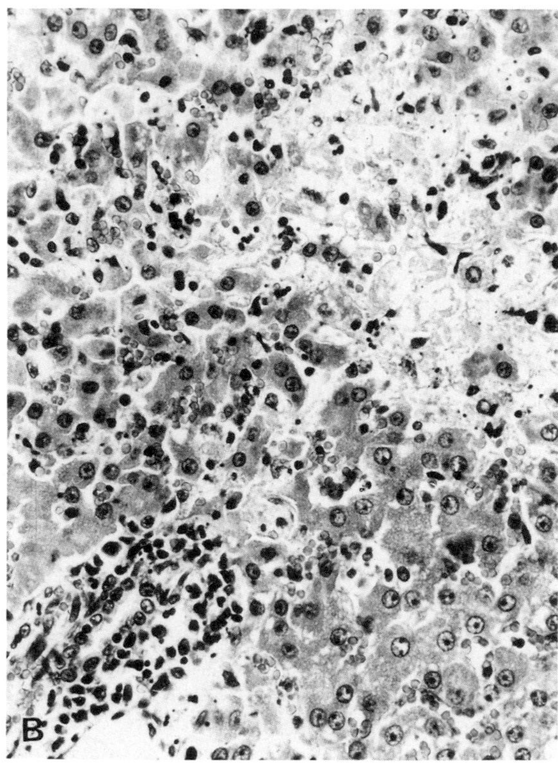

Fig. 2.21B Lytic necrosis. Toxoplasmosis. Kitten.

E. Focal Necrosis

Focal necrosis is very common in autopsy material. The lesions are microscopic or barely visible to the naked eye and are usually numerous. Their designation as focal depends on their size and on a random distribution relative to the acini. There is sometimes apparent a tendency for focal necroses to occur nearer to the axial portal vessels than to the periphery of the circulatory fields, and to be concentrated in some acinar agglomerates rather than others.

Focal necrosis occurs in many infections, parasitic migrations, and instances of biliary obstruction, and in these the designation focal hepatitis will often be more appropriate, since most are attended by some degree of focal inflammation. The infectious causes may be viral, such as equine herpesvirus-1 in the fetus, or bacterial. Many bacterial infections that are septicemic produce focal hepatic lesions consistently; examples are salmonellosis, tularemia, pseudotuberculosis, listeriosis in the fetus and newborn, and *Pasteurella haemolytica* septicemia in lambs. The focal necrosis may be the outcome of a Kupffer cell reaction, as in salmonellosis, or of bacterial embolism, as in pasteurellosis. The approximate cause can usually be determined by histologic examination.

In cattle, especially, focal necrosis in few or many visible foci is common at necropsy and is common enough to be important at slaughter; it is responsible for the descriptive appellation sawdust. The pathogenesis is not known and probably varies, but it may be caused by organisms from the gut that reach the liver in the portal blood. The lesion is not specific and consists of focal parenchymal necrosis with disruption of reticulin fibers and an infiltration of neutrophils and lymphocytes (Fig. 2.22); frank suppuration does not occur. This lesion is said to be most common in livers from feedlot-fattened cattle; whether or not it is a precursor of telangiectasis (see Vascular Factors in Liver Injury, Section IX of this chapter) remains conjectural.

Focal necrosis in biliary obstruction follows rupture of distended canaliculi or smaller cholangioles, with the formation of small bile lakes. The yellow pigment is readily visible microscopically and provokes small granulomas with giant cells.

Focal necroses are of very little functional significance for the liver, even when numerous. When they heal there is some scarring, but this too probably disappears in time. They are of diagnostic importance in some diseases such as salmonellosis, and of economic importance to the meat industry.

F. Periacinar Necrosis

The hepatocytes in the periacinar zone are particularly vulnerable to necrotizing insult because they are farthest from the source of incoming portal and arterial blood and are therefore last in line for oxygen and essential nutrients, and they contain the greatest concentration of

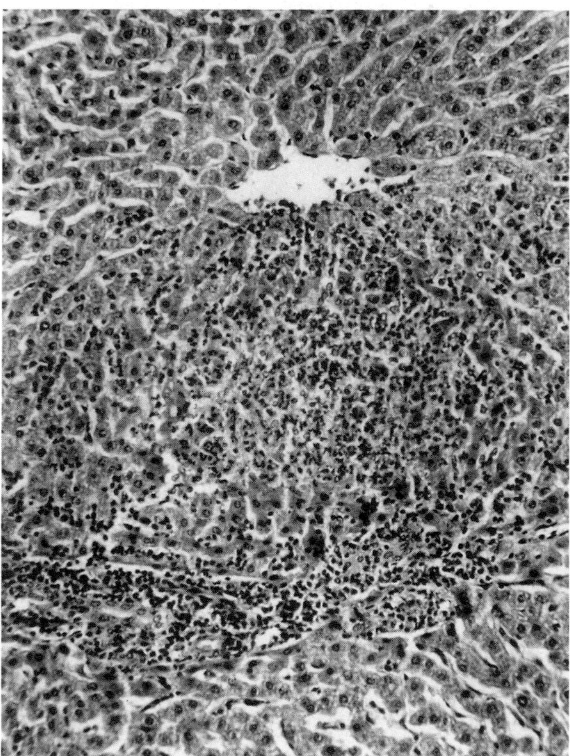

Fig. 2.22 Focal hepatitis—the so-called sawdust of cattle.

mixed-function oxidases which are capable of transforming certain exogenous compounds into reactive metabolites which may prove to be sufficiently toxic to kill the cells that produce them (see Toxic Liver Disease, Section XI of this chapter).

Severe viral infections, such as canine adenovirus (Fig. 2.23) and Rift Valley fever can produce periacinar necrosis, and the reasons for the increased susceptibility of the hepatocytes of this zone in these diseases are not obvious. It is possible that hepatocellular swelling and sinusoidal damage reduce effective perfusion of the periacinar hepatocytes, but it is also possible that these cells have greater intrinsic susceptibility to the viruses.

Periacinar degeneration and necrosis are seen commonly in animals that have died rather slowly. It is assumed that, in the agonal period, the hepatocytes in this zone are disproportionately disadvantaged as a result of the failing circulation, and that the damage is due to tissue hypoxia. This necrosis is more extensive if the animal is anemic. Periacinar necrosis is also seen in passive venous congestion of the liver and is described under Passive Venous Congestion (Section IX,C of this chapter).

The necrotic cells are usually replaced by stagnant blood, at least in the acute phase; therefore, in the liver with periacinar necrosis, there is usually a prominent **acinar pattern,** which takes the form of a fine, regular, pallid network of surviving, often fatty, hepatocytes in the periportal zone, which stands up above the red, collapsed areas adjacent to the hepatic venules (Figs. 2.14, 2.24A,B). But fatty change in the liver may also have a zonal distribution, and such livers may show a marked acinar pattern without having significant necrosis.

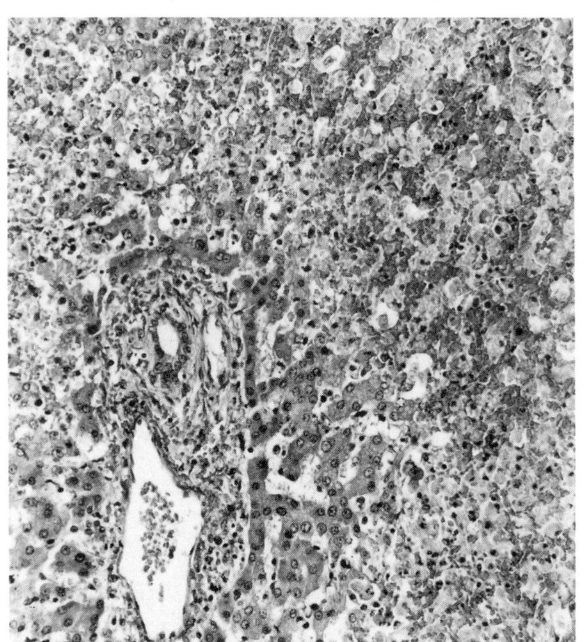

Fig. 2.23 Infectious canine hepatitis. Severe periacinar necrosis with periportal survival.

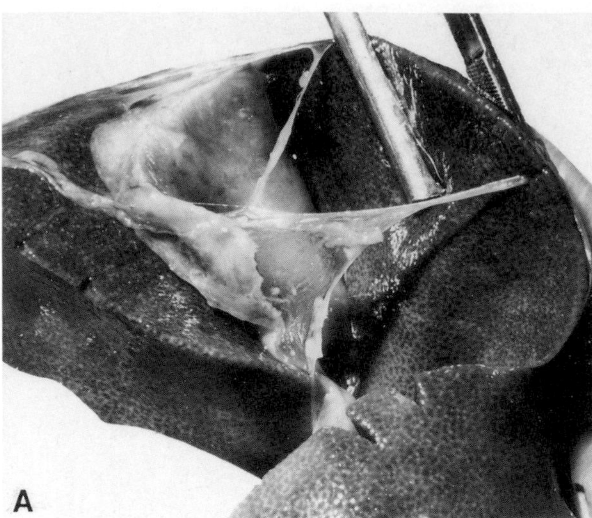

Fig. 2.24A Severe subacute passive congestion of liver, showing fibrin between lobes, and acinar pattern. Dog, congestive heart failure.

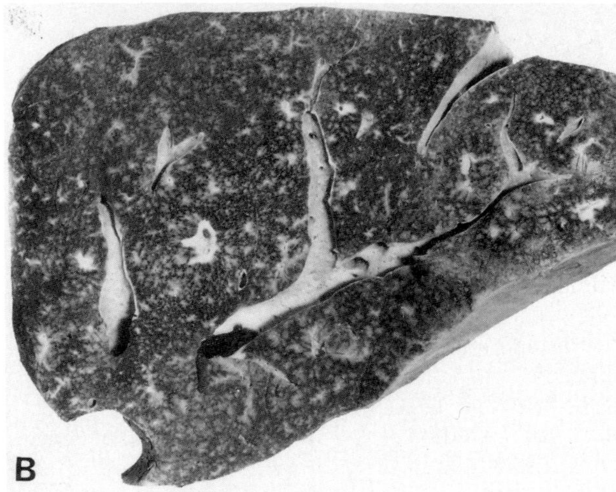

Fig. 2.24B Chronic passive congestion (nutmeg liver). Ox.

The zones of necrosis are usually coagulative in nature and may be restricted to the hepatocytes immediately surrounding the hepatic venules; this pattern gave rise to the time-honored designation centrilobular necrosis. Frequently, however, the areas of necrosis are joined to one another, thus cutting the conventional lobules into segments, and at the same time outlining the periphery of the circulatory fields of the hepatic acini (Fig. 2.25A). Some of these areas of necrosis extend up to larger portal triads, because the periphery of some acini may lie against the larger portal tracts (as the skin of a grape may lie against the major stem of the bunch). Often, the hepatocytes between the necrotic and more normal zones show hydropic degeneration or fatty change (Fig. 2.25B).

If the necrotizing insult is of short duration, quite exten-

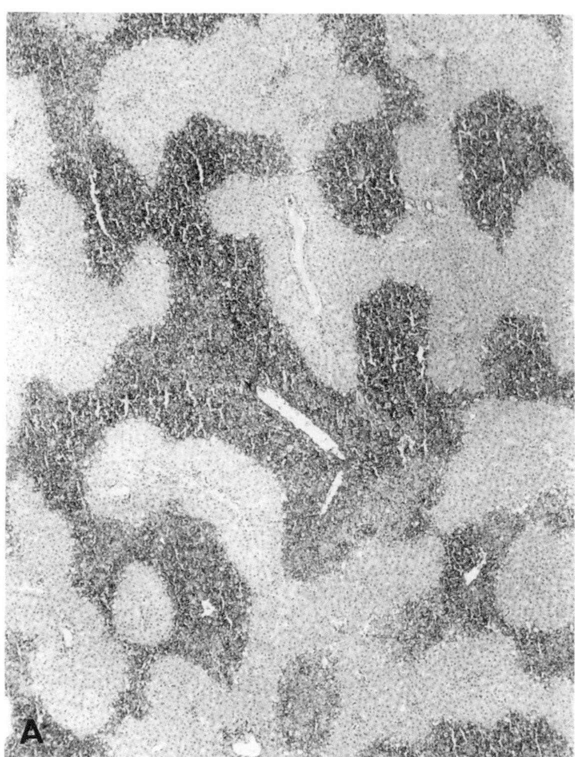

Fig. 2.25A Acini outlined by periacinar hemorrhagic necrosis. *Cestrum* poisoning. Sheep.

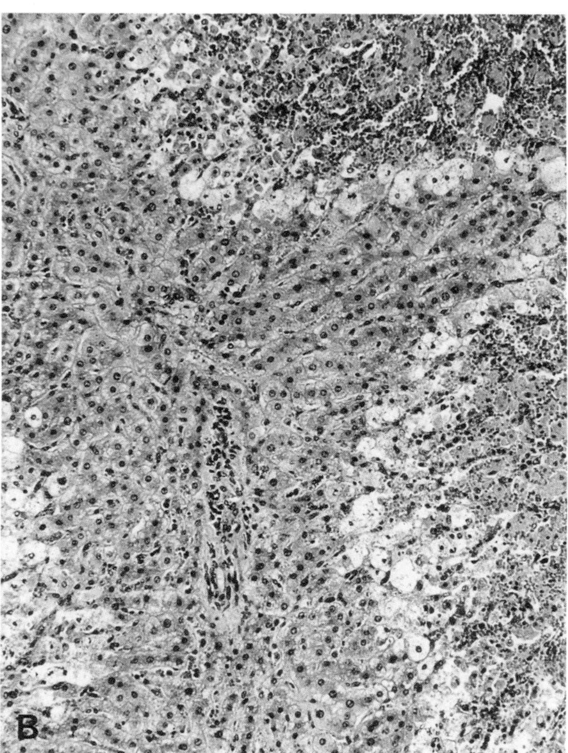

Fig. 2.25B Acute periacinar necrosis in *Cestrum parqui* poisoning. Ox. Necrotic zone bordered by hydropic hepatocytes.

sive periacinar necrosis may be followed by repair and complete restoration of normal structure and function within a few days. Severe periacinar necrosis may be followed shortly by cholangiolar cell proliferation and bile duct proliferation; this reaction seems to be related to the stimulus for hepatocellular proliferation, to which the cells of the finest branches of the bile ducts also seem susceptible. With restitution of the normal complement of hepatocytes, the proliferative response in the biliary tract subsides unless the original insult is continuous or repeated.

G. Midzonal Necrosis

The rarity of midzonal necrosis has in the past led to the contention that it was either an artefact or a stage on the way to periacinar necrosis. It is now established that some intoxications can produce selective midzonal necrosis, and the lesion has been reliably produced in experimental animals.

Acute midzonal necrosis may involve only a narrow, sharply defined band of hepatocytes, or it may be more diffuse within the acinus, so that periportal or periacinar degeneration may be superimposed on the more severe midzonal lesion. The acute phase of coagulative necrosis is followed by intense macrophage activity, which rapidly removes the dead cells and allows complete regeneration of normal structure.

H. Periportal Necrosis

The remarks just made about midzonal necrosis apply to coagulative periportal necrosis (Figs. 2.20, 2.26). It is a an uncommon lesion, perhaps more often seen than midzonal necrosis, and is caused by the same sort of complex interaction between specific types of hepatotoxins and the hepatic microsomal apparatus (see Toxic Liver Disease, Section XI of this chapter). It is usual to find, in the same liver, areas that show one or more of the patterns of zonal necrosis.

The various forms of zonal necrosis cannot reliably be distinguished from one another grossly, but one may expect to see in periportal necrosis a reversal of the pattern seen in periacinar necrosis; that is, in periportal necrosis, the surviving pale hepatocytes about the hepatic venules may appear as pale, raised islands in the meshes of a regular network of red, collapsed periportal tissue. Careful scrutiny may reveal the smallest hepatic venules at the center of the pale islands.

I. Paracentral Necrosis

Paracentral necrosis is a form of coagulative necrosis that involves an isolated complete hepatic acinus. Its characteristic pattern is revealed when the acinus is viewed in transverse section. It is possibly an ischemic lesion or infarct produced by an occlusion of a terminal portal ven-

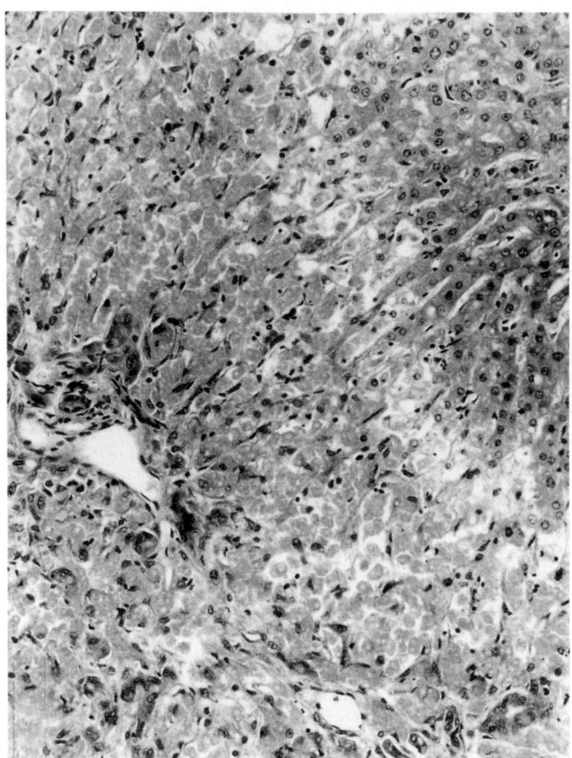

Fig. 2.26 Periportal necrosis in ngaione poisoning. Sheep. (Courtesy of A. A. Seawright.)

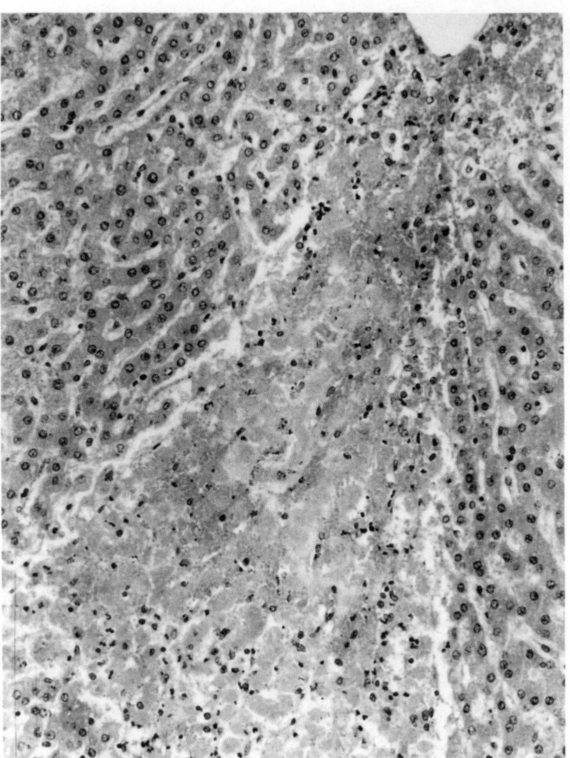

Fig. 2.27 Paracentral necrosis in ngaione poisoning. Sheep.

ule, such as may occur in disseminated intravascular coagulation. Its appearance in certain of the acute hepatotoxicities (Fig. 2.27) probably represents the death of a single complete acinus as a result of local vascular insufficiency, although, theoretically, high local microsomal enzyme activity or local deficiency of hepatocellular protective factors may play a part. Occlusion and rupture of a bile ductule or cholangiole is another potential cause of paracentral necrosis.

J. Massive Necrosis

Massive necrosis refers to events in individual acini, not to events in the liver as a whole. By accepted definition, every cell in the affected acinus is dead, including the hepatocytes of the limiting plate (Fig. 2.28). The definition is of some importance because the sequelae of this pattern of necrosis are quite distinct. There being no surviving parenchyma in the acinus, there is no source of cells for regeneration, and none to hold open the reticulin network of the acinus. The sequel to massive necrosis therefore is collapse of the reticulin and fibrous framework so that portal areas and hepatic venules are approximated, and the connective tissues condense and scarify. The definition is too restrictive because, about the periphery of such areas, it is possible to find acini showing necrosis of zonal distribution of both paracentral and periacinar patterns.

The distribution of massive hepatic necrosis of dietary origin in experimental animals, and occasionally spontaneously in others, clearly relates the lesion to vascular distributions in the organ, and the microscopic finding of zonal patterns of necrosis in many acini, not entirely destroyed, relates the necrosis to smaller units in the vascular fields. Massive hepatic necrosis can thus be defined as a process that destroys acinar agglomerates, usually very many contiguous ones, and produces lesser zonal injury to the periphery of surrounding acini. Collapse, condensation, and heavy scarring are characteristic (Fig. 2.29), the end result being known as postnecrotic scarring. The liver is not uniformly involved. Large areas of parenchyma remain intact and, adjacent to the necrotic areas, isolated acini and acinar agglomerates survive. From these, regeneration takes place concentrically to form giant hypertrophic nodules on axial portal vessels. Successive bouts of massive necrosis may occur, each with collapse and scarring as an inevitable sequel.

Massive hepatic necrosis may develop in three ways. It may in some parts of the organ represent the extreme degree of a periacinar (usually toxic) necrosis that in the remainder of the liver remains uniformly zonal. Acute vascular accidents may produce massive necrosis in which not only the parenchyma dies, but the supporting tissue as well, or it may be of dietetic origin.

A liver that is the seat of massive necrosis is of about normal size or small. Fine red threads of fibrin may be present on the surface, especially in the grooves between

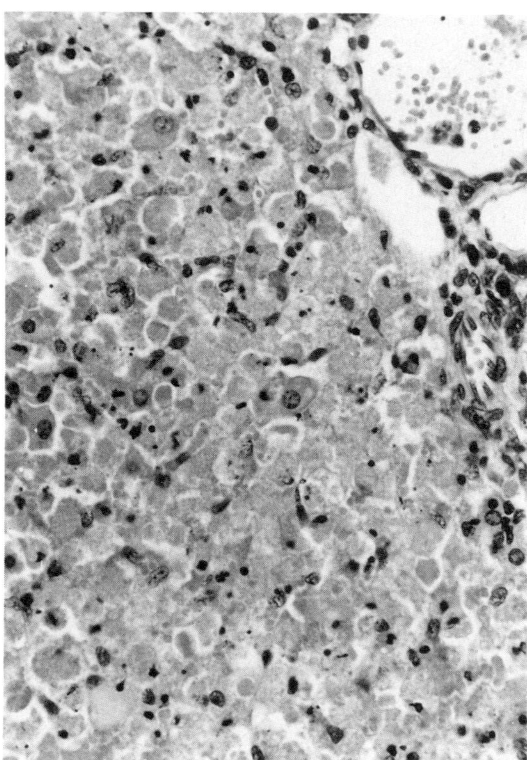

Fig. 2.28 Massive necrosis with destruction of the periportal limiting plate. Algal poisoning. Sheep. (Courtesy of A. R. B. Jackson.)

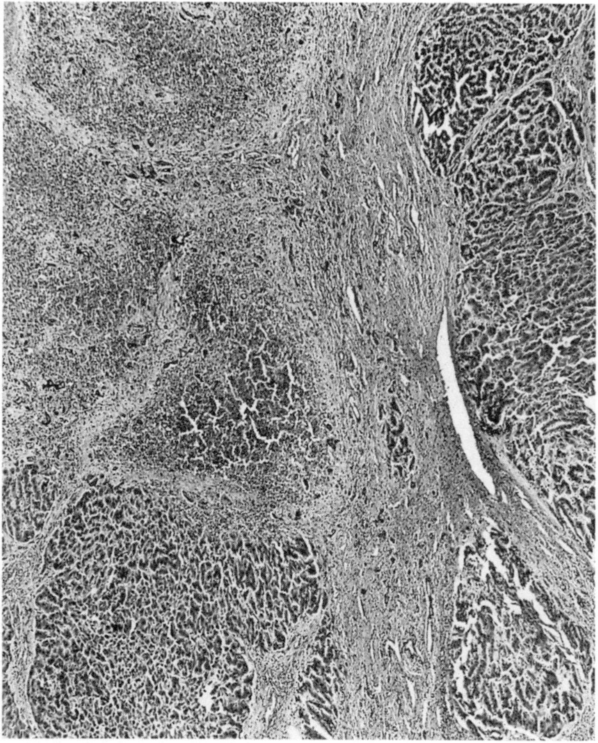

Fig. 2.29 Postnecrotic scarring and nodular regeneration. Ox.

the lobes. The organ presents a mosaic appearance of red, gray, or yellow areas intermingled with areas of dark redness. The mosaic pattern is occasionally broad, the intermingled colorful areas being some centimeters across, or the red hemorrhagic areas may be few and scattered. Usually, however, the mosaic pattern is finer (Fig. 2.30), the yellow areas of parenchyma forming irregular, coalescing patches that may not be more than 1 cm in diameter. The gray or yellow areas represent surviving tissue; the intermingled red areas represent areas of necrosis, hemorrhage, and collapse, and these are depressed a few millimeters below the surface. The mosaic pattern is present also on the cut surface and is especially striking in pigs, in which the lobules in necrotic areas appear as partially emptied blood cysts.

In the healing stage, the depressed areas of hemorrhage and necrosis are condensed, shrunken, and scarified, so that the surface of the liver is traversed by fine or heavy scars, which separate large nodules of regenerative hyperplasia (Fig. 2.31A,B). Further acute episodes may be superimposed, so that the presented lesion may be a mixture of acute massive necrosis and postnecrotic scarring. Continuing acute necrosis in areas of scarring is also commonly present, either because of continuance of the initial insult or as a consequence of the scarring itself.

When cells die of massive hepatic necrosis, the death is sudden and complete (coagulative); there is no evidence that they have passed through an initial stage of vacuolar degeneration. Examination of the lesion in the early stage reveals hemorrhage and pooling of blood close about the axial portal vessels, a picture superficially resembling periportal necrosis. Later, there is hemorrhage to replace all the dead parenchyma, but the early lesion, with its sudden necrosis and damming back of blood in the portal vessels,

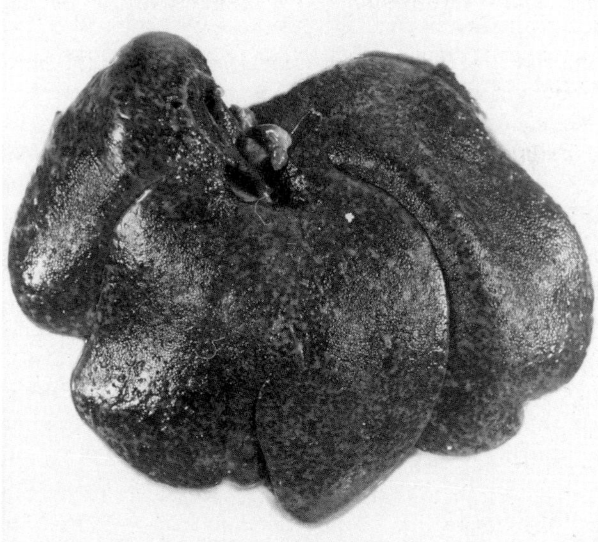

Fig. 2.30 Massive necrosis with darkening and early postnecrotic collapse. Hepatosis dietetica. Pig. (Courtesy of C. A. Grant.)

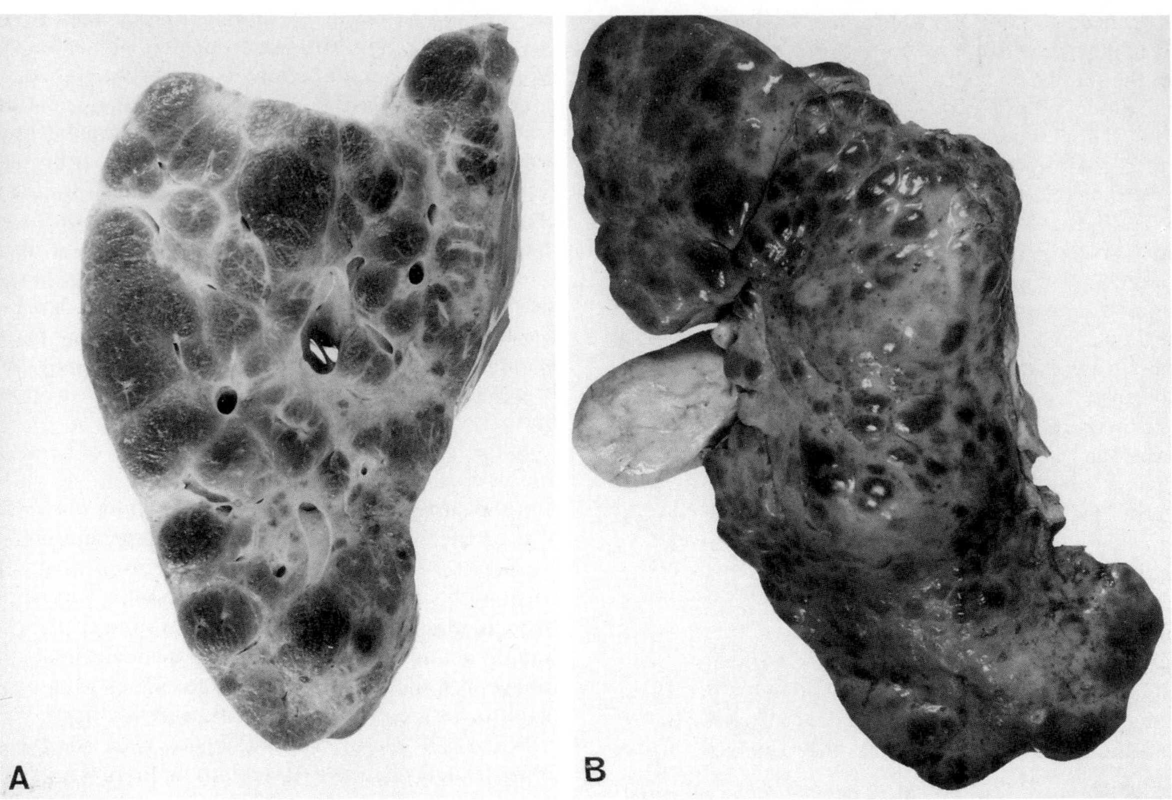

Fig. 2.31 (A) Cut surface to show postnecrotic scarring. Ox. (B) Capsular surface to show postnecrotic scarring. Ox.

is consistent with the idea that massive necrosis develops as a sudden destruction of all the cells (including sinusoidal lining cells) in acinar agglomerates, with complete cessation of intrasinusoidal blood flow in the affected areas. Sinusoidal microthrombosis is a likely cause of the latter.

Massive necrosis may appear with apparent randomness in the organ, but in less severe cases there is a tendency for it to preferentially involve the left lobe(s) of the liver; when the lesion is severe, portions of all lobes are involved. The relative restriction of some cases of massive necrosis to the left lobes is explained on the basis of streamlined portal flow. In rats, the usual experimental animal for producing dietary hepatic necrosis, the left lobes receive blood from the spleen and colon and are expected to be deficient in nutriment relative to the right lobe, which receives its blood from the small intestine. The occurrence of streamlining in domestic animals other than the dog is not established, but massive necrosis, or the scarring that results from it, is occasionally observed in sheep, cattle, and swine and is limited to, or most severe in, the left lobes.

Massive necrosis may also be seen in some areas of livers that are elsewhere more or less uniformly affected by zonal necrosis (usually periacinar). In these livers it is the portions compressed by adjacent viscera which are most prone to massive necrosis, and it is likely that relatively poor perfusion in these areas enhances the severity of the damage.

Hepatosis dietetica of swine is a polymorphous syndrome compounded of massive hepatic necrosis with its immediate or late effects, yellow-fat disease, degeneration of skeletal and cardiac muscle, serous effusions, ulceration of the squamous mucosa of the stomach, and fibrinoid necrosis of arterioles. All these lesions seldom occur in one animal; in practice, they occur alone or in any combination. They are known to be of nutritional origin, and the fact that the various lesions can occur separately indicates the complexity of the pathogenesis, which is discussed with diseases of muscle (in Muscles and Tendons, Volume 1, Chapter 2). Experimental observations have revealed the need for concurrent deficiencies of sulfur-containing amino acids, tocopherols, and trace amounts of selenium if hepatic necrosis is to develop. Selenium protects efficiently against the hepatic necrosis and massive effusions, and tocopherols are probably protective against all lesions of the syndrome. The pathogenesis is incompletely understood, but is in part related to the generation of free radicals, whose noxious effects are normally limited by a system of free-radical scavengers of which both vitamin E and selenium are important components. Vitamin E may exert its protection by combining directly with peroxides, whereas selenium is an integral part of reduced glutathione, which breaks down peroxides as they are formed. There is as yet no acceptable explanation for the sudden, catastrophic massive necrosis in livers conditioned by these deficiencies, but, once triggered, free-radical generation can be self-propagating, taking the form of a chain reaction which can rapidly degrade the lipoprotein membranes, which form so much of the hepatocyte complement of cytoplasmic organelles.

Hepatosis dietetica occurs in rapidly growing pigs fed diets largely of grain and containing protein supplements lacking in either quality or quantity. There is some evidence that in pigs that are nutritionally predisposed, a cold, damp environment or some other stress may precipitate the disease. Death usually occurs without signs of illness or after a short period of dullness. Melena, dyspnea, weakness, and trembling may be observed in some cases. Jaundice is indicative of a relapsing course.

Affected pigs are usually in good condition. The carcass is anemic if ulceration of the gastric mucosa has occurred, and in these cases, free and digested blood may be found in the stomach and intestine. Jaundice is not common, but yellow staining of adipose tissues (yellow-fat disease) is. In relapsing cases, hemorrhagic diathesis may occur, manifested mainly by hemorrhage into and about joints. Fluid containing much protein collects in the serous cavities in small volume. Fine strands of fibrin are present in the peritoneum.

Pulmonary edema accompanies myocardial lesions that consist of intramural and subendocardial hemorrhages with focal areas of hyaline degeneration. The changes in the liver dominate the autopsy findings. The massive hepatic necrosis is of the typical appearance described earlier (Fig. 2.32A,B), and in a number of cases, both acute and chronic lesions are found. The sites of severest injury are the dorsal parts on the diaphragmatic surface. The right lobe may escape and later undergo marked hypertrophy. The gallbladder is often edematous.

The histologic changes that occur in this syndrome are described elsewhere with the particular organs involved. Fibrinoid degeneration of small arteries occurs in some cases. The arterial degeneration may occur in any organ or in most organs but is relatively common only in the small vessels of the mesentery, gut, and heart (see mulberry-heart disease, in The Cardiovascular System, Volume 3, Chapter 1).

K. Necrosis of Sinusoidal Lining Cells

When hepatocytes are being destroyed by the elaboration of toxic molecules within their cytoplasm, it is to be expected that the sinusoidal lining cells may also suffer should the products of these biotransformations spill into the space of Disse. Lytic necrosis of these cells is in fact seen very early in the course of hepatotoxicities such as acute algal and ngaione poisoning, but the pathogenesis previously proposed remains unproven (Fig. 2.33A,B). The sinusoidal phagocytes are sometimes vulnerable by virtue of their role in clearing the portal blood of particulate or colloidal material; should these particles be toxic or infectious, Kupffer cell necrosis may occur alone, but more usually there is damage to surrounding hepatocytes as well.

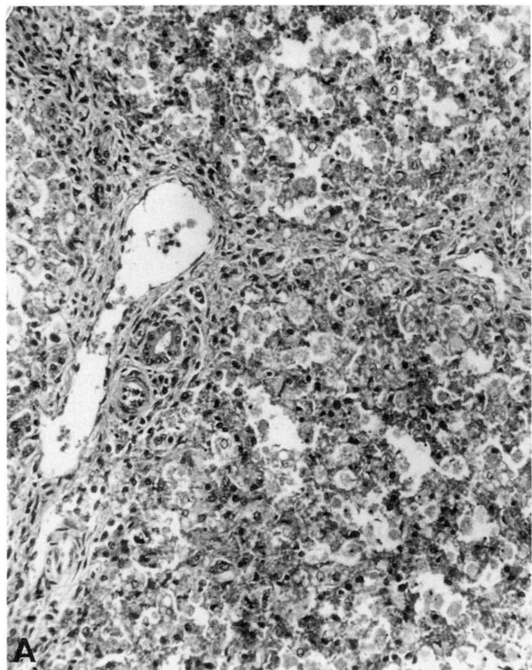

Fig. 2.32A Massive necrosis with hemorrhage and dissolution of parenchyma. Hepatosis dietetica. Pig.

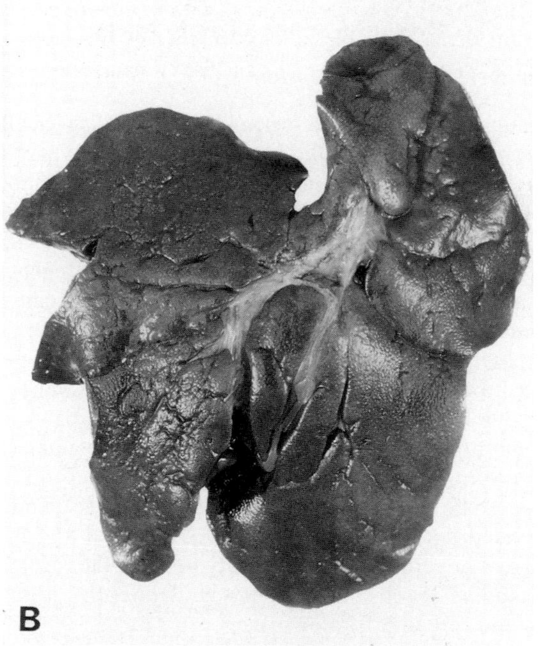

Fig. 2.32B Postnecrotic collapse of liver tissue in hepatosis dietetica. Pig.

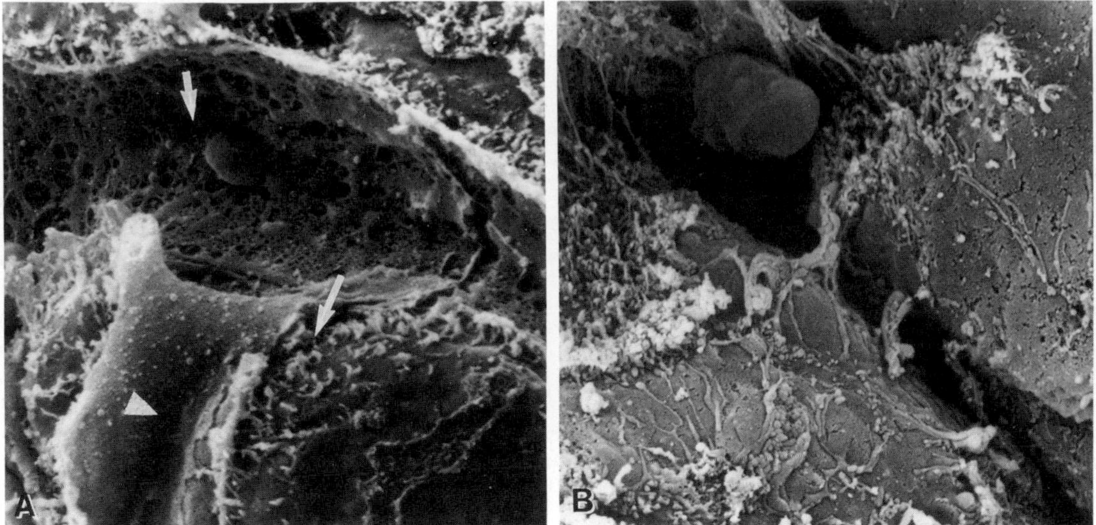

Fig. 2.33 (A) Scanning electron micrograph of mouse liver, perfused 15 min after intraperitoneal injection of toxin from *Microcystis aeruginosa*. Essentially normal structure of fenestrated endothelium (short arrow), sinusoidal lining cell (arrowhead) and space of Disse (long arrow). (B) As for (A); 30 min after injection. The endothelium has largely disintegrated; the underlying hepatocytes are still intact. (A and B courtesy of I. R. Falconer and *Aust J Biol Sci.*)

L. Necrosis of Bile Duct Epithelium

It is unusual for the bile duct epithelium to be singled out by specific necrogenic insults, but this is seen in intoxication by sporidesmin (see Chronic Heptotoxicity, Section XI,D of this chapter) and paraquat. Usually there is accompanying portal inflammation.

VI. Responses of the Liver to Injury

A. Hepatocellular Regeneration

As much as 70% of the liver can be removed surgically without particular upset, and in the course of a few weeks it is back to normal size, although not its original shape. The regeneration may be even more rapid following a toxic injury that destroys that much parenchyma, because in this circumstance a framework remains on which regeneration can take place, so the original conformation can be restored as well as the mass. The factors that regulate the proliferative response are still poorly understood, despite identification of circulating chalones involved in some sort of negative feed-back mechanism.

Regeneration must be regarded as a natural response of the liver to injury, but there are certain limitations on the process. To be complete, the affected areas of tissue must be provided with an adequate supply of blood and free drainage of bile; to be architecturally normal, the regenerating columns of cells must have as guidelines the original fibrous and reticulin framework.

In tissues which contain renewing cell populations, such as epidermis, gut, or bone marrow, stem cells are part of a proliferative compartment which is responsible for cell replacement. In an organ such as the liver in which differentiated cells have long life spans, the need for a stem cell compartment is not readily apparent; ordinarily, the differentiated cells remaining after injury divide and restore liver mass.

Nonetheless there are in the liver nonparenchymal epithelial cells, also called oval cells on account of the nuclear shape, which can be induced to proliferate and which may be a source of new hepatocytes or cholangiolar epithelium or even of epithelial tissues of ectopic type. The source and nature of the regenerative response will be influenced by the anatomic pattern and duration of the injury and, particularly in chemical intoxications, by the character of molecular interactions.

Focal loss of hepatocytes, as in focal necrosis, is repaired by proliferation of adjacent differentiated cells. Accelerated single-cell necrosis, such as occurs in chronic copper poisoning in sheep, is compensated by division of hepatocytes of seemingly random distribution. In the common periacinar necrosis, surviving hepatocytes, especially those in the periportal zone, can, after a delay of 24 hr or so, rapidly replace the lost cells. In periportal and midzonal necrosis, regeneration is provided by surviving cells in the acinus. Following massive necrosis or partial hepatectomy, cells everywhere in the liver contribute to the replacement of mass.

It may be appropriate to consider responses to physiologic demands as being under the same influences as reductions in hepatic mass. In the event of increased physiologic demand, the hepatic mass increases, either by hypertrophy of existing hepatocytes or by proliferative expansion of hepatocyte number when metabolic load cannot be accommodated by adaptive differentiation. Such adaptive changes usually occur in zonal patterns which reflect the normal functional heterogeneity of hepatocytes. When the inducing stimulus is removed, the surplus capacity is removed either by apoptosis or by atrophic reversion of cells to normal phenotype. It is not clear, however, whether the induced hypertrophic response differs biologically from regenerative proliferation or whether repair in the different circumstances is mediated by the same chemical signals.

Regeneration in livers subject to sustained or repetitive hepatocellular injury, such as occurs especially during exposure to intoxicants, has features which differ from the acute responses previously considered. Regeneration typically results in nodularity. The nodularity may be impressed on the liver by constricting bands of fibrous tissue. With some intoxicants, however, such as pyrrolizidine alkaloids, phomopsin, aflatoxin, and a variety of experimental carcinogens with alkylating properties, fibrosis is not limiting, and the nodules represent clones of cells which have avoided the toxic injury. The possible origins of such cells, which in these circumstances act as stem cells, include resistant hepatocytes and the oval cells of cholangioles. The proliferating hepatocytes may differ from normal hepatocytes in some of their enzymatic reactions, but there is evidence that they do redifferentiate, and that they can replace residual injured hepatocytes and restore the liver to normal if the initial intoxication is not continued.

B. Bile Duct Hyperplasia

It is improbable that the bile ducts are nothing more than ductular structures acting as conduits for the discharge of bile to the intestine, but very little is known of other functions, especially of the epithelial cells in the hierarchy of ductular structures. This hierarchy leads from extrahepatic ducts to large and small ducts in portal triads and to cholangioles, the canals of Hering, connecting them to the biliary canaliculi. Biliary hyperplasia is a characteristic reaction of the liver to particular types of insult, but much has still to be learned regarding the proliferative potentialities of these structures and the metabolic stimuli which provoke them.

Bile duct proliferation can occur quite independent of changes in the parenchyma, particularly when an irritant stimulus is centered on the triads, and it can also be independent of other changes in the triads, as least to the extent that there may be no more fibrosis then necessary to support the new ducts. Such pure bile duct proliferation may be a typical response to toxins such as alpha-naphthylisothiocyanate in experimental models or to physical biliary obstruction before infection complicates the picture. When the insults are removed, the excess of bile ducts may disappear completely. The most extravagant expressions of hyperplasia in the large ducts occur in hepatic coccidiosis and some forms of hepatic distomiasis; in the latter, the distinction between hyperplasia and neoplasia is blurred.

Proliferative activity in the larger intrahepatic ducts is not necessarily related to hepatic parenchymal injury except by coincidence. Proliferative activity of cholangioles is related to parenchymal injury and constitutes what is usually referred to as bile duct hyperplasia. The originating cells are not certainly identified but, in current knowledge, that role is ascribed to the oval, or perhaps other intercalated, cells in the cholangioles. Studies on isolated cells suggest that the intercalated cells are pluripotent and may differentiate into hepatocytes or cholangiolar epithelium; studies in experimental carcinogenesis or spontaneous hepatic disease in animals suggest that biliary, or more specifically cholangiolar, hyperplasia may be an attempt to regenerate parenchyma when the parenchymal cells themselves have lost this capacity. Illustrative examples from natural disease are provided by the toxicoses of phomopsin, pyrrolizidine alkaloids and aflatoxin, and by equine serum hepatitis and ovine white liver disease (Figs. 2.6, 2.7, 2.13).

C. Hepatic Fibrosis

Whereas regeneration is one characteristic reaction of the liver to chronic injury, fibrosis is another, and the combination of these is responsible for the coarse or fine

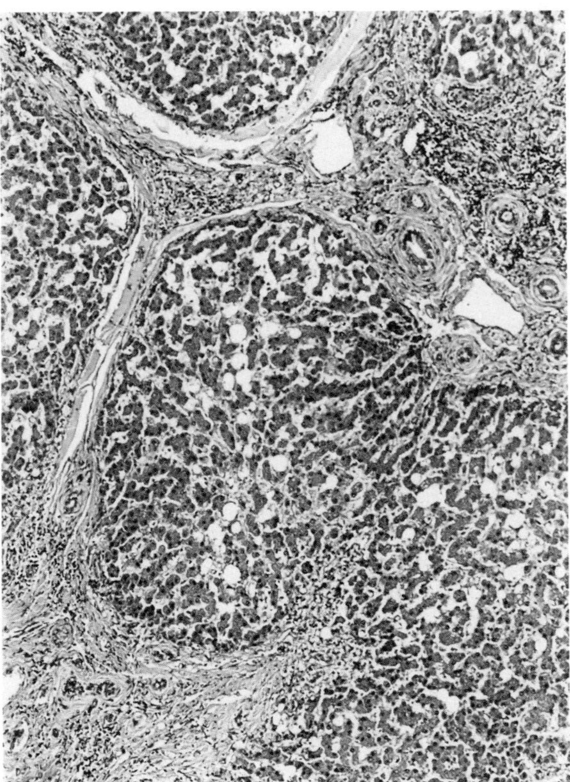

Fig. 2.34 Biliary fibrosis secondary to chronic cholangitis. Dog.

nodularities of chronic acquired hepatic disease. Any hepatic insult severe enough to cause hepatocellular necrosis with subsequent regeneration will result in some local fibrogenesis. In the earliest stages collagen is laid down in the space of Disse, and, at the same time, the sinusoidal endothelium tends to lose its fenestrae. Hence the relationship of hepatocyte to sinusoid comes to resemble that of other tissue cells to their capillaries. After recovery from mild insults, this immature collagen can be removed by enzymatic degradation. The balance is tipped in favor of progressive fibrosis when the insult continues to act, or when the initial damage is so severe that the scar that results is extensive enough to damage the parenchyma by progressive sclerosis.

The fibrosis may develop in a number of ways. It is, as elsewhere, a response to inflammation of the connective tissues of the liver, which include the portal and perivenular stroma and the liver capsule. In the event of inflammation in the portal triads, the fibrosis remains largely confined to these areas and is nominated as **biliary fibrosis** (Fig. 2.34). Fibrosis is also a response to primary parenchymal injury, and its manner of development and degree, and therefore its pattern, depends on the pattern and duration of the antecedent injury. In massive necrosis all parenchymal cells of a number of adjacent acini are destroyed, and the reticulin network collapses and condenses, so that surviving portal areas are approximated to produce broad, irregular bands of scar tissue. This form of fibrosis is called **postnecrotic scarring** and is due to condensation of preexisting stroma, plus a variable amount of fibroplasia and scarification (Figs. 2.29, 2.31A,B, 2.32B). The third general type of fibrosis is known as **diffuse hepatic fibrosis.** This is the outcome of a chronic parenchymal process, such as prolonged infiltration, or of repeated parenchymal injury, such as many episodes of zonal necrosis. The fibrosis is generated slowly to link portal areas and hepatic venules, intersecting the classical lobules to produce pseudolobulation. This pattern of fibrosis is particularly likely to provide conduits which allow portal and arterial blood to bypass the parenchyma. The resulting malnutrition, hypoxia, and deprivation of hepatotrophic factors are important in the genesis of the hepatocellular atrophy, which is almost always a concomitant of hepatic fibrosis.

Finally, fibrosis may develop around hepatic venules when the primary injury is in that region, and may be designated **periacinar fibrosis.** Good examples are seen in animals with prolonged passive venous congestion of the liver (Fig. 2.35A,B), especially when this is due to extracardiac sources of increased venous pressure, rather than to congestive heart failure. Otherwise, this pattern of fibrosis is a response to toxic injury; poisoning by pyrrolizidine alkaloids may cause it in ruminants, and extraordinary development of periacinar fibrosis may follow accidental exposure to nitrosamines in several species.

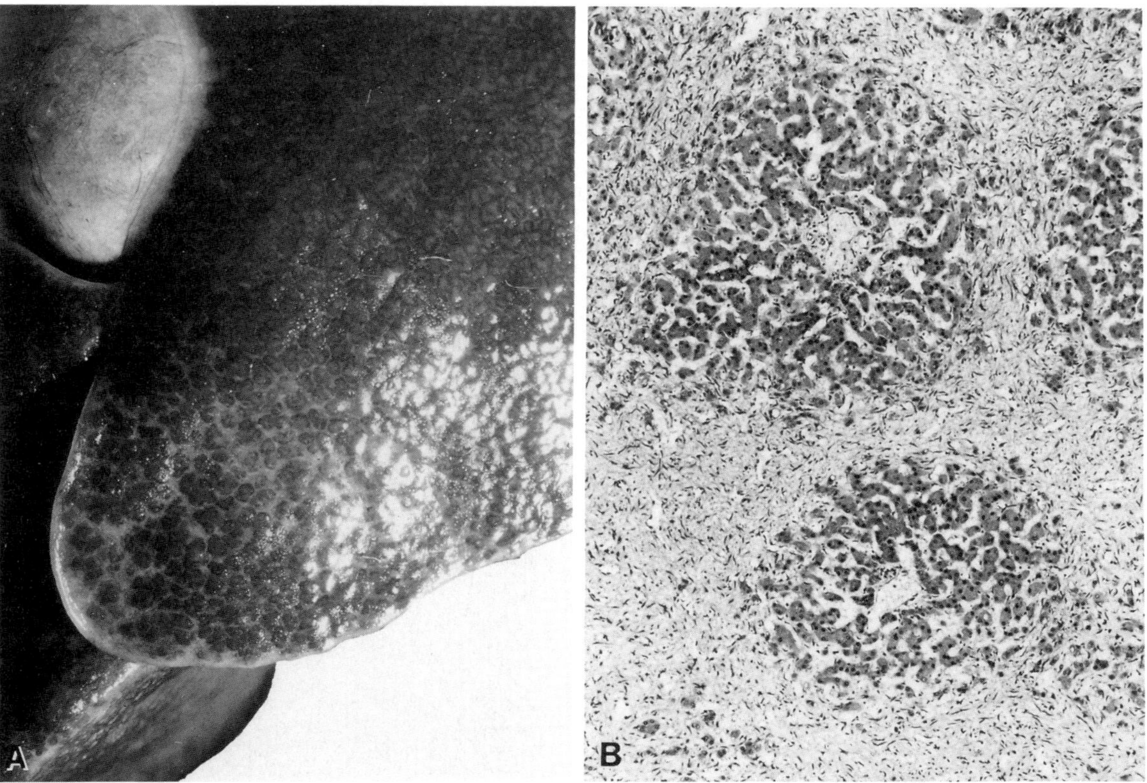

Fig. 2.35 (A) Periacinar fibrosis (cardiac fibrosis), most severe at the periphery of the lobe in chronic passive congestion. Chronic heartworm disease. Dog. (B) Section of (A).

D. Cirrhosis

Cirrhosis may be defined as a chronic disease of the liver characterized by fibrosis and regeneration, which results in disorganization of the hepatic architecture. The term is often used to describe livers that are tough due to postnecrotic collapse rather than to *de novo* collagen synthesis. Livers distorted by fibrosis rather than by true nodular regeneration are also said to be cirrhotic. The term cirrhosis, then, has a certain convenience of usage that is often offset by imprecise application, and we prefer to use the various designations of fibrosis, combined with the addition of nodular regeneration where appropriate.

E. Acquired Portosystemic Shunting

Any chronic liver disease which causes sufficient fibrosis or atrophy to significantly restrict the portal blood flow has the potential to cause the development of collateral portosystemic shunts. These are described under Vascular Factors in Liver Injury (Section IX of this chapter).

F. Idiopathic Chronic Liver Disease of Dogs

Because its cause is not known, it is convenient to describe here a liver disease of dogs that is characterized by obvious nodular regeneration combined with equally obvious atrophy and eventual liver failure. The cause is unknown, but it is tempting to ascribe it, at least in part, to repeated exposure to a hepatotoxin such as aflatoxin.

The gross impression of the liver is one of nodularity affecting most of the organ, most of the nodules being small, but some measuring 2–3 cm. In extreme cases (Fig. 2.36), some of the nodules are pedunculated and attached only by stalks of capsular tissue, and they are easily dislodged. The capsule over the nodules is of ordinary thickness, but between them it appears thickened and opaque. The margins of the lobes, where these are not incorporated in a nodule, are thin and leaflike and quite tough; this is in consequence of atrophy and may result in complete dissociation of the lobes at the hilus, each lobe then appearing to hang on its own stalk of vessels. Neither through consistency, resistance to cutting, nor by gross inspection is there any suggestion of fibrosis within the larger nodules: the toughness of the tissue between the nodules is probably due to condensation of preexisting stroma. The nodules may be of normal color and of liverlike consistency, or they may be yellowish, greasy, and soft or even pultaceous. The whole may be bile stained.

The microscopic picture is dominated by nodular regenerative hyperplasia, which causes compression and atrophy of remnants of severely fatty hepatic parenchyma (Fig. 2.37). The nodules may be microscopic in size and are then seen to be derived from portal units and of irregular distribution. They may be fatty from the outset or acquire fat later; compound nodules may be a mixture of units without fat and units moderately or severely fatty. There is a light fibrosis largely confined to portal areas. In

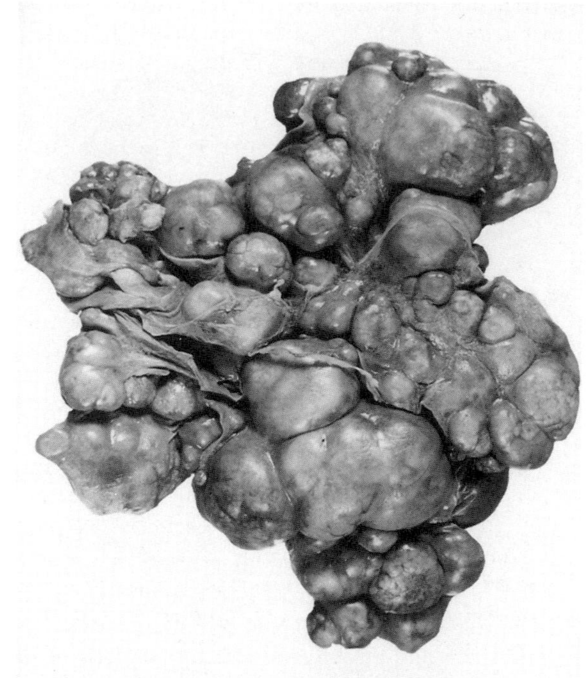

Fig. 2.36 The end result of diffuse fatty liver and nodular regeneration. Dog.

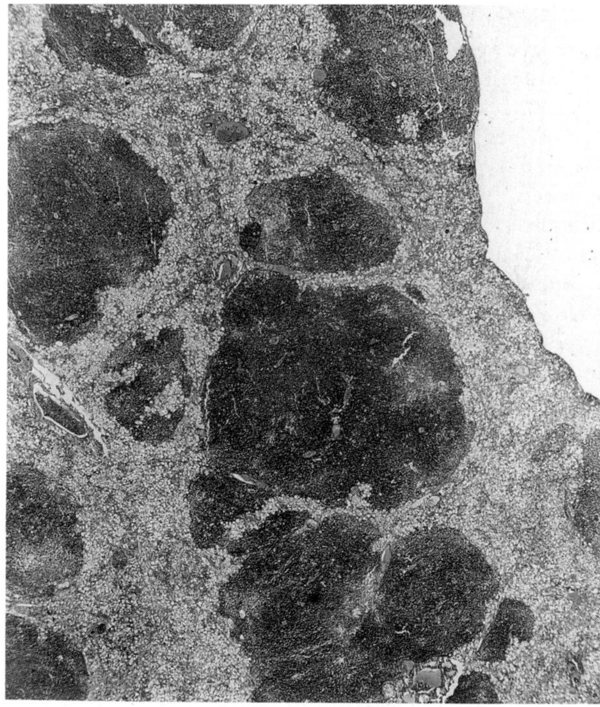

Fig. 2.37 Section of Fig. 2.38 to show diffuse fatty change and large nonfatty nodules.

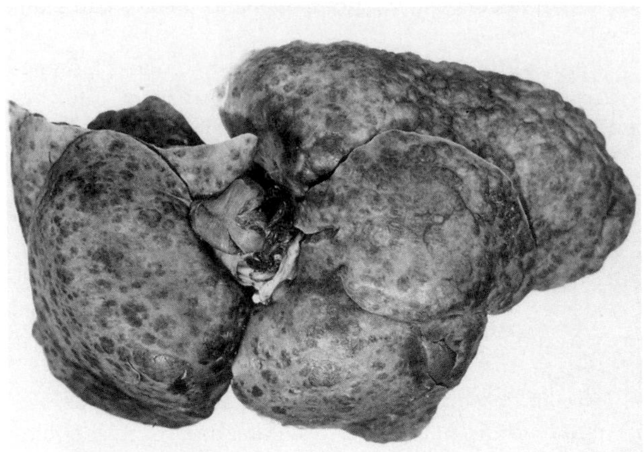

Fig. 2.38 Diffuse fatty liver with nodular regeneration. Dog.

the regenerative nodules, the fibrosis is irregular, but has a tendency to originate from the axial parent portal unit and to link up the veins. There is a fine fibrosis in the residual nonregenerative areas, but its pattern is obscured by compression and atrophy. Where the margins of the lobes are atrophic so that the capsule condenses into a leaflet, there is only mature condensed collagen, with perhaps a few atrophic remnants of bile ducts and blood vessels. It is worth emphasizing that *de novo* fibrogenesis is minimal in these organs and that they therefore do not qualify for the designation cirrhosis which is usually applied to them.

Livers of the type described are seen in animals dying after the age of at least 2 years, and because these are end-stage livers, it is difficult to be sure of the stages of their development. Earlier stages of the disease may be discovered incidentally in animals that have shown no clinical sign of liver disease (Fig. 2.38). In these cases the distribution of fatty change is very irregular, and the demarcation between original and regenerating parenchyma is quite difficult to discern; it may be more obvious on gross inspection than in sections.

Nodular hyperplasia of the liver, in which one or more nodules one to several centimeters in diameter project hemispherically from the surface, is common in old dogs, and is described under Hyperplastic Lesions (Section XII of this chapter). These nodules, which are often fatty, arise not in an organ that is otherwise normal, but in livers or portions of liver that are themselves the seat of fatty change, mild chronic congestion, and other features of slow architectural remodeling. The initiating cause may be in local perturbations of blood volume.

Bibliography

Bhathal, P. S., and Christie, G. S. A fluorescence microscopic study of bile duct proliferation induced in guinea pigs by 7-napthyl isothiocyanate. *Lab Invest* **20:** 480–487, 1969.

Crawford, M. A. *et al.* Chronic active hepatitis in 26 Doberman pinschers. *J Am Vet Med Assoc* **187:** 1343–1349, 1985.

Doige, C. E., and Lester, S. Chronic active hepatitis in dogs—a review of fourteen cases. *J Am Anim Hosp Assoc* **17:** 725–730, 1981.

Hoover, J. P. *et al.* Liver cirrhosis with calcification in a dog. *Comp Anim Pract* **19:** 24–26, 1989.

Johnson, G. F. *et al.* Chronic active hepatitis in Doberman pinschers. *J Am Vet Med Assoc* **180:** 1438–1442, 1982.

Mondelli, M. U., Manns, M., and Ferrari, C. Does the immune response play a role in the pathogenesis of chronic liver disease? *Arch Pathol Lab Med* **112:** 489–497, 1988.

Scheuer, P. J. Chronic hepatitis: A problem for the pathologist. *Histopathology* **1:** 5–19, 1977.

Scheuer, P. J., and Maggi, G. Hepatic fibrosis and collapse: Histological distinction by orcein staining. *Histopathology* **4:** 487–490, 1980.

Strombech, D. R., and Gribble, D. Chronic active hepatitis in the dog. *J Am Vet Med Assoc* **173:** 380–386, 1978.

Van den Ingh, T. S. G. A. M., and Rothuizen, J. Hepatoportal fibrosis in three young dogs. *Vet Rec* **110:** 575–577, 1982.

Vandersteenhoven, A. M., Burchette, J., and Michalopoulos, G. Characterization of ductular hepatocytes and end-stage cirrhosis. *Arch Pathol Lab Med* **114:** 403–406, 1990.

VII. Liver Failure

Hepatic failure is a syndrome that results from inadequate hepatic function. The mass of liver cells may be reduced below the critical amount, or the cell mass may be adequate, but fibrovascular disorganization has resulted in perfusion deficit and impaired liver cell function.

The physiologic functions of the liver have been outlined earlier. Failure of function may be single and specific, as illustrated by the deficiency of a single enzyme involved in, say, bile transport. In this case the clinical manifestation will be icterus unaccompanied, at least in the early stages, by any other signs of liver failure. More often, however, there is failure of multiple liver functions, and the resulting clinical syndrome is a complex metabolic catastrophe involving other systems.

To understand the clinical manifestations of hepatic insufficiency, a number of features must be borne in mind. First, the liver is possessed of a very large reserve of function, which is potentially increased by the powers of regeneration. Signs of insufficiency do not develop until the reserve is exhausted, and by that time the lesions are far advanced and usually irreversible. Equivalent degrees of reserve for all functions should not be expected. Second, the liver is a composite organ, and lesions of its substance involve several tissues, each of which may contribute some component to the clinical syndrome. Third, the signs of acute insufficiency differ from those of chronic insufficiency, although there is considerable overlapping. Fourth, the presenting signs may appear at first sight to be unrelated to hepatic disease and may be unaccompanied by other signs of hepatic failure.

A. Cholestasis and Icterus (Jaundice)

Jaundice, or discoloration of tissues and body fluids by an excess of bile pigments, is traditionally regarded as having two basic causes: overproduction of bilirubin, as in hemolytic disease, or impaired excretion of the pigment. The latter, cholestasis, may be conveniently subdivided into (1) failure of uptake or conjugation of unconjugated bilirubin, and (2) inability to excrete conjugated bilirubin. It is usual for these causes of jaundice to be combined to varying degrees in any animal with jaundice. In hemolytic disease, for example, the large amount of bilirubin presented to the liver for excretion may overload both the hepatocellular bile uptake and bilirubin conjugation mechanisms, as well as the intracellular and canalicular transport process. In addition, the anemia usually associated with severe hemolytic disease will compromise hepatocellular function and further hamper bilirubin excretion. Hepatocellular accumulation of bile salts in obstructive jaundice interferes with bile conjugation and transport by the smooth endoplasmic reticulum. For these reasons, it is difficult to predict the ratio of conjugated to unconjugated bilirubin in hyperbilirubinemia in most cases of jaundice.

The hepatocellular injury that causes failure of bile excretion may be nonspecific, as in severe necrotizing hepatotoxicity, or conversely, the injury may inhibit this function alone, leaving the hepatocyte with most other functions intact. One of the best examples of the latter type of injury in domestic animals is that of *Lantana* poisoning. In humans, this type of cholestasis is most often associated with idiosyncratic reactions to a wide variety of drugs, but this cause is rarely implicated in animals.

The mechanism of the cholestasis in *Lantana* poisoning is discussed later, but the details of most of the cholestatic diseases of animals remain to be worked out. There are two components of the hepatocyte cytoplasm that are likely targets for specific cholestatic insults. One is the smooth endoplasmic reticulum, in which bile conjugation and intracellular bile salt transport takes place; attention will be drawn to the changes that occur in this organelle in a wide variety of toxicities. The other is the contractile filamentous apparatus in the pericanalicular cytoplasm, which is part of the cytoskeleton and which is involved in active propulsion of bile along the canaliculi. Cholestasis has been produced by administration of cytochalasin, a toxin capable of specifically disorganizing these filaments.

Extrahepatic biliary obstruction initially causes increased pressure in bile ducts, with dilation and stasis of content in the smaller radicles in the portal triads. Shortly, however, the parenchymal changes are the same as in intrahepatic cholestasis. Brown bile pigment is present in canaliculi and hepatocyte cytoplasm. The canaliculi are distended and sometimes loculated. The bile plugs are homogeneous. In the hepatocyte cytoplasm, initially in periacinar zones and later in all zones, the pigment is present in large, irregular lysosomes. In long-standing cholestasis such as may occur with extrahepatic biliary obstruction, the hepatocytes become hydropic with a reticulated appearance to the cytoplasm and are coarsely impregnated with pigment. Cellular necrosis, possibly together with cholangiolar rupture, releases small lakes of bile, which become surrounded by macrophages and giant cells.

Rarely, jaundice may be due to congenital incompetence of hepatocellular uptake or transport of bile pigments. In mutant Southdown sheep there is deficiency in the uptake mechanism, and these animals, though showing few liver lesions, eventually develop chronic renal disease, the reason for which is not clear. Unconjugated bilirubin levels in the plasma are consistently elevated, but sufficient excretion takes place to prevent them from becoming icteric. They become photosensitized, indicating that phylloerythrin excretion is less efficient than that of bilirubin.

A similar defect in mutant Corriedales is in conjugated bilirubin excretion. There is also elevation of plasma bilirubin (just over half of which is conjugated), but there is no obvious jaundice. Nevertheless, phylloerythrin excretion in these Corriedales is also sufficiently impaired to produce photosensitization. There is impaired excretion of other conjugated metabolites, and there is pigmentation of the liver by polymerized residues of retained catecholamine metabolites. This pigment, resembling lipofuscin, accumulates in lysosomes in the pericanalicular cytoplasm.

The intensity of jaundice observed at autopsy is greatest in those diseases in which more than one of the classical causes of cholestasis are operating, as in chronic copper poisoning (see Chronic Hepatotoxicity, Section XI,D of this chapter). In this condition there is not only severe hemolysis but also widespread hepatocyte destruction, and some escape of bile into the sinusoids is likely as hepatocytes die and round up, thus rupturing the canaliculi.

Another factor influencing the intensity of jaundice is the duration of cholestasis. Maximal uptake of bile pigment by tissues takes 1–2 days, so cholestasis due to a single cause may be quite intense if the cause has been persistent. Conversely, complete failure of bile pigment excretion will have occurred in severe, acute fatal hepatic necrosis, but such animals at necropsy are only minimally icteric, due to the short duration of the cholestasis.

The recognition of jaundice at necropsy sometimes involves differentiation of bile staining of tissues from the yellow staining caused by accumulation of carotenoid pigments. These latter are limited to fat depots and are to be expected in certain species such as horses; sometimes there is breed influence, as seen in the yellow fat of Channel Island breeds of dairy cattle. The yellow discoloration of fat depots of older cats is less well understood; in animals fed ox liver, carotenoids may again be responsible; in others there may be some contribution by ceroid-type pigments. Distinction of the fatty pigments from bile depends on the absence of the former from pale, nonfatty tissues such as periosteum and dermal collagen.

B. Photosensitization

Photosensitization is an almost invariable accompaniment of nonhemolytic cholestasis of more than a few days' duration in herbivores that are kept in sunlight and that have been eating green feed. Photosensitization is the term applied to inflammation of skin (usually unpigmented) due to the action of ultraviolet light of wavelengths of 290 to 400 nm on fluorescent compounds that have become bound to dermal cells. These compounds may have been deposited unchanged in the skin after ingestion, the normal liver being incapable of excreting the native fluorescent compound. This is known as primary (type 1) photosensitivity and is seen, for example, after ingestion of hypericin in St. John's wort (*Hypericum perforatum*). Photodynamic agents may also be produced by aberrant endogenous metabolism (type 2 photosensitivity), the best example being congenital porphyria of cattle, which is due to accumulation of photodynamic porphyrins as a result of deficiency of uroporphyrinogen cosynthetase. The type of photosensitization we are concerned with here, and which is by far the most common, is hepatogenous (type 3) photosensitization, in which the photodynamic agent, phylloerythrin, is derived from chlorophyll by microbial transformation in the gastrointestinal tract of herbivores. This conversion occurs in normal animals in which the phylloerythrin is excreted in the bile by the same mechanism as are the bile pigments. Any instance of intrahepatic cholestasis or severe nonspecific hepatocellular injury in herbivores is therefore likely to result in photosensitivity if survival time is longer than a few days. It is possible, however, for mild photosensitization to appear in the absence of gross or microscopic evidence of cholestasis. This occurs unpredictably in animals on such apparently wholesome pastures as alfalfa, *Paspalum*, pangola, and *Panicum* grasses (see Chronic Hepatotoxicity, Section XI,D of this chapter).

If no hepatic changes can be discerned in photosensitized animals, the possibility of primary photosensitization must be considered, but hepatogenous photosensitization cannot be excluded unless adequate liver-function tests are performed.

C. Hepatic Encephalopathy

The neurologic manifestations of hepatic failure are variable and nonspecific; they range from dullness, through complete unawareness and compulsive and aimless movement, to mania and generalized convulsions. There is considerable variation in the clinical signs of hepatic encephalopathy between different species. Sheep rarely show more than dullness and central blindness, with perhaps some compulsive chewing movements and tremor. The picture in cattle is similar, but mania and aggression may also be seen, whereas frenzy is more often recorded in horses. The closer clinical observation accorded to cats and dogs may reveal more subtle behavioral changes, and inappetence and vomiting are commonly reported in carnivores with porto-systemic shunts. These signs usually indicate imminent death, the exceptions being portosystemic shunting (see Vascular Factors in Liver Injury, Section IX of this chapter) or deficiency of a urea-cycle enzyme. In these cases the less severe clinical syndrome of hepatic encephalopathy may occur intermittently for many months, and the clinical signs may disappear after appropriate dietary modification.

Ammonia retention is responsible for the major part of the clinical signs and the brain lesions (see diseases of The Nervous System, Volume 1, Chapter 3). The ammonia is largely of dietary origin and derived from digestion of food protein in the intestine or bacterial degradation of protein and urea in the large bowel. Ammonia accumulates in the general circulation and in the cerebrospinal fluid in both shunting and general liver failure, and some of the brain changes typical of hepatic encephalopathy have been reproduced by ammonia infusion. Further evidence of the importance of ammonia as a cause of hepatic encephalopathy is the fact that it occurs in the rare cases of hyperammonemia due to deficiency of a urea-cycle enzyme; in these animals, presumably, there is not much disorder of other liver functions. Nevertheless, the central nervous system derangement in liver failure is the result of a considerably more complex biochemical disorder than simple ammonia retention. The role of gamma-aminobutyric acid (GABA) and its neural receptors is probably significant in the development of the syndrome. An important inhibitory neurotransmitter within the brain, GABA is normally produced and absorbed from the large bowel, and is normally metabolized in the liver. Not only do GABA levels in plasma rise during hepatic failure, but also there is an increase in the concentration of the GABA receptor within the brain. Plasma GABA is normally excluded by the blood–brain barrier, but this restraint is somehow overcome in hepatic encephalopathy. There are many variably toxic amines, captans, and short-chain fatty acids which are normally removed from the portal blood in one passage through the liver after production in the large bowel. These may be responsible for the incompetence of the blood–brain barrier, and they may also act as false neurotransmitters.

It is probable that in the different species, the pathogenesis and manifestations of hepatic encephalopathy differ. The spongiform myelinopathy which occurs in most species appears not to do so in humans and horse, in which species instead the astrocytes show the most striking changes. In cases of complete liver failure, hypoglycemic convulsions may result from failure of glucose synthesis.

D. Hemorrhage and Liver Failure

Spontaneous hemorrhage is not often part of the syndrome of slowly developing liver failure; the implication is that in chronic liver disease, loss of the ability to synthesize clotting factors is of less significance than the other consequences of liver failure. There is, however, some impairment of hemostasis which is due to reduced synthesis of coagulation factors in parallel with the generalized impairment of protein synthesis by the liver. In acute necrotizing liver damage, however, a large proportion of the animal's blood volume is placed in intimate contact with a large area of damaged parenchyma and sinusoidal endothelium. This will trigger the usual thrombotic cascade, which will in turn initiate compensatory fibrinolysis. The end result of this sequence will be rapid consumption of clotting factors, which will be all the more profound because these are for the most part synthesized in the liver. Thus hemorrhagic diathesis will occur terminally in such animals, and be reflected at necropsy by widespread ecchymoses and petechiae, which may distract the observer from liver changes which macroscopically may well be less spectacular.

E. Nephropathy

Acute liver failure may be accompanied by oliguria and biochemical indications of renal failure. The kidneys are large, moist, and stained by bile pigments, which are present histologically in tubular epithelium and luminal casts. The renal component is referred to as **biliary nephrosis.** The mechanisms are not known but may represent a perfusion deficit with shunting of blood from cortex to medulla.

F. Edema

The liver is responsible for the synthesis of most plasma proteins, an activity which takes place on the polyribosomes of the rough endoplasmic reticulum, to be followed by discharge into the plasma in the space of Disse.

Reduced levels of plasma albumin occur in chronic liver disease reflecting impaired protein synthesis. It is an important factor in the pathogenesis of edema and ascites. Hypoalbuminemia is, however, less frequently a result of primary liver disease than it is of reduced synthesis in protein malnutrition, or excessive loss in urine or intestinal secretions.

Bibliography

Adler, M., Chung, K. W., and Schaffner, F. Pericanalicular hepatocytic and bile ductular microfilaments in cholestasis in man. *Am J Pathol* **98:** 603–616, 1980.

Engelking, L. R. Disorders of bilirubin metabolism in small animal species. *Compend Cont Ed (Pract Vet)* **10:** 712–723, 1988.

Hooper, P. T. Spongy degeneration in the central nervous system of domestic animals. III. Occurrence and pathogenesis—hepatocerebral disease caused by hyperammonemia. *Acta Neuropathol (Berl)* **31:** 343–351, 1975.

Manderino, D., and DeVries, J. G. Hepatic encephalopathy in dogs. *Mod Vet Pract* **66:** 975–984, 1985.

McGavin, M. D., Cornelius, C. E., and Gronwall, R. R. Lesions in Southdown sheep with hereditary hyperbilirubinemia. *Vet Pathol* **9:** 142–151, 1972.

Phillips, M. J. *et al.* Intrahepatic cholestasis as a canalicular motility disorder: Evidence using cytochalasin. *Lab Invest* **48:** 205–211, 1983.

Phillips, M. J., Poucell, S., and Oda, M. Biology of disease: Mechanisms of cholestasis. *Lab Invest* **54:** 593–608, 1986.

Popper, H. Pathologic aspects of cirrhosis. A review. *Am J Pathol* **87:** 228–264, 1977.

Roskams, T. *et al.* Neuroendocrine features of reactive bile ductules in cholestatic liver disease. *Am J Pathol* **137:** 1019–1025, 1977.

Rudolph, R., McClure, W. J., and Woodward, M. Contractile fibroblasts in chronic alcoholic cirrhosis. *Gastroenterology* **76:** 704–709, 1979.

Schaffner, F. *et al.* Mechanism of cholestasis VII.—Naphthylisothiocyanate-induced jaundice. *Lab Invest* **28:** 321–331, 1973.

Strombech, D. R., Meyer, D. J., and Freedland, R. A. Hyperammonemia due to a urea cycle enzyme deficiency in two dogs. *J Am Vet Med Assoc* **166:** 1109–1111, 1975.

Taboada, J., and Meyer, D. J. Cholestasis associated with extrahepatic bacterial infection in five dogs. *J Vet Intern Med* **3:** 216–221, 1989.

Thompson, K. G., Lake, D. E., and Cordes, D. O. Hepatic encephalopathy associated with chronic facial eczema. *N Z Vet J* **27:** 221–223, 1979.

Tyler, J. W. Hepatoencephalopathy. Part II. Pathophysiology and treatment. *Compend Cont Ed (Pract Vet)* **12:** 1260–1276, 1990.

VIII. Postmortem and Agonal Changes in the Liver

The liver, rich in nutrient for bacteria and freely exposed to agonal invaders from the intestine, undergoes postmortem decomposition very rapidly. Gas bubbles form in the blood vessels. The vessels and adjacent parenchyma are stained by hemoglobin. The substance of the organ becomes soft and claylike, and the formation of

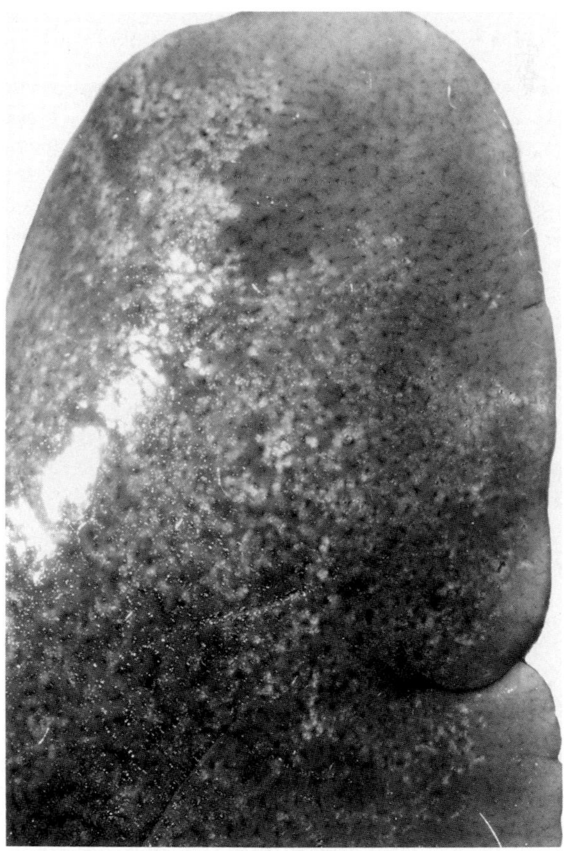

Fig. 2.39 Fine gas bubbles under hepatic capsule. Putrefaction. Dog.

putrefactive gases may make it foamy. On the capsular surface, irregular, pale foci are visible; they resemble infarcts or fatty areas but can be observed to increase in size and, microscopically, are without cellular reaction (Fig. 2.39). Bacilli are present in large numbers in such foci. Greenish-black pigmentation of the capsule and superficial parenchyma occur where the liver is in contact with gut. The lobes surrounding the gallbladder are stained brownish with bile.

There is much microscopic structural change in the liver approaching and immediately following death. In general, the confusing autolytic changes affect mainly the regions around the hepatic venules. Indeed, cytologic criteria of necrosis in periacinar necrosis are more reliably found in animals that have been allowed to die or that are killed in extremis. Shrinkage of liver cells and disappearance of many with widening of periacinar sinusoids is seen after death with hepatic congestion. Dissociation of liver cells may be complete, with every cell in every cord separated and free from adjacent cells so architectural patterns are lost. The least expression of this change affects periacinar cells first, and they become detached, rounded in contour, condensed, and hyperchromatic. The dissociation is seen particularly in feline parvovirus infection and leptospirosis, but it is related somewhat to postmortem change.

IX. Vascular Factors in Liver Injury

The dynamics of the liver cell population in health and disease are interwoven with the dynamics of its blood supply. Hepatic parenchyma manifests the usual degenerative changes of hydropic change, fatty degeneration, and necrosis. But very characteristic of the liver is the extraordinary rapidity with which necrosis develops in response to a wide variety of insults. Part of the explanation lies in the action of the liver in accumulating toxic compounds or degrading them into even more toxic fragments. The frequency with which necrosis develops suggests that there is often, or even inevitably, some additional influence that may transform a mild primary injury to, in cellular terms, a fatal or necrotizing injury. If there is such a complicating influence, it is likely to reside in deranged circulation in the sinusoids.

A. Hepatic Artery

The mammalian liver has a double blood supply, of which the hepatic artery is an important part. It distributes largely to the peribiliary capillary circulation of the portal triads, via which it also anastomoses with the portal vein. Its distribution of blood to the sinusoids is through these other vessels rather than directly. Anomalous origin of the arterial supply is common. It is difficult to ascribe a function to the hepatic artery in terms of parenchymal function, and its role may be no more than that of providing a reserve supply of oxygen. It is doubtful that any mammalian liver can survive complete interruption of its arterial supply, a feat difficult to achieve because of the abundance of potential collaterals. Obstruction developing rapidly enough to prevent other collaterals from developing leads to parenchymal necrosis in dogs, cats, and horses, and probably ruminants as well. The extent of necrosis depends on how completely the obstruction excludes collateral circulation and also on the oxygen tension of the portal blood. Oxygen tension varies between and within species and depends on the state of the general circulation, varying directly with blood pressure. In ischemic areas, bile flow ceases immediately, and a pattern of ischemic necrosis occurs that involves acinar agglomerates. The fate of animals with arterial occlusion and parenchymal ischemia is determined largely by bacteriologic factors; anaerobes, especially clostridia, proliferate rapidly, and their toxins can cause death.

Hepatic arterial occlusions occur rather commonly in animals but usually, as in parasitic infestations, involve small intrahepatic branches and are of little consequence. Large segments may be necrotic in cats as a result of thrombosis of the aorta and hepatic artery. Verminous arteritis may occlude the hepatic artery in horses.

B. Portal Vein

The portal vein, draining the splanchnic viscera, contributes most of the large volume of blood perfusing the liver. Available estimates indicate that, normally, approximately two thirds of hepatic blood flow is portal in origin. A feature of the portal flow is that in some animals, including the dog, it is streamlined, blood from the stomach and duodenum passing preferentially to the left lobes and that from the jejunum and ileum passing to the right lobes. In the dog, under stable conditions, this streamlining is consistent. Frequent shifts in streamlining occur with altered disposition of viscera so that only slight differences are expected in the perfusates in right and left lobes of the liver. These differences may, however, be critical in some types of liver injury, as has been suggested for the patterns of dietary hepatic necrosis. Streamlining may account for the different regional distributions sometimes observed with metastatic tumors and infections (Fig. 2.40). In the same sense, the umbilical vein usually delivers to the left lobe in preference to the right, and metastatic umbilical infections may be strictly localized to one lobe or the other.

The volume of portal blood flow is determined largely by events in the splanchnic circulation. From the hilus on, the portal vein demonstrates an extraordinarily high degree of branching, which tends to ensure an even distribution of portal blood flow while providing for a wide variety of flow patterns. The size of the liver or any segment of it is dependent on the volume of blood perfusing it, and the average blood flow per unit weight of tissue tends to be uniform. This emphasizes the correlation between portal flow and the shape and size of the liver or its lobes, but also that, ordinarily, hilar areas of the liver are no better perfused than the marginal areas. It follows from

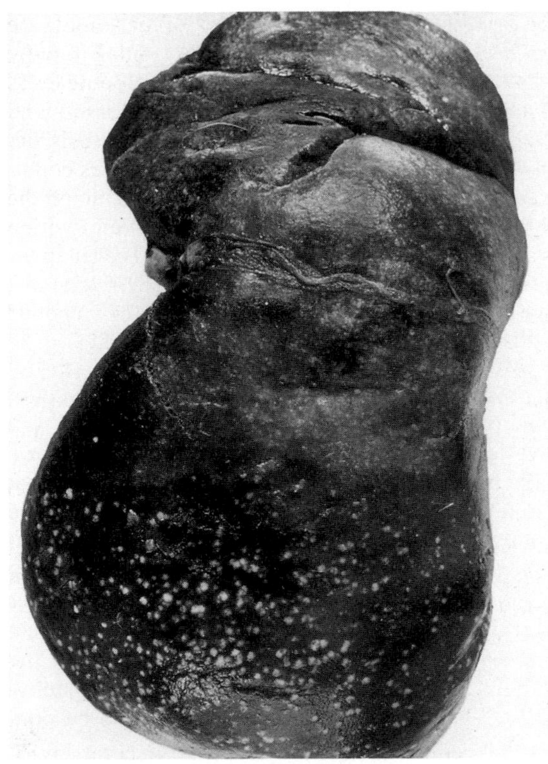

Fig. 2.40 Miliary abscesses in left lobe of liver. Neonatal listeriosis. Lamb.

the previous discussion of hepatotrophic factors that, if the volume of hepatic blood is increased to a portion of the liver, that portion will hypertrophy. Reduction in the volume of hepatic flow leads to atrophy of deprived segments of liver.

Obstruction of the portal vein, if sudden and complete, produces a condition akin to strangulation of the gut, and death occurs quickly without significant hepatic change. Obstruction of a large branch of the portal vein leads in cattle, sheep, and cats to acute ischemia of a wedge of tissue in which necrosis may be zonal or massive. Obstruction to many small portal radicles is common, with necrosis of many acini. It is evident that if a collateral supply develops and oxygenation remains adequate, obstruction of portal radicles will have no immediate effect on the hepatic parenchyma, save perhaps to make it more sensitive to toxic injury. There is, however, a long-term effect, probably nutritional. The parenchyma in the affected lobe, deprived of hepatotrophic factors, loses much of its regenerative power and atrophies fairly rapidly, allowing condensation and scarification of the stromal tissues.

Acute increase in pressure in the portal vein may occur in any severe episode of widespread acute hepatic necrosis; the cause appears to be simple obstruction of the sinusoidal flow by thrombosis and sinusoidal disruption. In such animals there is severe acute congestion of the liver, slight ascites, free fibrin accumulations in the abdomen (not the firm capsular adhesions seen in passive congestion), and distended portal lymphatics.

Obstruction of the extrahepatic portal vein is quite uncommon. Thrombosis is the usual event, and this may be caused by tumors, states of hypercoagulability, retrograde intravascular growth of hepatic neoplasms, and inflammation which may be infective or associated with pancreatitis. Atresia of the portal vein can be demonstrated in some cases of congenital portosystemic shunting, but there may be no increase in portal venous pressure. Portal vein obstructions of slow development are expected to lead to portal hypertension and its consequences.

Obstruction to intrahepatic portal vessels is a consequence of the common fibrosing lesions centered on the portal triads. The small portal vessels may be obliterated in the proliferative portal lesions, and new connections may be established, including small functional arteriovenous communications. Regenerative hepatic nodules may deform and compress the vessels, as may infiltrative carcinomas and the common lymphosarcomas.

C. Efferent Hepatic Vessels

For the purposes of this discussion, efferent hepatic vessels are taken to include the sinusoids, terminal hepatic venules or central veins, various-sized tributaries of the hepatic veins, and the vena cava.

In essence, the sinusoidal bed of the liver is a vast, continuous meshwork of interconnected blood spaces in which, potentially, blood can move in any direction, at least within a lobe. Probably, with normal activity, the path of the red cell through the liver is devious and variable and responsive to the many factors influencing intrahepatic pressure. This should not obscure the fact, however, that there is a basic pattern of flow, fairly direct between portal areas and central vein and associated with a basic pattern of pressure gradients and streamlines. It is the basic pattern of flow that determines metabolic gradients within acini and which, in association with metabolic differences, influences the zonal susceptibility of the liver to injury. The immediate importance of sinusoidal flow rates and directions is probably determined largely by oxygen tension.

Severe respiratory hypoxemia can produce pathologic changes in the liver. Acute anemia may also do so, with periacinar necrosis as the result. Low levels of oxygen saturation, as in chronic passive congestion, are also responsible for periacinar lesions, although necrosis in this condition is not blatant. More debated is the contribution of reduced sinusoidal flow and oxygen saturation on the zonal distribution of many toxigenic liver lesions, especially those producing the common periacinar necrosis. Any reduced blood perfusion would further place at a disadvantage any parenchymal cells already injured by direct toxic action. Reduced sinusoidal flow some hours after carbon tetrachloride injury has been demonstrated. Whether this is due to swelling of injured parenchymal cells is not clear; other mechanisms, including altered properties of sinusoidal endothelium, have not been assessed.

There are various anatomic patterns of fibrosis of the liver, not always clearly separable, but the pattern described in this chapter as diffuse fibrosis has, as one important feature, the transformation of the sinusoid to a more or less conventional capillary. The role of hepatic lipocytes in this transformation is discussed earlier; the significant outcomes include vascular short-circuits, deprivation of hepatocytes, and increased portal venous pressure.

The hepatic venules anastomose to form the hepatic veins and the efferent circulation. The structure of these vessels varies between species, but these are matters largely unexamined. Spiral sphincters of the hepatic vein are well developed in dogs, and sphincter spasm is invoked to explain the intense engorgement of the liver with certain anesthetics and in anaphylaxis in this species. It is likely that the rate and pattern of development of fibrosis in some types of liver injury are determined to some extent by the amount of stroma normally present in these vessels.

In some forms of hepatic injury there may develop in the hepatic venules irregular subintimal deposits of fibrous tissue; these may be regularly circumferential or asymmetric (Fig. 2.41). These deposits have been rather imprecisely termed **veno-occlusive disease,** no matter what their origin, or whether or not occlusion of the vessels is truly demonstrated. Veno-occlusive disease was first described in association with chronic pyrrolizidine alkaloid poisoning (see Toxic Liver Disease, Section XI of this chapter), but now the term is likely to be applied over-generously to chronic liver disease of any cause.

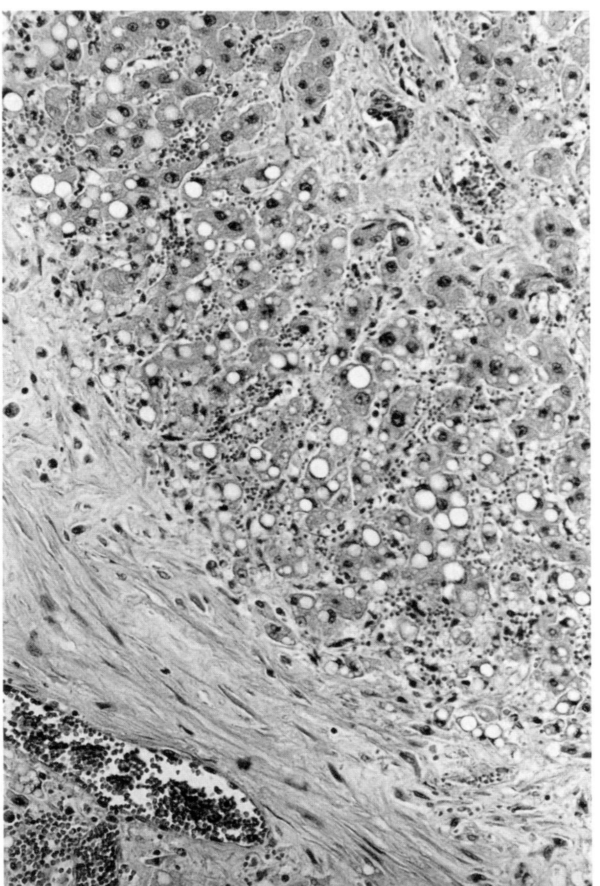

Fig. 2.41 Asymmetric perivenular fibrosis (veno-occlusive disease). Ox. *Senecio* spp. poisoning.

The principal problem of the efferent circulation is chronic obstruction of its outflow. Obstruction is seldom noted at the level of the hepatic veins, although this effect, due to suppurative phlebitis, is occasionally seen in cows, and space-occupying lesions in critical positions, such as around the vena cava in the mediastinum, occur in all species. Most cases by far are due to increased central venous pressure and passive congestion as a result of cardiac incompetence or constrictive pericarditis.

Passive venous congestion denotes an elevation of pressure in the hepatic veins and venules relative to the pressure in the portal venules. This may be due to congestive heart failure, or much less frequently, of partial obstruction of the larger hepatic veins or posterior vena cava by abscess or neoplasm. It is also seen when part of the liver is incarcerated as a result of diaphragmatic hernia, or when a lobe is subjected to chronic partial torsion. When the liver is simply engorged with blood as a result of anaphylaxis, shock, or other acute insult, it is said to be congested.

In the early stages, the liver is swollen, dark, and bloody on section, and there is little accentuation of the acinar pattern. There is usually excessive blood-tinged abdominal fluid, because the congested liver elaborates lymph at a vastly increased rate; this may be seen exuding from the capsule during life and distending hilar and gallbladder lymphatics in fresh carcasses. Because this lymph is rich in most clotting factors, it tends to clot on the liver capsule, and the lobes may be stuck together by wads of fibrin, which are often blood-tinged (Fig. 2.24A).

In passive congestion of longer duration, the capsular surface takes on a finely nodular texture and becomes thick and gray, and the fibrin deposits may become organized into flat, tough, capsular plaques (Fig. 2.42). In dogs and cats, the edges of the central lobes become rounded, whereas the margins of lateral and caudate lobes are sharpened by peripheral atrophy and fibrosis (Fig. 2.35A). If the cause of the congestion is still present, there is usually copious ascites at this stage. Slicing a chronically congested liver reveals a reticulated acinar pattern, which is often more obvious beneath the capsule than in deeper parenchyma. This pattern is known as nutmeg liver and is due to the contrast of the red color of periacinar necrosis and blood replacement with the pallid, slightly raised periportal tissue consisting of surviving but fatty hepatocytes (Fig 2.24B). This pattern may be mimicked by some forms of toxic periacinar necrosis or fatty change but should always be distinguishable from them by the presence of fibrous plaques in Glisson's capsule in the passively congested liver.

The microscopic picture in acute passive congestion is one of fairly uniform sinusoidal engorgement, with accom-

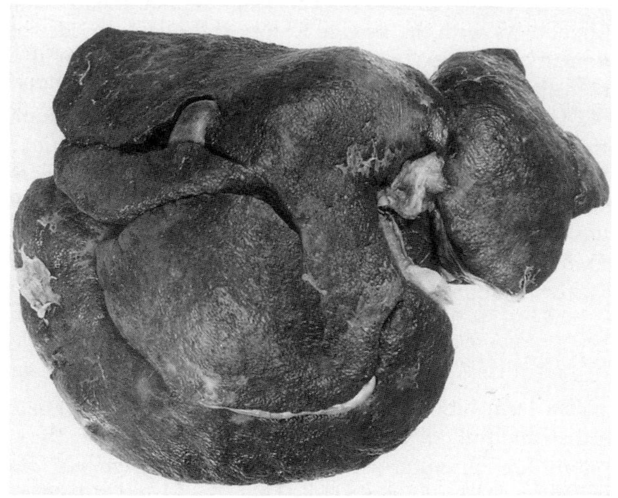

Fig. 2.42 Capsular irregularity and patchy fibrosis in chronic passive congestion. Dog.

panying distension of lymphatics in the stroma of hepatic veins, portal triads, and capsule. There follows rapidly fatty change, atrophy, and necrosis of periacinar hepatocytes; these cells are not replaced while poor sinusoidal circulation persists. The reticulum framework in the periacinar zone, however, remains, and erythrocytes tend to percolate into the spaces left by the hepatocytes, and may be trapped there when blood drains from sinusoids and veins in freshly fixed sections (Fig. 2.17). The intrahepatic network of lymphatics at this stage becomes very distended and may form extensive cavernous channels about hepatic veins and venules, in portal triads, and just beneath the capsule. Distension of the space of Disse may be seen, but rarely if ever in tissue well fixed soon after death, and is best regarded as a postmortem artefact. The parenchyma that lies against the larger portal areas is periportal in a geographic sense only, and not in a functional or circulatory sense. In fact, much of it is relatively peripheral in a circulatory sense, so there should be no surprise in finding that in a suitable plane of section, the zones of hemorrhage and necrosis cut back to involve the parenchyma against the larger portal tracts, thereby isolating small, viable clumps of tissue about the terminal portal venules.

Over longer periods, the stagnant blood and remnants of stroma in the periacinar zones are gradually replaced by fibrous tissue which links hepatic venules with one another and with the larger portal triads; simple and compound acini are outlined by periacinar fibrosis. This pattern of hepatic fibrosis is known as cardiac fibrosis (Fig. 2.35B).

Notwithstanding the statistical dominance of afflictions of the vena cava and those beyond, which result in increased central venous pressure, there are important associations of intrahepatic venules with disease, perhaps especially with portal hypertension. Acute inflammatory change and thrombosis of sublobular veins is typical of, for example, acute salmonellosis in many species, but these are terminal diseases without ongoing consequences for the liver.

It is not yet possible to assemble a catalog of specific injurious influences on the draining veins. Muscular transformations of central and sublobular veins are ascribed to increased, and pulsatile, intravascular pressures deriving from congenital or acquired arteriovenous shunting. Fibrous remodeling of these veins appears to be a distinctive feature of nitrosamine intoxication in domestic animals. Hepatic veno-occlusive disease in which fibrous proliferation transforms the centrilobular veins into closed drainage systems is a feature of pyrrolizidine toxicosis in humans ingesting these alkaloids in so-called bush tea. But it is also seen in consequence of prolonged chemotherapy and other interventions. In domestic animals, occlusive changes in terminal venules are notable only in poisoning by ragwort, *Senecio jacobea,* in cattle (Fig. 2.41).

D. Portosystemic Shunts

Congenital shunts have been described with the congenital anomalies. Acquired shunts may be difficult to identify postmortem. They are easily destroyed by routine dissection, and they are likely to be overshadowed by rather more dramatic liver changes than is the case with congenital shunts. To be classified as acquired, the shunts should be associated with evidence of portal hypertension, such as distension of the portal veins, and ascites. The shunts tend to develop between mesenteric veins and the posterior vena cava, right renal vein, or gonadal veins, and are multiple, taking the form of a plexus of tortuous, thin-walled vessels (Fig. 2.3). Esophageal shunts and varicosities which are of some significance in humans are not so in animals; indeed the varicose dilatations which develop in response to portal hypertension are not of themselves of significance, although indicative of portal hypertension.

Livers subject to secondary shunting are also small but, in addition, show variable nodularity and increase in proportion of fibrous tissue. The cause of the degeneration is rarely apparent; there may be chronic, diffuse, progressive inflammation, or simply nodular regeneration among bands of condensed stroma.

Multiple, tortuous, and apparently acquired portosystemic shunts may be found in a developmental disorder of unknown pathogenesis in dogs known as **hepatoportal fibrosis.** This distinctive form of developmental liver disease has been described in young dogs that develop portal hypertension and extrahepatic shunts relatively early in life. There is a variable amount of portal fibrosis and deficiency of smaller radicles of the portal veins. These animals are presented with hepatic encephalopathy and ascites, and the shunts are multiple and resemble those seen in acquired liver disease. The only clear distinctions of this condition from acquired hepatic shunts are the pattern of portal fibrosis, the absence of small portal venules, distension of the larger intrahepatic branches of the portal vein, and the immaturity of the animals. Grossly, the livers are small, show irregular capsular depressions, or are finely nodular throughout. The dogs are usually young and without a history of exposure to hepatotoxins. The inference is that they suffer from a form of hepatic **abiotrophy** as a developmental disorder, and portal hypertension supervenes when a critical amount of liver tissue has undergone atrophy.

E. Telangiectasis

Telangiectasis is a cavernous ectasia of groups of sinusoids that occurs in all species but is particularly common in **cattle.** The lesion is not functionally significant. Telangiectases occur throughout the liver as dark red areas, irregular in shape but well circumscribed, and ranging from pinpoints to many centimeters in size. Sectioned or capsular surfaces are depressed after death, and on cutting they appear as cavities from which the blood drains to reveal a delicate network of residual stroma and strands of atrophic hepatocytes. In bovine livers that bear early telangiectases, there are usually small foci of mononuclear cells that are intimately associated with a few degenerate hepatocytes in the center of the cluster. The reaction is reminiscent of cell-mediated immune reactions and suggests the possible pathogenic mode, whereby the removal of hepatocytes is sufficiently subtle as to cause no scarring, or to stimulate hepatocyte replacement, but merely leaves a parenchymal defect, which is occupied by expansion of the adjacent sinusoids.

Telangiectasis in livers of **cats** is quite common in older animals. As with the bovine lesion, there is no evidence clinically of related liver dysfunction. In cats, the cavities are rather more frequent in the subcapsular zone (Fig. 2.43A) and rarely exceed 2–3 mm in size. There are often other senile changes in these livers, such as chronic fatty change, nodular hyperplasia, and chronic cholangiohepatitis, but there is no evidence that these changes have any causal relationship to the telangiectasis, the focal lesions of which are to the naked eye indistinguishable from foci of extramedullary hematopoiesis.

F. Peliosis Hepatis

This term has been used for a long time to designate focal, blood-filled spaces in the liver in humans; these lesions are of unknown cause and were originally described in tuberculous patients and, more recently, in association with therapy by various steroids. There is a similarity between the changes of telangiectasis and peliosis, but to consider them identical is probably an error. One form of sinusoidal dilatation in cattle is named peliosis, specifically to differentiate it from bovine telangiectasis. This form, unlike telangiectasis, begins as a diffuse periportal sinusoidal dilatation (Fig. 2.43B) and develops in cattle poisoned by plants of the *Pimelea* genus. Since these changes are also found in these animals in spleen and in other organs with sinusoidal microcirculation, it seems that the lesions may be adaptive to progressive and

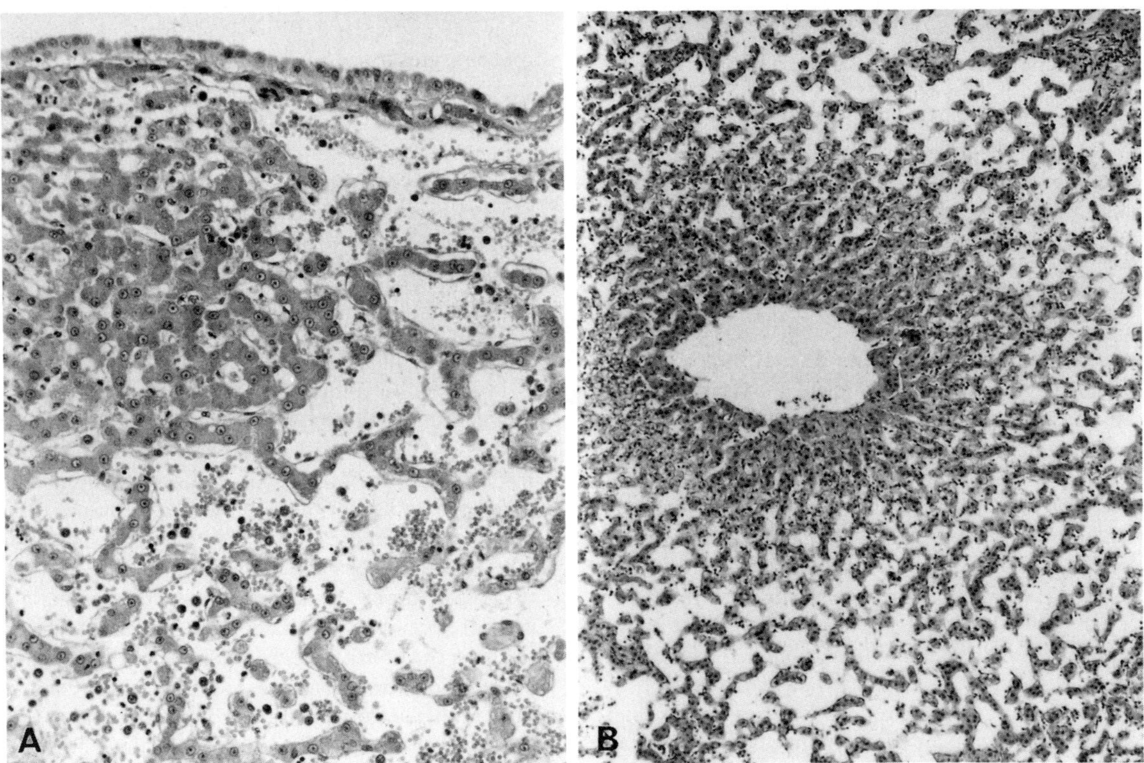

Fig. 2.43 (A) Subcapsular telangiectasis. Cat. (B) Periportal sinusoidal dilatation. Chronic *Pimelea* poisoning. Ox.

dramatic increases in total blood volume. In the late stages of the intoxication by *Pimelea,* the liver may resemble a huge, blood-filled sponge. The animals eventually die of a combination of hemodilutional anemia and circulatory failure.

G. Portal Hypertension

Blood received by the portal vein has already traversed the splanchnic capillary circulation and is of very low pressure. A sustained increase in portal venous pressure such as to induce collateral connections between the portal and other veins is almost always a consequence of intrahepatic lesions in which congenital or acquired anastomoses exist between the hepatic artery and portal vein branches. The common passive congestion of the liver is not associated with portal hypertension of significant degree. The complications of portal hypertension include portosystemic shunts, congestive splenomegaly, and ascites. Ascites is discussed in detail with The Peritoneum and Retroperitoneum (Chapter 4 of this volume); there are sources other than the liver for fluid which accumulates in the abdominal cavity.

Bibliography

Berger, B., and Whiting, P. G. *et al.* Congenital feline portosystemic shunts. *J Am Vet Med Assoc* **188:** 517–521, 1986.

Gosselin, S. J. *et al.* Occlusive disease of the liver in captive cheetah. *Vet Pathol* **25:** 48–57, 1988.

Greenway, C. V., and Oshiro, G. Intrahepatic distribution of portal and hepatic arterial blood flow in anaesthetized cats and dogs and the effect of portal occlusion, raised venous pressure, and histamine. *J Physiol (Lond)* **227:** 473–485, 1972.

Jensen, R. *et al.* Ischemia—a cause of hepatic telangiectasis in cattle. *Am J Vet Res* **43:** 1436–1439, 1982.

Kanel, G. C. *et al.* A distinctive perivenular hepatic lesion associated with heart failure. *Am J Clin Pathol* **73:** 235–239, 1980.

Kelly, W. R., and Seawright, A. A. *Pimelea* poisoning of cattle. *In* "Effects of Poisonous Plants on Livestock," R. F. Keeler, K. R. Van Kampen, and L. F. James (eds.), pp. 293–300. New York, Academic Press, 1978.

Lautt, W. W., and Greenway, C. V. Hepatic venous compliance and the role of liver as a blood reservoir. *Am J Physiol* **231:** 292–295, 1976.

Moore, P. F., and Whiting, P. G. Hepatic lesions associated with intrahepatic arterioportal fistulae in dogs. *Vet Pathol* **23:** 57–62, 1986.

Munson, L., and Worley, M. B. Veno-occlusive disease in snow leopards *(Panthera uncia)* from zoological parks. *Vet Pathol* **28:** 37–45, 1991.

Patnaik, A. K., Lieberman, P. H., and MacEwan, E. G. Splenosis in a dog. *J Small Anim Pract* **26:** 23–31, 1985.

Rand, J. S. *et al.* Portosystemic vascular shunts in a family of American cocker spaniels. *J Am Anim Hosp Assoc* **24:** 265–272, 1988.

Valentine, R. W., and Carpenter, J. L. Spleno–mesenteric–renal venous shunts in two dogs. *Vet Pathol* **27:** 58–60, 1990.

Van Den Ingh, T. S. G. A. M. *et al.* Congenital portosystemic shunts in three pigs and one calf. *Vet Pathol* **27:** 56–58, 1990

X. Inflammation of the Liver and Biliary Tract (Hepatitis)

The term hepatitis is reserved for hepatic lesions, focal or diffuse, that are known, or reasonably assumed to be caused by infectious agents, including parasites, or are lesions that reveal the full inflammatory response, irrespective of the cause. This definition allows us to include viral infections that are hepatotropic even though the lesions are necrotizing and not easily distinguishable, except by the presence of inclusion bodies, from toxic necrosis. The term hepatitis is sometimes used to describe the liver changes seen in some hepatointoxications, particularly when these changes include a leukocytic response to damaged cells.

There are, in inflammations of the liver, some reactions that are specifically hepatic but not specifically inflammatory. Edema of the liver occurs in diffuse hepatitis or diffuse cholangitis, but also in severe toxic injury and passive congestion, and is related to the usual permeability and hemodynamic changes, respectively. Grossly, edema is not evident unless it involves the gallbladder, as it often does, or the large extrahepatic bile ducts. Microscopically, edema is evident in the portal triads and sometimes in the adjacent parenchyma as a clear separation of the sinusoidal lining cells from the hepatic cords by fluid that is often rich in protein.

Mobilization of the Kupffer cells and their related macrophages in the portal units is a response to inflammation of the liver. This also occurs in many diseases of which hepatitis is not a part, the Kupffer cells merely participating in the monocyte–macrophage activity of engulfing circulating matter such as bacteria in subacute bacteremia, erythrocytes in the hemolytic anemias, or even breakdown products of hepatic cells in hepatic injuries of many causes. Active Kupffer cells increase in number and size, the nuclei become large and vesicular, and the cytoplasm is basophilic and may contain vacuoles or ingested particulate matter. In overwhelming infections, many of the Kupffer cells are dead, and only naked yeastlike nuclei may be present.

A diffuse sequestration of leukocytes (Fig. 2.44) in the sinusoids as hepatic leukocytosis occurs in many acute or subacute bacteremias, just as they become sequestered in the pulmonary vessels to produce one anatomic form of interstitial pneumonia. Whereas they are certainly of functional significance in the lung when numerous, they are probably not so in the liver. Hepatic leukocytosis may be difficult to distinguish from myeloid metaplasia, which develops when the liver attempts to assume the functions of an incompetent bone marrow.

Agents capable of causing hepatitis include viruses, bacteria, spirochetes, fungi, and helminths. They will be discussed in this order, excepting the fungi and spirochetes. The systemic mycoses frequently involve the liver, but these diseases have been discussed with other organs or systems. The spirochetal disease, leptospirosis, is discussed with The Urinary System (Chapter 5 of this volume). Hepatitis is a particularly common lesion in autopsy

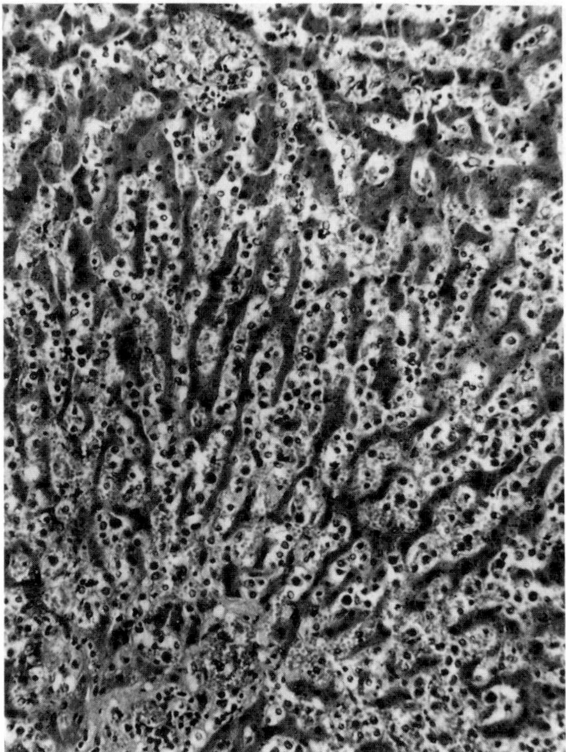

Fig. 2.44 Sinusoidal leukocytosis in pyometra. Bitch.

material, and in the livers of almost all adult animals there are traces of inflammation, usually insignificant in degree and obscure in pathogenesis.

The conventional signs of acute inflammation are those that occur in vascular connective tissue, which in the liver is restricted to portal triads and the surrounds of the bile duct. Inflammatory phenomena in these tissues are easily overlooked, but they are nonetheless important in hepatitis, which may be associated with subtle primary lesions in the parenchyma. This is often the case with viral infections. The capsule of the liver is well supplied with lymphatics, and exudation from these may be indicative of diffuse hepatic inflammation; the exudates are removed by normal visceral movements, and the residues on the surfaces of the liver must be looked for carefully. Within the parenchyma, the indicators of inflammation consist of aggregations of inflammatory cells in the sinusoids, lymphatic distension and edema in the portal triads, and the presence in the triads of a few leukocytes. In fetal hepatitis, care is necessary to distinguish inflammatory change from normal hematopoiesis.

Acute **diffuse hepatitis** is a common pathologic change in animals. Its epidemiologic characteristics are those of the infecting agent, which is usually viral, and it is, grossly, difficult to recognize in the absence of visible necrosis. In the dog, acute diffuse hepatitis is best exemplified in infectious canine hepatitis and toxoplasmosis. The herpesvirus infections of neonatal calves and foals produce acute hepatitis, as does Rift Valley fever in lambs.

The causes of **focal hepatitis** include those of focal necrosis, as discussed earlier. The foci may be few or numerous and may be acute or chronic in their characteristics, or granulomatous, and the reaction may be sufficient to cause swelling of the organ. Foci of hepatitis that lack specificity are common incidental findings microscopically. They are assumed to reflect Kupffer cell activity against enteric bacteria, but focal leukocyte reactions to cell death also occur in accelerated single-cell necrosis.

A. *Biliary Tract*

Inflammation of the gallbladder is **cholecystitis.** Inflammation of the bile ducts is **cholangitis.** Inflammation of the smallest bile ducts, the intrahepatic cholangioles, almost never occurs in animals, but when it does, it can be labeled **cholangiolitis.** The divisions are largely artificial. Cholecystitis may occur alone if the neck of the gallbladder is obstructed. Cholangiolitis may occur alone, and in humans is thought to be associated with altered permeability of the cholangioles for bile. It is more usual for inflammation in the biliary system in animals to involve all of it.

1. Cholangiohepatitis

Involvement of the periportal hepatic parenchyma by extension of inflammation from the ducts is almost inevitable, and the lesions can quite accurately be regarded as cholangiohepatitis. Cholangiohepatitis in animals is usually attributable to parasites, their effects aggravated by bacteria. It is also the specific lesion produced by the fungal toxin, sporidesmin.

Bacterial cholangiohepatitis is relatively uncommon. Its pathogenesis is similar to that of pyelonephritis, the main questions concerning whether the bacteria arrive hematogenously and descend in the ducts to produce inflammation, or ascend the ducts from the intestine, and whether in either event there is some predisposition. If bacterial cholangiohepatitis is to develop, as opposed to the mere presence of organisms in bile, then stasis in the biliary system is required. It is sometimes possible to demonstrate a mechanical obstruction to the flow of bile. This may be a tumor of the pancreas, or scar tissue derived from an inflammatory process in an adjacent viscus, such as granulomatous or suppurative gastritis, suppurative lymphadenitis of the hilar nodes, or a primary hepatic abscess situated at the hilus. There may be no obvious mechanical obstruction save that produced by the cholangitis itself.

Several bacterial species that produce bacteremic disease are eliminated in the bile, the Salmonellae being the best known example, and it may be assumed from this that there is a continuous normal portal–biliary circulation of enteric microorganisms. This in turn implies a mechanism whereby organisms can traverse the hepatocyte from the sinusoid to the canaliculus, and survive. The details of such process are unknown. Bacterial cholangiohepatitis is usually caused by nonspecific organisms, such as coliforms and streptococci, which are probably of enteric origin. Descending infections of hematogenous origin are at least feasible if there is relative stasis in the extrahepatic ducts, which allows time for bacterial proliferation. Of the specific infections, salmonellosis is a distinctive cause of fibrinous cholecystitis in cattle, especially calves.

What are clearly descending inflammations are occasionally observed in cattle. They take their origin in traumatic suppurative hepatitis and may extend directly from the suppurative focus or arise as seedings from inflamed intrahepatic lymphatics. Cholangiohepatitis of this origin may be restricted in its distribution to biliary fields, but it does in some cases become quite diffuse in the biliary system.

The course and pathologic changes in cholangiohepatitis vary greatly, from a fulminating suppurative infection to a persistent but mild inflammation that over a period of months or years leads to hepatic fibrosis of biliary distribution. Severe suppurative cholangiohepatitis may follow a short course to death, the effects being those of the infection itself, which may become septicemic, rather than of hepatic injury. At autopsy, the liver is swollen, soft, and pale, and its architecture is blurred. Few or many suppurative foci may be visible beneath the capsule and on the cut surface (Fig. 2.45). They are small, sometimes miliary in distribution, and not encapsulated. Lesions in other organs may be those of septicemia and jaundice. Microscopically, the larger ducts contain purulent exudate, and the smaller ones are disintegrated. Dense masses of neutrophils, liquefied or not, are present in the portal triads and infiltrate the degenerate parenchyma.

In subacute and chronic cholangiohepatitis, the inflammation is more proliferative than exudative. The liver is enlarged and may be of normal shape, or distorted owing to irregular areas of atrophy and regenerative hyperplasia. Its surface may be smooth or finely granular; the capsule is thickened and may bear fibrous villi or be adherent to adjacent viscera. Eventually, jaundice develops, and the organ is pigmented with bile. On the cut surface, the enlarged portal tracts are easily visible and accentuate the architecture of the organ. Eventually, the new fibrous tissue replaces the parenchyma, and in chronic diffuse cases in which the original infection persists, continuous fibroplasia may produce hepatic enlargement, the organ becoming huge, gray, and gristly. Alternatively, the chronic fibrosis may occur in wedge-shaped areas oriented to a small bile duct. The enlarged interlobular ducts may be readily visible and frequently contain plugs of inspissated secretion and debris. This lesion may be referred to as biliary infarction.

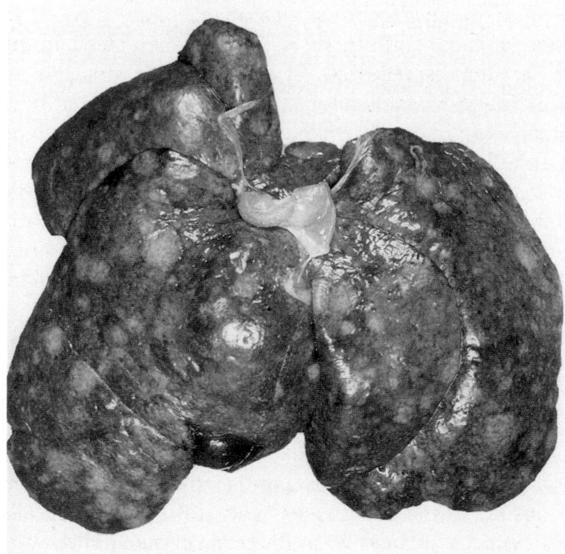

Fig. 2.45 Acute cholangiohepatitis. Dog.

Microscopically, the reaction remains centered on portal tracts (Fig. 2.46A). These are expanded in subacute cases by infiltration of leukocytes and macrophages and the proliferation of small ducts (Fig. 2.46B) and, in chronic cases, chiefly by organizing fibrous tissue and proliferating bile ducts. Encroachment on the parenchyma is minimal but inevitable (Fig. 2.46A). Continued degeneration of the periportal parenchyma probably is an additional stimulus to local fibroplasia, which, as well as thickening the smallest portal triads, extends along their length and links up with neighboring triads, thus subdividing the acini into segments. The hepatic venules and sublobular veins are involved. Regenerative nodules are not a prominent feature of cholangiohepatitis unless large areas of parenchyma have been destroyed, in which case the least-damaged lobes are expanded by coarse nodules.

Chronic cholangitis and cholangiohepatitis of ill-defined cause occur in mature cats, often in conjunction with a low-grade interstitial pancreatitis. The inflammatory portal infiltrate is dominated by lymphocytes (Fig. 2.46B, Fig. 2.58), but there is also scant participation by granulocytes, including eosinophils. These animals develop some portal fibrosis, bile ductular proliferation, and eventually, a degree of hepatic remodeling due to fibrosis. The condition has been observed to regress after prednisolone therapy and has been compared to primary biliary cirrhosis. In the cat and horse, however, the biliary and pancreatic ducts have a common entry to the duodenum, and simultaneous infectious inflammation of these systems is common.

Chronic active hepatitis is used to designate a pattern of chronic, progressive inflammation of the liver in humans, many cases of which follow hepatitis B virus infection. Identical liver changes, however, may occur in immune-mediated diseases, such as systemic lupus erythematosus, and in some idiosyncratic drug reactions. There is chronic inflammation of the portal tracts, extending into the periportal parenchyma, obliterating first the limiting plate and then more distant hepatocytes. In this process, known as piecemeal necrosis, individual and small groups of hepatocytes are isolated by fine, fibrous septa and small groups of inflammatory cells of various types. Piecemeal necrosis may eventually account for enough of the parenchyma to cause liver failure; nevertheless, nodular regeneration is not a regular feature, even of chronic cases.

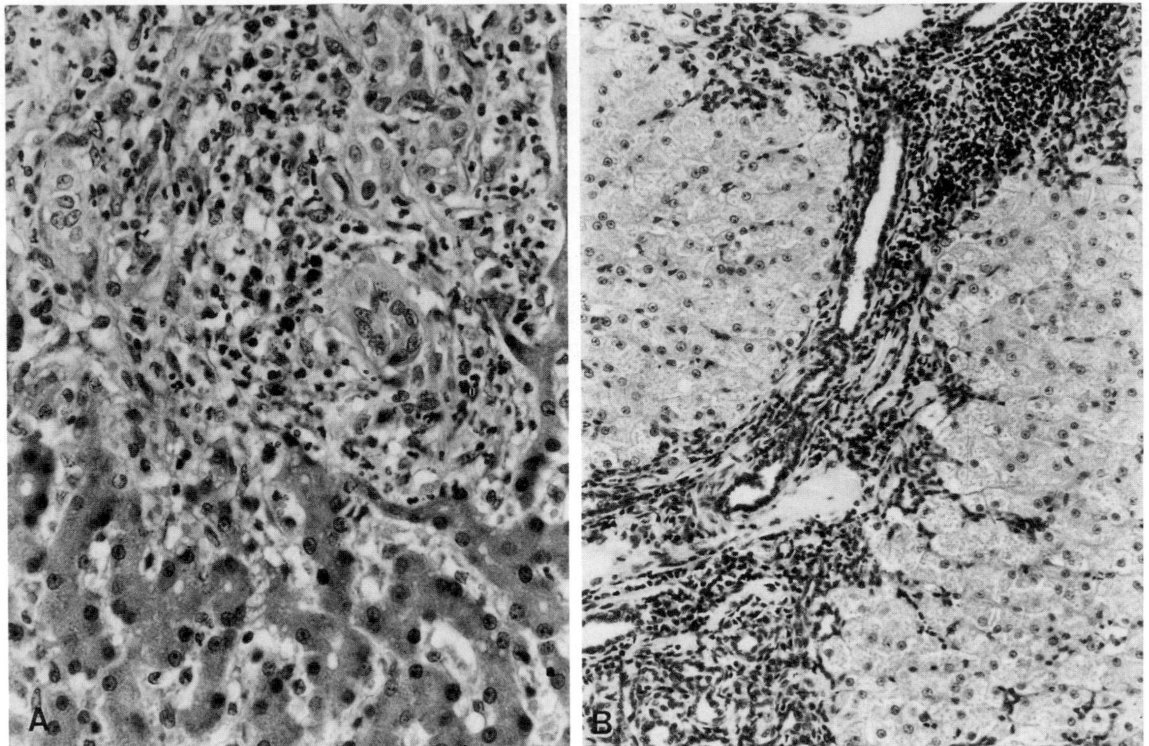

Fig. 2.46 (A) Cholangiohepatitis. Dog. Destruction of limiting plate. (B) Lymphocytic cholangiohepatitis. Cat.

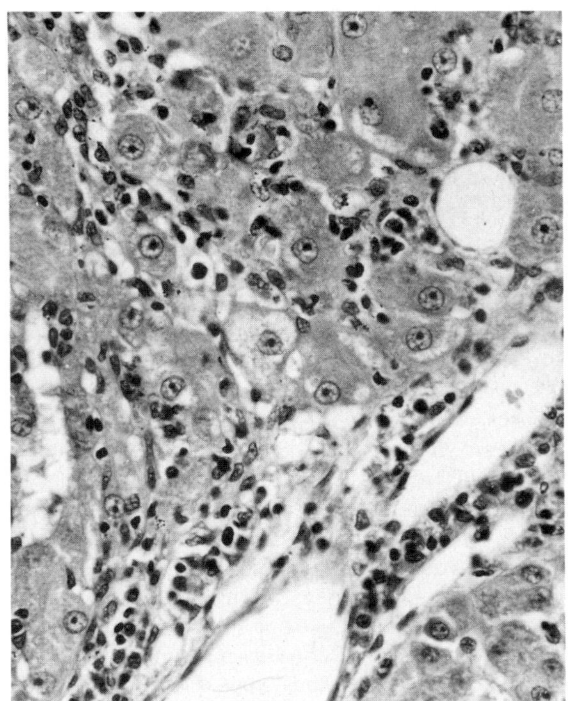

Fig. 2.47 Periportal piecemeal necrosis and inflammation. So-called chronic active hepatitis. Dog.

There is considerable overlap between the morphologic features of chronic active hepatitis as described in humans and of chronic cholangiohepatitis. There is increasing interest in hepatic disease in dogs with features resembling the human disease (Fig. 2.47), but stringent clinical, immunologic, and pathologic criteria will need to be applied before chronic active hepatitis can be established as a separate entity in animals.

There is a single report of **canine acidophil-cell hepatitis** as a cause of hepatic failure in dogs in the United Kingdom and Ireland. Histologically acidophilic periportal hepatocytes were present, and portal fibrosis developed. Experimental transmission to dogs and rats was included in the report.

Bibliography

Bennett, A. M. *et al*. Lobular dissecting hepatitis in the dog. *Vet Pathol* **20:** 179–188, 1983.

Collins, J. E., Dubey, J. P., and Rossow, K. D. Hepatic coccidiosis in a calf. *Vet Pathol* **25:** 98–100, 1988.

Jarrett, W. F. H., O'Neil, B. W., and Lindholm, I. Persistent hepatitis and chronic fibrosis induced by canine acidophil cell hepatitis virus. *Vet Rec* **120:** 234–235, 1987.

Johnson, G. F. *et al*. Chronic active hepatitis in Doberman pinschers. *J Am Vet Med Assoc* **180:** 1438–1442, 1982.

Lucke, V. M., and Davies, J. D. Progressive lymphocytic cholangitis in the cat. *J Small Anim Pract* **25:** 249–260, 1984.

Morrison, W. B. Cholangitis, choledocholithiasis, and icterus in a cat. *Vet Pathol* **22:** 285–286, 1985.

Rutgers, H. C., and Haywood, S. Chronic hepatitis in the dog. *J Small Anim Pract* **29:** 679–690, 1988.
Van Den Ingh, T. S. G. A. M., Rothuizen, J., and van Zinnicq Bergman, H. M. S. Destructive cholangiolitis in seven dogs. *Vet Q* **10:** 240–245, 1988.

2. *Biliary Tract Obstruction*

Cholelithiasis (gallstones) is seldom observed in animals. The stones usually form in the gallbladder and are composed of a mixture of cholesterols, bile pigments, salts of bile acids, calcium salts, and a proteinaceous matrix. Such stones of mixed composition are yellowish black or greenish black and are friable. There may be hundreds of small ones or a few large ones (Fig. 2.48). The large stones are usually faceted. The origin of these mixed gallstones is uncertain, but their development is probably secondary to chronic mild cholecystitis and related to disturbances of the resorptive activities of the gallbladder, whereby the bile salts are removed faster than the stone-forming compounds. Calculi seldom form in the ducts, although calcareous deposits often do so in fasciolosis of cattle. Gallstones are usually asymptomatic. Occasionally, they lodge in and obstruct bile ducts and cause jaundice. The larger stones may cause pressure necrosis and ulceration of the mucosa, local dilatations of the bile ducts, and saccular diverticula of the gallbladder.

Occasionally, particles of solid ingesta may find their way into the gallbladder; sand has been seen in sheep, and seeds, in pigs.

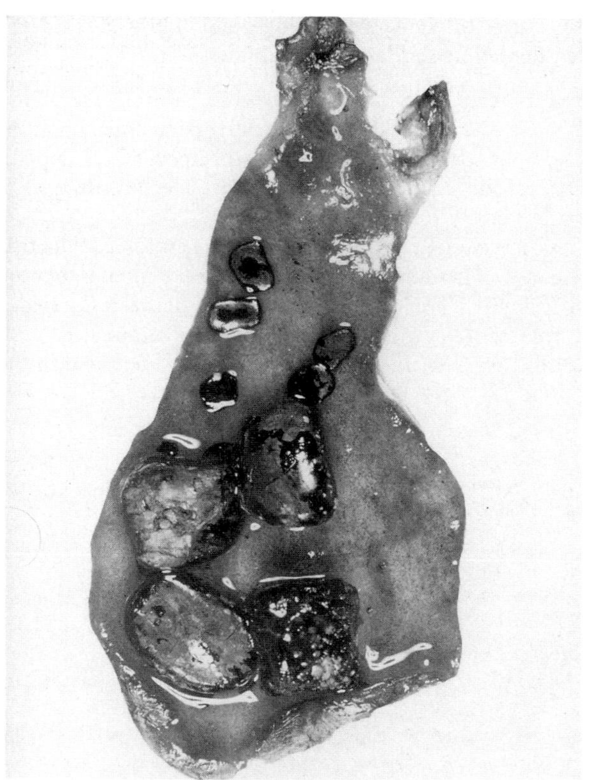

Fig. 2.48 Gallstones. Dog.

Biliary obstruction is rarely due to impacted gallstones. Usually it is due to cholangitis, the obstruction being produced by masses of detritus and biliary constituents, parasites, or cicatricial stenosis of the ducts. Adult ascarids may cause mechanical obstruction. Tumors of the pancreas and duodenum, and tumors and abscesses of the hilus of the liver and portal nodes, may cause compression stenosis of the ducts. Edematous swelling of the papilla in enteritis may also be of significance.

The consequences of biliary obstruction depend on the site and duration of the obstruction. When the main duct is involved, there is jaundice. When one of the hepatic ducts is involved, there is no jaundice, and depending on the efficiency of biliary collaterals, there may be no pigmentation of the obstructed segments of liver. The ducts undergo progressive cylindric dilatation, which may be extreme. The smallest interlobular ducts and the cholangioles proliferate. There is inflammation in the walls of the ducts and the portal triads, and this is probably due in part to chemical irritation by bile acids, but is due largely to secondary bacterial infections. These infections may be acute and purulent, or low grade; in the latter cases, bacteria may not be easily cultured. The cholangiohepatitis that almost inevitably follows has been described earlier (Fig. 2.49).

Inflammatory stenoses of larger ducts may recanalize via mucosal glands, which can proliferate and link to form a tortuous detour around the obstruction.

Rupture of the biliary tract or the gallbladder causes steady leakage of bile into the peritoneal cavity, the omen-

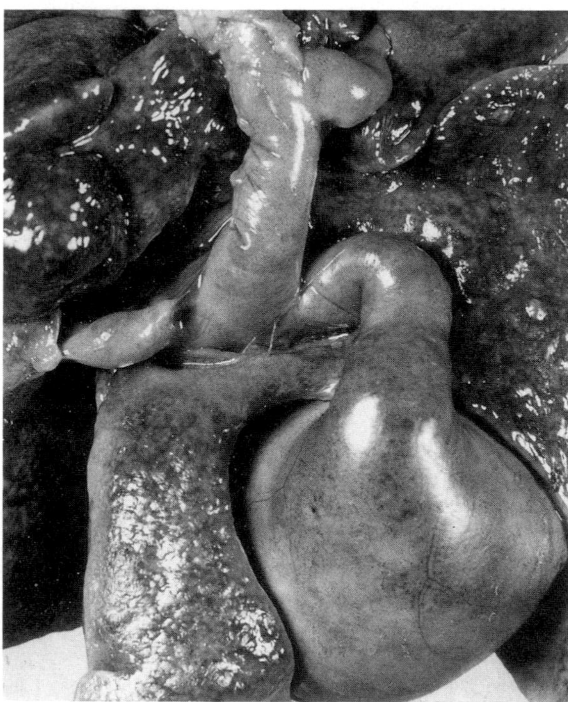

Fig. 2.49 Common bile duct obstruction and ascending cholangiohepatitis. Dog.

tum being unable to seal even small defects. The bile salts are very irritating and may cause acute chemical peritonitis. The peritoneal effusion that follows may remain sterile; more often it is infected by enteric bacteria, and severe diffuse peritonitis ensues. This may be rapidly fatal, particularly if clostridia are involved. Most perforations of the biliary tract are traumatic in origin.

Bibliography

Button, C. *et al.* Crystal-associated cholangiohepatopathy and photosensitisation in lambs in Victoria. *Aust Vet J* **64:** 176–180, 1987.

Johnston, J. K. *et al.* Cholelithiasis in horses: Ten cases (1982–1986). *J Am Vet Med Assoc* **194:** 405–409, 1989.

Mullowney, P. C., and Tennant, B. C. Choledocholithiasis in the dog: A review of a case with rupture of the common bile duct. *J Small Anim Pract* **23:** 631–638, 1982.

Prasse, K. W. *et al.* Chronic lymphocytic cholangitis in three cats. *Vet Pathol* **19:** 99–108, 1982.

Shibayama, Y. Factors producing bile infarction and bile duct proliferation in biliary obstruction. *J Pathol* **160:** 57–62, 1990.

Timbs, D. V., Durham, P. K., and Barnsley, D. G. C. Chronic cholecystitis in a dog infected with *Salmonella typhimurium*. *N Z Vet J* **22:** 100–102, 1974.

Van Der Leur, R. J. T., and Kroneman, J. Three cases of cholelithiasis and biliary fibrosis in the horse. *Equine Vet J* **14:** 251–253, 1982.

B. Virus Infections of the Liver

1. Infectious Canine Hepatitis

Canine adenovirus-1, the cause of infectious canine hepatitis, can cause severe disease in dogs and other canids and is ubiquitous, being excreted in the urine for long periods by infected animals. Vaccination has greatly reduced the frequency with which the disease occurs, and it is now rare in many countries in which it was endemic. Deaths from infectious canine hepatitis are usually sporadic, although small outbreaks occur among young dogs in kennels. Fatalities seldom occur among dogs older than 2 years. In areas where the disease is not controlled by vaccination, it is probable that most dogs in the general population contact the virus in the first 2 years of life and suffer either an inapparent infection or a mild febrile illness with pharyngitis and tonsillitis.

In more severe cases there is vomiting, melena, high fever, and abdominal pain. There may be petechiae on the gums; the mucous membranes are blanched, and only occasionally are they slightly jaundiced. Nervous signs of nonspecific character occur in a few cases. There is also a peracute form of the disease in which the animal is found dead without signs of illness, or after an illness of a few hours only. In convalescence, there may be a unilateral or bilateral opacity of the cornea caused by edema, which disappears spontaneously (Fig. 2.50A).

The virus of infectious canine hepatitis has special tropism for endothelium, mesothelium, and hepatic parenchyma, and it is injury to these that is responsible for the pathologic features of edema, hemorrhage (which is predominantly serosal), and hepatic necrosis. The histologic specificity of the lesions depends on the demonstration of large, solid intranuclear inclusion bodies in endothelium or hepatic parenchyma (Fig. 2.50B). Inclusions are occasionally observed in other differentiated cells but always have the same morphologic and tinctorial features, being deeply acidophilic with a bluish tint.

The morbid picture of spontaneously fatal cases is usu-

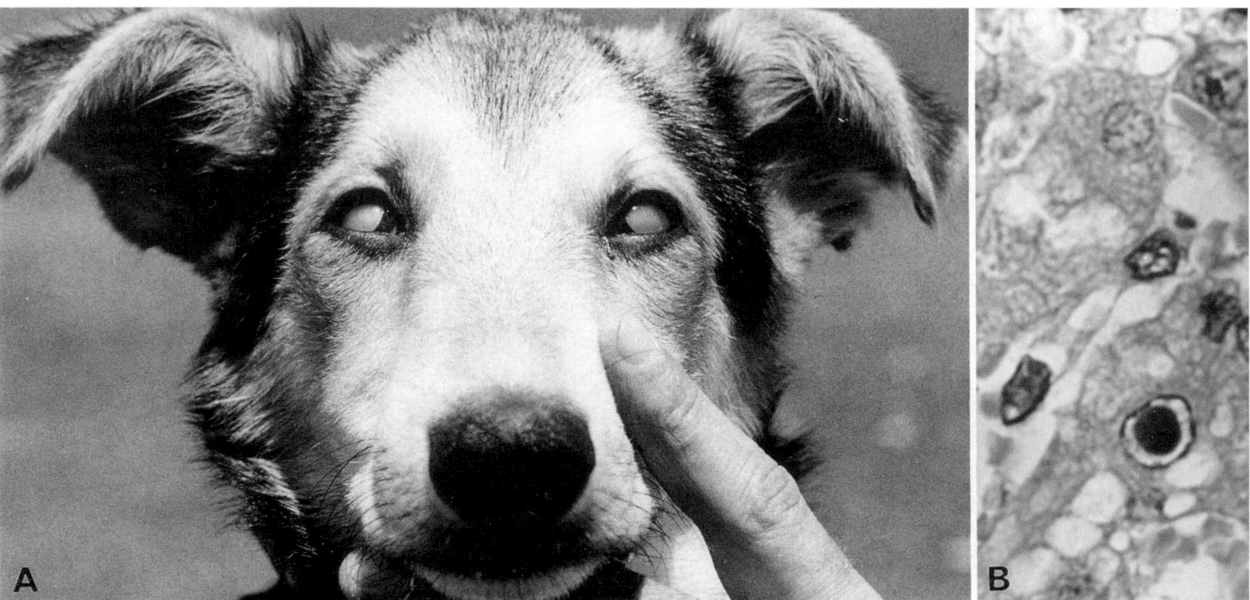

Fig. 2.50 (A) Corneal edema in convalescent stage of infectious canine hepatitis. (B) Infectious canine hepatitis. Intranuclear inclusion body in hepatocyte.

ally distinct enough to allow a diagnosis to be made grossly at necropsy. The superficial lymph nodes are edematous, slightly congested, and often hemorrhagic. Blotchy hemorrhages may be present on the serous membranes (Fig. 2.51A), and there is usually a small quantity of fluid, clear or bloodstained, in the abdomen. Hemorrhages on the serosa of the anterior surface of the stomach are usually linear, the so-called paintbrush type. Jaundice, if present, is slight. The mesenteries are slightly moist, and the serosa of the small intestine has a ground-glass appearance. The liver is slightly enlarged, with sharp edges, and is turgid and friable, sometimes congested, with a fine, uniform, yellowish mottling. Red strands of fibrin can be found on its capsule, especially between the lobes. In the majority of cases the wall of the gallbladder is edematous (Fig. 2.51B); when the edema is mild it may be detected only in the attachments of the gallbladder. In cases in which the gallbladder is edematous, it may also be darkened by intramural hemorrhages.

Gross lesions in other organs are inconstant. Small hemorrhagic infarcts may be found in the renal cortices of young puppies. Hemorrhages may occur in the lungs, and occasionally there are irregular areas of hemorrhagic consolidation in the diaphragmatic lobe. Hemorrhages in the brain occur in a small percentage of cases. These are capillary and venular hemorrhages best appreciated when darkened by formalin, and then, depending on their concentration, the affected portions of brain appear grayish or dark brown. Microscopic hemorrhages occur in any part of the brain, but when numerous enough to be grossly visible, they are confined to the midbrain and brain stem, avoiding the cerebral cortex and cerebellum (Fig. 2.52). Hemorrhagic necrosis of medullary and endosteal elements occurs in the metaphyses of long bones in young

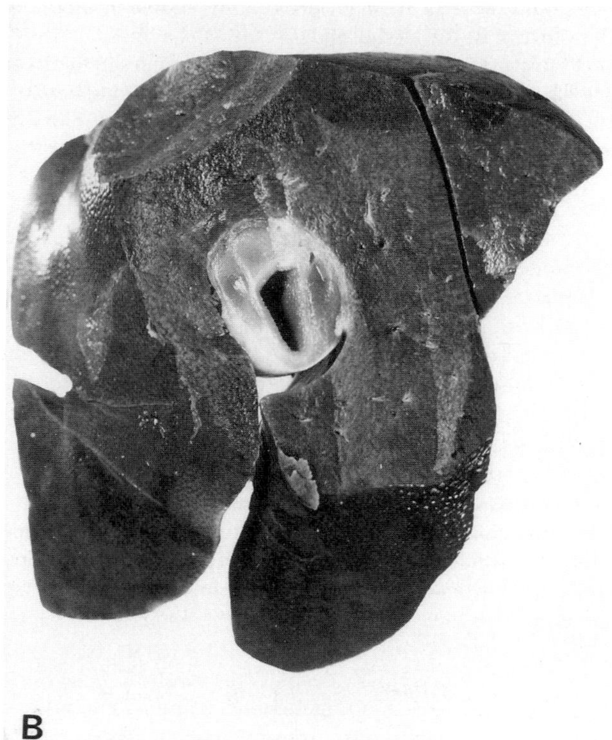

Fig. 2.51B Infectious canine hepatitis. Severe edema of gallbladder wall.

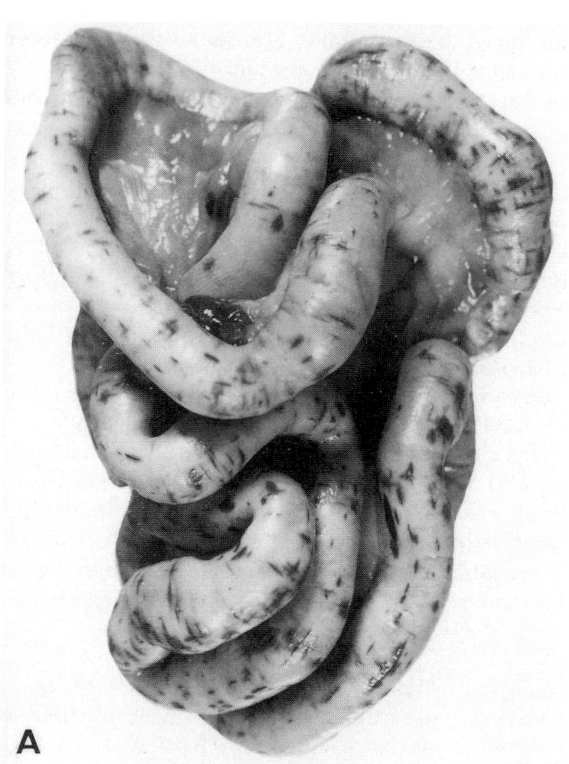

Fig. 2.51A Infectious canine hepatitis. Serosal hemorrhages over intestine.

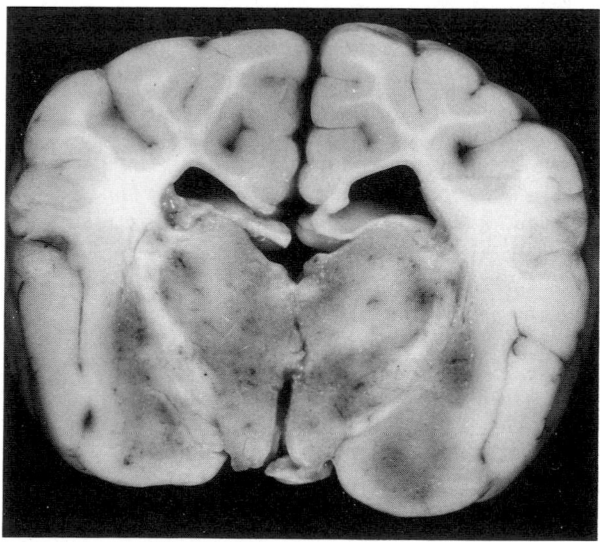

Fig. 2.52 Infectious canine hepatitis. Brain darkened by small hemorrhages, predominantly in midbrain.

dogs, and the hemorrhages are readily visible through the thin cortex of the distal ends of the ribs.

At low magnification, the histologic changes in the liver are quite reminiscent of the zonal necrosis of acute hepatotoxicities. There is an as yet unexplained susceptibility of the periacinar parenchyma to necrosis in this disease (Fig. 2.23). Close to the portal triads, the hepatocytes may be near normal in appearance, except for loss of basophilia and the presence of a scattering of inclusion bodies. In spontaneously fatal cases, most of the parenchyma of the peripheral and central portions of the acini is dead, the hepatocytes having undergone granular acidophilic coagulation necrosis, and in some of these, ghosts of inclusion bodies may be detectable. The margin between necrotic parenchyma and viable tissue is usually quite sharp, although in the viable tissue there are many individual hepatocytes undergoing apoptosis, most of them without inclusion bodies. Fatty changes are common but not constant. The dead cells do not remain long, so the sinusoids become dilated and filled with blood. The reticulin framework remains intact, an observation in keeping with the fact that in recovered cases, restitution of the liver is complete. Massive necrosis with collapse does not occur. As is typical of severe periacinar necrosis, the necrotic zones, initially eccentric areas about hepatic venules, extend and link to isolate portal units. Intranuclear inclusions can be found in Kupffer cells in variable numbers. Many of the Kupffer cells are dead, others are proliferating, and others are actively phagocytic in the removal of debris. Leukocytic reactions in the liver are mild and are directed against the necrotic tissue; mononuclear cells are present, but neutrophils, many degenerating, predominate. There is some collection of bile pigment, but it is moderate, in keeping with the short course of the disease.

Microscopic lesions in other organs are due largely to injury to endothelium. Inclusion bodies in endothelial cells can be difficult to find and are looked for with most profit in renal glomeruli, where endothelium is concentrated. Occasionally, they are found in the epithelium of collecting tubules. When areas of hemorrhagic consolidation of the lungs are present, there is hemorrhage, edema, and fibrin formation in the alveoli, and in these consolidated areas, inclusions are often common in alveolar capillaries and even in dying cells of the bronchial epithelium. Changes in the brain are essentially secondary to vascular injury and may be absent. Hemorrhages, if present, are from capillaries and small venules, and inclusions in endothelial nuclei can usually be found in vessels that have bled. Other endothelial and adventitial cells are hyperplastic and mixed with a few lymphocytes. Small foci of softening or demyelination may be present in relation to the hemorrhages.

The lymphoreticular tissues are congested, and inclusions may be found in the primitive reticulum cells of follicles, in the red pulp of the spleen, and in macrophages anywhere.

The detailed pathogenesis of infectious canine hepatitis has to be worked out. Many infections appear to be clinically silent, and other dogs recover after mild febrile disease with tonsillitis. The fulminating pattern of clinical disease and the possibility of convalescent phenomena need further examination. Some sudden deaths in this disease are associated with midbrain hemorrhage, and others occur with, at most, slight structural evidence of liver injury. Following oral exposure, which is probably the natural route of infection, virus multiplication occurs in the tonsils and leads to tonsillitis. The tonsillitis is sometimes quite severe and may be fatal, with extensive clear edema of the throat and larynx. Fever accompanies the tonsillitis and apparently precedes the viremic phase, which is of short duration and accompanied by a severe leukopenia. Hepatic necrosis develops at about the seventh day of experimental infection. The sequence of developments in the liver is not clear, but it is possible that virus proliferation occurs first in Kupffer cells. In surviving animals, hepatic regeneration occurs rapidly, and there do not appear to be any significant residual lesions. Small foci of hepatocellular necrosis involving one to several liver cells may still be present at 2 weeks, and foci of proliferated Kupffer cells may be detectable for another week or two, but progressive hepatic injury does not occur in the natural disease. Progressive hepatic injury does not seem to follow the acute phase of the natural disease, despite the fact that adenoviral antigen may be demonstrated immunohistochemically in Kupffer cells in dogs with various forms of chronic hepatitis. Focal interstitial nephritis occurs commonly, and the cellular infiltrates are persistent but not functionally significant. They consist of interstitial lymphocytic accumulations, especially about the corticomedullary junction and in the loose stroma of the pelvis.

Corneal edema is a late development (Fig. 2.50A). It may occur by the seventh day of infection but is usually delayed to between 14 and 21 days. Viral antigen can be detected in these eyes by fluorescent techniques, but not in the corneal structures. Inflammatory edema is present in iris, ciliary apparatus, and corneal propria, and inflammatory cells are abundant in the filtration angle and iris. The infiltrates are principally plasma cells, and there is evidence that the ocular lesion is a hypersensitivity reaction to viral antigen.

Originally it was assumed that the widespread tendency to hemorrhage in this disease was due to leakage from damaged vascular endothelium, coupled with an inability on the part of the damaged liver to replace clotting factors. Whereas these effects play a role, it is now known that the exhaustion of clotting factors is in large part due to their accelerated consumption, as the widespread endothelial damage is a potent initiator of the clotting cascade.

2. Wesselsbron Disease

This disease is caused by an arthropod-borne Flavivirus that according to serological surveys is widespread in Africa in various species of animals and birds. Various *Aedes* mosquitoes are the vectors. Humans are also susceptible to clinical and inapparent infection. The virus produces outbreaks of abortion and perinatal death in sheep. Susceptible adults rarely show clinical signs but may have a biphasic febrile response to infection; other clinical signs when present are of hepatitis and jaundice.

The lesions in lambs dying within 12 hr of birth consist mainly of widespread petechiae and gastrointestinal hemorrhage; longer survival allows jaundice to develop, and the liver becomes orange-yellow, enlarged, friable, and patchily congested. The bile in the gallbladder becomes thick and dark in some cases, but this may be due more to hemorrhage into the gallbladder than to hemolysis. Lymph nodes are rather constantly enlarged, congested, and edematous.

The most characteristic histologic changes are seen in the liver. There is no zonal pattern of hepatocellular damage as in infectious canine hepatitis; rather, there are randomly scattered foci of necrosis, with apoptosis and proliferation of sinusoidal lining cells. Mononuclear cells and pigment-filled macrophages accumulate in the portal stroma as well as in the sinusoids. In a variable proportion of cases, hepatocyte nuclei may contain eosinophilic, irregular inclusions. These are not accompanied by as much margination of nuclear chromatin as that associated with conventional viral inclusions, and their significance at this stage is obscure. In jaundiced animals there may be considerable canalicular cholestasis; whether or not this is the result of hemolysis does not appear to have been determined. Hepatocellular proliferation is apparent in the less acute cases. Lymphoid follicles in lymph nodes and spleen show pronounced lymphocyte necrosis and stimulation of lymphoblasts.

3. *Rift Valley Fever*

This is an arthropod-borne virus infection of ruminants and humans in Africa and is in many respects similar to Wesselsbron disease (Fig. 2.53). Rift Valley fever is, however, responsible for greater losses than the former infection. Morbidity and mortality may occur in adult sheep; death sometimes occurs in adult cattle, but it is chiefly a disease of the young, causing heavy mortality among lambs, kids, and calves and abortion in ewes, does, and cows.

The virus belongs to the Bunyaviridae and is transmitted by many species of mosquito of the genera *Culex* and *Aedes* in which transovarial passage can occur. Mosquitoes, once infected, remain so, and in them the virus is not pathogenic. High levels of viremia occur in sheep and cattle and are maintained for as long as 5 days. During epizootics, the virus may be spread by fomites, aerosols, and mechanically by other biting insects.

The infection in enzootic form is widespread in eastern and southern Africa but it has, in plaguelike proportions, extended to Egypt. Nonetheless, there is no explanation as to why the disease has remained confined to Africa.

In endemic situations, the disease in adults is usually mild, but in epidemics which extend to wholly susceptible host populations it may cause, in sheep and goats, severe illness with fever, vomiting, mucopurulent nasal discharge, and dysentery. The mortality rate is then very high in lambs and to 50% in adults. The disease in cattle is less severe, but pregnant animals abort, and the mortality rate in calves may reach 30%.

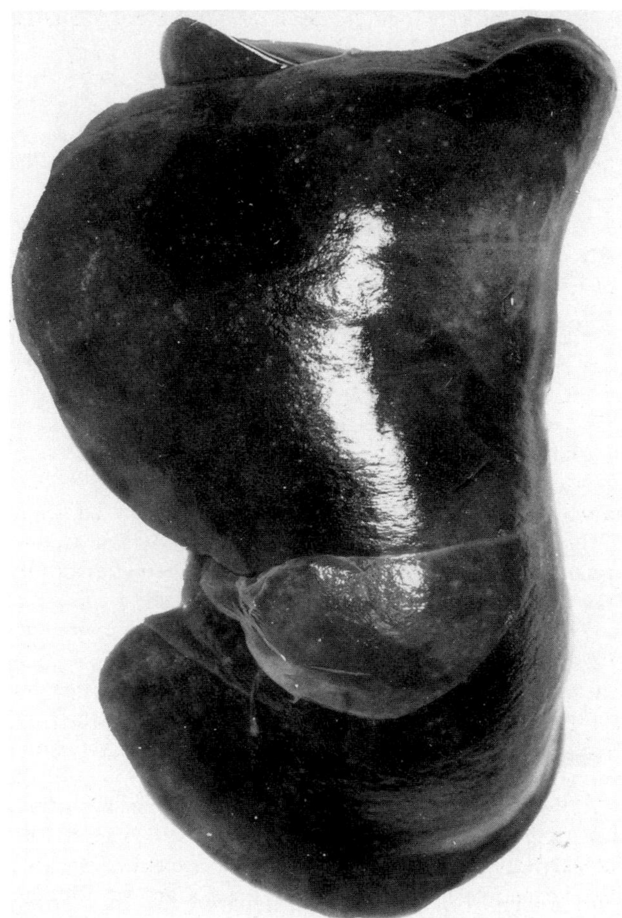

Fig. 2.53 Experimental Rift Valley fever. Sheep. (Courtesy of B. C. Easterday.)

As in Wesselsbron disease, the gross postmortem picture is dominated by widespread hemorrhage, ranging from serosal petechiae to severe gastrointestinal bleeding. The liver in the acute cases in neonatal lambs is similar to that in cases of Wesselsbron disease, being yellow, swollen, soft, and patchily congested or hemorrhagic. In older animals and in less acute cases, however, the liver tends to be darker and show scattered pale foci of necrosis 1–2 mm in diameter (Fig. 2.53). There may be fibrinous perihepatitis, edema of the gallbladder wall, and a moderate, blood-tinged ascites.

Within 12 hr of experimental infection of lambs, there are randomly distributed foci of hepatocellular necrosis in the liver. These foci include knots of inflammatory cells and prominent apoptotic bodies, and initially involve about half a dozen hepatocytes (Fig. 2.54). Within a few hours, however, these primary foci enlarge and may become almost confluent. In the meantime, the remaining parenchyma may rapidly undergo necrosis that spares

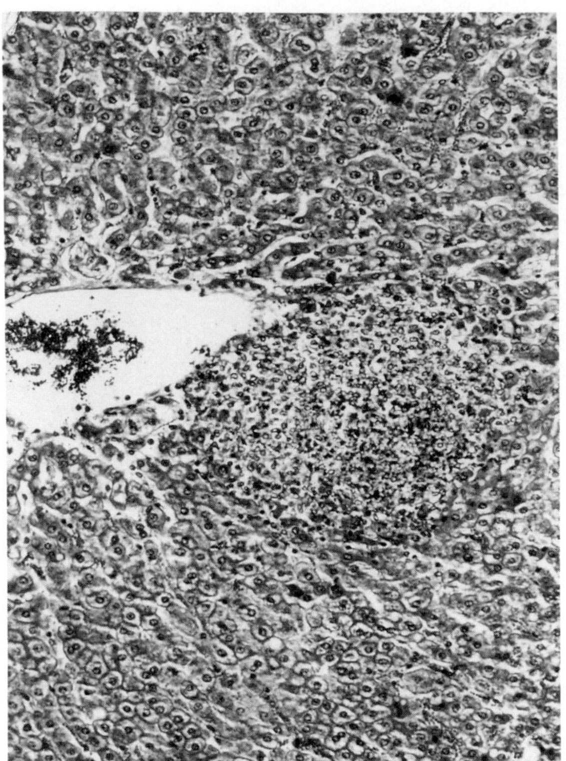

Fig. 2.54 Random focal necrosis in early Rift Valley fever. Lamb.

only a small rim of periportal hepatocytes. In naturally infected calves, the primary foci of necrosis undergo lysis more rapidly than the surrounding parenchyma; these foci thus have a striking washed-out appearance. Where the expanding foci of necrosis include portal triads, there may follow fibrinous vasculitis and thrombosis. Fibrin deposition in sinusoids is common, and so is mineralization of necrotic hepatocytes. Cholestasis is apparent in sections but is not a prominent feature.

Eosinophilic intranuclear inclusion bodies, often elongated, are sometimes seen in degenerate hepatocytes; there is associated nuclear vesiculation and chromatin margination. There is necrosis in germinal centers of lymphoid follicles in lymph nodes and spleen similar to that seen in Wesselsbron disease. Renal glomerular hypercellularity and necrosis have been described in the experimental disease.

Ultrastructural studies have shown condensation of degenerate hepatocytes, abundant apoptosis, and the presence of mummified, membrane-bound fragments of hepatocellular cytoplasm, but sinusoidal lining cells are not notably damaged; the Kupffer cells instead participate in the uptake of the dying hepatocytes. There is abundant fibrin in sinusoids in the vicinity of the primary foci of necrosis and also within hepatocytes and macrophages. The intranuclear inclusions are composed not of recognizable virus particles but of filaments. Virus is discernible occasionally in the cytoplasm, associated with tubular membranes.

It seems that the primary infection of the liver produces the primary necrotic foci, from which more virus spreads to damage neighboring parenchyma; the virus clearly has a marked preference for hepatocytes over other tissues. The hemorrhagic component of the syndrome is probably related to consumption of clotting factors; there is no direct evidence for the endothelial damage seen in infectious canine hepatitis.

It is now evident that there has been some confusion in early reports from Africa of liver diseases of ruminants. Some cases of phyto- and mycotoxicosis and of chronic copper poisoning have probably been ascribed to virus infection, and vice versa. It is also understandable that Rift Valley fever and Wesselsbron disease may have been mistaken for one another, but it is now held that these two diseases may be distinguished by careful pathologic examination as well as by isolation of the viruses. In summary, Rift Valley fever is characterized by obvious focal hepatic necrosis, on which is superimposed an almost massive periacinar and midzonal necrosis; cholestasis is not so prominent as it is in Wesselsbron disease. The liver lesions in the latter disease consist of smaller, randomly distributed foci of hepatocellular necrosis, more active reaction by the sinusoidal lining cells, and more obvious cholestasis.

4. *Equine Serum Hepatitis*

We are taking some liberty in including equine serum hepatitis, also known as Theiler's disease, under viral hepatitis, but we are impressed by its epidemiologic similarities to type B viral hepatitis of humans. The disease usually, but not invariably, occurs in horses that have been injected with equine serum or tissue emulsions and has a rather constant incubation period of 42–60 days, although this may be a few days shorter or a month longer. The disease was originally observed in horses passively immunized against African horse sickness and later in horses passively immunized against anthrax, tetanus, and equine encephalomyelitis. A high incidence has been observed in horses passively immunized against *Clostridium perfringens* toxins in an attempt to protect against grass sickness. Vaccines against equine herpesvirus-1 prepared from equine fetal tissue have produced the disease and, finally, the disease continues to be a problem where pregnant mare serum is routinely injected into mares at the time of breeding. In each of these situations, the inoculated serum or tissue is of equine origin, and although such an association holds for the great majority of cases, there are many, but usually sporadic, cases that have certainly not been inoculated with anything. The origin of the infection, if it is such, in these latter cases is not known. The incidence of equine serum hepatitis among inoculated animals is very variable. Attempts to reproduce the disease by experimental transmission have rarely been successful. The disease is seldom diagnosed in the absence of acute neurologic disturbances, and is fatal when these appear.

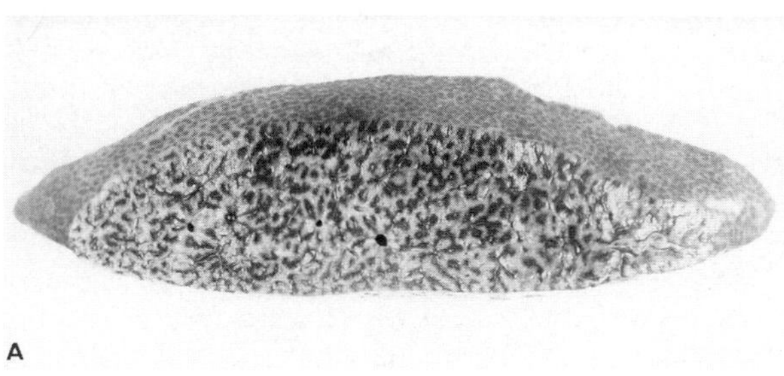

Fig. 2.55A Slice of liver from equine serum hepatitis. The reticular pattern suggests zonal necrosis.

There are observations, however, that indicate that recovery after transient illness with jaundice is common, and that recovery is in some instances incomplete, such horses remaining stupid and intractable.

The onset of the clinical syndrome is usually sudden, and the course short, death occurring in 6 to 24 hr or so. There is jaundice and neurologic disturbance, hyperexcitability, often with mania, continuous walking and pushing, apparent blindness, and ataxia. Death then occurs suddenly without a period of prostration.

At autopsy, icterus is present, there is moderate ascites, the spleen is normal or congested, and there may be petechial hemorrhages on serous membranes and renal cortices, and some congestion of the intestine with hemorrhage into its lumen. The characteristic lesions are hepatic. The liver usually is of normal size but may be slightly enlarged or shrunken, friable, and stained by bile pigments; its surface is mottled and may bear a few strands of fresh fibrin. The mottling is more evident on the cut surface, which appears as if severely congested and fatty (Fig. 2.55A).

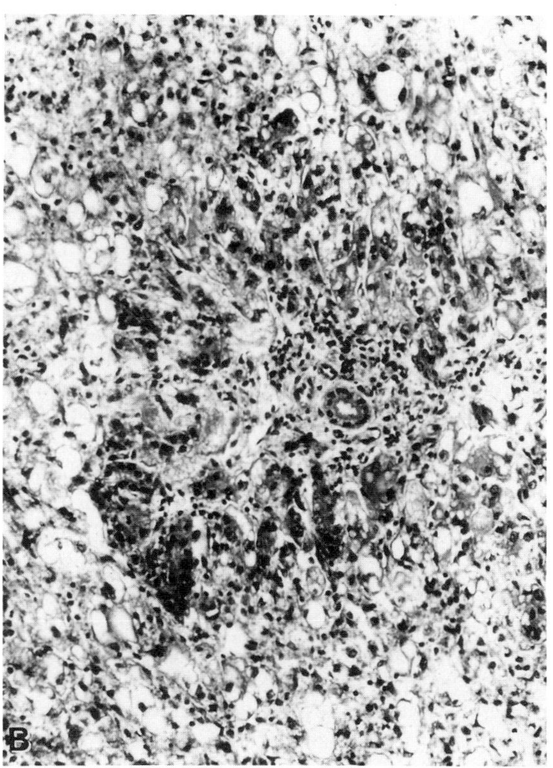

Fig. 2.55B Equine serum hepatitis. Section of the liver in (A) to show extensive periacinar degenerative changes, cellular infiltration, and periportal survival zone.

The hepatic lesion is considerably older than the clinical course would suggest. There are a few swollen and vacuolated hepatocytes against the portal units, or there may be no normal parenchymal cells (Fig. 2.55B). Severe fatty changes, usually as single, very large globules, affect most of the cells of the acini. Acute necrosis is not in evidence, but in the periphery of the acini, severely ballooned cells undergo dissolution to leave scattered fatty cysts, but most of them disappear to leave either sinusoids that are dilated and stuffed with blood or a condensed and distorted reticulin framework. There is no significant hemorrhage. Extensive deposits of bile pigments are present in Kupffer cells and hepatocytes. Leukocytes infiltrate diffusely but not in large numbers, lymphocytes, plasma cells, and histiocytes being present with a few neutrophils, many of which undergo necrobiotic changes. There is a diffuse but very slight fibroplasia, especially in the portal units. In some cases there is attempted regeneration, small irregular columns of regenerating cells being present in the portal areas, apparently derived from cholangioles. Healed lesions have not been reported.

Bibliography

Carmichael, L. E. The pathogenesis of ocular lesions of infectious canine hepatitis. I. Pathology and virological observations. *Pathol Vet* **1:** 73–95, 1964.

Carmichael, L. E. The pathogenesis of ocular lesions of infectious canine hepatitis. II. Experimental ocular hypersensitivity produced by the virus. *Pathol Vet* **2:** 344–359, 1965.

Coetzer, J. A. W. The pathology of Rift Valley fever. II. Lesions occurring in field cases in adult cattle, calves, and aborted foetuses. *Onderstepoort J Vet Res* **49:** 11–17, 1982.

Coetzer, J. A. W., and Ishak, K. G. Sequential development of the liver lesions in new-born lambs infected with Rift Valley fever virus. I. Macroscopic and microscopic pathology. *Onderstepoort J Vet Res* **49:** 103–108, 1982.

Coetzer, J. A. W., Theodoridis, A., and Van Heerden, A. Wesselsbron disease: Pathological, haematological, and clinical studies in natural cases and experimentally infected new-born lambs. *Onderstepoort J Vet Res* **45:** 93–106, 1978.

Coetzer, J. A. W., Ishak, K. G., and Calvert, R. C. Sequential development of the liver lesions in new-born lambs infected with Rift Valley fever virus II. Ultrastructural findings. *Onderstepoort J Vet Res* **49:** 109–122, 1982.

Gocke, D. J., Morris, T. Q., and Bradley, S. E. Chronic hepatitis in the dog: The role of immune factors. *J Am Vet Med Assoc* **156:** 1700–1705, 1970.

Rakich, P. M. *et al.* Immunohistochemical detection of canine adenovirus in paraffin sections of liver. *Vet Pathol* **23:** 478–484, 1986.

Robinson, M., Gopinath, C., and Hughes, D. L. Histopathology of acute hepatitis in the horse. *J Comp Pathol* **85:** 111–118, 1975.

Wright, N. G. Experimental infectious canine hepatitis. IV. Histological and immunofluorescence studies of the kidney. *J Comp Pathol* **77:** 153–158, 1967.

C. Bacterial Diseases of the Liver

Bacterial hepatitis is especially common, but, with a few important exceptions, is usually focally distributed, in these cases being of little significance clinically. Bacteria may gain entrance to the liver by direct implantation, as by foreign body penetrating from the reticulum; by invasion of the capsule from an adjacent focus of suppurative peritonitis; hematogenously via the hepatic artery or portal and umbilical veins; or via the bile ducts.

Excepting peracute septicemias, there are few specific bacterial infections that have a sustained or repeated bacteremic phase without producing hepatic lesions. There are, in addition, many cases of nonspecific bacteremia, especially portal in origin, in which focal hepatitis occurs. Because their differential diagnosis is of some importance, it is probably useful here to list those specific bacterial diseases in which focal hepatitis is expected or characteristic, but not constant. The specific infections may occur as fetal or perinatal infections. The list includes *Listeria monocytogenes* in fetal and neonatal lambs (Fig. 2.40), calves, and piglets; *Campylobacter fetus* subsp. *fetus* and *Flexispira rappini* in fetal and neonatal lambs; *Actinobacillus equuli* in foals; *Yersinia pseudotuberculosis* in lambs and occasionally in dogs and cats; *Y. tularensis* in lambs; *Pasteurella haemolytica* and *Haemophilus agni* in lambs; *Salmonella* spp. in all hosts (Fig. 2.21A), *Nocardia asteroides* in dogs; and the mycobacteria in all hosts.

1. Hepatic Abscess

Hepatic abscesses, quite apart from the lesions of the specific infections just given, are common, especially in cattle. They may arise by direct implantation with a foreign body from the reticulum or by direct invasion of the capsule from a suppurative lesion of traumatic reticulitis and may be single or multiple, but in either case they are often preferentially distributed to the left lobe. They may be hematogenous from portal emboli or by direct extension of an omphalophlebitis (Fig. 2.56). Arteriogenic abscesses via the hepatic artery may occur in pyemias but are quite uncommon.

Omphalogenic abscesses are more common in calves than in other species but occur in all. The bacterial flora is frequently mixed, but *Actinomyces (Corynebacterium) pyogenes,* streptococci, and staphylococci usually predominate or may be pure. Hepatic abscesses are not an inevitable sequel to omphalitis or even to omphalophlebitis, but they do not develop from navel infections in the absence of omphalophlebitis. There being no flow of blood in these vessels, involvement of the liver is by direct growth along the physiologic thrombus. Omphalophlebitis can be quite severe without extension to the liver. Hepatic abscesses of omphalogenic origin are often restricted to the left lobe (Fig. 2.40), but they may be restricted to the right (Fig. 2.56) or be diffuse in their distribution.

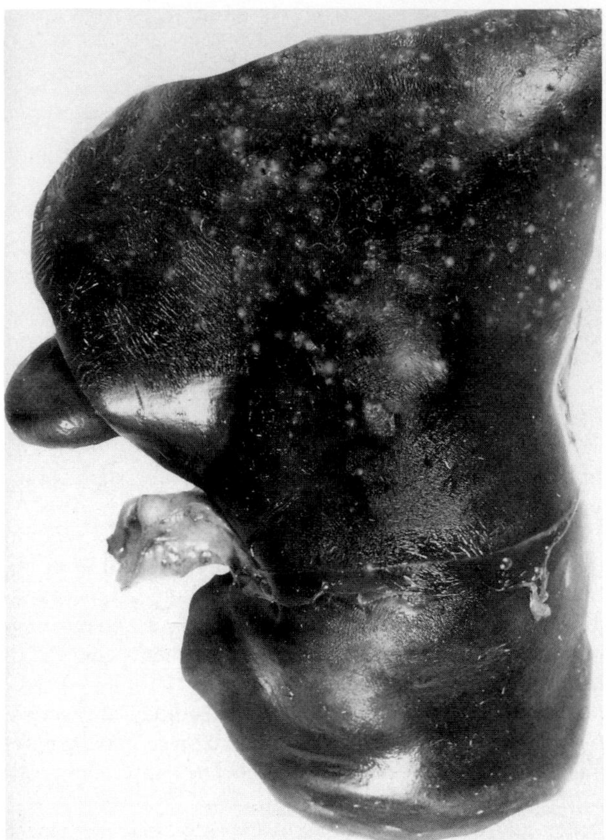

Fig. 2.56 Omphalophlebitis with miliary metastatic abscesses in right lobe. Calf.

Hepatic abscesses are also common and of much economic importance in cattle that have been fattened for slaughter. They are usually found at slaughter (Fig. 2.57A,B) but, when numerous, may be fatal after a few days of vague digestive illness. Their pathogenesis and character are discussed with rumenitis, to which they are a sequel (see The Alimentary System, Chapter 1 of this volume).

Hepatic abscesses of biliary origin occur in all animals. They are perhaps most frequent in pigs in which ascarids have migrated into the bile ducts. Cholangitic abscesses in horses, dogs, and cats are usually caused by enterobacteria as part of a fulminating ascending cholangiohepatitis that often is fatal after a short course (Figs. 2.45, 2.58).

The sequelae of hepatic abscessation are variable. Usually, they are insignificant and asymptomatic. Sterilization of the focus with either resorption and complete healing or encapsulation is common. Those near the surface of the liver regularly produce fibrinous and then fibrous inflammation of the capsule (Fig. 2.57A) and adhesion to adjacent viscera. They seldom perforate the capsule but do commonly break into hepatic veins to produce any one,

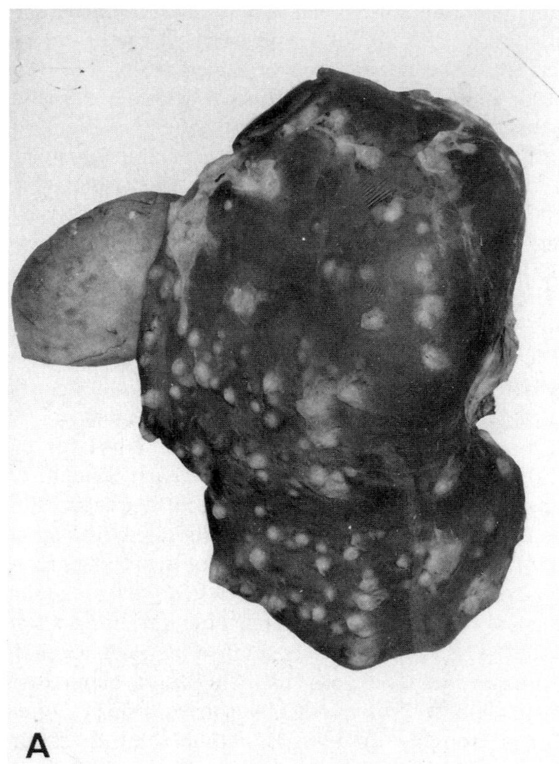

Fig. 2.57A Necrobacillosis of liver secondary to rumenitis. Ox.

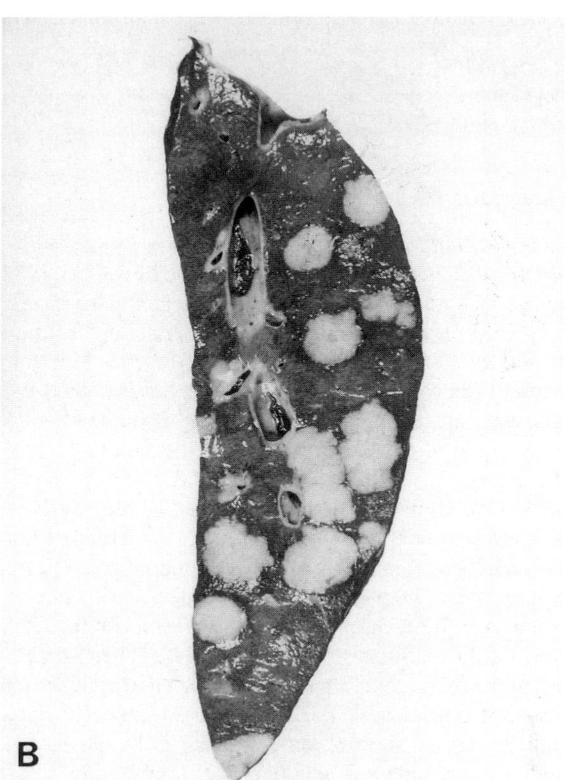

Fig. 2.57B Early hepatic necrobacillosis. Ox. (*Fusobacterium necrophorum* infection.) The pale areas of coagulative necrosis are bordered by acute inflammation.

or a combination of, thrombophlebitis of the vena cava, endocarditis, or pulmonary abscesses or embolism. Generalization is common, especially from omphalogenic abscesses of young animals. In adults, death may occur if the abscesses are multiple and fresh, and especially if they are necrobacillary in origin; death is probably the result of toxemia.

2. *Hepatic Necrobacillosis*

Occasionally, *Fusobacterium necrophorum* infection of the liver is observed following omphalophlebitis in lambs and calves, or as a complication of rumenitis in adult cattle. The hepatic lesions are multiple and typical of necrobacillary infection, being slightly elevated, rounded, dry areas of coagulation necrosis, sometimes a few centimeters in diameter (Fig. 2.57A,B) and surrounded by a zone of intense hyperemia. Affected neonates seldom live long enough for the necrotic foci to liquefy and assume the appearance of ordinary abscesses, but this may be seen in adult cattle. The histologic appearance of the foci in the stage of coagulative necrosis is quite characteristic. The necrotic amorphous central area is bordered by a zone of wholesale destruction of leukocytes, whose nuclear chromatin is dissipated in a finely divided form, and among which the filamentous fusobacteria are mostly concentrated. Outside this zone there is severe hyperemia and hemorrhage, and thrombosis of local vessels is common. The lesion in neonatal lambs is to be distinguished from that caused by *Campylobacter fetus* subsp. *fetus* and *Flexispira rappini*.

3. *Infectious Necrotic Hepatitis (Black Disease)*

Organisms of the genus *Clostridium* are notably circuitous in their means of producing disease. This is true of *C. novyi,* the type B strains of which are the cause of black disease (infectious necrotic hepatitis). This particular type of *C. novyi* produces three potent exotoxins, namely, alpha, the classical lethal toxin of the species; beta, which is a necrotizing and hemolytic lecithinase; and zeta, which is hemolytic. Black disease is essentially an intoxication produced by these exotoxins, and its development requires a combination of circumstances: a host that is not immune, a latent spore infection of tissue, and some agency to injure the liver sufficiently to produce an anaerobic environment in which the spores can germinate and proliferate. This combination of circumstances takes place most commonly in sheep, in which an environment suitable for germination of the organism is produced by immature wandering *Fasciola hepatica*.

Clostridium novyi is widely distributed in soil. Its distribution is possibly related to the movements of animals and is, as judged by the distribution of black disease, increasing. The spores are continually being ingested by

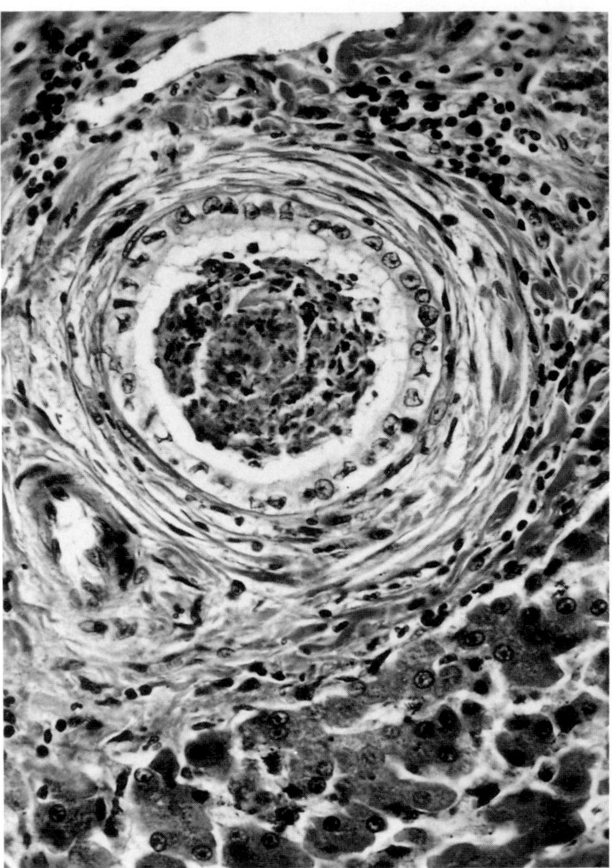

Fig. 2.58 Cholangitis. Cat. Bile duct contains exudate and is surrounded by fibrous tissue and mononuclear cells.

grazing animals in areas where black disease occurs, and some of them cross the mucous membranes, probably in phagocytes, and remain as latent infections in histiocytic cells, mainly in the liver, spleen, and bone marrow. The duration of latency in tissue is not known, but it can be many months, apparently. Many healthy sheep, cattle, and dogs harbor latent infections in their livers, the incidence of latent infections being much higher in animals that come from areas in which the disease is endemic.

Black disease is principally a disease of sheep. It occurs in cattle, perhaps with a higher incidence than is generally appreciated. It is occasionally seen in horses. The distribution of black disease as an enzootic malady parallels the distribution of the common fluke *Fasciola hepatica,* which is in turn determined by the distribution of the snails that act as intermediate hosts for the flukes. In Bessarabia and France, it is endemically related to the distribution of *Dicrocoelium dendriticum,* the lancet liver fluke. Cases of sporadic distribution may be related to *Cysticercus tenuicollis,* or a provoking agency may not be detectable.

Deaths in sheep from black disease occur rapidly and usually without warning signs. Illness, if observed, is brief and characterized by reluctance to move, drowsiness, rapid respiration, and quiet subsidence. Affected animals are usually in good nutritional condition. Postmortem decomposition occurs rapidly. The name of the disease is derived from the appearance of flayed skins, the dark coloration being caused by an unusual degree of subcutaneous venous congestion. Frequently there is edema of the sternal subcutis, and airways contain stable foam. The serous cavities contain an abundance of fluid, which clots on exposure to air: the fluid is usually straw colored, but that in the abdomen may be tinged with blood. The volume of fluid in the abdomen and thorax may vary from about 50 ml to 1.5 L. The pericardial sac is distended with similar fluid in amounts to ~300 ml. Subendocardial hemorrhages in the left ventricle are almost constant. Patchy areas of congestion and hemorrhage may be present in the pyloric part of the abomasum and in the small intestine.

The typical and diagnostic lesions occur in the liver and are always present. They are usually clearly evident on the capsular surface, the diaphragmatic surface especially, but the organ may have to be sliced carefully to find them. Usually the liver will contain lesions of acute or chronic fascioliasis, or other migratory parasites (see preceding sections). It is also, in consequence of hydropericardium, congested. The lesion of black disease, and occasionally there are several, is a yellowish-white area of necrosis 2–3 cm in diameter, surrounded by a broad zone of intense hyperemia, roughly circular in outline, and extending hemispherically into the substance of the organ (Fig. 2.59A). There may be a coagulum of fibrin on the capsular surface overlying the necrotic area. Occasionally, the essential lesions are rectilinear in shape or very irregular. The lesions appear homogeneous on the cut surface, but some contain poorly defined centers of soft or cheesy material.

The histologic evolution of the hepatic lesions begins with the necrotic and hemorrhagic tracts caused by wandering immature flukes. These are sinuous tunnels ~0.5 cm in diameter that contain blood, necrotic hepatic cells, and the leukocytes, chiefly eosinophils, attracted by the flukes. About the tunnels is a narrow zone of coagulative necrosis, also produced by the flukes. As usual, the necrotic tissue is demarcated by a thin zone of scavenger cells, chiefly neutrophils. If latent spores are present in the necrotic areas, they quickly vegetate and are visible in sections as large, gram-positive bacilli. The vegetative organisms by means of their exotoxins cause necrosis of the surrounding tissue (Fig. 2.59B), including the eosinophils of the fluke tunnel. As the area of necrosis expands, the bacterial proliferation keeps pace so that bacilli can be found in all parts of the necrotic focus but not in the surrounding viable tissue. Usually they are concentrated at the advancing margin of the lesion, just inside a zone of infiltrated neutrophils. At about the time of death and immediately afterward, the bacilli scatter in the liver and to other organs.

4. Bacillary Hemoglobinuria

Bacillary hemoglobinuria is a counterpart of black disease. The cause is *Clostridium haemolyticum,* which may

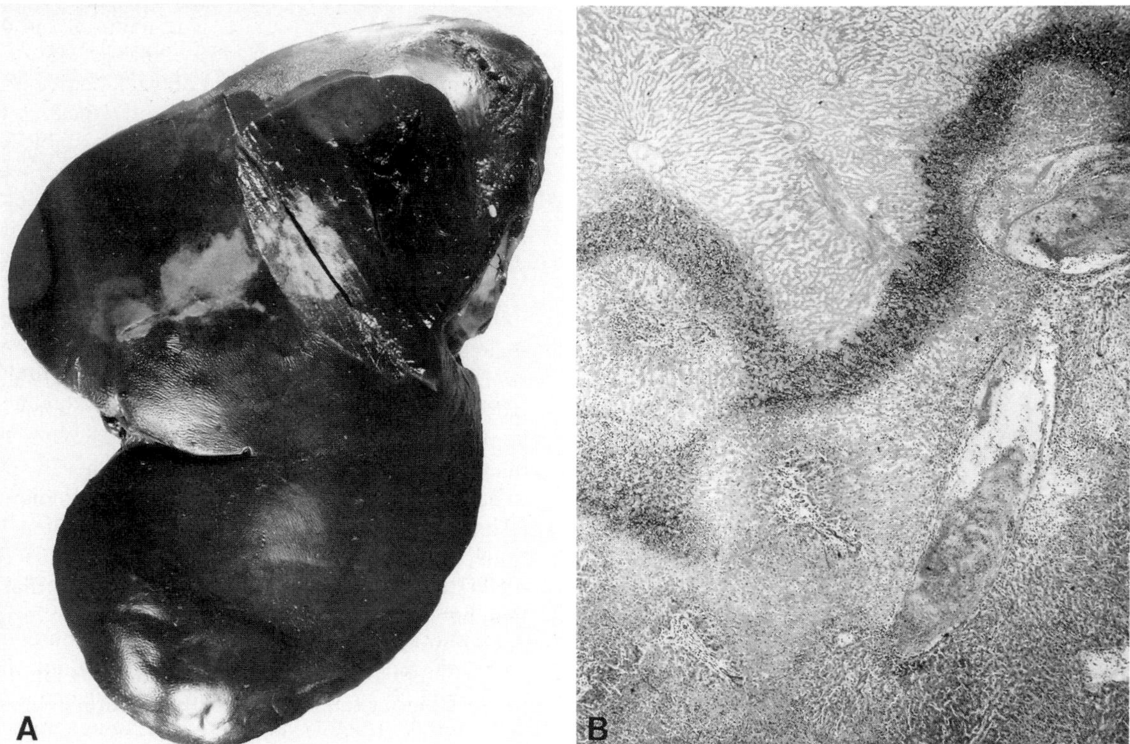

Fig. 2.59 (A) Infectious necrotic hepatitis (black disease); sheep. Irregular pale area of necrosis in right lobe. (B) Section of (A). Vascular thrombosis, and area of coagulative necrosis isolated by a zone of acute inflammatory infiltrate.

quite properly be regarded as a toxigenic type of *C. novyi*, both species producing the beta toxin, which is a necrotizing and hemolytic lecithinase. The pathogenesis of the two diseases is comparable, both of them depending on a focus of hepatic injury within which latent spores can germinate. Bacillary hemoglobinuria as an endemic malady exists only in areas where *Fasciola hepatica* abounds, and it is probable that flukes are the main cause of the initiating lesion. The disease does occur sporadically where there are no flukes and may be prompted by other parasites or other diverse focal lesions, which are smudged out in the expanding areas of necrosis. There is scant information on the ecology of the organism, but it is clear that it has its own environmental requirements, and the disease will not persist in areas where these requirements are not met. The spores will remain in the livers of cattle for several months after removal from pastures where the disease is endemic. Spores may persist in the bones of cadavers for 2 years. Spores of this and other sporulating anaerobes can frequently be demonstrated in the liver, where they are probably retained in Kupffer cells.

Bacillary hemoglobinuria occurs in cattle and sheep. It is characterized clinically by intravascular hemolysis with anemia and hemoglobinuria, but, perhaps reflecting variety in exotoxins between strains of the organism, hemolysis may not be a feature. The essential lesion is hepatic and similar to that of black disease but is much larger and usually single. It has been described as an infarct secondary to portal thrombosis, and although this may occur in isolated cases, it is scarcely a creditable pathogenesis for a disease of endemic occurrence. Thrombosis does occur in the affected areas but can be a result rather than a cause of the initial lesion and is found more frequently in the hepatic venules than in branches of the portal vein. There is severe anemia, the kidneys are speckled reddish or brown by hemoglobin, and the urine is of port wine color. The peritoneal vessels are injected, and in some cases there is severe, dry, fibrinohemorrhagic peritonitis.

5. Bacillus piliformis *Infection*

Bacillus piliformis infection has been known for a long time as Tyzzer's disease, a cause of severe losses in laboratory rodents; however, it has also been reported in foals, dogs, and cats. Although the disease is probably initiated by an intestinal infection, lesions in the gut are less specific and constant than those in the liver, which consist of focal hepatitis and necrosis.

Affected foals usually die between the ages of 1 and 4 weeks; often they are found dead after a short illness. The liver shows pale foci as much as a few millimeters across; these are represented microscopically by randomly distributed foci of coagulative necrosis with moderate polymorphonuclear inflammatory infiltrate. This lesion in itself is not diagnostic; its specificity depends on the presence of the causal organism in hepatocytes in the periphery of the necrotic zones. *Bacillus piliformis* can at present be

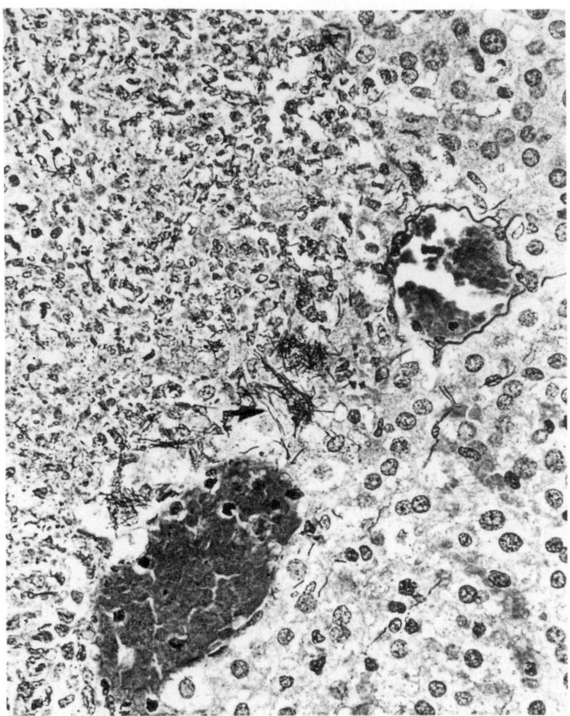

Fig. 2.60 *Bacillus piliformis* infection (Tyzzer's disease). Focal hepatitis; organisms in bundles in hepatocytes at margin of lesion (arrow). Warthin–Starry stain.

isolated only with difficulty on artificial media, so diagnosis is usually based on the demonstration of the large, long bacilli in the cytoplasm of degenerate and also otherwise apparently normal hepatocytes at the periphery of the necrotic zones. The organisms are Gram-negative and are best delineated with silver-impregnation techniques such as that of Warthin–Starry, but they may be seen with routine stains such as Giemsa, particularly when the material is fresh. The bacilli tend to lie in sheaves or bundles (Fig. 2.60). There may also be colitis sufficiently severe to cause diarrhea, but not so severe as that seen in rabbits with this disease.

Only a few cases of Tyzzer's disease have been reported in dogs and cats, and it seems likely that some form of immunologic inadequacy is necessary to allow infection in these species. The liver lesions are essentially the same as those in foals and rodents, and there is also enteritis involving the small intestine.

Bibliography

Gay, C. C. Infectious necrotic hepatitis (black disease) in a horse. *Equine Vet J* **12:** 26, 1980.

Janzen, E. D., Orr, J. P., and Osborne, A. D. Bacillary hemoglobinuria associated with hepatic necrobacillosis in a yearling feedlot heifer. *Can Vet J* **22:** 393–394, 1981.

Scanlan, C. M., and Edwards, J. F. Bacteriologic and pathologic studies of hepatic lesions in sheep. *Am J Vet Res* **50:** 363–366, 1990.

Scanlan, C. M., and Hathcock, T. L. Bovine rumenitis–liver abscess complex: A bacteriological review. *Cornell Vet* **73:** 288–297, 1983.

Timbs, D. V., Durham, P. K., and Barnsley, D. G. C. Chronic cholecystitis in a dog infected with *Salmonella typhimurium*. *N Z Vet J* **22:** 100–102, 1974.

Turk, M. A. M., Gallina, A. M., and Perryman, L. E. *Bacillus piliformis* infection (Tyzzer's disease) in foals in northwestern United States: A retrospective study of 21 cases. *J Am Vet Med Assoc* **178:** 279–281, 1981.

D. Helminthic Infections of the Liver and Bile Ducts

A variety of helminths (cestodes, nematodes, trematodes) and even the degenerate arachnid *Linguatula serrata* produce inflammation of liver and bile ducts, and indeed, they are as a group the most common cause of hepatic inflammation. Some of these parasites have the biliary system as their final habitat, and these are the ones to be discussed in detail here. The others produce hepatic lesions in the course of their natural or accidental migrations, and the lesions are discussed with the parasites under the organ (for most of them the gut) that is their final habitat. It is useful to describe here the lesions produced by larvae in transit.

The initial lesion produced by wandering larvae is traumatic. Sinuous tunnels permeate the parenchyma and of-

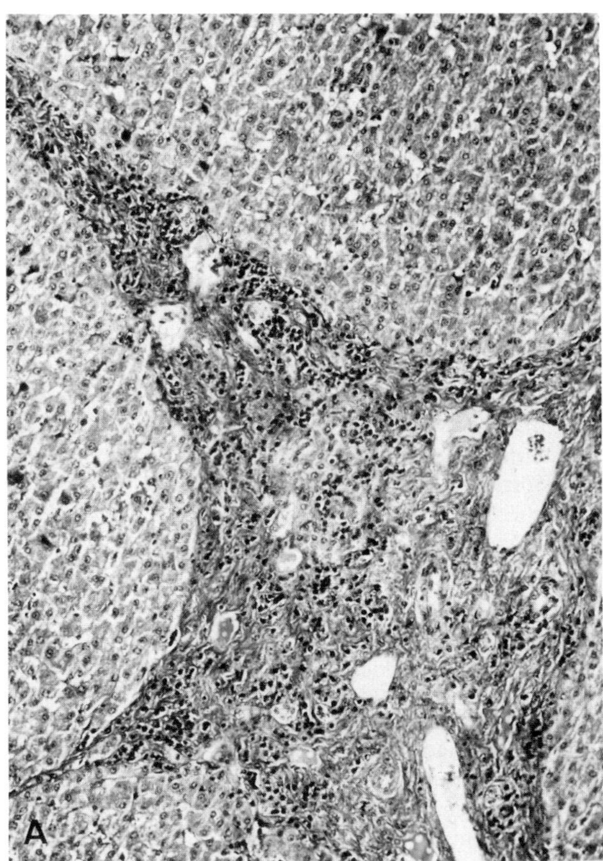

Fig. 2.61A Eosinophils infiltrating portal tissues. Larval migration. Pig.

ten breach the capsule. In the tunnels there are free red cells, degenerating hepatocytes, and leukocytes, chiefly eosinophils, which react to the parasites. Bordering the tunnel is a narrow zone of coagulation necrosis of parenchyma with infiltrated neutrophils at its margin. Eosinophils also infiltrate the portal triads (Fig. 2.61A). The necrotic parasitic tracts heal by scarification, and the fibroblastic tissue, infiltrated with eosinophils, is eventually incorporated into the portal units (interstitial hepatitis) (Fig. 2.61B). Most larvae escape from the liver but some eventually become encapsulated in the liver in abscesses containing numerous eosinophils. The abscesses may caseate and come to resemble tubercles, and eventually many are heavily mineralized to form permanent pearly nodules. In sheep, the most common cause of this type of hepatitis (aside from liver fluke) is *Cysticercus tenuicollis* in its wandering phase. Lambs may die of severe hemorrhagic hepatitis caused by very heavy infections of this parasite, and in pigs, an aberrant host, *C. tenuicollis* can produce a very intense inflammatory reaction.

In pigs, larvae of *Ascaris suum* and *Stephanurus dentatus* produce similar but distinct patterns of focal interstitial hepatitis. The ascarids produce their distinctive accentuation of the stroma (milk spots) when quite small larvae are immobilized by the host's inflammatory reaction; thus the foci are relatively small. The fibrotic lesion produced by *S. dentatus* larvae, on the other hand, is less focal and more in the nature of a track, and there are usually small, inflamed, capsular craters where the larvae have emerged from the liver to migrate to their preferred perirenal site. There will be obvious portal phlebitis at the hepatic hilus when infection by *S. dentatus* has been by the oral route (Fig. 2.62), and in these livers the parenchymal lesion is more severe in this vicinity.

Migration tracks left by larval strongyles are common under the liver capsule in young horses and are probably related to the dense, discrete fibrous tags that are almost universally found on the diaphragmatic surface of the liver of mature horses. The range of strongyle species capable of causing these lesions has not been defined. There are other and more devious means by which parasites produce hepatic lesions; the hydatid intermediate stages of *Echinococcus* encyst in the liver and may destroy much of it (Fig. 2.63A,B); the larvae of *Ascaris suum* in cattle add to the usual insult by causing portal phlebitis and small areas of infarction; the adults of *Ascaris* in all species, but especially in pigs, may migrate into the bile ducts (Fig. 2.64); and the eggs of schistosomes enter in the portal blood to lodge in the intrahepatic portal vessels and provoke granulomatous inflammation.

1. Cestodes

Stilesia hepatica and *Thysanosoma actinioides,* the fringed tapeworm, are the only cestodes that belong in

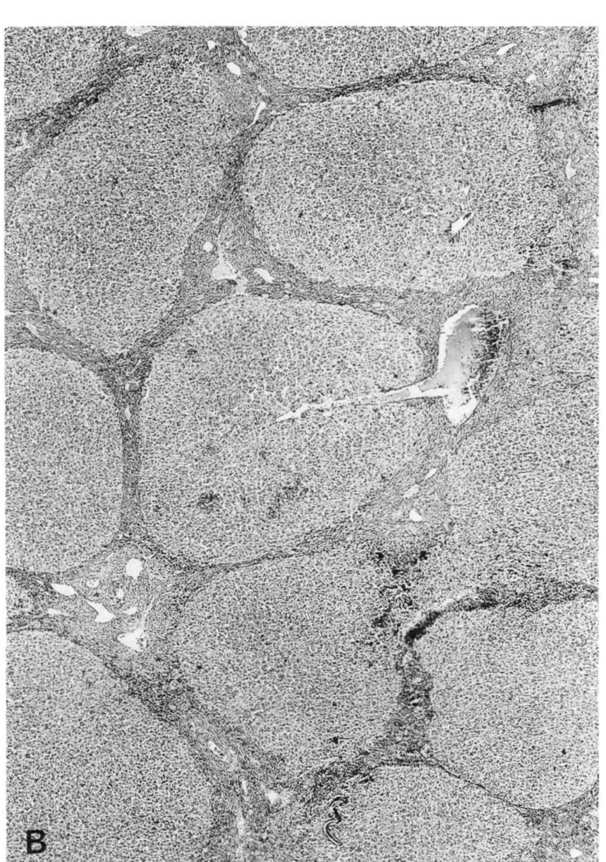

Fig. 2.61B Portal fibrosis following larval migration. Pig.

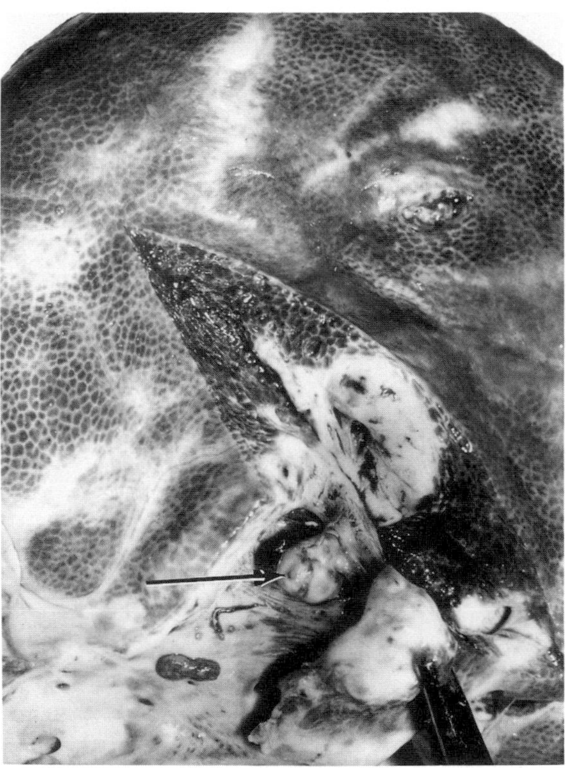

Fig. 2.62 Portal phlebitis and interstitial hepatitis produced by *Stephanurus dentatus* larvae after oral infection. Fresh and organizing thrombi in portal vein (arrow). Pig.

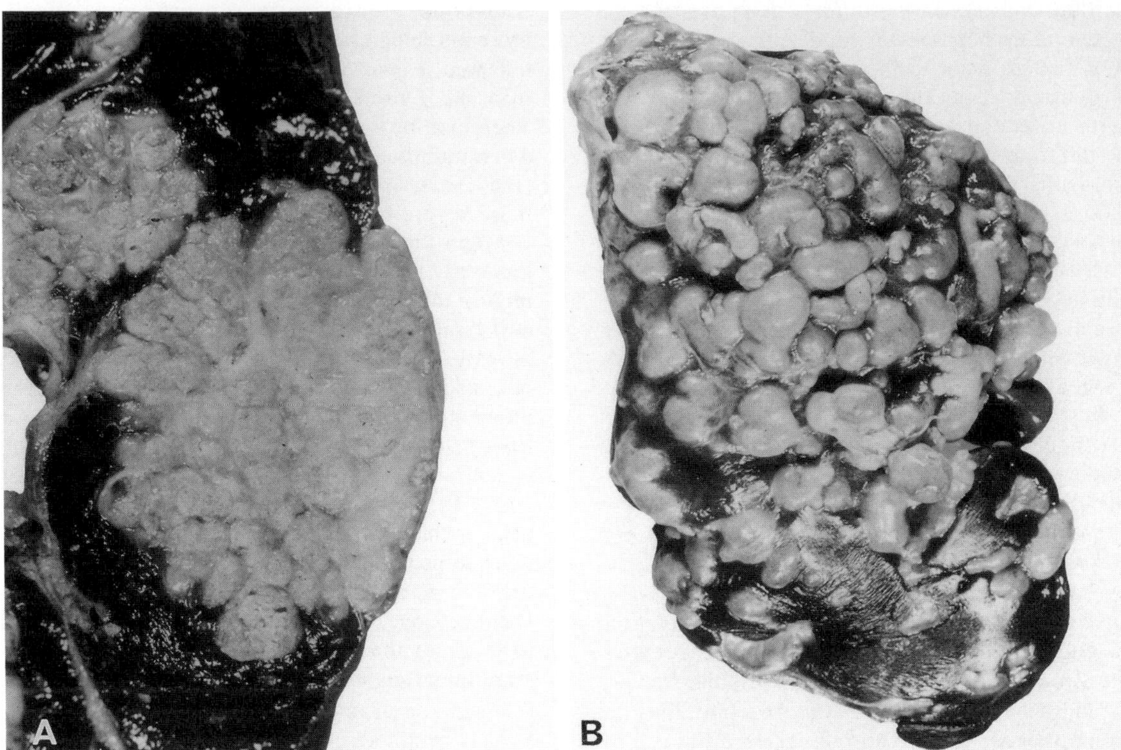

Fig. 2.63 (A)Degenerate *Echinococcus granulosus*. Mineralizing membranous debris and fibrosis. Ox. (B) *Echinococcus granulosus*. Severe hydatid liver disease. Sheep.

the bile ducts. They are parasites of ruminants, *Stilesia* occurring in Africa, *Thysanosoma,* in North America. The life cycles of the parasites are not completely known but probably involve oribatid mites as intermediate hosts. *Thysanosoma actinioides* may also be found in the pancreatic ducts and small intestine. Usually, the infestations are light but, even when heavy, are not of much significance. Very heavy infestations by *S. hepatica* occur without signs of illness, though the bile ducts may be nearly occluded, slightly thickened, and dilated. Saccular dilations of the ducts may occur and be filled with worms. The fringed tapeworm is perhaps more pathogenic, and unthriftiness may accompany heavy infestations. The cysticerci and hydatids which, in the intermediate stages, invade the liver are discussed with The Alimentary System (Chapter 1 of this volume).

2. Nematodes

Capillaria hepatica (*Hepaticola hepatica*) is the one nematode that in the adult phase inhabits the liver. It is a slender worm, morphologically resembling the whipworms, and it lives in the parenchyma rather than in the bile ducts. The usual hosts of the adult stage are rodents, but sporadic infestations are observed in dogs. These worms are not highly pathogenic. The adults provoke some traumatic hepatitis, and the eggs, which are deposited in clusters, provoke the development of localized granulomas. The eggs are readily recognized by their ovoid shape and polar caps. The granulomas can be seen through the capsule or in the substance of the liver as yellowish streaks or patches. The eggs cannot escape from the liver unless they are eaten by a predator. Predators, however, act only as transport hosts, and the ingested eggs are passed in the feces. Larvae develop in the eggs only in the external environment, and the cycle is completed when the mature larvae in the eggs are eaten by a suitable host.

3. Trematodes

A variety of trematodes (flukes) are parasitic in the livers of animals. They belong to the families Fasciolidae (*Fasciola hepatica, F. gigantica, Fascioloides magna*), Dicrocoeliidae (*Dicrocoelium dendriticum, D. hospes, Platynosomum concinnum,* and Opisthorchiidae (*Opisthorchis tenuicollis, O. sinensis, Pseudamphistomum truncatum*). The diseases produced are known collectively as distomiasis.

Fasciola hepatica, the common liver fluke of sheep and cattle, is the most widespread and important of the group. Patent infestations can develop in other wild and domestic animals and in humans. These flukes are leaf shaped and ~2.5 cm long in sheep and slightly larger in cattle. They are found in the bile ducts. Being hermaphroditic, only one fluke is necessary to establish a patent infestation, and each adult may produce 20,000 eggs per day. The longevity of the adult flukes is amazing and is potentially as great as

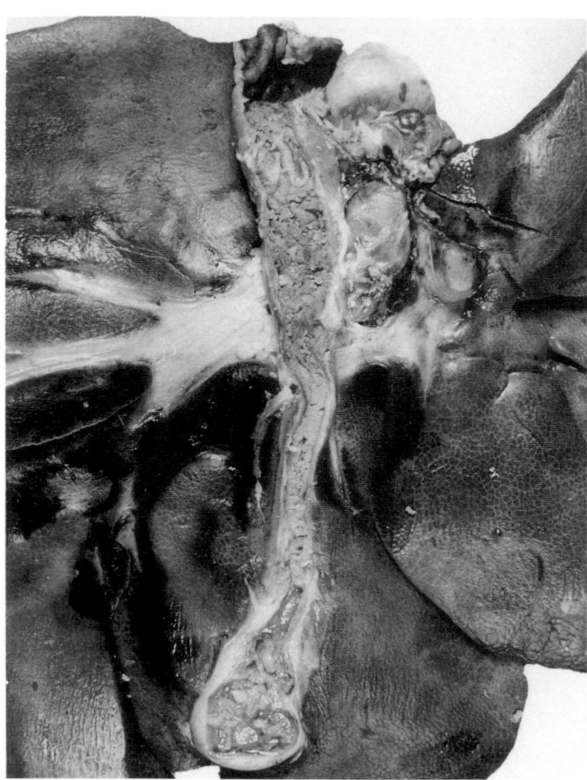

Fig. 2.64 Cholangitis and cholecystitis secondary to *Ascaris suum* invasion. Pig.

or greater than that of the host; they have been known to survive for 11 years, and it seems that they can produce eggs all this time. The eggs are eliminated in bile, and on pasture, in conditions of suitable warmth and moistness, hatch a larva (miracidium) in ~9 days. If the environmental temperature is low, the incubation period may be delayed for some months. The miracidium can survive only in moisture. It is actively motile and penetrates the tissues of the intermediate host, which is an aquatic snail. Different snails serve this purpose in different countries, but all of them belong to the genus *Lymnaea*.

Each miracidium, on penetrating a snail, develops into a mother sporocyst that reproduces, probably parthenogenetically, giving rise to a small number of the second generation, the redia. Each redia gives birth to either redia or cercariae, or to the two successively. Cercariae, the larval stage of the third (sexual) generation, first appear 1–2 months after the miracidium penetrates. Cercariae continue to escape daily for the life of the snail, but even so, total cercarial production is only 500–1000. They actively escape from the snail and are attracted to green plants, where they encyst and become infective metacercariae in 1 day. These can remain infective for 1 month in summer and to 3 months in winter. The developmental events from egg to this stage take 1–2 months under favorable conditions.

Infestation occurs by ingestion. Excystment occurs in the duodenum. The young flukes penetrate the intestinal wall and cross the peritoneal cavity, attaching here and there to suck blood and penetrate the liver through its capsule; a few no doubt pass in the portal vessels or migrate up the bile duct. They wander in the liver for a month or more before settling down in the bile ducts to mature, which they do in 2–3 months. Some may, by accident, enter the hepatic veins and systemic circulation to lodge in unusual sites; intrauterine infestations are on record. Lesions caused by aberrant flukes are quite common in bovine lung. They consist of resilient nodules just under the pleura of the peripheral parts of the lung. They range in diameter from about one to many centimeters and consist of thinly encapsulated abscesses situated at the ends of bronchi (Fig. 2.65). The content is slightly mucoid, unevenly coagulated brown fluid; in some lesions the reaction is predominantly caseous. The location of the lesion suggests that it begins as a peripheral bronchiectasis which later becomes sealed off. The fluke persists in the debris, but is small and hard to find.

The essential lesions produced by *Fasciola hepatica* occur in the liver and may be described, first, as those produced by the migratory larvae, and second, as those produced by the mature flukes in the bile ducts; the two often intermingle. There is the further incidence of peritonitis, which is produced by the young flukes on their way to the liver and, perhaps also, by some that break out through the capsule.

Usually there is no obvious reaction to the passage of

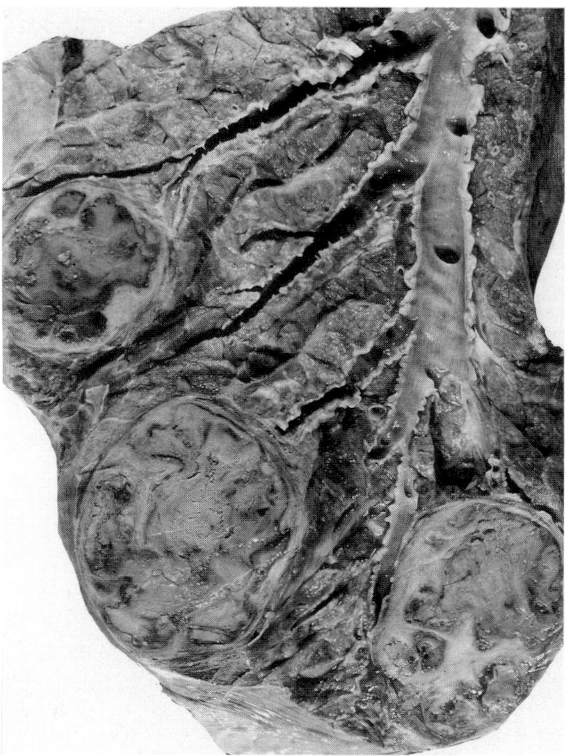

Fig. 2.65 Three caseous abscesses at the ends of bronchi, due to aberrant flukes. Ox.

young flukes through the intestinal wall and across the peritoneal cavity, except for small hemorrhagic foci on the peritoneum, where the flukes have been temporarily attached. Few or many parasites may be found in any ascitic fluid and attached to the peritoneum of the diaphragm and the mesenteries. When the infestations are heavy and repeated, such as may be observed in sheep, cattle, and swine, peritonitis occurs. The young flukes at this stage are less than 1 mm long. The peritonitis may be acute and exudative or chronic and proliferative. It is usually concentrated on the hepatic capsule (Fig. 2.66), especially its visceral surface, but may be restricted to the parietal peritoneum or to the visceral peritoneum, including the mesenteries of the gut. In acute cases there are fibrinohemorrhagic deposits on the serous surfaces, and in chronic cases there may be fibrous tags, with adhesions or a more or less diffuse thickening by connective tissue. Many young flukes can be found microscopically in the fibrinous deposits, and in the diffuse peritoneal thickenings, there are tortuous migration tunnels containing blood, debris, and the young parasites (Fig. 2.67). In cases with involvement of the visceral peritoneum, young flukes can be found in enlarged mesenteric lymph nodes.

The acute lesions in the liver caused by the wandering flukes are basically traumatic, but there is an element of coagulation necrosis, which is possibly related to toxic excretions of the flukes. The migratory pathways are tortuous tunnels that appear on cross section as hemorrhagic foci 2–3 mm in diameter. If the tunnels are followed, a young fluke less than 1 mm long can be found at the ends. When the infestation is heavy, the liver may appear to be permeated by dark hemorrhagic streaks and foci. Older tunnels from which the debris has been cleared may appear as light yellow streaks due to infiltration of eosinophils (Fig. 2.66). Microscopically, fresh tunnels are filled with blood and degenerate hepatocytes and are soon infiltrated by eosinophils. Later, histiocytes and giant cells arrange themselves about the debris and remove it, and healing occurs by granulation tissue, which is rich in lymphocytes and eosinophils. In light infestations the scars may disappear, but in heavy infestations they may fuse with each other and with portal areas to produce a moderate irregular fibrosis. There may, as yet, be no change in the bile ducts. Probably, most of the young flukes reach the bile ducts, but some do not, and they become encysted in the parenchyma. One or more flukes may be present in each cyst, which consists of a connective-tissue capsule and a dirty brown content of blood, detritus, and excrement from flukes. The cysts ultimately caseate and may mineralize or be obliterated by fibrous tissue. These cysts are most frequent on the visceral surface, where they cause bulging of the capsule.

Heavy infestations by immature flukes may cause death

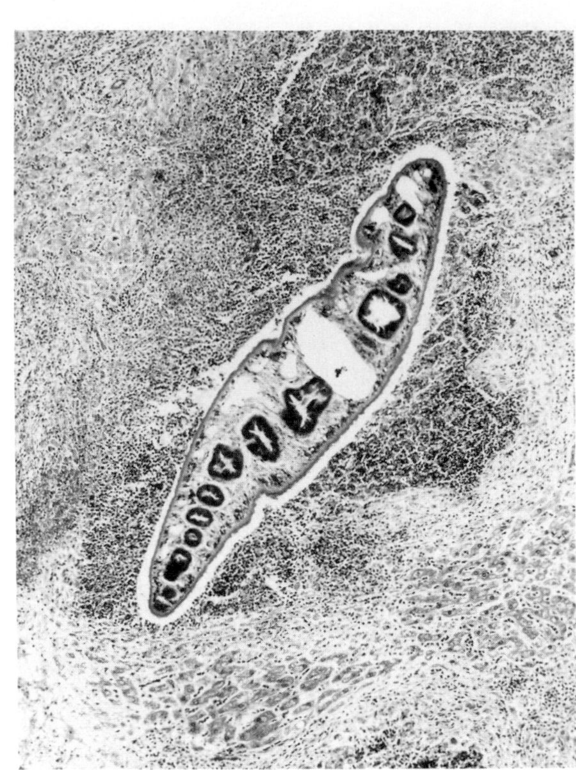

Fig. 2.67 Immature fluke, accompanied by acute inflammation. Sheep.

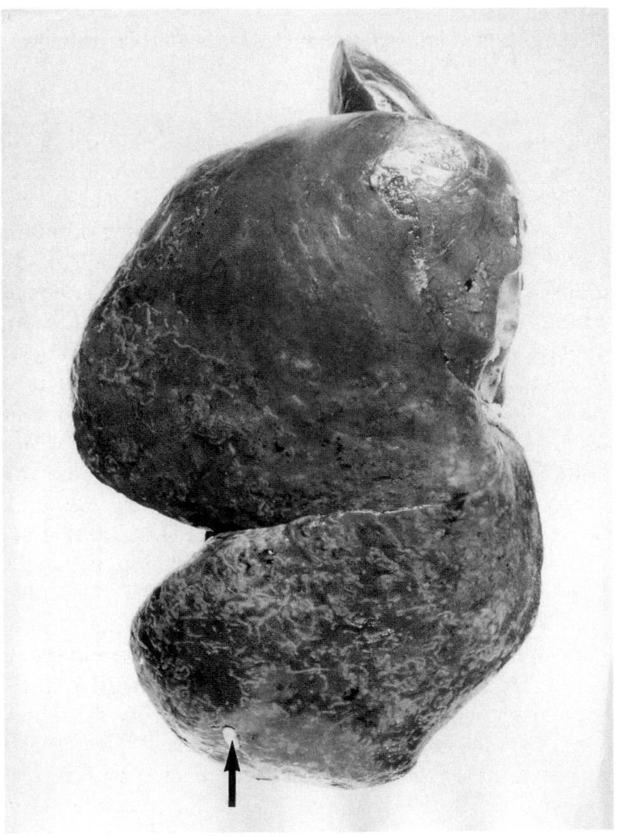

Fig. 2.66 *Fasciola hepatica*. Sheep. Tracks of immature flukes in acute infestation. Lesions concentrated in left lobe. Degenerate cysticercus (arrow).

in the stage of acute hepatitis. Such an outcome is not common, but occurs in sheep. It is estimated that 10,000 metacercariae ingested over a short period are necessary to produce acute death in sheep. Death may occur suddenly or after a few days of fever, lassitude, inappetence, and abdominal tenderness. This is also the stage of the parasitism in which black disease occurs (see preceding sections).

The mature flukes are present in the larger bile ducts and cause cholangiohepatitis. The relative importance of different factors in their pathogenicity is not known, but they cause mechanical irritation by the action of their suckers and scales, cause obstruction of the ducts with some degree of biliary retention, predispose to bacterial infections, suck blood, and probably produce toxic and irritative metabolic excretions.

The biliary changes occur in all lobes but are usually most severe in the left (Fig. 2.68A), and the right may be moderately hypertrophied. From the hilus, the bile ducts on the visceral surface stand out as whitish, firm, branching cords that in extreme instances may be an inch in diameter and allow detectable fluctuation over extended segments or in localized areas of ectasia (Fig. 2.68B). This dilatation of the ducts in sheep, swine, and horses is largely mechanical and is due to distension by masses of flukes and bile. It is permitted by the relative paucity of new connective tissue formation in the walls of the ducts in these species; this in turn is probably related to the rather mild catarrhal type of inflammation in the lumina of the ducts. In cattle, desquamative and ulcerative lesions in the large bile ducts are more severe than those in other species, and there is a correspondingly greater proliferation of granulation tissue in and about the walls of the ducts. The walls of the ducts in cattle are, in consequence, much thickened, and the lumen is irregularly stenotic and dilated and lined largely by granulation tissue. This contributes the typical pipe-stem appearance to the ducts in cattle; the connective tissue may be, in addition, mineralized, sometimes so heavily that it cannot be cut with a knife. The bile ducts contain dirty dark brown fluid of a mucinous or tough consistency, formed from degenerate floccular bile, pus, desquamated cells and detritus, clumps of flukes, and small masses of eggs in dark brown granular aggregates.

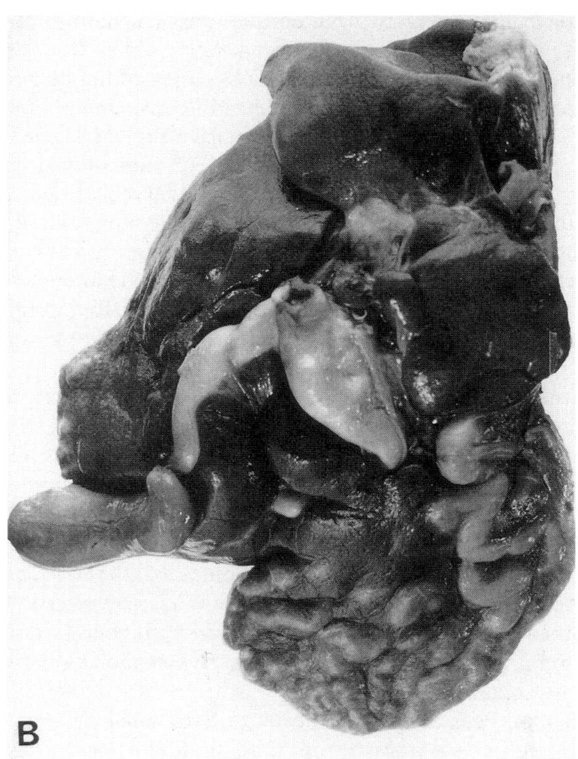

Fig. 2.68B Chronic fascioliasis. Sheep. Bile duct ectasia, atrophy of left lobe, hypertrophy of right lobe.

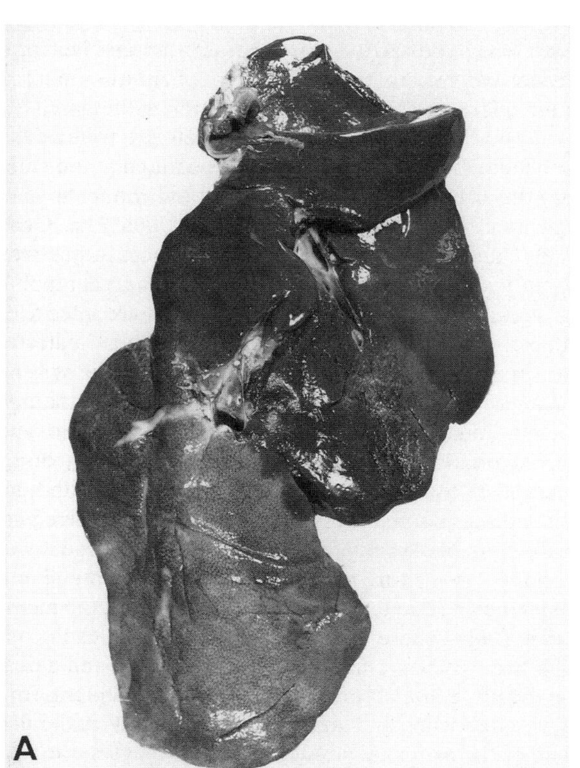

Fig. 2.68A Subacute *Fasciola hepatica* infestation, sheep. Early cholangiohepatitis and cholestasis in left lobe.

Although the lesions are most obvious in ducts large enough to contain the flukes, there is, with time and severe or repeated infestations, progressive inflammation in the smaller portal units due to direct irritation by the flukes, superimposed infections, and biliary stasis. The course of events is as described earlier for subacute and chronic cholangiohepatitis. The proliferating connective tissue and bile ductules in individual portal areas extend to join each other and the scars left over from the migratory phase, so that inflammatory fibrosis may obliterate parenchyma in many foci. In such livers, the left lobe, which is the one most severely affected, may be atrophied, indurated, and irregular.

The development of a cholangiohepatitis of the degree described depends on long-standing or heavy infestations. Lesions of lesser severity, or those less fully developed, are associated with light infestations of short duration. They may then be recognized only by local dilatations of the ducts, or even these may not be readily apparent. In such mild infestations, the fact of past or present parasitism may be suggested only by the detection of characteristic black iron–porphyrin pigments, grossly visible in the hilar nodes. It also contributes to the character of the biliary contents.

Chronic debility with vague digestive disturbances is common in chronic fascioliasis and, among sheep, deaths are common. Clinically and at postmortem there are, in addition to the essential lesions, more or less severe anemia, moderate anasarca, and cachexia. Jaundice is seldom seen.

Fasciola gigantica displaces *F. hepatica* as the common liver fluke in many parts of Africa and in nearby countries, Southeast Asia and the Hawaiian Islands. It is 2–3 times as large as *F. hepatica,* but its life cycle and pathogenicity are comparable.

Fascioloides magna is the large liver fluke of North America. It is a parasite of ruminants and lives in the hepatic parenchyma, not in the bile ducts, although in tolerant hosts, Cervidae, the cysts in which it localizes communicate with the bile ducts to provide an exit for ova and excrement. The life cycle of this parasite generally parallels that of *Fasciola hepatica*. The young flukes are very destructive as they wander in the liver. In cattle, they wander briefly, producing large necrotic tunnels before becoming encysted. The cysts, enclosed by connective tissue, do not communicate with bile ducts but form permanent enclosures for the flukes, their excreta, and ova. The cysts, which may be 1–2 inches in diameter, are remarkable for the large deposits of jet black, sooty iron–porphyrin pigment they contain (Fig. 2.69), and except for the flukes and soft contents, they superficially resemble heavily pigmented melanotic tumors. Commonly, these flukes pass from the liver to the lungs of cattle, to produce lesions of similar character. In sheep, this parasite wanders continuously in the liver, producing black, tortuous tracts, which may be 2 cm in diameter, and extensive parenchymal destruction. Even a few flukes may kill a sheep.

The dicrocoelid flukes inhabit both biliary and pancreatic ducts. *Eurytrema pancreaticum* prefers the pancreas (and is described in Chapter 3 of this volume), but in heavy infestations can be found in the bile ducts. *Dicrocoelium* and *Platynosomum* prefer the bile ducts. These are small, narrow flukes 0.5–1.0 cm long and may easily be mistaken for small masses of inspissated bile pigment. They are not highly pathogenic, and even in heavy infestations, there may be no signs of the toxemia observed in infestations by *Fasciola hepatica*. These flukes may occur as mixed infestations.

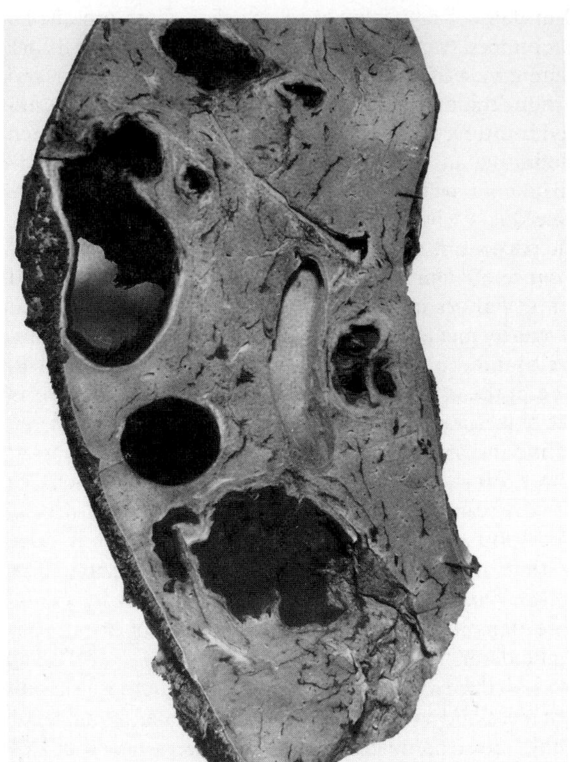

Fig. 2.69 Destructive pigmented lesions produced by *Fascioloides magna*. Ox.

Platynosomum fastosum is a parasite of cats in North America and the Amazonian regions of South America. The life cycle involves snails and lizards and presumably an arthropod. The infested livers are enlarged, friable, and may be bilestained. There is catarrhal inflammation of biliary passages, but it is not severe, and the walls may not be much thickened. The ducts are dilated and easily visible. There are vague digestive disturbances, and heavy infestations may cause complete anorexia and death.

Dicrocoelium hospes is found in cattle in countries south of the Sahara. Little is known of it, but it is presumed to be comparable in all respects to the better known *D. dendriticum* (the lancet fluke), which is common in Europe and Asia and sparsely distributed in the Americas and North Africa. This fluke is no more fastidious in its choice of final hosts than many other species of flukes, and depending on opportunity, it can infest all domestic species, with the possible exception of cats. It is, however, of most importance as a parasite of sheep and cattle, in which it inhabits the bile ducts. Other domestic species and rodents are important as reservoirs.

The life cycle of *Dicrocoelium dendriticum* differs in some details from that of *Fasciola hepatica*. The eggs are embryonated when laid and do not hatch until swallowed by one of the many genera of land snails that are the first intermediate hosts. In the snails, the mother sporocyst produces a second generation of daughter sporocysts, which in turn produce cercariae. The cercariae leave the snail in damp weather and are expelled from the snail's lung, clumped together in slime balls. The slime balls are not infective until the cercariae are swallowed by, and encyst in, the ant *Formica fusca*; other ants may be involved in different countries. The cycle is completed when the definitive hosts swallow the ants. The route of migration of the larvae from the gut to the liver is probably via the bile ducts from the duodenum.

The pathologic changes in the liver produced by *Dicrocoelium dendriticum* are those of a cholangiohepatitis that is less severe than that produced by *Fasciola hepatica*. The severity and diffuseness of the hepatic lesion is determined by the number of lancet flukes present, and they may be in the thousands. The dilated ducts are darkened by the flukes and their eggs. Even in early infestations, there may be some scarring of the organ at its periphery. In heavy infestations of long standing, there is extensive biliary fibrosis, producing an organ that is indurated, scarred, and lumpy, and that at the margins may bear areas that are shrunken and completely sclerotic. The histologic changes are the same as those in fascioliasis, with perhaps a more remarkable hyperplasia of the mucous glands of the large ducts.

The opisthorchid flukes are parasites in the bile ducts of carnivores. They may also occur in swine and humans, and one species, *Opisthorchis sinensis* (*Clonorchis sinensis*), is an important human parasite. There is some uncertainty regarding the proper classification of these flukes, and some of those given may not be valid species. The life cycles, where known, include molluscs as the first intermediate hosts and freshwater fish as the second.

Metorchis conjunctus is the common liver fluke of cats and dogs in North America and is important as a parasite of sled dogs in the Canadian Northwest Territories. The first intermediate host is the snail *Amnicola limosa porosa,* and the second is the common suckerfish *Catostomus commersonii*. The cercariae actively burrow into the musculature of the fish to encyst and become infective. The immature flukes crawl into the bile ducts from the duodenum and mature in ~28 days. Infestations may persist for more than 5 years. *Metorchis albidis* has been described in a dog from Alaska; *Parametorchis complexus,* in cats in the United States of America; and *Amphimerus pseudofelineus,* in cats and coyotes in the United States of America and Panama; the life cycles are not known but are presumed to include fish.

Opisthorchis felineus is the lanceolate fluke of the bile ducts of cats, dogs, and foxes in Europe and Russia. It is particularly common in eastern Europe and Siberia and is more sparse in other areas. *Opisthorchis sinensis* is well documented as the Oriental or Chinese liver fluke; it is endemic in Japan, Korea, southern China, and Southeast Asia. There are additional species of *Opisthorchis* in humans and animals, but they are less well known than the species cited. The first intermediate hosts for the miracidia of *O. tenuicollis* and *O. sinensis* are snails of the genus *Bithynia,* and several genera of cyprinid fishes can act as second intermediate hosts.

Pseudamphistomum truncatum occurs in carnivores and humans sporadically in Europe and Asia. Its life cycle is as for *Opisthorchis*.

The opisthorchid flukes, so far as known, resemble *Dicrocoelium* in migrating up the bile ducts to their habitat. This may be the reason that they are more numerous in the left than in the right lobes of the liver. They can probably live in the liver for as long as the host lives. The pathologic effects are comparable to those of *D. dendriticum*. Light infestations may be asymptomatic, and heavy infestations may cause jaundice, chronic cholangiohepatitis, and severe biliary fibrosis. Both in humans and animals, adenomatous and carcinomatous changes of the biliary glands have occurred in association with these parasites; the association is probably more than coincidental.

Bibliography

Anderson, P. J., Berrett, S., and Patterson, D. S. P. Resistance to *Fasciola hepatica* in cattle. II. Biochemical and morphological observations. *J Comp Pathol* **88:** 245–251, 1978.

Arundel, J. H., and Hamir, A. N. *Fascioloides magna* in cattle. *Aust Vet J* **58:** 35–36, 1982.

Ross, J. G., Todd, J. R., and Dow, C. Single experimental infections of calves with the liver fluke, *Fasciola hepatica* (Linnaeus 1758). *J Comp Pathol* **76:** 67–81, 1966.

Rushton, B., and Murray, M. Hepatic pathology of a primary experimental infection of *Fasciola hepatica* in sheep. *J Comp Pathol* **87:** 459–470, 1977.

Taylor, D., and Perri, S. F. Experimental infection of cats with the liver fluke *Platynosomum concinnum*. *Am J Vet Res* **38:** 51–54, 1977.

Watson, T. G., and Croll, N. A. Clinical changes caused by liver fluke *Metorchis conjunctus* in cats. *Vet Pathol* **18:** 778–785, 1981.

Weensvoort, P., and Over, H. J. Cellular proliferations of bile ductules and gamma-glutamyl transpeptidase in livers and sera of young cattle following a single infection with *Fasciola hepatica*. *Vet Q* **4:** 161–172, 1982.

E. Miscellaneous Inflammatory Disease

Focal or diffuse **fetal hepatitis** characterizes a number of intrauterine fetal infections (see Diseases of the Pregnant Uterus, in Volume 3, Chapter 4). Whether caused by bacteria or viruses, focal necrosis is often present and bacteria or viral inclusions can often be identified (Fig. 2.70). Frequently, however the lesions are subtle and diffuse and without necrosis, and the inflammatory process may be difficult to distinguish from hematopoiesis. There is inflammatory edema of the connective tissues of the portal triads with distension of lymphatics there and beneath Glisson's capsule. A preponderance of mature granulocytes in the portal triads and in the adventitia of hepatic veins helps to distinguish inflammatory infiltrates from hematopoietic foci, which are predominantly in sinusoids.

Giant-cell hepatitis, which occurs in humans in a variety of congenital and neonatal infections, in association with some metabolic disorders such as galactosemia and in

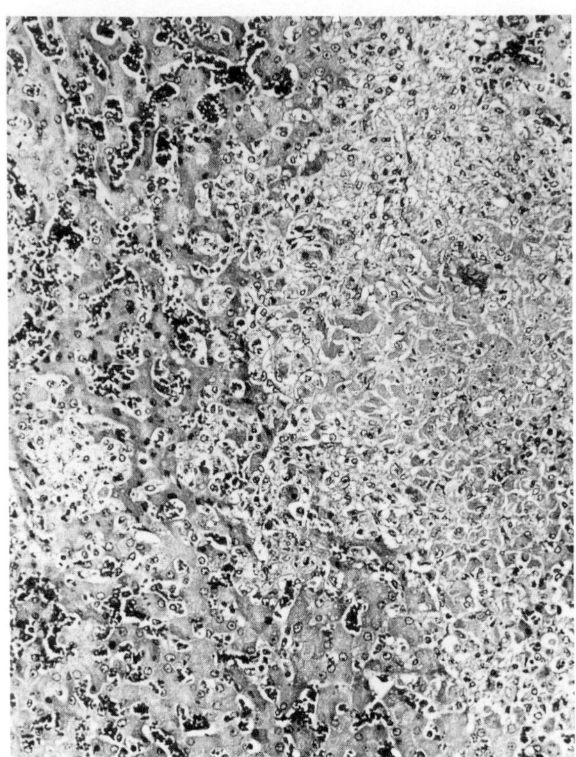

Fig. 2.70 Focal coagulative necrosis in equine herpesvirus-1 infection. Foal.

some cases of Down's syndrome, may not be properly described as hepatitis. An alternative title is neonatal giant-cell transformation and response to liver damage associated with conjugated hyperbilirubinemia. This is an uncommon lesion in animals but is recorded in cats, calves, and aborted foals. There is good evidence for maternal leptospirosis in some cases in foals.

The liver is deeply bilestained. Histologically, the acinar structure is effaced, and the blood vessels, engorged. The hepatocytes are large and syncytial and may contain 10 or more nuclei. The pale or ballooned cytoplasm contains bile pigments, and cytoplasmic invaginations into hepatocyte nuclei are common. Inflammatory cells are not conspicuous.

Hypertrophic liver cirrhosis in calves is described from Germany and occasionally observed elsewhere. It may not be a pathologic entity. Death may occur in liver failure within a few days to weeks of birth, or the disease may be discovered at slaughter for veal. The liver is moderately enlarged with rounded borders, very firm, but smooth on the surface and gray. Histologically, there is some biliary hyperplasia, but the lesion is dominated by diffuse fibrosis infiltrated in the early stages by mononuclear inflammatory cells. No cause has been identified. Early lesions may be found in unborn or aborted calves.

Protozoal hepatitis is due mainly to *Toxoplasma, Neospora,* and *Leishmania,* described elsewhere. Hepatic coccidiosis, expressed as acute cholangiohepatitis similar to that in mink and rabbits, is observed in isolated cases in the goat, calf, and dog. These presumably aberrant infections do not develop to the sexual stages, and the organisms are unclassified.

Bibliography

Doll, K. *et al.* Leberzirrhosen bei jungen Kälberin. *Tierärztl Prax* **17:** 149–156, 1989.

Lipscomb, T.P. *et al.* Intrahepatic biliary coccidiosis in a dog. *Vet Pathol* **26:** 343–345, 1989.

Wilkie, I.W. *et al.* Giant-cell hepatitis in four aborted foals: A possible leptospiral infection. *Can Vet J* **29:** 1003–1004, 1988.

XI. Toxic Liver Disease

A. Hepatic Biotransformations

There are many intoxications to which the liver is more susceptible than other tissues. Immediately there arises a paradox: the liver has an acknowledged central role in detoxification and excretion of xenobiotic substances, yet it may undergo almost complete necrosis when exposed to compounds that leave the rest of the body virtually untouched. Attempts to resolve this paradox have, naturally, assumed an association between this susceptibility and the more unique aspects of liver function. The biotransformation of xenobiotics is itself a well-developed, although not unique, function of hepatocytes, and it is now known that a large class of toxins are hepatotoxic because, in transformation of these substances into excretable metabolites, the liver converts them to intermediate reactive radicals that are much more toxic than the parent molecules. If the original compound is of relatively low toxicity, as is the case with carbon tetrachloride as an example, it follows that the liver will suffer much more damage than any other tissue because the toxic metabolite, which is usually unstable and short-lived, tends to damage only the cytoplasm of the cell in which it is produced. The usual periacinar location of such liver injury is related to the relatively high concentration in this zone of the microsomal mixed-function oxidases responsible for these biotransformations.

Compounds that are hepatotoxic tend to be fat soluble rather than water soluble, because the latter are more readily eliminated by the kidney. Many of the biotransformations effected by the microsomal enzymes are directed to the conversion of lipophilic substances to water soluble substances for renal clearance.

When death accompanies acute toxic hepatic necrosis, pulmonary congestion and edema are often observed as well. A possible reason for this phenomenon is that sufficient toxic intermediate metabolites and fibrin degradation products are swept from the liver to damage the lung. Apart from the probable occurrence of overflow of toxic pyrrolic metabolites from the liver after large doses of pyrrolizidine alkaloids, there is little experimental support for this suggestion. Lung tissue has been shown to possess its own complement of mixed-function oxidases and is therefore capable of performing its own suicidal biotransformations.

When the role of intermediary metabolism in hepatotoxicity was recognized, it soon became apparent that the activity of the responsible enzymes could be increased (induced) by exposure to a range of nontoxic xenobiotics or to intrinsic compounds such as steroid hormones. This increase should lead to increased susceptibility to certain hepatotoxins. Some toxins have been demonstrated to depress these enzymes, thus conferring some protection against the acute hepatotoxicity of other toxins. It has been shown, for example, that a small dose of carbon tetrachloride will prevent death in rats given a normally lethal dose of the same toxin shortly afterward, carbon tetrachloride in this instance having the opposite of a cumulative effect. This protection is due to the small prior dose's binding with and inactivating the enzymes of the mixed-function oxidase system, in particular, the terminal heme cytochrome P-450. This inactivation and subsequent protection may explain the apparently anomalous results of some dosage trials, in which a larger amount of toxic material given in divided doses may cause less liver damage than a small amount given as a single dose.

Other factors such as nutritional status may be involved. Prolonged starvation, for example, may result in the catabolism of microsomal protein and hence reduction of enzyme activity, thus conferring some resistance to this sort of hepatotoxicity. On the other hand, well-nourished animals, after a short fast sufficient only to deplete glycogen stores, may be very susceptible to hepatotoxicity. It has been suggested that glycogen in the cytoplasm may exert a protective effect against toxic reactive radicals by trapping them before they damage the more vital membranous components of the cell.

During discussion earlier of massive necrosis, there was mention of the importance of reduced glutathione and the selenium–vitamin E status of the liver cell in relation to dietary hepatic necrosis, and the ability of the membranes of the cell to cope with toxic endogenous free radicals. It is therefore reasonable to expect that livers deficient in these factors will be more susceptible to those hepatotoxins which are degraded to toxic intermediates.

With so many variables involved, it is not surprising that the outcome of naturally occurring exposure to this class of hepatotoxins is unpredictable. Both the severity and pattern of the liver lesions depend on the sum of the variables and on the tempo of metabolic reactions triggered by the episodes of intoxication. The complexity of these interactions is exemplified by experimental manipulation of the pattern of necrosis produced by **ngaione,** a furanosesquiterpene component of essential oils from species of Myoporaceae. Administration of this toxin to normal animals at certain dose rates produces, in a high proportion of cases, a distinctive pattern of midzonal necrosis (Fig. 2.71), a lesion previously described. If prior to intoxication the animals have had their microsomal mixed-function oxidases induced by administration of barbiturate or dichlorodiphenyltrichloroethane (DDT), the predominant distribution of necrosis produced by ngaione is periportal (Figs. 2.20, 2.26). On the other hand, if the activity of the enzymes has been chemically suppressed, the ngaione-induced lesion is predominantly periacinar. The explanation of this phenomenon rests on the fact that the activity of the microsomal enzymes is always greater in the periacinar zone, even after induction or suppression, and assumes that ngaione and related compounds are degraded by microsomes by rate-limited processes whose efficiency is proportional to the concentration of the mixed-function oxidases present in the cell. Accordingly, if the concentration of enzyme is high (as in the periacinar hepatocytes in the normal animal), the parent compound is completely degraded to nontoxic metabolites so rapidly that there will be accumulation of insufficient toxic intermediates to damage the cell. In the normal animal, then, necrosis will occur only in those midzonal hepatocytes that have enzyme sufficient to produce toxic intermediates, but insufficient to completely degrade these to safe levels. The periportal hepatocytes will not be damaged because they have not enough enzyme to produce sufficient toxic intermediates from the parent compound. In the induced animal, enough enzyme is present in periacinar and midzonal cells for complete detoxification, and the necrosis is then periportal. In the enzyme-suppressed liver, only the periacinar hepatocytes retain enzyme activity sufficient to produce lethal concentrations of the toxic

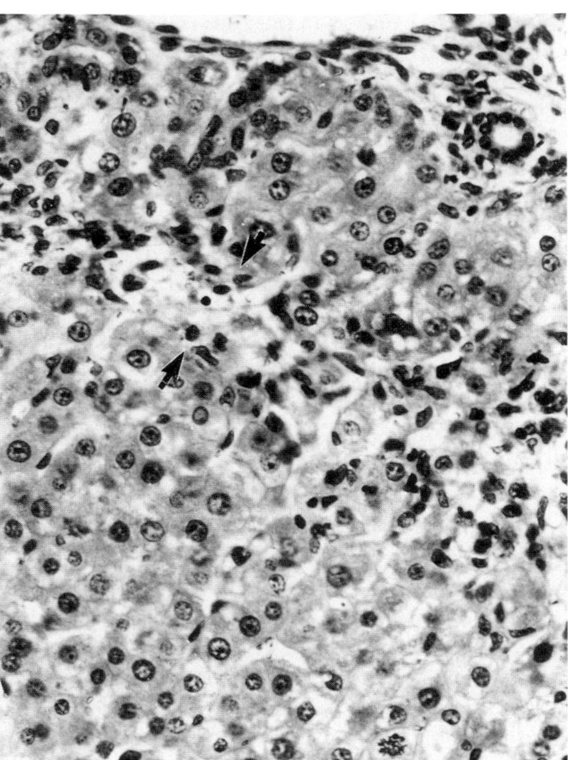

Fig. 2.71 Midzonal necrosis. The necrotic hepatocytes have been removed (arrows) during recovery phase after ngaione poisoning. Sheep. (Courtesy of A. A. Seawright.)

intermediate; the necrosis in this case is therefore periacinar. This explanation may apply to those naturally occurring instances of periportal and midzonal toxic hepatic necrosis that appear from time to time.

Rarely, biotransforming enzymes may be more concentrated in the periportal than in the other zones, leading consistently to periportal necrosis on exposure to compounds that are degraded by them to toxic intermediates. The classic example of this is the effect of allyl formate or allyl alcohol on rat liver. Both these substances are metabolized to acrolein by alcohol dehydrogenase, a microsomal enzyme that is more concentrated in the periportal hepatocytes. Acrolein is an alkylating aldehyde capable of producing lethal membrane damage. The necrosis can be prevented by pretreatment with pyrazole, which inhibits alcohol dehydrogenase.

B. Preferential Uptake of Hepatotoxins

There are other reasons for the peculiar vulnerability of the liver to some toxins; these depend on the capacity of the organ to selectively concentrate certain intrinsic compounds and xenobiotics. There are transport systems that greatly facilitate the entry of bile acids into the hepatocytes, and it follows that if these mechanisms promote the uptake of toxins, then the liver will be preferentially damaged by such agents. This mechanism has been established as part of the basis of the hepatoxicity of phalloidin, the toxic polypeptide from *Amanita,* and there is evidence that the hepatotoxicity of other water-soluble toxins, such as atractylosides, may depend on similar mechanisms. As will be described later, the hepatotoxic component of chronic copper poisoning of ruminants is certainly the result of the peculiar avidity of the liver for this element, particularly in sheep.

In the following sections, the hepatotoxicities will be somewhat arbitrarily separated into **acute** and **chronic.** Although it is recognized that the difference between acute and chronic hepatotoxicity is often simply a matter of dose-rate, it is convenient to categorize the sources according to the syndrome of liver damage they most commonly produce.

Bibliography

Clawson, G. A. Mechanisms of carbon tetrachloride hepatotoxicity. *Pathol Immunopathol Res* **8:** 104–112, 1989.

Comporti, M. Biology of disease. Lipid peroxidation and cellular damage in toxic liver injury. *Lab Invest* **53:** 599–623, 1985.

Freeman, B. A., and Crapo, J. D. Biology of disease: Free radicals and tissue injury. *Lab Invest* **47:** 412–426, 1982.

Gopinath, G., and Ford, E. J. H. Location of liver injury and extent of bilirubinemia in experimental lesions. *Vet Pathol* **9:** 99–108, 1972.

McGavin, M. D., and Knake, R. Hepatic midzonal necrosis in a pig fed aflatoxin and a horse fed moldy hay. *Vet Pathol* **14:** 182–187, 1977.

Pass, M. A. The relationship of drug metabolism to hepatotoxicity with some examples in sheep. *Vet Annual* **22:** 129–134, 1982.

Reid, W. D. Mechanism of allyl alcohol-induced hepatic necrosis. *Experientia* **28:** 1058–1061, 1972.

Russo, M. A., Kane, A. B., and Farber, J. L. Ultrastructural pathology of phalloidin-intoxicated hepatocytes in the presence and absence of extracellular calcium. *Am J Pathol* **99:** 159–174, 1980.

Ying, T. S., Sarma, D. S. R., and Farber, E. The sequential analysis of liver cell necrosis. *Am J Pathol* **99:** 159–174, 1980.

Zieve, L. *et al.* Hepatic regenerative enzyme activity after pericentral and periportal lobular toxic injury. *Toxicol Appl Pharmacol* **86:** 147–158, 1986.

C. Acute Hepatotoxicity

It is emphasized that the outcome of acute exposure to hepatotoxins is often an unpredictable product of many factors. The same factors operate in chronic hepatotoxicity but are compounded by variations in rates of exposure and by adaptive responses of the liver. For example, continuous exposure to a toxin may maintain detoxification mechanisms at such a pitch as to enable the liver to handle concentrations of toxin that would cause severe damage if administered intermittently.

The histologic changes in acute toxic hepatic injury are rather stereotyped. They range from single-cell necrosis, through confluent coagulative and shrinkage zonal necrosis, to massive hemorrhagic destruction that includes sinusoidal lining cells. The histology of these acute intoxications is usually characterized by severe periacinar necrosis (Figs. 2.25B, 2.72A,B). Rarely, the pattern of necrosis may be periportal (Figs. 2.20, 2.26) or midzonal (Fig. 2.71). The characteristics of these injuries are described under Patterns of Hepatic Necrosis (Section V of this chapter). Depending on the metabolic status of the animal, there may be variably severe fatty or hydropic change in hepatocytes adjacent to the necrotic zones (Figs. 2.25, 2.72A), and the necrotic cells may accumulate calcium, but these variations on the general theme have little diagnostic or pathogenetic specificity. In sublethally injured cells there may be spectacular clumping of smooth endoplasmic reticulum (Fig. 2.8), particularly in the periacinar zones. This change is not specific.

The clinical and gross characteristics of fatal acute intoxications are rather consistent, regardless of the origin of the toxin. The animal dies after a brief period of dullness, anorexia, colic, and a variety of neurologic disturbances, including convulsions; these are attributed to hepatic encephalopathy (see Liver Failure, Section VII of this chapter). Postmortem examination reveals a slight excess of clear, yellow abdominal fluid, which contains sufficient fibrinogen to form a loose, nonadherent clot. The liver may be deep reddish purple and obviously swollen in very heavily intoxicated cases, with prominent edema of the gallbladder wall and its attachments, and there is distension of lymphatics of the serosa of the gallbladder and of the porta hepatis. In fatal cases where the toxic dose more nearly approaches the 50% lethal dose (LD_{50}), there is less severe hemorrhage, and the liver is paler and shows more obvious acinar pattern.

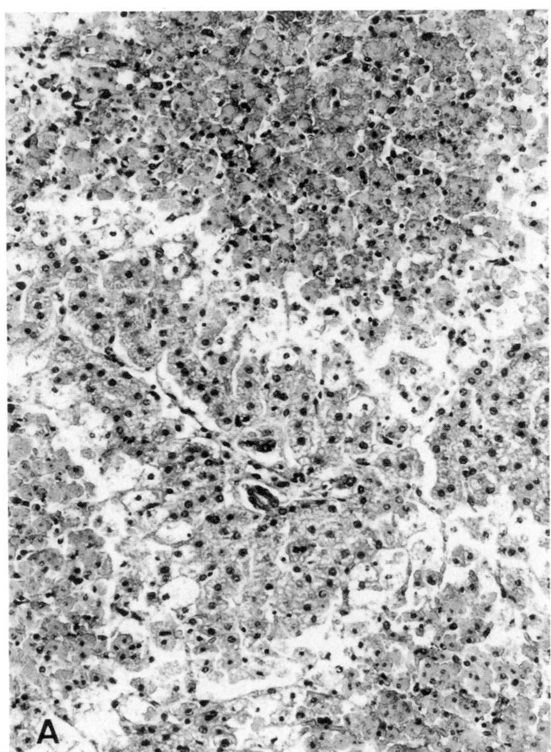

Fig. 2.72A Acute coagulative and hemorrhagic periacinar necrosis in *Cestrum parqui* poisoning. Ox. The periportal and the necrotic zones are separated by a margin zone of hydropic hepatocytes.

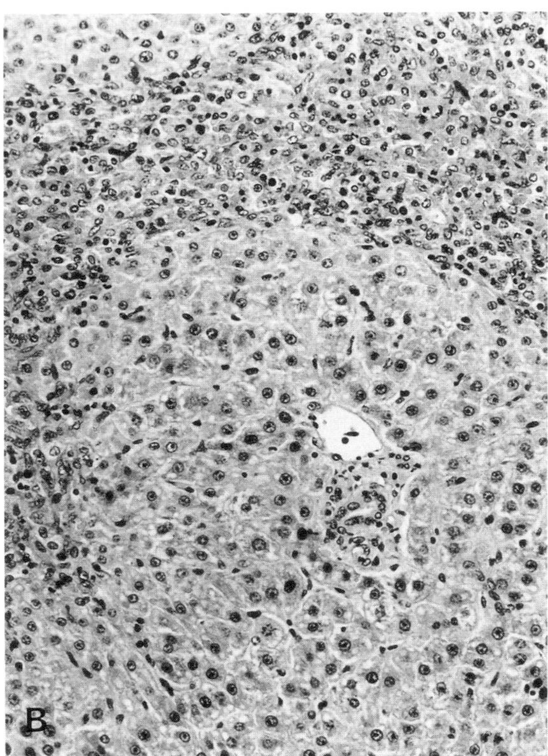

Fig. 2.72B *Cestrum* poisoning. Ox. Repair of the periacinar injury 4 days after sublethal intoxication.

In acute fatal hepatotoxicities there is almost always widespread hemorrhage terminally; petechiae and ecchymoses are seen most consistently on serous membranes, especially on the epi- and endocardium. Diffuse hemorrhage into the gut, particularly the duodenum in ruminants, is also common, as are hemorrhages into the wall of the gallbladder. The hemorrhage in these organs is probably related to damage done by toxic metabolites excreted in the bile. Hemorrhages elsewhere are due to excessive consumption of clotting factors by the disrupted sinusoids on the one hand and, on the other, to failure of the damaged liver to replace those factors.

Photosensitization is not a feature of the acutely fatal hepatotoxicities, unless it occurs in the recovery phase in sublethally intoxicated herbivores; in these it is likely to be relatively mild and transient.

The causes of acute hepatotoxicity include administered drugs, but phytotoxins may produce spectacular losses in free-ranging herbivores; usually the victims are ruminants either that are under some nutritional stress or that have been introduced suddenly to new grazing; herds and flocks of traveling stock are particularly prone to this sort of accident. Other factors involving the plant, such as stage of growth, are of paramount importance in determining toxicity. An extreme example of this is poisoning by *Xanthium pungens* (Noogoorah burr) in Australia, in which the toxin is greatly concentrated in the cotyledons. Since the seeds are rarely eaten, even by cattle, field intoxications occur only when this plant is eaten shortly after germination.

The botanical range of plants capable of producing acute hepatotoxicity is extremely broad, toxic genera being found in families as diverse as the relatively primitive Cycadaceae and blue-green algae, through the Compositae and Solanaceae. The toxic compounds are probably also as diverse, but in many cases, these remain to be identified. An exhaustive review of the toxicity of these plants would be repetitive; instead, some of the better known and more representative examples are discussed, with comments on special features where appropriate.

1. Blue-Green Algae

These microscopic plants growing as a bloom on lakes and ponds may be highly toxic. Outbreaks of poisoning are not common, but they occur in many countries and may be responsible for heavy mortality among animals or birds that take the algae when drinking. Most well-documented cases have involved *Microcystis aeruginosa*, a bloom that may poison after the algae have been piled by wind against the shores of expanses of water that have accumulated phosphates and nitrates as runoff from fertilized soils (Fig. 2.33A,B). Other toxic species are included in the genera *Anabaena* and *Aphanizomenon*, but the nomenclature of this group of plants is confused. Not all isolates of *Microcystis* are toxic. It is not known to what extent natural poisoning is caused by the algae themselves in their various stages of growth and decay, or to what extent it may be caused by saprophytic bacteria. Some deaths are too sudden to be due to liver damage and are probably the result of the fast-death factor that has been found in some blooms. The syndrome is one of collapse and prostration, with hyperesthesia that may be manifested as convulsions and death within a few minutes; there are no specific lesions in this form of the toxicosis.

Most work has been done on the hepatotoxin, which is a polypeptide whose amino acid content seems to be variable. It is possible that this toxin uses bile acid transport mechanisms to enter the hepatocyte, and that it may not need microsomal metabolism to exert its effect. Mice can be completely protected from a lethal dose of microcystin by prior administration of either rifampin or cyclosporin-A, both of which block bile acid uptake by hepatocytes. Likewise, sodium deoxycholate and bromsulfothalein, which inhibit uptake of microcystin by isolated rat hepatocytes, also protect these cells from damage by the toxin.

The mechanism of cell damage includes disorganization of cytoskeletal filaments, which is probably responsible for distortion of hepatocyte cell membranes *in vitro,* and for the dissociation of hepatocytes seen early in intoxication *in vivo*.

The toxin is released when the algae disintegrate, which may occur spontaneously in water, or after application of copper sulfate, or in the rumen or stomach after ingestion. Ruminants are most commonly poisoned, but poisoning has been reported in horses, dogs, and domestic poultry.

The distribution of the necrosis is usually periacinar to massive but is occasionally periportal or rarely, midzonal. The pattern may vary within one liver and from case to case. In subacute intoxications, the liver is severely fatty, and necrosis is limited to individual hepatocytes or small groups of them instead of being zonal. Phagolysosomes and bile pigments accumulate in the cytoplasm, and there is slight biliary proliferation and fibrosis.

2. Cycadales

Members of this order have been responsible for chronic hepatotoxicity and neurotoxicity in cattle, but acute hepatotoxicity has been reported in sheep that have eaten the seeds or young leaves of species of Zamiaceae. The toxin responsible is methylazoxymethanol, which is the aglycone of various nontoxic glycosides, including cycasin and macrozamin, in these plants. The toxin is split from the glycoside in the gut, and its hepatotoxicity is the result of further metabolism in hepatic microsomes; the pattern of necrosis is thus periacinar. The metabolites of the aglycone are apparently potent alkylating agents, and the chronic liver lesions reflect this; there is megalocytosis (which is not so persistent as that of pyrrolizidine alkaloid poisoning), nuclear hyperchromasia, cholestasis, fatty change, and varying degrees of diffuse fibrosis. Cytosegresome formation and cytoplasmic invaginations into nuclei are apparently not a prominent feature. There is fairly consistent tubular nephrosis.

Chronic cycad poisoning of cattle causes a chronic nervous disorder characterized by a progressive proprioceptive deficit. This is due to axonopathy in upper spinocerebellar and lower corticospinal tracts. The axonopathy, morphologically subtle at first, may progress eventually to frank Wallerian degeneration. Two neurotoxic agents have been isolated from cycads; neither is methylazoxymethanol. Cattle affected by the neurologic syndrome often have some degree of chronic liver injury.

3. Solanaceae

There are many species of genus *Cestrum. Cestrum diurnum* is a cause of enzootic calcinosis in cattle; the other known toxic species all produce similar hepatic disease. Speciation within the genus is uncertain, partly due to hybridization. The species named as hepatotoxic are *C. parqui, C. laevigatum,* and *C. aurantiacum.*

Cestrum spp., the ink-berry plants, cause acute hepatotoxicity in the field in South America, southern and central Africa, and Australia. Cattle are more frequently poisoned than are other species, but sheep and goats are susceptible, and fowl may be if they eat the fruit. The young leaves and unripened berries are the most toxic parts of the plant. There are no records of chronic liver disease caused by this plant, and photosensitization is rarely seen. The toxin is water soluble and has recently been identified as an atractyloside. The pattern of necrosis is consistently periacinar (Figs. 2.25B, 2.72A,B).

4. Compositae

The toxin of *Xanthium pungens,* the cocklebur, is concentrated in the cotyledons. Pigs and cattle are the subject of most intoxications, usually after rain has allowed germination following a period of feed scarcity. The clinical signs and lesions are not specific, being those described for acute hepatotoxins in general. The toxin carboxyatractyloside is present in the achenes and cotyledons and is responsible for the field intoxications: it is therefore not surprising that the liver pathology of experimental *Xanthium* and *Cestrum* intoxications are identical.

Helichrysum blandowskianum is hepatotoxic to cattle and has caused sudden deaths with periacinar necrosis in the field in southern Australia. The toxin has not been identified.

Three species of Compositae in South Africa, *Asaemia axillaris, Athanasia trifurcata,* and *Lasiospermum bipinnatum,* have been associated with field outbreaks of acute hepatotoxicity, but it seems that they are more often responsible for more chronic disease with photosensitivity. Experimental intoxications by all three of these species have in some animals produced midzonal as well as periacinar necrosis; a periportal distribution is typical of *Lasiospermum* in sheep.

5. Ulmaceae

Trema aspera, the poison peach, has caused severe losses in cattle in Australia. The syndrome is acute, there is no photosensitization, and mildly intoxicated animals may recover completely. The toxic principle is a glycoside, designated trematoxin. The pattern of necrosis is consistently periacinar and is identical in appearance to that of *Cestrum* and *Xanthium* poisoning (Fig. 2.72A,B).

The gross and microscopic lesions of experimental poisoning by *Trema, Xanthium pungens,* and *Cestrum parqui* have been shown to be identical in all morphologic respects in the same group of sheep.

6. Myoporaceae

The variation in pattern of zonal necrosis (Figs. 2.20, 2.26, 2.27, 2.71) seen in intoxication by the Myoporaceae has been discussed earlier. Species so far incriminated are *Myoporum deserti, M. acuminatum, M. insulare,* and *M. tetrandum* of Australia, and *M. laetum* of New Zealand. The toxic oils are contained in the leaves and branchlets, but within the species there is variation in the chemical characters and toxicity of the oils; not all strains of toxic species are toxic. There is some delay between ingestion and absorption of the furanosesquiterpenoid oils, the best known of which is ngaione, which are responsible for intoxication, so 24–48 hr may elapse before signs of toxicity appear. Some animals live long enough to become photosensitized; others may die much more rapidly, with pulmonary edema. The edema appears to be a direct effect of the toxin after metabolism by alveolar lining cells.

Livers from intoxicated sheep may show a striking, broad pattern of variable congestion and even infarction, which is superimposed on the more regular acinar pattern of zonal necrosis. Microscopically these livers show acute fibrinoid necrosis of portal vessels, which suggests that the coarser lesions may have a vascular basis.

7. Carbon Tetrachloride

The toxin carbon tetrachloride has been mentioned already as the archetype of toxic metabolism, in which necrogenic membranous lipoperoxidation follows the evolution of a highly reactive radical from the parent molecule after microsomal transformation. Carbon tetrachloride has been intensively studied in the development of laboratory animal models of hepatic necrosis, fatty liver, and hepatic fibrosis and remodeling, but it has also been used for many years as a fasciolicide. Under certain conditions there have been severe losses, usually of sheep, following administration of recommended anthelmintic doses. Part of the early loss after drenching is due to respiratory dysfunction when the chemical is delivered into the pharynx or trachea.

Much effort has been exerted to define the factors leading to increased susceptibility to delayed mortality from hepatic disease. Hepatic factors such as induced microsomal metabolism and impaired antioxidant capacity may be important in the toxicity in sheep under field conditions. Additional nutritional factors, however, may be involved; for example, high intake of protein after dosing may produce a concentration of ammonia in the portal blood that is too high for the damaged liver to detoxify, resulting in death from ammonia intoxication.

Very severe acute carbon tetrachloride poisoning produces severe periacinar to massive liver necrosis. In less severe intoxications there may be more obvious fatty change in hepatocytes surrounding the necrotic zones than that seen in other acute hepatotoxicities, so that, grossly, the liver may be very pale and swollen. In these animals there are degenerative changes in renal tubular epithelium. Photosensitization after intoxication is slight or does not occur, and survival beyond a few days should allow complete restoration of normal hepatic histology. Hexachlorethane, tetrachlorethylene, and chloroform are other chlorinated hydrocarbons with apparently similar hepatotoxic properties, but these agents are little used now as medicinal agents.

8. Cresols

The tarred walls and floors of piggeries and the clay pigeons used as targets by gun clubs are occasionally responsible, by virtue of contained cresols, for poisoning of pigs. The poisoning may be acute, with severe periacinar necrosis the only significant lesion; or it may be chronic, with jaundice, ascites, and severe anemia added to the pathologic picture.

9. Phosphorus

White phosphorus is still used for vermin control. It is mixed with fat in order to promote absorption, and much of the dose is transported to the liver shortly after ingestion. A small amount may be lost by vomition, for elemental phosphorus is directly irritant to the gastrointestinal tract. The mechanism of phosphorus hepatotoxicity is uncertain; it is apparent that metabolism to a toxic intermediate is not necessary, but there is some dispute on the involvement of lipoperoxidation in the hepatocellular injury. There is evidence that protein synthesis is impaired early and that this is responsible for the lipid accumulation that is so prominent a feature.

A few hours after ingestion of phosphorus there is severe colic and vomition, due to the irritant nature of the element. If the animal survives this acute phase there may be apparent recovery for a few days, followed by jaundice and other signs of liver failure, and death by about the fifth day. At autopsy there is severe icterus and fatty liver, the latter sometimes being predominantly periportal in distribution. Hepatocellular necrosis is not often a prominent feature histologically, notwithstanding the evidence of liver failure. Fatty change is also seen in the myocardium and distal nephrons.

10. Iron

Iron–dextran complexes have been widely used in the treatment and prevention of anemia in suckling swine. Very occasionally, severe losses may occur in animals with marginal vitamin E–selenium deficiency; in these cases there is, apparently, iron-catalyzed lipoperoxidation in hepatocytes and muscle. The result of this, as far as the liver is concerned, is sudden massive necrosis similar in many respects to that of hepatosis dietetica. Large amounts of potassium escape into the circulation from the liver and muscle, and sudden death may result from the cardiotoxicity of this ion. At autopsy, there is staining of the subcutaneous tissues and lymph nodes near the site of injection, and there are lesions in the liver or skeletal muscles. The liver is of normal size, and of normal color or pale, depending on whether or not the animal is anemic. The presence of an underlying necrosis may be indicated only by the numerous small or large hemorrhages present on the capsular and cut surface (Fig. 2.73). Insoluble iron compounds with the staining reactions of hemosiderin are found in mesenchymal cells in many tissues, the largest amounts being in macrophages of the local lymph nodes and in the Kupffer cells.

Death in piglets from hepatic necrosis occurs about 10 hr after administration, but saccharated iron may, in the same circumstances, produce acute widespread muscle necrosis at about 24 hr rather than hepatic necrosis. The myocardium is not affected.

Acute hepatotoxicity is reported in young foals due to administration of a proprietary paste of iron and yeast products, given as a dietary supplement within a few hours of birth. Not all foals so treated became sick, but those which were, developed severe acute periacinar necrosis, resembling the disease in piglets.

11. Sawfly Larvae

This acute hepatotoxicity of cattle and, to a lesser extent, sheep, is of particular interest in that the toxin is present in an insect, the larva of the sawfly *Lophyrotoma interruptus*. This larva is parasitic on the leaves of the tree *Eucalyptus melanophloia,* and heavy infestations may occur in parts of northeastern Australia. On completion of feeding, masses of larvae sometimes accumulate at the base of the tree where they may die and decompose. Cattle in particular find these masses attractive, perhaps as a result of nutritional stress. The hepatotoxin is an octapeptide, which produces acute periacinar necrosis with no specific features. Whether or not the larvae synthesize the toxin, or concentrate it from the tree, has not been determined. Recently, however, a similar intoxication by the blue-black birch sawfly, *Arge pullata* from birch trees, has been recognized in sheep and goats in Denmark. The production of such similar intoxications from unrelated substrates suggests that this class of insect manufactures the hepatotoxin *de novo*.

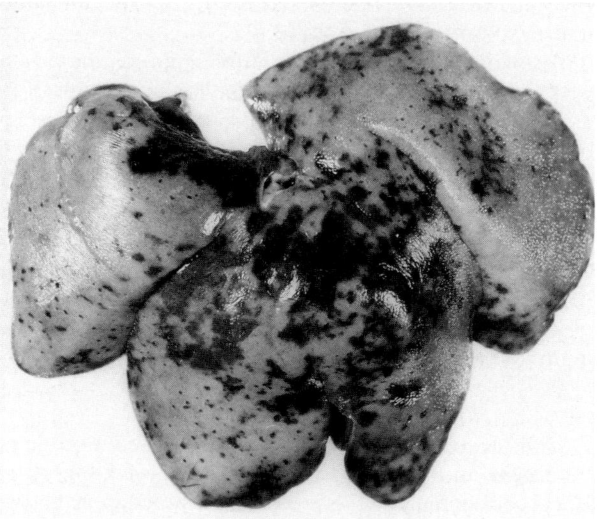

Fig. 2.73 Early massive necrosis with random hemorrhage and pallor. Iron dextran poisoning. Pig.

Bibliography

Acland, H. M. *et al.* Toxic hepatopathy in neonatal foals. *Vet Pathol* **21:** 3–9, 1984.

Baker, D. C., and Green, R. A. Coagulation defects of aflatoxin-intoxicated rabbits. *Vet Pathol* **24:** 62–70, 1987.

Falconer, I. R. *et al.* Liver pathology in mice in poisoning by the blue-green alga *Microcystis aeruginosa. Aust J Biol Sci* **34:** 179–187, 1981.

Harvey, R. B. *et al.* Progression of aflatoxicosis in growing barrows. *Am J Vet Res* **49:** 482–487, 1988.

Hermansky, S. J. *et al.* Evaluation of potential chemoprotectants against microcystin-LR hepatotoxicity in mice. *J Appl Toxicol* **11:** 65–74, 1991.

Hirono, I. Cycasin. *In* "Naturally Occurring Carcinogens of Plant Origin—Toxicology, Pathology and Biochemistry," I. Hirono, (ed.), pp. 1–19. 1987. Kodansha Ltd and Elsevier Science Publishers.

Hooser, S. B., *et al.* Toxicity of microcystin-LR, a cyclic heptapeptide hepatotoxin from *Microcystis aeruginosa,* to rats and mice. *Vet Pathol* **26:** 246–252, 1989.

Hooser, S. B. *et al.* Microcystin-LR-induced ultrastructural changes in rats. *Vet Pathol* **27:** 9–15, 1990.

Jackson, A. R. B. *et al.* Clinical and pathological changes in sheep experimentally poisoned by the blue-green alga *Microcystis aeruginosa. Vet Pathol* **21:** 102–113, 1984.

Jarrett, I. V., and Chinnock, R. J. Outbreaks of photosensitisation and deaths in cattle due to *Myoporum* aff. *insulare* R. Br. toxicity. *Aust Vet J* **60:** 183–186, 1983.

Ketterer, P. J. *et al.* Canine aflatoxicosis. *Aust Vet J* **51:** 355–357, 1975.

Polzin, D. J. *et al.* Acute hepatic necrosis associated with the administration of mebendazole to dogs. *J Am Vet Med Assoc* **179:** 1013–1016, 1981.

Runnegar, M. T. C., Gerdes, R. G., and Falconer, I. R. The uptake of the cyanobacterial hepatotoxin microcystin by isolated rat hepatocytes. *Toxicon* **29:** 43–51, 1991.

Seawright, A. A., and Hrdlicka, J. The effect of prior dosing with phenobarbitone and β-idethylaminoethyl diphenylpropyl acetate (2KF525A) on the toxicity and liver lesion caused by ngaione in the mouse. *Br J Exp Pathol* **53:** 242–252, 1972.

Seawright, A. A., Filippich, L. J., and Steele, D. P. The effect of carbon disulphide used in combination with carbon tetrachloride on the toxicity of the latter drug for sheep. *Res Vet Sci* **15:** 158–166, 1973.

Seawright, A. A. *et al.* Toxicity of *Myoporum* spp. and their furanosesquiterpenoid essential oils. *In* "Effects of Poisonous Plants on Livestock," R. F. Keeler, K. R. Van Kampen, and L. F. James (eds.), pp. 241–150. New York, Academic Press, 1978.

D. Chronic Hepatotoxicity

In contrast to the acute intoxications, lesions with a fair degree of specificity are produced by many of the more chronic hepatotoxicities. In addition to the individually specific features, the chronic intoxications produce a range of changes common to them. These include accelerated necrobiosis, fibrosis of various patterns, bile duct hyperplasia, nodular regeneration, and some degree of cholestasis. Many also produce megalocytosis of hepatocytes. Some of these hepatotoxins are potent carcinogens, and some are teratogens, but this is not an important consequence in domestic animals. Clinical signs of hepatic failure may include photosensitization, nervous dysfunction, and jaundice. Most of the toxins responsible for chronic hepatotoxicity may produce acute nonspecific zonal or massive necrosis if experimentally administered at dose rates higher than those to which animals are likely to be exposed in the field, although such acute toxicity is occasionally observed in field cases of the diseases.

The association between illness and death in animals and the ingestion of moldy feed has been known by veterinary diagnosticians for a long time. Developments in commerce, science, and technology since the 1950s have enormously expanded the potential scale of mycotoxic disease and have provided the techniques necessary for identification and assay of toxic metabolites. The target organs for the action of mycotoxins vary with the toxic metabolite, and there are species differences in susceptibility. Some of the syndromes of intoxication are sufficiently distinctive in clinical signs and pathologic changes to allow firm diagnosis, but others are not, and the subclinical effects are not well defined for any of them. Reference to defined mycotoxicoses is made in relation to target organs in several other chapters in these volumes.

1. Aflatoxin

The **aflatoxins** are a group of bisfuranocoumarin compounds produced as metabolites mainly by *Aspergillus flavus, A. parasiticus,* and *Penicillium puberulum*. The metabolites are designated by spectral qualities, and the major ones are B_1, B_2, G_1, and G_2. Many others may be produced in minor amounts in fungal colonies or as metabolic products of the major toxins in animals. The most significant and best studied of the aflatoxins is B_1 because of its relative abundance and its potency as a hepatotoxin.

Strains of *Aspergillus* differ in the varieties and amounts of individual toxins produced, indicating that the biosynthesis of the toxins is genetically determined. The production of toxins also varies under different conditions of fungal growth, being influenced by the quality of the substrate, temperature, relative humidity and moisture content of the substrate, and microbial competition. Thus the toxicity of moldy feedstuffs is impossible to assess without measurement of toxin production. Aflatoxins can be produced on growing crops in the field, but much greater levels are likely to accumulate in stored or unharvested mature grains, particularly if they are damaged by moisture. A variety of feeds other than grains, ranging from legume stubbles to bread, may be the substrate in outbreaks of aflatoxicosis.

Aflatoxins are metabolized by the hepatic mixed-function oxidase system to a variety of toxic and nontoxic metabolites, the proportions of which vary with the species and age of animal involved. There is very much species variation in susceptibility to the toxin, and as much or more variation with age. The LD_{50} of aflatoxin B_1, in 2-day-old ducklings, for example, is reported to be double that for 1-day-old birds, and the same sort of variation seems to hold for mammals. This age susceptibility has important implications in suckling animals, for toxic metabolites of aflatoxins may be excreted in the milk. Sheep and adult cattle are quite resistant to the toxin, whereas dogs, pigs, and calves are sensitive and may be fatally intoxicated by a dose rate of less than 1.0 mg per kilogram body weight.

The toxic effects of aflatoxin B_1 are related principally to the binding of its toxic metabolites to macromolecules, in particular, to nucleic acids and nucleoproteins. It is not surprising, therefore, that the toxic effects include carcinogenesis, teratogenesis, mitotic inhibition, and immunosuppression. Protein and RNA synthesis are inhibited at higher dose rates, which probably accounts for the necrotizing effects and fatty change seen at these rates.

Prolonged exposure to low concentrations of the toxin may produce merely reduced growth rates and moderate enlargement of the liver without any significant hepatic signs. The enlargement may be partly due to hypertrophy of hepatocellular smooth endoplasmic reticulum and some degree of fatty change. As the level of aflatoxin in the ration increases (in young pigs, e.g., to 1.0 mg per kilogram ration), the liver may show all or none of the following changes: pallor, enlargement, bile staining, increased firmness due to fibrogenesis, and fine nodular regenerative hyperplasia. There may also be edema of the gallbladder and bile-tinged ascites in more severe cases. Even under experimental conditions, some individuals may show minimal liver lesions, whereas their fellows, under the same levels of exposure, die of liver failure. Histologically, affected livers show obvious increase in size of some hepatocytes and their nuclei (megalocytosis), focal necrosis, and cytosegresome formation. Bile ductules proliferate early (Fig. 2.9), and reticulin and collagen deposition occurs throughout the acinus according to no distinct pattern. Fatty change in affected livers is variable in extent and occurrence, and bile pigments accumulate in canaliculi and hepatocytes in more severely affected livers. Minor degrees of megalocytosis may be seen in proximal tubular epithelium in the kidney. The changes produced resemble those of pyrrolizidine alkaloid toxicosis.

At higher dose rates of aflatoxin, most periacinar hepatocytes disappear and are replaced by an ill-assorted mixture of inflammatory cells, fibroblasts, and primitive vascular channels. The liver may be much smaller than normal, particularly in young animals, due presumably to mitotic inhibition, and focal hepatocellular necrosis is more obvious or may be supplanted by zonal (periacinar) necrosis. Fatty change in these livers may be severe and uniformly distributed.

Acute, fulminating liver necrosis is sometimes seen in dogs that eat moldy bread, dog food, or garbage, which may contain very high concentrations of the toxin. Younger animals are much more susceptible and may die within a few hours; the gross postmortem picture is dominated by widespread hemorrhage and massive hepatic necrosis.

2. Phomopsin

There are two distinct manifestations of toxicity associated with *Lupinus* spp.; discussed here is the condition formerly known as lupinosis, which is a mycotoxic liver disease. The teratogenic and neurotoxic effects of some of the isoquinoline alkaloids from the plants themselves are discussed in Volume 1 with Bones and Joints (Chapter 1) and The Nervous System (Chapter 3).

The fungus *Phomopsis leptostromiformis* is parasitic on green *Lupinus* plants, but it becomes saprophytic after the host dies. Phomopsins (A or B) are produced if the lupin stubble is moistened, and such stubbles may remain toxic for months. Severe acute liver damage has been described in sheep on very toxic stubbles in Western Australia, but in many of these cases it has been difficult to separate the toxicity of the lupins from that of copper, which in this area is often concentrated in ovine livers (see Copper, Section XI,D,10 of this chapter).

The usual syndrome of phomopsin poisoning is subacute to chronic. Inappetence occurs soon after experimental administration of the toxin is begun; liver damage is clinically inapparent for several days, although there is early hydropic change and accelerated necrobiosis among hepatocytes. An increase in mitotic activity is soon apparent, although the liver has by this time become smaller. The mitotic activity is in fact largely ineffectual, as close examination reveals that many mitotic figures are abnormal (Fig. 2.74A). There is either clumping or dispersal of chromatin, and there appears to be mitotic arrest at late metaphase. Remaining hepatocytes swell, their cytoplasm becomes granular, and their nuclei, vesicular. With progression, hepatic fibrosis occurs, predominantly diffuse in distribution, and by this stage there is usually clinical icterus and anorexia. There will be variably severe fatty change, dependent to a large degree on the fat reserves of the animal (Fig. 2.74B). There is also accumulation of complex pigment in macrophages in portal stroma and about hepatic venules; this granular material contains lipofuscin, ferric iron, and copper at least. Bile duct proliferation is also a prominent feature of the chronic disease.

The liver continues to shrink, presumably as a result of continued mitotic inhibition and progressive fibrosis. The organ is small, tough, and has a finely granular surface and texture. It is pale grayish orange but usually retains its shape. In naturally occurring cases, however, discontinuous intake of the toxin may produce a liver grossly distorted by asymmetric nodular regeneration and fibrosis. The atrophic changes are most severe in the left lobe.

Photosensitization occurs in phomopsin-poisoned sheep; it may be severe if the animals have access to green feed while under the influence of the toxin.

Phomopsin poisoning in cattle causes most losses when the animals are lactating or heavily pregnant; in these animals the syndrome is essentially one of ketosis, to which such cows would be predisposed by the anorexia that is an obvious clinical feature of this intoxication. Pregnant sheep are less likely to have access to toxic lupin roughage during late gestation; otherwise, ketosis triggered by phomopsin would be expected just as often as in cattle.

Chronic hepatic fibrosis with fine, nodular regeneration may occur infrequently in cattle due to chronic phomopsin poisoning. Similar liver changes may also be seen in horses, in which there may also be hemolytic anemia of unknown pathogenesis.

3. Sporidesmin

The mycotoxin sporidesmin is produced by the fungus *Pithomyces chartarum*; the most important substrate is dead ryegrass (*Lolium perenne*) that has been moistened in warm weather. Intoxication causes chronic liver damage and severe hepatogenous photosensitivity (facial eczema) and is a serious cause of loss of sheep and, to a lesser extent, cattle on the North Island of New Zealand. Sporadic and subclinical intoxication occurs irregularly on the South Island and in southern Australia and South Africa. Sporidesmin intake in conjunction with ingestion of *Tribulus terrestris* causes another hepatogenous photosensitivity **(geeldikkop)**; this is similar to but distinct from facial eczema, and is described in Section XI,D, 6 of this chapter.

Sporidesmin is concentrated in the fungal spores, and the toxigenicity of pasture is related to the density of the spores in it. Sporidesmin is not specifically hepatotoxic. Administration of the toxin does produce rapid disorganization of hepatic cell organelles and triglyceride accumulation, but these are mild and nonspecific changes. If administered in suitable dosage, the toxin causes permeability alterations in many tissues and will, for example, produce corneal edema on local application. The hepatobiliary lesions are due to the excretion of unconjugated sporidesmin in bile and its concentration there. Sporidesmin is also excreted in urine, and if the dose is high enough, edema and mucosal hemorrhage occur in the bladder. The hepatic lesion is due to irritation of mesenchymal tissues in the portal triads and surrounding the bile ducts. If the concentration of sporidesmin is high enough, the biliary epithelium undergoes necrosis, and diffusion of toxin produces irritative lesions and necrosis in the adjacent blood vessels.

The liver in acute forms of the disease is enlarged, with rounded edges, and is finely mottled and discolored yellowish green by retained bile pigments, although the discoloration may be blotchy. There is mild edema and

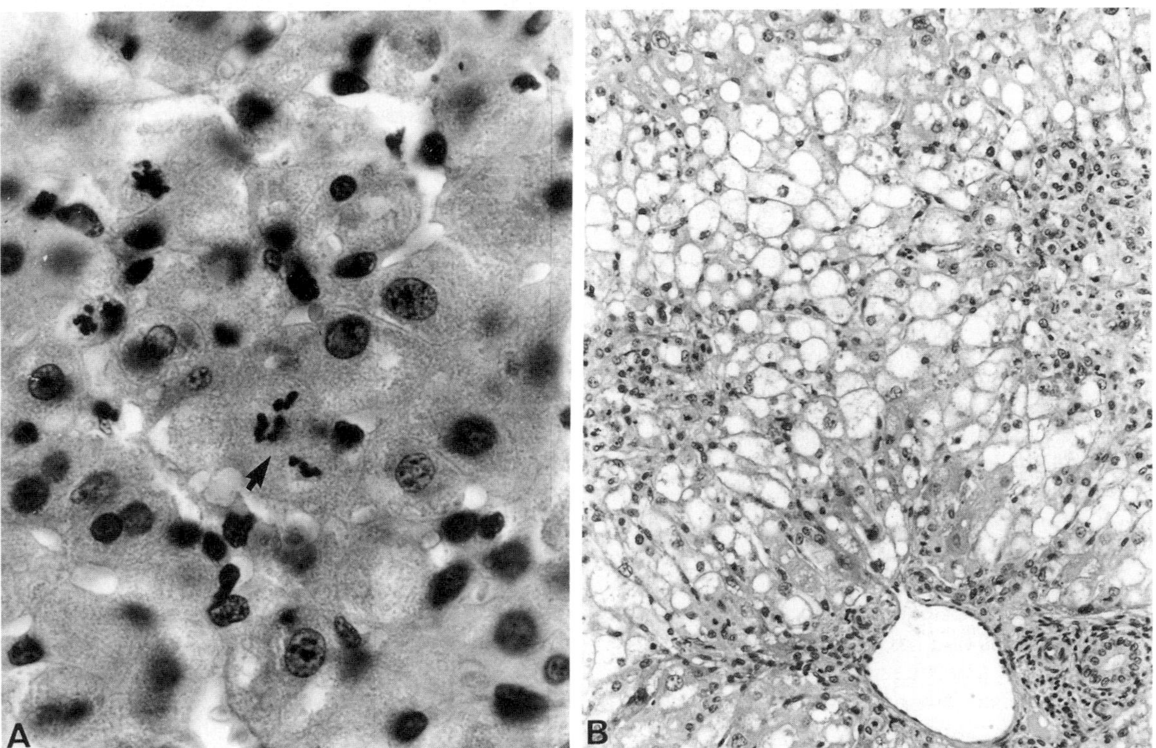

Fig. 2.74 (A) Subacute phomopsin poisoning. Sheep. Numerous and abnormal mitotic figures (arrow). (B) Phomopsin poisoning (lupinosis). Sheep. Zonal fatty change, periacinar collapse and periportal megalocytosis. (A and B courtesy of J. G. Allen.)

congestion of the wall of the gallbladder, which may be distended with bile of normal quality or with mucin (white bile). The extrahepatic ducts are thickened and prominent, and there is edema of the adventitia. The ductal changes may extend to the papilla of Vater and can be traced by the naked eye deeply into the parenchyma. In more chronic cases, alterations of size and pigmentation of the liver are variable. Pale areas of capsular thickening, which may be elevated or depressed, are visible. On cut surfaces they extend deeply as wedge-shaped areas in which biliary fibrosis has produced an exaggerated acinar pattern, and the parenchyma is pale and atrophic; these areas are related to occluded bile ducts and are sometimes referred to as biliary infarcts.

The liver is firm and cuts with increased resistance. The intrahepatic ducts are conspicuous. There is irregular stenosis of their lumens; some are occluded by cellular debris and inspissated bile or mucin, and in some, cicatrization of the new fibrous tissue causes complete atresia. Occlusion of the ducts causes the parenchyma served by them to undergo atrophy, necrosis, and fibrosis. The livers of animals that have survived an attack of cholangiohepatitis of this genesis are distorted in shape and size by large nodules of regeneration and persistent areas of atrophy and fibrosis. The atrophy and fibrosis may affect either lobe, but usually the left most severely (Fig. 2.75).

Histologically, the changes are those of an acute cholan-

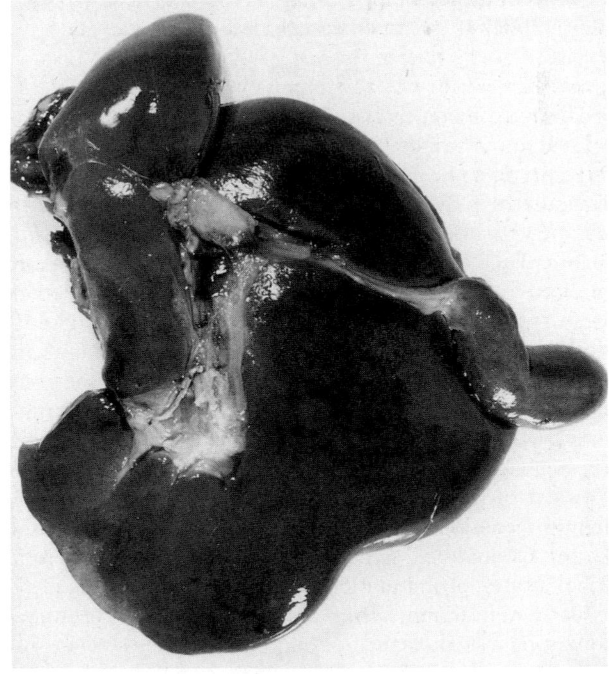

Fig. 2.75 Chronic sporidesmin poisoning (facial eczema). Atrophy of left lobe with hypertrophy of right and caudate lobes. (Courtesy of W. J. Hartley.)

gitis or cholangiohepatitis to which there is a minimum of leukocytic reaction. There is extensive necrosis of the lining of the larger intrahepatic ducts and the extrahepatic ducts, the epithelium being cast off as debris mixed with a few leukocytes. There is edema of the adventitia of the ducts, with active fibroplasia and scarring. Inflammatory cells are present, but not in large numbers, and they are chiefly lymphocytes and histiocytes. Injury to the smaller radicles of the bile ducts is less severe, but fibrosis and collagenization are active. The portal tracts are enlarged by fibrous tissue and by the active generation of new bile ducts that follows.

In more severe intoxications there may be coagulative necrosis of blood vessel walls in the portal triads; when this is incomplete, the most damaged segment of the vessel tends to be that adjacent to the nearest injured bile duct. Both arteries and veins may be affected, and it is possible that the so-called bile infarcts are related to vascular insufficiency as well as to impaired bile drainage. Changes in the hepatic parenchyma are minimal and secondary to those in the portal triads. In acute cases, there may be extensive pigmentation of hepatocytes and Kupffer cells by bile pigments, but this is irregular in distribution in the liver. Inspissated bile can be found in the bile ducts and as plugs in the canaliculi. There is some necrosis of hepatocytes adjacent to inflamed portal areas, and other areas of necrosis, focal in type and distribution and probably the result of biliary obstruction, may be numerous.

Other morbid alterations include great enlargement of the adrenals produced by cortical hypertrophy; sclerotic intimal plaques in the arteries, veins, and lymphatics in the hilus of the liver; and a tendency for the newly formed bile ductules to recanalize occluded ducts.

4. Pyrrolizidine Alkaloids

The pyrrolizidine alkaloids have been found in plants belonging to various unrelated botanical families, principally the Compositae, Leguminosae, Boraginaceae, and particularly in the genera *Senecio, Crotalaria, Heliotropium, Cynoglossum, Amsinckia, Echium,* and *Trichodesma*. There are, widely distributed in the world, many hundreds of species within these genera. Contained in these species is a huge range of pyrrolizidine alkaloids; more than 100 have been chemically defined, and about 30 of these have been shown to be toxic. Most of the toxic plant species contain more than one of the alkaloids, the toxic varieties of which are all esters of one of three amino alcohol bases (necines) or acids (necic acids). These toxins all must be metabolized to highly reactive pyrroles by dehydrogenation of the unsaturated necine ring of the parent alkaloid before they can express their full effects. Other routes of metabolism are ester hydrolysis and N-oxidation, both of which are detoxification pathways. However, N-oxides may prove toxic if ingested in this form from the plant, because they are reduced to the alkaloid form by microbial action in the gut.

The toxic pyrroles are electrophilic and can cause alkylation reactions with amino acids, nicotinamide, and guanine and adenine derivatives. At lower dose rates, the cell component most sensitive to these reactions is the nucleus. These alkylation products may dissociate in the cell, and it is possible that such dissociation may provide derivatives which are themselves alkylating agents, which may be the basis for cellular injury continuing after intake of the parent alkaloid has ceased.

Other pyrrole–nucleophile complexes, notably the S-derivatives, are relatively stable, and methods have been developed to detect these in tissue or serum samples. These methods involve reactions which produce pyrrolic esters, which may be detected by various chromatographic methods, which thus enable retrospective diagnosis of the poisoning, even in fixed tissue samples.

Thus the toxicity of an alkaloid for a given organ depends on three factors: the rate at which the parent alkaloid is converted to the pyrrolic derivative, the proportion of the alkaloid so converted, and the reactivity or binding capacity of the pyrrole. The rate, extent, and qualitative nature of these conversions vary with the species, age, and sex of the animal intoxicated as well as with the metabolic and mitotic status of its target cells; these variables in some measure explain the difficulty in predicting the outcome of pyrrolizidine alkaloid poisoning in an individual. In ruminants, an additional complicating factor may be the degree to which the toxins are degraded in the rumen before they have had a chance to be absorbed. Nevertheless, there are some consistent differences in species susceptibility to these toxins; pigs, for example, may be as much as 200 times more susceptible than sheep or goats, with cattle and horses being only about 15 times more resistant than pigs. These differences account for the fact that sheep can be used to graze out stands of *Senecio* that would be lethal to cattle.

The most characteristic effect of these toxins on the liver is the induction of nuclear and cytoplasmic gigantism (megalocytosis) (Fig. 2.6); this is related to an antimitotic effect, the mechanism of which is not yet clarified. It is not due to inhibition of DNA synthesis; indeed, continued nucleoprotein synthesis, combined with mitotic inhibition, accounts for the great increase in size of the nucleus and, probably, the basophilia of the cytoplasm that develops. Megalocytosis is not a change specific for pyrrolizidine alkaloidosis; it is seen in intoxication by other alkylating agents such as nitrosamines and aflatoxins. Nevertheless, the most florid examples of this change are produced by the pyrrolizidine alkaloids. The onset of megalocytosis is delayed by an interval determined by the mitotic activity of the organ. Thus, experimentally, animals that have had hepatocytes removed by hepatectomy or by acute hepatotoxic insults will develop megalocytosis more rapidly and to a more severe degree than controls.

The volume of affected cells may be increased as much as 20 times. Their nuclei are enlarged and single, the nuclear membrane stains strongly with basic dyes and is sharp, the chromatin is scant and fragmented, the nucleolus is enlarged, and frequently, there are globular cytoplasmic invaginations within the nuclei (Figs. 2.6, 2.76). The cytoplasmic volume is increased, the margins are condensed and sharp, the peripheral part of the cytoplasm is usually pale, and a diffuse central zone is rich in the basophilic granules of nucleic acids. Acidophilic spherical cytosegresomes are also a common but less specific finding. The enlarged cells are closely apposed, so sinusoids may not be evident. Small extravasations of bile may be present between them. Many of these megalocytes are in different stages of dying, but they die slowly, individually, and not as a tissue. These changes affect all the cells of the acinus, but in the early stages, periportal hepatocytes may be relatively spared. Occasionally, a whole acinus may escape, so a paracentral cluster of cells of normal size may be found adjacent to some hepatic venules.

In severe pyrrolizidine alkaloid poisoning, the liver becomes smaller while its hepatocytes get larger; cells must obviously be lost to balance this equation. They are not replaced, owing to the mitotic inhibition, and the remaining megalocytes suffer reduced function. The evidence that megalocytes are not very good hepatocytes lies in the fact that liver failure occurs long before the liver mass falls below the 30% theoretically necessary to sustain life.

The sequential hepatic changes in domestic species receiving small or intermittent doses of alkaloids have not been studied, but intermittent doses are probably responsible for the many livers in which nodular regenerative hyperplasia occurs. The nodules are diffusely but not uniformly distributed in the liver and consist of cells that are morphologically normal or that are small and contain fatty vacuoles. The origin of these cells and their relation to preexisting architecture are not clear. They may also fall victim to later alkaloid intoxication.

Concurrent with the development of megalocytosis, there is some fibroplasia and proliferation of bile ducts in the portal triads. The fibroplasia is minimal in sheep, moderate in horses, and may be marked in cattle (Fig. 2.77). As a rule, it is only in cattle that the fibrous tissue infiltrates along the sinusoids to dissect lobules, separate individual cells, and link up with the walls of efferent veins. A special form of fibrosis has been produced about the hepatic veins by pyrrolizidine alkaloid poisoning. This takes the form of sometimes asymmetric masses of exuberant young fibrous tissue which tend to obliterate the hepatic venules, hence the appellation veno-occlusive disease. This was originally described in human bush tea poisoning, and was subsequently reproduced in primates and other experimental animals, but it may also occur in some field cases of bovine pyrrolizidine alkaloidosis. The amount of bile duct proliferation may be much greater than that of fibrosis. Its stimulus is not known, but it may be an abortive attempt at regeneration, and it may in the terminal stages account for almost half the weight of the liver. In fatal cases in cattle, the primary hepatocyte injury is abetted by the vascular complications of chronic hepatic

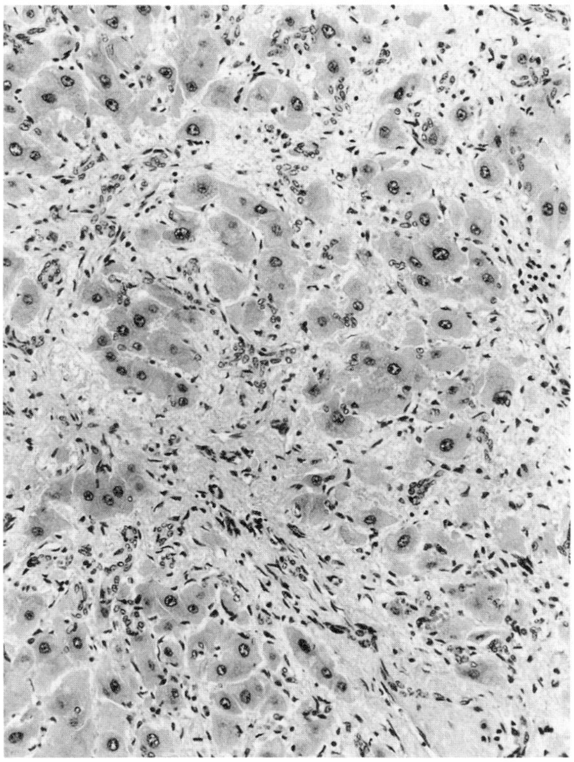

Fig. 2.76 Megalocytosis and diffuse fibrosis in *Crotalaria* poisoning. Ox. Fibrous septa have subdivided the acini.

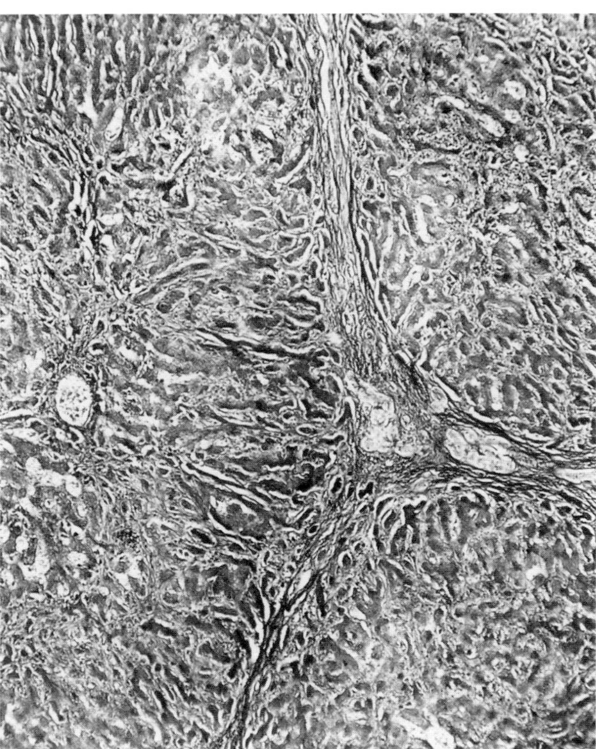

Fig. 2.77 Diffuse fibrosis of liver in chronic *Senecio* poisoning. Ox.

fibrosis and remodeling. The livers are very tough and nodular (Fig. 2.78A,B), and the nodules have variably efficient biliary drainage, so there may be a very striking color pattern, ranging from fatty yellow through green and brown. Ascites is present due to portal hypertension, which may also produce severe mesenteric edema and diarrhea; rectal prolapse may accompany the latter. Moderate jaundice and photosensitization are usual.

The disease in sheep is always protracted as a consequence of the relative resistance of this species; indeed, clinical signs may not be seen until after a second season's exposure. The shape of these failed livers is normal, but they are small, grayish yellow, fairly smooth, and toughened by condensation of normal stroma rather than by fibroplasia. If the liver copper content was high before intoxication, there will in the terminal stages of the disease probably be enough copper released to trigger an episode of intravascular hemolysis. In this case the carcass will be intensely jaundiced, and the urinary tract, stained with hemoglobin. The relationship of chronic copper poisoning to pyrrolizidine alkaloid poisoning is subsequently discussed; the plants most often implicated are *Heliotropium europaeum* and *Echium plantagineum*.

Liver failure produced in horses by these alkaloids is characterized pathologically by much the same sort of picture as that seen in cattle; clinically there is usually severe nervous disorder, such as head pressing and compulsive walking. In the past this gave rise to the colloquial names walkabout and walking disease. This is regarded as hepatic encephalopathy, rather than evidence of any specific neurotoxic property of the alkaloids.

Acute poisoning by the pyrrolizidine alkaloids is unusual; because of the unpalatability of the plants, the amount of toxin naturally ingested is usually too small to produce acute effects. However, the seeds are also toxic, and the small seeds of *Amsinkia* may, depending on harvesting technique, heavily contaminate other harvested grains used in prepared pig and poultry foods. Experimentally, it produces periacinar necrosis with hemorrhage and laking of blood in the affected zones and endothelial damage to the hepatic venules and smaller hepatic veins. The morphology of the acute lesion is not clearly different from that produced by a variety of other hepatotoxins and is associated with biochemical disturbances similar to those produced by carbon tetrachloride. Small zones of necrosis and hemorrhage may occur in natural poisonings in horses especially, and less commonly in cattle, but necrosis of tissue can be entirely absent in these species, as it usually is in sheep, and it does not contribute to the natural evolution of the typical lesions.

The metabolites of pyrrolizidine alkaloids affect tissues other than the liver; death in some instances may be due to renal damage and in others, to pulmonary vascular and interstitial lesions. Variation in the source of the toxin and in the species of target animals accounts for the differences in susceptibility of the different tissues, but as a generaliza-

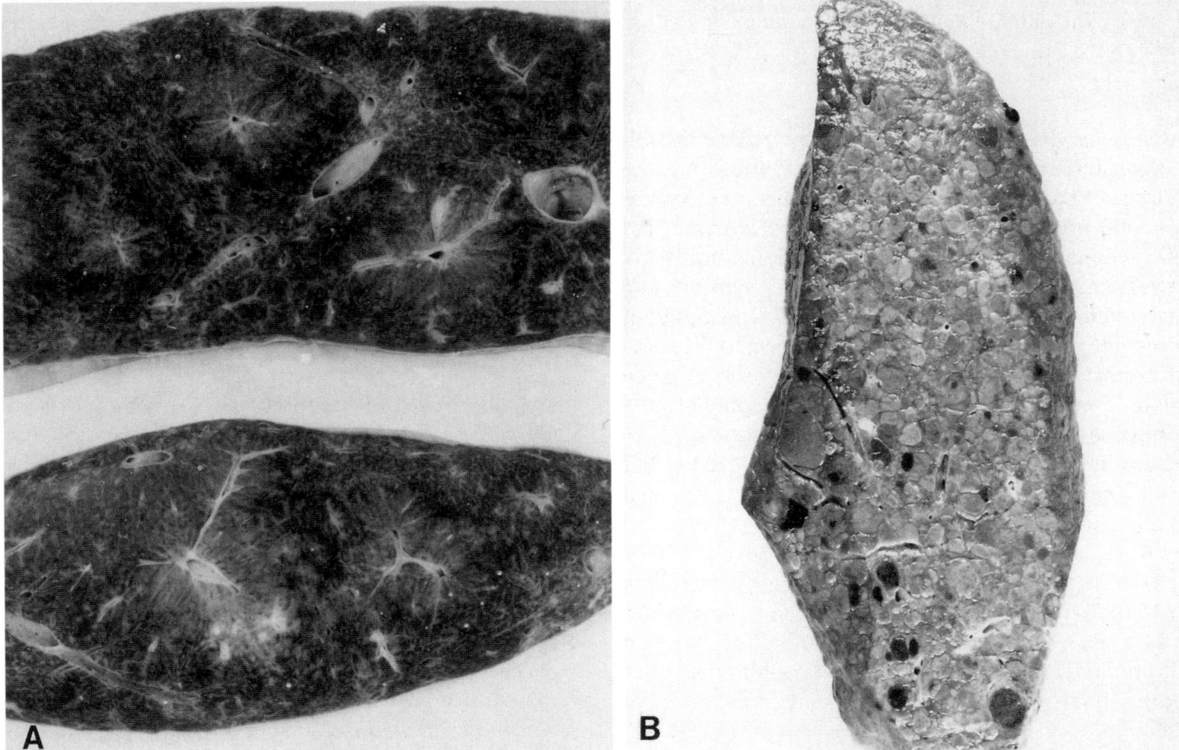

Fig. 2.78 (A) *Senecio* poisoning. Calf. Diffuse fibrosis, mimicking nutmeg liver of chronic congestion. (B) Liver, bovine. *Heliotropium* poisoning. Fibrosis and nodular regeneration. Some nodules stained by bile.

tion, it may be stated that the alkaloids from *Crotalaria* affect the widest range of tissues in most animals.

The pulmonary toxicity of pyrrolizidine alkaloids in rats is well recognized, and lung lesions occur that are characterized by severe vascular engorgement and edema. It should not be assumed that all hepatotoxic pyrrolizidine alkaloids produce lung lesions or that all animal species are equally susceptible to this type of lung injury. Jaagsiekte has been described in horses eating *Crotalaria dura,* and *C. crispata* produces similar lesions. Sheep develop pulmonary signs after eating *C. globifera* and *C. dura,* and pigs after eating *Senecio jacobaea* (Fig. 2.79). The reference to jaagsiekte implies a morphologic similarity to pulmonary adenomatosis of sheep that is not warranted. The experimental feeding of *C. spectabilis* to rats or the injection of the alkaloid monocrotaline, extracted from the plant, produces progressive pulmonary disease and cor pulmonale, with necrotizing vasculitis of the pulmonary arterioles. These lesions in the rat, which are of hypertensive nature, are secondary to changes in the alveolar septa, and this is probably the site of initial injury in domestic species. Monocrotaline produces septal edema and degeneration of all cells and the elastic tissue of rat alveolar septa.

There is considerable hyperemia, hemorrhage, and alveolar edema with migration of septal cells. There is progressive deposition of reticulin and collagen in the alveolar septa. Emphysema occurs in pigs and is an outstanding feature of the pulmonary disease of horses. The essential reactive lesion is diffuse fibrosis of alveolar and interlobular septa, with patchy epithelialization occurring more slowly (Fig. 2.79).

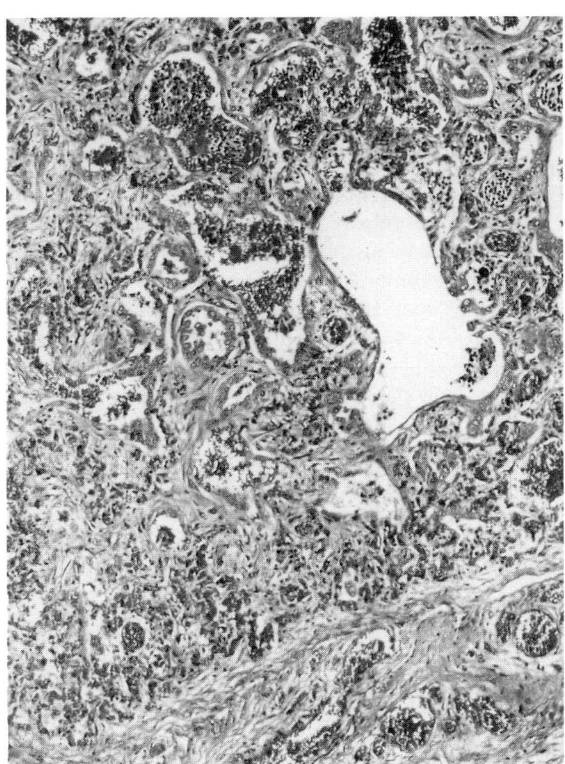

Fig. 2.79 Pulmonary congestion and hemorrhage, septal fibrosis, and epithelial metaplasia. *Senecio* poisoning. Pig.

5. Lantana

Lantana camara contains at least two cholestatic poisons, the triterpenes lantadene A and B, of which A is the more toxic. Like the other toxins described here, lantadene A will produce severe acute zonal necrosis of the liver if given in artificially large doses. The naturally occurring disease, however, is a subacute or chronic one characterized by anorexia, severe icterus, constipation, polyuria, dehydration, and photosensitization; this intoxication is most commonly seen in cattle, and rarely in sheep and goats. The latter species are quite susceptible to the toxin but are less likely to eat the plant.

Heavily intoxicated cattle can die within 2 days, but most fatal cases run a course of about 2 weeks. Ruminal stasis and anorexia appear early, along with polyuria due to nephrosis. Photosensitization is usually severe after 2 days, and the animals become severely dehydrated as a result of the renal lesion and disinclination to drink. The static rumen is a reservoir of toxin, and should rumen activity recommence, more toxin is released to the lower alimentary tract, where it is absorbed and perpetuates the intoxication.

Bile retention is present in poisoned animals, the jaundice being more severe in chronic cases, which have had more time for bile pigments to bind to tissues. The liver is enlarged, pale, and stained yellow, orange, or greenish gray by bile pigment. The gallbladder is enlarged, often spectacularly so, and is filled with pale, sometimes slightly mucoid bile. The gallbladder distension is partly explained by specific paralysis of this organ by lantadene A. The large bowel contains dark, dry feces, and the kidneys are slightly enlarged and wet on section, and, especially in the more chronic cases, the cortex is pale, and the medulla, hyperemic.

The most consistent histologic finding in the liver is hepatocellular enlargement and fine cytoplasmic vacuolation (Fig. 2.7), together with some degree of bile accumulation in canaliculi, hepatocyte cytoplasm, and Kupffer cells. The canalicular cholestasis is usually more severe in the periacinar zones, whereas the cytoplasmic vacuolation is often more pronounced in the periportal hepatocytes. There is usually some bile duct proliferation, and in some cases there will be a high incidence of focal coagulative necrosis or hepatocellular dissociation. There is also much apoptosis and cytosegresome formation in the periportal zone. The severity of the liver changes may be much less than expected from the intensity of the icterus and photosensitization; in these cases, electron microscopy will show an apparent increase in volume of smooth endoplasmic reticulum and a quite characteristic form of collapse of many bile canaliculi. Other canaliculi are distended and have damaged microvilli. Since much of the bilirubin that accumulates in the plasma of such animals is conjugated, it seems that the cholestasis is due in large measure to direct interference with canalicular transport of bile. Whether or not this is related to direct damage to the contractile apparatus of the hepatocellular cytoskeleton (see Cholestasis, Section VII,A of this chapter) has not been determined.

The renal lesion is a nonspecific tubular nephrosis, ranging in severity from mild vacuolar change to patchy tubular necrosis and extensive tubular cast formation. The role of the hyperbilirubinemia in the production of the renal damage has not been assessed. Severe myocardial necrosis can be produced in sheep by *Lantana* poisoning and may be responsible for the early deaths in cattle.

The cholestatic agent in *Lippia rehmanni,* icterogenin, is chemically identical to lantadene A.

6. *Tribulosis (and Other Crystal-Associated Cholangiohepatopathy)*

Photosensitizing liver diseases have caused enormous loss of sheep in South Africa, and it is now apparent that the most important of these, **geeldikkop,** is due to the interaction between sporidesmin and a component of *Tribulus terrestris*. The same association is also recognized in Australia. The sporidesmin may be produced on a variety of substrates (including *Tribulus*); facial eczema, the disease it produces in the absence of *Tribulus,* has been described. It seems that *Tribulus* by itself rarely if ever produces changes in the liver, but an unidentified component of the plant, together with the mycotoxin, produces liver lesions that are histologically distinct from those produced by sporidesmin alone.

The gross lesions of geeldikkop are similar to those of facial eczema in that there is generalized icterus, and the liver is discolored by bile pigment and either slightly swollen or distorted, according to the duration of the disease. In poisoning by sporidesmin alone, however, there is more obvious edema and fibrosis of bile ducts, and bile infarcts in the parenchyma are more common. In geeldikkop, the most characteristic gross finding is the presence of a white, semifluid accumulation of fine, crystalline material that can be expressed from the cystic duct and larger intrahepatic ducts. The gallbladder mucosa is also partly covered with a fine, crystalline deposit.

The most consistent histologic abnormality in geeldikkop is the presence in bile ducts of varying amounts of crystalline material (Fig. 2.80). The crystals are fine, flat, and are deposited in affected ducts, and, less commonly, in hepatocytes themselves and in renal tubules. There may be associated bile ductular proliferation in severe cases, but often the degree of histologic hepatocellular damage is mild compared to the severity of the photosensitization. It is unlikely that the cholestasis is solely due to mechanical obstruction by the crystals, since photosensitization can occur in such outbreaks in animals whose livers show very little cholangitis and contain very few crystals. The severity of peribiliary fibrosis is more variable and probably depends on the relative contribution of sporidesmin to the intoxication. There is some hepatocellular degeneration, including cytosegresome formation and apoptosis, and there is fairly uniform swelling of cytoplasm. Bile pigment accumulates in Kupffer cells and hepatocyte cytoplasm, but not to any marked extent in canaliculi. Focal necrosis of the gallbladder mucosa is often present. The severity of the hepatic lesion increases with the duration of exposure.

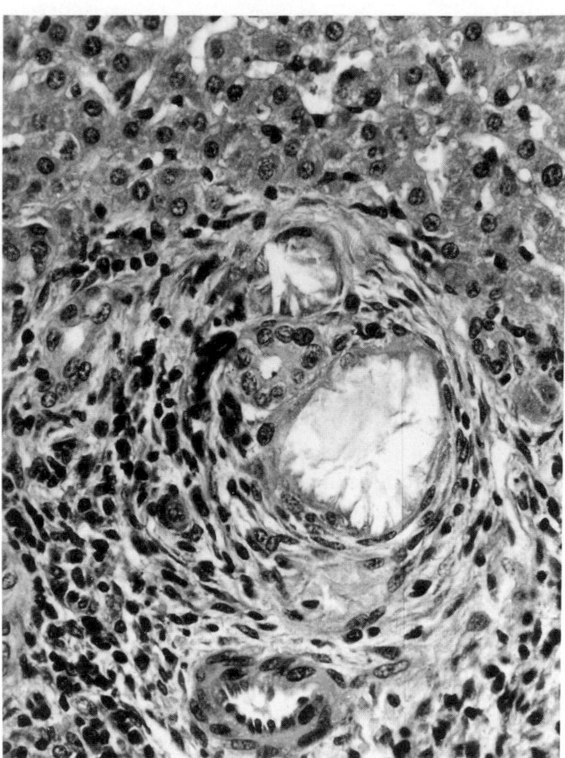

Fig. 2.80 Chronic cholangitis and plugging of bile duct by lipophilic crystalloid material. Photosensitivity disease of sheep on Pangola grass. Similar reaction to that seen in geeldikkop.

The identity of the biliary crystals is not known; they persist in paraffin sections, and solvent studies have shown that they are not cholesterol, cholic acid, glycocholate, or taurocholate. They may be related to the steroidal sapogenins present in these plants.

Crystal-associated cholangiohepatopathy is not specific for *Tribulus* intoxication. Similar changes occur in ruminants intoxicated by *Agave lecheguilla, Narthecium* spp., *Nolena texana,* and the pasture species *Brachiaria decumbens* and the *Panicum,* especially *P. coloratum,* the klein grass; candidate mycotoxicoses have not been identified for any of these intoxications. Crystal deposition is not reported in horses poisoned on klein grass. Young green oats, *Avena sativa,* infected by the toxic fungus, *Drechslera campanulate,* are reported to cause hepatopathy with crystal formation in goats.

It is apparent that neither *Tribulus* nor *Panicum* stands are at all times dangerous, so there is the possibility of involvement of endophytic fungi, which may render them toxic under certain conditions. However, *Agave lechegu-*

illa contains a crystalline steroidal sapogenin which is similar if not identical to the crystals extracted from the biliary tract of sheep experimentally intoxicated with this plant. Similarly, crystals from the bile of lambs naturally photosensitized on a *Panicum* pasture have been shown by mass spectrometry to be very similar to the crystals from *A. lecheguilla*. It is not established whether *Panicum* spp. at certain times contain the crystals or a precursor compound from which crystals are produced by hepatic metabolism. Other plants reported to occasionally produce unexpected photosensitivity include *Digitaria, Cooperia pedunculata, Nidorella foelida,* and *Chloris,* and such valuable pasture genera as *Medicago, Trifolium,* and *Avena*.

7. *Nitrosamines*

Epizootics of poisoning by dimethylnitrosamine occurred in Norwegian cattle, sheep, and fur-bearing animals, from 1957 to 1962. The toxin was present in herring meal and was thought to be a reaction product of trimethylamine and other lower amines with sodium nitrite, added as a preservative, the reacting amines being products of decomposition. Animals consumed several pounds of the toxic meal each day before becoming ill.

At autopsy, there was moderate anasarca and signs of hemorrhagic diathesis. Livers affected acutely were enlarged and firm, with mottled discoloration and sometimes a nutmeg appearance. In chronic intoxication, the liver was small, granular, and very firm. A number of animals recovered after a prolonged convalescence, and in these there was atrophy and fibrosis of the left and caudate lobes, and the right lobe was hyperplastic and hemispheric. Histologically, in acute cases, there was widespread hemorrhagic necrosis of periacinar distribution and an unusual degree of intimal and subendothelial reaction in sublobular and hepatic veins. The chronic lesion was dominated by extensive fibrosis of periacinar distribution, with obliterative changes in many central and sublobular veins.

The hepatocellular changes in chronic nitrosamine poisoning are not specific; they are essentially those described with the other alkylating agents. There is megalocytosis, nuclear vesiculation and nucleolar prominence, cytoplasmic intranuclear inclusions, and variable fatty change and cytoplasmic bile accumulation.

This intoxication has little veterinary importance now that it is easily prevented; most interest in these compounds is based on their use as research tools in molecular pathology. They have great carcinogenic potential, but this was not evident in the accidental poisonings.

8. *Indospicine*

Legumes of the genus *Indigofera* for some years have been known to contain the toxic amino acid indospicine (6-amidino-2-hexanoic acid), which is a structural analog of arginine, and which was shown in early experimental work to be hepatotoxic for rats and other species. The dose rates necessary to cause chronic liver injury in these species were, however, quite high, and field cases of intoxications were seen only in cattle grazing *I. spicata,* which has the highest naturally occurring concentrations of indospicine. More recently, in Australia, a serious outbreak of fatal liver disease occurred in dogs which had been fed meat from horses which had been grazing *I. linnaei,* a plant native to the arid zones of Australia, which has been known to produce in horses a chronic neurological disorder known as Birdsville horse disease. The disease in horses is not associated with liver damage, although these animals do accumulate indospicine in most tissues, and muscle concentrations typically reach between 20 and 30 μg/kg.

Dogs fed indospicine-contaminated meat for several weeks may develop progressive liver damage, which begins as vacuolation of a narrow band of periacinar hepatocytes, followed shortly by accumulation of mononuclear inflammatory cells in this zone and in the stroma of the hepatic venules. Progression of the lesion is marked by piecemeal necrosis of a widening zone of periacinar hepatocytes, disorganization, vacuolation due to hydropic and fatty change, and accumulation of ceroid pigment in macrophages (Fig. 2.81). Moderate periacinar fibrosis is seen in later stages, as well as pronounced canalicular cholestasis: by this stage, affected animals begin to show icterus, inappetence, and depression. Bile ductular proliferation is not a marked feature. Death is attended by the usual signs

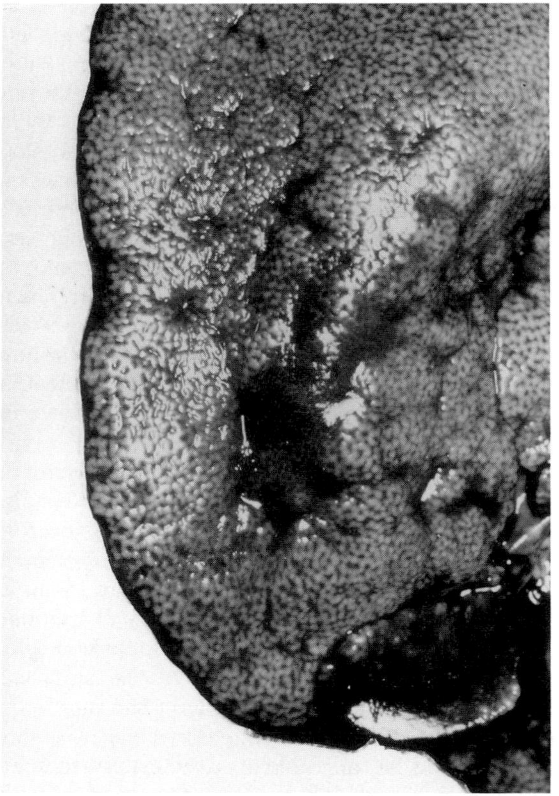

Fig. 2.81 Acinar fatty and hydropic change, alternating with postnecrotic collapse. Indospicine poisoning. Dog.

of hepatoencephalopathy and tendency to bleed spontaneously. There is no evidence of direct neurologic damage as is seen in horses.

This intoxication is remarkable by virtue of its unpredictability. Experimental intoxication by pure indospicine has been shown to validly reproduce the naturally occurring intoxication caused by horsemeat feeding; however, liver failure can be produced by either means in only a small proportion of dogs so exposed. On the other hand, milder degrees of liver damage are reliably produced by both methods. Thus it seems an idiosyncratic response is superimposed on a more consistent effect of the toxin: the nature of the accompanying inflammatory response suggests that the former may be immunologically mediated. This has yet to be established, as has the proposal that the mechanism of the intoxication is due to competitive inhibition of arginine.

The biology of the canine intoxication is also remarkable in that it is, like saw-fly larva poisoning, a rare example of a naturally occurring hepato-intoxication acquired through the food chain.

9. Trifolium hybridum *(Alsike Clover)*

Sporadically but fairly commonly, transient outbreaks of photodynamic dermatitis in sheep, cattle, and horses grazing on trefoils, medics, and clover occur. These outbreaks are probably examples of hepatogenous photosensitivity for which a basic hepatic lesion has not been described, except in two instances. Massive hepatic necrosis, sometimes with signs of photosensitivity, occurs in sheep, in restricted areas of California. The association with pastures dominated by birdsfoot trefoil (*Lotus tenuis*) may be only coincidental. **Alsike clover** is hepatotoxic for horses and probably for other species, but information is available for the horse only.

The effects of alsike clover poisoning in horses are cumulative, and it is only after exposure to the plant for a year or more that signs of hepatic insufficiency may develop. The toxic principles have not been isolated. Signs of poisoning may develop only in the exceptional circumstance in which alsike is greatly predominant in pastures and in the hay prepared therefrom. It is suggested that the toxic principle is in highest concentration in the flowering stage and that it is preserved in haying.

There remains some doubt whether alsike is toxic to the hepatic parenchyma. Degenerative parenchymal changes consisting of atrophy, fatty degeneration, and necrosis may be seen at autopsy, but these changes are minimal and are largely confined to lobules which are shrunken and compressed by fibrous tissue of biliary distribution. The liver is enlarged, sometimes greatly so, pale in color, and tough or rubbery in consistency. The surface is smooth, but its appearance is mottled. The mottling is clear on the cut surface and is caused by bands of grayish fibrous tissue, distinctly visible to naked eye, surrounding and compressing each lobule. Near the margins of the liver and in some other areas, scar tissue may completely replace the parenchyma. Microscopically, there is a benign proliferation of fibrous tissue and of well-formed bile ducts in the portal areas unaccompanied by signs of inflammation and, usually, unaccompanied by parenchymal damage. In the early stages, the proliferation of bile ducts is often greater than the proliferation of the fibrous tissue, but later the proportions are reversed. The proliferating tissue extends slowly to connect adjacent portal triads circumscribing areas which correspond to conventional lobules. The fibrous tissue does not permeate along the sinusoids, and there is a gradual and uniform constriction of the parenchyma.

The development of a relatively pure biliary fibrosis in alsike clover poisoning without evidence of antecedent parenchymal damage suggests that the toxin is only mildly irritating, that it is excreted in bile, and that it exerts its stimulating effect locally in the portal triads.

The liver is the only organ in which significant structural alterations occur in this disease. There is jaundice and emaciation, but ascites is absent. The clinical signs are referable to hepatic injury, there being jaundice, and neurological disturbances, either excitement or mania in irregular episodes, or long periods of extreme dullness, anorexia, apparent blindness, forced wandering, head pushing, and yawning. Photodynamic dermatitis is a complication.

10. Copper

Copper alone of the heavy metals seems to have a selectively toxic effect on the liver, and there is significant variation in species susceptibility. Sheep as a species are most prone to copper poisoning, with some breeds being more susceptible than others. Bedlington terriers are also unusually susceptible. In these dogs and sheep, toxic amounts of copper can accumulate in the liver while dietary copper levels are not excessive by standards for other species. Copper poisoning does occur in cattle and pigs, but in these species it is due to abnormally high intake of the element.

Chronic copper poisoning of sheep occurs as a result of the presence of three environmental factors acting alone or in concert. First, excessive copper intake may occur as a result of contamination of pasture or prepared feed; the latter is difficult to avoid when feed mills are preparing rations for different species and is probably partly responsible for the observation that housed sheep are more prone to copper poisoning than animals at pasture. Second, increased copper accumulation occurs as a result of increased availability of dietary copper; this happens when dietary levels of molybdenum are unusually low. Molybdenum, in the presence of sufficient sulfate, forms insoluble complexes with copper in the gut and liver, making the copper biologically inert. Subterranean clover growing on calcareous soils in southern Australia may be relatively deficient in molybdenum, and in these areas, British breeds of sheep are known to be more susceptible than Merinos to chronic copper poisoning. A breed of sheep from the Hebridean island of North Ronaldsay has apparently adapted to a seaweed diet low in both copper and molybdenum but rich in zinc. Zinc is also capable of interfering with copper uptake, and these sheep, while avoiding copper deficiency, are exquisitely susceptible to chronic copper poisoning when transferred to normal pasture. Other hepatotoxins constitute the third environmental factor that predisposes sheep to outbreaks of chronic copper poisoning. The most important of these are pyrrolizidine alkaloids (from *Heliotropium* or *Echium*) in eastern Australia, and phomopsin from lupins in western Australia and, possibly, South Africa.

The basis for chronic copper poisoning in sheep is the peculiar avidity of the liver for copper, coupled with the very limited rate at which this species can excrete the element in the bile. After intraportal injection of a copper isotope, practically all the radioactivity is removed during the first passage through the liver. Most of the copper is sequestered in hepatocellular lysosomes, where it does little damage at concentrations of 200–300 parts per million (ppm) dry weight. As the concentration rises, there is presumably more interaction between other cell components and the copper. There is some evidence that lysosomal membranes lose integrity and allow copper and lysosomal hydrolases to damage the rest of the cytoplasm. By the time the liver copper concentration has reached 300 ppm or more, there is a histologically apparent increase in hepatocellular turnover, with single hepatocytes undergoing apoptosis within a dense knot of neutrophils. At still higher copper levels, the apoptotic rate increases, while all cells become swollen and their nuclei vesicular. The mitotic rate increases, presumably to keep pace with the accelerated loss of hepatocytes, and large macrophages appear in the sinusoids and stromal spaces about the vessels (Fig. 2.82). These cells contain eosinophilic, granular debris, which consists of copper-containing lipofuscins.

Sheep with liver copper concentrations in excess of 1000 ppm may be clinically and hematologically normal, so long as the increasing mitotic rate produces enough new hepatocytes to take up the copper released by dying cells. At this stage, however, there will be elevated levels of liver-specific enzymes in the plasma. As soon as the rate of hepatocellular loss exceeds the replacement rate, the plasma copper levels begin to rise. Eventually, the blood copper concentration is high enough to damage circulating erythrocytes, and intravascular hemolysis ensues. The effect of the hemolysis on the liver is to accelerate the rate of hepatocellular necrosis; thus, copper enters the circulation at an increasing rate. The clinical syndrome then is one of paroxysmal intravascular hemolysis and liver failure, in which a sheep may pass from apparent good health to death within ~6 hr.

The association of chronic copper poisoning with phomopsin and pyrrolizidine alkaloid poisoning has already been noted. The relationship is understandable in the light of the critical role hepatocellular mitosis plays in sheep in delaying the onset of the hemolytic crisis. It is to be expected that any agent that interferes with the mitotic process will provoke the crisis at an earlier stage of copper accumulation. There is good field evidence that less specific stresses, such as brief starvation, may also precipitate the crisis in susceptible sheep.

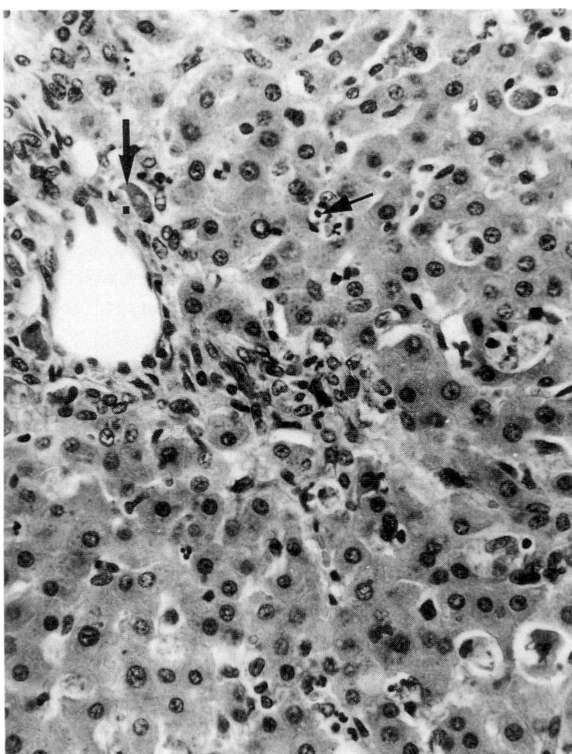

Fig. 2.82 Liver in prehemolytic phase of chronic copper poisoning. Apoptosis (small arrow), focal leukocyte aggregation, and pigmented macrophages in sinusoids and stroma (large arrow). Sheep.

The carcass is discolored by deep jaundice, superimposed on which is the reddish color imparted by free hemoglobin. Often there is a brownish hue as well, because a proportion of the hemoglobin is oxidized to methemoglobin. The kidneys are deep reddish brown, and the urine, deep red, as a result of hemoglobinuria. The liver is slightly soft and swollen, and deep orange. The bile is dark and granular, and the spleen is engorged, dark, and soft. The histologic changes of the preclinical stages are present in the liver and are somewhat obscured by the periacinar necrosis of hypoxemia and the bile accumulations of hemolytic disease. The histology may be further confused by the presence of changes induced by other toxins, should these have been involved.

During the hemolytic crisis, some of the copper is lost from the disintegrating liver; some passes into the urine, and kidney copper concentration rises to 1000 ppm or more. Kidney copper levels therefore give a truer indication of a prior hemolytic crisis due to chronic copper poisoning than does elevation of liver copper alone.

The events described in sheep also occur in chronic copper poisoning in pigs and cattle, and acute intravascular hemolysis may be seen, especially in calves. Usually, however, there is less of the acute terminal chain reaction in these species, and there is more evidence of chronic liver damage with extensive portal fibrosis and biliary hyperplasia within the triads.

Acute copper poisoning is most often seen in ruminants after accidental administration of single large doses of copper, by either the oral or the parenteral routes. The liver lesion is a nonspecific acute periacinar necrosis, and intravascular hemolysis may occur if plasma copper levels are sufficiently elevated. Acute gastroenteritis will be produced by oral dosage and may also be seen after sufficiently large parenteral doses of copper.

Chronic copper toxicosis in **Bedlington and West Highland white terriers** differs from the disease in sheep in that the susceptibility to it is inherited within the breed as an autosomal recessive character. The canine disease is not characterized by a hemolytic finale, as in sheep; hemolysis, if it occurs, is never a prominent part of the disease.

Affected dogs are usually presented with signs of progressive liver failure; ill thrift, wasting, ascites, nervous signs, and less consistently, jaundice. Grossly, the livers are fibrotic and pale, and in later stages, finely nodular. The most characteristic feature of the histology is the presence of numerous golden brown, refractile granules in most hepatocytes, and darker pigment in Kupffer cells. These granules are autophagolysosomes that contain ferric iron and copper (Fig. 2.83A), but their ultrastructure and other histochemical reactions suggest that they consist mostly of lipofuscin. The hepatic lesion has been described as chronic active hepatitis, because scanty periportal infiltrates of inflammatory cells (Fig. 2.83B) and prominent piecemeal necrosis are present. It seems likely that the inflammatory infiltrates are a reaction to accelerated hepatocyte turnover. The pattern of fibrosis is complex; it seems to be a mixture of portal and diffuse types. Most hepatocytes are swollen, and many contain fat.

Hepatic copper concentrations in these animals may be very high; as much as 12,000 ppm by dry weight has been recorded, and levels higher than 5000 ppm are not uncommon. Thus it would seem that these dogs have much more effective copper-binding mechanisms in their hepatocellular lysosomes than do sheep. This disease has been proposed as a model of hepatolenticular degeneration (Wilson's disease) of humans, but there are differences between the two copper-storage diseases. In the human condition, there are lowered levels of plasma ceruloplasmin; this is not seen in Bedlingtons, nor are the fairly specific brain lesions of Wilson's disease.

11. Drug-Induced Hepatotoxicity

Idiosyncratic drug-induced hepatotoxicity has not been reported in animals so frequently as it has in humans, in which the unexpected and atypical response to a drug is reputed to be the most common cause of massive hepatic

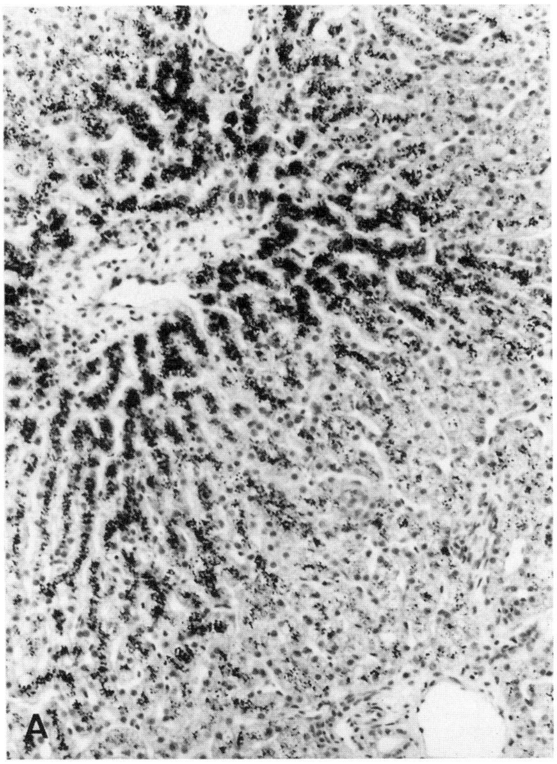

Fig. 2.83A Section of the liver in (B), stained with rhodanine for copper. Predominantly periacinar distribution of lysosomal copper.

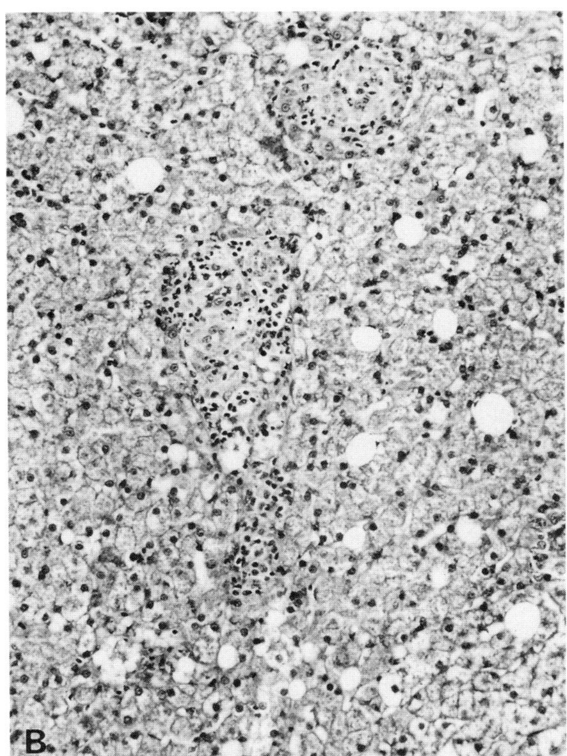

Fig. 2.83B Liver of Bedlington terrier. Infiltrate of inflammatory cells and granular macrophages in portal stroma, and random fatty change.

necrosis. Severe periacinar hepatic necrosis has been associated with use of the anthelmintic mebendazole in dogs; signs of hepatic failure appear within 2 weeks after exposure. Drug-induced hepatotoxicity may be mediated by allergic phenomena, which are characterized by granulomatous infiltrates containing eosinophils; this does not seem to be the case with mebendazole. It is likely that susceptibility to this type of intoxication is related to production of atypical drug metabolites, but if this is the case, the delayed onset of some cases is not explained.

The drug-induced hepatopathies that occur most frequently are associated with long-term anticonvulsant therapy. Anticonvulsant drugs alone or in combination do cause perturbations of hepatocyte metabolism but in only a small percentage of cases is there progression to fibrosis, nodularity, and failure.

Idiosyncratic reactions to sulfonamides occur in dogs producing syndromes of either cutaneous drug eruption, polyarthritis, and fever, or hepatitis/hepatic necrosis. Trimethaprim-sulfadiazine has been associated with each syndrome. Doberman pinschers appear to be unusually sensitive to the sulfadiazine in this drug combination. This may be related to the limited capacity to detoxify hydroxylamine metabolites of sulfonamides that has been demonstrated in ~50% of Dobermans.

Bibliography

Baker, D. C. *et al.* Hound's-tongue *(Cynoglossum officinale)* poisoning in a calf. *J Am Vet Med Assoc* **194:** 929–930, 1989.

Bath, G. F. Enzootic icterus—a form of chronic copper poisoning. *J S Afr Vet Assoc* **50:** 3–14, 1979.

Bridges, C. H. *et al.* Kleingrass (*Panicum coloratum* L.) poisoning in sheep. *Vet Pathol* **24:** 525–531, 1987.

Bunch, S. E. *et al.* Toxic hepatopathy and intrahepatic cholestasis associated with phenytoin administration in combination with other anticonvulsant drugs in three dogs. *J Am Vet Med Assoc* **190:** 94–198, 1986.

Crible, A. E., and Spielberg, S. P. An *in vitro* investigation of predisposition to sulphonamide idiosyncratic toxicity in dogs. *Vet Res Commun* **14:** 241–252, 1990.

Elmes, M. E. *et al.* Metallothionein and copper in liver disease with copper retention—A histopathological study. *J Pathol* **158:** 131–137, 1989.

Fuentealba, I., Haywood, S., and Foster, J. Cellular mechanisms of toxicity and tolerance in the copper-loaded rat. II. Pathogenesis of copper toxicity in the liver. *Exp Mol Pathol* **50:** 26–37, 1989.

Glastonbury, J. R. W. *et al.* A syndrome of hepatogenous photosensitisation, resembling geeldikkop, in sheep grazing *Tribulus terrestris*. *Aust Vet J* **61:** 314–316, 1984.

Gooneratne, S. R. *et al.* Intracellular distribution of copper in the liver of normal and copper-loaded sheep. *Res Vet Sci* **27:** 30–37, 1979.

Hardy, R. M. *et al.* Periportal hepatitis associated with the use of a heartworm–hookworm preventive (diethylcarbamazine-oxibendazole) in 13 dogs. *J Am Anim Hosp Assoc* **25:** 419–429, 1989.

Haywood, S. *et al.* Copper toxicosis and tolerance in the rat. *Exp Mol Pathol* **43:** 209–219, 1985.

Haywood, S., Rutgers, H. C., and Christian, M. K. Hepatitis and copper accumulation in Skye terriers. *Vet Pathol* **25:** 408–414, 1988.

Hegarty, M. P. *et al.* Hepatotoxicity to dogs of horse meat contaminated with indospicine. *Aust Vet J* **65:** 337–340, 1988.

Hooper, P. T. Cycad poisoning in Australia—etiology and pathology. *In* "Effects of Poisonous Plants on Livestock," R. F. Keeler, K. R. Van Kampen, and L. F. James (eds.), pp. 337–347. New York, Academic Press, 1978.

Hooper, P. T. Pyrrolizidine alkaloid poisoning—pathology with particular reference to differences in animal and plant species. *In* "Effects of Poisonous Plants on Livestock," R. F. Keeler, K. R. Van Kampen, and L. F. James (eds.), pp. 161–176. New York, Academic Press, 1978.

Hooper, P. T., and Scanlan, W. A. *Crotalaria retusa* poisoning of pigs and poultry. *Aust Vet J* **53:** 109–114, 1977.

Howell, J. McC., Gooneratne, S. R., and Gawthorne, J. M. Wilson's disease. *Comp Pathol Bull* **16:** 3–4, 1984.

Ishmael, J., Gopinath, C., and Howell, J. McC. Experimental chronic copper toxicity in sheep. Histological and histochemical changes during the development of the lesions in the liver. *Res Vet Sci* **12:** 358–366, 1971.

Ishmael, J. *et al.* Experimental chronic copper toxicity in sheep. Biochemical and haematological studies during the development of lesions of the liver. *Res Vet Sci* **13:** 22–29, 1972.

Jago, M. V. *et al.* Lupinosis: Response of sheep to different doses of phomopsin. *Aust J Exp Biol Med Sci* **60:** 239–251, 1982.

Johnson, G. F. *et al.* Cytochemical detection of inherited copper toxicosis of Bedlington terriers. *Vet Pathol* **21:** 57–60, 1984.

Kellerman, T. S. *et al.* Photosensitivity in South Africa. IV. The experimental induction of geeldikkop in sheep with crude steroidal saponins from *Tribulus terrestris*. *Onderstepoort J Vet Res* **58:** 47–53, 1991.

King, T. P., and Bremner, I. Autophagy and apoptosis in liver during the prehemolytic phase of chronic copper poisoning in sheep. *J Comp Pathol* **89:** 515–530, 1979.

Koppang, N. The toxic effects of dimethylnitrosamine in sheep. *Acta Vet Scand* **15:** 533–543, 1974.

Kumaratilake, J. S., and Howell, J. McC. Lysosomes in the pathogenesis of chronic copper poisoning. *J Comp Pathol* **100:** 381–390, 1989.

Ludwig, J. *et al.* The liver in the inherited copper disease of Bedlington terriers. *Lab Invest* **43:** 82–87, 1980.

MacLachlan, G. K., and Johnston, W. S. Copper poisoning in sheep from North Ronaldsay maintained on a diet of terrestrial herbage. *Vet Rec* **111:** 299–301, 1982.

Mason, J. The biochemical pathogenesis of molybdenum-induced copper deficiency syndromes in ruminants: Towards the final chapter. *Irish Vet J* **43:** 21–22, 1990.

Nation, P. N. Alsike clover poisoning: A review. *Can Vet J* **30:** 410–415, 1989.

Newberne, P. M. Chronic aflatoxicosis. *J Am Vet Med Assoc* **163:** 1262–1267, 1973.

Pass, M. A., Gemmel, R. T., and Heath, T. J. Effect of *Lantana* on the ultrastructure of the liver of sheep. *Toxicol Appl Pharmacol* **43:** 589–596, 1978.

Pass, M. A. *et al.* Lantadene A toxicity in sheep. A model for cholestasis. *Pathology* **11:** 89–94, 1979.

Peterson, J. E. Biliary hyperplasia and carcinogenesis in chronic liver damage induced in rats by phomopsin. *Pathology* **22:** 213–222, 1990.

Seaman, J. T. Pyrrolizidine alkaloid poisoning of sheep in New South Wales. *Aust Vet J* **64:** 164–167, 1987.

Seawright, A. A., and Allen, J. G. Pathology of the liver and

kidney in *Lantana* poisoning of cattle. *Aust Vet J* **48:** 323–331, 1972.
Seawright, A. A. *et al.* Pyrrolizidine alkaloidosis in cattle due to *Senecio* species in Australia. *Vet Rec* **129:** 198–199, 1991.
Su, L. C. *et al.* A defect of biliary excretion of copper in copper-laden Bedlington terriers. *Am J Physiol* **243:** G231–G236, 1982.
Thornburg, L. P. *et al.* Hereditary copper toxicosis in West Highland white terriers. *Vet Pathol* **23:** 148–154, 1986.
Thornburg, L. P. *et al.* Hepatic copper concentrations in purebred and mixed-breed dogs. *Vet Pathol* **27:** 81–88, 1990.
Twedt, D. C., Sternlieb, I., and Gilbertson, S. R. Clinical, morphological, and chemical studies on copper-toxicosis of Bedlington terriers. *J Am Vet Med Assoc* **175:** 269–275, 1979.
Valdivia, E. *et al.* Alterations in pulmonary alveoli after a single injection of monocrotaline. *Arch Pathol Lab Med* **84:** 64–76, 1967.

XII. Hyperplastic and Neoplastic Lesions of Liver and Bile Ducts

Hepatobiliary tumors are quite common in animals and are probably, excepting lymphomas, the most common of visceral tumors in cats, cattle, sheep, and dogs. It also seems, again excepting lymphomas, that primary tumors are more common than secondary tumors, perhaps due to the infrequency of gastrointestinal neoplasms and to euthanasia of animals before primary tumors elsewhere have disseminated as fully as they might.

The classification of tumors of the liver and bile ducts presents some difficulty in terms of deciding whether a tumor is benign or malignant, or of hepatocellular or cholangiocellular origin. With respect to the first difficulty, tumors of orderly and benign appearance may metastasize. The second difficulty is perhaps artificial, and a histogenetic classification requires a clearer statement than can presently be made on the embryogenic relationships of the hepatocytes, oval cells, and bile duct epithelium. There is no record of tumor of the extrahepatic bile ducts in animals, but it is possible that some carcinomas thought to arise from the pancreatic ducts may actually arise from the distal portions of the bile duct.

Ectopic and metaplastic lesions in the gallbladder are rarely observed. Ectopic tissue includes hepatocyte nodules attached to or within the wall, and pancreatic islands which may include islets of Langerhans. Gastric ectopia, distinguishable readily by the presence of chief and parietal cells, may form plaques or large polyps. Ectopia of cardiac or pyloric mucosa is mimicked by metaplastic changes.

Hyperplastic nodules are common in old dogs and have been reported but are rare in swine. The lesions in dogs do not have a breed or sex predisposition, but their incidence increases sharply with age. The nodules are usually multiple and randomly distributed throughout the lobes (Fig. 2.84). Nodules do develop in fibrotic livers, but the common hyperplastic nodules of old dogs regularly develop in nonfibrotic livers. An association with proliferation and hypertrophy of the perisinusoidal fat-storing cells, the Ito cells, and the presence of ceroid pigment with lipid in macrophages and lipogranulomas has been shown.

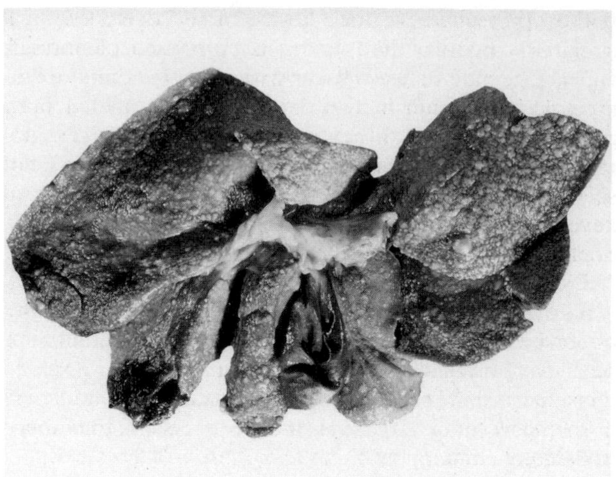

Fig. 2.84 Early nodular regeneration. Dog. This lesion may follow gradual hepatocellular loss.

The nodules are spherical and vary in size from 2 mm to 3 cm or more. They can be sharply distinct from the surrounding parenchyma, being either lighter than the surrounding liver, the cells containing increased amounts of fat or glycogen, or darker because the sinusoidal vessels are distended with blood, but some nodules are the same color as the surrounding tissue and can be identified only by examination of a washed or blotted slice under a strong light.

The hyperplastic nodules grow expansively, but do not induce a fibrous capsule; they do cause compression and atrophy of the surrounding parenchyma. The hepatocytes making up the nodule are normal in appearance although slightly larger than their unaffected colleagues. The sinusoids of the nodules are often dilated, and foci of hematopoiesis are common. Necrosis and hemorrhage in hyperplastic nodules are rare.

The hallmark of the hyperplastic nodule, in contrast to the hepatic adenoma and hepatocellular carcinoma, is that it retains a modified lobular structure and contains recognizable portal areas. However, this feature is easy to miss in needle biopsies, and the differentiation between hyperplastic nodules and other benign and malignant hepatic cell tumors can be difficult. The radial orientation of the hepatic plates around afferent veins is usually absent.

Although there is an association between drug administration and nodule formation in humans and experimental animals, none has been shown with the natural disease in dogs.

The **myelolipoma** is an unusual tumor or tumorlike metaplastic lesion that develops in the livers of cats, both domestic and captive wild felidae. They develop as multiple growths in one or more lobes varying from 0.5 to 5 cm in diameter. Their high fat content makes them lighter in color than the surrounding liver; they are yellow to orange.

If they project above the surface of the liver, they are irregularly nodular. The lesion is composed of normal-appearing, mature fat cells with a variable admixture of myeloid cells, both mature and immature cells of both granulocytic and erythrocytic series being present. In domestic and captive wild cats, similar lesions have been seen in the spleen. These were judged to be separate developments of the same process. Metastasis to other organs has not been reported.

Cystic hyperplasia of the mucus-producing glands in the walls of the gallbladder and larger bile ducts is occasionally observed in dogs (Fig. 2.85). The hyperplastic nodules are sessile or polypoid, and the cysts contain mucin. Some of these may be the result of chronic inflammation. Mucosal hyperplasia in the large bile ducts is observed frequently in the long-standing mild cholangiohepatitis of fluke infestation. The hyperplasia is of microscopic dimensions, but in some instances it appears histologically to be atypical. Localized, polypoid foci of cystic hyperplasia are specific changes in cattle poisoned by highly chlorinated naphthalene.

True neoplasms of the liver and bile ducts are best designated as either hepatocellular or cholangiocellular. Hepatocellular tumors predominate in cattle and sheep, and cholangiocellular tumors predominate in dogs and cats. Other species rarely have primary hepatic tumors. With the exception of the occasional association of liver tumor with certain flukes and the rare adenoma seen in the bovine liver with chronic pyrrolizidine poisoning, hepatobiliary tumors in domestic animals are not successors to antecedent liver disease. There are none of the associations between viruses, chemical carcinogens, mycotoxins, and drugs such as synthetic steroids and hepatobiliary tumors as are known to occur in humans.

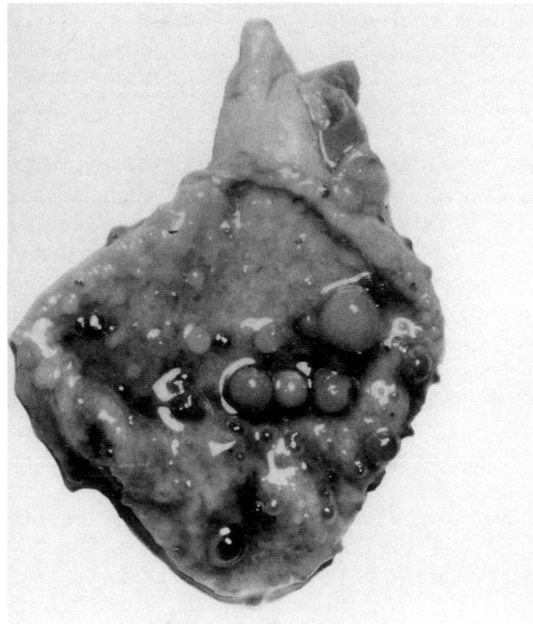

Fig. 2.85 Cystic mucosal hyperplasia. Gallbladder. Dog.

A. Hepatocellular Tumors

Hepatocellular adenomas (hepatomas) are usually single, and they may be 15 cm or more in diameter. The smaller ones project as smooth nodes, but some of the larger specimens are lobate, and some, pedunculated (Fig. 2.86A). They are soft and light brown or yellowish; some are pigmented by bile, the remainder of the liver not being pigmented. Demarcation is fairly sharp and sometimes provided by a connective-tissue capsule. Histologically, the cells do not differ clearly from normal hepatocytes, are arranged in cords or tubules (which may be irregular) (Fig. 2.86B), and often contain small amounts of fat. There are no portal tracts, bile ducts or cholangioles, or hepatic venules, and no suggestion of acini. Bile pigments may be present. In sheep and cattle, hematopoietic foci may be found in the adenomas.

Hepatocellular carcinomas are uncommon. As a general rule, hepatocellular tumors in dogs and cats are more likely to be malignant than benign; in the ox and sheep, the opposite applies. The primary tumor is usually single. Small intrahepatic metastases may surround the primary, having developed in the portal lymph nodes. Malignant tumors cannot be clearly distinguished from adenomas. Several features suggest malignancy, including the absence of pedunculation or clear demarcation and the presence of a varied coloration of the cut surface produced by hemorrhage, necrosis, fatty change, and bile pigmentation. Invasion of portal vessels, sometimes clearly evident

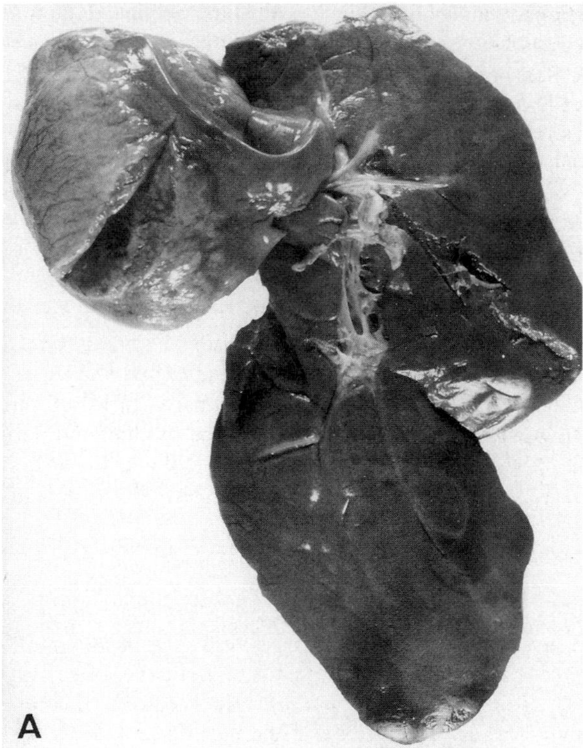

Fig. 2.86A Hepatoma in caudate lobe. Sheep.

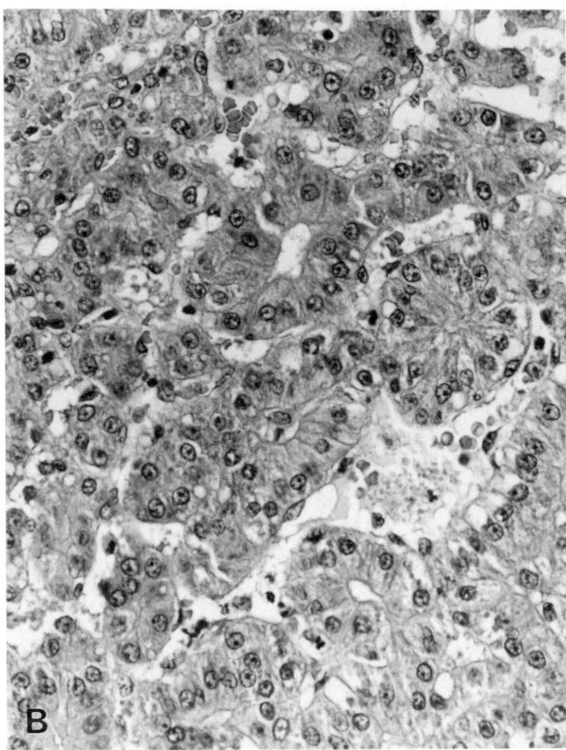

Fig. 2.86B Hepatoma of glandular acinar form. Dog.

grossly, is decisive. Some of these tumors in cattle are scirrhous, hard, and white. Carcinomas occasionally penetrate the capsule to implant on the peritoneum. Hematogenous metastases occur first in the lungs, and some appear to arrive in masses to impact in relatively large vessels.

Free venous invasion is typical of the hepatocellular tumors, and intravascular spread may extend to the large hepatic veins and vena cava. Retrograde growth in the portal veins may extend to the spleen and the stomach, and the resulting portal hypertension and varicose venous shunts assist further spread in portal fields. Spontaneous rupture is common and may cause fatal hemoperitoneum.

Hepatocellular carcinomas may be clearly composed of hepatocytes that have granular acidophilic cytoplasm, a large nucleus with a distinct membrane, and acidophilic nucleoli. Some tumors are composed of cells in which the cytoplasmic volume is small and its quality hard to determine, and these tumors are difficult to distinguish from those of cholangiocellular origin. These also tend to grow in diffuse sheets or as trabeculae, cords, or alveolar masses, a few to many cells thick. In some trabecular areas, canaliculi or acini are formed, and these spaces may contain bile. A feature of some hepatocellular tumors is the presence of giant cells, quite conspicuous by virtue of a large nucleus, multilobed nuclei, or multiple nuclei.

B. Cholangiocellular Tumors

Cholangiocellular adenomas are seen mainly in old dogs and cats. The smaller specimens may be solid on the cut

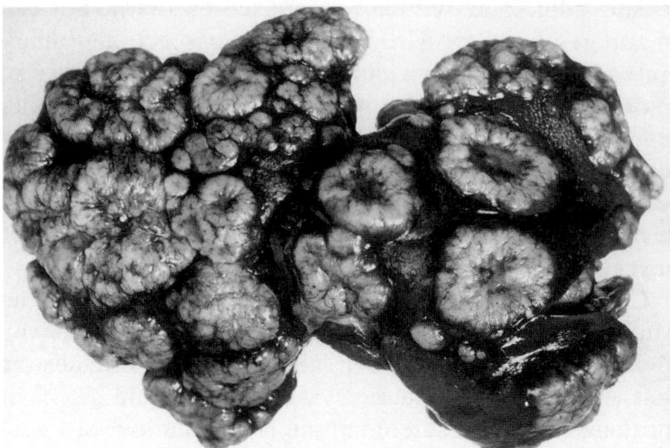

Fig. 2.87 Multiple umbilicated foci of cholangiocellular carcinoma. Cat.

surface and white, but the large specimens, and many of the small ones, are cystic, forming small or large blisters that contain a clear watery fluid. Their volume may be greater than that of the lobe they occupy. Whether these are truly neoplasms or represent acquired or congenital cystic lesions can be argued with little confidence. If any bile is present in the fluid, the tumors should probably be regarded as cysts; if the content is clearly mucinous, the cysts are probably neoplastic.

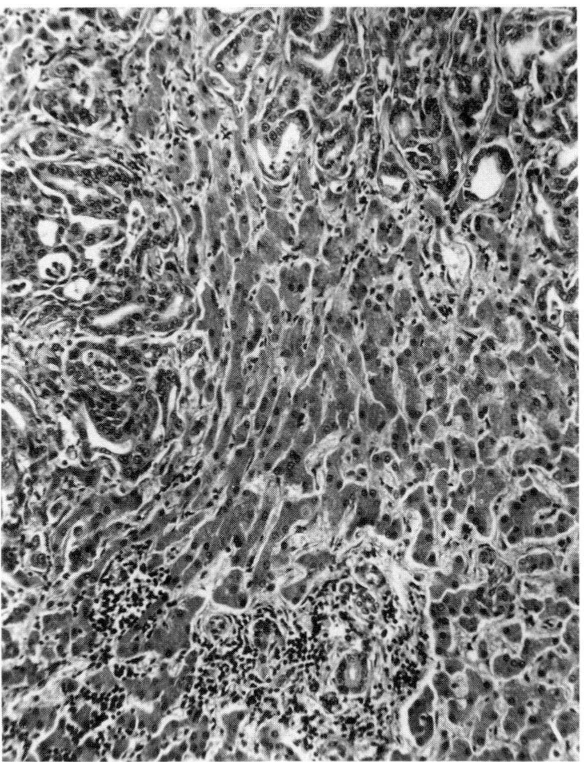

Fig. 2.88 Infiltrative cholangiocellular ompressing hepatocellular plates. Dog.

The solid specimens are composed of a large number of tubules lined by a single layer of respectable biliary epithelium. The stroma varies in amount. There is no sign of active invasion of the parenchyma. The **cystadenomas** are multilocular and lined by a mucosa resembling that of the bile ducts; it may, however, be flattened by pressure, or it may in some areas be papillary. The septal stroma is collagenous. Adenomas of the gallbladder are seldom observed, and then chiefly in cattle.

Cholangiocellular carcinomas are a curious group because in dogs and cats, the species usually affected, the tumors are almost always multiple or diffuse, suggesting that whatever incites them acts diffusely (Fig. 2.87). Solitary ones do occur. The multiple nodules of tumor might represent intrahepatic lymphogenous metastases, but the possibility of multicentric origin must be entertained. Hematogenous metastases are distinctly unusual, but deposits in the regional nodes are common. In cats especially, there is a tendency to invade Glisson's capsule and implant on the peritoneum.

The livers so affected are usually otherwise normal, and in these there is no suggestion as to cause. In humans, the relatively high incidence of bile duct carcinoma in some regions is related to chronic infestation with opisthorcid flukes, especially *O. viverrini* and *Clonorchis sinensis*, and coexistence of fluke and tumor has been observed in carnivores. The biliary changes usually associated with these flukes is of the nature of hyperplastic or adenomatoid proliferation of the epithelium and submucosal glands with goblet-cell metaplasia. There is minimal inflammatory change in the absence of superimposed bacterial infection.

Cholangiocellular tumors can usually be distinguished from the hepatocellular variety by their multiplicity, firmness, whitish color produced by more or less abundant stroma, and the typical umbilication of those that involve the capsule. Even multiple nodules may not cause much enlargement of the liver, but the diffuse variety may cause great enlargement, although with retention of shape, and severe bile pigmentation.

Microscopically, cholangiocellular carcinoma is usually distinctly adenocarcinomatous, producing ductules and acini, and sometimes papillary formations (Fig. 2.88). The cells are cuboidal or columnar, with a small amount of clear or slightly granular cytoplasm. The nuclei are small and fairly uniform, and the nucleoli are not prominent. The tubules do not contain bile, but in well-differentiated specimens may contain mucin.

Primary intrahepatic cholangiocellular carcinoma can be difficult, and often impossible, to distinguish from secondary tumors, especially those of pancreatic origin. Mucus secretion and intrasinusoidal permeation are more typical of biliary origin. Distinction from hepatocellular carcinoma of trabecular pattern may be assisted by demonstration of bile, bile canaliculi, and cytoplasmic organelles in tumors of hepatocellular origin.

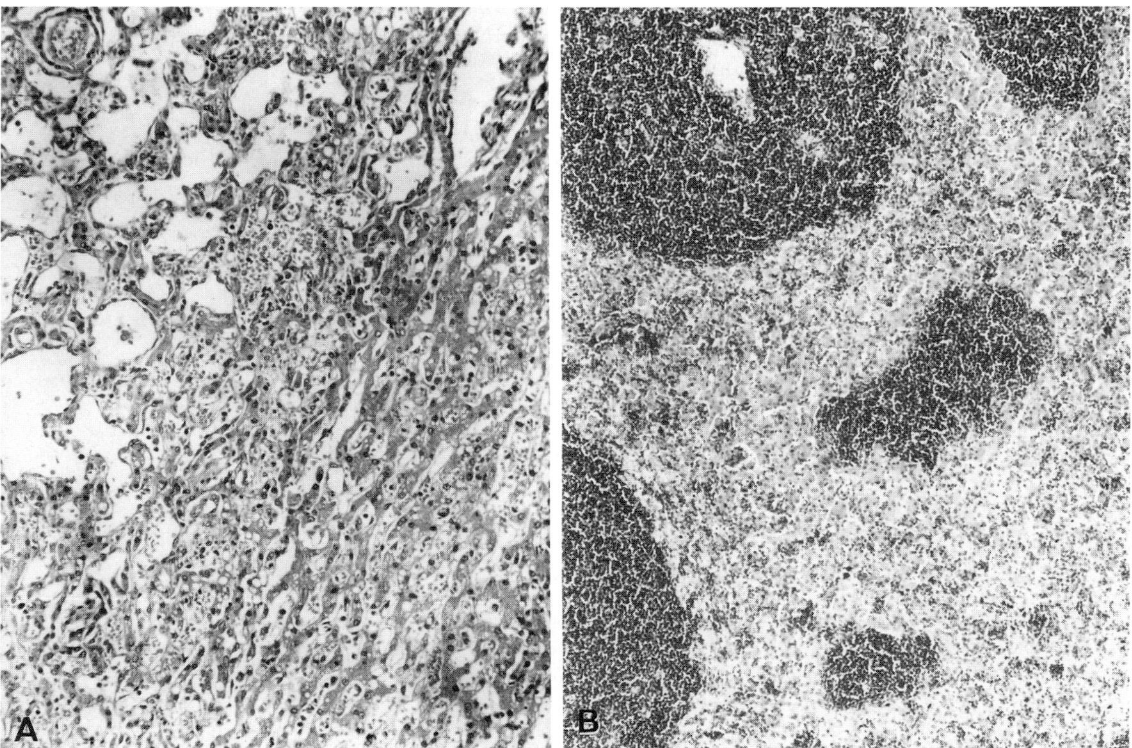

Fig. 2.89 (A) Hemangiosarcoma. Dog. Attenuation and isolation of hepatocytes by invading cells. (B) Lymphoma. Dog. The malignant infiltrate is heaviest in the stroma of triads and hepatic venules.

C. Mesodermal Tumors

Primary mesodermal tumors of the liver are quite uncommon. Benign tumors of smooth muscle are occasionally observed in the gallbladder of dogs and oxen. Primary hemangiosarcomas are rarely seen in dogs and cattle; hemangiosarcoma of the liver should always be considered metastatic until proven otherwise by diligent search. Some of these tumors are solitary, large, and grayish white, with scattered hemorrhagic areas, and others are ill-defined and cavernous. The latter may rupture into the peritoneal cavity to produce severe hemorrhage. Microscopically, it may be impossible to find malignant cells in or lining cavernous areas. At the margins of the tumor, there is a distinctive pattern of growth in which small, solid nodules of malignant cells may be found, or these cells can be found forming capillary structures or invading along preexisting sinusoids. The latter phenomenon is particularly characteristic. As the cells invade along the sinusoids, perhaps in single file, they initially produce little distortion of the hepatic cords. Behind them the sinusoids are spread widely apart, and individual hepatocytes or portions of cords are isolated and appear to be floating freely, surrounded by a thin layer of connective tissue and neoplastic cells. Some of the malignant cells manifest phagocytic properties, and in some there is a suggestion of reproduction by amitosis.

D. Metastatic Tumors

Metastatic tumors of the liver are of wide variety. Some of the carcinomas and sarcomas come via the lungs and hepatic artery. These may be multiple but are seldom numerous; some thyroid and mammary carcinomas are exceptions. Malignancies arriving via the portal vein, such as **pancreatic carcinoma,** may practically replace the liver before producing clinical signs, one of which may be icterus, caused either by extrahepatic bile duct obstruction, or by intrahepatic cholestasis, or both.

Except for the pigment of **melanomas** and the blood of **hemangiosarcomas,** the type of metastatic tumor cannot be distinguished by its gross appearance. Sarcomas do tend to form a few large, smooth-surfaced nodules, and carcinomas do tend to form more nodules and to be umbilicate when in contact with Glisson's capsule. Hemangiosarcomas (Fig. 2.89A) come from the spleen, usually, and may virtually replace the liver with small, blood-filled caverns. Their microscopic appearance is the same as that of the primary tumors (see the preceding sections). **Lymphomatosis** is common (Fig. 2.89B), especially when the spleen is involved. The hepatic infiltration may be in discrete nodules 2 cm or more in size, but it is usually diffuse in the connective tissues of the portal triads. Diffuse infiltration of the liver in myeloproliferative disorders and mast-cell leukemia may cause extreme enlargement of the organ; the infiltrates localize preferentially in the sinusoids.

Bibliography

Anderson, W. A., Monlux, A. W., and Davis, C. L. Epithelial tumors of the bovine gall bladder. A report of eighteen cases. *Am J Vet Res* **19:** 58–65, 1958.

Becker, F. F. Hepatoma—nature's model tumor. A review. *Am J Pathol* **74:** 179–210, 1974.

Bergman, J. R. Nodular hyperplasia in the liver of the dog: An association with changes in the Ito cell population. *Vet Pathol* **22:** 427–438, 1985.

Fabry, A., Benjamin, S. A., and Angleton, G. M. Nodular hyperplasia of the liver in the beagle dog. *Vet Pathol* **19:** 109–119, 1982.

Farber, E., and Sarma, D. S. R. Chemical carcinogenesis: The liver as a model. *Pathol Immunopathol Res* **5:** 1–28, 1986.

Leblanc, B. *et al.* Lymphomatoid granulomatosis in a beagle dog. *Vet Pathol* **27:** 287–289, 1990.

Patnaik, A. K., Hurvutz, A. I., and Lieberman, P. H. Canine hepatic neoplasms: A clinicopathologic study. *Vet Pathol* **17:** 553–564, 1980.

Patnaik, A. K. *et al.* Canine hepatocellular carcinoma. *Vet Pathol* **18:** 427–438, 1981.

Patnaik, A. K. *et al.* Canine bile duct carcinoma. *Vet Pathol* **18:** 439–444, 1981.

Patnaik, A. K. *et al.* Canine hepatic carcinoids. *Vet Pathol* **18:** 445–453, 1981.

Trigo, F. J. *et al.* The pathology of liver tumors in the dog. *J Comp Pathol* **92:** 21–39, 1982.

ACKNOWLEDGMENTS

The help of the following is gratefully acknowledged: Paul Fabbri for photographic prints, Rosemary Murray for typing, and John Pearson for revision of the text on Platyhelminths.

CHAPTER 3 The Pancreas

K.V.F. JUBB
University of Melbourne, Australia

I. General Considerations

The pancreas is tucked away with the duodenum in the upper abdomen where it is relatively well protected against trauma and where it is not readily accessible to the clinician. For these reasons, destructive processes of the pancreas, with the exception of acute pancreatic necrosis, which can be shockingly painful, are revealed as metabolic disturbances, digestive abnormalities, or biliary retention. There are large reserves of endocrine and exocrine function in the pancreas, and metabolic disturbances do not become manifest until a large proportion of the organ or of the islets of Langerhans is lost. Pancreatic disease which is not associated with pain can therefore remain clinically silent for long periods.

The pancreas develops from two primordial outpouchings, dorsal and ventral, from the entodermal lining of that portion of the embryonic gut destined to become the duodenum.

The ventral diverticulum arises in relation to, or from, the primitive hepatic diverticulum. As a result of unequal growth of the duodenal wall, the hepatic and ventral pancreatic anlagen are rotated so that the ventral and dorsal anlagen are brought into apposition and fuse. As the ventral anlage grows in the surrounding mesenchyme, a duct forms and arborizes under the inductive influence of the mesenchyme, and acinar cells differentiate from this ductal epithelium very early in organogenesis. The ventral anlage is destined to become the right lobe of the definitive pancreas, and the dorsal anlage, to become the left lobe.

The duct systems of the two pancreatic anlagen also fuse to produce an anastomotic network. There are differences between and within species as to which of the embryonic ducts is predominant in the developed pancreas. The accessory pancreatic duct, derived from the dorsal anlage, does not persist in small ruminants and in the majority of cats; it is the major duct in the dog, the lesser duct in the horse, and the only duct in the pig and ox. The pancreatic duct, derived from the ventral anlage, is the only duct in small ruminants and most cats; it is the main duct in the horse, and is the lesser duct, and occasionally absent, in the dog.

The islet cells are also derived from larger ducts. The relative contribution of the dorsal and ventral duct anlagen to the distribution of islets in the organ is unknown, but differing rates of contribution may account for different densities of islets in regions of the pancreas and, possibly, for the variable mix of cell types within islets.

The differentiation of islet cells begins even earlier than that of acinar cells in the developing embryo. Uncertainty still surrounds their origin and whether they are derived from ductal epithelium, and thereby from entoderm, or from accompanying cells migratory from neural crest mesenchyme or neurectoderm. Different functional types of islet cells may have different origins.

The cells of the islets are best distinguished by immunochemical techniques, although the beta cells are well revealed by certain stains such as aldehyde fuchsin. Six distinct cell types have been identified with specific secretory products. The alpha cells, which produce glucagon, are typically located at the periphery of islets and constitute about 15% of cells in the islets in which they are present; they are not, however, uniformly distributed among islets. The beta cells, which produce insulin, are present in all islets; they are distributed throughout the islet, composing about 70% of the cell population.

The delta cells are also present in all islets in low numbers; there are two subtypes, one of which produces somatostatin, and the other produces vasoactive intestinal polypeptide. Gamma cells, which produce pancreatic polypeptide, and the enterochromaffin cells, which produce serotonin, are sparsely and variably distributed. It is notable that, with the exception of alpha and beta cells, which are confined to the pancreas, the other islet cells have histochemical and functional counterparts in the gastrointestinal tract, and they may have a common derivation from entoderm or from neural crest.

The pancreas is a lobulated structure, the lobules separated by fine connective tissue septa. Generally, each lobule receives blood from a single arterial branch, and much of the circulation to the acinar tissue is supplied by a portal system of capillaries which emerge from the sinusoids of the islets. In the horse, most of the acinar circulation follows this portal system. In other species, lobules which do not contain islets and exocrine tissue distant from islets are perfused directly from arterial branches. The arrangement of sinusoids in the islets allows the different types of islet cells to modulate the functions of others, and the acinar portal circulation allows the islet hormones to exert trophic or inhibitory effects on acinar cells. Insulin, in particular, and pancreatic polypeptide are trophic for acinar tissue, and somatostatin and glucagon are inhibitory. The circulatory arrangements and the complex interplay of hormones must influence the common pathological changes of atrophy and of diffuse and nodular hyperplasia, and possibly also the pathogenesis and distribution of pancreatic necrosis.

The acinar pancreas is a labile organ. It synthesizes much more protein on a weight-for-weight basis than does any other tissue and consumes a correspondingly large amount of precursor substrate. The response of the exocrine pancreas to changing nutrient intake is rapid, and adaptation to new diets can produce dramatic alterations in the composition of exocrine secretion. Protease secretion is a reflection, in part, of dietary protein levels, and amylase secretion is influenced by the level of dietary carbohydrate and by plasma levels of cortisol and insulin. The influence of diet on lipase secretion is less clear, apparently because it is to some extent dependent on dietary protein levels.

Hypertrophy of the pancreas produced by acinar cell hypertrophy and hyperplasia is a response to diets high in protein and energy; when these are withdrawn, the pancreas reverts by apoptosis and necrobiosis; when the reduction in protein and energy intake proceeds to suboptimal levels, there is atrophy of cells and of the organ. These responses focus attention on the acinar cells and their metabolic machinery. However, the embryologic differentiation of the exocrine pancreas depends on the inductive influences of the surrounding mesenchyme, and it is reasonable to suppose that the structural and functional integrity of the mature pancreas will also depend on this mesenchymal, including vascular, environment. Indeed, there is some evidence from experimental copper deficiency that atrophy and loss of acinar tissue is a consequence of changes in stroma and basement membranes.

The pancreas has not received a commensurate share of the attention given to the liver and its responses to injury, notwithstanding the close embryologic association and a number of parallels in cytodifferentiation, both embryologically and in experimental carcinogenesis, between intrahepatic ducts and pancreatic ducts. The acinar cells will respond to injury as do other parenchymal cells, and complete restitution from remaining acinar cells may replace minimal losses. Extensive or persistent injury may not be repaired by acinar reconstitution, and the cellular responses may involve ductular epithelium and interstitial cells, in ways reminiscent of intrahepatic bile ducts and their responses in chronic liver injury. The potential of the pancreatic ductular epithelium for reactive or reparative differentiation toward acinar cells, islet cells, or hepatocytes is recognized. The limits imposed on these alternative processes are not recognized but, as in the liver, are probably determined by the integrity of the blood supply and excretory ducts and on competitive fibrogenesis.

Bibliography

Bencosme, S. A., and Liepa, E. Regional differences of the pancreatic islet. *Endocrinology* **57**: 588–593, 1955.

Fitzgerald, P. J. The problem of the precursor cell of regenerating pancreatic acinar epithelium. *Lab Invest* **9**: 67–85, 1960.

Go, V. L. W. *et al* (ed.). "The Exocrine Pancreas: Biology, Pathobiology, and Diseases." Raven Press, New York, 1986.

Henderson, J. R., and Daniel, P. M. A comparative study of the portal vessels connecting the endocrine and exocrine pancreas, with a discussion of some functional implications. *Q J Exp Physiol* **64**: 267–275, 1979.

Nickel, R. *et al.* "The Viscera of Domestic Mammals." Springer-Verlag, New York, 1973.

Nielsen, S. W., and Bishop, E. J. The duct system of the canine pancreas. *Am J Vet Res* **15**: 266–271, 1954.

Noden, D. M., and de Lahunta, A. "The Embryology of Domestic Animals: Developmental Mechanisms and Malformations." Williams & Wilkins, Baltimore, Maryland, 1985.

O'Brien, T. D. *et al.* Immunohistochemical morphometry of pancreatic endocrine cells in diabetic, normoglycaemic, glucose-intolerant and normal cats. *J Comp Pathol* **96**: 357–369, 1986.

Rao, M. S. *et al.* Role of periductal and ductular epithelial cells of the adult pancreas in pancreatic hepatocyte lineage: A change in the differentiation commitment. *Am J Pathol* **134**: 1069–1086, 1989.

Rao, M. S. *et al.* Differentiation and cell proliferation patterns in rat exocrine pancreas: Role of type I and type II injury. *Pathobiology* **58**: 37–43, 1990.

Scarparelli, D. G. Multipotent development capacity of cells in the adult animal. *Lab Invest* **52**: 331–333, 1985.

Williams, D. A. Exocrine pancreatic disease. *In* "Textbook of Veterinary Internal Medicine," S. D. Ettinger (ed.), pp. 1528–1554. Philadelphia, Pennsylvania, W.B. Saunders, 1989.

Williams, J. A., and Goldfine, E. D. The insulin–acinar relationship. *In* "The Exocrine Pancreas: Biology, Pathology, and Diseases V," V. L. W. Go *et al.* (eds.), pp. 347–360. Raven Press, New York, 1986.

A. Anomalies of the Pancreas

A variety of anomalies occur in the pancreas but, with the exception of hypoplasia and congenital aplasia of islets of Langerhans, they are of no significance. Variations of the disposition of the ducts are common in dogs. Accessory or ectopic portions of pancreas are observed in dogs. These are probably produced by dislocation of portions of the duodenal buds and are found as small nodules in the submucosa or muscularis of the stomach, intestine, and gallbladder, in the parenchyma of the liver and spleen, and in the mesentery. The ectopic tissue is of normal integrity and presumably functional, though the entry of ducts into an adjacent viscus cannot always be demonstrated. Islet cell tissue may or may not be present. In cats, pancreatic bladders which resemble gall bladders and which are formed by dilation of a duct are recorded. More severe malformations of the pancreas occur as part of generalized malformations which are incompatible with life. Cystic pancreatic ducts may occur with polycystic kidneys and cystic bile ducts in various species. Animals affected die in uremia.

Hypoplasia of the pancreas occurs in dogs and calves. The defect is of the acinar tissue; the islet cell tissue may be quantitatively and qualitatively normal, although in some canine cases, which are not diabetic, islets may be difficult to demonstrate, even with special stains. The hypoplastic pancreas in the **calf** is small, pale, loosely textured, and has indefinite margins. Microscopically, the islets are normal, but the acinar tissue is present as small separated groups of cells in glandular arrangement. Some of these cell groups are well differentiated with zymogen granules and no acinar lumen, but in most of them the cells are small, dark, and of indifferent type, arranged as glands with a patent lumen. The ducts are normal. Clinically, steatorrhea and diarrhea are observed.

In **dogs,** hypoplasia of the pancreas usually is not revealed until the affected animals are about 1 year of age. These animals then develop steatorrhea and quickly become emaciated in spite of a voracious appetite. The late onset of signs of pancreatic insufficiency is probably to be attributed to decompensation, and it is perhaps noteworthy in this respect that the onset of steatorrhea is often preceded by an intercurrent illness. At postmortem, these dogs are potbellied because the intestines are greatly dilated. Of those that are allowed to die, many have intestinal accidents. The intestinal veins are congested, and the intestinal lumen contains bulky, fatty stool. The abdomen is devoid of fat, and the clearness of the mesenteries allows the flimsy tissue of the hypoplastic pancreas to be recognized (Fig. 3.1). The main ducts and their larger tributaries can be seen and recognized by the naked eye. Many of the smaller ducts are recognizable grossly with the aid of transillumination. The ducts are of normal size, length, and configuration. Surrounding the axial ducts is a narrow thin veil or sheet of pink acinar tissue. In a small proportion of dogs, the pancreas may appear normal but microscopically contains nodules of acinar tissue in a gland with abundant fat. The relationship of this lesion to the more common type is unclear. Usually the acinar tissue forms small fasciculi, each of which would probably correspond to a lobule in a normoplastic gland (Fig. 3.2A,B). The cells are small, of an indifferent nature, stain darkly, and do not assume a glandular interstitial tissue. Cases of hypoplasia of the pancreas in dogs tend to be grossly similar, but histologically there may be evidence of continuing regression of ducts and acini. Others have interpreted this condition as pancreatic atrophy because of the degeneration which is present in acinar cells. In these cases, the distinction between atrophy and hypoplasia is difficult.

Pancreatic hypoplasia has been observed in several breeds of dogs. It is most frequent in the German shepherd, in which there is good evidence for a genetic basis, but the causes and pathogenesis may not be the same in all cases.

Aplasia of islet tissue, causing diabetes mellitus, has been reported in dogs aged 2–3 months. The distribution of islets in the normal pancreas is irregular, and it is necessary to examine tissue from many parts of the organ in order to establish the diagnosis.

Occasionally, foci of other tissues are incorporated in the pancreas and, with the exception of hepatocyte foci, are not of pathologic significance. Hepatocytes may appear in the pancreas during attempted regeneration follow-

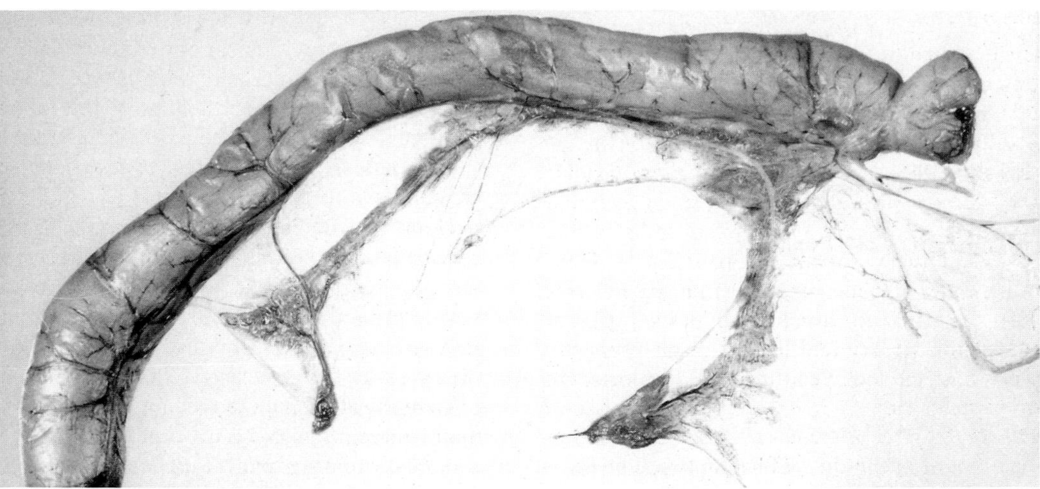

Fig. 3.1 Hypoplasia of acinar pancreas. Dog. Gross appearance showing normal duct system with condensed endocrine tissue.

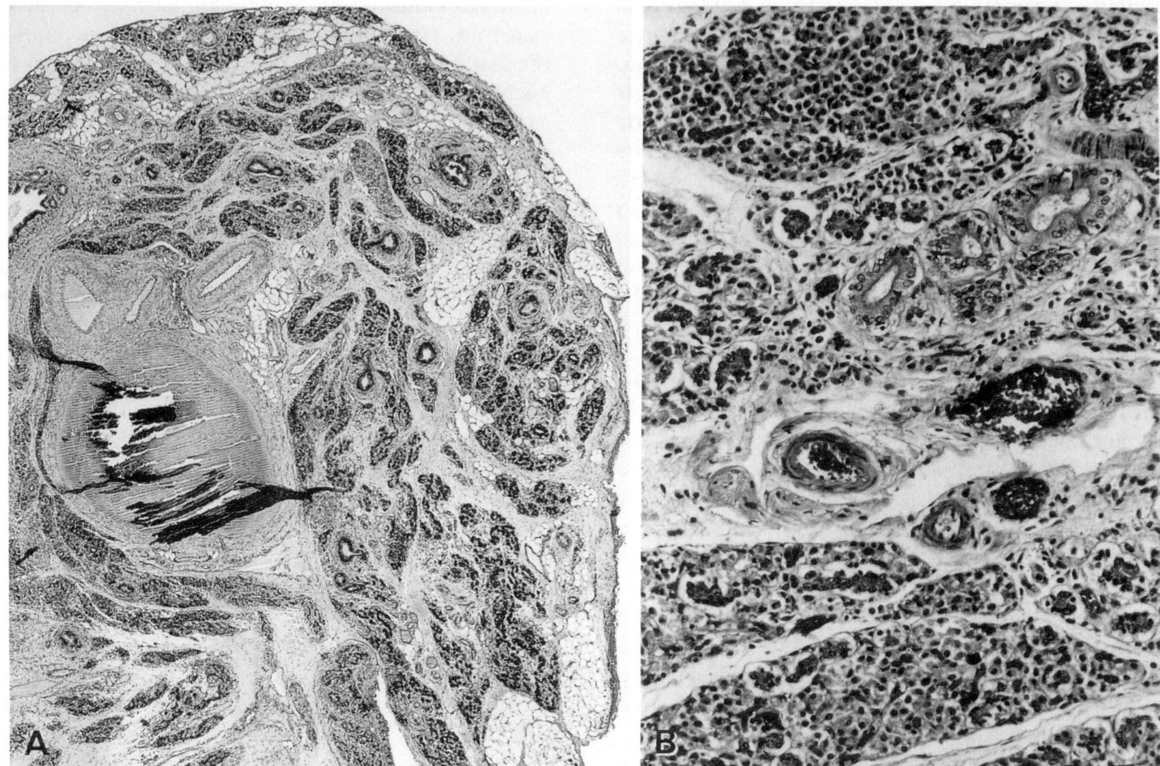

Fig. 3.2 (A) Microscopic appearance of pancreatic hypoplasia. (B) Islet tissue, intercalated and interlobular ducts are condensed.

ing submassive lobular injury and are thought to arise from pluripotent ductular cells.

Bibliography

Baker, E. Congenital hypoplasia of the pituitary and pancreas glands in the dog. *J Am Vet Med Assoc* **126**: 468, 1955.

Barron, C. N. Ectopic pancreas in the dog. A report of three cases. *Acta Anat (Basel)* **36**: 344–352, 1959.

Bolydreff, E. B. Report of an accessory pancreas on the ileum of a dog. *Anat Rec* **43**: 47–51, 1929.

Hashimoto, A. *et al.* Juvenile acinar atrophy of the pancreas of a dog. *Vet Pathol* **16**: 74–80, 1979.

Westermark, E. The hereditary nature of canine pancreatic degenerative atrophy in the German shepherd dog. *Acta Vet Scand* **21**: 389–394, 1980.

B. Regressive Changes in the Pancreas

The exocrine pancreas is susceptible to many adverse influences. The classical morphologic types of cellular degeneration occur in many febrile, toxic and cachectic illnesses but these appear to be of little clinical importance.

1. Degeneration, Autolysis, and Atrophy

Degenerative changes should not be confused with postmortem autolysis. Autolysis occurs rapidly after death. Advanced autolysis with a patchy distribution is rather common in histologic material and is produced by rough handling of the organ at postmortem with rupture of cells and liberation of enzymes. The autolyzed tissue stains a slate-gray color with hematoxylin, resists eosin, and has a washed-out appearance.

A **lipofuscin pigment** is responsible for the khaki color sometimes observed in the canine pancreas. It has been produced by prolonged tocopherol deficiency. The intestinal musculature is similarly pigmented. The pigment, in the form of small brown granules, is present in the basal portions of the cytoplasm of the acinar cells, in the myocytes of the intestine, and in a number of other locations, such as the pigment epithelium of the retina where it is distinguishable from pigments normally present.

Lipomatosis of the pancreas is occasionally observed in cats and swine. It is usually part of a general obesity but may be restricted to the pancreas. The adipose tissue accumulates in the interstitium and disperses the parenchyma, creating a false impression, microscopically, of a severe reduction in glandular tissue. There may be some pressure atrophy, but lipomatosis is without clinical significance for the pancreas.

Atrophy of the pancreas occurs commonly but is seldom appreciated. It may be a primary atrophy or it may be secondary to other pancreatic lesions. Primary atrophy is a diffuse change, which does not produce any alteration of the gross form of the organ, and microscopic changes may be subtle and easily missed on routine examination.

The acinar atrophy of kwashiorkor, a syndrome of protein–calorie deficiency in children, is well documented, and similar histomorphologic changes, although not necessarily of the same causation, are widespread in animals. Probably most of these are reflections of protein–calorie deficiency, of starvation, of the inanition of chronic disease, or of the maldigestion of gastrointestinal mucosal injury, and as such, they will be accompanied by atrophy of other tissues, especially of the liver. Specific nutritional deficiencies also occur, including deficiencies of essential amino acids and of the trace elements zinc, copper, and selenium. These may be simple deficiencies of the elements, or the deficiency may be conditioned by other dietary ingredients, such as excess iron or molybdenum in the conditioning of copper deficiency, or excess calcium in the conditioning of zinc deficiency.

The molecular pathogenesis of pancreatic atrophy cannot be detailed but may directly involve acinar intracellular metabolism or indirectly do so from changes in the interstitium. The progress of atrophy begins with depletion of acidophilic zymogen granules and later development of cytoplasmic basophilia. There is progressive shrinkage of the cytoplasm and, finally, dissociation of cells to produce a microscopic picture in which there is no acinar or glandular arrangement but, instead, a diffuse sheet of small, dark-staining cells without polarity (Fig. 3.3A,B).

Secondary pancreatic atrophy is the result of concurrent pancreatic disease, usually duct obstruction with fibrosis. As a consequence, secondary atrophy affects the pancreas nonuniformly, although the entire organ may be involved, the affected parts of the organ are reduced in size, misshapen, coarsely nodular, and tough. On section, the affected portions consist largely of fibrofatty tissue in which accessory structures, such as nerves, vessels, ducts, and islets of Langerhans are condensed. The islets, except for being concentrated in smaller areas, appear normal.

Spontaneous obstruction of the ducts, with the exception of the developmental stenosis that is occasionally seen in cats, is usually accompanied by some degree of inflammation and interstitial fibrosis, especially after repeated bouts of pancreatic necrosis. Therefore, the atrophy induced by duct obstruction is often compounded by the atrophy of pressure and ischemia induced by interstitial scar tissue. Under these circumstances, the islet tissue may also be affected. When the extra-pancreatic ducts are obstructed experimentally by ligation, complete atrophy of the exocrine portion of the gland ensues. The islets are spared, and interstitial inflammation and fibrosis do not develop.

Pancreatic lithiasis, the calculi consisting mainly of calcium carbonate and calcium phosphate, may be found incidentally in cattle but is rare in other species. The calculi are associated with, and may be a consequence of, inflammation, such as is caused by flukes, where these occur. The calculi are never large, but they may be numerous like sand grains. Obstruction of the pancreatic duct is probably not complete, with ectasia accompanied by

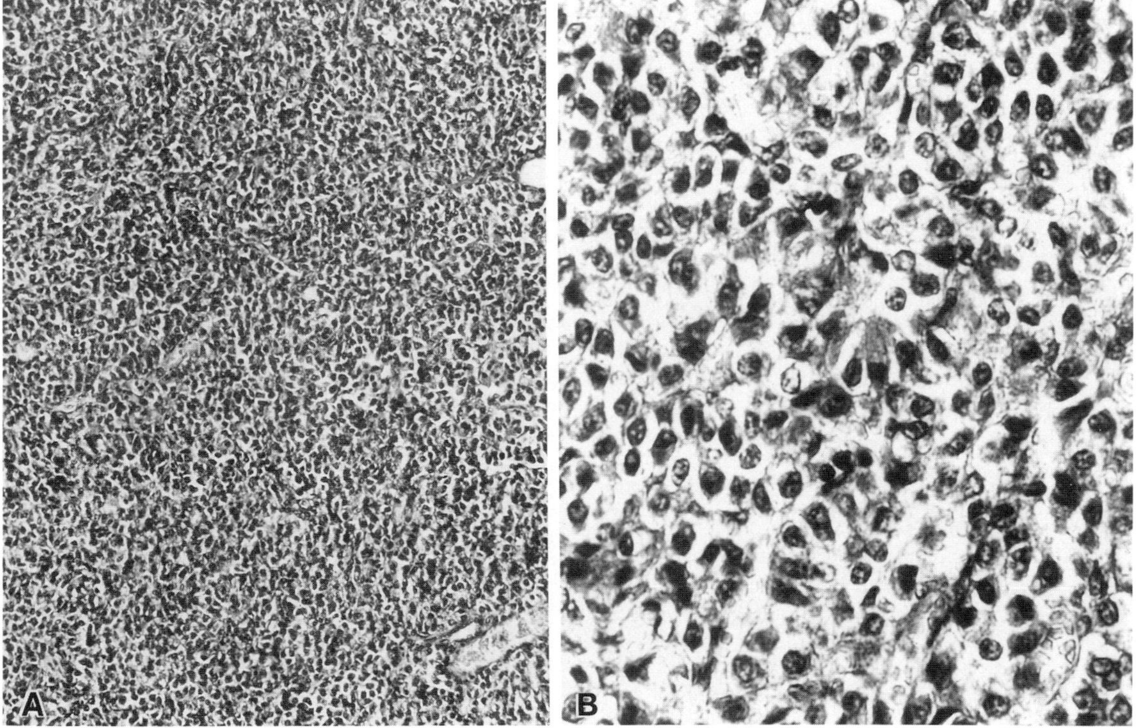

Fig. 3.3 (A) Nutritional atrophy of pancreas. Pig. (B) Detail of (A) showing absence of cytoplasmic granularity with vacuolation.

inflammatory contractures and cystic dysplasia of mucosal glands.

Bibliography

Dalgaard, J. B. Pancreolithiasis in cattle. *Skand Vet Tidskr* **35**: 362–364, 1945.

De Caro, A. *et al.* The human pancreatic stone protein. *Biochimie* **70**: 1209–1214, 1988.

Eppig, J. J., and Leiter, E. H. Exocrine pancreatic insufficiency syndrome in CAA/J mice. *Am J Pathol* **86**: 17–30, 1977.

Fell, B. F. *et al.* Observations on the pancreas of cattle deficient in copper. *J Comp Pathol* **95**: 573–590, 1985.

Pound, A. W., and Walker, N. I. Involution of the pancreas after ligation of the pancreatic ducts. 1. Histological changes. *Br J Exp Pathol* **62**: 547–558, 1981.

Simpson, K. W. *et al.* Effects of exocrine pancreatic insufficiency and replacement therapy on the bacterial flora of the duodenum in dogs. *Am J Vet Res* **51**: 203–206, 1990.

Szabo, T. *et al.* Pancreatic atrophy in the canine : An entity of exocrine–endocrine dissociation. *Mt. Sinai J Med* **45**: 503–508, 1978.

2. Acute Pancreatic Necrosis

Acute pancreatic necrosis is an important disease of dogs. It is reported to occur rarely in horses and swine, but adequate distinction is not always drawn between pancreatic necrosis, pancreatitis, and atrophy. The designation of pancreatic necrosis is preferred to one of pancreatitis to indicate more precisely the basic necrotizing character of the lesion. Even this designation is not wholly satisfactory because the major morphologic changes are not in the parenchyma of the organ, but rather in the interstitial and peripancreatic adipose tissue.

There are two acute, potentially catastrophic diseases of the pancreas in dogs and humans, which are not always separated or, indeed, easy to separate in autopsy material. They are acute pancreatic necrosis and acute hemorrhagic pancreatitis. The former is common in the dog, and the latter, quite unusual. Descriptions of the disease in humans do not allow conclusions as to relative frequency, but the ratios are probably reversed. Acute pancreatic necrosis is perilobular, the injury and inflammation concentrated at the periphery of affected pancreatic lobules with more or less extensive involvement of surrounding adipose and other mesenchymal tissues; the duct system and centrilobular tissue is intact in the acute disease. Acute hemorrhagic pancreatitis is initially periductular and centrilobular, the lesions enlarging and becoming confluent to involve most of the pancreas and are soon complicated by extensive hemorrhage and sepsis.

It is doubtful whether recovery from acute pancreatic necrosis in dogs ever occurs. The term chronic relapsing pancreatitis is sometimes applied by the pathologist to the

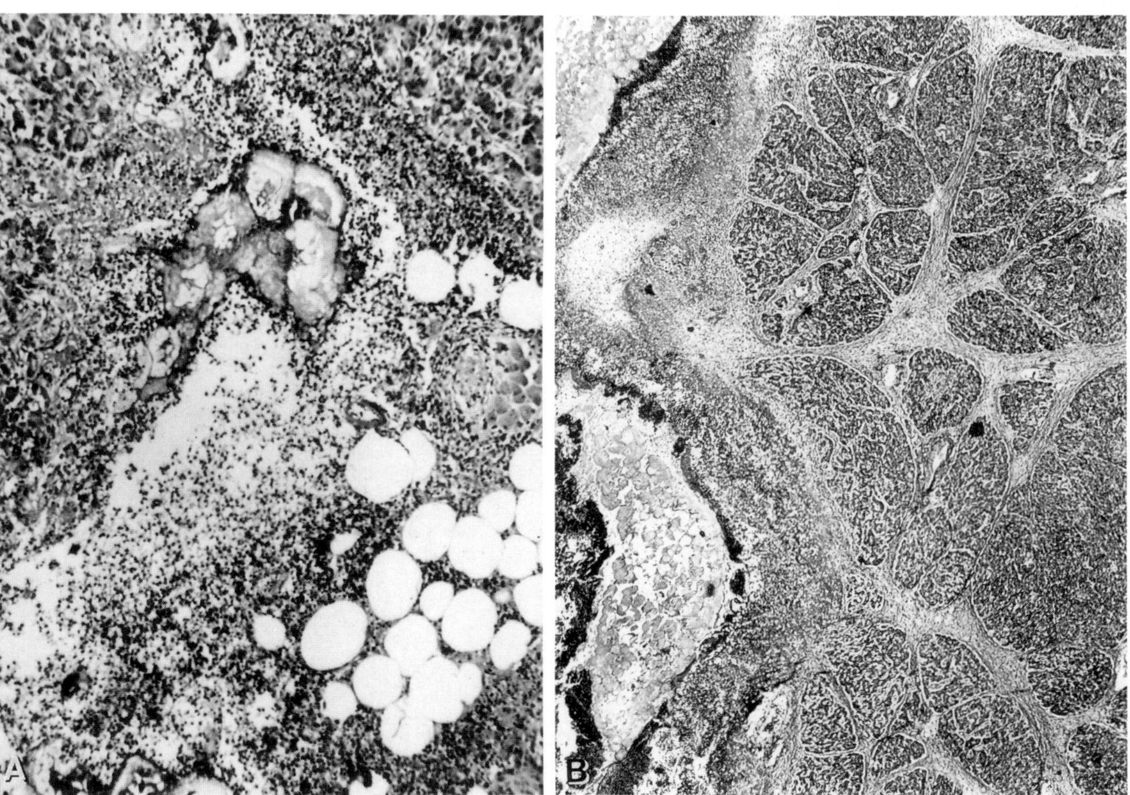

Fig. 3.4 (A) Acute pancreatic necrosis. Dog. The severe inflammatory reaction is centered on pancreatic fat, with relative sparing of acinar tissue (upper right). (B) Acute necrosis in pancreas, which also shows postnecrotic scarring. Dog.

prolonged disease, but there is doubt as to whether this is really a relapsing disease. Rather, it appears that if the animal survives the initial acute episode, as it usually does, the necrotizing process smolders continuously and often asymptomatically until there is almost no pancreas left. There is seldom any difficulty in finding microscopic areas of acute necrosis in these chronically affected organs, even in the terminal stage when the dog dies or is destroyed because it has diabetes mellitus or steatorrhea and cachexia. Whether the apparently relentless course is due to persistence of the primary pathogenetic mechanism or to a self-perpetuating property of the lesion is not known. The initial lesion is often localized to one portion of the gland, and the smoldering foci are often multiple, of random distribution, affect the periphery of the remnants, and tend to avoid the parenchyma, which has survived in the original focus, and which is undergoing fibrous enclosure and atrophy.

The initial acute episode of pancreatic necrosis may or may not be clinically apparent. It occurs mainly in obese females and when clinically expressed is characterized by signs of severe abdominal pain and cardiovascular collapse in shock. Death may follow in 2–3 days. Of diagnostic significance, elevation of lipase and amylase in serum and abdominal fluid occurs, and abdominal fluid may also contain droplets of fat released from damaged adipose tissue. Not all cases are clinically apparent, and the disease may pass unnoticed until terminally, when signs of exocrine and endocrine insufficiency develop as a consequence of the unrelenting destruction. Pancreatic necrosis is a common cause of diabetes mellitus in dogs since the acute reactions destroy islets as well as acinar tissue.

The pathogenesis of acute pancreatic necrosis in dogs is obscure, excepting perhaps those cases which follow surgical manipulation of the pancreas and those which follow prolonged corticosteroid therapy. Dogs which are fed diets high in fat and low in protein develop acute pancreatic necrosis, which is histogenetically comparable to the spontaneous disease and, of the models available for producing this type of pancreatic injury, those involving dietary manipulation may be the most rewarding. The fact that the lesions involve the periphery of the lobules, which is also the periphery of the circulatory fields, suggests a role for hypoperfusion, and possibly reperfusion, in the pathogenesis; this could account for development of the disease after prolonged hypotension and surgical procedures.

Regardless of the primary mechanism of pancreatic necrosis, there is general agreement that the visible lesions are produced by the proteolytic enzymes of the organ. By what means they are activated and released from intracellular compartments remains hypothetical. The enzymes may become activated while still within acini, or there may be rupture of canaliculi or acini with release of enzymes into the stroma and activation there. In experimental diet- and hyperstimulation-induced pancreatic necrosis, activation occurs intracellularly, following fusion of lysosomes and zymogen granules; lysosomal proteases, such as cathepsin B, are apparently responsible for activation of trypsinogen.

Whatever the mechanism and site of initial enzymic activation, pancreatic damage is amplified by oxygen-derived free-radical production, which contributes to the organ edema by effects on endothelial cell membranes, and by sequential activation of the arsenal of pancreatic enzymes, both by trypsin and by inflammatory products. Liberated lipases initiate fat hydrolysis, but pro-elastase and prophospholipase activation appear to be particularly important in exacerbating the lesion. Consumption of plasma protease inhibitors, especially alpha-macroglobulins, permits activation of the kinin, coagulation, fibrinolytic, and complement cascade systems by free proteases, leading to the clinical systemic signs of disseminated intravascular coagulation and shock.

In fatal cases of acute pancreatic necrosis there is, at postmortem, a small quantity of fluid in the abdominal cavity. The fluid contains droplets of fat and is often blood-stained. Hemorrhages may be present in the omentum, but extensive hemorrhage is not a feature of the lesion. Numerous chalky areas of fat necrosis surrounded by a halo of reddening are present adjacent to the pancreas and in the mesentery. At a greater distance from the pancreas, areas of fat necrosis may be found as far away as the ventral mediastinum to which, presumably, the enzymes are conveyed in lymphatics. The whole of the pancreas

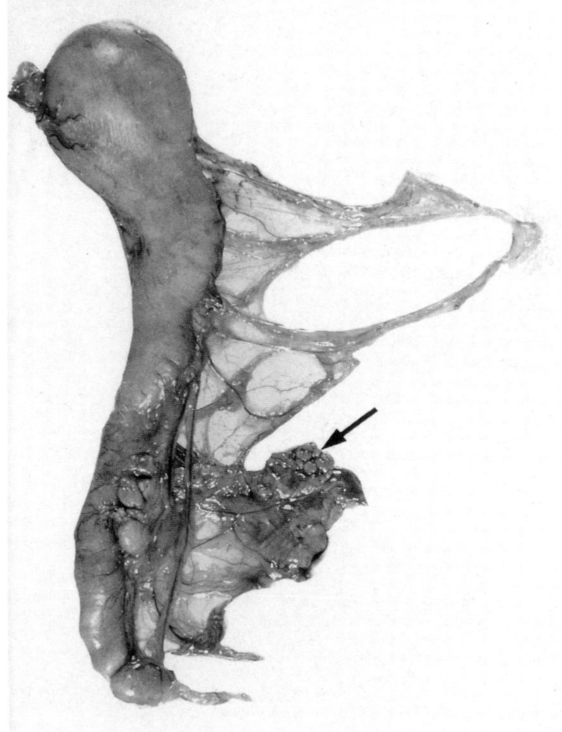

Fig. 3.5 Postnecrotic scarring of pancreas. Dog. Only nodular remnants are left (arrow).

may be edematous, swollen, and soft, or the edematous swelling may be confined to localized areas of more severe change. The necrotizing process may occur in the midportion of the gland opposite the ducts, or in one of the branches. Yellowish or hemorrhagic fibrinous adhesions pass from the affected surface of the pancreas to the omentum and visceral surface of the liver. The cut surface presents a variegated appearance due to merging of whitish areas of fat necrosis and grayish-yellow areas of parenchymal necrosis; one or other appearance may predominate. The texture is unusually greasy. The areas of parenchymal necrosis are softened and may be liquefied.

The microscopic picture includes necrosis of adipose tissue, necrosis of parenchymal tissue, edematous separation of stroma, necrosis and thrombosis of blood vessels, and reactionary inflammatory infiltrate (Fig. 3.4A,B). The infiltrating leukocytes form a border zone at the boundary of necrotic and viable tissue. The necrotic fat has the usual histologic characters. Necrosis of the pancreatic parenchyma begins at the periphery of the lobules. Small foci of acinar tissue, separate from the stroma, become shrunken and acidophilic, and undergo coagulative necrosis. The collagenous stroma resists digestion for some time. With the onset of parenchymal necrosis, the septal tissues are further distended with fluid, in which much fibrin may be precipitated. Occlusion of capillaries by fibrin thrombi occurs at the margin of the necrotic areas. Venous thrombosis, sometimes with inflammation or necrosis of the wall of the vessel, occurs adjacent to and distant from the lesion; similar changes may occur in the small arteries, but these, as a rule, are less susceptible to injury. Widespread venous and arterial thrombosis is observed as a terminal development in many organs.

The end result of the necrotizing process, provided that the acute episodes are not fatal, is almost complete destruction of the organ (Fig. 3.5). Depending on the stage at which the pancreas is observed, it may be irregular in conformation and knobby, or reduced to a few distorted lobules adjacent to where the ducts enter the duodenum. In some cases, the remnants of the organ are too small to be visible, but they may still be palpable in areas indicated by a slight puckering of the mesentery. In spite of the severity of the active process, scar tissue is minimal, and adhesions are absent or minor. Microscopically, a few small rounded lobules remain, and are compressed and atrophic. The interstitial tissue is increased, but this is probably due as much to condensation of stroma as to fibroplasia. The vessels and nerves are also condensed into the small area of the pancreatic remnant. Islets of Langerhans often cannot be identified. Other changes may be present at autopsy, their nature depending on whether the animal has steatorrhea or diabetes mellitus.

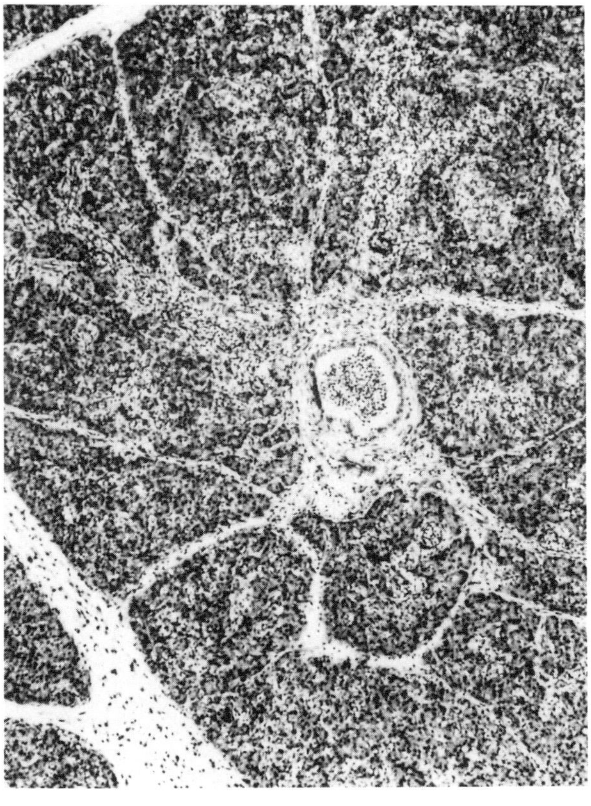

Fig. 3.6 Acute interstitial pancreatitis. Cat. Reaction is centered on duct.

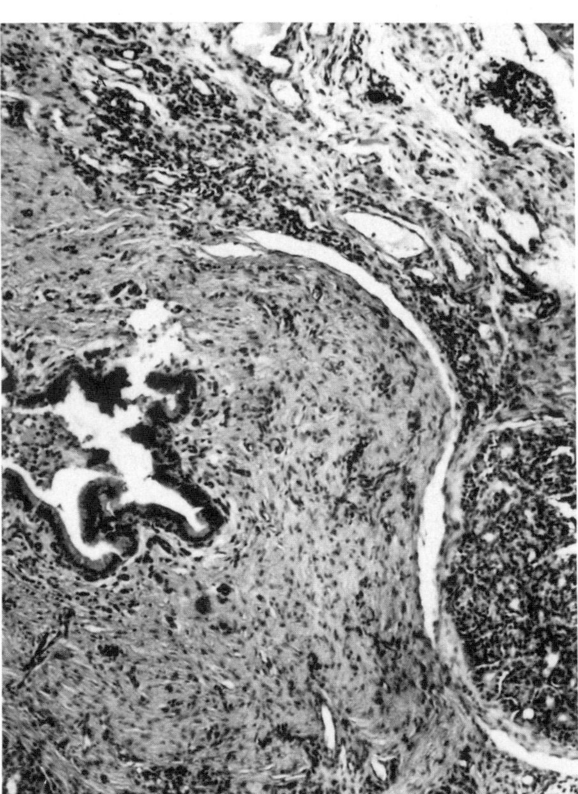

Fig. 3.7 Chronic interstitial pancreatitis. Cat. Note heavy fibrosis around duct.

C. *Inflammation of the Pancreas*

1. Pancreatitis

Acute hemorrhagic pancreatitis characterized by centrilobular and periductal necrosis is an important human disease associated in about 80% of cases with biliary calculi or alcohol abuse. A similar lesion is occasionally observed in dogs, but predisposing conditions have not been identified. It is likely that the initiating event is reflux of duodenal content into the main pancreatic duct, causing ductal inflammation and leakage and activation of enzymes. The pancreas is edematous and hyperemic initially, and the lobular tissue becomes friable and hemorrhagic. The extensive hemorrhage and exudate may obscure the pancreatic tissue. The necrosis and saponification of adipose tissue may also be obscured by the hemorrhage. Liquefaction of the necrotic tissue leaves large lakes of debris, and infection by enteric organisms may cause abscessation.

Acute pancreatitis, in which there is suppuration or the formation of abscesses, is seldom seen, but it can arise by direct extension from a neighboring focus of infection, as it occasionally does from peritonitis and from perforated esophagogastric ulcers of swine. Suppurative lesions of lymphohematogenous origin are rare. Generalized **granulomatous infections** have a lesser tendency to avoid the pancreas, but the metastatic lesions are usually microscopic and minor. Destructive granulomatous pancreatitis is part of multisystemic eosinophilic epitheliotropic syndrome of horses, and pyogranulomatous pancreatitis occurs in the coronavirus disease, feline infectious peritonitis. **Acute interstitial pancreatitis** is common in systemic toxoplasmosis, especially in cats (Fig. 3.6). Grossly the organ is slightly swollen by diffuse interlobular edema, or a hemorrhagic and necrotizing process may accompany a similar process in the duodenum.

Chronic interstitial pancreatitis is the form of inflammation that is usually seen in animals. It is seldom of clinical significance but is occasionally responsible for death. The lesion is not uncommon in cats, is occasionally observed in horses, and is rarely observed in other species. It arises usually by spread to the interstitial tissue of an inflammatory process which begins in the ducts (Fig. 3.7). When of this pathogenesis, the causes are nonspecific, with the exception of some parasitic trematodes, the microbes present being normal inhabitants of the gut. As an alternative to ascending inflammation of the ducts, pancreatitis which begins in the interstitial tissue is common in horses but of no significance; these lesions are produced by the larvae of *Strongylus equinus,* which pass part of their developmental cycle in and about the pancreas. *Stephanurus dentatus* may encyst in the pancreas of pigs following its intrahepatic migration. The abscesslike le-

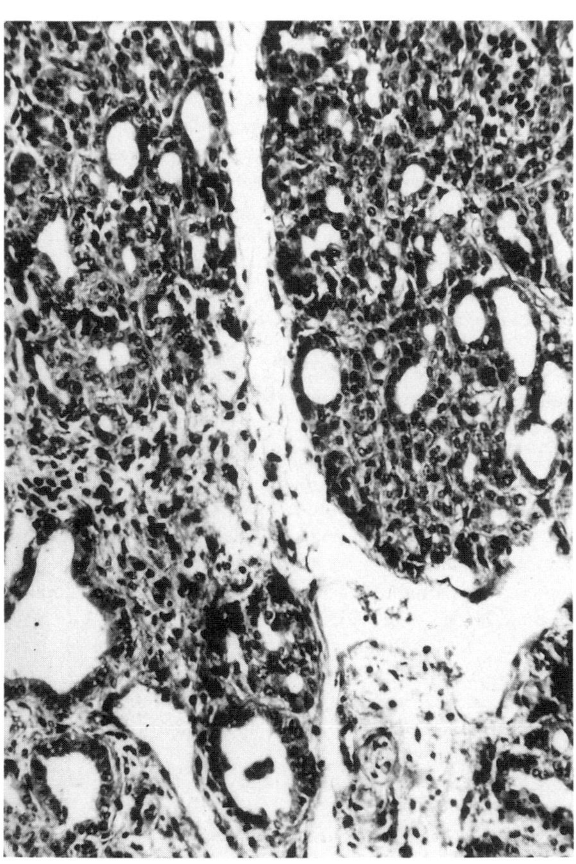

Fig. 3.8 Atrophy of acinar tissue and dilation of ducts in vitamin A deficiency. Calf.

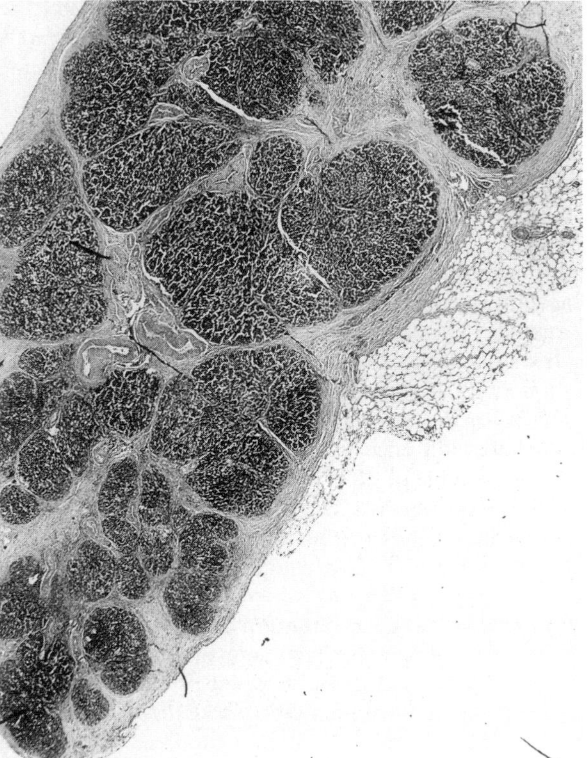

Fig. 3.9 Chronic interstitial pancreatitis. Cat.

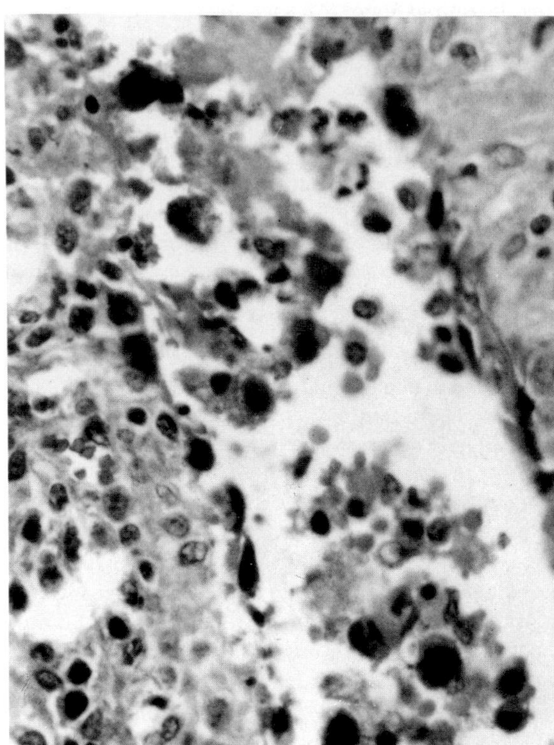

Fig. 3.10 Adenovirus inclusions in pancreatic duct. Foal. Combined immunodeficiency.

sions produced apparently are of no significance. With the exception of parasitic infestations and the predispositions offered by metaplastic changes in the epithelium of the ducts in vitamin A deficiency (Fig. 3.8), the primary causes of chronic interstitial pancreatitis are not known. In cats, in which species the pancreatic and biliary ducts fuse before entering the duodenum, cholangitis frequently, and perhaps always, coexists with inflammation of the pancreatic ducts. The same may occur in horses.

In chronic interstitial pancreatitis, the organ may be reduced in size or enlarged. In horses, the tendency is for enlargement to occur and the organ to be replaced by a tough mass of scar tissue, which merges with surrounding attachments. Flattened remnants of pancreatic tissue may be present near the surface of the mass. When incised, the tortuous and eccentrically dilated ducts are readily apparent. In some of them, there is inflammatory exudate or pus, and in others, a large amount of slightly opaque mucus, which makes the cut surface slimy.

In cats, the pancreas is usually reduced in size, firm, gray, and irregular. Through the capsule, but particularly on the cut surface, clear retention cysts are often visible. Fibrosis may not be recognizable on gross inspection, but there are exceptional cases in which the whole organ is converted into a shrunken, distorted, fibrous remnant. Histologically, the ducts contain a catarrhal exudate and are surrounded by heavy fibrosis (Fig. 3.7). Localized stenoses occur and, in other segments, microcysts. The epithelium of the ducts is hyperplastic or metaplastic and may be squamous. The fibrous tissue spreads from around the ducts to the interlobular stroma and subdivides many of the lobules (Fig. 3.9). The acinar tissues atrophy as a response to enveloping fibrosis. The islets of Langerhans are well preserved. The stromal tissues are permeated by leukocytes, chiefly of mononuclear variety. The chronically inflamed ducts are a potential site for the development of pancreatic **calculi,** but these are rarely seen; they are more frequent in cattle than in other species. The calculi are small, seldom larger than 4–5 mm, white, hard, composed of carbonates and phosphates, and thousands may be present.

Focal pancreatitis, in which small clusters of acinar cells undergo necrosis, is a frequent microscopic finding in systemic infections by viruses with epitheliotropic properties. They include canine parvovirus, canine distemper virus, adenoviruses in several species (Fig. 3.10), and the virus of foot-and-mouth disease. This form of pancreatitis is not significant to the course of these infections, except for foot-and-mouth disease virus in ruminants, in which diabetes mellitus may occur in delayed convalescence.

Bibliography

Anderson, N. V. Pancreatitis in dogs. *Vet Clin North Am* **2:** 79–97, 1972.

Emanuelli, G. *et al.* Experimental acute pancreatitis induced by platelet-activating factor in rabbits. *Am J Pathol* **134:** 315–326, 1989.

Feldman, B. F. *et al.* Biochemical and coagulation changes in a canine model of acute necrotizing pancreatitis. *Am J Vet Res* **42:** 805–809, 1981.

Freudiger, U. Diseases of the exocrine pancreas in the cat. *Berl Munch Tierarztl Wochenschr* **102:** 37–43, 1989.

Hendricks, J. C. *et al.* Reflux of duodenal contents into the pancreatic duct of dogs. *J Lab Clin Med* **96:** 912–916, 1980.

Joubert, L. *et al.* Pancréatite aigue necrosante stéatorrhéique d'allure enzootique, chez le porc d'engrais. *Rev Med Vet* **115:** 453–490, 1964.

Kazacos, E. A., and Van Vleet, J. F. Sequential ultrastructural changes of the pancreas in zinc toxicosis in ducklings. *Am J Pathol* **134:** 581–595, 1989.

Lindsay, S., Entenman, C., and Chaikoff, I. L. Pancreatitis accompanying hepatic disease in dogs fed a high-fat, low-protein diet. *Arch Pathol* **45:** 635–638, 1948.

Lombardi, B., Estes, L. W., and Longnecker, D. S. Acute hemorrhagic pancreatitis (massive necrosis) with fat necrosis induced in mice by D,L-ethionine fed with a choline-deficient diet. *Am J Pathol* **79:** 465–478, 1975.

Longnecker, D. S. Pathology and pathogenesis of diseases of the pancreas. *Am J Pathol* **207:** 100–121, 1982.

Manabe, T., and Steer, M. L. Protective effects of PGE_2 on diet-induced acute pancreatitis in mice. *Gastroenterology* **78:** 777–781, 1980.

Panabokke, R. G. An experimental study of fat necrosis. *J Pathol Bacteriol* **75:** 319–331, 1958.

Perry, T. T. Role of lymphatic vessels in the transmission of lipase in disseminated fat necrosis. *Arch Pathol* **43:** 456–465, 1947.

Rimaila-Parnanem, E., and Westermark, E. Pancreatic degenerative atrophy and chronic pancreatitis in dogs. *Acta Vet Scand* **23:** 400–406, 1982.

Robert, A. *et al.* Prevention by prostaglandins of caerulein-induced pancreatitis in rats. *Lab Invest* **60:** 677–691, 1989.

Schoenberg, M. H. *et al.* Oxygen free radicals in acute pancreatitis of the rat. *Gut* **31:** 1138–1143, 1990.

Steer, M. L., and Meldolisi, J. The cell biology of experimental pancreatitis. *N Engl J Med* **316:** 144–150, 1987.

Thordal-Christensen, A., and Coffin, D. L. Pancreatic diseases in the dog. *Nord Vet Med* **8:** 89–114, 1956.

2. *Parasitic Diseases of the Pancreas*

Ascarids may invade the pancreatic ducts from the intestine in swine and dogs. A variety of trematodes, including *Dicrocoelium dendriticum, Opisthorchis felineus, Opisthorchis (Clonorchis) sinensis,* and *Metorchis conjunctus,* occur in the pancreatic ducts. Their presence there in numbers large enough to provoke interstitial pancreatitis betokens an overflow from the biliary ducts where they belong and with which they are described.

Flukes of the genus *Eurytrema* accept the pancreatic ducts as their primary habitat, although they may, simultaneously, infest the biliary tract. A number of species have been named in the genus, but their distinction as species is uncertain. *Eurytrema pancreaticum* of ruminants is probably the most important species, as it is common in parts of Asia, Madagascar, and South America; *E. coelomaticum* is common in cattle in Brazil; *E. fastosum* infests carnivorous animals in the same geographical areas as does *E. pancreaticum.* Pigs can be infested with the species from either herbivores or carnivores.

Infestation of the pancreatic ducts by these trematodes leads to chronic interstitial pancreatitis. *Eurytrema pancreaticum* has some preference for the left lobe of the pancreas. The acinar tissue may be almost destroyed and replaced by fibrofatty tissue; the islets survive much better. *Eurytrema (Concinnum) procyonis* is found in the main pancreatic duct of small carnivores and is usually associated with some periductal fibrosis but with minimal changes in the parenchyma of the gland. In areas in which the fluke occurs, as many as 10% of cats may be infested, and with heavy infestations, the main duct may be greatly dilated and much of the gland, shrunken, pale, and fibrotic.

Bibliography

Burggraaf, H. Pancreas-diastomatose (fascioliasis of the pancreas). *Tijdschr Diergeneeskd* **62:** 399–407 and 469–481, 1935. *(Eurytrema).*

Florence, R. Existence chez les bovins de Madagascar de l'*Eurytrema pancreaticum. Bull Soc Pathol Exot Filiales* **32:** 446–447, 1939.

Fox, J. J. *et al.* Pancreatic function in domestic cats with pancreatic fluke infection. *J Am Vet Med Assoc* **178:** 58–60, 1981.

Pinto, C. Variacoes morfologicas observadas no "*Eurystrema fastotum*" (Kossack, 1910). *Campo, Rio de J* **6:** 50–52, 1935. (Morphologic types of *E. fastotum* in cats.)

Purves, G. B. The species of *Eurytrema* in domestic ruminants. *Vet Rec* **11:** 583–584, 1931.

Purves, G. B. Further parasites of domestic animals in Malaya. *Vet Rec* **11:** 761, 1931. (Includes *Eurytrema rebelle* in the cat.)

Tang, C. C. Studies on the life history of *Eurytrema pancreaticum* (Janson, 1889). *J Parasitol* **36:** 559–573, 1950.

D. ***Neoplastic and Similar Lesions of the Exocrine Pancreas***

Nodular hyperplasia of the pancreas is a common finding in old dogs, cats, and cattle. In most instances, there is no sign of an antecedent injury. The hyperplasia involves the exocrine tissue only, occurs in many foci, and may involve whole lobules or only portions of them. Grossly, the hyperplastic lobules project as flat elevations from the contour of the organ, are whiter than the surrounding tissue, and are palpably hard. The histologic picture provides a mosaic and should be interpreted cautiously because the hyperplastic nodules cannot always be readily distinguished from adenomas. The hyperplasia seldom involves a whole lobule uniformly; instead there are one or more nodules in the lobules. The hyperplastic nodules are not encapsulated and do not compress the surrounding parenchyma. The morphology of the cells in each nodule is rather uniform, and there is always some resemblance to acinar structure. The cells may appear as enlarged counterparts of normal exocrine cells with a bulky, brightly acidophilic cytoplasm, or they may be of indifferent character, producing a low cuboidal lining for glandular spaces, or they may form small indifferent clusters without a lumen. The mosaic appearance is due to the irregular admixture of nodules of diverse architecture.

Adenomas of acinar and ductular origin, when distinguished from nodular hyperplastic lesions, are extremely rare. **Adenocarcinomas** occur with some frequency in dogs and less often in cats. There may be a greater tendency for adenocarcinomas to arise centrally within the gland, and those that compromise biliary drainage lead to early clinical signs. The neoplasms may be more or less spherical and circumscribed, or they may have some resemblance to masses of scar tissue. On cross section, the yellow lobulated structure of normal glands is replaced by grayish scirrhous tissue, in which there may be some areas of necrosis and hemorrhage. Some of these tumors may contain cysts with a mucinous content and, histologically, localized ductular arrangements which may be well differentiated and difficult to distinguish from the duct response to incomplete obstruction.

Pancreatic adenocarcinomas often have an aggressive behavior, with implantation on the peritoneum and metastatic disease common. Metastases to the liver are usual, either as small nodules or a few large ones. Local lymph nodes may also contain metastases, and direct invasion of the duodenal wall is frequent. These neoplasms have a tendency to provoke much scirrhous stroma. It is not possible to correlate closely the histologic structure with behavior. Some well-differentiated specimens may metastasize widely. The whole spectrum of adenocarcinomatous structure, from diffuse groups of anaplastic cells to well-differentiated structures which mimic normal acini or

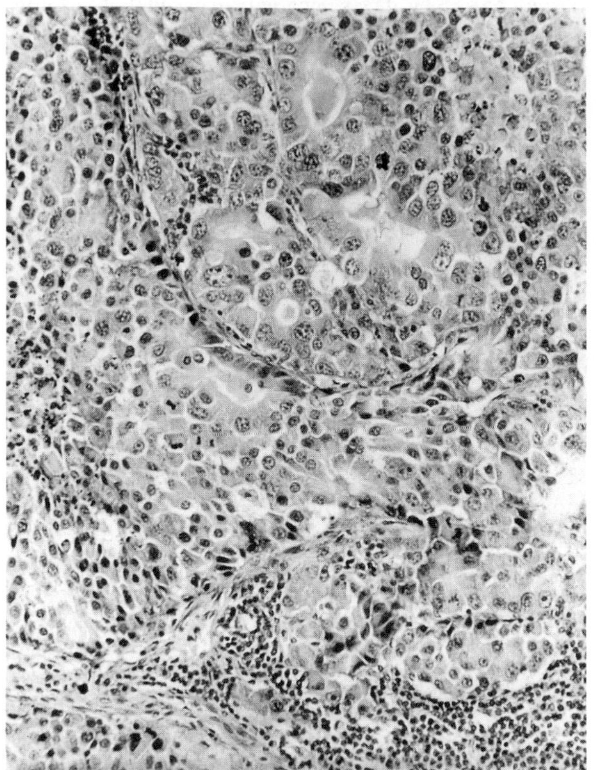

Fig. 3.11 Pancreatic adenocarcinoma. Dog. There is necrosis of acinar tissue and a mononuclear cell infiltration. Tumor is forming tubular structures. Karyomegaly and mitotic figures are present.

ducts, can be found (Fig. 3.11). An attempt is usually made to distinguish tumors of acinar origin from those which arise from ducts. The distinction is rather arbitrary because the degree and direction of differentiation are unpredictable, and ductular cells are known to have pluripotent capacity. However, there are some tumors in which the neoplastic glandular structures are lined by cuboidal or columnar cells which have a clear cytoplasm and secrete mucus and which resemble the epithelium of ducts. Tumors of probable acinar origin are composed of small hyperchromatic cells, which tend to form distorted glandular arrangements. Tumors that cannot easily be distinguished from normal acinar tissue are clearly of acinar origin and may be associated with areas of fat necrosis within and adjacent to both primary and metastatic tumor foci.

The incidence of acinar pancreatic neoplasia in humans has increased over the last decade and, experimentally, carcinogens have been identified that induce neoplasia in animals. Nitrosamines are potent pancreatic acinar carcinogens in hamsters, and enzyme-altered foci and hyperplastic and dysplastic nodules develop progressively after exposure. Selenium deficiency enhances carcinogenesis in this model. Methylxanthine-containing beverages are thought to increase the risk of acinar neoplasms in humans. To date, chemicals that induce spontaneous acinar or ductular neoplasms in dogs and cats have not been identified.

Bibliography

Moulton, J. E. "Tumors in Domestic Animals," University of California Press, Berkeley, California, 1990.

Popp, J. A. Tumors of the liver, gallbladder, and pancreas. *In* "Tumors in Domestic Animals 3rd Ed." J. E. Moulton (ed.), University of California Press, Berkeley, California, 1990.

II. Islets of Langerhans

Reference is made earlier in this chapter to certain properties of the islets which are of interest to the pathologist. The beta cells and their responsibilities in carbohydrate metabolism, however, are the matters of prime concern. Tumors of islet cell type which produce excessive gastrin effects are rare in domestic animals. The beta cells appear to be uniformly distributed in the islets, which is at variance with the distribution of other cell types except the delta cells.

The cells of pancreatic islets normally release amines and polypeptides which serve to regulate intermediary metabolism either in the conventional hormonal mode or as local trophic or paracrine influences. The syndromes which may result from dysplastic islet cells reflect either quantitative changes in the secretion of individual polypeptides, or the aberrant secretion of more than one peptide, or the secretion of peptides of abnormal functional characteristics.

Pancreatic **islet hyperplasia** in domestic animals probably occurs with greater frequency than currently assumed, because variability in islet density with age and in different regions of the pancreas limit the ability to detect subtle proliferative responses. Islet cell hyperplasia is described in a number of laboratory species, including monkeys, mice, rats, and hamsters. It can be induced through hormonal mechanisms, either as compensatory hyperplasia in surviving islets following destruction of a portion of the gland, or as a consequence of hormonal antagonism by iatrogenic or naturally occurring hyperadrenocorticoidism. Nesidioblastosis, the term used to describe combined ductular and islet cell proliferation common in childhood pancreatitis, and which leads to hyperinsulinism, is not a commonly recognized entity in domestic animals, although a similar condition has been induced experimentally by administration of nitrosamines to hamsters, and nesidioblastosis has been described in dogs with islet cell neoplasms.

Bibliography

Bencosme, S. A., and Leipa, E. Regional differences of the pancreatic islet. *Endocrinology* **57:** 588–593, 1955.

Furuoka, H. *et al.* Immunocytochemical component of endocrine cells in pancreatic islets of horses. *Jpn J Vet Sci* **51:** 35–43, 1989.

Nelson, R. W. Disorders of the endocrine pancreas. *In* "Textbook of Veterinary Internal Medicine." S. J. Ettinger (ed.),

Vol. 1: 1676–1720. Philadelphia, Pennsylvania, W. B. Saunders, 1989.

Zucker, P. F., and Archer, M. C. Alterations in pancreatic islet function produced by carcinogenic nitrosamines in the Syrian hamster. *Am J Pathol* **133:** 573–577, 1988.

A. Degenerative Lesions of the Islets of Langerhans: Diabetes Mellitus

Necrosis of the islets occurs in acute pancreatic necrosis. Their progressive destruction, along with the acinar tissue, is a common cause of diabetes mellitus in dogs. Atrophy of the islets occurs as a result of fibrosis in chronic interstitial pancreatitis, but because the islet tissue is more resistant to atrophy of this cause than is the acinar tissue, diabetes mellitus is seldom a complication of pancreatitis. Insular insufficiency is possible from extensive neoplastic destruction of the pancreas. Amyloidosis of the islets, causing remarkable enlargement of them, is occasionally observed in cats (Fig. 3.12). The amyloid is restricted to the islets and may not be found in other tissues. Amyloidosis of the islets is regularly associated with diabetes in cats, but whether the amyloid deposits cause or result from the diabetic state is not known. In dogs with diabetes mellitus which is not the result of pancreatic necrosis, varying degrees of sclerosis of the islets can sometimes be readily seen. Sclerosis is, however, occasionally observed in minor degrees in old nondiabetic dogs, so its significance is difficult to assess. The sclerotic process in diabetic dogs may replace whole islands or parts of them and may be so condensed as to assume to some extent the appearance of hyalin. As with amyloidosis, it is undetermined whether sclerosis is a cause or an effect of diabetes mellitus.

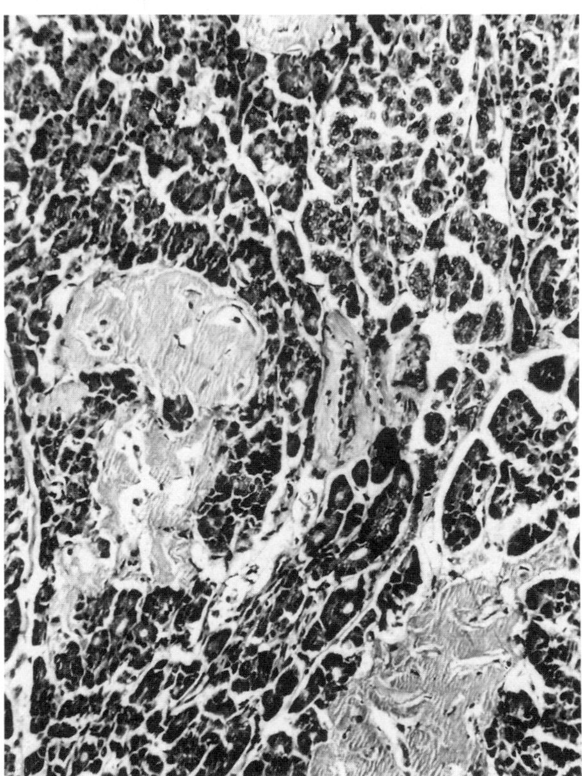

Fig. 3.12 Diabetes mellitus. Amyloidosis of islets of Langerhans. Cat.

A number of viruses are known to replicate in the pancreas but, with the exception of the diabetes mellitus which may be seen in chronic foot-and-mouth disease of cattle, are not known to be significant in islet disease. Congenital aplasia of islet tissue is referred to with anomalies of the pancreas.

Diabetes mellitus is due to inadequate insulin action. The inadequacy of action may be due to deficient production of insulin, or to failure of insulin as an effector hormone in peripheral tissues, or to antagonism by other hormones. Diabetes mellitus is therefore not a single disease but a syndrome in which all cases share some common metabolic, clinical, and pathologic features.

Insulin is an anabolic hormone with direct effects on carbohydrate, protein, and fat metabolism. It promotes the uptake by cells of glucose to form intracellular glycogen; it directs amino acids to protein synthesis instead of to gluconeogenesis; and it promotes the uptake of fatty acids by adipose tissue to form storage triglycerides. Inadequate insulin action leads therefore to a general catabolic state. There is increased gluconeogenesis from glycogen and protein leading to hyperglycemia; protein synthesis is reduced leading to wasting of tissues; and hyperlipidemia results from increased lipolysis and diminished uptake of free fatty acids in adipose tissue. The hyperglycemia increases the filtered load of glucose in primary urine to levels in excess of the tubular transport mechanism, leading in turn to glycosuria, osmotic diuresis, and thirst. The excess of fatty acids presented to the liver is metabolized via acetyl-coenzyme A, in the absence of glucose, to form the ketoacids. The ketoacids, acetoacetic and beta hydroxybutyric, and acetone dissociate to produce ketoacidosis.

The complex of metabolic disturbances, if uncontrolled by therapy or unless partially suppressed by residual insulin action, leads to hyperosmolarity, profound dehydration, acidosis, and other electrolyte disturbances, which result in neurologic derangements and coma.

Diabetes mellitus is not a disease of sudden onset or of all-or-none expression. The normal pancreas contains a substantial reserve of beta cells and insulin-producing capacity, which may have to be reduced to 20% of normal before the catabolic processes become dominant. The anabolic effects of insulin are exerted on many tissues and through numerous metabolic steps, not all of which are deranged equally or simultaneously as insulin effect declines. **Reduced glucose tolerance is a feature that is early and common to all types of diabetes mellitus.**

The classification of diabetes mellitus into its different types continues to evolve as new knowledge is gained. The reference classification is that used for the human condition, noting that it is not directly applicable to domestic animals. In the human classification, **type I** diabetes mellitus is generally equatable with juvenile-onset and insulin-dependent diabetes, in which insulin secretion is reduced or nonexistent. **Type II** diabetes is generally equatable with adult onset or non-insulin-dependent diabetes in which levels of insulin in the pancreas are approximately normal, but the target cells in peripheral tissues that respond to insulin are deficient in insulin-receptor activity, or the intracellular machinery that responds to insulin is defective. There is evidence that within type II diabetes there are examples also of aberrant synthesis of insulin or failure of the release response to changing glycemic levels. A third category of diabetics are those affected by **secondary diabetes,** arising as a consequence or complication of other disease.

Type I, or insulin-dependent, diabetes of humans is the result of reduced output of insulin from the islets, which in turn, is the result of depleted numbers of beta cells. No doubt there will be various ways in which beta cells can be selectively destroyed; alloxan and streptozotocin intoxication are examples. However, the emphasis in the human disease is on selective immune-mediated destruction. There are genetic linkages which confer high and low levels of susceptibility to type I diabetes, but the initiating factors are unknown. Presumably, susceptible individuals are exposed to a foreign antigen structurally similar to a component of beta cell cytoplasm and which provokes a cell-mediated immune response. Autoantibodies are also produced, but it is doubtful whether they contribute to the cellular injury; they are important in identifying those who are likely to develop type I diabetes. Viruses are candidate sources for the foreign protein.

The beta cells must possess some properties which make them especially vulnerable to immune injury. They do appear to be particularly susceptible to cytokine injury, such as by interleukin-1 that is secreted by activated macrophages; they are unusually susceptible to membrane injury by free radicals, and, when damaged, they express an excess of major histocompatability complex (MHC) molecules, which are able to promote cytotoxic T-lymphocyte activity.

The immune destruction of beta cells in humans proceeds slowly, and years may elapse between the triggering event and the onset of clinical diabetes. During this progress, some islets will have lost all beta cells, some will show infiltrates of lymphocytes with a few monocytes, and some will be normal. Ultimately all beta cells are lost, and the inflammatory infiltrates disappear.

Diabetes of this pathogenesis is not established in domestic animals. That autoantibodies occur in diabetic dogs is noted, as is the occasional observation of insulitis. Foot-and-mouth disease virus may be responsible in this way for diabetes in ruminants.

Early-onset diabetes in animals occurs in dogs which are presented clinically at a few months of age. These are not examples of selective beta cell destruction but instead examples of islet hypoplasia. A few small, shrunken islets may be present, but usually none can be identified. Scattered endocrine cells may be present, as they normally are, in the interacinar tissue. This would suggest that islets had differentiated, perhaps imperfectly, and then had undergone accelerated degeneration. This supposition takes into account the facts that differentiated islet cells with synthetic activity are present very early in organogenesis, prior to acinar cell differentiation, and that the islet secretions are trophic for acinar tissue. The exocrine pancreas in dogs without islets shows moderate atrophy consistent with withdrawal of trophic influences.

Islet hypoplasia tends to affect purebred dogs, and pedigree analysis of keeshonds and golden retrievers suggests a heritable cause.

Destruction of islets concurrently with other pancreatic tissues in the pancreatic necrosis syndrome is a common cause of insulin-responsive diabetes in adult dogs. Affected animals are those with the chronic relapsing pattern of pancreatic necrosis, such animals also presenting with evidence of exocrine deficiency.

Human **type II** diabetes is non-insulin dependent, usually develops in the adult and is a common and important disease. Genetic influences are important, but genes of the MHC complex are not involved. Other, constitutional factors such as obesity, exercise, and diet are important. Type II diabetes is probably not a single etiologic entity. The levels of insulin in the pancreas are about normal, but release of insulin from beta cells in response to glucose load is impaired, or the released insulin may not be consumed in peripheral tissues. Peripheral insulin resistance may be due to deficient insulin receptors or intracellular mediators of insulin action. The hyperglycemia and glucose intolerance may in these cases be accompanied by levels of plasma insulin which are above normal.

The roles of hyporesponsiveness of beta cells to blood glucose levels and of peripheral resistance to insulin, other than in cases of antagonistic endocrinopathy, are not established in domestic animals. Obesity in dogs and cats is associated with reduced glucose tolerance and insulin resistance, but such animals are usually normoglycemic, and there is not evidence that they progress to overt clinical diabetes; transient periods of hyperglycemia may, however, occur during episodes of intercurrent disease or stress. Insulin resistance is demonstrable in the lipemic syndromes of obese horses and cats, described with diseases of the liver (Chapter 2 of this volume).

Abnormal control of islet secretion appears to be central to the development of non-insulin dependent diabetes in desert rodents such as the sand rat (*Psammomys obesus*), spiny mouse (*Acomys hirinus*), and tuco-tuco (*Ctenomys talarum*). These arid-zone rodents develop diabetes when fed laboratory chow *ad lib,* suggesting that metabolic overload in these animals may lead to diabetes by direct effect on beta cells or indirectly by disturbed paracrine homeostasis within the islets. It is possible that the observed degranulation and degeneration of beta cells represents exhaustion atrophy.

The majority of cases of diabetes in cats is associated with islet abnormalities and perhaps corresponds most closely with human type II diabetes. The common morphologic feature in the islets is the deposition of amyloid, and this occurs also in spontaneously diabetic monkeys (*Macaca nigra*). This is endocrine-associated amyloid, and it is not related to systemic or secondary amyloidosis—although the two may coexist in some cats. The amyloid is deposited between capillaries and islet cells, and the fibrils are closely associated with the cell membranes of beta cells. Terminally, most islets are affected, and most of the islet space is occupied by amyloid. Those islets which are least affected tend to be in lobes in which the beta cells are normally present in lesser numbers.

There is substantial homology in the peptide units of islet amyloid polypeptide in human and feline islet amyloid and in the amyloid deposits in human and canine insulomas. The polypeptide occurs in normal beta cells of many species and may be cosecreted with insulin. There is evidence that the peptide might be inhibitory of glucose-stimulated insulin secretion and of glycogenesis from glucose in muscle.

The presence of amyloid in the islets of normoglycemic cats is an indicator of prediabetes.

The pathogenesis of **secondary diabetes** reflects antagonisms between insulin and other hormones. The antagonisms are exerted in peripheral tissues, but those which are conducive to sustained hyperglycemia may overburden the beta cells and exhaust them.

Endogenous progesterone is diabetogenic in the bitch, and persistent corpora luteal action in pseudopregnancy may initiate postestrus diabetes in the bitch. Pyometra sometimes coexists with the clinical diabetes. The effects of progesterone are indirect; it stimulates release of growth hormone, which inhibits insulin-receptor activity and intracellular responses to insulin. Progestogens administered to cats are also diabetogenic in that species, in which the effects appear to be direct and due to the glucocorticoidlike activity of progesterone.

Pituitary tumors, as a source of unregulated production of growth hormone, cause diabetes in dogs, cats, and horses. The adenomas in dogs and cats are of acidophil cells. In horses, diabetes has been associated with acidophil cell tumors of the anterior lobe and with adenomas of the pars intermedia.

Insulin-resistant diabetes is the most consistent expression of hyperadrenocorticoidism in cats and is common also in dogs, in which it may be a consequence of exogenous glucocorticoid administration.

The lesions of diabetes mellitus in cats and dogs are comparable. Apart from emaciation, and possibly dehydration, the principal lesion at autopsy is a remarkably yellow fatty liver. The pancreas may appear normal or reveal the lesions of postnecrotic scarring or pancreatitis. Lipemia may be evident as a milkiness of the serum.

Microscopic lesions can usually, but not always, be found in the pancreas. In addition to the insular changes described earlier, there may be vacuolation of the islet cells and, with it, vacuolation of the epithelium of the

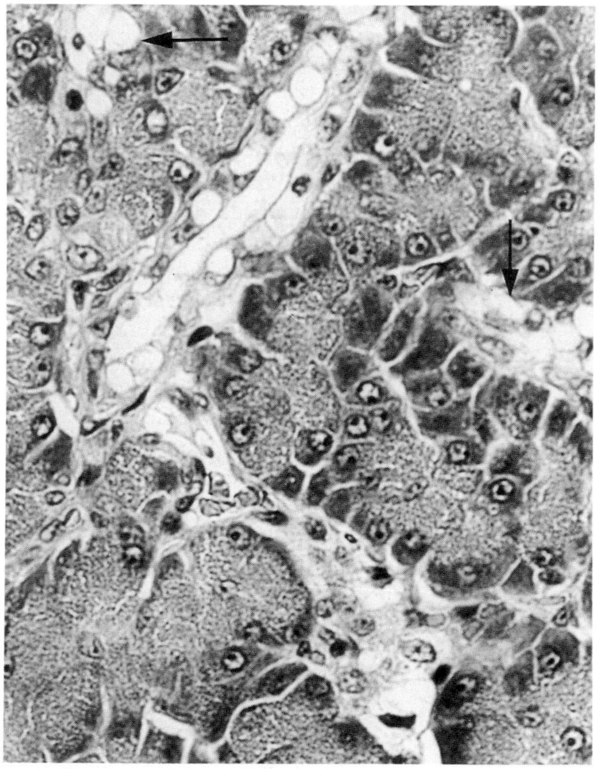

Fig. 3.13 Vacuolar (glycogen) degeneration of islet (arrows) and ductal epithelium. Dog.

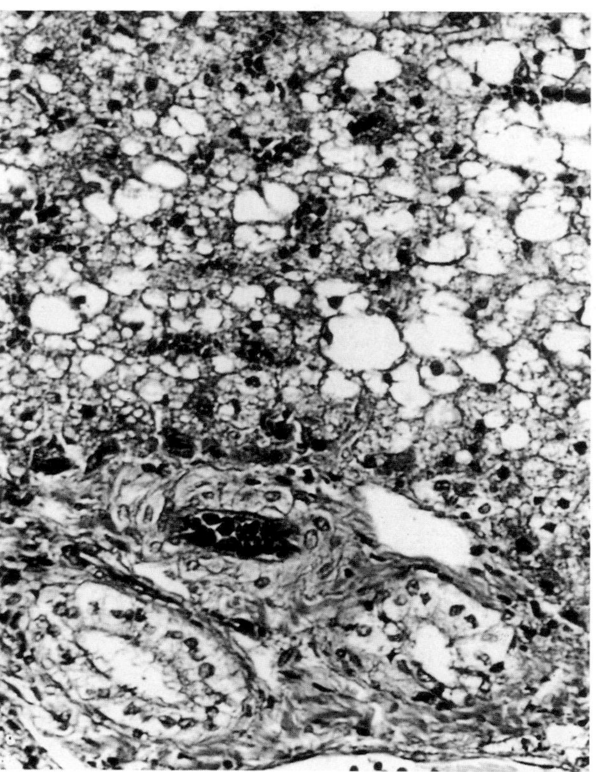

Fig. 3.14 Severe hepatic lipidosis with vacuolation of bile duct epithelium. Dog.

smaller ducts (Fig. 3.13). The vacuolation in routine sections is due to the accumulation of glycogen and is a specific lesion for diabetes mellitus, but is thought to be present only in acutely developing severe cases. Glycogen nephrosis, which is present as a vacuolar change in the renal epithelium, is also highly specific for diabetes. The glycogen is deposited chiefly in Henle's loop and the distal convoluted tubule and mainly in the nephrons of the inner cortex. As well as the severe hepatic lipidosis (Fig. 3.14), there is fatty degeneration of the epithelium of the proximal convoluted tubules. Fat emboli are occasionally present in the glomerular capillaries.

In long-standing diabetes, diffuse or nodular glomerulosclerosis may develop. Periodic acid–Schiff-positive basement membrane material accumulates, causing hyaline thickening of the capillary basement membranes and sclerosis of lobules in the glomerular tufts. Diffuse thickening of the mesangium develops and may lead to glomerular obliteration (Fig. 3.15). The increased accumulation of basement membrane, at least in insulin-dependent diabetics, may be related to an inherent defect in somatic cells, which leads to an increased rate of cell turnover with duplication of basement membranes. The lesion which is most obvious in glomerular capillaries also involves capillaries in other tissues and the basement membranes of Bowman's capsule and convoluted tubules.

The complicating vascular lesions and infections which are so important in humans are rare in domestic animals although emphysematous cystitis develops occasionally (see The Urinary System, Chapter 5 of this volume), and some dogs present with secondary bacterial infections of respiratory and urinary tracts and of the skin. The relative lack of complications in animals is probably related to the severity and duration of the disease. The course of the disease in dogs is ordinarily fairly short, but the exceptional natural case and some experimental ones may survive for 2 years or more, and show, in addition to diffuse glomerulosclerosis, retinal capillary aneurysms. The latter are suitably demonstrated only in retinal spreads.

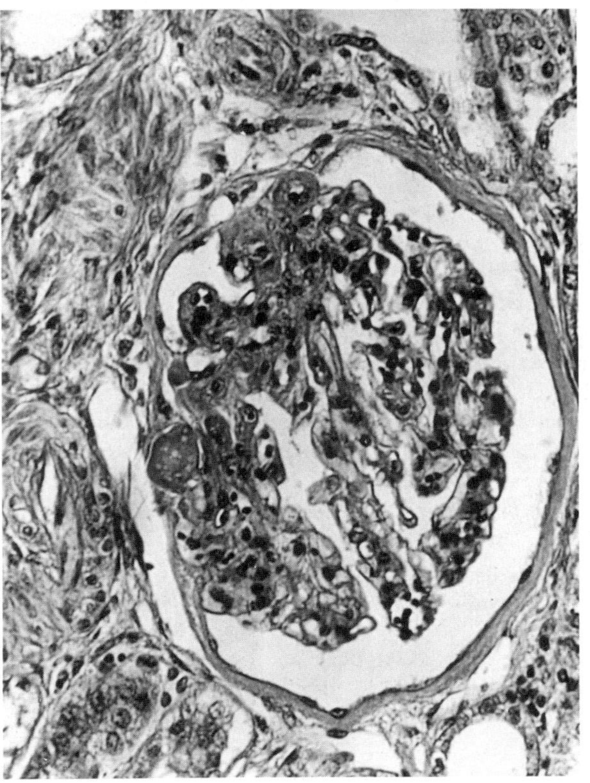

Fig. 3.15 Diffuse and nocular hyalinization of glomerulus. Dog. Basement membranes are thickened, and there is a capsular adhesion.

Cataract formation is an early and common complication of diabetes in the dog, and it may be the presenting sign. Cataracts do not occur in cats, suggesting that their lens metabolism differs from that in dogs. Glucose readily enters the lens from aqueous humor. Persistent elevation of glucose saturates the normal anaerobic glycolytic pathway, the excess glucose then being converted by the activity of aldose reductase to sorbitol and fructose. The latter two saccharides cannot diffuse freely through the lens capsule. They act osmotically, causing influx of water, which leads to swelling and degeneration of the lens fibers.

The biochemical mechanism leading to cataract may also operate in peripheral nerves. Peripheral and autonomic neuropathies are common and important in diabetic humans, but they are rarely reported in animals. The changes are a mix of degeneration and regeneration distally affecting motor and sensory nerves. The neuropathy is reversible if blood sugar levels are controlled.

Bibliography

Atkins, C. E. *et al.* Morphologic and immunocytochemical study of young dogs with diabetes mellitus associated with pancreatic islet cell hypoplasia. *Am J Vet Res* **49:** 1577–1581, 1988.

Dahme, E. *et al.* Diabetische Neuropathie bei Hund und Katze—eine bioptischelectronmikroscopische Studie. *Tierarztl Prax* **17:** 177–188, 1989.

Eigenmann, J. E. Diabetes mellitus in elderly female dogs; recent findings on pathogenesis and clinical implications. *J Am Anim Hosp Assoc* **17:** 805–812, 1981.

Foulis, A. K. The pathogenesis of beta cell destruction in type I (insulin-dependent) diabetes mellitus. *J Pathol* **152:** 141–148, 1987.

Harrison, L. C. *et al.* MHC molecules and beta-cell destruction. Immune and nonimmune mechanisms. *Diabetes* **38:** 815–818, 1989.

Howard, C. F. Longitudinal studies on the development of diabetes in individual *Macaca nigra*. *Diabetologia* **29:** 301–306, 1986.

Ihle, S. L., and Nelson, R. W. Insulin resistance and diabetes mellitus. *Compend Cont Ed Pract Vet* **13:** 197–203, 1991.

Jarrett, I. G. Alloxan diabetes in sheep. *Aust J Exp Biol Med Sci* **24:** 95–102, 1946.

Kramer, J. W. *et al.* Inherited, early onset, insulin-requiring diabetes mellitus of Keeshond dogs. *Diabetes* **29:** 558–569, 1980.

Marmor, M. *et al.* Epizootiologic patterns of diabetes mellitus in dogs. *Am J Vet Res* **43:** 465–470, 1982.

Nelson, R. W. *et al.* Glucose tolerance and insulin response in

normal-weight and obese cats. *Am J Vet Res* **51:** 1357–1362, 1990.
O'Brien, T. D. *et al.* Immunohistochemical morphometry of pancreatic endocrine cells in diabetic, normoglycaemic glucose-intolerant and normal cats. *J Comp Pathol* **96:** 357–369, 1986.
Patz, A., and Maumenee, A. E. Studies on diabetic retinopathy. I. Retinopathy in a dog with spontaneous diabetes mellitus. *Am J Ophthalmol* **54:** 532–541, 1962.
Velasquez, M. T., Kimmel, P. L., and Michaelis, O. E. Animal models of spontaneous diabetic kidney disease. *FASEB J* **4:** 2850–2859, 1990.

B. Neoplasms of the Islet Cells

Pancreatic islet tumors are uncommon and have been described mainly in dogs, affecting principally older animals. Islet cell tumors may be benign or malignant and, although usually solitary, may be multiple, which makes the distinction between hyperplastic and adenomatous lesions difficult.

Grossly, islet tumors are characterized by their firm-to-hard consistency, well-defined borders and homogeneous nature, and distinctive pale grayish-purple color. Although the tumors are well circumscribed, and some well encapsulated, this is not a reliable indicator of benign behavior, because islet carcinomas may appear thus but have metastases in adjacent lymph nodes and also commonly in the liver.

Microscopically, islet tumors, whether benign or malignant, form architectural patterns that are closely reminiscent of normal islets. Cells are arranged in a typical neuroendocrine pattern, forming trabecular, pseudoacinar, or glandular patterns separated by a delicate fibrovascular stroma (Fig. 3.16A,B). Stromal deposits of islet-associated polypeptide with characteristics of amyloid may be present.

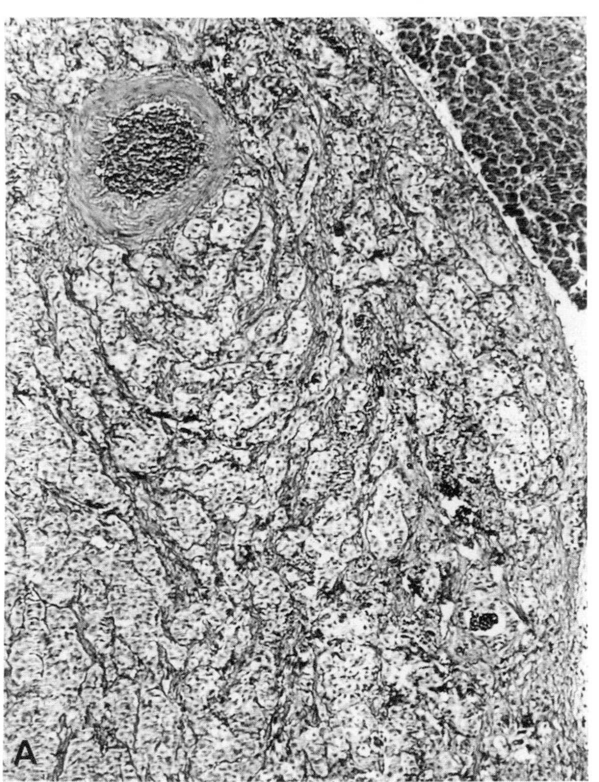

Fig. 3.16A Islet cell tumor compressing acinar pancreas.

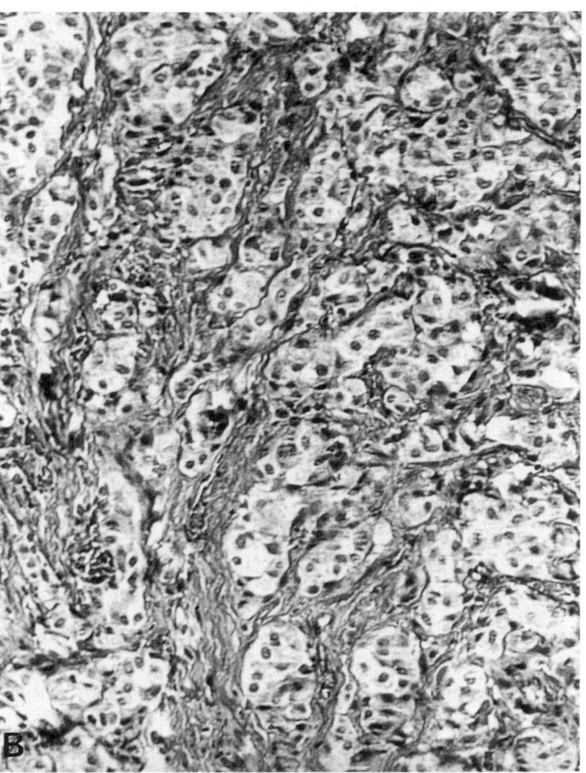

Fig. 3.16B Detail of (A): islet cell tumor compressing acinar pancreas.

Polypeptide hormones are produced by islet cells and by other neuroendocrine cells [amine precursor uptake and decarboxylation (APUD) cells] in the pancreas and adjacent gastric and duodenal tissues. In humans, 16 peptide hormones have been identified in association with pancreatic endocrine cell neoplasia. In domestic animals, only four syndromes have been documented, but a greater number of peptides have been identified by immunocytochemical studies. Not all islet tumors are associated with clinical manifestations of hormone excess, and there is a poor correlation between the immunohistochemical profile of islet tumors and clinical disease. Most islet tumors comprise a variety of peptide-producing cells and, with few exceptions, this composition is reiterated in metastases.

1. Insulinoma.

Most of the functional pancreatic islet tumors described in domestic animals are associated with a syndrome of hyperinsulinism, hypoglycemia, and neurologic signs, attributable to the tumors containing a high proportion of functional beta cells. Animals develop episodic hypoglycemia, often in relationship to periods of fasting, stress, or exercise, and this leads to neurologic signs of confusion, stupor, seizures, and coma. Chronically, a peripheral neuropathy may also develop. Injections of glucose result in a rapid response. Even small tumors may cause profound clinical signs, so that care should be taken in searching for the pancreatic tumor that is responsible. In dogs, islet cell tumors that are classified functionally as insulinomas can be shown by immunocytochemical means to be complex, with immunoreactivity to other peptides present within the neoplasms.

2. Gastrinomas.

Islet cell tumors are rarely responsible for the production of polypeptides with gastrin activity, but these have been described in dogs. Gastrin is not normally produced in pancreatic islets but in the gastric and duodenal mucosa, where it stimulates glandular secretion. The clinical syndrome caused by hypergastrinemic states is known as the Zollinger–Ellison syndrome. Excess gastrin causes gastric hypersecretion leading to gastric hyperacidity and mucosal hyperplasia of the antral region, and gastric and duodenal ulceration. Affected dogs present with clinical signs of anorexia and severe weight loss, associated with vomiting and diarrhea.

3. Glucagonoma.

A syndrome of hyperglycemia, vacuolar hepatopathy, and skin erythema with superficial necrotizing dermatitis has been recognized in humans associated with islet tumors that secrete excessive glucagon. A similar condition has been described in dogs, but the diagnosis is complicated by the usual coexistence of diabetes mellitus in these animals. The relationship of glucagonemia to the clinical disease remains to be resolved, because hepatic and cutaneous lesions of an identical nature can be found in dogs in which no pancreatic tumor can be identified.

Vipomas and somatostatinomas are described in humans but have not as yet been identified in domestic animals.

Bibliography

Braund, K. G. *et al.* Peripheral neuropathy associated with malignant neoplasms in dogs. *Vet Pathol* **24:** 16–21, 1987.

Fix, A. S., and Harms, C. A. Immunocytochemistry of pancreatic endocrine tumors in three domestic ferrets (*Mustela putorius furo*). *Vet Pathol* **27:** 199–201, 1990.

Friesen, S. R. Tumors of the endocrine pancreas. *New Engl J Med* **306:** 580–589, 1982.

Gross, T. L. *et al.* Glucagon-producing pancreatic endocrine tumors in two dogs with superficial necrolytic dermatitis. *J Am Vet Med Assoc* **197:** 1619–1622, 1990.

Happe, R. P. *et al.* Zollinger–Ellison syndrome in three dogs. *Vet Pathol* **17:** 177–186, 1980.

Hawkins, K. L. *et al.* Immunocytochemistry of normal pancreatic islets and spontaneous islet cell tumors in dogs. *Vet Pathol* **24:** 170–179, 1987.

Huxtable, C. R., and Farrow, B. R. H. Functional neoplasms of the canine pancreatic-islet beta-cells: A clinicopathological study of three cases. *J Small Anim Pract* **20:** 737–748, 1979.

Johnson, S. E. Pancreatic APUDomas. *Sem Vet Med Surg (Small Anim)* **4:** 202–211, 1989.

O'Brien, T. D. *et al.* Canine pancreatic endocrine tumors: Immunohistochemical analysis of hormone content and amyloid. *Vet Pathol* **24:** 308–314, 1987.

O'Brien, T. D., Westermark, P., and Johnson, K. H. Islet amyloid polypeptide and calcitonin gene-related peptide immunoreactivity in amyloid and tumor cells of canine pancreatic endocrine tumors. *Vet Pathol* **27:** 194–198, 1990.

CHAPTER 4 The Peritoneum and Retroperitoneum

IAN K. BARKER
University of Guelph, Canada

I. General Considerations

The peritoneal cavity is incompletely divided into compartments by the mesentery, omentum, and ligaments, which are composed of double serosal membranes. Its surface area is greater than that of the skin. The normal peritoneum is a smooth, shiny membrane that is semipermeable to the movement of water and small solute molecules. There is just enough fluid present in the cavity to keep it moist. Normal peritoneal fluid is in osmotic equilibrium with the plasma, but does not contain fibrinogen or other high-molecular-weight proteins, and does not clot. The peritoneal cavity has a dynamic circulation, driven by intestinal motility and respiratory excursions, which can disperse fluid (and particulate contaminants) completely throughout the abdominal and pelvic cavities within minutes to hours.

Fluid and suspended particulates leave the abdominal cavity by two general routes. Most fluid drains via small stomata into the lymphatic lacunae of the diaphragm, and thence via the sternal lymph nodes to the right lymphatic duct, or via mediastinal lymph nodes to the thoracic duct. Less is taken up through the omentum and abdominal viscera, and drains via visceral lymphatics and lymph nodes to the thoracic duct. On the omentum of many species are small milky spots, focal aggregates of lymphoid tissue and fixed phagocytes that are not covered by mesothelium, and that sample the peritoneal contents. Omental lymph drainage originates at them.

The peritoneal surface is covered by a single layer of squamous mesothelial cells, which have microvilli on their surface. Mesothelial cells are fragile, in that they will slough after exposure to such mild insults as air, physiological saline, intestinal dilation, and ischemia of relatively short duration. However, they regenerate quickly; within a few hours, rounded primitive mesenchymal cells, which differentiate to mesothelium, can cover a defect in the peritoneal surface.

Mesothelial cells have high fibrinolytic activity, which normally protects against formation of adhesions. If they are damaged and inflammation is initiated, fibrin effusion and inflammatory cell emigration from the well-vascularized subserosal stroma of the omentum and visceral peritoneum may be rapid and profuse. Fibrinous adhesions may occur among the abdominal viscera, the mesenteries, and omentum. Neovascularization and fibroplasia from the subserosal stroma follow quickly, organizing adhesions. Entrapment of bacteria by fibrin, and adhesion of the omentum and mesentery, with the normal partial subdivision of the abdominal cavity by serosal structures, can result in localization of sepsis within the abdomen. However, peritonitis can also be more or less generalized. Omental bursitis is an example of peritonitis localized within a compartment, and the peritonitis of traumatic reticulitis also is frequently localized by fibrin and adhesions. Blood or fluid in the abdomen may occasionally be confined within a serosal space, but is usually generalized. Vascularized adhesions of the omentum may provide the circulation to ischemic tissue in the abdomen.

The peritoneal membrane forms ligaments between organs that it surrounds, and in some cases these ligaments, particularly the nephrosplenic ligament in the horse, are involved in bowel entrapments. Normal openings, such as the epiploic foramen, and congenital or acquired defects in the double layer of peritoneum making up the mesentery, can also be involved in entrapments (see Intestinal Obstruction Section VI,F, and Intestinal Ischemia and Infarction, Section VI,H, in The Alimentary System, Chapter 1 of this volume).

The **retroperitoneum** is the areolar and adipose connective tissue immediately outside the peritoneal lining of the abdominal cavity. The most significant part extends along the dorsum from the diaphragm to the anus. It is continuous cranially with the retropleura and mediastinum, and ventrally with the potential space between the serosal layers of the mesenteries. Its actual volume is small, except when adipose tissue accumulates, as it normally does in the dorsal retroperitoneum, pelvic cavity, omentum, and mesenteries. In the emaciation of inanition and protein–energy malnutrition, the fat depots of the omentum, mesenteries, and retroperitoneum undergo serous atrophy, as do those in the subcutaneous tissues, the thorax, and the marrow cavities (Fig. 4.1).

There appear to be no absolute barriers to movement of fluid within the retroperitoneal space of dogs; it may travel in the fascia around the dorsal and ventral aspects of the sublumbar muscles, to gain access to the fascial planes of the abdominal wall. Suppurative processes of the retroperitoneum of dogs may drain on the flank, by passing along the fascial planes of the abdominal and the iliopsoas muscles, to emerge in the lumbodorsal triangle, cranial-ventral to the tuber coxae.

Antemortem and postmortem effusions and discoloration in the peritoneal cavity should be distinguished. Some fluid accumulates in the peritoneal cavity after death, and this becomes stained with hemoglobin as soon as erythrocytes in the serosal vessels lyse. Such fluid does not clot and often is also present in other serous cavities. Diffusion of bile pigments through the wall of the gall bladder, the bile ducts, or the duodenum also will stain adjacent viscera.

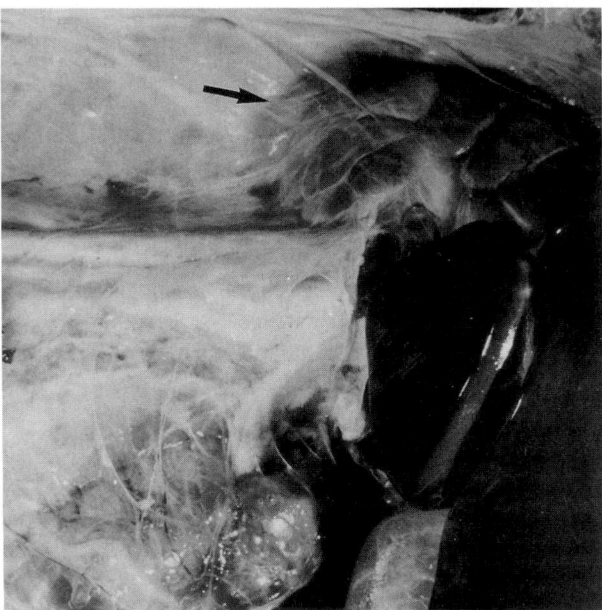

Fig. 4.1 Serous atrophy of fat. Calf. Protein–energy malnutrition. Note dark liver (right) and lack of normal perirenal (arrow) and retroperitoneal fat.

Bibliography

Abernethy, N. J. *et al.* Lymphatic drainage of the peritoneal cavity in sheep. *Am J Physiol* **260:** F353–F358, 1991.

Brownlow, M. A., Hutchins, D. R., and Johnston, K. G. Reference values for equine peritoneal fluid. *Equine Vet J* **13:** 127–130, 1981.

Grindem, C. B. *et al.* Peritoneal fluid values from healthy foals. *Equine Vet J* **22:** 359–361, 1990.

Hosgood, G. The omentum—The forgotten organ: Physiology and potential surgical applications in dogs and cats. *Compend Cont Ed Pract Vet* **12:** 45–51, 1990.

Hosgood, G. *et al.* Intraperitoneal circulation and drainage in the dog. *Vet Surg* **18:** 261–268, 1989.

Johnston, D. E., and Christie, B. A. The retroperitoneum in dogs: Anatomy and clinical significance. *Compend Cont Ed Pract Vet* **12:** 1027–1033, 1055, 1990.

Leak, L. V., and Rahil, K. Permeability of the diaphragmatic mesothelium: The ultrastructural basis for "stomata." *Am J Anat* **151:** 557–594, 1978.

Raftery, A. T. Mesothelial cells in peritoneal fluid. *J Anat* **115:** 237–253, 1973.

Schaffner, T. *et al.* Macrophage functions in antimicrobial defense. *Klin Wochenschr* **60:** 720–726, 1982.

Whitaker, D., Papadimitriou, J. M., and Walters, M. N-I. The mesothelium: Its fibrinolytic properties. *J Pathol* **136:** 291–299, 1982.

II. Anomalies

Congenital anomalies of the peritoneal membranes are rare; they are associated most frequently with embryonic remnants of vitelline structures. A **persistent vitelline or omphalomesenteric duct** may form a fibrous ligament, or **vitelloumbilical band,** between the intestine or Meckel's diverticulum and the umbilicus. The remnant may be partial, not reaching the umbilicus, and may be attached to the mesentery or to a loop of intestine. Either form of band may become involved in herniation and obstruction or strangulation of the intestine (see Displacements, Section VI,G, and Intestinal Ischemia and Infarction, Section VI,H in Chapter 1 of this volume, The Alimentary System).

A **mesodiverticular band** is the result of a **persistent vitelline artery.** The band is a fold of mesentery, occasionally carrying a patent vitelline artery in its free edge, that extends from the cranial mesenteric artery, or from a spot partway down the mesenteric veil, to the antimesenteric side of the intestine (to the site of Meckel's diverticulum). The pocket formed between this fold and the normal mesentery may entrap intestine; defects may develop in it which permit strangulation of intestinal loops. Occasionally, double (left and right) mesodiverticular bands are present. Rarely, fibrous cords of mesenteric tissue may be found that do not appear to be part of embryonic remnants of vitelline structures.

The **falciform ligament,** which in its free margin may contain the remnant of the umbilical vein as the round ligament, varies in size among species and individuals; it is typically largest in young animals. There is potential for entrapment or strangulation of bowel, if a large, persistent falciform ligament is perforated.

External hernias are the result of abnormal openings in the abdominal wall, which permit passage of the abdominal contents. They may be congenital or acquired. Congenital defects resulting in hernias are of several kinds. They include abnormally increased size of normal openings such as the inguinal canal; persistence of fetal openings, as in umbilical hernia; and defects in closure of the abdominal cavity, as in schistosomus reflexus or congenital diaphragmatic hernia (see External Hernia, Section VI,G,5 of The Alimentary System, Chapter 1 of this volume).

Congenital pleuroperitoneal diaphragmatic hernias are very rare; they are most common in dogs. They usually involve a defect in the muscle of the left dorsal quadrant of the diaphragm, as is the case in humans and rabbits. These presumably result from failure of the left pleuroperitoneal fold to fuse with the septum transversum; the reason for the particular susceptibility of the left side is unknown. The lesion in some breeds of dogs may have an autosomal recessive mode of inheritance. Some congenital pleuroperitoneal defects in small animals may be more extensive, to the point that virtually the entire diaphragm is missing. The margins of the diaphragmatic defect are smooth, and a large mass of abdominal viscera, often including stomach, spleen, liver, small intestine, and omentum, may pass into the thoracic cavity through the opening. Most small animals born with these defects probably die at, or shortly after, birth. Surprisingly, in large animals, some such lesions, which seem to be congenital, may be clinically silent for a considerable period. The others produce respiratory difficulty, or abdominal pain, if incarceration of herniated viscera occurs.

Peritoneopericardial diaphragmatic hernias are more commonly seen in small animals than are pleuroperitoneal hernias, perhaps because the animals live longer. They are triangular and ventral, and presumably result from abnormal development of the septum transversum. They are sometimes associated with cardiac anomalies, malformations of the sternum and costochondral junctions, or umbilical hernias. Myelolipomas have been reported in the liver of two cats with peritoneopericardial hernias; the relationship to the diaphragmatic defect, if any, is obscure. Though various portions of the liver, spleen, omentum, and small intestine may herniate into the pericardial sac, these lesions often are clinically silent but occasionally are associated with dyspnea, failure to thrive, vomition, etc. These lesions rarely become complicated and life threatening.

The differentiation of congenital from acquired and postmortem diaphragmatic hernia is discussed subsequently.

III. Traumatic Lesions of the Abdomen and Peritoneum

Physical trauma to the abdomen is common. Among the sequelae are hemorrhage; peritoneal sepsis; uremia due to the escape of urine into the abdomen; and dysfunction of traumatized organs.

External forces applied to the abdominal wall, if focused, may cause perforation, with laceration of underlying viscera. If a projectile or sharp object is involved, there may be penetrating wounds of solid viscera, or perforation of hollow organs. Peritonitis may ensue if sepsis is introduced from the external environment, or by leakage from damaged gut.

Blunt trauma to the abdomen, if sufficiently forceful, will result in contusion of abdominal viscera; avulsion of organs from supporting mesenteries or ligaments, and from their vascular supply; and perhaps laceration of the capsule of solid organs such as the liver, spleen, and kidney. Hollow organs, such as the stomach, gallbladder, and urinary bladder may rupture, releasing their contents into the abdominal cavity. The momentary increase in intra-abdominal pressure resulting from such trauma may cause acquired hernias, forcing viscera through natural apertures such as the inguinal canal, weak points such as the perineum, or through lacerations in the diaphragm, or in the abdominal wall, with eventration. In small animals, trauma associated with automobile accidents is the commonest cause of abdominal hernias.

In abdominal trauma, contusions and perforation or laceration may be evident on the underside of the skin, and in subcutaneous tissues. Anatomic relationships should be sought between any internal abnormalities and such lesions. Animals with a lacerated liver or spleen may be pale from internal hemorrhage. Contusion or laceration of the kidney results in subcapsular, retroperitoneal, or peritoneal hemorrhage. The spleen is contracted in exsanguinated animals. The source of hemorrhage may be subtle slits or crevasses in the capsule of the involved organ, or the laceration may be obvious. Massive trauma may fragment or pulp the liver or spleen. Portions of spleen, in particular, may implant and persist ectopically elsewhere in the abdomen (splenosis), and may be encountered as an incidental finding. The presence of bile from a ruptured gall bladder is obvious as a muddy brown or green-black deposit over the viscera. Urine in the abdominal cavity, if not suspected, may be mistaken for ascitic fluid, and lacerations of the contracted urinary bladder may be small and difficult to detect. If the pregnant uterus is ruptured, fetuses may be distributed in the abdomen. They will die and cause peritonitis, if the dam survives and they are not removed.

Endogenous forces also may result in herniation. The additional weight of intestinal contents in pregnancy, especially when complicated by an event such as hydrops amnios, may cause ventral hernia. Straining to defecate, or at parturition, may also cause herniation; the former is associated with perineal hernias in dogs; the latter, with acquired diaphragmatic hernias in horses. Tympany of the large bowel in horses, or of the forestomachs in ruminants, may also cause defects in the abdominal wall or diaphragm. Antemortem lesions must be differentiated from postmortem tears due to bloating of viscera. The presence of hemorrhage in the torn muscle, or strangulation of herniated gut, is evidence for the former.

Acquired diaphragmatic hernia is usually a sequel to trauma such as an automobile accident, kick, etc., and should be sought in animals known to have suffered such an event. The diaphragm is weaker than the abdominal wall. If, at the moment of impact to the abdomen, the glottis is open, a very high pressure differential may be generated between the abdominal and pleural sides of the diaphragm, which is relieved by laceration.

In small animals, the diaphragmatic muscle, rather than the tendinous part, tends to tear, but otherwise the location and orientation of the lesion is a function of events at the moment of impact. Almost any of the abdominal viscera may herniate into the thorax through the defect, but liver and small bowel do so most commonly. The lesion may be clinically silent for a considerable period, sometimes years, but sooner or later results in respiratory difficulty, hydrothorax, ascites, chylothorax, gastric tympany, and intestinal obstruction. At surgery or necropsy, acute diaphragmatic laceration is obvious. If chronic, the margin of the laceration is usually thickened by fibroplasia and smooth, but rarely there may be adhesion to the viscera. Differentiation of such lesions from congenital hernias is based on the age, clinical history, and any evidence of scarring or adhesions at the margin of the diaphragmatic defect.

In horses, acquired lesions usually involve the area where the tendinous portion meets the pars costalis, whereas postmortem laceration of the diaphragm in the horse is most common at the ventral midline, in the xiphoid area (Fig. 4.2). Most horses with acquired diaphragmatic hernias develop abdominal pain, rather than respiratory signs.

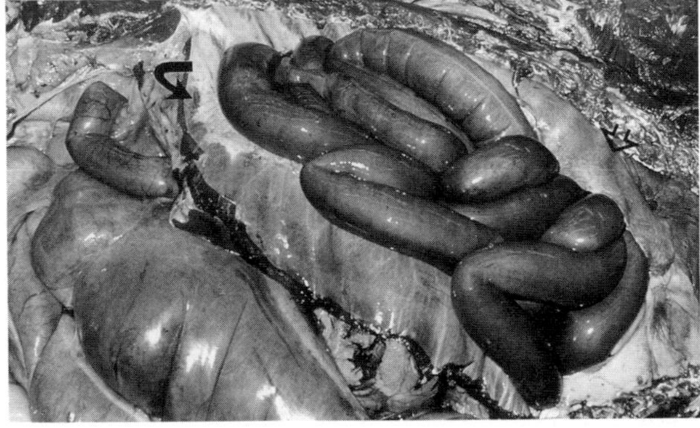

Fig. 4.2 Acquired diaphragmatic hernia. Horse. Loops of small intestine have passed through the diaphragmatic laceration into the thoracic cavity compressing lung (open arrow). Diaphragm (curved arrow).

Bibliography

Boudrieau, R. J., and Muir, W. W. Pathophysiology of traumatic diaphragmatic hernia in dogs. *Compend Cont Ed Pract Vet* **9:** 379–385, 1987.

Bristol, D. G. Diaphragmatic hernias in horses and cattle. *Compend Cont Ed Pract Vet* **8:** S407–S412, 1986.

Corley, J. R., and Bertone, A. Diaphragmatic hernia in a horse. *Equine Pract* **12:** 28–31, 1990.

Freeman, D. E., Kock, D. B., and Boles, C. L. Mesodiverticular bands as a cause of small intestinal strangulation and volvulus in the horse. *J Am Vet Med Assoc* **175:** 1089–1094, 1979.

Hay, W. H., Woodfield, J. A., and Moon, M. A. Clinical, echocardiographic, and radiographic findings of peritoneopericardial diaphragmatic hernia in two dogs and a cat. *J Am Vet Med Assoc* **195:** 1245–1248, 1989.

Koch, D. B., Robertson, J. T., and Donawick, W. J. Small intestinal obstruction due to persistent vitelloumbilical band in a cow. *Am J Vet Res* **173:** 197–200, 1978.

Kolata, R. J. Trauma in dogs and cats: An overview. *Vet Clin North Am: Small Anim Pract* **10:** 515–522, 1980.

Levine, S. H. Diaphragmatic hernia. *Vet Clin North Am: Small Anim Pract* **17:** 411–430, 1987.

Perdrizet, J. A., Dill, S. G., and Hackett, R. P. Diaphragmatic hernia as a cause of dyspnoea in a draft horse. *Equine Vet J* **21:** 302–304, 1989.

Schulman, A. J. *et al.* Congenital peritoneopericardial diaphragmatic hernia in a dog. *J Am Anim Hosp Assoc* **21:** 655–662, 1985.

Valentine, B. A. *et al.* Canine congenital diaphragmatic hernia. *J Vet Intern Med* **2:** 109–112, 1988.

Waldron, D. R., Hedlund, C. S., and Pechman, R. Abdominal hernias in dogs and cats: A review of 24 cases. *J Am Anim Hosp Assoc* **22:** 817–823, 1986.

Wilson, G. P., and Hayes, H. M. Diaphragmatic hernia in the dog and cat: A 25-year overview. *Sem Vet Med Surg (Small Anim)* **1:** 318–326, 1986.

IV. Abnormal Contents in the Peritoneal Cavity

Foreign material is commonly found in the peritoneal cavity. Materials of endogenous origin, such as ingesta or urine, indicate an abnormality of another organ.

Ingesta is frequently found in the peritoneal cavity of horses and cattle, seldom in swine, sheep, and goats, and rarely in dogs and cats. The site of perforation or rupture in the stomach or intestine is usually easy to find, especially when the animal dies before there is time for peritonitis to develop. Such is the case, for instance, in gastric rupture in the horse, and sometimes in perforating abomasal ulcer in cattle. Once peritonitis has developed and matted the intestines and mesenteries, the primary site of perforation may be very difficult to detect, especially as severe peritonitis itself may tie down or devitalize segments of the intestinal wall and promote leakage of content.

Points of predilection for antemortem leakage should be examined for defects at necropsy. These include any devitalized segment of small or large bowel; segments of obstructed bowel, which perhaps have undergone impaction with pressure necrosis, or tympany and rupture; and the ruptured stomach of the horse and perforated abomasum of the cow. Cecal rupture following overload or impaction usually occurs on the medial side. Rectal perforation will also cause contamination of the abdomen with feces, and these lesions may be hard to find.

Rectal perforation is most commonly secondary to accidental injury during palpation. Most tears occur about 25–30 cm from the anus, in the peritoneal portion of the rectum, on the dorsal aspect. Tears which perforate the muscularis have the potential for contamination of the peritoneal cavity. The less severe of these have an intact serosa, with formation of a subserosal diverticulum, or a fistula into the potential space of the mesorectum. These may result in perineal abscessation or fistulation, pelvic cellulitis, or rectal diverticulae, among other complications. Often they perforate the mesorectum, causing gross fecal contamination of the peritoneum.

Postmortem rupture of a viscus must be differentiated from an ante-mortem lesion. The rumen, stomach, or large bowel of putrefied, bloated carcasses may rupture. Autolysis of the abomasum may release gastric contents in calves and lambs fed milk replacers. The margins of the defect in the viscus are not hemorrhagic, and the peritoneal surfaces show no indication of inflammation.

Hemoperitoneum is the presence of blood in the peritoneal cavity. The amount present at death is not necessarily an indication of the volume of bleeding during life, because the blood may be removed quite rapidly via diaphragmatic lymphatics. The blood in the cavity may be fluid or partially clotted. Animals may die from hemorrhage into the peritoneal cavity, but the outcome will depend on the rate and volume of bleeding, the site of hemorrhage, the cause, and the initial state of the animal.

Hemoperitoneum is seen most commonly in the dog and cat as a result of traumatic injury to the liver, spleen, and kidney. Manual efforts at artificial resuscitation, if vigorous, may rupture the liver. Splenic hemangiosarcomas, which bleed into the abdomen, are common in dogs past middle age. Spleen and liver which are enlarged and tensed by infiltrating leukemic cells, fat, or amyloid are predisposed to rupture; the volume of hemorrhage in these cases may be very small. Rupture of the liver, and hemorrhage, may occur in infectious canine hepatitis.

In several species, anticoagulant rodenticides, such as warfarin, may cause hemorrhage which results in unclotted blood in the abdomen. Calves born of cows which have been fed moldy sweet-clover hay bleed from the umbilical vessels into the peritoneal cavity, as well as elsewhere. Manual ablation of a corpus luteum is a source of hemorrhage in cattle. In cattle and horses, laceration of the uterus or rupture of a uterine artery at parturition can result in a fatal hemorrhage. In horses, hemoperitoneum may be due to hemorrhage from a granulosa-thecal cell tumor of the ovary, and in all species any friable intra-abdominal or retroperitoneal neoplasm may occasionally rupture and bleed, if traumatized.

Hemorrhage on or beneath the peritoneum, without free blood in the cavity, may occur in acute bacterial toxemias and in other conditions which interfere with vascular integrity or hemostasis. Peritoneal hemorrhage must be differentiated from hemorrhagic peritonitis, which is an important lesion in some diseases. Subserosal hemorrhage and hemomelasma ilei occur occasionally on the intestine of the horse, associated with trauma to vessels by migrating strongyles. Rarely, subserosal hematomas may cause intestinal obstruction. Hemorrhage into an omental or mesenteric cyst can cause sudden abdominal enlargement without free blood in the abdomen.

Bibliography

Embertson, R. M., Hodge, R. J., and Vachon, A. M. Near-circumferential retroperitoneal rectal tear in a pony. *J Am Vet Med Assoc* **188:** 738–739, 1986.

Evans, K. *et al.* Hemoperitoneum secondary to traumatic rupture of an adrenal tumor in a dog. *J Am Vet Med Assoc* **198:** 278–280, 1991.

Gatewood, D. M. *et al.* Intra-abdominal hemorrhage associated with a granulosa-thecal cell neoplasm in a mare. *J Am Vet Med Assoc* **196:** 1827–1828, 1990.

Kobluk, C. N., and Smith, D. F. Intramural hematoma in the jejunum of a mare. *J Am Vet Med Assoc* **192:** 379–380, 1988.

Sanders-Shamis, M. Perirectal abscesses in six horses. *J Am Vet Med Assoc* **187:** 499–500, 1985.

Watkins, J. P. *et al.* Rectal tears in the horse: An analysis of 35 cases. *Equine Vet J* **21:** 186–188, 1989.

A. *Ascites (Hydroperitoneum)*

Ascites is the accumulation of excess fluid, usually a transudate or modified transudate, in the peritoneal cavity. Ascitic fluid is generally watery, clear, or straw colored, and contains few leukocytes but many desquamated mesothelial cells. The serosal lining is normal, unless fluid has been present for weeks, when the serosa may appear cloudy.

Ascites can be viewed most simply as the result of diminished removal, or overproduction, of peritoneal fluid. Logical pursuit of the cause of ascites should lead to the primary problem, of which ascites is but a sign.

Reduced removal of fluid from the peritoneal cavity is due to obstruction of the primary route of lymphatic drainage through the diaphragm. The limited area for lymphatic absorption and the small size of the stomata on the diaphragmatic serosa explain the ease and rapidity with which peritoneal drainage can be blocked.

Obstruction of diaphragmatic lymphatics as a cause of ascites is best exemplified in peritoneal carcinomatosis. Metastases of carcinomas usually implant most extensively on the diaphragm in the region of the lymphatic stomata, and colonization of the lymphatic vessels there is easily demonstrated microscopically. The neoplastic cells are carried to the anterior abdomen by the normal peritoneal fluid circulation. Carcinomatous implants on the peritoneum, in addition to obstructing diaphragmatic lymphatics, may produce fluid. This has been argued for papillary adenocarcinoma of the ovary which, in the bitch, provides the best example of implantation and ascites.

Ascites also may develop if there is obstruction to sternal lymphatic flow cranial to the diaphragm. This may occur in lymphomatosis of adult cattle, when there is massive neoplastic involvement of the cranial mediastinal and sternal lymph nodes.

Overproduction of peritoneal lymph is mainly related to altered hydrostatic pressure gradients in the hepatic and portal circulation. The exception is rare **chylous ascites,** which results when the cisterna chyli is ruptured. Its origin is indicated by the milkiness of the fluid, due to the presence of chylomicrons.

The balance of oncotic and hydrostatic pressure, which regulates fluid exchange between blood vessels and interstitial tissue, depends on the relative retention of large molecules within the circulation. Vascular injury in the portal field, which allows increased permeability to plasma protein, substantially alters the balance of forces and favors transudation. Small amounts of ascitic fluid may be generated under these circumstances in a variety of systemic illnesses, such as the clostridial intoxications, endotoxemia, acute uremic syndromes in ruminants and pigs, and in the exudative diathesis of pigs deficient in vitamin E.

Ascites resulting from overproduction of fluid is usually an expression of hepatic lymphedema. Increased prehepatic portal venous pressure alone usually does not to lead to ascites; if present, such fluid is low protein, being derived from intestinal and mesenteric interstitial fluid. Acute portal vein obstruction causes intestinal infarction and death, but not ascites. Slowly developing portal hypertension of prehepatic, hepatic, or hepatic venous origin may cause transient ascites, which resolves with the development of collateral portal–postcaval venous shunts within a few weeks. However, portal hypertension of cardiac origin does not result in portocaval shunts, because the elevation in central venous pressure permits no pressure gradient between the portal and postcaval systems.

The *sine qua non* of hepatic ascites is that there be increased resistance in the intrahepatic or posthepatic circulation, with edema of the liver. The exception is the increase in portal blood flow caused by hepatic arteriovenous fistulae or anastomoses, which are rare, and usually the result of a congenital defect; in this circumstance, hydrostatic pressure at the level of the hepatic sinusoids is elevated by the arterialization of the portal flow.

The usual conditions causing increased hepatic or posthepatic resistance to blood flow are fibrosis or cirrhosis of the liver, and congestive heart failure. In cirrhosis, intrahepatic resistance may be compounded by the development of arteriovenous anastomoses in the fibrous septa around nodules; these arterialize the hepatic–portal circulation, further elevating hydrostatic pressure.

There are a variety of additional causes of increased hepatic resistance to blood flow. These include primary neoplasms of the liver, especially cholangiocellular carcinomas, which tend to be diffuse and infiltrative; secondary tumors, especially lymphosarcomas, which widely infiltrate the liver; extensive infestation with hydatid cysts; and chronic biliary trematodiasis, or other causes of chronic cholangiohepatitis and portal fibrosis. Tumors or abscesses in or compressing the hepatic vein as it leaves the liver, or obstructions in the caudal vena cava cranial to the entry of the hepatic vein, will cause posthepatic obstruction.

When the liver is congested, there is an increased flow of hepatic lymph, which has a high concentration of protein. The bulk of hepatic lymph comes from the space of Disse, which is separated from the sinusoidal lumen only by a fenestrated endothelium that is freely permeable to plasma constituents, including large protein molecules. Hence, the formation of hepatic lymph is not regulated by plasma oncotic pressure, but is sensitive to small changes in hydrostatic pressure in the sinusoids. This accounts for the frequency with which ascites is associated with those diseases which cause increased central and hepatic venous pressure, or increased intrahepatic resistance to blood flow.

If the capacity of the hepatic lymphatics cannot handle the excess, then lymph, high in protein, oozes from the hepatic capsule, presumably from the rich lymphatic plexus there, and it may spill from the efferent lymphatics which pass from the porta hepatis to the cisterna chyli. In hepatic ascites these efferent lymphatics become very large, numerous, and thick walled.

The fluid which enters the peritoneal cavity is continually in flux. Gross ascites will develop only when the normally high capacity to drain fluid from the abdomen is exceeded by the rate of production, and this requires an increase in renal retention of sodium and water. The resultant expansion of plasma volume permits the development of edema and ascites in congestive heart failure, and ascites in hepatic disease. In cirrhosis, intrahepatic portal hypertension may activate a hepatic baroceptor reflex that switches on the renin–angiotensin system, and stimulates sympathetic pathways that also promote renal sodium and water retention. The resulting expansion of plasma volume further increases hydrostatic pressure in the hepatic sinusoids, driving lymph production to the point that ascitic fluid accumulates. Secondarily, reduced effective vascular volume, associated with sequestration of fluid in ascites, expansion of the splanchnic circulation, and other systemic circulatory events, also causes sodium retention, via the renin–angiotensin pathway, with aldosterone secretion, and by parallel mechanisms. In heart failure, activation of the renin–angiotensin system is expected, due to reduced effective vascular volume. However, in only a minority of cases of congestive failure in dogs and cats is there ascites.

Hypoproteinemia due to reduced hepatic synthesis may occur in severe liver disease. Normally, oncotic forces are subsidiary to hydrostatic forces at the level of the sinusoid in affecting the formation of lymph. However, in cirrhosis, once advanced capillarization of sinusoids occurs, the free permeability of the hepatic vascular system to the flow of

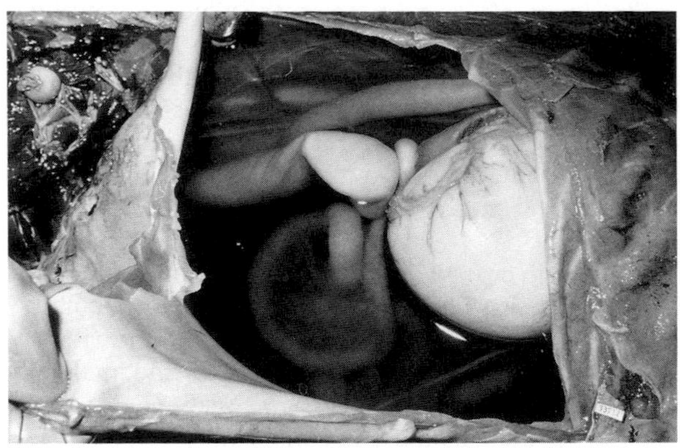

Fig. 4.3 Ascites in a dog with profound hypoproteinemia due to enteric protein loss from lymphangiectasia.

large molecules is reduced. In this circumstance, reduced plasma oncotic pressure due to hypoalbuminemia will promote continued hepatic lymph formation and ascites; it will also promote fluid flux to the peritoneum across the splanchnic capillary bed.

Hypoproteinemia of nonhepatic origin is associated most commonly with protein-losing enteropathy, such as Johne's disease, or with protein-losing nephropathy, as in glomerular amyloidosis or other glomerulopathy. Severe hypoproteinemia will reduce plasma oncotic pressure, promoting edema and permitting transudate to accumulate in serous spaces, including, but not exclusively, in the peritoneal cavity (Fig. 4.3).

Effusion of fluid, sometimes massive, in the peritoneal cavity, thorax, and ventral body wall is part of the postmortem picture in sheep and cattle which die of urethral obstruction, and the fluid may have a distinct uriniferous odor. The pathogenesis of this fluid accumulation is uncertain. Although in a few cases there is a rupture of the lower urinary tract which might permit leakage, in many cases a rupture cannot be demonstrated. Renal uremia also is associated with similar fluid accumulations in cattle; this is evident in some which die with renal amyloidosis, and a contributing factor here is probably hypoproteinemia due to prolonged massive proteinuria. Acute toxic nephrosis may also be accompanied by massive effusions, and, as is usually the case with ascites of urinary tract disease, the mesenteries and retroperitoneum are also saturated.

Bibliography

Crowe, D. T., and Crane, S. W. Diagnostic abdominal paracentesis and lavage in the evaluation of abdominal injuries in dogs and cats: Clinical and experimental investigations. *J Am Vet Med Assoc* **168:** 700–705, 1976.

Crowe, D. T. *et al.* Chronic peritoneal effusion due to partial caudal vena caval obstruction following blunt trauma: Diagnosis and successful surgical treatment. *J Am Anim Hosp Assoc* **20:** 231–238, 1984.

Floras, J. S. *et al.* Increased sympathetic outflow in cirrhosis and ascites: Direct evidence from intraneural recordings. *Ann Int Med* **114:** 373–380, 1991.

Johnson, S. E. Portal hypertension. Part I. Pathophysiology and clinical consequences. *Compend Cont Ed Pract Vet* **9:** 741–748, 1987.

Kopcha, M., and Schultze, A. E. Peritoneal fluid. Part I. Pathophysiology and classification of nonneoplastic effusions. *Compend Cont Ed Pract Vet* **13:** 519–526, 1991.

Moore, P. F., and Whiting, P. G. Hepatic lesions associated with intrahepatic arteriovenous fistulae in dogs. *Vet Pathol* **23:** 57–62, 1986.

Rocco, V. K., and Ware, A. J. Cirrhotic ascites. *Ann Int Med* **105:** 573–585, 1986.

Unikowsky, B., Wexler, M. J., and Levy, M. Dogs with experimental cirrhosis of the liver but without intrahepatic hypertension do not retain sodium or form ascites. *J Clin Invest* **72:** 1594–1604, 1983.

B. Abdominal Fat Necrosis

Necrosis of mesenteric or other abdominal or retroperitoneal fat is a common finding at autopsy. The pathogenesis is poorly understood, but there appear to be a number of causes.

In **pancreatic necrosis,** enzymatic necrosis of fat is always seen, and peripancreatic necrosis of fat may be the initial morphologic change. In acute pancreatic necrosis, discrete foci or confluent masses of white necrotic adipose tissue are surrounded by a zone of intense hyperemia with fibrin deposited on the surface. Such lesions may be limited to the peripancreatic fat, or are distributed throughout the abdominal cavity. Free droplets of fat can be found in the peritoneal fluid, which is likened to chicken soup.

Microscopically the acute lesion is made up of necrotic fat cells containing acidophilic, opaque, amorphous, or lacy substance, or basophilic fibrillar or granular mineralized material. Masses of degenerating neutrophils and necrotic debris are present. Fibroplasia and vacuolated macrophages are features of the chronic lesion along with necrotic fat and occasionally dystrophic mineralization.

The lesion is attributed to release of proteolytic and lipolytic enzymes from the necrotic acinar pancreas. Degeneration of neutrophils may aid the ongoing process. Lipase released from degenerating fat cells probably also contributes to necrosis of fat.

Widespread or isolated **focal necrosis of abdominal and retroperitoneal fat** is found frequently in sheep, and sometimes in horses, pigs, and other animals. This necrotic fat usually is seen only at the chronic stage, in the form of small dry, firm, or gritty plaques. A flat white color distinguishes the plaques from surrounding normal fat. There usually is no grossly apparent inflammatory reaction, and microscopically the lesions resemble the chronic lesion previously described, with occasional macrophages containing large lipid vacuoles and necrotic debris encapsulated by connective tissue. The pathogenesis of this form of fat necrosis has not been explained. The focal lesion may be due to avascular necrosis of fat from pressure ischemia. This is perhaps due to differences in the texture or composition of the fat, or some circulatory deficit in the small capillaries that nourish the large masses of fat, since the lesion is most common in very fat animals. It is also possible that the lesions are initiated by intracellular lipolytic disturbances associated with accelerated mobilization of fat to meet metabolic demands.

The third form, not uncommon and perhaps the most interesting, is **massive fat necrosis in cattle.** This condition has been reported most frequently in Channel Island breeds, and occurs in excessively fat cattle. Both sexes are affected, but probably not clinically before the second year of life. The disease has several significant features. Although it is often seen as an incidental lesion, it can be fatal, usually by intestinal obstruction, or by complications such as compression of the ureters. There also may be obstruction of the pelvic canal, causing dystocia or other gynecologic problems. As well, the hard lumps of necrotic fat may be mistaken for fetal structures, lymphoid tumors, and other abdominal masses on rectal palpation. Clinical signs most commonly are due to intestinal obstruction, as the gut is compressed by the firm lumps of necrotic fat (Fig. 4.4). Affected animals may exhibit anorexia, diarrhea, constipation, colic, or bloat. They may become emaciated prior to death.

The necrosis may occur in any portion of the omental, mesenteric, and retroperitoneal fat, and it is sometimes seen in intermuscular and subcutaneous fat, as well. In the early stage there is acute inflammation, and the hard necrotic masses are surrounded by a zone of hyperemia; the overlying peritoneum may be necrotic, perhaps with adhesions to adjacent viscera. The masses may vary from small nodules to large solid masses which are encapsulated by fibrous tissue, and which on cut section are firm, dry, and caseous, or sometimes moist, oily, and deep yellow. The surfaces of such masses may be molded to the contours of adjacent organs.

Because of the unusual bulk of the necrotic tissue, and because necrotic fat is sometimes found in abnormal locations, such as under the serosa of the intestine, the condition has been called lipomatosis, but the lesions are not hyperplastic or neoplastic.

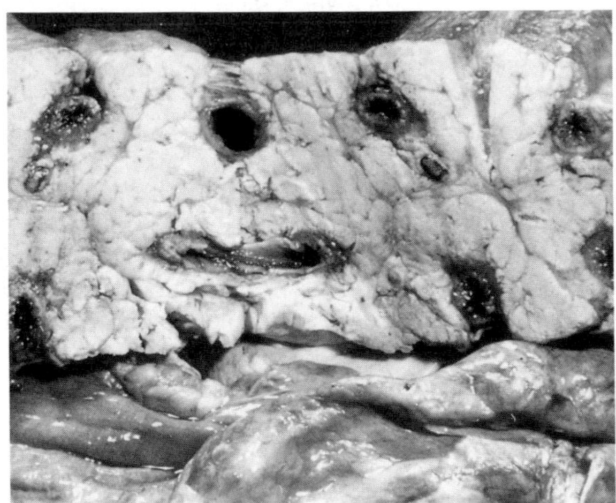

Fig. 4.4 Mass of fat enclosing intestinal loops in abdominal fat necrosis. Ox.

On microscopic examination the tissue resembles a mixture of acute and chronic fat necrosis with few neutrophils, a few lymphocytes and plasma cells, and many macrophages and giant cells, with some interstitial fibrosis. Elongate clefts and mineral may be present in macrophages and giant cells.

The pathogenesis of this diffuse lipogranulomatosis in cattle is not clear, but there is evidence of a dietary cause, somewhat similar to that of steatitis as it occurs in horses, pigs, and other species. The different lesions in cattle may be due to the chemical composition of their fat. The lesion is possibly related to production in the rumen of high levels of saturated fatty acids, which form long-chain compounds that are solid at normal body temperature. Release of lipases from damaged adipocytes, or ischemic necrosis, may result in the formation of soaps, cholesterol, or other crystalline material, to which the body reacts. This provokes the inflammatory response, with the accumulation of the foreign material in giant cells and macrophages, and fibrosis.

Steatitis (yellow-fat disease) occurs in many species of animal except ruminants, affecting the abdominal and retroperitoneal fat, along with other adipose tissue. It is caused by a diet high in polyunsaturated fat and low in tocopherols, allowing oxidation of fatty acids. Peroxidation creates free radicals, which damage tissue and provoke the characteristic inflammatory response in the adipose tissue. Several types of steatitis, all vitamin E responsive, occur in newborn or young, as well as in mature animals. Ceroid-lipofuscin, which is not present in all forms of steatitis, is responsible for the yellow color, and often fills the macrophages which are a feature of this form of steatitis (see Panniculitis, Volume 1, Chapter 5).

Bibliography

Danse, L. H. J. C., and Steenbergen-Botterweg, W. A. Enzyme histochemical studies of adipose tissue in porcine yellow fat disease. *Vet Pathol* **11:** 465–476, 1974.

Danse, L. H. J. C., and Verschuren, P. M. Fish oil-induced yellow fat disease in rats. 1. Histologic changes. *Vet Pathol* **15:** 114–124, 1978.

Freeman, B. A., and Crapo, J. D. Biology of disease. Free radicals and tissue injury. *Lab Invest* **47:** 412–426, 1982.

Ito, T. A pathological study on fat necrosis in swine. *Jpn J Vet Sci* **35:** 299–310, 1973.

Ito, T. *et al.* Pathological studies on fat necrosis (lipomatosis) in cattle. *Jpn J Vet Res* **30:** 141, 1968.

Johnson, R., and Dunstan, R. Abdominal fat necrosis in a heifer. *Compend Cont Ed Pract Vet* **7:** S103,S110, 1985.

Kirby, P. S. Steatitis in fattening pigs. *Vet Rec* **109:** 385, 1981.

Kroneman, J., and Wensvoort, P. Muscular dystrophy and yellow fat disease in Shetland pony foals. *Neth J Vet Sci* **1:** 42, 1968.

Maeda, T. Studies on fat necrosis of beef cattle in Japan. I. Occurring aspects. II. An area study of the outbreak of fat necrosis. *Bull Fac Agric, Tottori* Univ **30:** 205–210, 211–217, 1978.

Moreau, P. M. *et al.* Disseminated necrotizing panniculitis and pancreatic nodular hyperplasia in a dog. *J Am Vet Med Assoc* **180:** 422–425, 1982.

Platt, H., and Whitwell, K. E. Clinical and pathological observations on generalized steatitis in foals. *J Comp Pathol* **81:** 499–506, 1971.

Rumsey, T. S. *et al.* Chemical composition of necrotic fat lesions in beef cows grazing fertilized Kentucky-31 tall fescue. *J Anim Sci* **48:** 673–682, 1979.

Shimada, Y., and Morinaga, H. Studies on bovine fat necrosis. I. Epidemiological observations. *J Jpn Vet Med Assoc* **30:** 584–588, 1977.

Wensvoort, P., and Steenbergen-Botterweg, W. A. Nonextractable lipids in the adipose tissue of horses and ponies affected with generalized steatitis. *Tijdschr Diergeneeskd* **100:** 106–112, 1975.

Vanselow, B. A., and McCausland, I. P. Steatitis in two donkey foals. *Aust Vet J* **57:** 304–305, 1981.

Vitovec, J., Proks, C., and Valvoda, V. Lipomatosis (fat necrosis) in cattle and pigs. *J Comp Pathol* **85:** 53, 1975.

V. Inflammation of the Peritoneum: Peritonitis

Damage to the serosa of the peritoneal lining, and subsequent inflammation, is very common in the large domestic animals, and less common in dogs and cats. Peritonitis may be classified as primary or secondary; as acute or chronic; as local or diffuse; as septic or nonseptic; and on the basis of the type of exudate, which may be serofibrinous, fibrinopurulent, purulent, hemorrhagic, or granulomatous. Differences in distribution, type of exudate, and duration of the lesion can be more or less anticipated from the source and the etiology. Most cases of peritonitis in domestic animals are secondary; that is, they arise as complications of other events in the abdomen, rather than arising *de novo,* probably by hematogenous spread. The causes of peritonitis are numerous and varied, so only some of the more common and important of them will be considered.

Chemical peritonitis may be induced by a variety of agents. The intraperitoneal instillation of a number of therapeutic agents causes a mild, and usually inconsequential, peritonitis. However, experimental antibiotic lavage of the abdomen has been associated with serosal damage and formation of adhesions. Talc, formerly used as surgical glove powder, and starch, now used for that purpose, may provoke granulomatous peritonitis. Characteristic starch granules may be recognized in phagocytes within granulomas, forming a Maltese cross in polarized light, and pink by periodic acid–Schiff stain. Barium sulfate which accidentally spills into the abdomen is highly irritant, causing a potentially fatal hemorrhagic peritonitis, often complicated by intercurrent sepsis, the effects of which may be potentiated. Survivors will have extensive adhesions, and granulomas in which barium is seen in macrophages and giant cells.

The most devastating forms of chemical peritonitis are endogenous, and are caused by bile and pancreatic enzymes. The peritonitis caused by bile is intense, and if complicated by sepsis, may be rapidly fatal. There is very little exudate unless the leakage is minor and infected, and then it may become purulent. Biliary peritonitis is readily recognized by the typical staining. The peritonitis of pancreatic necrosis is also acute and is rather common in dogs, rare in horses, and virtually never occurs in other species. The reaction about the pancreas, particularly its head, is liquefactive and purulent, and the exudate mats the lesser omentum to the pancreas and the adjacent liver and other organs. This local peritoneal reaction resolves completely if the animal survives, and only very minor adhesions or slight puckering of the mesentery persist, with fibrosis in the pancreas. The peritoneal exudate is usually scant, but is distinctive because, as well as pus, it contains white droplets of fats and soaps released from the adipose tissue by the pancreatic enzymes. Leakage of chyle from a ruptured lymphatic into the abdomen may induce a mild granulomatous serositis.

Bacterial peritonitis may occur if bacteria reach the peritoneum by direct implantation. This is usually as a result of perforating lesions (Fig. 4.5), from a contaminated external surface, either a hollow viscus in the gastrointestinal or urogenital tract, or from the skin. It is most commonly associated with the lesions previously described, which are the source of peritoneal contamination by ingesta. In females, the abdominal cavity is open to the exterior through the reproductive tract, and infection may enter the abdomen through the uterine tube, as well as by rupture of the uterus or laceration of the vagina. Cystitis and rupture of a contaminated bladder may also result in peritonitis.

Bacterial peritonitis is also common as an extension from inflammation localized in an abdominal viscus or the

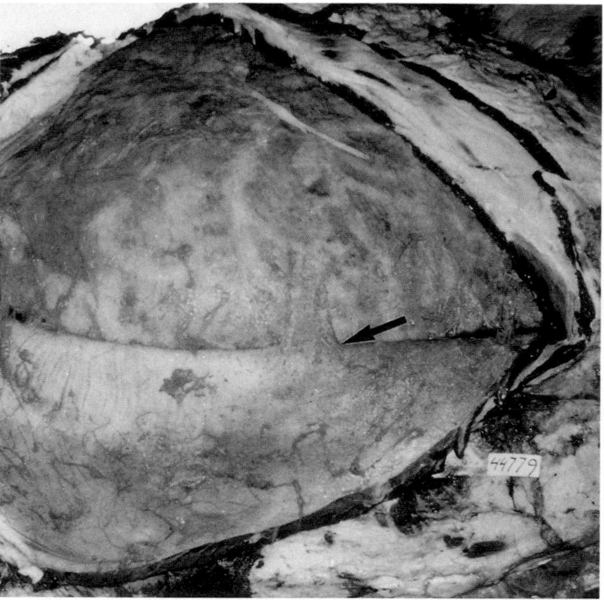

Fig. 4.5 Acute diffuse fibrinous peritonitis. Calf. Perforating abomasal ulcer. A tenacious sheet of fibrin is present between the omentum and the abdominal wall (arrow).

umbilicus, or as a typical part of the syndrome in a number of specific bacteremic diseases. Acute serofibrinous peritonitis may occur by extension through the wall of a gangrenous intestine or uterus prior to rupture; death from toxemia may intervene before rupture occurs. Secondary peritonitis occasionally results by extension from retroperitoneal infection, or in ruminants from omental bursitis. In those cases in which peritonitis develops by direct extension, there is little difficulty in ascertaining its origin, even when the process becomes diffuse.

The sources of peritonitis are so varied that a detailed consideration cannot be given to them here. Instead, some of the features of peritonitis in the different species are given, with an indication of the specific diseases in which peritonitis may occur. The nature of peritonitis in specific infections is discussed more fully with the those diseases, in other chapters. The consequences of peritonitis are discussed in the next section.

A. *Consequences of Peritonitis*

Acute generalized peritonitis is a catastrophic sequel in many local diseases of the abdominal cavity, but it may be a relatively insignificant secondary event in the generalized infections, though useful to pathologists as part of the suite of lesions used in diagnosis. Obviously, peritonitis does not significantly affect the outcome of an *Escherichia coli* septicemia, or clostridial infections such as blackleg or braxy.

Within the first few hours of generalized peritonitis, there may be intestinal hypermotility. However, paralytic ileus, mediated by autonomic innervation, soon supervenes. The development of ileus has the advantage that exudates are no longer distributed by intestinal movements. But there is also the disadvantage that fibrinous adhesions develop between loops of intestine, which may, if the animal recovers, produce fibrous adhesions and their sequelae.

The systemic effects of generalized peritonitis are related largely to detrimental effects on cardiovascular function, circulatory homeostasis, and acid–base balance. These are partly the result of sequestration of fluid and plasma protein in the peritoneal exudate; sequestration of fluid and electrolyte in amotile gut; and loss of intestinal absorptive function. Endotoxin, and exotoxins such as those produced by clostridia, may be absorbed into the circulation, directly through the peritoneum or via the lymphatic drainage. These cause increased vascular permeability, shock, and other detrimental cardiovascular effects. Death from toxemia may result before obvious peritonitis develops. Sepsis may spread via the lymphatics to the pleura and the sternal or mediastinal nodes, or it will attain the general circulation, causing septicemia.

Not all cases of generalized peritonitis are immediately fatal. Depending on the nature of the exudate, the lesions may resolve completely, be converted to diffuse adhesions, or persist in some localized areas as chronic active or adhesive peritonitis.

Peritoneal insult, with the initiation of inflammation by mediators released from local mast cells and other mesenchymal elements, results in massive outpouring of fibrinogen and chemotaxis of neutrophils. Tissue thromboplastin polymerizes fibrin. Damage to, or loss of, the peritoneal lining may diminish the fibrinolytic activity of mesothelium, and its capacity to produce a plasminogen activator; hence, normal fibrinolytic mechanisms are inhibited. Fibrin adheres to the denuded subserosal stroma, which is edematous, congested, or hemorrhagic. The lesion heals by fibroplasia and neovascularization, which extend from the subserosa into the fibrin framework. Mesothelium differentiates from mesenchymal elements in the subserosa, and covers the surface from below, rather than centripetally; hence, reconstitution of the mesothelium is not affected by the size of the defect. In uncomplicated situations, the wound has been debrided by phagocytes, fibroplasia and collagen deposition is well under way, and mesothelial reconstitution accomplished, by about 5–8 days after the insult.

If the bridges of fibrin between damaged serosal surfaces persist beyond 3–4 days after the original insult, usually related to failure of fibrinolysis, they become organized by connective tissue, and fibrous adhesions form. Contraction of connective tissue as it matures, and in response to tension, may result in close apposition and adhesion of adjacent structures, or stenosis, if fibrous bands surround or compress a hollow viscus. The effect is impaired motility, obstruction, or circulatory embarrassment. Fibrous adhesions may remodel and occasionally will separate, but often persist as scars on the serosa.

Formation of adhesions seems to be promoted by ischemia, increasing severity of tissue necrosis, foreign material such as sutures on the serosa, and by sepsis; the common factor may be that all increase the inflammatory reaction.

The duration of peritonitis may be a significant question in cases such as iatrogenic rectal perforation, and its assessment requires careful gross and microscopic examination of the serosal surface and the adherent exudate. The proliferation and degree of differentiation of fibroblasts in the exudate and in the edge of any wound, and the presence and degree of differentiation of regenerating mesothelial cells, will give some indication of the age of the lesion. The thickness of granulation tissue over the old serosa may give an indication of the duration of chronic peritonitis.

Bibliography

Baxter, G. M., Broome, T. E., and Moore, J. N. Abdominal adhesions after small intestinal surgery in the horse. *Vet Surg* **18:** 409–414, 1989.

Dean, P. W., Robertson, J. T., and Jacobs, R. M. Comparison of suture materials and suture patterns for inverting intestinal anastomosis of the jejunum in the horse. *Am J Vet Res* **46:** 2072–2077, 1985.

Elkins, T. E. *et al.* A histologic evaluation of peritoneal injury and repair: Implications for adhesion formation. *Obstet Gynecol* **70:** 225–228, 1987.

Ellis, H. The hazards of surgical glove dusting powders. *Surg Gynecol Obstet* **171:** 521–527, 1990.

Gfeller, R. W., and Sandors, A. D. Naproxen-associated duodenal ulcer complicated by perforation and bacteria- and barium sulfate-induced peritonitis in a dog. *J Am Vet Med Assoc* **198:** 644–646, 1991.

Hosgood, G. L., and Salisbury, S. K. Pathophysiology and pathogenesis of generalized peritonitis. *Probl Vet Med* **1:** 159–167, 1989.

Kipnis, R. M. Cholelithiasis, gallbladder perforation, and bile peritonitis in a dog. *Canine Pract* **13:** 15–27, 1986.

Lundin, C. *et al.* Induction of peritoneal adhesions with small intestinal ischaemia and distention in the foal. *Equine Vet J* **21:** 451–458, 1989.

O'Leary, J.–P. *et al.* The role of feces, necrotic tissue, and various blocking agents in the prevention of adhesions. *Ann Surg* **207:** 693–698, 1988.

Rappaport, W. D. *et al.* Antibiotic irrigation and the formation of intra-abdominal adhesions. *Am J Surg* **158:** 435–437, 1989.

Sullins, K. E. Intestinal adhesion reduction. *In* "The Equine Acute Abdomen," N. A. White, II (ed.), pp. 245–250. Philadelphia, Pennsylvania, Lea & Febiger, 1990.

B. Peritonitis in Horses

Diffuse peritonitis in horses is usually acute and fatal; this is perhaps associated in part with the small omentum, and a poor capacity to wall off contaminated areas. In most cases, clinical peritonitis is caused by rupture or perforation of the stomach or intestine. Copious purulent peritonitis may be seen in *Rhodococcus equi* infection of foals, which may also cause purulent mesenteric lymphadenitis. Intestinal infection of foals by *Actinobacillus equuli* causes fibrinous mesenteric lymphadenitis and peritonitis. Castration may cause an acute diffuse nonseptic peritonitis as a response to hemorrhage into the abdominal cavity, whereas peritoneal lavage with solutions containing povidone-iodine may cause severe diffuse chemical peritonitis. Seminoperitoneum, due to laceration of the vagina at breeding, is an unusual cause of acute diffuse nonseptic peritonitis; sperm are present in the cytoplasm of neutrophils. Chronic diffuse peritonitis is virtually never recorded in horses, other than in a rare animal with nocardiosis.

Acute or chronic local peritonitis does occur occasionally from surgical or castration wounds; from other penetration from the skin; and from streptococcal abscess in the mesentery. It may be secondary to local verminous lesions: from suppurative gastritis in habronemiasis, or from perforating *Gasterophilus* or *Anoplocephala*. Migrating *Strongylus equinus* or *S. edentatus* larvae cause retroperitoneal lesions in the flank, perirenal fat, and diaphragm; perihepatitis with fibrous tags on the liver capsule; and a chronic diffuse thickening and inflammation in the mesentery, omentum, and hepatorenal ligament, with occasional caseous nodules. Large strongyles returning to the gut may cause focal peritoneal lesions on the ileum, cecum, and colon. Penetrating wounds caused by ingested foreign bodies are very rare in horses, but may be responsible for chronic focal peritonitis involving the stomach.

Bibliography

Beroza, G. A. *et al.* Cecal perforation and peritonitis associated with *Anoplocephala perfoliata* infection in three horses. *J Am Vet Med Assoc* **183:** 804–806, 1983.

Bertone, J. J., and Dill, S. G. Traumatic gastropericarditis in a horse. *J Am Vet Med Assoc* **187:** 742–743, 1985.

Biberstein, E. L., Jang, S. S., and Hirsh, D. C. *Nocardia asteroides* infection in horses: A review. *J Am Vet Med Assoc* **186:** 273–277, 1985.

Dart, A. J., Hutchins, D. R., and Begg, A. P. Suppurative splenitis and peritonitis in a horse after gastric ulceration caused by larvae of *Gasterophilus intestinalis*. *Aust Vet J* **64:** 155–158, 1987.

Gay, C. C., and Lording, P. M. Peritonitis in horses associated with *Actinobacillus equuli*. *Aust Vet J* **56:** 296–300, 1980.

Hinschcliff, K. W., MacWilliams, P. S., and Wilson, D. G. Seminoperitoneum and peritonitis in a mare. *Equine Vet J* **20:** 71–73, 1988.

Mair, T. S., Hillyer, M. H., and Taylor, F. G. R. Peritonitis in adult horses: A review of 21 cases. *Vet Rec* **126:** 567–570, 1990.

Schneider, R. K. *et al.* Response of pony peritoneum to four peritoneal lavage solutions. *Am J Vet Res* **49:** 889–894, 1988.

Schumacher, J. *et al.* Peritonitis following castration in 3 horses. *Equine Vet Sci* **7:** 220–221, 1987.

Schumacher, J. *et al.* Effects of castration on peritoneal fluid in the horse. *J Vet Int Med* **2:** 22–25, 1988.

C. Peritonitis in Cattle

Acute diffuse fibrinopurulent peritonitis is common in cattle, and is usually the result of perforation of a viscus, especially the reticulum or uterus. Both may also result in local acute, and then chronic, peritonitis, with adhesions. Traumatic reticuloperitonitis (hardware disease) may be part of, or evolve to include, septic reticulopericarditis, if the offending foreign body advances far enough. Disordered motility of the forestomachs, manifest clinically as vagus indigestion, may follow scarring of traumatic reticuloperitonitis.

Cattle seem to have a relatively high capacity to localize and wall off septic foci within the peritoneal cavity. Abscesses may develop from such foci, which have been contained by local chronic peritonitis. Sometimes these may become quite large; they usually contain creamy pus, from which *Actinomyces pyogenes* is most commonly isolated. Perforation of the abomasum or intestine is more likely to give diffuse fibrinous or fibrinohemorrhagic peritonitis, but occasionally they, too, will cause local chronic peritonitis and abscessation.

Extension of infection from the umbilicus of the neonate produces fibrinopurulent peritonitis, which is not localized, but is most severe along the ventral abdominal wall, adjacent to associated liver abscesses, or up the urachus to the bladder. Fibrinous peritonitis may be an expression of polyserositis in neonatal calves with septicemic colibacillosis. Serofibrinous peritonitis, sometimes with very copious exudate (and with similar lesions on other serous membranes) is typical of sporadic bovine encephalomyelitis. Diffuse fibrinohemorrhagic peritonitis occurs in most cases of clostridial hemoglobinuria, and in some cases of blackleg and septicemic pasteurellosis; a more localized peritonitis of this type occurs in some cases of clostridial enterotoxemia caused by *Clostridium perfringens* type B and type C and in braxy.

Tuberculosis causes white nodular granulomas (pearls) as large as several centimeters in diameter; actinobacillosis, although rather rare, produces the usual heavily scarified granulomas, especially about the peritoneum of the forestomachs.

Bibliography

Floyd, J. G. *et al.* Periabomasal abscess in a cow. *J Am Vet Med Assoc* **192:** 663–664, 1988.

Palmer, J. E., and Whitlock, R. H. Perforated abomasal ulcers in adult dairy cows. *J Am Vet Med Assoc* **184:** 171–174, 1984.

Weaver, D. A. Duodenal perforation and abdominal abscess in a cow. *J Am Vet Med Assoc* **195:** 1603–1605, 1989.

D. *Peritonitis in Sheep*

Peritonitis of specific cause is uncommon in sheep, except for the very local reaction which accompanies penetration of the intestine by the larvae of *Oesophagostomum columbianum*. The uterus is probably the usual site in adults from which infection spreads to the peritoneum; the antecedent lesion in most cases is postpartum septic metritis. The peritonitis is fibrinopurulent and bloody. Serofibrinous peritonitis is a potential feature of any disease caused by *Mycoplasma*.

E. *Peritonitis in Goats*

Mycoplasma mycoides may cause acute fibrinous peritonitis in goats, although acute death from septicemia, or arthritis and mastitis are more common. Paratuberculosis (Johne's disease) frequently produces a nodular granulomatous lymphangitis in the mesentery and sometimes caseous or calcified lymphadenitis.

F. *Peritonitis in Swine*

A few filmy strands of fibrin frequently overlie the intestine and the borders of the mesentery in many acute infectious diseases of swine, and in conditions which result in vascular damage, such as edema disease and vitamin E/selenium-responsive conditions; this does not qualify as peritonitis.

Diffuse fibrinopurulent peritonitis is common in pigs (Fig. 4.6); the intestines may be so matted that they cannot be dissected. *Actinomyces pyogenes, Escherichia coli* or a miscellany of organisms are frequently present in these, and in some the inflammatory process can be traced to castration wounds. In such cases, the peritonitis may be localized to the inguinal and pelvic regions; adhesions and death from intestinal obstruction may occur. Occasionally, *A. pyogenes* produces discrete encapsulated abscesses as profuse implants on both visceral and parietal peritoneum.

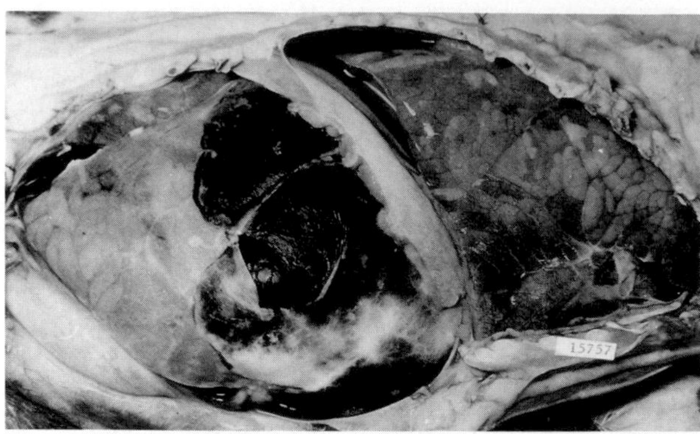

Fig. 4.6 Fibrinous polyserositis. Pig. *Escherichia coli* septicemia.

A serofibrinous peritonitis, with fibrinous arthritis and exudation on other serous surfaces, is indicative of Glasser's disease, caused by *Haemophilus parasuis*. *Mycoplasma hyorhinis* and possibly other mycoplasmas may produce a serofibrinous peritonitis that becomes fibrous, with adhesions to a thickened serous membrane; this disease is to be distinguished from Glasser's disease, and from septicemias due to *Streptococcus suis* type 2. Small, firm, lemon-yellow nodules, and flattened disks of inspissated fibrin often are found free in the peritoneal cavity in chronic *Mycoplasma* infections.

Rectal strictures in swine cause marked dilation of the colon and cecum. The serosa is frequently thickened, white, and covered with fibrin tags, resembling infectious serositis. The thickening is probably caused by subserosal edema and fibrosis in the intestinal wall.

Stephanurus dentatus larvae cause subserosal focal hepatitis and a mild reaction with edema in the perirenal fat and retroperitoneal tissue, and sometimes in the mesentery and local lymph nodes, as they move to the kidney. In intestinal anthrax in swine there is acute gelatinous hemorrhagic peritonitis very typically localized to the mesentery between the intestine and the mesenteric node, the distribution of the lesion being due to the lymphatic spread of the infection from the intestine.

Tuberculous peritonitis in swine is localized and characterized by adhesions to the spleen.

G. *Peritonitis in Dogs*

Fibrinohemorrhagic peritonitis, usually slight and easily overlooked, is common in infectious canine hepatitis. The peritoneum, especially that covering the intestine, is gray and granular like ground glass, and there are a few red strands of fibrin, most of them about the liver. There is edema of the intestinal subserosa and frequently petechiae or larger hemorrhages. In parvovirus infection, similar lesions may be present on the serosa of affected segments of intestine.

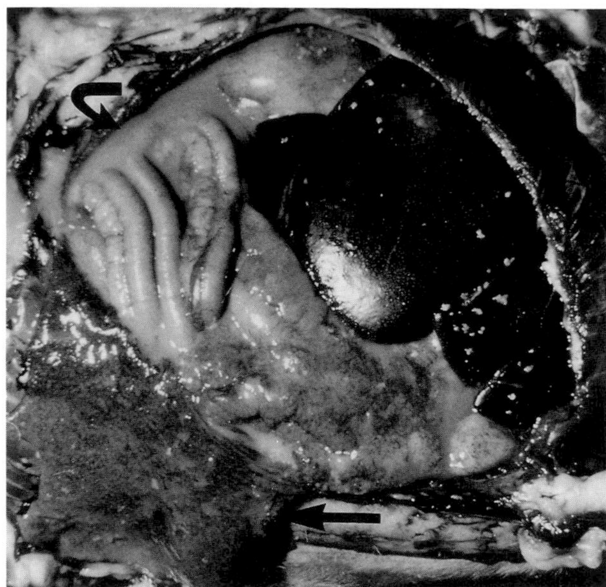

Fig. 4.7 Nocardial peritonitis. Dog. The peritoneum of the reflected abdominal wall (arrow) and the omentum is granular due to adherent microcolonies of *Nocardia*. Note excess, cloudy peritoneal fluid (curved arrow).

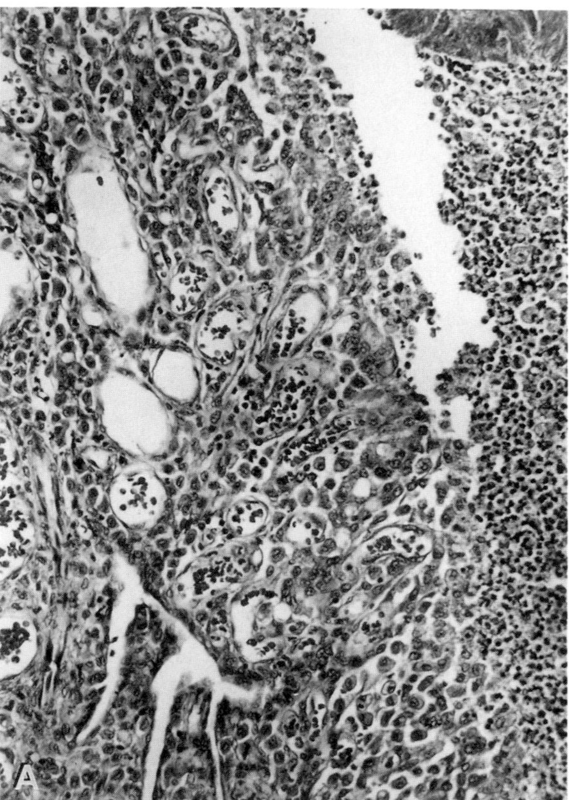

Fig. 4.8A Nocardial peritonitis. Dog. Thin-walled capillaries on peritoneal surface.

Suppurative peritonitis in the dog is uncommon; it has been observed in puppies as an extension from umbilical and hepatic abscesses caused by streptococci. Septic peritonitis involving a variety of agents, often including *E. coli* and anaerobes, may follow surgical contamination of the abdomen; a penetrating wound or perforation of the gut; rupture of the urinary bladder; or rupture of pancreatic, hepatic, or prostatic abscesses. Putrid peritonitis occurs when the uterus ruptures, either as a result of pyometra or septic metritis with fetal putrefaction.

Nocardiosis produces very characteristic peritonitis (Fig. 4.7), though it more commonly causes pleuritis. Sometimes there are pyogranulomas, but most frequently there is a profuse, pink mush on the peritoneum. The color is from blood in the copious cellular exudate; the blood is derived from a tremendous proliferation of thin-walled capillaries on serous surfaces (Fig. 4.8A), which are thickened, red, and edematous. Microscopic pyogranulomatous lesions are evident on the peritoneal surfaces (Fig. 4.8B). *Actinomyces* spp., most commonly *A. viscosus*, may produce similar gross lesions, often with small yellow sulfur granules free in the exudate, or in granulomas. The granulomas may be large and adherent, involving the omentum, mesenteries, and affected mesenteric lymph nodes (Fig. 4.9). Chronic pyogranulomatous or granulomatous peritonitis occurs in the rare cases of eumycotic mycetoma and phycomycosis which involve the abdominal cavity. There is usually thickening and fibrosis of the serosa of affected segments of gut, with marked formation of adhesions, and the development of firm granulomatous masses on the gut wall and in the mesenteries and omentum. In cases of granulomatous peritonitis, fungal culture should be carried out, as well as attempts at isolation of *Nocardia* and *Actinomyces*.

Sclerosing encapsulating peritonitis, a characteristic pathologic syndrome, occurs rarely in the dog. Affected animals have borborygmus, vomition, and ascites. The syndrome gets its name from the thick layer of granulation tissue that lines the abdominal cavity, or parts of it, and covers or encapsulates the organs that are involved. The effect is to produce one or more thick-walled cystic spaces, incorporating some or most of the abdominal cavity and its organs, forming a cocoonlike structure. Within the space is a large volume of clear or serosanguinous, but relatively acellular, fluid, and perhaps a few strands of more or less organized fibrin. The involved organs are often atrophic or misshapen due to the thick fibrous capsule on their surface. Vessels resembling portocaval shunts are described in animals in which the liver was severely affected, implying the development of portal hypertension due to disordered intrahepatic circulation.

Microscopically, the capsule which covers organs, and lines the wall of the peritoneal cavity, is composed of a thick layer of progressively maturing granulation tissue. There are a few scattered aggregates of mixed inflammatory cells and foamy macrophages, and a few adipocytes, invested in the capsular stroma. But there is no exudation of inflammatory cells from the surface, which is composed

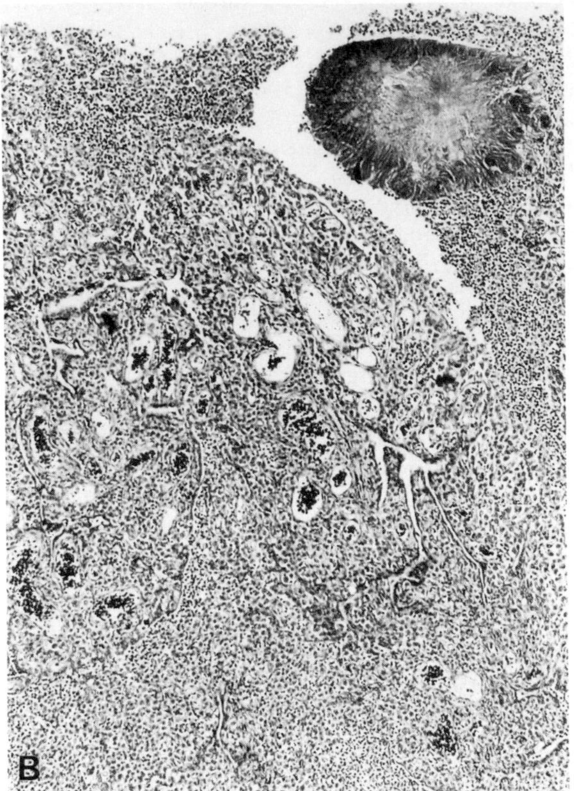

Fig. 4.8B Nocardial peritonitis. Dog. Pyogranulomatous inflammation. Bacterial colony (top right) is surrounded by neutrophils.

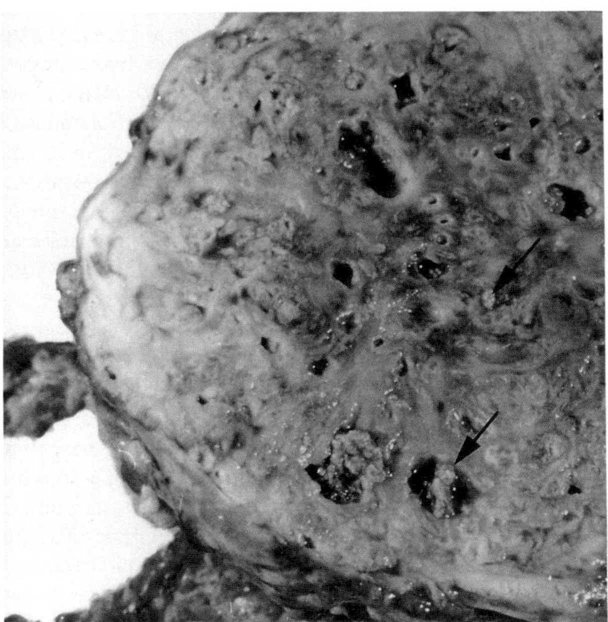

Fig. 4.9 Granulomatous mass involving the mesentery and omentum. Dog. *Actinomyces* peritonitis. Sulfur granules shell out of pyogranulomatous foci on the cut surface (arrows).

of granulation tissue of variable maturity, and may be covered by a single layer of mesothelium. The etiology is unknown, but it seems nonseptic. A similar syndrome in humans is considered a possible complication of peritoneal dialysis, which is not implicated in dogs.

Bibliography

Boothe, H. W., Lay, J. C., and Moreland, K. J. Sclerosing encapsulating peritonitis in three dogs. *J Am Vet Med Assoc* **198:** 267–270, 1991.

Clark, D. M. *et al.* Clostridial peritonitis associated with a mast cell tumor in a dog. *J Am Vet Med Assoc* **188:** 188–190, 1986.

Edwards, D. F., Nyland, T. G., and Weigel, J. P. Thoracic, abdominal, and vertebral actinomycosis. *J Vet Int Med* **2:** 184–191, 1988.

Greenfield, C. L., and Walshaw, R. Open peritoneal drainage for treatment of contaminated peritoneal cavity and septic peritonitis in dogs and cats: 24 cases (1980–1986). *J Am Vet Med Assoc* **191:** 100–105, 1987.

Hardie, E.M. Peritonitis from urogenital conditions. *Probl Vet Med* **1:** 36–49, 1989.

Hosgood, G., and Salisbury, S. K. Generalized peritonitis in dogs: 50 cases (1975–1986). *J Am Vet Med Assoc* **193:** 1448–1450, 1988.

Miller, R. I. Gastrointestinal phycomycosis in 63 dogs. *J Am Vet Med Assoc* **186:** 473–478, 1985.

Valentine, B. A., and Porter, W. P. Multiple hepatic abscesses and peritonitis caused by eugonic fermenter-4 bacilli in a pup. *J Am Vet Med Assoc* **183:** 1324–1325, 1983.

Walker, R. L. *et al.* Eumycotic mycetoma caused by *Pseudallescheria boydii* in the abdominal cavity of a dog. *J Am Vet Med Assoc* **192:** 67–70, 1988.

H. Peritonitis in Cats

Foul-smelling peritonitis occurs when the uterus ruptures due to pyometra or fetal putrefaction. Peritonitis also occurs from penetrating wounds or by extension from retroperitoneal tissues, and occasionally septic peritonitis is caused by anaerobes such as those associated with catbite abscesses. Nocardial and actinomycotic peritonitis similar in appearance to the disease in dogs may complicate feline leukemia virus infection in cats and the myeloproliferative diseases.

Bibliography

Scott, P. C. *et al.* Suppurative peritonitis in cats associated with anaerobic bacteria. *Aust Vet J* **61:** 367–368, 1984.

The group of feline coronaviruses which includes the **feline infectious peritonitis** (FIP) viruses is closely related to transmissible gastroenteritis virus of swine, and to canine coronavirus. In cats the various coronavirus strains have a spectrum of virulence, from asymptomatic enteric infection, through symptomatic enteric infection (see The Alimentary System, Chapter 1 of this volume), to virulent systemic infection, which is expressed as FIP. The antibodies produced against FIP virus cannot be distinguished readily from those stimulated by the other feline coronaviruses. In comparison to their enteric counterparts, the FIP virus strains have less tropism for the gut. They replicate in macrophages, which disseminate the virus to many parts of the body, and this is central to their virulence.

Feline infectious peritonitis has a worldwide distribution, but the disease is sporadic, and has a low prevalence, despite the fact that exposure of cats to coronaviruses seems common. Young cats, most commonly between 6 months and 3 years of age, tend to be affected. Though morbidity is typically low, occasional outbreaks of disease may occur; mortality approaches 100%.

Although FIP may be acquired by exposure to exogenous virus, probably by the oro-nasal route, it may also arise by unpredictable mutation of an endogenous enteric coronavirus. Virus replicates in tonsil or gut, and subsequently in regional lymph nodes. Enteric infection may produce mild, subclinical blunting and fusion of villi. The viremia that follows primary replication results in infection of macrophages in many tissues, especially those with a rich vasculature or sinusoidal circulation, and many fixed phagocytes. A secondary viremia associated with infected macrophages occurs.

Several factors in the host–parasite interaction influence the prevalence of disease and its clinical expression. Once the virus is disseminated systemically in macrophages, the outcome is the result of the type and efficacy of the host immune response. This in turn may be affected by factors such as age at exposure; innate genetic susceptibility and immune competence; the presence of circulating antibody to coronavirus; stressors; glucocorticoids and other causes of immunosuppression, particularly concurrent infection with feline leukemia virus (FLV) and feline immunodeficiency virus (FIV).

If a strong cell-mediated immune response is generated, and activates macrophages, FIP virus replication is terminated, and disease does not occur. If no cell-mediated immunity develops, even though antibody is produced, macrophages producing virus accumulate around vessels and in the interstitium of the serous surfaces and tissues throughout the body, generating the effusive, or wet form of FIP. This syndrome has a rapid clinical course, progressing to death in 1–12 weeks. If there is a weak or ineffective cell-mediated immune response, the noneffusive, or dry, clinical syndrome ensues, with a less florid macrophage response in tissue, and poorer virus production. This form of the disease has a more prolonged clinical course, which may extend for 1–6 months. Though often described as distinct entities, the wet and dry forms of FIP are the extremes of a continuum of clinicopathologic syndromes. Effusive disease occurs more commonly than the noneffusive.

Some animals which successfully abort the progress of the infection with a strong cell-mediated response may remain persistently infected; in some of these, infection may recrudesce to produce disease weeks or months later. Animals with preexisting antibody to coronavirus may be more susceptible to disease, due to enhanced primary infection of macrophages as a result of increased uptake of virus in phagocytosed antigen–antibody complexes. Infection with FLV or FIV may sufficiently impair cell-mediated immune competence that it permits full expression of effusive FIP, or recrudescent infection; 20–50% of animals with FIP are reported to be infected with feline leukemia virus. Impairment of T-suppressor cell activity may explain in part the exaggerated antibody response to FIP virus.

Preexisting antibody to coronavirus, and excessive non-neutralizing antibody production, promote formation of antigen–antibody complexes. These are taken up by macrophages, further enhancing infection, and they are deposited in the wall of small vessels. Complement fixation by the antigen–antibody complex enhances phagocytosis of virus by macrophages, and promotes neutrophil chemotaxis, with concomitant local tissue destruction. Arthus reactions occur in the walls of small venules and arterioles, especially in the serosal surfaces and parenchymatous organs, such as kidney and liver. The cellular infiltrates around vessels are often characterized as pyogranulomatous, on account of the mixed population of neutrophils, macrophages, and other round cells, though they never evolve to true granulomas.

Vascular lesions permit the effusion of protein-rich fluid into the serous spaces, causing the wet form of FIP. Endothelial damage also results in disseminated intravascular coagulation in the terminal stages of the disease, with thrombocytopenia and evolution of fibrin split products.

Cats with the effusive form of FIP are typically depressed, inappetent, and lose body condition. They may develop abdominal distension due to the accumulation of fluid. Pleural effusion also is present in ~25% of cases, and may cause dyspnea. Cardiac tamponade due to pericardial effusion is rare. In contrast to animals with noneffusive FIP, ocular and central nervous signs are unusual. These cats are hypergammaglobulinemic, and may have leukocytosis and neutrophilia, though some, in the terminal stages, or if infected with FLV, may be lymphopenic. Most go on to die; very few recover, after passing through a phase of noneffusive disease.

Cats with noneffusive FIP have a chronic disease of insidious onset, also characterized by weight loss, fever, and depression. They frequently develop signs specific to organs severely affected by vascular lesions. These may include ocular disease; central nervous disorders such as ataxia, posterior paresis, head tilt, specific nerve palsies, nystagmus, and behavioral changes; renal failure; and hepatic or pancreatic insufficiency.

Cats dying of FIP are emaciated. At necropsy, the separation of the syndromes is arbitrary, based on the extent of serous effusion, and the organ distribution of inflammatory foci. In the effusive form, visceral lesions are sometimes minimal, and in the noneffusive form, peritonitis may be mild or not obvious on gross examination. All serous surfaces throughout the body may be involved in the inflammatory response, and pleurisy with pleural effusion is present in many cases of effusive FIP.

Peritonitis is present in most animals, although marked effusion is not found in those with the dry form. As much

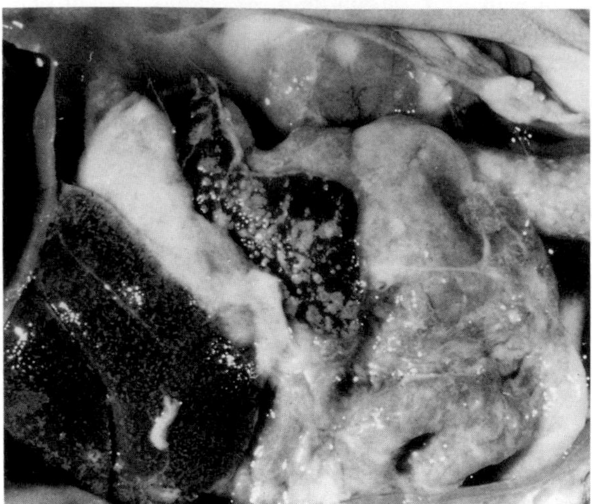

Fig. 4.10 Feline infectious peritonitis. Exudative lesion with fibrin on mesentery and viscera, and granulomas in liver, spleen, kidney, and wall of large and small intestine.

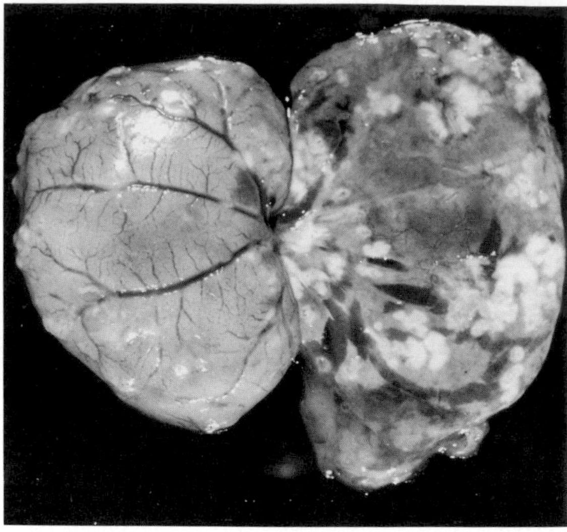

Fig. 4.11 Feline infectious peritonitis. Focal pyogranulomatous lesions involving renal cortex and reflected capsule.

as 1 liter of abdominal exudate may be present in cats with effusive FIP. The fluid is usually viscous, clear, and pale to deep yellow, although it may be flocculent and contain strands of fibrin. The serosal surfaces may be covered with fibrin, giving them a granular appearance. Fibrin is frequently prominent over the visceral peritoneum (Fig. 4.10), and fragile adhesions may be present. There are white foci of necrosis or raised plaques or nodular cellular infiltrations on the serosa, and extending into the organs or wall of the intestine. These vary in size from a few millimeters to a centimeter in diameter. The omentum may be contracted into a mass in the cranial abdomen, and adherent to itself and other abdominal surfaces. Mesenteries may be thickened and opaque.

The kidneys may be enlarged and nodular, with few or many, small to large, white, firm nodules protruding from the cortex (Fig. 4.11). Hepatitis and pancreatitis of variable degree may also be present, characterized by small, white foci of inflammation in these organs. The tunica vaginalis may be affected, resulting in periorchitis in entire males. Fibrin is usually less prominent in the thorax, but firm white foci may be present under the pleura, and the lungs may be dark and rubbery. Hydropericardium and epicarditis occur less frequently. Abdominal and thoracic lymph nodes may be enlarged and have a lobulated pattern on cut surface.

In cats with noneffusive FIP, there may be inflammatory foci in the abdominal or thoracic organs as described, or lesions may be restricted to the eyes and nervous system. The lesions in the eyes may appear as a diffuse uveitis or chorioretinitis, progressing to panophthalmitis; fibrin is often present in the anterior chamber. Lesions in the central nervous system can involve the leptomeninges, spinal cord, or brain, but usually are visible grossly only on the leptomeninges, as thickening or white streaks. Occasionally, acquired hydrocephalus may accompany inflammatory obstruction of the third or fourth ventricles.

The characteristic microscopic lesion is a generalized vasculitis and perivasculitis, especially of venules (Fig. 4.12), with a focal mixed inflammatory reaction. This lesion occurs in the serous membranes, in the connective

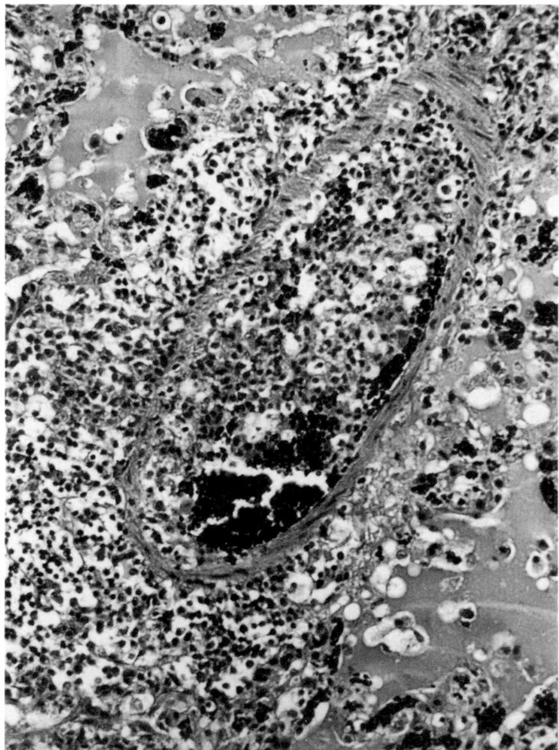

Fig. 4.12 Feline infectious peritonitis. Vasculitis and perivasculitis in the lung. There is severe pulmonary edema.

tissue of the parenchymatous organs, the eye, and the meninges. Neutrophils, lymphocytes, plasma cells, and macrophages accumulate in and around affected vessels. The endothelium swells, and medial necrosis may be evident, with narrowed vascular lumina; thrombosis may occur. The proportion of neutrophils in the reaction varies, and some lesions may be composed mainly of a mixture of mononuclear cells, or histiocytes. Fibroplasia is variable; occasionally, adventitial fibrosis occurs with little cellular infiltrate. The vascular lesion results in the serofibrinous and cellular exudate on the serosal surfaces, and the nodules visible on the surfaces and deeper in solid organs. The small random necrotic foci found in the parenchyma of the liver in some cases may be due to thrombophlebitis and infarction.

The microscopic changes on the omentum, mesentery, and serosal tissues vary in severity. The mild changes are proliferation of mesothelial cells, slight fibrin exudate with fibroblast proliferation, and scattered neutrophils and mononuclear cells. The severe changes result in a thick layer of fibrin adherent to the serosa, with necrosis and/or hypertrophy of mesothelium. Large numbers of neutrophils, mononuclear cells, and necrotic debris may be embedded in the fibrin. The vasculitis may extend from the serosa into the intestine, affecting the muscularis, myenteric ganglia, the submucosa, and the mucosa, which may be segmentally infarcted.

Lesions in various organs are caused by the vascular damage which occurs in the capsule and stromal connective tissue. They may be found throughout the body. Subcapsular infiltrations occur particularly in the liver, lung, and pancreas, and perivasculitis can develop deep in the parenchyma, especially in the kidney. In addition to focal lung lesions, there may be diffuse interstitial pneumonia, sometimes most severe close to the visceral pleura. Similarly, severe focal or generalized lymphoplasmacytic interstitial nephritis may develop. In the spleen and lymph nodes there is histiocytosis, and either depletion or hyperplasia of lymphoid follicles.

Cellular infiltrations in the spinal or cerebral meninges, the choroid plexuses, ependyma, and perivascular spaces tend to be more mononuclear and diffuse, with only occasional focal perivasculitis. Degenerative and necrotic lesions in the parenchyma of the central nervous system appear to be related to the vasculitis. Ocular lesions are common, but usually subclinical (see The Eye and Ear, Volume 1, Chapter 4).

Effusive FIP must be differentiated from bacterial peritonitis and pyothorax in particular, whereas the noneffusive form must be distinguished in some of its manifestations from lymphosarcoma, steatitis, mycotic infections, and toxoplasmosis. The combination of characteristic gross and microscopic lesions usually poses no diagnostic challenge when a complete necropsy is possible. Feline infectious peritonitis may be more difficult to diagnose on the basis of the vasculitis in biopsies, or in highly selected fixed-tissue submissions. Isolation of the agent is not routinely attempted.

Bibliography

Evermann, J. F. *et al.* Biological and pathological consequences of feline infectious peritonitis virus infection in the cheetah. *Arch Virol* **102:** 155–171, 1988.

Grahn, B. H. The feline coronavirus infections: Feline infectious peritonitis and feline coronavirus enteritis. *Vet Med* **86:** 376–393, 1991.

Hayashi, T. *et al.* Pathology of noneffusive type feline infectious peritonitis and experimental transmission. *Jpn J Vet Sci* **42:** 197–210, 1980.

Hoskins, J. D. Coronavirus infection in cats. *Compend Cont Ed Pract Vet* **13:** 567–586, 1991.

Jacobse-Geels, H. E. L., Daha, M. R., and Horzinek, M. C. Antibody, immune complexes, and complement activity fluctuations in kittens with experimentally induced feline infectious peritonitis. *Am J Vet Res* **43:** 666–670, 1982.

Kellner, S. J., and Litschi, B. Augenveränderungen bei der Felinen Infektiösen Peritonitis. *Kleintierpraxis* **34:** 261–266, 1989.

Montali, R. J., and Strandberg, J. D. Extraperitoneal lesions in feline infectious peritonitis. *Vet Pathol* **9:** 109–121, 1972.

Pedersen, N. C. Feline infectious peritonitis. *In* "Comparative Pathobiology of Viral Diseases, Vol II," R. G. Olsen, S. Krakowka, and J. R. Blakeslee, Jr. (eds.), pp. 115–136. Boca Raton, Florida, CRC Press, 1985.

Pedersen, N. C. Virologic and immunologic aspects of feline infectious peritonitis virus infection. *Adv Exp Biol Med* **218:** 529–550, 1987.

Stoddart, M. E. *et al.* The sites of early viral replication in feline infectious peritonitis. *Vet Microbiol* **18:** 259–271, 1988.

Tamke, P. G. *et al.* Acquired hydrocephalus and hydromyelia in a cat with feline infectious peritonitis: A case report and brief review. *Can Vet J* **29:** 997–1000, 1988.

Weiss, R. C. Feline infectious peritonitis and other coronaviruses. *In* "The Cat. Diseases and Clinical Management, Vol. I," R. G. Sherding (ed.), pp. 333–355. New York, Churchill Livingstone, 1989.

Weiss, R. C., and Scott, F. W. Pathogenesis of feline infectious peritonitis: Pathologic changes and immunofluorescence. *Am J Vet Res* **42:** 2036–2048, 1981.

Wolfe, L. G., and Griesemer, R. A. Feline infectious peritonitis: Review of gross and histopathologic lesions. *J Am Vet Med Assoc* **158:** 987–993, 1971.

VI. Parasitic Diseases of the Peritoneum

Most of the parasites found in the peritoneal cavity are there in the normal course of migrations to another site, or as an accident. Only a few larval and adult helminths use the abdominal cavity as their normal habitat.

Cysticerci (*Cysticercus tenuicollis* in ruminants; *C. pisiformis* in lagomorphs) may be found on the peritoneum during their normal development; they are nonpathogenic, and excite virtually no tissue response, beyond a thin, bland fibrous capsule. Rarely, cysticerci have been encountered in the abdomen of carnivores, which are abnormal hosts. Spargana, elongate larval forms of *Spirometra* spp., may encyst in a bland fibrous capsule in the peritoneal cavity of carnivores and swine. Tetrathyridia, the larvae of the tapeworm *Mesocestoides*, may proliferate extensively in the abdominal cavity of carnivores, where they cause a characteristic pyogranulomatous peritonitis, or parasitic ascites.

Fasciola hepatica larvae can cause acute and chronic peritonitis in cattle and sheep; the inflammation involves the parietal peritoneum and sometimes the visceral peritoneum, especially that of liver, spleen, and omentum. The changes may consist of many tags of fibrin or a more diffuse thickening, and the young flukes may be found in the inflammatory lesions both on and beneath the peritoneum.

Dioctophyma renale seems not so well adapted to canids as to mustelids. In dogs, worms may not complete their migration from the duodenum to the right kidney. As a result, they sometimes initiate chronic perihepatitis, in which reaction characteristic ova, if not the worm or its remnants, may be found.

Stephanuris dentatus, in the course of its migrations through the liver and peritoneal cavity to the kidneys in pigs, may cause local hemorrhage, peritonitis, and perihepatitis.

Strongylus edentatus and *S. equinus* pass through the liver and the ligaments and lumen of the peritoneal cavity in their migration. Fibrous tags on the liver, particularly the diaphragmatic aspect, are sequelae of *S. edentatus* migration. The larvae of both species may be found in the retroperitoneal tissues of the dorsal abdomen in horses, and in the mesenteries and omentum, where they sometimes incite eosinophilic granulomas.

Ascarids of all species occasionally may cause obstruction and rupture of the small intestine or bile duct, so that they may be found in the abdomen as a terminal event.

Some parasites use the peritoneal cavity as their final habitat. *Setaria* spp., onchocercid filarioid nematodes, inhabit the peritoneal cavity of many domestic and wild ungulates, such as horses, cattle, buffalo, camels, sheep, goats, swine, deer, and antelope. They are commonly found at autopsy in cattle and horses in endemic areas.

Some species of *Setaria* have a cosmopolitan distribution and may be found in several species of wild and domestic ungulates (*S. equina* in Equidae, *S. labiatopapillosa* in cattle, buffalo, and perhaps deer and antelope), whereas others are restricted geographically (*S. digitata,* Asia) perhaps by the distribution of intermediate hosts.

Adult *Setaria* usually do not cause significant peritoneal lesions in their normal host. There are rare reports of occlusion of the uterine tube by *S. labiatopapillosa* in cattle. As well, adult *S. labiatopapillosa* in the peritoneal cavity, or in the vaginal space around the testis, may incite granulomatous peritonitis or periorchitis if they die; remnants of the dead nematode may be detected in sections of the granulomatous reaction. Adult *S. digitata* may be found occasionally in abnormal locations, such as the heart, lungs, and mesenteric lymph nodes, where they incite eosinophilic granulomas. The larval form of *S. digitata* can produce mild adhesive peritonitis and granulomas in the retroperitoneum and bladder of cattle. The larvae of *S. equina, S. digitata,* and perhaps others which normally spend part of their time in the central nervous system, may occasionally penetrate the neural parenchyma and cause lesions.

The sheathed microfilariae deposited by the adult females in the peritoneal cavity are found in the blood. The intermediate host may be a mosquito, or for some *Setaria* spp., biting flies (*Haematobia* and *Stomoxys* spp.). The microfilariae develop into infective larvae in 2–3 weeks. They are released from the feeding arthropod and enter the final host.

Setaria digitata is normally found as an adult in the peritoneal cavity of cattle and buffalo in Asia. The migration of larvae in the brain and spinal cord of aberrant hosts, such as horses, camels, sheep, and goats, causes a neurologic disease, called lumbar paralysis or kumri in Asia. The migrating larvae apparently cause little or no damage in the natural host. The location of the lesions is variable, as are the clinical signs produced. Characteristically, the neurologic signs are ataxia, weakness, or paralysis. The severity of the signs varies from slight weakness to quadriplegia, depending on the number and location of the wandering parasites; however, affected animals may remain bright and alert.

The lesions produced are fundamentally traumatic; the inflammatory component is less conspicuous. A careful gross examination of brain and spinal cord may reveal the areas of damage as brown foci or streaks. The lesions tend to be focal, and may be difficult to find. Apart from the foci of malacia, the remainder of the nervous system may be normal.

The most obvious feature of the microscopic lesions is the microcavitation caused mechanically by migrating larvae; hemorrhage is variable. Surrounding the areas of cavitation, there is loss of myelin, gitter cell formation, and fragmentation of axons. Gemistocytic astrocytes are present in older lesions. Occasionally the parasites can be found in section and identified, but the cerebral lesions produced by aberrant parasitic migration, irrespective of the parasite, are distinctive and suggest the diagnosis. They differ from more conventional lesions in that all neural structures (myelin, axis cylinders, nerve cells, and glia) are involved; the patterns of damage are random; and eosinophils are usually the most common inflammatory cell. Neutrophils and macrophages are also often present, along with mild meningitis and vascular cuffing.

The term cerebrospinal nematodiasis has been applied to nervous diseases resulting from aberrant larval migrations (see The Nervous System, Volume 1, Chapter 3). Many parasites such as *Strongylus vulgaris* may be occasional culprits. Only *Setaria digitata,* and a few other nematodes, such as *Angiostrongylus cantonensis* in dogs, *Parelaphostrongylus* (formerly *Pneumostrongylus) tenuis* and *Elaphostrongylus cervi* in abnormal cervid or other ungulate hosts, and *Baylisascaris procyonis* in rodents and lagomorphs, produce the syndrome with any frequency. *Setaria* species which may occur normally in cervids have been reported to cause cerebrospinal nematodiasis in deer; however, *Elaphostrongylus* larvae produce similar signs and lesions, and differentiation may be difficult.

Setaria digitata larvae may invade the eye of horses, via the optic nerve, as do the microfilariae of *S. equina*. Here they may cause endophthalmitis.

Bibliography

Anderson, R. C. The pathogenesis and transmission of neurotropic and accidental nematode parasites of the central nervous system of mammals and birds. *Helminthol Abstr* **37:** 191–210, 1968.

Baharsefat, M. *et al.* The first report of lumbar paralysis in sheep due to nematode larvae infestation in Iran. *Cornell Vet* **63:** 81–86, 1973.

Frauenfelder, H. C., Kazacos, K. R., and Lichtenfels, J. R. Cerebrospinal nematodiasis caused by a filariid in a horse. *J Am Vet Med Assoc* **177:** 359–362, 1980.

Fujita, J. *et al.* Heterotopic parasitism of *Setaria digitata* (Linstow, 1906) in the heart of a cattle. *Jpn J Vet Sci* **47:** 999–1001, 1985.

Innes, J. R. M., and Pillai, C. P. Kumri—so-called lumbar paralysis—of horses in Ceylon (India and Burma), and its identification with cerebrospinal nematodiasis. *Br Vet J* **111:** 223–235, 1955.

Manspeaker, J. E., Haaland, M. A., and Nepote, K. H. Occlusion of a bovine oviduct by *Setaria labiatopapillosa*. *Vet Med: Small Anim Clin* **78:** 109–111, 1983.

Osborne, C. A. *et al. Dioctophyma renale* in the dog. *J Am Vet Med Assoc* **155:** 605–620, 1969.

Powe, T. A., and Powers, R. D. Periorchitis after tetramisole treatment in bulls implanted with *Setaria labiatopapillosa*. *J Am Vet Med Assoc* **186:** 588–589, 1985.

VII. Miscellaneous Lesions

Cysts of the peritoneum are rather common but insignificant. Those associated with genital adnexa are described with those systems. Cysticerci have been mentioned; *Echinococcus granulosus* may develop cysts on the peritoneum following the rupture of a mature hydatid into the abdomen. Small cysts, sometimes multiple, which are observed in the omentum, may be either inclusion cysts or local lymphatic ectasia; they are inert.

The normal squamous mesothelial cells of the serosa may undergo metaplasia to a cuboidal or columnar type resembling epithelium. Such metaplasia is probably the mildest response of the peritoneum to irritation but may also be a response to estrogen. Inflammatory metaplasia leading to ossification may occur in peritoneal scars, especially in swine. It may also be found in the mesenteries and the dorsal retroperitoneum without obvious antecedent change, although ossification may occur following fat necrosis as well. The newly formed bones are flat and of variable size and shape and are usually found in adipose tissue.

VIII. Neoplastic Diseases of the Peritoneum

Primary tumors of the peritoneum may arise from the serosa itself, from the subserous connective tissues, and from various differentiated tissues such as nerve sheaths. Tumors arising from the serosa are called **mesotheliomas,** sometimes termed malignant. The qualification is unnecessary, as virtually all are malignant, although the malignant behavior is usually expressed as implantation rather than metastasis.

Mesotheliomas are rare. They occur with greatest frequency in cattle and dogs but are reported occasionally in horses, cats, pigs, and other species. Interest in mesotheliomas has increased since the association between asbestos fiber and mesothelioma was discovered in humans. This association has not been confirmed in animals, though ferruginous bodies, suggestive of asbestos exposure, have been found in the lungs of some urban dogs with mesothelioma, and an association has been made between mesothelioma in dogs and exposure of owners to asbestos. In domestic animals, mesothelioma is notable because it occurs most frequently as a congenital neoplasm in fetal or young cattle (Fig. 4.13A,B).

Mesotheliomas arise from the cells of the serous linings of pericardial, pleural, and peritoneal cavities, and they may involve all three locations. Only in swine are they apparently mainly pleural.

They usually appear as multiple firm, sessile, or pedunculate nodules, from a few millimeters to 6–10 cm in diameter, or as villous projections, on a thickened mesentery

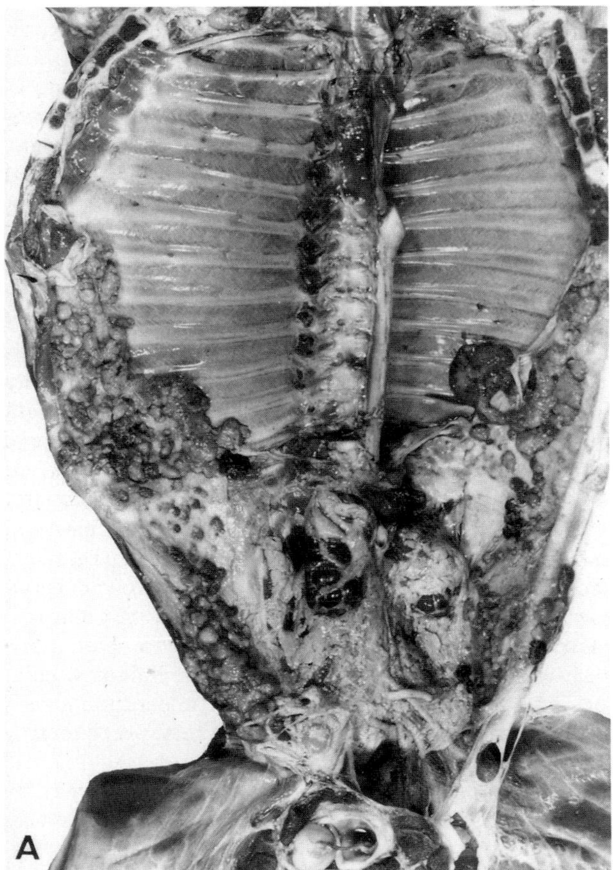

Fig. 4.13A Congenital mesothelioma. Calf. Tumor nodules are confined to peritoneal cavity.

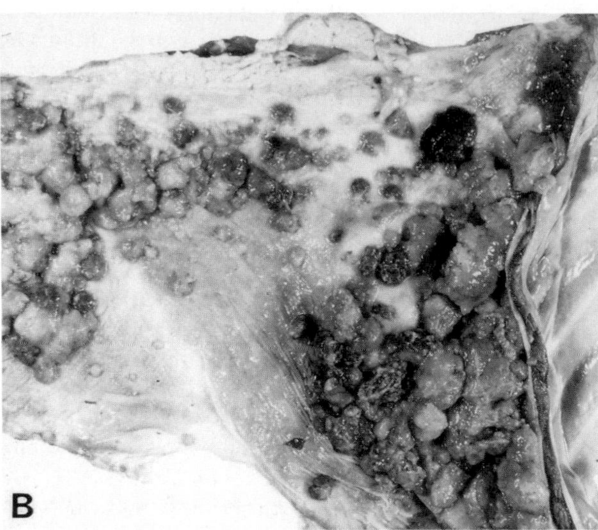

Fig. 4.13B Close-up of (A) showing nodules of mesothelioma on peritoneum.

or serosal surface; fibrous or sclerosing forms, which are more plaquelike, have occasionally been reported as well. The tumor frequently is associated with a milky or blood-tinged effusion, and in sclerosing tumors in which adhesions occasionally occur, the lesion might resemble chronic granulomatous peritonitis. Ascites as the result of blocked lymphatics usually is present with peritoneal tumors.

Mesotheliomas of the pleura, pericardium, or peritoneum may assume a variety of histologic patterns. However, they usually appear predominantly papillary, and resemble adenocarcinoma, or as spindle cells resembling fibrosarcoma.

The most common tumor is a solid mass made up of single layers of dark, plump cuboidal, columnar, or rounded epithelioid neoplastic mesothelial cells with a distinct border and abundant pink cytoplasm, over a proliferating fibrocellular stroma. Mitotic figures are typically not numerous. Some tumors have atypical cells with marked anisokaryosis and prominent nucleoli, or large multinucleate cells. The mesothelial cells form loops and festoons in a papillary pattern, or line cystic spaces and tubular structures. There may be a mucinous matrix in this acinar pattern. These mesotheliomas, which resemble adenocarcinoma, can mimic implantation of a true carcinoma so completely that adequate differentiation may rest on very careful examination for, and exclusion of, a primary focus of carcinoma. Special stains to eliminate secretory granules, characteristic of some adenocarcinomas, or electron-microscopic examination, may be required to identify the cell type.

Mesotheliomas that are predominantly fibrous may resemble fibrosarcomas. In the sclerosing forms there may be a thick fibrous serosa with adhesions, and large anaplastic cuboidal cells may be found in clusters or lining cystic spaces within the fibrous tissue.

Lipomas are the most frequently encountered tumors of the peritoneal interstitium. These benign tumors are well known in horses, in which they usually originate in the mesenteries. They may reach enormous size, but their significance is that they tend to become pedunculated and may cause acute strangulation obstruction when the pedicle winds about a loop of intestine. In cut section, the core of some of these tumors is friable and necrotic, probably from ischemia; only the superficial centimeter or so remains viable, perhaps nourished by diffusion from the peritoneal environment (Fig. 4.14). In the dog, lipomas arise in the omentum, rather than the mesenteries, and they settle on the abdominal floor. They may become very large, but tend not to be pedunculated. They do not, therefore, cause acute distress and, although they may appear malignant histologically, metastases are unusual. They, too, may develop a pseudocapsule and central areas of necrosis.

Other tumors of the subserosal connective tissues, including myxomas, fibromas, and their malignant counterparts, are rare, although fibrosarcomas are observed in dogs, and an omental fibrosarcoma has been reported in a horse. Neurofibromatosis of cattle may involve the abdominal nerves and plexuses, and ganglioneuromas are also observed in this species. Extramedullary pheochromocytomas are observed in cattle and dogs, and nonchromaffin paragangliomas occur in dogs, the latter usually in association with similar tumors elsewhere.

Secondary tumors of the peritoneum are not common, but may occur in any abdominal neoplasia. These arise mainly by direct implantation, rather than by lymphogenous or hematogenous metastasis. Carcinomas are much more common than sarcomas. Secondary carcinomas must be differentiated from mesothelioma. They may be very scirrhous and, when accompanied by ascites, may resemble chronic peritonitis; a relative or complete absence of adhesions is often a helpful distinguishing feature at autopsy. There are obviously many possibilities for the origin of secondary tumors; several common types are listed.

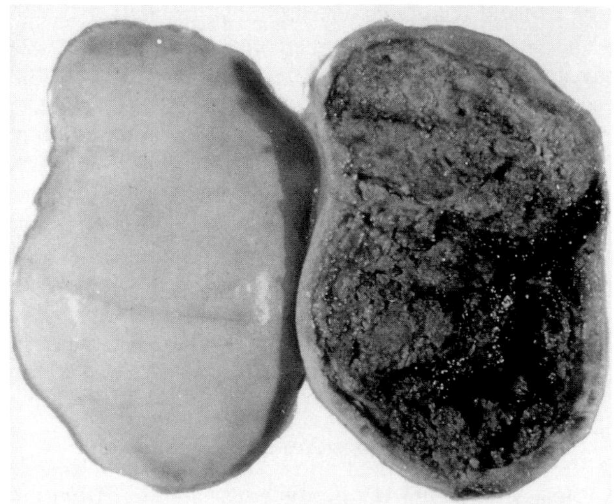

Fig. 4.14 Pedunculate lipoma (transected) from mesentery. Horse. Note necrotic core and thin capsule of viable tissue.

Ovarian carcinomas have already been mentioned as a cause of ascites, and in the differential diagnosis of mesothelioma. Implants of ovarian carcinoma tend to be papillary. Bile duct carcinomas and pancreatic adenocarcinomas tend to be scirrhous, as do intestinal adenocarcinomas in cattle and sheep. Squamous cell carcinomas of the equine stomach form rather discrete implants, which may resemble nodules of mesothelioma, or granulomas; they may be differentiated enough to be recognizably keratinized on gross inspection. Transitional cell tumors developing in cattle with enzootic hematuria implant locally on the pelvic surfaces, and rectal adenocarcinoma in dogs also tends to confine its implants to the pelvic peritoneum. Malignant melanomas of perineal origin in horses produce flattish black smudges on the peritoneum, or in the mesenteries, as may occasional metastatic melanomas in dogs.

Bibliography

Ackerman, L. J., and Silver, J. N. Abdominal liposarcoma in a dog. *Mod Vet Pract* **65:** 470, 1984.

Dubielzig, R. R. Sclerosing mesothelioma in five dogs. *J Am Anim Hosp Assoc* **15:** 745–748, 1979.

Forbes, D. C., and Matthews, B. R. Abdominal mesothelioma in a dog. *Can Vet J* **32:** 176–177, 1991.

Glickman, L. T. *et al.* Mesothelioma in pet dogs associated with exposure of their owners to asbestos. *Environ Res* **32:** 305–313, 1983.

Harbison, M. L., and Godleski, J. J. Malignant mesothelioma in urban dogs. *Vet Pathol* **20:** 531–540, 1983.

Harvey, K. A. *et al.* Omental fibrosarcoma in a horse. *J Am Vet Med Assoc* **191:** 335–336, 1987.

Hashimoto, N., Oda, T., and Kadota, K. An ultrastructural study of malignant mesotheliomas in two cows. *Jpn J Vet Sci* **51:** 327–336, 1989.

Leder, J. A., Franco, D. A., and Langheinrich, K. A. Metastatic ovarian cystadenocarcinoma in a gilt. *Aust Vet J* **67:** 467, 1990.

Magnusson, R. A., and Veit, H. P. Mesothelioma in a calf. *J Am Vet Med Assoc* **191:** 233–234, 1987.

Raflo, C. P., and Nuernberger, S. P. Abdominal mesothelioma in a cat. *Vet Pathol* **15:** 781–783, 1978.

Ricketts, S. W., and Peace, C. K. A case of peritoneal mesothelioma in a thoroughbred mare. *Equine Vet J* **8:** 78–80, 1976.

Smith, D. A., and Hill, F. W. G. Metastatic malignant mesothelioma in a dog. *J Comp Pathol* **100:** 97–101, 1989.

Thrall, D. E., and Goldschmidt, M. H. Mesothelioma in the dog: Six case reports. *J Am Vet Radiol Soc* **19:** 107–115, 1978.

Trigo, F. J., Morrison, W. B., and Breeze, R. G. An ultrastructural study of canine mesothelioma. *J Comp Pathol* **91:** 531–539, 1981.

IX. Diseases of the Retroperitoneum

Problems in the retroperitoneum may originate in the stroma of the space itself, from organs in the space, or may extend from adjacent organs.

Retroperitonitis may arise from sepsis involving the pelvic or abdominal urogenital tract, or the mesenteric root; from penetrating wounds; and from migrating grass awns or other foreign bodies. Frequently, it will evolve to form a fluctuant abscess or draining fistula in the flank, based on the anatomic path of least resistance for advancing phlegmon in the soft tissue of the region, discussed earlier. The lesion is usually a poorly encapsulated sinus or abscess, with a wall of granulation tissue, and containing liquid pus. It may extend to involve adjacent vertebrae in periostitis or osteomyelitis. A foreign body may be encountered on exploration, or the lesion may be traced back to a primary septic focus in the abdomen, perhaps a renal or perirenal abscess; an ovarian stump with a remnant of unresorbed suture; or an abscess or pyogranuloma in the root of the mesentery. Usually, a mixed flora will be isolated. If *Actinomyces* spp. are implicated, there may be a frankly granulomatous lesion with sulfur granules in the abdomen or the flank.

Non-neoplastic retroperitoneal masses include hematomas, or accumulations of urine, following trauma to the caudal abdominal or pelvic area. Hemorrhage may dissect widely in this area, and the origin will usually be difficult to detect. Rupture of retroperitoneal hematomata may be fatal. Retroperitoneal hemorrhage in newborn calves is often an indication of fracture of the spinal column due to rotation during assisted calving. Renal and perirenal cysts, and pseudocysts or capsular cysts, may also be encountered, usually incidentally.

Neoplasms of the retroperitoneal space may be protean in type, but reflect the main organs and tissues of the region. They include lipomas, fibrosarcomas, lymphosarcomas, osteosarcomas, and nonchromaffin paragangliomas, as well as primary renal adenocarcinomas and adrenal tumors. Occasional highly malignant adenocarcinomas of obscure histogenesis and origin occur in the dorsal retroperitoneum in dogs.

Tumors metastatic to the region include those commonly involving the sublumbar lymph nodes, such as lymphosarcoma, and transitional cell, prostatic, colonic, perianal gland, and anal gland malignancies. Metastatic involvement of the sublumbar chain of lymph nodes frequently stimulates periosteal reaction on the ventral aspect of adjacent vertebral bodies. Occasionally, tumors metastatic to the region will lyse vertebral bodies or transverse processes, and they may occasionally gain the spinal canal. Lytic and osteophytic reactions must be distinguished from the effects of osteomyelitis.

Bibliography

Johnston, D. E., and Christie, B. A. The retroperitoneum in dogs: Retroperitoneal infections. *Compend Cont Ed Pract Vet* **12:** 1035–1045, 1990.

Roush, J. K., Bjorling, D. E., and Lord, P. Diseases of the retroperitoneal space in the dog and cat. *J Am Anim Hosp Assoc* **26:** 47–54, 1990.

ACKNOWLEDGMENTS

The assistance of Edward Eaton, Carol Lee Ernst, Judy Henry, and Gary Smith in the preparation of the manuscript and illustrations is gratefully acknowledged. Grant Maxie and A. van Dreumel are thanked for critically reviewing the text.

CHAPTER 5 The Urinary System

M. GRANT MAXIE
Ontario Ministry of Agriculture and Food, Canada

With a contribution by
John F. Prescott
Ontario Veterinary College, Canada

THE KIDNEY

I. General Considerations

The kidney is the central organ involved in the maintenance of a constant extracellular environment in the body. The vital homeostatic functions performed by the kidney include excretion of waste products, maintenance of normal concentrations of salt and water in the body, regulation of acid–base balance, and production of a variety of hormones (erythropoietin, renin, prostaglandins), including metabolism of vitamin D to its active form, 1,25-dihydroxycholecalciferol. The essential requirements for normal renal function are adequate perfusion with blood (pressure greater than 60 mm Hg), adequate functional renal tissue, and normal elimination of urine from the urinary tract.

Failure of the urinary mechanism occurs if there is inadequate perfusion (**prerenal failure**), inadequate processing (**renal failure**), or inadequate discharge (**postrenal failure**). The outcome so far as the composition of body fluids is concerned is always approximately the same; there is imbalance of salt and water, and of acids and bases, and there is retention of wastes. The most commonly used index of failure is the amount of urea retained. Urea itself is rather harmless, but if other urinary functions are sufficiently disturbed, a fairly consistent set of clinical signs emerges, and the syndrome is called **uremia.**

Water and salt are, quantitatively and in an evolutionary sense, the most important constituents of body fluids. The assumption during evolution of a terrestrial existence and homeothermy by mammals imposed a need to conserve water and salt and simultaneously excrete large quantities of metabolites. Homeothermy, with sustained high body temperatures, imposed a sustained high metabolic rate, a need for control of the peripheral circulation, and structural modifications to the integument. Carbon dioxide is very soluble in water, and highly diffusible, and responsibility for its excretion has been transferred from the integument of aquatic and amphibian ancestors to the respiratory system of mammals; as the end product of fat and carbohydrate metabolism, carbon dioxide presents no problem of elimination to the renal excretory mechanism. Nitrogenous wastes, and a multitude of other organic compounds and inorganic substances, impose a substantial load on the renal mechanism. Mammals excrete urea which is highly soluble, diffusible, and osmotically active; excretion of wastes and conservation of water in mammals require concentrating mechanisms capable of raising the osmotic pressure of urine above that of blood. The extracellular fluid and plasma of the body are dialyzed through the kidney many times in a day, producing copious amounts of primary urine, of which almost all is reabsorbed. Although this system effectively rids the body of wastes, it requires a large expenditure of energy and a dependable renal blood supply.

Renal blood flow is normally high, as much as 25% of the cardiac output. The kidneys are not given to reactive hyperemia, although blood flow may be increased by the action of pyrogens in febrile states. Pathologists are concerned particularly with the causes and consequences of reduced renal perfusion. Peripheral and splanchnic blood flow may be sacrificed in the event of crisis, but renal blood flow is diminished only in order to preserve circulation to the prime priorities of cardiac output, the heart and the brain. Renal oxygen consumption, relatively small in relation to renal blood flow, is high relative to that of other tissues and is equal to about 10% of whole body consumption. Most of the oxygen consumed by the kidney is expended in the interests of resorption of essential solutes, a predominantly cortical function, and the consequences of reduced perfusion are largely borne by the cortex.

A unique feature of renal blood flow is that it varies little over a wide range of arterial pressures, thus ensuring a stable glomerular filtration rate (GFR). The kidneys possess intrinsic mechanisms by which they vary their vascular resistance in order to maintain constant glomerular filtration. Renal blood flow, on which the function of nephrons depends, is normally directed predominantly toward the outer cortical nephrons rather than to the inner cortical, or juxtamedullary nephrons, but may be redistributed between the two areas. Reduction in perfusion is a common occurrence in the kidney, affects primarily the cortex, and may lead to atrophy of tubular epithelium and tubular dilation, to necrosis of tubular epithelium, or to more or less extensive necrosis of the renal cortex. Blood flow to juxtamedullary nephrons is maintained more effectively than is flow to outer cortical nephrons, and blood may be directed from the outer cortex to the inner cortex under conditions of reduced renal blood flow. Preservation of blood flow to juxtamedullary nephrons serves to maintain function of the nephrons that are able to conserve water, and hence aid in maintaining circulating blood volume, and that are able to concentrate urine, and hence to eliminate waste products economically.

The glomerulus produces ultrafiltrate as the net result of the difference between the high systemic blood hydrostatic pressure and the low proximal tubular hydrostatic pressure. Urinary ultrafiltrate is isosmotic with plasma, and there is essentially zero colloid osmotic pressure in ultrafiltrate to favor diffusion. The glomerular basement membrane is semipermeable, and dissolved substances and particles in suspension move across the glomerular capillaries at rates determined by size, shape, and electrical charge. Malfunction of the glomerulus may be due to inadequate glomerular blood flow and/or structural alterations which decrease or increase its permeability. The outcome of glomerular injury is influenced by the limited capacity in the glomerulus for disposal of deposits, the capillary obstruction which results from swelling of endothelial and mesangial cells, the production of basement-membrane-like material by injured mesangial cells, and permeability changes in basement membranes.

The principal function of the kidney is the regulation of salt and water balance; this requires a system of monitors and feedbacks in order to achieve fine regulation. The renin–angiotensin system regulates sodium balance, and the hypothalamus and antidiuretic hormone control osmotic and volume regulation. The structural basis of the renin–angiotensin system is provided by the juxtaglomerular apparatus; to maintain **glomerulotubular balance,** the GFR is adjusted locally and continually to changes in the chloride concentration of tubular fluid. Generally, and over the longer term, the renin–angiotensin system stimulates the adrenal glands to produce aldosterone to assist in the retention of sodium and therefore of water.

The formation of primary urine requires that substances from plasma must pass freely across the glomerular membrane and into the tubules. Once within the tubules, the substances are, in a strict sense, outside the body. Many of the filtered substances are retrieved by a system of selective reabsorption that requires special machinery and energy. The function may be defective, allowing essential substances to be wasted in the urine. This occurs when enzymes are genetically deficient, or cortical epithelial cells are injured, or, because plasma levels of filterable substances are unusually high or the glomerulus is unusually permeable, the quantity of the material to be reabsorbed exceeds the transport capacity of the epithelial cells. Myriad tubular functions are carried out sequentially, and the structure of the tubule varies along its length corresponding to the function to be performed; at least 12 functionally and anatomically distinct segments are described.

Terrestrial mammals have a need to conserve water while eliminating high loads of waste, and a need therefore to concentrate urine above the tonicity of plasma. This function is provided by the loop of Henle; juxtamedullary nephrons have long loops, and cortical nephrons have short loops. Some species have predominantly long loops and some, predominantly short loops; those animals with a preponderance of long loops have greater concentrating ability. Although the deep or juxtamedullary nephrons are the first to develop and are active while centrifugal development of the rest of the cortex is underway, neonatal nephrons have immature functional capacity and a relative inability to conserve sodium. Neonatal pigs, in particular, are thus very susceptible to dehydration. In calves, in contrast to most other neonates, renal functional capacity approaches that of adult cattle within 2–3 days of birth.

According to the **intact nephron** or adaptive nephron hypothesis, nephron function is an all-or-none phenomenon. In progressive renal disease, the remaining nephrons respond by hyperplasia and hypertrophy, since new nephrons cannot be formed following renal maturation. Glomerular filtration and tubular function then increase concomitantly, and glomerulotubular balance and homeostasis are maintained. All of the renal components are interdependent, and if one component is irreversibly damaged, function of the other components is impaired: glomerular disease can cause decreased peritubular perfusion and tubular atrophy; tubulointerstitial disease can cause glomerular obsolescence. There is a tendency for all forms of chronic renal disease to destroy all four components of the kidney, resulting in chronic renal failure and shrunken scarred **end-stage kidneys;** differentiation of the initiating cause may be impossible. Interstitial inflammation and fibrosis may be primary events, but they also commonly accompany primary diseases of the glomeruli and tubules. Chronic generalized renal disease in dogs frequently was ascribed in the past to interstitial nephritis, and leptospirosis was espoused as the most common cause. Because of vaccination, canine leptospirosis is no longer predominant, and chronic renal disease in dogs as it now occurs is the end result of a wide variety of causes.

A. Anatomy

The renal collecting system is derived from the ureteral bud (metanephric duct), a diverticulum of the mesonephric (wolffian) duct, and consists of the ureter, pelvis, calyces, and collecting ducts. Nephrons develop from the metanephric blastema and attach to the growing ends (ampullae) of the collecting system. The uriniferous tubule consists of the nephron and the collecting tubule. The renal calyces are the cup-shaped recesses of the pelvis, which enclose conical masses of medulla pyramids. The apex of a pyramid is referred to as a papilla, and its tip is fenestrated by collecting ducts (area cribrosa). The fornix is the uppermost blind end of a calyx or pelvis.

The kidneys of domestic animals can be classified as **unipyramidal** (unilobar) or **multipyramidal** (multilobar). Cats, dogs, small ruminants, and horses have unipyramidal kidneys. In cats, one lobe is present, and papillary ducts open into a calyx on a single renal papilla. In dogs, small ruminants, and horses, there is complete or partial fusion of several lobes and a single crestlike papilla (renal crest). Pigs have multipyramidal kidneys in which there are several distinct renal lobes, pyramids, and their respective papillae. Extensions of renal cortex between the pyramids are known as the renal columns of Bertin. Simple papillae occur in central pyramids, and compound papillae in pyramids at the renal poles; this is of pathogenetic significance because compound papillae are more susceptible to ascending infection. The kidneys of cattle are also multipyramidal, but have distinct external lobation, with each lobe having one pyramid. The renal calyces of cattle join directly to form the ureter without forming a pelvis. Note the difference between a renal lobe and a renal lobule. A renal lobule consists of a medullary ray and its associated nephrons. Medullary rays are seen histologically as lighter-staining linear areas in the cortex, and consist of collecting tubules, thick ascending limbs, and the terminal straight portions of the proximal tubules. Interlobular arteries course between lobules.

On sagittal section of a kidney, subdivisions of cortex and medulla may be distinguished, particularly in dogs and sheep. The cortex has a darker outer zone, and a paler inner zone, which in mature dogs often has prominent pale streaks due to the presence of fat in collecting ducts. Outer and inner zones may be seen in the medulla of canine kidneys, and the outer zone may be further subdivided into outer and inner bands (stripes), due to the presence of the thick segments of the descending and ascending limbs of the loop of Henle, respectively. The inner zone of the medulla (papilla) contains the thin segments of the loop of Henle (Fig. 5.1A). Mucous glands are large and prominent in the medulla of equine kidneys, and mucus and crystals are normally present in the equine renal pelvis.

The functional unit of the kidney is the **nephron,** which

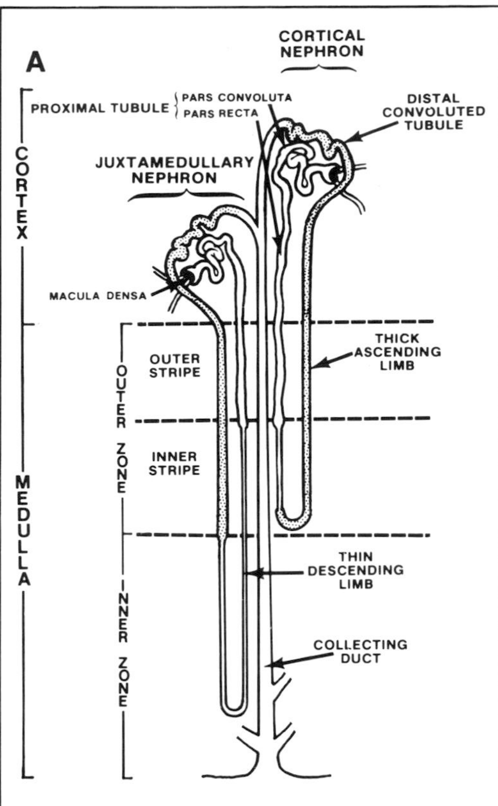

Fig. 5.1A Diagram showing components of cortical and juxtamedullary nephrons and their location in zones of the kidney.

consists of the renal corpuscle, proximal tubule, loop of Henle, and distal tubule. The glomerulus and Bowman's capsule compose the renal corpuscle. The following approximate numbers of nephrons are present in each kidney: human, 1,000,000; dog, 400,000; cat, 200,000. The number of nephrons is fixed at birth in most mammals, although nephrogenesis may continue for several weeks after birth in animals with a short gestation period such as dogs, cats, and pigs.

Renal diseases may primarily affect one of four subdivisions of the kidney, namely blood vessels, glomeruli, tubules, and interstitium.

1. Vascular Supply

Although the kidneys constitute only about 0.5% of body weight, they receive 20–25% of cardiac output. In multilobed kidneys, the renal artery divides in the pelvic region to form interlobar arteries that run in the renal columns between lobes up to the corticomedullary junction, where they branch to form arcuate arteries. These arteries run along the corticomedullary junction parallel to the capsule and terminate by radiating interlobular arteries into the cortex. Glomerular afferent arterioles are given off by the interlobular arteries, and give rise to several lobules of capillary loops within the glomerulus. The capillaries later rejoin to form the glomerular efferent arteriole and then divide again to form a peritubular capillary plexus. The efferent arterioles of the juxtamedullary nephrons branch to form descending vasa recta (straight vessels), which enter the medulla. The ascending vasa recta reform from the medullary capillary plexus and form a countercurrent exchange system with their closely associated descending vasa recta. The glomerular capillary tufts are perfused at high pressure, which favors filtration; the capillary bed rising from the efferent arterioles is low pressure, favoring reabsorption.

Because the renal artery and its branches are end-arteries, occlusion of any branch leads to infarction. Interference with glomerular capillary flow markedly alters peritubular blood flow, especially in the medulla. The medulla is particularly sensitive to ischemia because of its relative avascularity and the low hematocrit in medullary capillaries.

Intrarenal blood flow is finely controlled by complex mechanisms, which are still being elucidated. The **juxtaglomerular apparatus** consists of the afferent and efferent arterioles adjacent to their respective glomerulus, the macula densa of the corresponding distal convoluted tubule, and a collection of cells (lacis or nongranular cells) at the glomerular hilus between the arterioles. Myoepithelial cells (juxtaglomerular or granular cells) of the afferent arteriole wall contain renin. When afferent arteriolar blood pressure, and hence GFR, decreases, an intrinsic afferent arteriolar myogenic response and **tubuloglomerular feedback** mechanisms are activated; the tubular fluid chloride concentration is decreased at the macula densa, causing dilation of the afferent arteriole and constriction of the efferent arteriole to increase the GFR, as follows. Renin is released and this proteolytic enzyme cleaves angiotensinogen, an $(\text{alpha})_2$ globulin of plasma, to form angiotensin I. Angiotensin I is subsequently cleaved by angiotensin I-converting enzyme to form angiotensin II, one of the most potent pressor agents known, and angiotensin III. Angiotensin III and, to a lesser extent, angiotensin II also initiate adrenocortical synthesis of aldosterone, which aids, over the longer term, in increasing afferent arteriolar perfusion by stimulating resorption of sodium from the distal convoluted tubules and collecting ducts, resulting in water retention and expansion of the extracellular fluid volume. Both angiotensin II and III induce prostaglandin synthesis. Angiotensin II also stimulates the secretion of antidiuretic hormone (ADH, vasopressin). These events, in concert with angiotensin-mediated efferent arteriolar constriction, are sensed by the macula densa, and the tubuloglomerular feedback mechanism previously detailed is reversed, leading to afferent arteriolar constriction, decreased glomerular filtration rate, and hence restoration of **glomerulotubular balance.** These mechanisms of blood pressure sensing and tubuloglomerular feedback result in maintenance of glomerular filtration pressure within fine limits over a broad range of systemic arterial blood pressure. The renin system is intimately interrelated with adenosine, atrial natriuretic factor, endothelin, vasopressin, the renal kallikrein–kinin system, renal sympathetic nerves, and prostaglandins to autoregulate intrarenal blood flow and modulate tubular salt and water transport. The contribution of these various factors to control of renal blood flow varies between normal and abnormal states; for example, prostaglandins are apparently of little significance in maintaining intrarenal blood flow under normal circumstances, but become important during periods of hypotension.

The renal venous system begins with formation of venules from the peritubular vasa recta, and then closely parallels the arterial system. Veins in the outer cortex drain into stellate veins, which in cats are present on the capsular surface and are prominent, and thence into interlobular veins. Veins within the kidney have very thin walls and are susceptible to compression.

Lymphatics occur in the renal cortex and medulla. One set of lymphatics drains the cortical and medullary interstitium and follows the pattern of the vascular system; another set of lymphatics drains the capsular area. Lymphatic flow increases after urinary obstruction and in interstitial disease.

2. *Glomerulus*

The glomerulus is a vascular–epithelial structure designed for the ultrafiltration of plasma. It develops embryologically by the invagination of a capillary-rich mesenchymal mass into the Bowman's space, an epithelium-lined sac. The visceral epithelium covers the glomerular capillaries to become an essential part of the filtration membrane, and the parietal epithelium, or Bowman's capsule, lines the urinary space which receives glomerular ultrafiltrate. The arterioles enter and leave the glomerulus at the vascular pole, and urine enters the proximal tubule at the urinary pole of the glomerulus. The glomerular filtration membrane consists of three layers: capillary endothelium containing fenestrae of 50–100 nm diameter; glomerular basement membrane (GBM), which is 100–300 nm thick and consists of a central electron-dense lamina densa and peripheral electron-lucent layers, the lamina rara interna and externa; and visceral epithelial cells (podocytes). The podocytes have complex interdigitating trabeculae whose foot processes (pedicels) are embedded in the lamina rara externa of the GBM. The pedicels are separated by 25–50 nm wide filtration slits, which are bridged by thin slit diaphragms with pores of 6–9 nm diameter. Glomerular basement membrane is produced continuously by the podocytes, and is continuous below these cells, but does not completely encircle the glomerular capillaries; endothelial cells and mesangium are in direct contact.

A large volume of glomerular ultrafiltrate is formed as a product of the high hydrostatic pressure of arteriolar blood, and the selective permeability of the filtration membrane. The entire plasma volume is filtered about 100 times per day. The glomerulus is highly permeable to water and small solutes, but virtually excludes albumin (molecular weight ~70,000, radius 3.6 nm) and higher molecular weight plasma proteins from the filtrate. The GBM is a size-dependent barrier to filtration, prohibiting passage of particles with radius greater than 3.5 nm. The filtration membrane also excludes particles from filtration on the basis of charge. Thus, anionic molecules such as albumin are repelled by virtue of the presence of negatively charged sialoglycoproteins in the lamina rara interna and externa and the negatively charged cell coats of the endothelial and epithelial cells. Obviously then, changes in porosity or charge of the filtration membrane alter glomerular permeability and can lead to proteinuria, a hallmark of glomerular damage. A small amount of albumin normally passes through the filter but is rapidly resorbed in the proximal tubules. The glomeruli of neonates are permeable to colostral protein for a few days.

The **mesangium** is the central region of the glomerulus, which forms a supporting framework about which the glomerular capillaries ramify. The mesangial matrix is basement-membrane-like periodic acid–Schiff (PAS)-positive glycoprotein, and the mesangial cells are phagocytic, contractile cells, which are derived from vascular smooth muscle cells. These cells function in phagocytic removal of deposited macromolecules, removal of GBM, and may modulate intraglomerular blood flow; mesangial cells both respond to and produce a variety of cytokines. Mesangial cell hyperplasia and increased mesangial matrix (mesangial sclerosis) are common changes in glomerular disease.

3. Tubules

The kidney functions by producing a large volume of protein-free glomerular filtrate from which are resorbed the constituents that the body needs. Thus, about 99% of the sodium chloride and water filtered are resorbed. This system effectively rids the body of wastes, which are filtered by the glomeruli and not resorbed by the tubules. Structure of a tubule segment is correlated with its function. Thus, cells of the proximal convoluted tubule have a well-developed brush border and numerous mitochondria. Energy for the sodium pump in this actively resorptive area is provided by mitochondrial oxidative phosphorylation; this area is, therefore, especially vulnerable to ischemia. Also, toxins are frequently resorbed by or secreted by the proximal tubule, causing chemical injury.

About 90% of the hydrogen ion excretion by the kidney occurs in the proximal tubule. The proximal tubule actively resorbs large quantities of sodium and chloride, and water passively follows; hence, 60–80% of the glomerular ultrafiltrate which enters the proximal tubule is resorbed isotonically. Tubules and peritubular capillaries are in close apposition to allow rapid removal of resorbed sodium chloride and water. Sodium is cotransported with glucose and amino acids. Hydrogen ions are accompanied by sodium bicarbonate as counterion. Proximal tubules are not responsive to aldosterone or vasopressin. In addition to salt and water, proximal tubules resorb glucose, amino acids, calcium, phosphate, uric acid, proteins, and potassium. Many substances, e.g., glucose, amino acids, and water-soluble vitamins, are threshold substances, which are almost completely resorbed until a certain concentration is reached in the glomerular filtrate, at which concentration the transport maximum is exceeded, and the substance appears in the urine. Overloading of the resorptive capacity of the proximal tubules in conditions such as diabetes mellitus also overwhelms the resorptive capacity of distal tubules and leads to **osmotic diuresis.** Interference with the production, release, or action of ADH on the distal nephron and collecting ducts, as occurs in pituitary or renal diabetes insipidus, results in obligatory **water diuresis** and excretion of hypo-osmotic urine and hence polyuria. Proximal tubules secrete hydrogen ions, organic acids, *p*-aminohippurate, penicillin, and some iodinated radioopaque materials.

The long loops of Henle of the juxtamedullary nephrons penetrate deep into the medulla and assist in making the renal medulla the only hypertonic tissue in the body. Urine-concentrating ability is directly proportional to the length of the loop of Henle; desert-dwelling rodents have very long loops of Henle, whereas baby pigs have short loops and are thus very susceptible to dehydration. The loops of Henle serve as countercurrent multipliers and the capillaries as simple countercurrent exchangers, with the flow in each occurring in opposite directions. The source of the solute gradient that becomes greater toward the tip at the papilla is the loop of Henle (active process). The gradient is preserved by the vasa recta countercurrent exchanger (passive process). Sodium chloride is pumped (chloride active, sodium passive) from the ascending limb of the loop of Henle into the interstitium, in turn drawing water from the descending limb, and progressively increasing the solute concentration in the descending limb. The ascending limb is impermeable to water; thus, the tubular fluid becomes dilute and may be hypotonic. More salt may be resorbed from the collecting ducts, further diluting the fluid. Water diuresis occurs when a state of water excess exists and ADH is not released from the neurohypophysis. If antidiuresis is required, ADH is released and renders the epithelium of the collecting tubule highly permeable to water, reducing the volume of tubular fluid entering the hypertonic medulla. This remaining fluid is then concentrated to three to four times the blood osmolality (280 mOsm/l) during passage to the tip of the papilla. The water resorbed in the medulla is passively transported into the ascending vasa recta and removed. The solute concentration of the medulla is about one half due to sodium, and one half due to urea. During antidiuresis, ADH renders the cortical portions of the collecting ducts permeable to water but not urea, thus increasing the urea concentration of the luminal fluid. Antidiuretic hormone increases the permeability of the medullary portions of the collecting ducts to urea and water; urea then diffuses from collecting tubule to interstitium until luminal urine and interstitial concentrations are equal. Tubules are not functionally mature in the kidneys of most neonates; thus, they cannot generate hypotonic urine and hence conserve solute in the medulla; inability to produce a medullary solute gradient limits their capacity to concentrate urine.

It is generally believed that there is little if any further modification of urine once it leaves the tip of the papilla. However, urea may be conserved by moving across the renal papillary epithelium from the pelvic urine. Either osmotic diuresis or water diuresis may result in **medullary solute washout** due to increased tubular flow rates and hence decreased efficiency of the countercurrent multiplier, the loop of Henle. The quantities of urea and sodium chloride resorbed are decreased due to decreased tubular fluid transit time; hence, the medullary solute gradient decreases as does urine concentrating ability. The same mechanism is operative in chronic renal disease, in which there are high tubular flow rates in the small number of hypertrophic tubules present.

Although body buffers and pulmonary control of carbon dioxide excretion are the first line of defense in protecting the pH of the extracellular fluids, it is the action of the kidneys that ultimately corrects acid–base balance. The kidneys excrete the excess alkali or acid responsible for the disturbance; thus, the kidneys correct metabolic alkalosis by excreting an alkaline urine containing the excess bicarbonate. The kidneys correct metabolic acidosis by increasing resorption of filtered bicarbonate, excreting titratable acids (secrete hydrogen ions), and by producing ammonia.

4. Interstitium

The interstitium normally contains peritubular capillaries and a few fibroblasts, and interstitial tissue is usually obvious only around interlobar, arcuate, and interlobular arteries. Expansion of the cortical interstitium is abnormal, and may occur as a result of edema, cellular infiltration, or fibrosis. The glycosaminoglycan content of the medullary interstitium increases with age and ischemia. Specialized interstitial cells produce prostaglandins, particularly prostaglandin E_2 (PGE_2) and $PGF_{2\alpha}$.

B. Examination of the Kidneys

1. Gross Examination

The systematic gross inspection of a kidney entails observation of its size, shape, color, and consistency. The kidneys are usually equal in size and about three vertebrae long. Renal enlargement may occur due to addition of blood, edema fluid, fat, urine in the pelvis or tubules, or swollen or hypertrophic nephrons. Acute inflammation causes renal enlargement due to addition of fluid and cells, whereas chronic inflammation causes scarring and loss of substance. The kidneys are usually bean- or horseshoe-shaped, although the bovine kidney is lobated externally. Focal lesions, such as those caused by infarction or pyelonephritis, may markedly distort the renal outlines, whereas more generalized diseases such as glomerulonephritis do not. The normal renal color is brown-red, except in mature cats, in which the cortices are yellow due to their high fat content. The fat content in cats is apparently hormonally determined; pregnant females and sexually inactive old males have the most fat, pseudopregnant females and castrated males have somewhat less, estrous females and sexually active males have moderate amounts, and anestrous females have little or no renal fat. Kidneys autolyze fairly rapidly after death, particularly in fat animals in a warm environment. Pulpy kidneys occur due to clostridial enterotoxemia in sheep, and may be difficult to distinguish from advanced autolysis.

The urinary system may be maintained intact during examination, or the kidneys may be removed from the carcass. The kidney should not be severed from the ureter until the absence of hydronephrosis has been established. Each kidney is cut in the sagittal plane, and the cut surface is examined. The normal cortex to medulla ratio in this plane is about 1:2 or 1:3. The cortex normally accounts for 80% of the renal mass, a fact which is better appreciated in a coronal, than in a sagittal, section. Diffuse diseases of the kidney usually respect the integrity of the medulla. Pyelonephritis is peripelvic with involvement of the medulla. A pale cut surface suggests the deposition of fat or acute early nephrosis; if the surface is pale and wet, there is edema and diffuse tubular dilation. Focal glomerular lesions do not cause glomerular prominence, but diffuse lesions, such as amyloidosis or diffuse glomerulitis, very often do. Removal of the renal capsule is essential for examination of the outer surface of the cortex. The capsule should strip easily and leave a smooth surface underneath. Tearing of the cortex may indicate fibrous adhesions of scarring, except in the horse, which normally has trabeculae attached to the capsule.

2. Histologic Examination

The kidney must be trimmed so that a section from capsule to papilla is available. The section should first be examined subgrossly for evidence of localized lesions, e.g., infarcts, abscesses, granulomas, pyelitis, mineralization, neoplasm, scars, or medullary loss. The section is then scanned at low power, and lesions are noted. Glomeruli are normally distributed randomly throughout the cortex with approximately three to four present per 40× field. Tubules should be tightly packed with little intervening connective tissue. Goat and sheep glomeruli are more cellular than those of most species. Horses have the largest glomeruli of domestic animals (about 200 μm diameter) and the only glomeruli that are visible grossly. Glomeruli in neonatal kidneys are small and hyperchromatic, particularly in the outer cortex. Nephrons may be seen in the S stage of development in the outer cortex of fetuses and in neonates with ongoing centrifugal renal development, such as dogs, cats, and pigs.

After scanning the section, the four basic elements of the kidney should be systematically examined, namely glomeruli, tubules, interstitial tissue, and blood vessels, to determine which structure is primarily injured.

Reactions of **glomeruli** to injury consist basically of combinations of cellular proliferation, leukocytic infiltration, thickening of the basement membrane, and hyalinization or sclerosis. Epithelium of the proximal tubule may be present in the glomerular urinary space in acute nephrosis or, more commonly, due to squeezing of the kidney during gross examination, especially if the kidney is autolytic; this change is termed infraglomerular reflux. Hyaline casts in tubules usually indicate increased glomerular permeability.

Tubules, especially proximal convoluted tubules, are the kidney elements most susceptible to ischemia and many toxins; degenerative changes are nonspecific in character and usually not diagnostic of the causative condition. The proximal convoluted tubule is the longest cortical part of the nephron; hence, proximal tubules compose the bulk of the cortex. Proximal tubules are more eosinophilic than the other tubules and have a brush border that may be seen in rapidly fixed preparations and which is well demonstrated by the PAS stain. Delay in fixation leads to sloughing of apical cytoplasm into tubular lumina (potocytosis). Cells of the distal tubule do not have a brush border, are flatter and more numerous in cross section of the tubule than are those of the proximal tubule, and the tubular lumina are larger.

Cortical tubules and capillaries are closely associated in order to facilitate fluid resorption, and **connective tissue** is normally visible in the cortex only near arteries. Hence cortical fibrosis is a significant finding, especially in an animal with renal insufficiency. Fibrosis may cause tubular obstruction and hence create retention cysts proximally.

Blood vessel changes may occur in various systemic states as in other organs, e.g., arteriolosclerosis in diabetes mellitus, or arteritis in malignant catarrhal fever.

The **renal medulla** should be closely examined because this is the site of urine concentration and the accumulation of protein casts. Tubules and ducts are normally separated by more connective tissue and ground substance in the medulla than in the cortex. Tubulointerstitial mineralization is common in renal disease and may be seen along with cortical mineralization in cases of hypercalcemic nephropathy. The papilla should be examined carefully for evidence of papillitis, an early lesion in pyelonephritis, for amyloid, and for papillary necrosis. Inclusion bodies are often prominent in pelvic transitional epithelium in canine distemper; distemper inclusions must be differentiated from nonspecific epithelial inclusions.

C. Renal Biopsy

Percutaneous needle biopsy of kidneys is useful to evaluate renal disease in domestic animals, and is of particular use in cases of acute glomerulonephritis, nephrotic syndrome, asymptomatic proteinuria, and acute renal failure. It is usually possible to obtain 10–20 glomeruli using a TruCut or a Franklin–Silverman biopsy needle in an adult dog; a minimum of approximately five glomeruli is necessary to characterize a glomerular lesion. The main hazard of the technique is arterial puncture and hemorrhage, which on rare occasions is fatal.

In addition to the usual hematoxylin and eosin staining of paraffin sections of kidney, several other techniques are useful:

1. The PAS stain, which stains glomerular and tubular basement membranes and mesangial matrix. Thin sections (3 μm) must be used. The PAS–methenamine–silver technique is an improvement of this stain.
2. Silver impregnation of basement membranes and of leptospires.
3. Other special stains for fibrin, amyloid, and lipids. Microscopic resolution of glomerular lesions is markedly improved by the use of 1-μm thick methacrylate-embedded sections.
4. Immunofluorescence studies for localization of immunoglobulins, complement, fibrin-related compounds, and foreign antigens, especially in glomeruli.
5. Immunoperoxidase techniques, for localization of a wide variety of antigens.
6. Electron microscopy, particularly for characterizing glomerular basement membrane deposits.

Bibliography

Abrahamson, D. R. Structure and development of the glomerular capillary wall and basement membrane. *Am J Physiol* **253:** F783–F794, 1987.

Bacallo, R., and Fine, L. G. Molecular events in the organization of renal tubular epithelium: From nephrogenesis to regeneration. *Am J Physiol* **257:** F913–F924, 1989.

Banks, W. J. Urinary System. *In* "Applied Veterinary Histology," 2nd Ed. Baltimore, Maryland, Williams & Wilkins, 1986.

Barnes, J. L., and Hevey, K. A. Glomerular mesangial cell migration. Response to platelet secretory products. *Am J Pathol* **138:** 859–866, 1991.

Barsanti, J. A., and Finco, D. R. Protein concentration in urine of normal dogs. *Am J Vet Res* **40:** 1583–1588, 1979.

Berliner, R. W. Mechanisms of urine concentration. *Kidney Int* **22:** 202–211, 1982.

Bernstein, L. M. "Renal Function and Renal Failure." Baltimore, Maryland, Williams & Wilkins, 1965.

Blantz, R. C. *et al.* Physiologic adaptations of the tubuloglomerular feedback system. *Kidney Int* **38:** 577–583, 1990.

Bovee, K. C. (ed.). "Canine Nephrology." Philadelphia, Pennsylvania, Harwal Publishing, 1984.

Brenner, B. M, and Rector, F. C., Jr. (eds.). "The Kidney," 3rd Ed. Philadelphia, Pennsylvania, W.B. Saunders, 1986.

Brown, E. M. Urinary system. *In* "Textbook of Veterinary Histology," 3rd Ed., H.-D. Dellman and E. M. Brown (eds.), 264–285, Philadelphia, Pennsylvania. Lea & Febiger, 1987.

Bulger, R. E., Cronin, R. E., and Dobyan, D. C. Survey of the morphology of the dog kidney. *Anat Rec* **194:** 41–66, 1979.

Burkholder, P. M. Functions and pathophysiology of the glomerular mesangium. *Lab Invest* **46:** 239–241, 1982.

Cheville, N. F. Kidney. *In* "Cell Pathology," 2nd Ed. 559–587 Ames, Iowa, Iowa State University Press, 1983.

Chou, S. Y., Porush, J. G., and Faubert, P. F. Renal medullary circulation: Hormonal control. *Kidney Int* **37:** 1–13, 1990.

Cotran, R. S., Kumar, V., and Robbins, S. L. The kidney. *In* "Robbins Pathologic Basis of Disease," 4th Ed. 1011–1081 Toronto, W.B. Saunders, 1989.

Cuttino, J. T., Jr. *et al.* Renal medullary lymphatics: Microradiographic, light, and electron microscopic studies in pigs. *Lymphology* **18:** 24–30, 1985.

Darmady, E. M., and MacIver, A. G. "Renal Pathology." London, Butterworths, 1980.

Eriksson, L. Renal corticopapillary concentration gradient in calves. *Acta Vet Scand* **13:** 197–205, 1972.

Ettinger, S. J.(ed.). "Textbook of Veterinary Internal Medicine," 3rd Ed. Toronto, 1893–2141 W.B. Saunders, 1983.

Fettman, M. J., and Allen, T. A. Developmental aspects of fluid and electrolyte metabolism and renal function in neonates. *Compend Cont Ed Pract Vet* **13:** 392–403, 1991.

Golden, A., and Maher, J. F. "The Kidney. Structure and Function in Disease," 2nd Ed. Baltimore, Maryland, Williams & Wilkins, 1977.

Heptinstall, R. H. "Pathology of the Kidney," 3rd Ed. Boston, Massachusetts. Little, Brown, 1983.

Hoffman, E. O., and Flores, T. R. High-resolution light microscopy in renal pathology. *Am J Clin Pathol* **76:** 636–643, 1981.

Jackson, E. K. Adenosine: A physiological brake on renin release. *Annu Rev Pharmacol Toxicol* **31:** 1–35, 1991.

Jamison, R. L., and Maffly, R. H. The urinary concentrating mechanism. *N Engl J Med* **295:** 1059–1067, 1976.

Jeraj, K., Osborne, C. A., and Stevens, J. B. Evaluation of renal biopsy in 197 dogs and cats. *J Am Vet Med Assoc* **181:** 367–369, 1982.

Johns, E. J. Role of angiotensin II and the sympathetic nervous system in the control of renal function. *J Hypertension* **7:** 695–701, 1989.

King, P. A., and Goldstein, L. Renal excretion of nitrogenous compounds in vertebrates. *Renal Physiol* **8:** 261–278, 1985.

Knepper, M., and Burg, M. Organization of nephron function. *Am J Physiol* **244:** F579–F589, 1983.

Leaf, A., and Cotran, R. "Renal Pathophysiology." New York, Oxford University Press, 1976.

Monaghan, M. L. M. A morphometric study of the bovine glomerulus. *Res Vet Sci* **40:** 271–272, 1986.

Nash, A. S. Renal biopsy in the normal cat: Development of a modified disposable biopsy needle. *Res Vet Sci* **40:** 246–251, 1986.

Schmidt-Nielsen, B. Excretion in mammals: Role of the renal pelvis in the modification of the urinary concentration and composition. *Fed Proc* **36:** 2493–2503, 1977.

Solez, K., Racusen, L. C., and Walker, W. G. Morphologic classification of renal disease and the realities of clinical nephrology: Do we need a new approach? *Acta Pathol Microbiol Immunol* (Suppl.) **4:** 11–16, 1988.

Sonnenberg, H. Mechanisms of release and renal action of atrial natriuretic factor. *Acta Physiol Scand* **139** (Suppl. 591): 80–87, 1990.

Stein, J. H. Regulation of the renal circulation. *Kidney Int* **38:** 571–576, 1990.

Striker, L. J. *et al.* Mesangial cell turnover: Effect of heparin and peptide growth factors. *Lab Invest* **64:** 446–456, 1991.

Takemura, N. *et al.* Atrial natriuretic peptide in the dog with mitral regurgitation. *Res Vet Sci* **50:** 86–88, 1991.

Zollinger, H. U., and Mihatsch, M. J. "Renal Pathology in Biopsy. Light, Electron, and Immunofluorescent Microscopy and Clinical Aspects." New York, Springer-Verlag, 1978.

D. Renal Disease, Renal Failure, and Uremia

Renal disease, which encompasses any deviation from normal renal structure or function, is usually subclinical. Severe renal disease may lead to renal failure, which is typically divided into acute and chronic forms. **Acute renal failure** is characterized by rapid onset of oliguria or anuria and azotemia; it may result from acute glomerular or interstitial injury or from acute tubular necrosis, and is often reversible. **Chronic renal failure** is the end result of many chronic renal diseases, is usually irreversible, and is characterized by prolonged duration of signs of uremia.

Clarification of terminology is in order. **Uremia** literally means urine in the blood. It is a clinical syndrome of renal failure, caused by biochemical disturbances, and is often accompanied by extrarenal lesions. **Azotemia,** which is sometimes incorrectly used synonymously, is a biochemical abnormality characterized by elevation of blood urea and creatinine, but without obligatory clinical manifestations of renal disease. Azotemia may be of renal or of extrarenal origin. **Prerenal azotemia** results from renal hypoperfusion, due to conditions such as congestive heart failure, shock, or hemorrhage. **Postrenal azotemia** occurs as a result of urinary obstruction.

The evolution from normal renal function to uremia over the course of progressive renal disease occurs through four overlapping stages. In the stage of **diminished renal reserve,** the GFR is about 50% of normal, and the animal is asymptomatic but is susceptible to additional renal insults. At the stage of **renal insufficiency,** GFR is 20–50% of normal, the animal is azotemic and becomes polyuric. In the stage of **renal failure,** GFR is only 20–25% of normal, the kidneys cannot maintain homeostasis, and uremia ensues, with its attendant gastrointestinal, cardiovascular, respiratory, and skeletal complications. In **end-stage renal disease,** GFR is less than 5% of normal, and the animal is in the terminal stages of uremia.

The biochemical disturbances of uremia reflect changes in the normal renal functions directed to regulation of fluid volume, regulation of electrolyte and acid–base balance, excretion of waste products, and metabolism of hormones. The clinical signs may be related to the renal disease itself, as with pyuria or renal pain; to the effects of reduced renal function, as with metabolic acidosis or dehydration; or to the compensatory responses to renal dysfunction, as with hyperparathyroidism.

Interference with **fluid volume regulation** may result in either dehydration or anasarca. Dehydration due to reduced renal concentrating ability may be related to lesions of the renal medulla and juxtamedullary nephrons. Vomition, and sometimes diarrhea, often exacerbates the dehydration. Anasarca, caused by reduction in the volume of glomerular filtrate in diffuse renal disease or by activation of the renin–angiotensin system, occurs infrequently. A more common cause of edema is hypoproteinemia due to loss of protein through injured glomeruli.

Disturbances in **electrolyte balance** include excesses and deficits of plasma sodium, potassium, and calcium. The handling of these substances by the kidney is complex, even in health; in disease it is often paradoxical and involves disordered tubular function, compensatory mechanisms, and endocrine imbalances. Excesses of plasma sodium, potassium, and calcium contribute to anasarca, cardiotoxicity, and hypercalcemic nephropathy respectively, whereas deficits may cause dehydration, muscular weakness, tetany, and osteodystrophy.

Several aspects of the uremic syndrome contribute to **acid–base imbalance** and metabolic acidosis. Compensatory hyperventilation may occur. The main factors leading to acidosis in uremia are a reduced capacity of distal and collecting tubules to produce ammonia, increased retention of hydrogen ions, and increased utilization, with impaired reabsorption, of bicarbonate ions. The term **uremic acidosis** encompasses simultaneous azotemia, anion retention, and acidosis; **renal tubular acidosis** (discussed under Specific Tubular Dysfunctions, Section V,D of The Kidney in this chapter) describes acidosis without retention of urea or anions.

Failure to excrete metabolic wastes, such as urea and creatinine, is the basis for tests of renal function; elevated levels indicate reduced glomerular filtration. However, azotemia occurs only after the loss of 75% or more of the GFR and is thus an insensitive indicator of renal disease. Tests of concentrating ability, such as the water deprivation test, are also of limited usefulness because concentrating ability is not affected until at least two thirds of the renal mass has become nonfunctional.

Disturbances in endocrine function are important causes of signs and lesions in uremic animals. Retention of phosphate, due to reduced glomerular filtration, causes depression of ionized calcium, deficiency of $1{,}25(OH)_2D_3$, increased synthesis and secretion of parathyroid hormone (PTH), and development of secondary hyperparathyroidism (see Renal Osteodystrophy, Volume 1, Chapter 1). Reduced renal catabolism of PTH, and end-organ resistance to PTH, may contribute to hyperparathyroidism. Most uremic animals have hyperphosphatemia, and normocalcemia or hypercalcemia. Sometimes hypercalcemia and hypophosphatemia occur in uremic dogs, possibly because of lack of feedback inhibition of PTH release. Similar changes occur in some uremic horses and may be related to decreased renal excretion of calcium.

Nonregenerative **anemia** in uremic animals is of uncertain pathogenesis and may result from a combination of factors, including decreased renal production of erythropoietin and inhibitory effects of increased serum PTH concentrations (see The Hematopoietic System, Volume 3, Chapter 2). A bleeding disorder associated with a platelet factor III abnormality may exacerbate the anemia. Renal metabolism of vitamin D is sometimes impaired in animals with diffuse renal disease, and may add an element of osteomalacia to renal osteodystrophy. Abnormal glucose metabolism occurs occasionally in uremic dogs, and may be a result of peripheral resistance to insulin-mediated uptake of glucose or to reduced breakdown of insulin by diseased kidneys.

As well as the metabolic disturbances attributable to particular biochemical derangements, there is in uremic animals a nonspecific effect of **uremic toxins.** This is probably due to the combined action of toxic products of protein catabolism and the various chemical and endocrine imbalances previously described. These toxins include phenols, indoles and guanidines, potassium, sulfate and phosphate ions, absorbed degradation products of intestinal bacteria, and PTH. They are thought to be responsible for the profound malaise which characterizes the uremic syndrome.

The cause of death in uremia probably varies from case to case. Metabolic acidosis, hyperkalemia, or hypocalcemia may be severe enough to be fatal.

Gross lesions in uremia are divisible into those that caused uremia and those that resulted from it. The former are usually intrarenal, but may not be in prerenal and postrenal azotemia. Lesions which are the result of uremia are mainly, but not exclusively, extrarenal.

Most forms of prerenal azotemia have a common basis of reduced renal blood flow and glomerular filtration. This occurs in a variety of circumstances, including severe dehydration, massive hemorrhage especially into the upper intestinal tract, congestive heart failure, and shock of any cause. Reduced renal flow in these conditions is part of an adaptational mechanism which diverts blood to vital organs such as brain and heart. When the diversion is severe or prolonged, intrarenal mechanisms which channel renal flow away from cortical nephrons to juxtamedullary nephrons may produce patchy or diffuse cortical ischemia and necrosis (see Renal Cortical Necrosis, Section III,D of The Kidney in this chapter). In such cases, if the animal survives, prerenal azotemia may be superseded by uremia of renal origin originating in cortical necrosis.

Postrenal azotemia is always due to obstruction to the outflow of urine, and hence is oliguric or anuric. The causes are those which, if intermittent or incomplete, may lead to hydronephrosis or, if sudden and complete, may lead to rupture or leakage of the lower urinary tract.

A form of extrarenal uremia, distinct from those mentioned, occurs in newborn animals, especially pigs, and is characterized by very high levels of blood urea. The kidneys of newborn pigs, dogs, and cats are functionally immature, and incapable of producing hypertonic urine. Normally this is of no consequence, because milk provides enough fluid to excrete, in hypotonic urine, the small amount of waste produced. However, when these newborn animals are anorectic, they lack both nutrients and fluid, and begin to catabolize tissue proteins and purines. Being unable to excrete the excess solute from protein and purine breakdown, their blood urea and uric acid reach very high levels. Since anorexia is usually associated with fever, vomition, or diarrhea, fluid loss is very rapid. In pigs, the excess solute is deposited in the inner medulla as streaks of light yellow urate precipitates (Fig. 5.1B), which disappear during histologic processing. Pigs apparently are unique among mammals in that they do not reabsorb urates from glomerular filtrate; this accounts for their concentration in the medulla. It is not clear whether baby pigs also have an immature liver which fails to convert uric acid to allantoin.

The **nonrenal lesions** of uremia occur inconstantly and

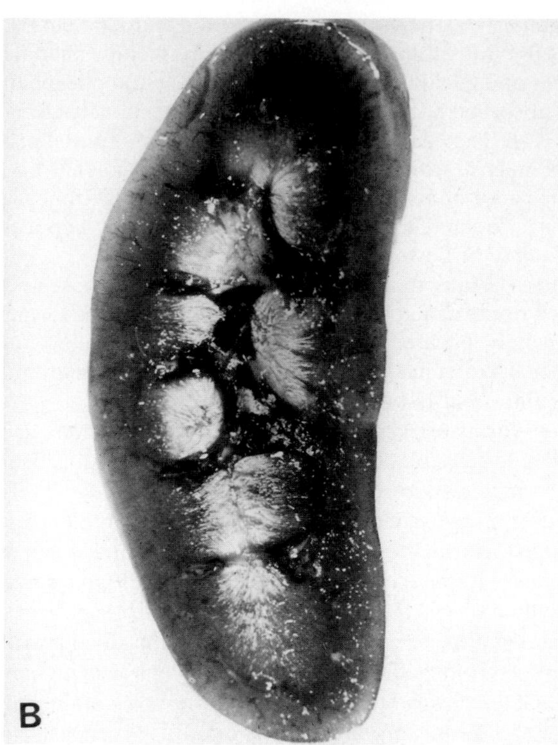

Fig. 5.1B Urate calculi in medulla and pelvis of dehydrated piglet. Some calculi were transferred to the cortical surface when the kidney was sliced.

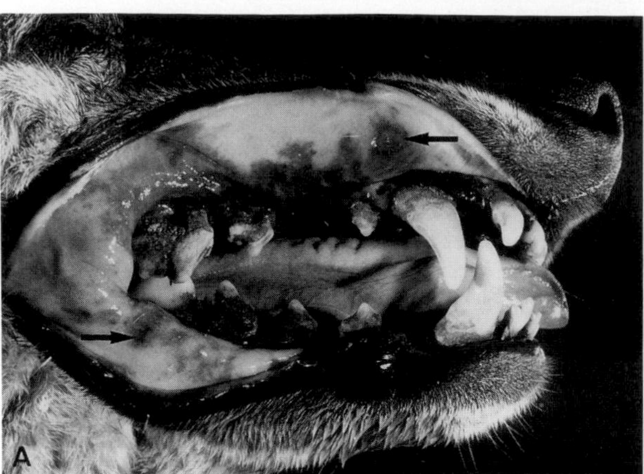

Fig. 5.2A Uremia. Dog. Ulcers of buccal mucosa (arrows).

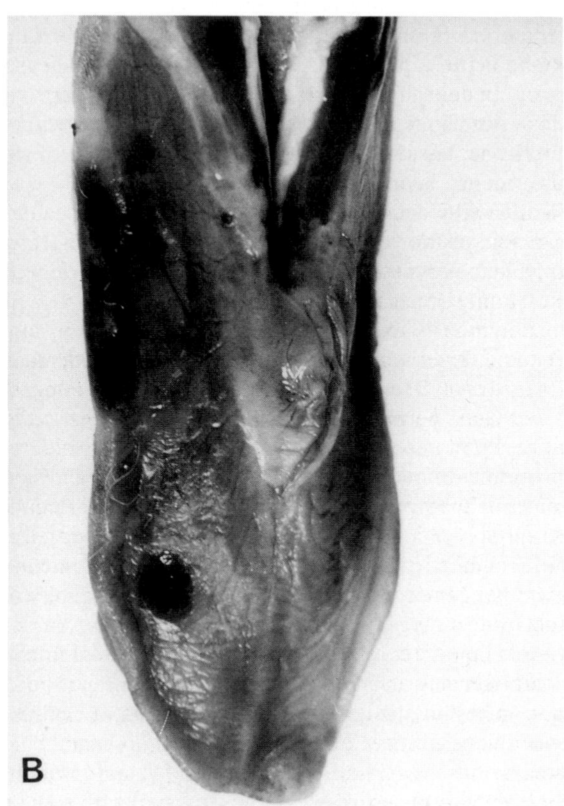

Fig. 5.2B Uremia. Dog. Ulcers on lateral margin and ventral surface of tongue.

unpredictably, though they tend to be seen most often in dogs, especially those with chronic rather than acute renal failure. Many animals dying with uremia are cachectic. This is probably caused by the anorexia, vomition, and diarrhea which often occur, and which necessitate body tissue catabolism to supply energy. Besides this general lack of condition, several distinctive lesions may develop in the gastrointestinal, cardiovascular, respiratory, and skeletal systems (see also these systems).

Ulcerative, necrotic stomatitis occurs in dogs and cats, and there is usually a foul-smelling brown film coating the tongue and buccal mucosa (Fig. 5.2A,B). Like the gastrointestinal changes, oral lesions are more common in chronic than in acute uremia. The pathogenesis of the ulcers is not always clear, but some are associated with fibrinoid necrosis of arterioles, and some are related to bacterial production of ammonia from urea in the saliva. Large areas of the gastric mucosa are often swollen, suffused with red-black blood, and partly ulcerated. This lesion, often called gastritis, is initially noninflammatory, though opportunist bacteria may infect the ulcerated mucosa. Mucosal infarction occurs secondary to arteriolar necrosis. Mineralization of the middle and deep zones of the gastric mucosa is common. Necrosis and mineralization of the muscular coats are sometimes present. Intestinal lesions resemble those in the stomach, but they are less frequent, less severe, and without mineralization. Gastrointestinal lesions probably account for much of the vomition, diarrhea, and melena of uremic dogs. Intestinal intussusceptions sometimes develop in dogs with gastrointestinal lesions. Cats may have gastrointestinal lesions similar to those of dogs but, in uremic cattle, colitis is more common, and the stomach and proximal intestine are edematous. The liver shows inconstant degenerative changes, and there may be acinar dilation of the pancreas with inspissation of secretion. The hyperamylasemia and hyperlipasemia which occur in some uremic dogs are apparently the result of concurrent pancreatitis rather than of reduced renal clearance of the enzymes.

Arterial lesions found in animals with acute renal insufficiency (arterial hyaline degeneration) or with chronic renal failure (hyperplastic arteriolosclerosis) are discussed elsewhere (Diseases of the Vascular System, Volume 3, Chapter 1). Lesions of various organs, such as uremic gastric infarction, may result from arterial degeneration and thrombosis. Arteriolar lesions in the myocardium sometimes cause ischemia and degeneration. Arterial degeneration is perhaps most frequent in acute uremia due to tubular necrosis. In chronic uremia, the left ventricle is often hypertrophied and dilated. Hypertension is common in canine nephritis, and ventricular hypertrophy may be initiated or exaggerated by the hypertension. Lesions in the circulatory system are unusual, except in the dog, but arterial degeneration may occur in the intestines in cattle with acute nephrosis and contribute to the colonic lesions of acute uremic syndromes in this species. In cattle with urethral calculi, a pericardial effusion may be part of the anasarca. In dogs, hydropericardium with dull granulation of the pericardium may occur. Edematous distension of retroperitoneal tissue, expressed particularly as perirenal edema, occurs in pigs and cattle; the underlying renal lesion is usually acute tubular necrosis caused by ochratoxin or *Amaranthus retroflexus* in pigs, and oak poisoning in cattle (see Nephrotoxic Tubular Necrosis, Section V,B of The Kidney in this chapter).

Most animals dying in uremia develop terminal pulmonary edema. The mechanism is obscure, and the edema is not always associated with significant pulmonary congestion; increased permeability of alveolar capillaries is the most likely pathogenesis. In a few animals, acute pneumonia develops terminally. It may be associated with aspiration of gastric content, and its fulminant nature possibly is related to the immunosuppression which develops in uremia. Pulmonary mineralization occurs in chronically uremic dogs. Mineral is deposited in the walls of the alveolar ducts and pulmonary arterioles. Dull granulations of the visceral pleura may be present over the cranial lobes. Occasionally in uremia, spectacular pulmonary lesions develop. They may be visible in radiographs as lines of increased density spreading out from the hilus, and these features are those of interstitial edema. At autopsy the lung is edematous and resilient, and the alveolar spaces contain much fibrin in the edema fluid. Leukocytes are present but may be a response to accidental superimposed infection. Mineralization is extensive with impregnation particularly on reticulin of alveolar walls, which are widened (Fig. 5.3A). The lesion is referred to as uremic lung or **uremic pneumonitis;** it is not common, and when it occurs it may be patchy.

Perhaps the most constant lesion in the dog is mineralization beneath the parietal pleura in the cranial intercostal spaces (Fig. 5.3B). It is preceded by necrosis of the subpleural connective tissue with extension to intercostal muscle and overlying pleura. Once mineralization has oc-

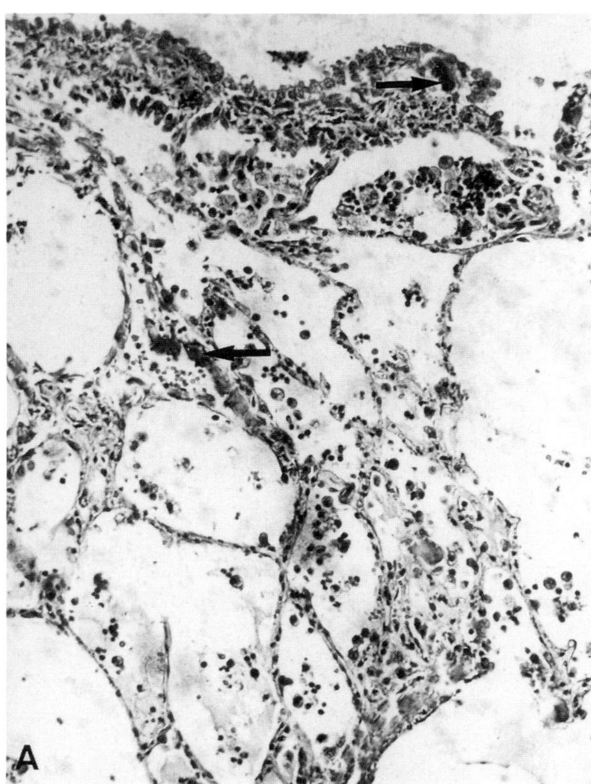

Fig. 5.3A Uremia. Dog. Mineralization of alveolar and bronchiolar wall (arrows), mild edema, and intra-alveolar cellular exudate.

curred and the pleura is repaired, the lesion appears as gray-yellow thickenings, horizontally wrinkled. The cranial intercostal spaces are involved first; when deposition is extensive, many more spaces may be affected.

The pathogenesis of diffuse tissue mineralization in uremia is not clear. There are at least two types of mineral deposit, and serum concentrations of calcium, magnesium, phosphate, and carbonate probably determine the type of calcium phosphate compound that is formed. When calcium is higher than magnesium, apatites are formed, whereas the opposite relationship favors deposition of amorphous calcium phosphate. The regularity with which certain tissues and organs are mineralized is no doubt related to local characteristics such as tissue glycosaminoglycans, local pH, and cellular factors.

The effects of chronic uremia on the skeleton are discussed with renal osteodystrophy (Volume 1, Chapter 1) and the parathyroid glands (Volume 3, Chapter 3). Enlarged parathyroids are common in dogs with chronic renal failure; osseous lesions are less so.

Uremic encephalopathy is apparently an uncommon complication of uremia in domestic animals. It has been reported clinically in dogs, and was evident as multifocal spongiform encephalopathy in a Holstein heifer with severe, chronic interstitial nephritis.

The **renal lesions** of uremia are varied but, if the syn-

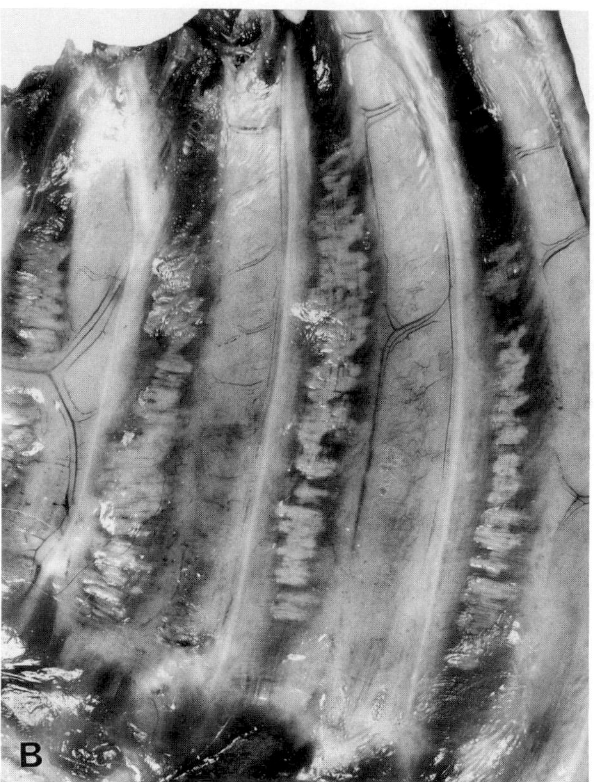

Fig. 5.3B Necrosis and mineralization beneath intercostal pleura between cranial ribs.

drome is chronic, certain common changes tend to occur. The end result is a fibrosed, mineralized kidney with sclerosed glomeruli, and sometimes areas of hyperplastic and hypertrophic tubules. Often this can be diagnosed only as **end-stage kidney.** Severe mineralization occurs late in the course of renal failure and may diffusely involve glomerular and tubular basement membranes, or be deposited at the corticomedullary junction. In the latter case, temporary ischemia with reflow involving the straight part of the proximal tubule, which is at the periphery of the postglomerular circulation, may be responsible. Dietary phosphate restriction may inhibit renal mineralization and its attendant inflammation, scarring, and loss of nephrons. Interstitial fibrosis and glomerulosclerosis are slowly progressive lesions, which are common in the end stages of many renal diseases. Hyperplasia and hypertrophy of tubules are inconstant changes that probably precede the onset of renal failure. Azotemia develops when glomerular filtration is reduced to 75% of normal. Until this time, adaptive changes in intact nephrons maintain renal function at an adequate level as other nephrons are incapacitated. The glomerulus is probably the limiting factor in this compensatory mechanism, since it has a relatively limited ability to increase its function. It seems unlikely that uremia provides a suitable environment to permit or encourage compensatory hyperplasia, and it is likely that enlargement of nephrons is an early response to a reduction in renal mass rather than an adaptation to uremia.

Regardless of the initiating cause, **chronic renal failure tends to be progressive.** Progression occurs because of persistence of the primary disease problem and/or the addition of other renal insults or complications, such as urinary tract infection, systemic hypertension, and intrarenal deposition of mineral. As well, endogenous factors that often develop as compensatory mechanisms may contribute to perpetuation of renal failure. These factors include glomerular capillary hypertension and hyperfiltration, renal hypertrophy, increased renal oxygen consumption, and increased renal ammoniagenesis. Surviving nephrons may also be injured as a result of altered phosphate metabolism, altered lipid composition, and by increased activity of the coagulation system. High dietary protein intake increases renal blood flow and GFR, possibly through the actions of mediators such as glucagon, growth hormone, prostaglandins, the renin–angiotensin system, biogenic amines, and a hepatic-derived renal vasodilator known as glomerulopressin; restricting protein intake can minimize renal hemodynamic changes and slow the progression of chronic renal failure. Glomerular hyperperfusion can lead to glomerulosclerosis and proteinuria. Compensatory hyperfunction of renal tubules in a failing kidney can lead to increased renal ammoniagenesis, increased renal ammonia concentration, activation of the third component of complement, and complement-mediated inflammation and injury; such tubulointerstitial lesions may be progressive.

Also to be considered when assessing renal disease in a mature or aged animal are **normal aging changes** that occur in the absence of any specific renal insult; these background changes may lead to decreased renal reserve, but usually not to renal failure. In aged dogs for example, renal weight is reduced by 20–30% due to decreased size and number of nephrons. In humans, GFR decreases with age because the renal fraction of cardiac output decreases and because of intrarenal vascular changes such as coalescence of glomerular capillaries in juxtamedullary glomeruli and atrophy of arterioles of cortical glomeruli. Glomerular mesangial volume increases, proximal tubule volume and length decrease, and interstitial connective tissue increases. Changes in the ground substance of medullary connective tissue can reduce medullary hyperosmolality and hence renal concentrating ability. Aged animals with purely senescent renal changes have decreased compensatory abilities, such as hypertrophy, and are hence very susceptible to renal insults. Proteinuria may be taken as an indicator of increased glomerular permeability, but there is no sensitive and specific test for quantifying renal aging at present.

Bibliography

Allen, T. A., and Roudebush, P. Canine geriatric nephrology. *Compend Cont Ed Pract Vet* **12:** 909–917, 1990.

Black, D. A. K. A perspective on uremic toxins. *Arch Intern Med* **126:** 906–909, 1970.

Bohle, A. *et al.* The pathogenesis of chronic renal failure. *Pathol Res Pract* **185:** 421–440, 1989.
Bricker, N. S. On the pathogenesis of the uremic state. An exposition of the "trade-off hypothesis." *N Engl J Med* **286:** 1093–1099, 1972.
Cheville, N. F. Uremic gastropathy in the dog. *Vet Pathol* **16:** 292–309,1979.
Comty, C. M., Cohen, S. L., and Shapiro, F. L. Pericarditis in chronic uremia and its sequels. *Ann Intern Med* **75:** 173–183, 1971.
Divers, T. J. Chronic renal failure in horses. *Compend Cont Ed Pract Vet* 5: S310–S317, 1983.
Finco, D. R., and Rowland, G. N. Hypercalcemia secondary to chronic renal failure in the dog: A report of four cases. *J Am Vet Med Assoc* **173:** 990–994, 1978.
Gottschalk, C. W. Function of the chronically diseased kidney. The adaptive nephron. *Circ Res* **28** & **29** (Suppl. II): 1–13, 1971.
Harris, C. L, and Krawiec, D. R. The pathophysiology of uremic bleeding. *Compend Cont Ed Pract Vet* **12:** 1294–1298, 1990.
Hebert, L. A., and Bay, W. H. On the natural tendency to progressive loss of remaining kidney function in patients with impaired renal function. *Med Clin North Am* **74:** 1011–1024, 1990.
LeGeros, R. Z., Contiguglia, S. R., and Alfrey, A. C. Pathological calcifications associated with uremia. Two types of calcium phosphate deposits. *Calcif Tissue Res* **13:** 173–185, 1973.
Malluche, H., and Faugere, M. C. Renal bone disease 1990: An unmet challenge for the nephrologist. *Kidney Int* **38:** 193–211, 1990.
Monaghan, M. L. M. *et al.* Ageing changes in the bovine kidney. *J Comp Pathol* **96:** 699–710, 1986.
Moon, M.L., Greenlee, P.G., and Burk, R. L. Uremic pneumonitis-like syndrome in ten dogs. *J Am Anim Hosp Assoc* **22:** 687–691, 1986.
Oldrizzi, L. *et al.* "Progressive Nature of Renal Disease: Myths and Facts." Contributions to Nephrology, Vol. 75. Basel, S. Karger, 1989.
Petrites-Murphy, M. B. *et al.* Role of parathyroid hormone in the anemia of chronic terminal renal dysfunction in dogs. *Am J Vet Res* **50:** 1898–1905, 1989.
Polzin, D. J. The effects of ageing on the canine urinary tract. *Vet Med* **85:** 472–482, 1990.
Polzin, D. J., and Osborne, C. A. Current progress in slowing progression of canine and feline chronic renal failure. *Compan Anim Pract* **2:** 52–62, 1988.
Polzin, D., Osborne, C., and Adams, L. Nutritional management of chronic renal failure. *Sem Vet Med Surg (Small Anim)* **5:** 187–196, 1990.
Schoots, A. *et al.* Uremic toxins and the elusive middle molecules. *Nephron* **38:** 1–8, 1984.
Slatopolsky, E. *et al.* The parathyroid–calcitriol axis in health and chronic renal failure. *Kidney Int* **38** (Suppl. 29): S41–S47, 1990.
Summers, B. A., and Smith, C. A. Renal encephalopathy in a cow. *Cornell Vet* **75:** 524–530, 1985.
Tennant, B., Bettleheim, P., and Kaneko, J. J. Paradoxic hypercalcemia and hypophosphatemia associated with chronic renal failure in horses. *J Am Vet Med Assoc* **180:** 630–634, 1982.
Tvedegaard, E., Falk, E., and Nielsen, M. Uremic arterial disease in rabbits with special reference to the coronary arteries. *Acta Pathol Microbiol Immunol Scand* (Sect A) **93:** 81–88, 1985.

II. Anomalies of Development

The embryology of mammalian kidneys involves the sequential development of three successive but overlapping structures: the pronephros, mesonephros, and metanephros. The first two become vestigial, but act as inducers of the definitive kidney, the metanephros. Pronephric tubules, arising in the intermediate mesoderm of the cervical region, form the pronephric duct by fusion and extension of their caudal ends. This duct opens into the cloaca and, although the pronephric tubules are not functional in mammalian embryos, the utilization of their duct by the mesonephric tubules gives them potential significance in the genesis of renal anomalies. Mesonephric tubules develop from thoracic mesoderm caudad to the pronephros. The mesonephros is functional in mammalian embryos but degenerates before birth. In males, some of the caudal tubules persist as efferent ducts of the epididymis, and the duct itself is utilized as the vas deferens. In females, cystic remnants of mesonephric tubules in the mesovarium may form the epoophoron and paroophoron, and remnants of the duct are known as Gartner's duct.

The formation of the metanephros, the definitive kidney, begins with the development of a ureteral bud from the mesonephric duct immediately cranial to its junction with the cloaca. The bud, accompanied by vessels and nerves, grows into a mass of mesenchymal cells, the metanephric blastema, and it is on the interaction of these two structures that normal renal and ureteral development depend. As the bud grows into the blastema, it makes a specific number of successive, dichotomous divisions. The tubes formed by early divisions of the ureteral bud dilate and become the pelvis and calyces of the kidney. Tubes formed by later divisions develop into collecting ducts, and the last divisions give rise to collecting tubules. As the blind end of each collecting tubule, the ampulla, grows into the metanephric blastema, it induces compact masses of cells to form about it. These masses soon cavitate, become S-shaped, and unite with the side of the ampulla, which continues to advance and divide.

The cavitated cell masses develop into nephrons. Connection of the lumens of the nephron and the collecting tubule occurs very soon after the cell mass cavitates. Glomerular development involves the formation of a lateral invagination in the S-shaped mass by mesenchymal cells, which differentiate into endothelial and mesangial cells and become linked with the renal vasculature.

The complicated formation of the kidney provides for many patterns of malformation. The interaction of ureteral bud and metanephric blastema involves mutual inductions, and malformations of renal tissue often are accompanied by ureteral anomalies.

The incidence of urinary tract anomalies is not known for most species. Survey results from large numbers of lambs suggest that anomalies occur much more often than is commonly believed.

Bibliography

Crocker, J. F. S., Brown, D. M., and Vernier, R. L. Developmental defects of the kidney. A review of renal development and experimental studies of maldevelopment. *Pediatr Clin North Am* **18:** 355–376, 1971.

Dennis, S. M. Urogenital defects in sheep. *Vet Rec* **105:** 344–347, 1979.

A. Abnormalities in the Amount of Renal Tissue

Lack of renal tissue may be complete or partial and is called agenesis or hypoplasia, respectively.

Renal agenesis may be caused by developmental failure of the pronephros, mesonephros, or ureteral bud, by absence or complete unresponsiveness of the metanephric blastema, or by complete degeneration of the metanephric blastema. Partial degeneration, or partial responsiveness of the blastema to the inductive influences of the ureteral bud, probably produces renal dysplasia. The presence of even a fragment of recognizable metanephric tissue necessitates this diagnosis.

Agenesis may be unilateral or bilateral. As is the case with all renal anomalies, agenesis may be associated with other urogenital deformities. Unilateral renal agenesis is compatible with normal life if the other kidney is normal; however, contralateral dysplasia, or even hypoplasia, may be present, in which case renal failure ultimately develops. The ureter may be absent or malformed, with a blind end that terminates in connective tissue at the renal site. Bilateral agenesis is inconsistent with postnatal life. Renal agenesis occurs infrequently in all species, except when there is a familial incidence, as in some beagles, Shetland sheepdogs, and Doberman pinschers, and in Large White pigs. Bilateral agenesis may account for some stillbirths, but this can be assessed only by careful examination of fetuses.

Hypoplastic kidneys are small, but most abnormally small kidneys, even in young animals, are not hypoplastic. The limited size of hypoplastic kidneys is associated with a reduced number of histologically normal lobules and calyces. Renal hypoplasia is a quantitative defect caused by reduced mass of metanephric blastema or by incomplete induction of nephron formation by the ureteral bud. When the amount of blastema is normal, but there is malfunction of the ureteral bud, renal dysplasia probably develops. Most of the small kidneys diagnosed as hypoplastic are probably dysplastic or scarred. The term cortical hypoplasia should be avoided since it is inconsistent with established concepts of renal embryology and anatomy. Renal hypoplasia is rare. It may be unilateral or bilateral. When unilateral, contralateral hypertrophy is expected.

Bilateral hypoplasia probably always leads to renal failure, and this often complicates or precludes the diagnosis because of the secondary changes that develop. Several forms of renal hypoplasia occur in humans but, because of the confusion of terminology, the variations and incidence of the condition in animals cannot be assessed. Kidneys suspected of being hypoplastic should be weighed along with their mates and examined for evidence of dysplasia and hypertrophy. In humans, in the absence of acquired disease, a decrease in size of one kidney by more than 50% or reduction of total renal mass by more than one third is taken as evidence of hypoplasia.

Details regarding **excess renal tissue** are not well documented. Duplication of ureters and kidneys occurs in cattle, pigs, and dogs, but it is not clear whether total renal mass is increased.

Bibliography

Andrews, F. M. *et al.* Bilateral renal hypoplasia in four young horses. *J Am Vet Med Assoc* **189:** 209–212, 1986.

Brownie, C. F., Tess, M. W., and Prasad, R. D. Bilateral renal agenesis in two litters of Shetland sheepdogs. *Vet Hum Toxicol* **30:** 483–485, 1988.

Burk, D., and Beaudoin, A. R. Arsenate-induced renal agenesis in rats. *Teratology* **16:** 247–259, 1977.

Chevalier, R. L. Renal response to ureteral obstruction in early development. *Nephron* **56:** 113–117, 1990.

Mack, C. O., and McGlothlin, J. H. Renal agenesis in the female cat. *Anat Rec* **105:** 445–450, 1949.

Mason, R. W., and Cooper, R. Congenital bilateral renal hypoplasia in Large White pigs. *Aust Vet J* **62:** 413–414, 1985.

Robbins, G. R. Unilateral renal agenesis in the beagle. *Vet Rec* **77:** 1345–1347, 1965.

B. Anomalies of Renal Position, Form, and Orientation

The kidneys develop in the pelvis and migrate to their sublumbar location, meanwhile rotating so that the ureter attains its normal orientation. During this movement the blood supply shifts from the iliac arteries to the aorta. Various disruptions of this procedure may occur. Vitamin A deficiency in sows may cause anomalies such as those to be described.

Malposition of the kidneys **(renal ectopia)**, observed more frequently in swine than in dogs or cats, is usually caudal, with the kidney in the pelvic or inguinal position. One or both kidneys may be displaced. The kidneys may be normal or abnormally small. The renal arteries arise close to the bifurcation of the aorta or from the iliacs. The

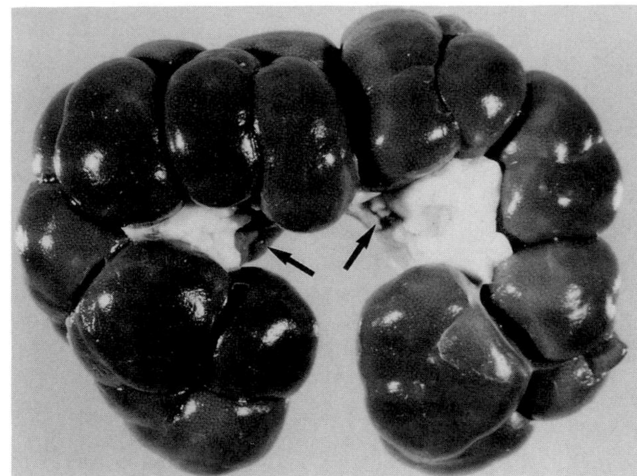

Fig. 5.4 Horseshoe kidney. Calf. Ureters have been severed (arrows).

ureter is short but may be kinked and thereby predisposed to hydronephrosis and pyelonephritis, or may empty into the genital tract, causing urinary incontinence.

Fetal lobulations, normal in embryos and cattle, may persist owing to failure of fusion of individual renal segments. They are not of pathologic significance.

Horseshoe kidney, seen in all species, results from a fusion of the cranial or caudal poles of the kidneys (Fig. 5.4). The fusion may involve only a small portion of the capsule or parenchyma or be sufficient to produce a common pelvis. The ureters are not involved, and their disposition depends on whether the cranial or caudal poles are fused. Such kidneys function normally.

Bibliography

Kaufmann, M. L. *et al.* Renal ectopia in a dog and a cat. *J Am Vet Med Assoc* **190:** 73–77, 1987.

O'Handley, P., Carrig, C. B., and Walshaw, R. Renal and ureteral duplication in a dog. *J Am Vet Med Assoc* **174:** 484–487, 1979.

Pitts, W. R., and Muecke, E. C. Horseshoe kidneys: A 40-year experience. *J Urol* **113:** 743–746, 1975.

Story, H. E. A case of horseshoe kidney in the domestic cat. *Anat Rec* **86:** 307–319, 1943.

C. Renal Dysplasia

Renal dysplasia is disorganized development of renal parenchyma due to anomalous differentiation. Lesions may be gross or microscopic. Renal dysplasia is usually congenital, but in cats, dogs, and pigs, which have an active subcapsular nephrogenic zone at birth, dysplasias may be caused by disease in the early neonatal period until differentiation of the nephrogenic tissue is completed. The quantitative changes that continue until maturity are not susceptible to dysplastic influences.

The causes of renal dysplasia are ill defined, but there are indications that inheritance is not important, if the familial renal diseases of dogs and the polycystic diseases are excluded. An autosomal dominant form of cystic renal dysplasia has been reported in Suffolk sheep. Most human cases are associated with intrauterine ureteral obstruction, and some cases in pigs and calves probably have the same cause; rapid growth and the increased activity of the intrarenal renin–angiotensin system in the fetus may cause greater susceptibility to permanent renal injury. Renal dysplasia in kittens is caused by fetal infection with panleukopenia virus; in puppies, by neonatal infection by canine herpesvirus; and in calves, is associated with fetal infection by bovine virus diarrhea virus. Other teratogenic agents undoubtedly can produce renal dysplasia in these and other species. Renal dysplasia in pigs has been attributed to hypovitaminosis A.

There is considerable variation in the appearance of those dysplastic kidneys which are grossly abnormal. Most of them are small, which accounts for their frequent misdiagnosis as hypoplastic. They are usually misshapen and fibrosed with thick-walled cysts and dilated tortuous ureters (Fig. 5.5). One or both kidneys may be affected. If the lesion is unilateral, the ipsilateral ureter should be examined for anomalous valves, diverticula, or atresia. If both kidneys are involved, scrutiny of the bladder and lower urinary tract is indicated. Some dysplastic kidneys may be only slightly irregular in contour (Fig. 5.6) or may appear normal, in which case microscopic examination is required for diagnosis. Dysplasias caused by teratogenic viruses usually are included in this group. Considerable emphasis has been placed on the size of renal arteries in dysplasias, but changes should be interpreted with caution

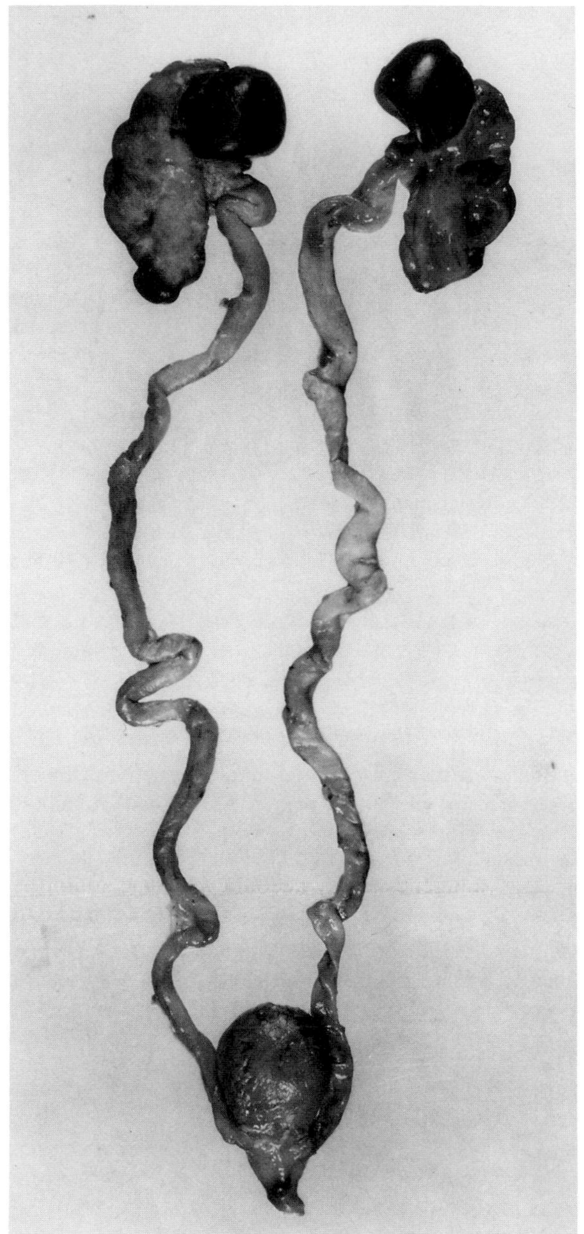

Fig. 5.5 Renal dysplasia. Pig. Dilated ureters lead to fibrotic malformed kidneys.

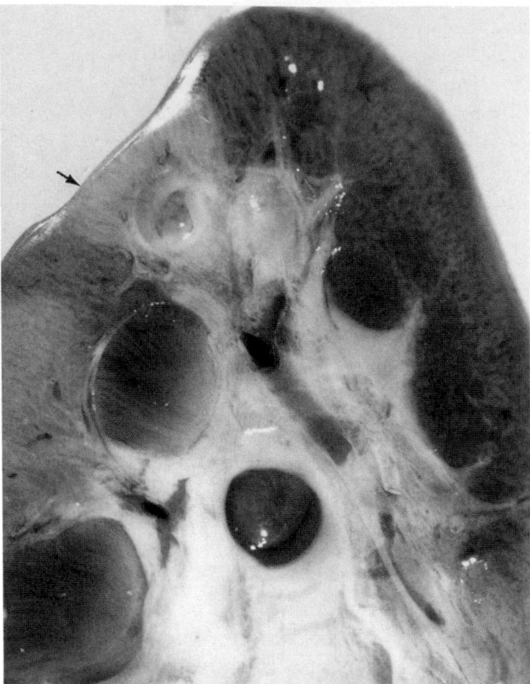

Fig. 5.6 Focal renal dysplasia (arrow). Pig.

since degenerative lesions in the renal parenchyma may be accompanied by vascular atrophy. Extrarenal anomalies, such as imperforate anus, may occur in association with renal dysplasia.

The microscopic criteria of renal dysplasia are the presence of structures inappropriate to the stage of development of the animal, or the development of structures that are clearly anomalous. Among the former are areas of undifferentiated mesenchyme in cortex or medulla (Fig. 5.7A), and groups of immature glomeruli (small glomeruli

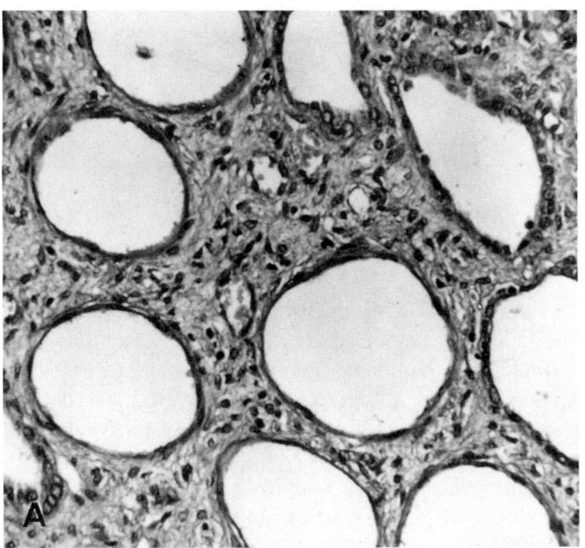

Fig. 5.7A Loose intertubular mesenchyme and dilated medullary tubules in renal dysplasia. Calf.

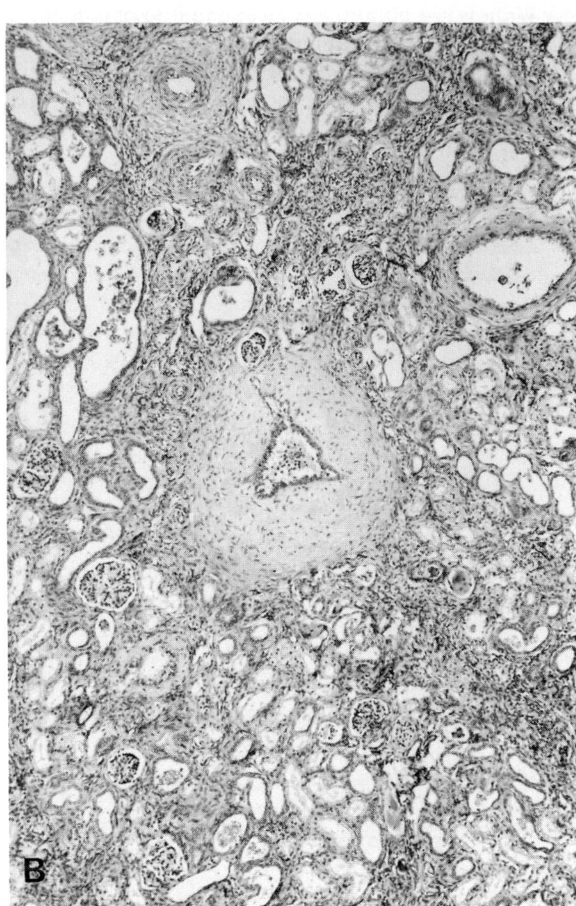

Fig. 5.7B Renal dysplasia. Calf. Thick-walled primitive duct in renal cortex is lined by cuboidal epithelium. (Slide courtesy of S. Groom.)

with peripheral nuclei and inapparent capillaries) in the cortex of adolescent or adult animals. Anomalous structures include collecting tubules ending blindly in cortical connective tissue, or primitive ducts lined by cuboidal or columnar epithelium and surrounded by concentric layers of mesenchyme (Fig. 5.7B). Cartilage nodules, which are found in some dysplastic human kidneys, are rarely if ever present. This absence is probably a function of the stage of development at which metanephric injury occurs. Cartilage nodules imply injury to uncommitted mesenchyme, that is, to nephrogenic cord before its interaction with the ureteral bud. Other anomalous structures clearly are nephrogenic, and represent improper interaction of ureteral bud and mesenchyme. There is some support for the opinion that only primitive ducts and cartilage nodules are prima facie evidence of dysplasia, on the grounds that all other lesions may be produced by acquired renal disease. Some of the more prominent gross lesions of dysplastic kidneys, such as fibrous cysts, dense medullary fibrosis, and fibrous wedges extending from pelvis to cortex probably are regressive changes due to obstruction or infarction. Because ureteral anomalies are often concomitant, dysplastic kidneys are abnormally susceptible to pyelonephritis. Otherwise there is little or no evidence of infection in the renal parenchyma. The dark nuclei of improperly differentiated nephrogenic tissue should not be misinterpreted as lymphocytes.

Renal dysplasia with gross changes usually causes uremia. When lesions are bilateral, this is explicable in terms of reduced functional renal mass. With unilateral dysplasia, systemic hypertension induced by constriction of arteries in the affected kidney may be responsible.

Bibliography

Dunham, B. M. *et al.* Renal dysplasia with multiple urogenital and large intestinal anomalies in a calf. *Vet Pathol* **26:** 94–96, 1989.

Jones, T. O. *et al.* A vertically transmitted cystic renal dysplasia of lambs. *Vet Rec* **127:** 421–424, 1990.

Kilham, L., Margolis, G., and Colby, E. D. Congenital infections of cats and ferrets by feline panleukopenia virus manifested by cerebellar hypoplasia. *Lab Invest* **17:** 465–480, 1967.

Percy, D. H. *et al.* Lesions in puppies surviving infection with canine herpesvirus. *Vet Pathol* **8:** 37–53, 1971.

Picut, C. A., and Lewis, R. M. Microscopic features of canine renal dysplasia. *Vet Pathol* **24:** 156–163, 1987.

Zicker, S. C. *et al.* Bilateral renal dysplasia with nephron hypoplasia in a foal. *J Am Vet Med Assoc* **196:** 2001–2005, 1990.

D. Renal Cysts

Cystic diseases of the kidney include various conditions characterized by one or more grossly visible cystic cavities in the renal parenchyma. No satisfactory classification of renal cysts exists, but an acceptable compromise would be based on mode of inheritance, or lack thereof, the presence of lesions in other organs, and the clinical course in affected animals.

Some prefatory remarks about renal cysts are in order. Cysts can arise during organogenesis, and may be associated with histologic criteria of renal dysplasia. In humans, most dysplastic kidneys are cystic, and most cystic diseases of childhood are dysplasias. Cysts can arise in nephrons and collecting tubules after the end of nephrogenesis. Examples are provided by steroid-induced cysts in various species, and atypical cysts in patients undergoing long-term hemodialysis. Cysts can develop in any part of the nephron, including the glomerular space, or in the collecting system. In glomerulocystic disease, they develop only in Bowman's space, but this exclusivity is exceptional. There is no evidence that cysts are caused by failure of nephrons to unite with the collecting system. Analyses of their content indicate that they are part of functional nephrons, and that their activity is consistent with their location in the nephron.

Three mechanisms, which are not mutually exclusive, may lead to the formation of renal cysts: (1) renal cysts may be caused by obstructive lesions; examples are the acquired retention cysts of chronic renal disease, some dysplastic cysts, and possibly those of glomerulocystic disease; (2) a fundamental change, of unknown origin, may occur in the tubular basement membrane and result in formation of saccular or fusiform dilations of the tubules; and (3) disordered growth of tubular epithelial cells may lead to focal hyperplastic lesions and cyst formation. Enhanced renal cystogenesis occurs in humans with primary aldosteronism or primary renal potassium wasting, perhaps as a consequence of chronic hypokalemia and tubular obstruction by proliferating tubular epithelial cells. Renal cysts are dynamic structures, and their growth may be modified by pharmacologic means.

Many chemicals, such as long-acting corticosteroids, diphenylamine, polychlorinated biphenyls, 5,6,7,8-tetrahydrocarbazole-3-acetic acid, alloxan, diphenylthiazole, and nordihydroguaiaretic acid, cause renal cysts in experimental animals. Corticosteroids induce hypokalemia, and cyst formation is prevented by injections of some potassium salts, but in general the mechanisms of cyst development are not known. It seems possible that some of the therapeutic, prophylactic, and pollutant chemicals to which animals are exposed could be responsible for sporadic cases of renal cysts.

Renal cysts vary in size from the barely visible (Fig. 5.8A) to structures which exceed that of the organ itself (Fig. 5.8B). Most lie within these limits, and although they are more numerous in the cortex than medulla, this may simply reflect the relative volumes of the two regions. The cyst wall is clear or opaque depending on the amount of surrounding connective tissue. The content is watery. Cysts are lined by flattened or cuboidal epithelium, which

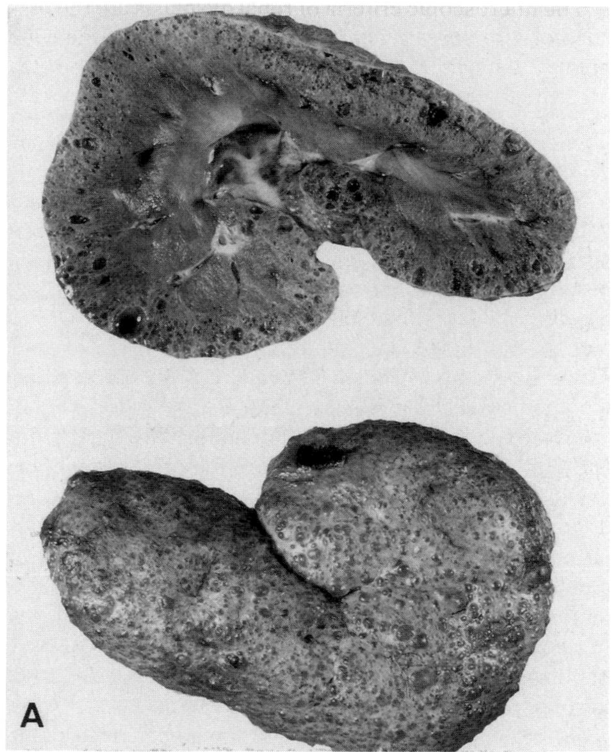

Fig. 5.8A Polycystic kidney. Horse 8 years old.

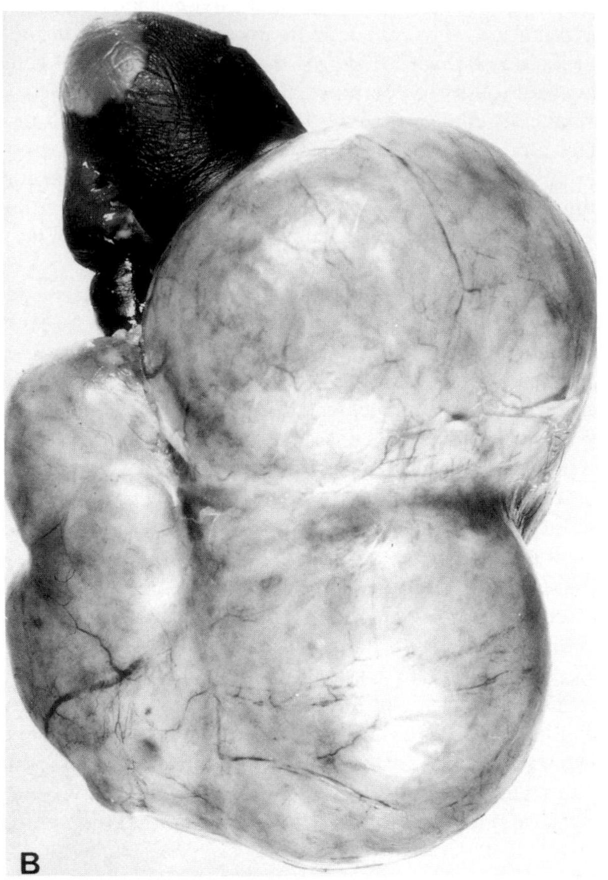

Fig. 5.8B Renal cysts involving each pole of the kidney. Pig.

grossly is smooth and shiny. A few cysts are more or less divided by thin trabeculae, but most are unilocular and roughly spherical, ovoid or fusiform.

Simple renal cysts occur in all species but are most common in pigs and calves. There are different patterns of occurrence in pigs, but it is not clear whether similar patterns exist in other animals. The usual finding in pigs is one or a few unilocular cortical cysts, about 1–2 cm across, that bulge from the renal surface or are exposed when the kidney is sliced. They are usually bilateral, and are incidental findings in young pigs. Affected kidneys are discarded in abattoirs. Although usually regarded as sporadic occurrences, these lesions may be examples of a cystic renal disease which is inherited as an autosomal dominant trait. Polygenic inheritance may determine the number of cysts in animals with the dominant gene. In this condition, few cysts are present at birth, but they gradually increase in number, and there may be 80–90 by 1 year of age. Cysts occur in different parts of the kidney and nephron. Signs of renal failure are not seen, but the condition has similarities to a human cystic disease in which renal failure develops in adults—a similar course in mature swine is not inconceivable.

Occasionally areas containing many small cysts occur in one lobe of a bovine kidney or one pole of an equine kidney. They are not significant clinically.

Congenital forms of **polycystic kidney disease** (PKD) associated with cystic bile ducts, bile duct proliferation, and sometimes pancreatic cysts occur in pigs, lambs, calves, puppies, kittens, and foals. A genetic cause is proposed in some species (autosomal recessive in Cairn terriers) but rejected in others; a similar syndrome in children is inherited as an autosomal recessive trait. The disease in domestic animals is manifest by stillbirths or death in renal failure during the first few weeks of life. Grossly the kidneys are large and pale, and contain numerous 1- to 5-mm cysts that involve both cortex and medulla. Bile duct cysts range from barely visible to 3 cm across, and the gallbladder and biliary system often are distended with bile, which discolors the liver. Polycystic liver disease also occurs in adult humans with the autosomal dominant form of PKD; renal cysts develop bilaterally, are of proximal or distal tubular origin, can reach 3–4 cm diameter, and lead to hypertension or renal failure by the fourth to fifth decade of life. Syndromes resembling both the autosomal dominant and autosomal recessive forms of human PKD have been described in related cats; Persian cats appear to be disproportionately affected. Polycystic kidney disease has also been reported as a sporadic event in adult horses and ferrets.

Uremic medullary cystic disease complex is a group of progressive renal disorders of children that leads to chronic renal failure as a result of formation of corticomedullary cysts, cortical tubular atrophy, and interstitial fibrosis. A similar syndrome has been identified in a Shetland sheepdog.

Glomerulocystic disease is seen occasionally in stillborn foals and collie dogs. Cysts, barely visible, are present only in Bowman's spaces. Their significance in foals is not known. In dogs, uremia develops.

Acquired cysts of the kidney do develop when tubules are obstructed by scar tissue. They are multiple and small, rarely exceeding 1.0 cm in diameter. Most are located in convoluted tubules and Bowman's spaces. Hyperplastic collecting tubules sometimes are grossly visible as elongated cysts in the medulla of dogs with renal failure. These acquired cysts are distinguishable from primary cysts in that they occur in kidneys with extensive scarring.

Perinephric pseudocysts occasionally develop uni- or bilaterally as a collection of fluid, which may be urine, blood, lymph, or transudate, in the space between the renal capsule and the renal reflection of the peritoneum; the space is not lined by epithelium and is thus a pseudocyst rather than a true cyst. Potential causes include trauma, surgery, neoplasia, venous congestion, and hypertension. Affected cats are usually old and have concomitant chronic renal disease.

Bibliography

Abdinoor, D. J. Perinephric pseudocysts in a cat. *J Am Anim Hosp Assoc* **16:** 763–767, 1980.

Avner, E. D. Renal cystic disease. Insights from recent experimental investigations. *Nephron* **48:** 89–93, 1988.

Bertone, J. J. *et al.* Monitoring the progression of renal failure in a horse with polycystic kidney disease: Use of the reciprocal of serum creatinine concentration and sodium sulfanilate clearance half-time. *J Am Vet Med Assoc* **191:** 565–568, 1987.

Biller, D. S., Chew, D. J., and DiBartola, S. P. Polycystic kidney disease in a family of Persian cats. *J Am Vet Med Assoc* **196:** 1288–1290, 1990.

Chalifoux, A. *et al.* Glomerular polycystic kidney disease in a dog (blue merle collie). *Can Vet J* **23:** 365–368, 1982.

Kaspareit-Rittinghausen, J. *et al.* Hereditary polycystic disease associated with osteorenal syndrome in rats. *Vet Pathol* **26:** 195–201, 1989.

Ramsay, G. *et al.* Polycystic kidneys in an adult horse. *Equine Vet J* **19:** 243–244, 1987.

Torres, V. E. *et al.* Association of hypokalemia, aldosteronism, and renal cysts. *N Engl J Med* **322:** 345–351, 1990.

Webster, W. R., and Summers, P. M. Congenital polycystic kidney and liver syndrome in piglets. *Aust Vet J* **54:** 451, 1978.

Wells, G. A. H., Hebert, C. N., and Robins, B. C. Renal cysts in pigs: Prevalence and pathology in slaughtered pigs from a single herd. *Vet Rec* **106:** 532–535, 1980.

Wijeratne, W. V. S., and Wells, G. A. H. Inherited renal cysts in pigs: Results of breeding experiments. *Vet Rec* **107:** 484–488, 1980.

Wulfson, M. A. Pyelocaliceal diverticula. *J Urol* **123:** 1–8, 1980.

E. Familial Renal Disease

Familial renal diseases are documented or suspected in many dog breeds, and they are a major cause of chronic renal failure in young animals. **Familial nephropathy** occurs in the following breeds: bull terrier, chow chow, cocker spaniel, Doberman pinscher, Lhasa Apso, Norwegian elkhound, Samoyed, Shih Tzu, soft-coated Wheaten terrier, and standard poodle. **Juvenile nephropathy,** which is suspected of being familial, occurs in at least 20 other dog breeds, including perhaps most prominently the malamute, miniature schnauzer, keeshond, and German shepherd. The mode of inheritance has been established in the bull terrier (autosomal dominant), cocker spaniel and Shih Tzu (autosomal recessive), and Samoyed (sex linked); nephropathy is probably autosomal recessive in soft-coated Wheaten terriers. Pedigree analysis of other affected breeds may lead to the addition of more breeds to the list. Control programs are being undertaken by several breed societies.

Familial glomerulonephritis of Finnish Landrace sheep is discussed with other glomerulonephritides. Progressive renal fibrosis occurs in mutant Southdown sheep with hyperbilirubinemia. Specific tubular dysfunctions in dogs are discussed with Diseases of Tubules (Section V of The Kidney in this chapter).

The canine familial renal diseases are characterized by renal failure, mostly in immature or young adult dogs, which is not associated with primary renal inflammation. For most breeds, only terminal clinical signs and end-stage lesions are described—inheritance, pathogenesis, and early morphologic changes are not reported. The age of onset of renal failure varies from a few weeks to several years but, in most cases, is 4–18 months. This wide age range and the lack of morphologic specificity hinder the definition of these diseases since there is a danger that any noninflammatory renal lesion in a dog of an appropriate breed will be diagnosed as familial.

It is probable that some of the chronic interstitial nephritides formerly attributed to leptospirosis were familial renal diseases. The possibility that these diseases are examples of renal dysplasia seems unlikely since primitive ducts are not present. Glomeruli with the appearance of immaturity must be interpreted cautiously, particularly when they are found in areas of scarring.

Available evidence suggests that lesions primarily involve either glomeruli or interstitium around glomeruli. Interstitial lesions are fibrous, and may be segmental or generalized. The fibrotic segments often contain apparently immature glomeruli, and this pattern is found frequently, but not exclusively, in Lhasa Apso and Shih Tzu dogs; the radial conformation of these scars is suggestive of an ischemic origin. Such asynchronous differentiation of nephrons may be the result of acquired scarring and mechanical inhibition of maturation. Whether familial renal diseases are expressions of dysplasia is a moot point. The *sine qua non* of dysplasia (primitive ducts, cartilage nodules—see Dysplasia (Section II,C of The Kidney in this chapter) is rarely met in affected kidneys; expanding the definition of dysplasia to include the presence of immature glomeruli greatly, and perhaps illegitimately, expands the number of affected cases of juvenile renal disease characterized as being dysplastic. Until etiopathogenesis of these syndromes is better defined, they might better be termed nephropathies.

Brief descriptions of some of the more clearly defined syndromes follow.

1. Samoyed Hereditary Glomerulopathy

The disease occurs in both sexes but is much more common and severe, and has an earlier onset and more rapid course, in males than in females. Affected males develop proteinuria and wasting at 2–3 months of age, azotemia after 5 months, renal failure after 7 months, and die by 15 months of age. Females first show signs of renal disease in middle or old age, but these may be preceded by mild, persistent proteinuria lasting for several years. The disease is inherited as an X-linked dominant trait; severe disease occurs in about 50% of male offspring of carrier dams.

Glomerular lesions consist of membranoproliferative glomerulonephropathy, progressing to glomerulosclerosis; fibrin may be present in the urinary space. As well, there may be thickening of basement membranes of Bowman's capsules and tubules, periglomerular and interstitial fibrosis, and mild interstitial infiltration by mononuclear inflammatory cells. The pathognomonic transmission electron microscopic change, which precedes light microscopic changes, is multilaminar splitting of the lamina densa of the GBM (Fig. 5.9A,B); electron-dense particles are present occasionally between the split layers. Scanning electron microscopy reveals effacement of foot processes and the presence of microvilli and globular projections on podocytes. Proteinuria is initially selective (primarily albumin) but becomes nonselective as the GBM lesion becomes more severe. An abnormal NC1 domain of collagen type IV is present at birth in affected dogs, and may result in inadequate cross-linking of collagen type IV in the GBM and hence progressive wear and tear caused by filtration pressure.

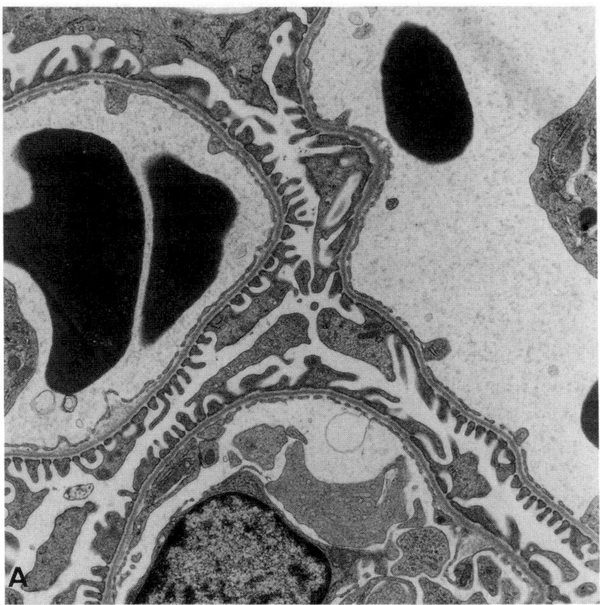

Fig. 5.9A Normal glomerulus showing epithelial (podocyte) foot processes, fenestrated endothelium, and trilaminar basement membrane. (Courtesy of B. Horney.)

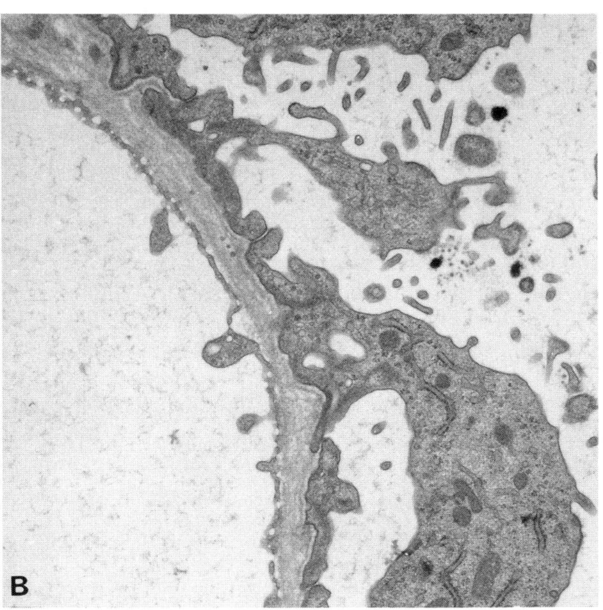

Fig. 5.9B Samoyed hereditary glomerulopathy. Male, 4 months. Multilaminar, irregular splitting of basement membrane. (Courtesy of B. Horney.)

The glomerular lesions in Samoyed hereditary glomerulopathy closely resemble those in human hereditary nephritis, which also has a male predominance. The nerve deafness and ocular abnormalities that occur in Alport's syndrome, a form of human hereditary nephritis, are not features of the disease in Samoyeds. The inheritance and lesions characteristic of familial nephropathy in bull terriers are also similar to those of human hereditary nephritis.

2. Familial Glomerulonephritis of Doberman Pinschers

Dogs of both sexes are affected, and signs, including polyuria, polydipsia, and weight loss, first develop at a few weeks to several years of age. Most animals are younger than 1 year. Prolonged survival is possible; dogs showing signs at a few months may live for many years.

This disease occurs in Doberman pinschers in North America. The variability in the rate of progression of the disease could indicate degrees of expressivity of the defect or reflect differences in exposure to exogenous or endogenous factors which injure the genetically predisposed kidney. Immune complexes have been identified in glomeruli of some dogs; this may reflect trapping of circulating complexes in the defective GBM or, alternatively, *in situ* formation of complexes in the defective GBM.

Grossly, the kidneys are light brown, slightly small, and have diffuse, fine, subcapsular pits, which appear as radial streaks on cut surface. There may be fine white stippling of the subcapsular surface due to the protein-filled tubules and lipid in epithelial cells in the subacute stage of the disease (Fig. 5.10A,B). A few bitches have concomitant agenesis of the right ureter and kidney, with or without contralateral compensatory hypertrophy. The association of renal agenesis is probably coincidental.

Microscopically there is membranoproliferative glomerulonephritis, which begins as focal segmental mesangial thickening and accentuation of glomerular lobulation

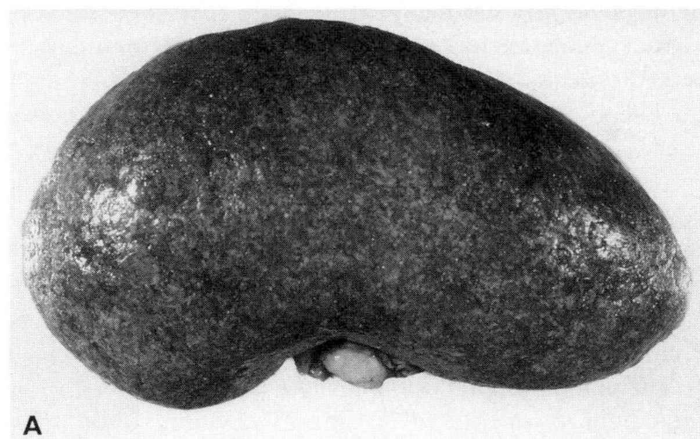

Fig. 5.10A Familial renal disease. Doberman pinscher. White stippling due to protein-filled tubules and lipid in tubular epithelium.

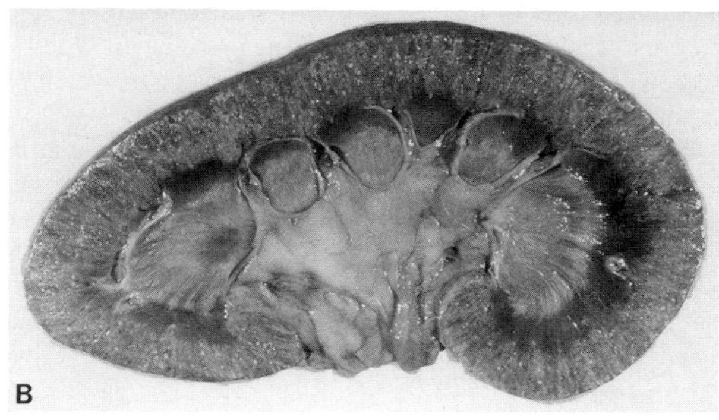

Fig. 5.10B Familial renal disease. Doberman pinscher. Cut surface of kidney shown in (A).

(Fig. 5.11). These early lesions are sometimes present at birth, sometimes at several months. Glomerular changes progress to segmental or diffuse mesangial proliferation with increased mesangial matrix and glomerular adhesions and sclerosis. Sclerotic glomeruli appear as shrunken tufts at the vascular pole of cystic Bowman's spaces. The cysts may be visible grossly; they are associated with the progressive tubulointerstitial disease and are secondary to glomerular lesions. The interstitial lesions consist of fibrosis and monocyte infiltrations around diseased nephrons and in the medulla. In severely affected kidneys,

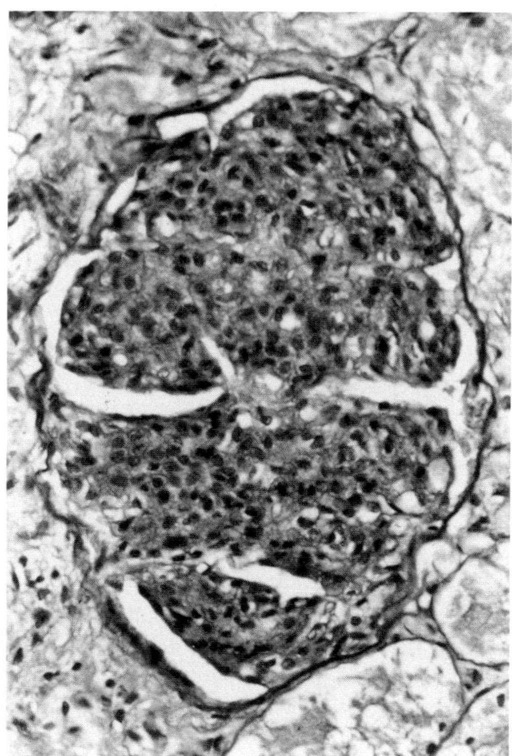

Fig. 5.11 Proliferative glomerulonephritis. Doberman pinscher, 12 weeks old.

compensatory hypertrophy and hyperplasia of tubules occur in adaptive nephrons.

Ultrastructurally, there is irregular multifocal thickening of the GBM with lamellation of the lamina densa and the presence of electron-dense particles within intramembranous lucent foci. In some affected dogs, there is marked attenuation of the lamina densa plus intramembranous or subendothelial deposition of matrix that contains collagen fibers. These ultrastructural lesions resemble those in Samoyeds and humans with hereditary nephropathy.

3. Familial Renal Disease in Norwegian Elkhound Dogs

The disease occurs in both sexes. Signs of renal failure begin as early as 3 months, but dogs with lesions may be clinically normal at 5 years of age. Animals showing early onset and rapid progression of renal failure may be dwarfed. There are no specific biochemical characteristics. Dwarfism in Norwegian elkhounds may be chondrodysplastic (see Bones and Joints, Volume 1, Chapter 1). The disease is reproducible in breeding trials using dogs from appropriate strains, but the mode of transmission is not known.

Grossly, there are light gray streaks, and occasionally wedge-shaped lesions, in the cortex. As the disease progresses, the kidneys become contracted, pale, and tough from abundant cortical and medullary fibrosis.

Histologic changes begin as periglomerular fibrosis with hypertrophy and hyperplasia of parietal epithelium and progress to more or less diffuse fibrosis of cortex and medulla. The lesion is generalized, but not all glomeruli are necessarily involved. Wedge-shaped areas containing severe lesions are consistent with vascular injury, but there is no evidence of vascular abnormalities. As fibrosis progresses, constriction of normal nephrons occurs, and there is a progressive loss of glomeruli. In microdissected kidneys, small saccular dilations are demonstrable in distal tubules and collecting ducts in the early phase of the disease. Late in the course, marked dilation and hyperplasia of collecting ducts occurs; this is a nonspecific lesion in chronic renal disease. There is no evidence of inflammation until renal disease is well established, at which time occasional, randomly distributed foci of mononuclear cells develop.

In contrast to the hereditary glomerulopathies in Samoyeds and Doberman pinschers previously discussed, the lesion in Norwegian elkhounds is primarily a noninflammatory tubulointerstitial nephropathy.

Bibliography

Booth, K. A case of juvenile nephropathy in a Newfoundland dog. *Vet Rec* **127:** 596–597, 1990.

Brown, C. A. *et al.* Suspected familial renal disease in chow chows. *J Am Vet Med Assoc* **196:** 1279–1284, 1990.

Chew, D. J. *et al.* Juvenile renal disease in Doberman pinscher dogs. *J Am Vet Med Assoc* **182:** 481–485, 1982.

Cuppage, F. E., Shimamura, T., and McGavin, M. D. Nephron

obstruction in mutant Southdown sheep. *Vet Pathol* **16:** 483–485, 1979.
Finco, D. R. *et al.* Familial renal disease in Norwegian elkhound dogs: Morphologic examinations. *Am J Vet Res* **38:** 941–947, 1977.
Hill, G. S., Jenis, E. H., and Goodloe, S. The nonspecificity of the ultrastructural alterations in hereditary nephritis. *Lab Invest* **31:** 516–532, 1974.
Hood, J.C. *et al.* Hereditary nephritis in the bull terrier: Evidence for inheritance by an autosomal dominant gene. *Vet Rec* **126:** 456–459, 1990.
Hoppe, A. *et al.* Progressive nephropathy due to renal dysplasia in Shih Tzu dogs in Sweden: A clinical pathological and genetic study. *J Small Anim Pract* **31:** 83–91, 1990.
Jansen, B. S. *et al.* Scanning electron microscopy of cellular and acellular glomeruli of male dogs affected with Samoyed hereditary glomerulopathy and a carrier female. *Can J Vet Res* **51:** 475–480, 1987.
Jones, B. R. *et al.* Chronic renal failure in young Old English sheepdogs. *N Z Vet J* **38:** 118–121, 1990.
Morton, L. D. *et al.* Juvenile renal disease in miniature schnauzer dogs. *Vet Pathol* **27:** 455–458, 1990.
Picut, C. A., and Lewis, R. M. Comparative pathology of canine hereditary nephropathies: An interpretive review. *Vet Res Commun* **11:** 561–581, 1987.
Robinson, W. F., Huxtable, C. R., and Gooding, J. P. Familial nephropathy in cocker spaniels. *Aust Vet J* **62:** 109–112, 1985.
Thorner, P. *et al.* The NC1 domain of collagen type IV in neonatal dog glomerular basement membranes. *Am J Pathol* **134:** 1047–1054, 1989.

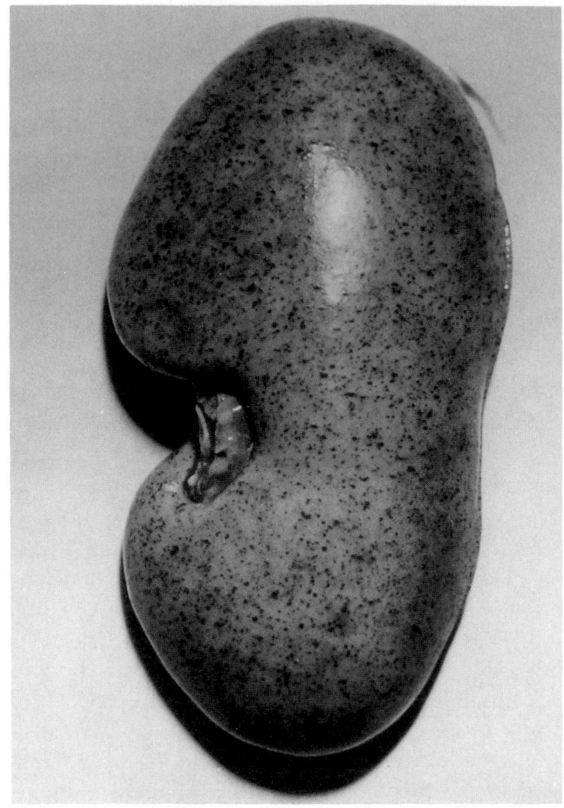

Fig. 5.12 Renal cortical petechiae. African swine fever. (Courtesy of C. Brown.)

III. Circulatory Disturbances and Diseases of the Blood Vessels

A. Renal Hyperemia

Active hyperemia is seen in acute nephritis but especially in the acute septicemias and bacterial intoxications. The kidney is swollen and uniformly dark, although in some cases the hyperemia may be largely restricted to the medulla. Microscopically, all vessels, especially capillaries, are filled with blood. Very acute congestion with intertubular hemorrhages occurs in clostridial enterotoxemia of lambs and calves.

Passive hyperemia (congestion) follows the usual principles. Affected kidneys are enlarged and dark, and the capsular vessels are injected. On section, the corticomedullary junctional zone is dark and prominent, and there is engorgement of visible tributaries.

B. Renal Hemorrhages

Hemorrhages are especially common in the renal cortex in a variety of bacteremias and viremias and sometimes in healthy slaughtered animals. Petechiae are very common in piglets dead of any cause. Many or few pinpoint hemorrhages occur beneath the capsule in hog cholera, African swine fever, and porcine salmonellosis (Fig. 5.12). In porcine erysipelas, the hemorrhages tend to be larger and more irregular in size and shape. Severe hemorrhage in the wall of the renal pelvis and the medulla sometimes occurs in hog cholera, in other acute infections of swine, and in the hemorrhagic diatheses; the hemorrhage occurs from the congested medullary vessels. Extensive subcapsular hemorrhage is not uncommon in clostridial enterotoxemia of calves; it produces a black cast molded to the shape of the cortex.

C. Renal Infarction

Infarcts of the kidney are common lesions of localized coagulation necrosis produced by embolic or thrombotic occlusion of the renal artery or of one of its branches. The sequelae depend on whether the obstructing material is septic or bland and on the size and number of the vessels obstructed (Fig. 5.13). Bland thrombi produce typical infarcts; septic thrombi produce abscesses that may heal, sequestrate, or discharge into the pelvis. Thrombosis of a trunk of a renal artery will produce total or subtotal necrosis of the kidney, the extent of the latter depending on the presence and efficiency of parahilar and capsular collaterals. If an arcuate artery is obstructed, there is necrosis of a wedge of both cortex and medulla; if an interlobular vessel is involved, infarction is limited to the cortex. The ease and the frequency with which the kidneys are infarcted depend on their vascular architecture being of the

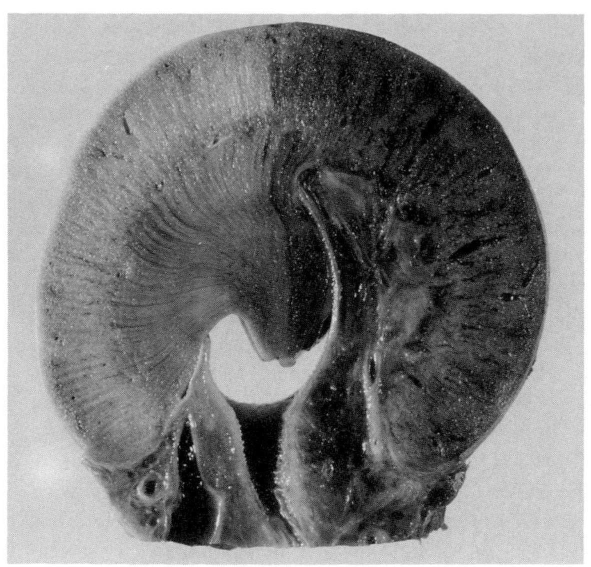

Fig. 5.13 Infarction of half kidney following ligation of one of two renal arteries. Dog. (Courtesy of B. P. Wilcock.)

end-artery type and on the large volume of blood which continually traverses them.

Soon after total obstruction of a vessel, the related wedge of tissue is swollen and intensely cyanotic, and it is congested by the blood that oozes into the vessels from collaterals. There is no sharp line between the infarcted zone and the adjacent normal tissue because in the narrow boundary zone, there is an outer part in which blood continues to ooze slowly and an inner part which is more or less well served by diffusion from the viable tissue. In the outer part of the marginal zone, the red cells survive and circulation may be reestablished, but this zone persists for the first 2–3 days; it is usually referred to, apparently erroneously, as the zone of reactive hyperemia. The limit of useful diffusion determines the actual limit of the infarct, and it is here that dehemoglobinization begins, neutrophils accumulate, and the area of total necrosis begins. The dehemoglobinization begins from the periphery at about 24 hr and may be complete in 2–3 days, the infarcted area then being white (Fig. 5.14A). Before decoloration begins, the area that will be affected is outlined by a thin but distinct white line of leukocytes.

The sequence of degenerative changes in the infarcted tissue reflects the specialization and sensitivity of the various structures. At the outer margins, only a few proximal tubules show epithelial necrosis. More centrally, every proximal tubule is dead, and inside the zone of diffusion, everything is dead (Fig. 5.14B). In the peripheral dead zone, there may in a week or so be some revascularization along preformed channels. The necrotic zone is progressively replaced by fibrous tissue, and healed infarcts persist as pale gray-white scars, wedge-shaped and much depressed below the surface. The scars may be difficult

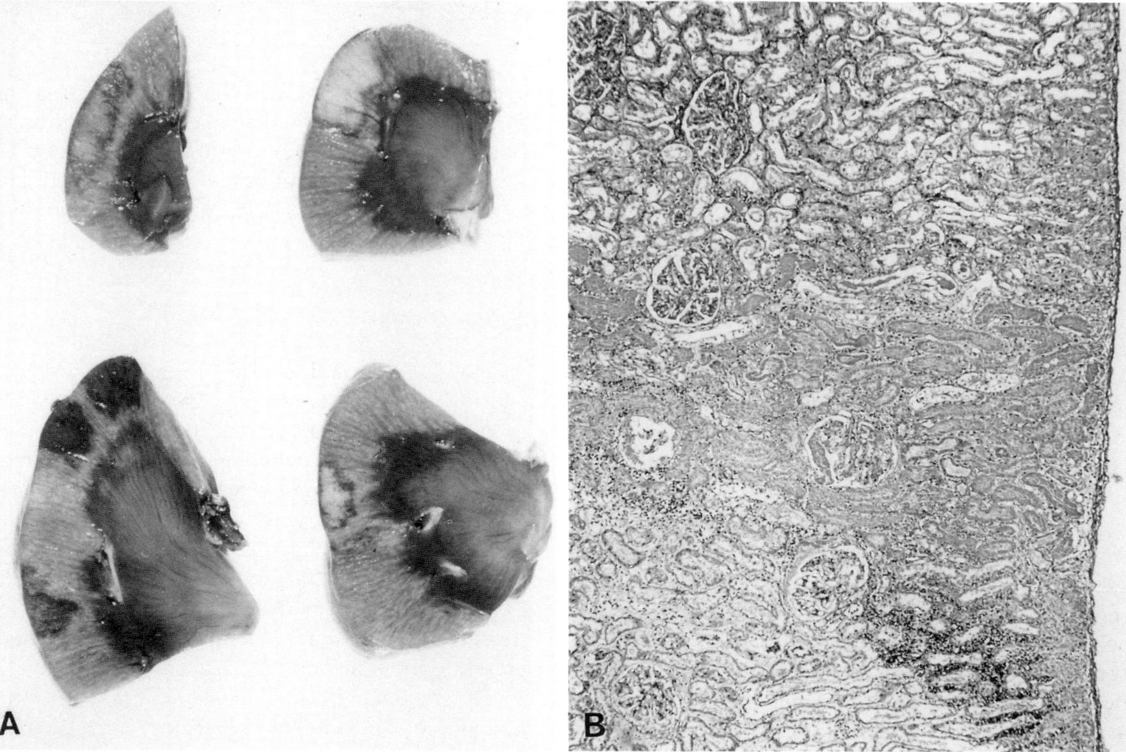

Fig. 5.14 (A) Renal infarcts. Cow. Dark (hemorrhagic) infarcts are about 1 day old. Those with dehemoglobinized centers are 2–3 days old. (B) Renal infarct. Sheep.

or impossible to distinguish grossly from focal healed pyelonephritis.

Minute emboli which lodge in the glomerular or intertubular capillaries may produce small infarcts which are not detectable macroscopically. Because of the small size of such infarcts, there may be adequate diffusion across the infarcted zone so that leukocytes do not accumulate, epithelial necrosis is minimal and soon repaired, and circulation is reestablished. Commonly, infarcts of various ages in a kidney indicate recurrent embolic episodes.

Primary vascular disease of the kidneys in animals is of little significance. Renal arteriosclerosis is not rare as an incidental finding in cattle, and arteritis is occasionally observed as polyarteritis nodosa or in systemic disease such as malignant catarrhal fever. A variety of degenerative proliferative arterial changes occur in chronic diffuse inflammatory disease, but they are probably secondary although exaggerated by the hypertension that is expected to develop.

D. Renal Cortical Necrosis and Acute Tubular Necrosis

Acute tubular necrosis and renal cortical necrosis are grouped together here for purposes of discussion; acute tubular necrosis is also discussed later with Diseases of Tubules (Section V of The Kidney in this chapter). These lesions occur infrequently in animals, but may, if severe, cause acute renal failure and death. Either variety of renal necrosis is usually a manifestation of hypoperfusion, or shock, which may be classified as cardiogenic, hypovolemic, septic, or neurogenic. Outbreaks of renal cortical necrosis occur in kennels of dogs, but the causative circumstances have not been traced. Renal cortical necrosis and acute tubular necrosis occur in cattle in a variety of endotoxemic conditions, such as mastitis or metritis, and in gastrointestinal diseases, such as severe enteritis and grain overload. In horses, this often provides the fatal outcome to azoturia. Bilateral cortical necrosis is a rare complication of esophagogastric ulceration in swine, and apparently results from hemorrhagic shock.

In acute tubular necrosis, there is patchy necrosis of segments of both proximal and distal tubules with involvement also of the basement membranes; necrotic tubular epithelial cells become casts, which cause tubular blockage and oliguria. Other contributors to oliguria are tubular backleak through disrupted tubular basement membranes, compression of medullary tubules by blood vessels dilated with trapped red cells, reflex constriction of afferent arterioles, and decreased glomerular membrane permeability. In renal cortical necrosis, the whole or part of both cortices is involved, and there is destruction of both tubules and glomeruli. It appears probable that these lesions represent differences in degree and that they result from patchy or complete renal ischemia.

The usual balance between the renin–angiotensin and the eicosanoid systems that maintains fine regulation of intrarenal blood flow is disrupted during ischemia. During hypotension, perfusion of outer cortical nephrons is reduced, while perfusion of inner cortical nephrons is maintained; that is, intrarenal blood flow is redistributed toward the inner cortex and medulla. This reaction occurs because the vasoconstrictive effects of angiotensin II and adrenergic stimulation are unopposed in the outer cortex, whereas in the inner cortex, prostaglandins modulate vasoconstriction; PGE_2 is produced in the medulla in response to ischemia, travels in tubular fluid to the area of the juxtaglomerular apparatus, and has a local vasodilatory effect on afferent arterioles of juxtamedullary nephrons.

The duration of ischemia is of obvious importance for the pathogenesis of necrosis. Complete ischemia of less than 2 hr duration can be expected to be followed by good reflow if cardiac output and blood pressure are restored to normal, whereas total ischemia of longer duration may be followed by patchy reflow or complete failure of reflow in the cortex, medulla, or both. Reflow is inhibited primarily because of vascular congestion by red cells swollen by plasma water uptake, and perhaps also by ischemia-induced swelling of endothelial cells of glomeruli, vasa recta, and peritubular capillaries, and by swelling of parenchymal cells. This **no-reflow phenomenon** may make an important contribution to renal ischemia and acute renal failure.

Another mechanism by which renal cortical necrosis occurs is via the generalized Shwartzman reaction, an

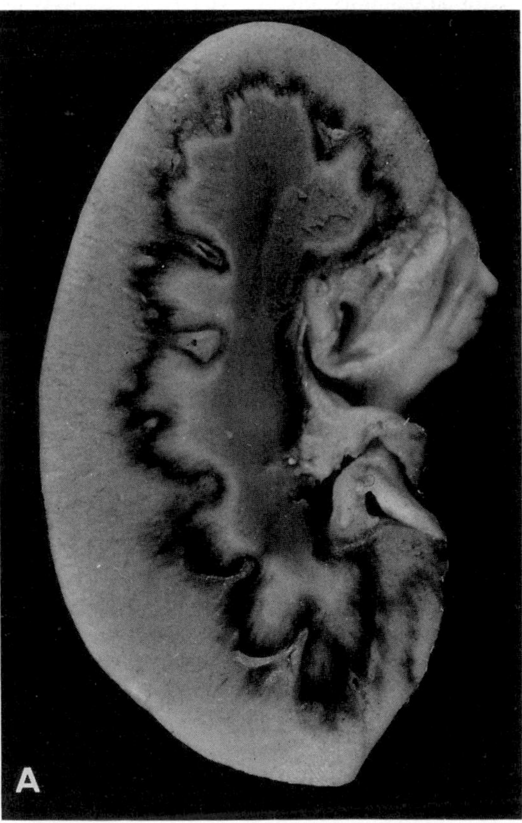

Fig. 5.15A Renal cortical necrosis. Pig. Pale cortex is delineated by hemorrhagic zone, which emphasizes the vascular supply.

example of disseminated intravascular coagulation, which is often due to Gram-negative endotoxemia. Endothelial injury in glomerular and peritubular capillaries leads to microthrombosis and hemorrhagic renal cortical necrosis. This severe degree of renal damage is usually rapidly fatal, but minimal lesions of this pathogenesis are common in a number of bacteremic diseases and visible as petechial or larger hemorrhages in the cortex.

The cellular destruction that occurs in ischemic renal injury begins with a decreased ability to produce adenosine triphosphate (ATP) and hence an increase in membrane permeability that allows influx of calcium into the cell. Excess free cytosolic calcium activates phospholipases that further increase membrane permeability and lead to membrane disruption and generation of toxic lipid by-products. Increased intracellular calcium also interferes with mitochondrial respiration and causes increased production of free radicals that further injure cell membranes and mitochondria. Unfortunately, reperfusion can be deleterious because reoxygenation increases the production of free radicals.

The gross appearance of the kidneys other than those with hemorrhagic renal necrosis varies considerably from case to case; it is probably determined by the severity, distribution, and duration of the ischemia and the quality of the reflow. In acute tubular necrosis, the cortices are finely mottled or flecked by small yellow foci of necrosis. In renal cortical necrosis, the cortices may be totally affected (Fig. 5.15A) or the injury may be patchy (Fig. 5.15B); pigs tend to develop a turkey-egg pattern marked by hemorrhagic glomeruli, but die before marked necrosis is evident, whereas cattle sometimes develop a distinctive patchy cortical necrosis (Fig. 5.16A,B). The reaction is the same as that previously described for infarction. A narrow subcapsular rim of viable tissue may remain. The affected areas of cortex are pale, almost white, slightly swollen, and stop sharply at the corticomedullary junction. The irregular areas of cortical infarction may be outlined by hemorrhage. The medulla may be normal, but in some cases, there is severe congestion of the inner stripe of the outer medulla or of the whole of the medulla so that it is swollen and resembles a blood clot.

The histologic appearance of a kidney with acute tubular necrosis includes irregular necrosis of the proximal tubules, often with disruption of the tubular basement membranes. Hyaline and granular casts may be present, particularly in distal tubules and collecting ducts. There may be interstitial edema as a result of tubular leakage. Preferential damage occurs to the pars recta and thick

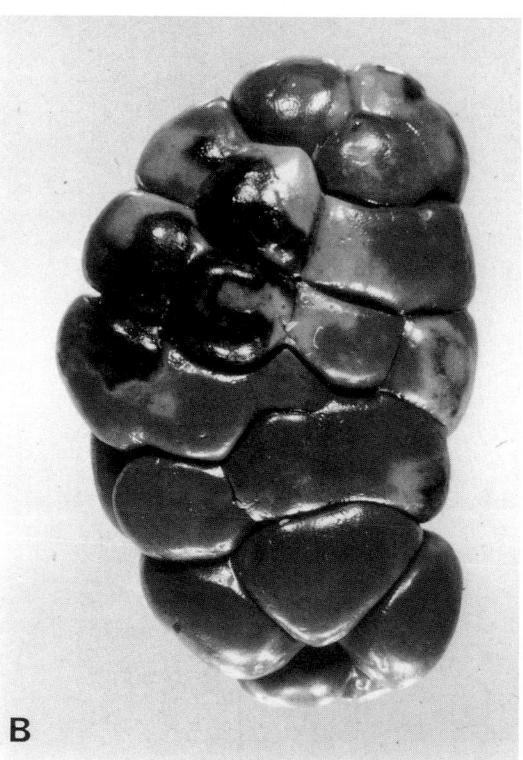

Fig. 5.15B Renal cortical necrosis. Cow. Note recent hemorrhagic and older dehemoglobinized areas of infarction.

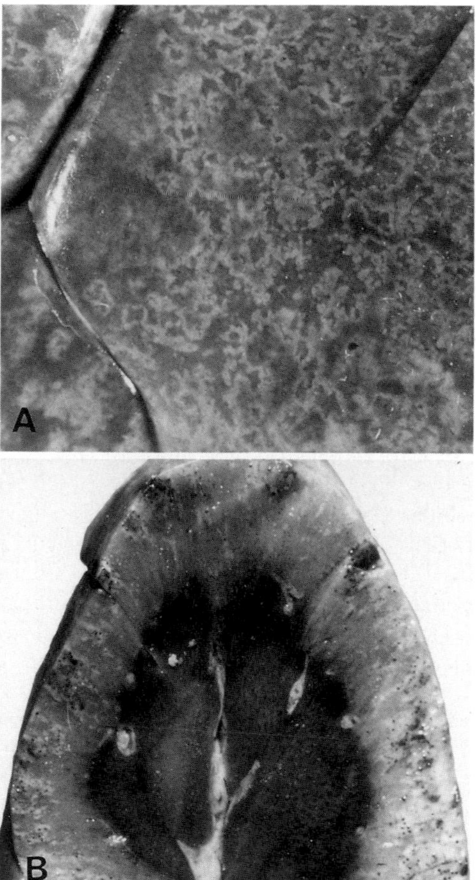

Fig. 5.16 (A) Capsular surface of kidney. Renal cortical necrosis associated with metritis and mastitis. Cow. (B) Cut surface of kidney shown in (A). Note predominance of lesions in outer cortex.

ascending limb primarily because of their location in the poorly perfused outer medulla. If the animal survives the ischemic episode, evidence of regeneration may be seen in ~1 week, namely tubules lined by flattened epithelial cells with hyperchromatic nuclei and occasional mitoses. In cases of severe ischemia and renal cortical necrosis, various patterns of infarction may be seen, with glomeruli and vessels, as well as tubules, being necrotic. Microthrombi may be seen in capillaries, and hemorrhage may be present in glomeruli. The medulla is usually preserved.

Bibliography

Bonaventre, J. V. Mediators of ischemic renal injury. *Annu Rev Med* **39:** 531–544, 1988.

Davies, D. J. The patterns of renal infarction caused by different types of temporary ischaemia. *J Pathol* **102:** 151–162, 1970.

Divers, T. J. *et al.* Acute renal failure in six horses resulting from haemodynamic causes. *Equine Vet J* **19:** 178–184, 1987.

Frega, N. S. *et al.* Ischemic renal injury. *Kidney Int* **10:** S17–S25, 1976.

Hani, H., and Indermuhle, N. A. Bilateral renal cortical necrosis associated with esophagogastric ulceration in pigs. *Vet Pathol* **17:** 234–237, 1980.

Hellberg, P. O. A., Kallskog, O., and Wolgast, M. Nephron function in the early phase of ischemic renal failure. Significance of erythrocyte trapping. *Kidney Int* **38:** 432–439, 1990.

Johnston, W. H., and Latta, H. Glomerular mesangial and endothelial cell swelling following temporary renal ischemia and its role in the no-reflow phenomenon. *Am J Pathol* **89:** 153–166, 1977.

Kreisberg, J. I. *et al.* Effects of transient hypotension on the structure and function of rat kidney. *Virchows Arch Cell Pathol* **22:** 121–133, 1976.

Mason, J. The pathophysiology of ischaemic acute renal failure. A new hypothesis about the initiation phase. *Renal Physiol* **9:** 129–147, 1986.

McDougal, W. S. Renal perfusion/reperfusion injuries. *J Urol* **140:** 1325–1330, 1988.

Montgomery, S. B. *et al.* The regulation of intrarenal blood flow in the dog during ischemia. *Circ Shock* **7:** 71–82, 1980.

Myers, B. D., and Moran, S. M. Hemodynamically mediated acute renal failure. *N Engl J Med* **314:** 97–105, 1986.

Rashid, H. A. *et al.* Renal cortical necrosis: A model for the study of juxtamedullary nephron physiology. *J Appl Physiol* **37:** 228–234, 1974.

Richman, A. V., Gerber, L. I., and Balis, J. U. Peritubular capillaries. A major target site of endotoxin-induced vascular injury in the primate kidney. *Lab Invest* **43:** 327–332, 1980.

Sheehan, H. L., and Davis, J. C. Minor renal lesions due to experimental ischaemia. *J Pathol Bacteriol* **80:** 259–270, 1960.

Stein, J. H. *et al.* Mechanism of the redistribution of renal cortical blood flow during hemorrhagic hypotension in the dog. *J Clin Invest* **52:** 39–47, 1973.

Wardle, E. N. Endotoxinaemia and the pathogenesis of acute renal failure. *Q J Med* **44:** 389–398, 1975.

E. Renal Medullary Necrosis

Under certain circumstances, medullary necrosis is the primary manifestation of renal injury. As noted, when renal hypotension occurs, cortical necrosis usually predominates due to redistribution of arterial flow to juxtamedullary nephrons. However, medullary vessels are damaged by greater than 2 hr of ischemia, and there may hence be failure of both medullary and cortical reflow after temporary ischemia, and both medullary and cortical necrosis result. In the case of venous occlusion, the elevated intrarenal blood pressure maintains the patency of lower-resistance cortical vessels but not of higher-resistance medullary vessels; hence, medullary infarction predominates.

Prostaglandin synthetase, which occurs in the kidney primarily in the medulla, may be inhibited by nonsteroidal antiinflammatory drugs (NSAIDs), such as aspirin, phenacetin, and phenylbutazone, resulting in decreased production of PGE_2 and loss of its vasodilatory effect on arterioles of juxtamedullary nephrons. This pathogenetic sequence causes the papillary necrosis characteristic of **analgesic nephropathy** in humans, and which also occurs in animals, especially in dehydrated horses treated with phenylbutazone (Fig. 5.17). Chronic interstitial nephropathy is an associated lesion in affected humans; cortical atrophy follows obstruction of collecting ducts.

Dehydration is involved in the pathogenesis of papillary necrosis in racing greyhounds. Papillary necrosis occurs in lambs and calves which are dehydrated when treated with phenothiazine, and the necrosis is again apparently

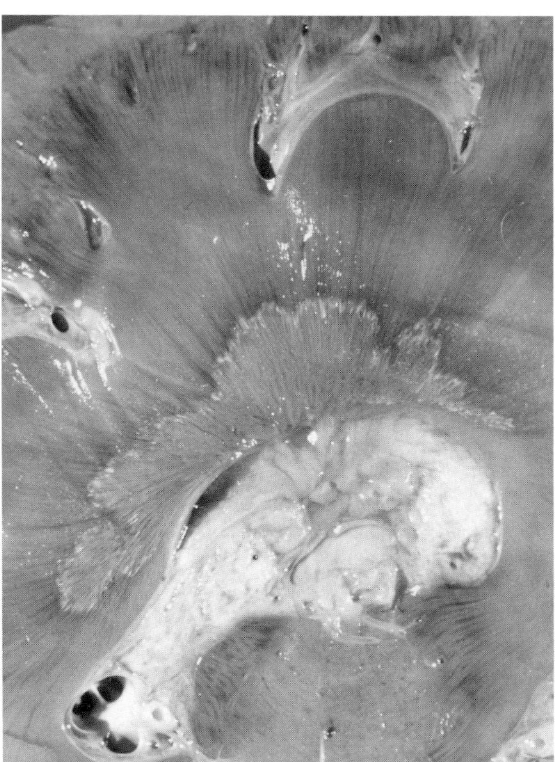

Fig. 5.17 Papillary necrosis. Horse. Lesion developed following intestinal resection and treatment with nonsteroidal antiinflammatory agents.

due to ischemia. Accidental ingestion of a combination of monensin and roxarsone has caused renal medullary necrosis in normally hydrated dogs and pups. Diabetes mellitus is not the important pathogenetic factor in animals that it appears to be in humans.

Papillary necrosis is a common consequence of urinary obstruction in animals. Pyelonephritis is also a common cause of papillary necrosis in animals, and fulminating pyelonephritic infections may produce necrosis of the papilla with scant inflammatory reaction in the early stages. The long thin-walled vessels supplying the medulla are easily occluded by compression, which could be caused by edema of the papillary interstitium alone. Compression of vessels is probably the mechanism by which amyloidosis causes papillary necrosis in cats. Deposition of amyloid mainly in the renal medulla, without or with little concomitant glomerular deposition, occurs often in cats and occasionally in cattle (see Amyloidosis, Section IV,F of The Kidney in this chapter).

The gross lesions of medullary necrosis vary greatly in their extent and stage of development (Figs. 5.17, 5.18). Acute papillary infarction may be an incidental finding in an animal dead of other causes, such as dehydration and electrolyte imbalances in neonatal diarrhea. Massive medullary infarction would no doubt be part of acute renal failure leading to death. In an animal which survives an episode of medullary necrosis, medullary scarring occurs, the papilla may slough, and secondary cortical scarring is seen. The sloughed papilla may remain in the pelvis and may become mineralized. Microscopic lesions cover the usual range of necrosis and scarring. Sequelae to medullary necrosis are based on the loss of the ability to concentrate urine, and include chronic renal failure and uremia.

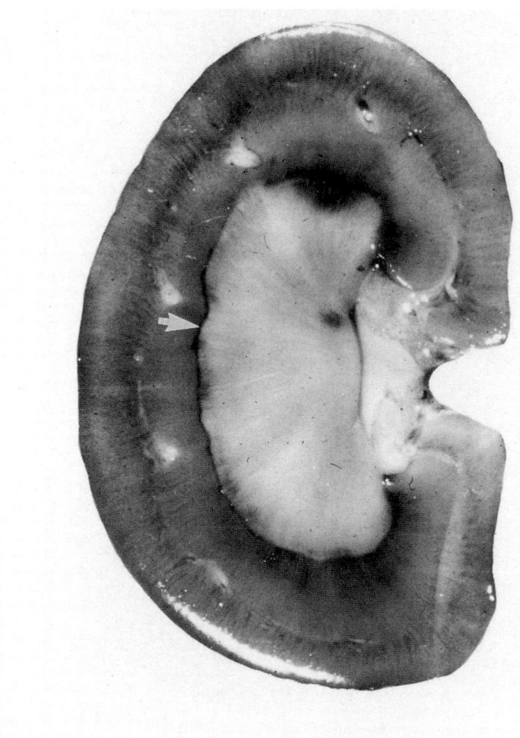

Fig. 5.18 Renal medullary necrosis. Dog. Necrotic inner zone of medulla is outlined by a thin line of hemorrhage (arrow).

Bibliography

Baum, N. H., Moriel, E. and Carlton, C. E. Renal vein thrombosis. *J Urol* **119:** 443–448, 1978.

Behm, R. J., and Berg, I. E. Hematuria caused by renal medullary crest necrosis in a horse. *Compend Cont Ed Pract Vet* **9:** 698–703, 1987.

Bennett, W. M., and DeBroe, M. E. Analgesic nephropathy—a preventable renal disease. *N Engl J Med* **320:** 1269–1271, 1989.

Duggin, G. G. Mechanisms in the development of analgesic nephropathy. *Kidney Int* **18:** 553–561, 1980.

Hazlett, M. J. *et al.* Monensin/roxarsone contaminated dog food associated with myodegeneration and renal medullary necrosis in dogs. *Can Vet J* **33:** (in press), 1992.

Lenz, S. D., and Carlton, W. W. Diphenylamine-induced renal papillary necrosis and necrosis of the pars recta in laboratory rodents. *Vet Pathol* **27:** 171–178, 1990.

Salisbury, R. M., McIntosh, I. G., and Staples, E. L. J. Mortality in lambs and cattle following the administration of phenothiazine. 2. Laboratory investigations. *N Z Vet J* **17:** 227–233, 1969.

Tobin, T. *et al.* Phenylbutazone in the horse: A review. *J Vet Pharmacol Ther* **9:** 1–25, 1986.

Wolf, D. C., Lenz, S. D., and Carlton, W. W. Renal papillary necrosis in two domestic cats and a tiger. *Vet Pathol* **28:** 84–87, 1991.

F. Hydronephrosis

Hydronephrosis is dilation of the renal pelvis and calyces associated with progressive atrophy and cystic enlargement of the kidney. The cause is some form of urinary obstruction, which may be complete or incomplete, existing at any level from the urethra to the renal pelvis. The obstruction may be caused by anomalous development of the lower urinary passages, or it may be acquired. Acquired causes include urinary calculi in any location, prostatic enlargement in the dog, cystitis especially if it is hemorrhagic, compression of the ureters by surrounding inflammatory or neoplastic tissue, displacement of the bladder in perineal hernias, and acquired urethral strictures. Depending on the site of obstruction, hydronephrosis may be unilateral or bilateral, and there may be some degree of hydroureter and dilation of the bladder.

The pathogenesis of hydronephrosis is based on the persistence of glomerular filtration in the presence of urinary obstruction, plus the development of ischemic lesions. Even with sudden complete obstruction, glomerular filtration continues, since filtrate diffuses into the renal interstitium and perirenal spaces, where it is drained by lymphatics and veins. Continued filtration creates increased pressure throughout the nephrons, collecting ducts, and calyces and pelvis, and shearing forces develop between the compressible parenchyma and the resistant connective tissues of the trabeculae. Pressure atrophy and

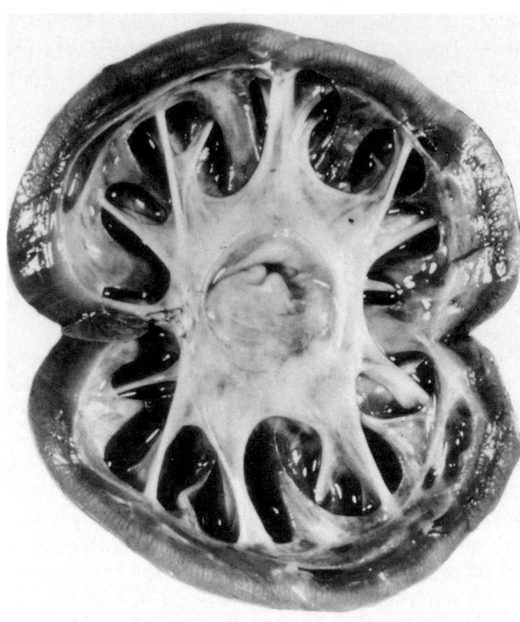

Fig. 5.19 Hydronephrosis. Sheep. Chronic lesion shows loss of medulla, cortical atrophy.

apoptosis of tubular epithelium occurs; hence, tubular function and concentrating ability diminish. As well, blood vessels are compressed, particularly hilar veins and inner medullary vessels, leading to papillary ischemia and necrosis. Glomerular filtration progressively decreases due to intrarenal vasoconstriction, and nephrons atrophy and are replaced by scar tissue.

The degree of development of hydronephrosis depends on whether or not it is bilateral, the completeness of the obstruction, and on other complications of obstruction. The development of an extensive degree of hydronephrosis requires that it be unilateral (Fig. 5.19). Bilateral obstruction, which includes obstruction localized to the bladder or urethra, results in early death from uremia. Unilateral obstruction will produce the greatest degree of hydronephrosis, especially if the obstruction is incomplete or intermittent because glomerular filtration will be little suppressed, and such kidneys may be massively enlarged. If an obstruction is removed within about 1 week, renal function returns. After about 3 weeks of complete obstruction or several months of incomplete obstruction, irreversible renal damage occurs. If hydronephrosis is unilateral, the remaining kidney, if normal, compensates adequately. Urinary stasis predisposes to infection; hence, pyelonephritis may be superimposed on hydronephrosis or vice versa.

Early gross changes consist of progressive dilation of

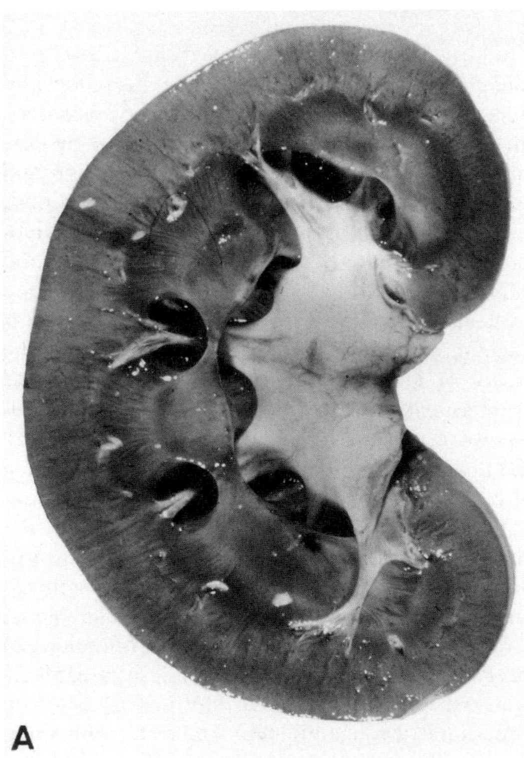

Fig. 5.20A Hydronephrosis. Sheep. Early lesion showing swollen kidney and dilation of calyces.

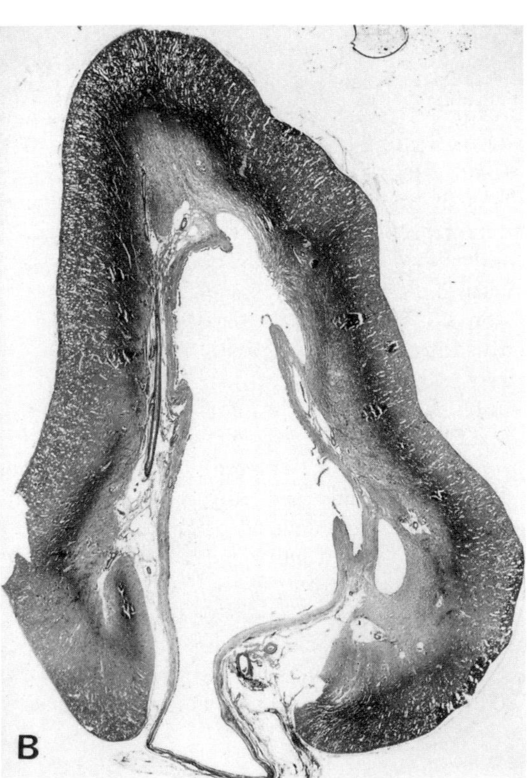

Fig. 5.20B Early hydronephrosis. Pig. Pelvis and cortical tubules are dilated. There is a discontinuous zone of congestion at corticomedullary junction.

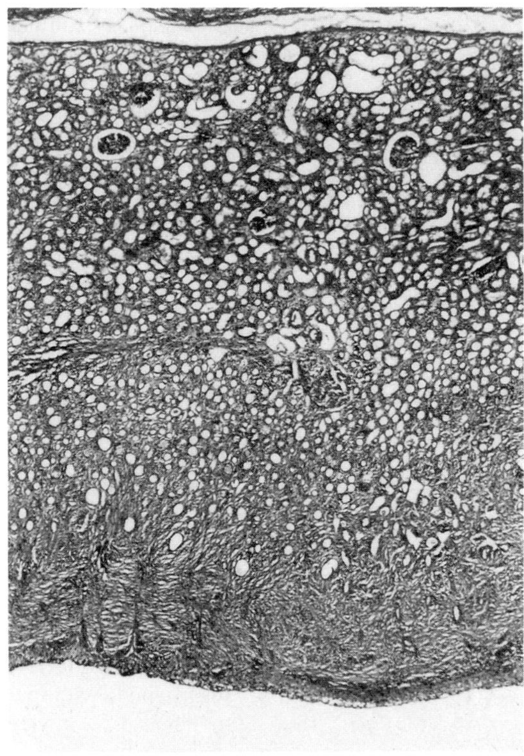

Fig. 5.21 Section through cortex and medulla of kidney with chronic hydronephrosis. Note fibrosis of medulla (below) and dilation of tubules.

the pelvis and calyces with blunting of the apices of the pyramids (Fig. 5.20A,B). Eventually these may become excavated to form multilocular cysts communicating with the pelvis and separated by an intricate series of ridges which represent original septa (Fig. 5.19). In advanced cases, the kidney may be transformed into a thin-walled sac with only a thin shell of atrophic cortical parenchyma.

The microscopic changes begin with dilation of the proximal convoluted tubules, and shortly there is dilation also of the distal and straight segments. The latter persists, with atrophy of the epithelium, but the dilation of the proximal tubules subsides; these portions then atrophy, become separated, and are replaced by light, diffuse cortical fibrosis (Fig. 5.21). The glomeruli persist for a long time, flattened and spread apart. Various degrees of ischemia up to infarction may develop patchily in the cortex if the obstruction is sudden and complete; the infarcts are venous in origin. There is progressive destruction of the pyramids by liquefaction necrosis, which spares the pelvic epithelium and tissue in a narrow zone immediately beneath. The necrotic tissue, to which there is no reaction, is liquefied and removed, and the pyramids are gradually destroyed.

Bibliography

Breitschwerdt, E. B. *et al.* Bilateral hydronephrosis and hydroureter in a dog associated with congenital urethral stricture. *J Am Anim Hosp Assoc* **18:** 799–803, 1982.

Chambers, J. N., Selcer, B. A., and Barsanti, J. A. Recovery from severe hydroureter and hydronephrosis after ureteral anastomosis in a dog. *J Am Vet Med Assoc* **191:** 1589–1592, 1987.

Gobe, G. C., and Axelsen, R. A. Genesis of renal tubular atrophy in experimental hydronephrosis in the rat. *Lab Invest* **56:** 273–281, 1987.

Greene, J. A., Thornhill, J. A., and Blevins, W. E. Hydronephrosis and hydroureter associated with a unilateral ectopic ureter in a spayed bitch. *J Am Anim Hosp Assoc* **14:** 708–713, 1978.

Hall, M. A., Osborne, C. A., and Stevens, J. B. Hydronephrosis with heteroplastic bone formation in a cat. *J Am Vet Med Assoc* **160:** 857–860, 1972.

Holmes, M. J., O'Morchoe, P. J., and O'Morchoe, C. C. C. The role of renal lymph in hydronephrosis. *Invest Urol* **15:** 215,219, 1977.

Nagle, R. B., and Bulger, R. E. Unilateral obstructive nephropathy in the rabbit. II. Late morphologic changes. *Lab Invest* **38:** 270–278,1978.

Skye, D. V. Hydronephrosis secondary to focal papillary hyperplasia of the urinary bladder of cattle. *J Am Vet Med Assoc* **166:** 596–598, 1975.

Yarger, W. E., Schocken, D. D., and Harris, R. H. Obstructive nephropathy in the rat. Possible roles for the renin–angiotensin system, prostaglandins, and thromboxanes in postobstructive renal function. *J Clin Invest* **65:** 400,412, 1980.

IV. Glomerular Disease

The specific glomerular diseases discussed here are **glomerulonephritis** and **glomerular lipidosis.** Glomeruli may also be significantly affected in a variety of systemic diseases, such as **amyloidosis,** which is also discussed, systemic lupus erythematosus, diabetes mellitus, bacterial endocarditis, and in various forms of vasculitis. Glomerular disease is of importance because, first, interference with glomerular blood flow, as well as decreasing the formation of ultrafiltrate, impairs peritubular perfusion and hence may cause loss of the entire nephron; and second, glomerular permeability may be altered, leading particularly to proteinuria. The terms glomerulonephritis (GN) and glomerulonephropathy are used interchangeably, and imply that secondary tubulointerstitial and vascular changes accompany the primary glomerular disease. The term glomerulitis is used when inflammation is restricted to glomeruli, as may occur in acute septicemias. Glomerulonephritis, which is usually of immune origin, is a common form of renal disease in domestic animals, and is a common antecedent of end-stage kidneys and renal failure, particularly in dogs and cats.

The clinical presentations of any renal disease are of limited variety, and clinicopathologic findings in animals with glomerular disease usually have no specificity. Thus, hematuria, proteinuria, oliguria, hyposthenuria, and azotemia occur in glomerular and other renal diseases; only proteinuria, occurring in the absence of urinary tract inflammation, is particularly indicative of glomerular damage, namely increased glomerular permeability. Marked proteinuria, as occurs in chronic glomerulonephritis and in amyloidosis, can lead to development of the **nephrotic**

syndrome, which as a clinical syndrome is characterized by hypoalbuminemia, generalized edema, and hypercholesterolemia; edema is less common in dogs than in humans with the nephrotic syndrome. The edema is the result of decreased plasma colloid osmotic pressure, stimulation of the renin–angiotensin–aldosterone system, and release of antidiuretic hormone in response to hypovolemia. The hepatic response to hypoproteinemia is apparently a generalized increase in production of proteins, including lipoproteins, leading to hyperlipoproteinemia and hypercholesterolemia. Proteinuria due to glomerular disease may be highly selective or poorly selective; that is, albumin or albumin plus globulins respectively appear in the urine. In summary, GN can be expressed clinically as acute or chronic renal failure, or as the nephrotic syndrome.

The following terms are generally accepted for the description of glomerular disease, and are often appended to the histologic diagnosis:

generalized, involves all glomeruli to some extent;
focal, involves only some glomeruli;
diffuse (global), involves the whole glomerulus;
segmental (local), involves only part of the glomerulus; and
mesangial, affects primarily the mesangial area.

Classification of GN in humans is relatively advanced and complex, based on extensive clinicopathologic correlations, clinical outcomes, and responses to therapy. The following simple classification system is currently in use for glomerulonephritis in domestic animals:

membranous, basement membrane thickening predominates;
proliferative, cellular proliferation predominates (Fig. 5.11);
membranoproliferative (mesangiocapillary, mesangioproliferative), both changes are present (Fig. 5.22A,B); and
glomerulosclerosis, progressive hyalinization sometimes resulting in glomerular obsolescence, in which the glomerulus is a shrunken, eosinophilic, hypocellular mass (Fig. 5.23).

Glomeruli at different stages of lesion development may occur in the same kidney, and the type of glomerular reaction may not be uniform among glomeruli.

A. Histologic Changes in Glomerulonephritis

Glomeruli commonly exhibit a spectrum of histologic changes. In view of the large renal reserve, it is important to correlate clinical and histologic findings in order to determine the clinical importance of glomerular changes. For example, in sheep and goats, GN is often generalized and well developed histologically, but is usually of little functional significance. Conversely, histologic glomerular changes may be slight, but clinical disease may be marked,

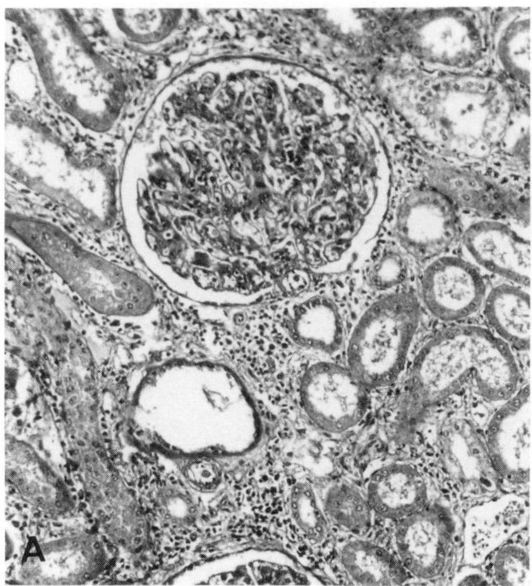

Fig. 5.22A Membranoproliferative glomerulonephritis and interstitial nephritis. Horse. Equine infectious anemia.

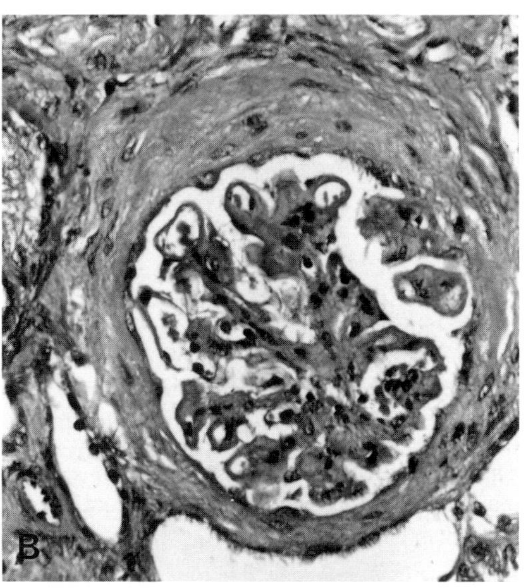

Fig. 5.22B Membranoproliferative glomerulonephritis. Dog. Marked thickening of Bowman's capsule.

as occurs in **minimal change disease,** wherein a mild ultrastructural lesion is accompanied by marked proteinuria.

Glomeruli may be nonspecifically involved in renal reactions such as renal cortical necrosis, previously discussed, and may be secondarily involved in tubulointerstitial diseases such as pyelonephritis. Septic emboli frequently lodge in the glomerular and peritubular capillary beds and cause focal glomerulitis and focal interstitial nephritis in diseases such as porcine erysipelas and in actinobacillosis of foals (Fig. 5.24A). Generalized glomerulitis, not necessarily associated with other renal change, is seen in acute septic disease and is characterized by

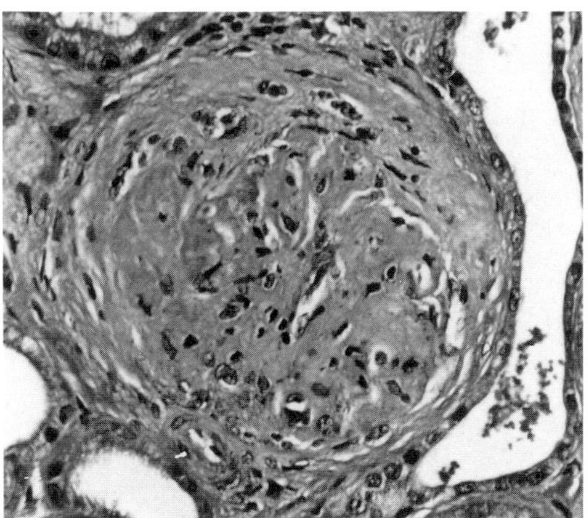

Fig. 5.23 Obsolescent glomerulus in chronic glomerulonephritis. Dog.

increased glomerular cellularity involving either or both epithelial and endothelial cells. Inclusions are common in glomerular endothelium in infectious canine hepatitis (Fig. 5.24B).

Basic inflammatory reactions of exudation, necrosis, and thrombosis occur in glomeruli as elsewhere, but some changes are typically glomerular.

Cellularity of the glomerular tuft may be increased by proliferation of endothelial, epithelial, or mesangial cells. This assessment is usually subjective. Proliferation of endothelial versus mesangial cells may be difficult to distinguish, and the term endocapillary GN is then applied. Mesangial cells in glomeruli of dogs usually occur singly or in pairs; hence, at least three mesangial cells must be in close proximity before the term mesangial hyperplasia is applied. In response to fibrin exudation into the urinary space in severe glomerular damage, monocytes invade, parietal epithelial cells proliferate, and **glomerular crescents** are formed. Some of the cells, possibly monocytes, undergo metaplasia to fibroblasts and produce collagen. In humans, crescents are most commonly seen in cases of rapidly progressive extracapillary GN, but they are indicative only of severe glomerular damage, and not pathognomonic of any one disease.

Neutrophils and monocytes may accumulate within glomerular capillaries and infiltrate the glomeruli, and may accompany cellular proliferation in GN.

The **swelling of foot processes** and their subsequent retraction is a reversible reaction of the visceral epithelial cells, and apparently occurs in response to basement membrane damage and protein leakage.

Glomerular capillary walls may be thickened in routine hematoxylin and eosin-stained sections due to endothelial or epithelial swelling and/or **thickening of the glomerular basement membrane** (GBM). The GBM itself is not visible unless special stains, such as PAS or PAS–methenamine–silver, are employed on thin (1–3 μm) sections. Electron microscopy is required to characterize

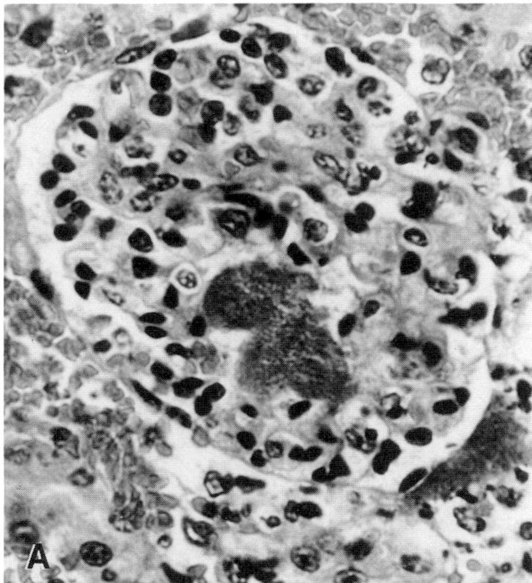

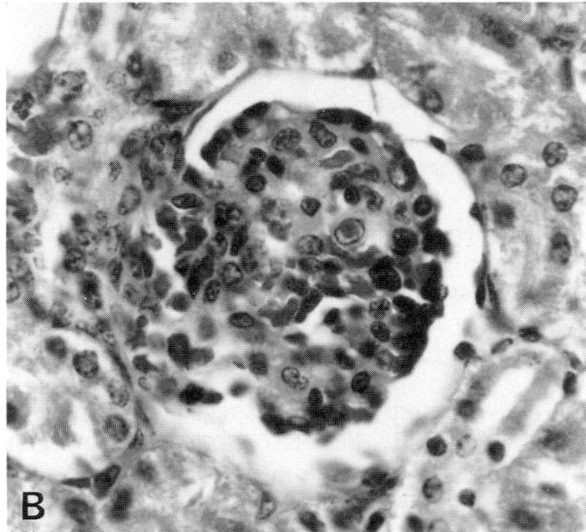

Fig. 5.24 (A) Embolic nephritis. Foal. Colonies of *Actinobacillus equuli* in glomerular and intertubular capillaries. (B) Glomerulus. Infectious canine hepatitis. Intranuclear inclusion body in endothelial cell.

properly the morphology of the thickening, which may be regular, as occurs in diabetic glomerulosclerosis, or irregular as with deposition of electron-dense material in subendothelial, intramembranous, or subepithelial (epimembranous) locations. These electron-dense deposits are usually immune complexes. Thickened peripheral capillary walls are particularly prominent in cases of membranous GN, and are referred to as wire loops; subepithelial immune complexes (humps) may become separated by projections (spikes) of basement membrane, and eventually surrounded by and incorporated within the membrane (Fig. 5.25A). This marked thickening of the GBM is somewhat paradoxically associated with marked proteinuria, probably as a result of changes in the charge and pore size of the GBM. In membranoproliferative GN, thickening of the GBM may be due to infiltration and splitting by

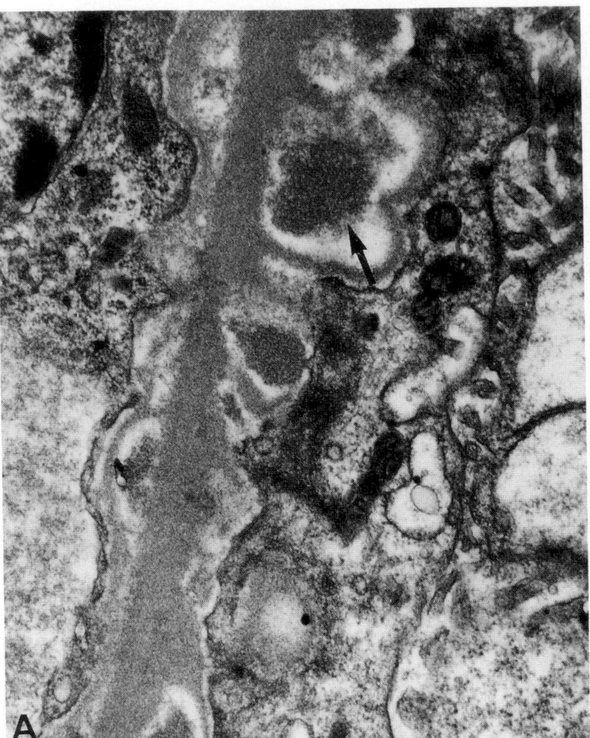

Fig. 5.25A Membranous glomerulonephritis. Dog. Dense deposits on subepithelial side of basement membrane. Some separated by spikes of membrane; others completely surrounded (arrows). (Courtesy of B. Horney.)

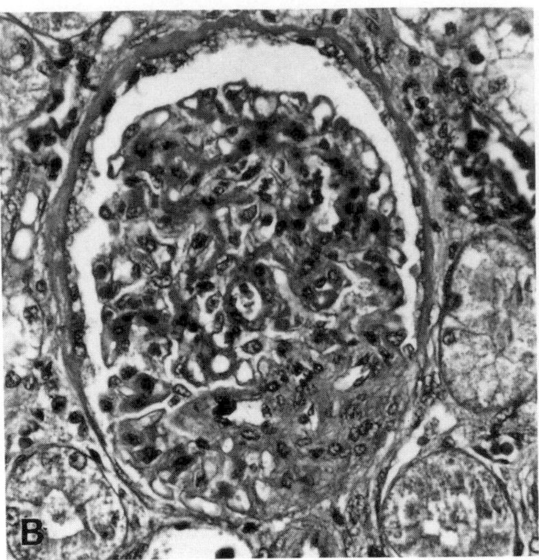

Fig. 5.25B Glomerulosclerosis and glycogen nephrosis in diabetes mellitus. Dog.

mesangial processes and matrix, and is seen with silver stains as a characteristic double-contoured glomerular basement membrane or tram-tracks, a change which is also termed reduplication.

As seen by light microscopy, **hyalinization,** or accumulation of homogeneous, eosinophilic, PAS-positive, basement membranelike material, is common in the mesangial areas in GN, especially in chronic cases. This mesangial sclerosis may be reversible but, if irreversible and progressive, may lead to obsolescence of the glomerulus. Hyaline material is commonly deposited in the mesangium in diabetes mellitus and amyloidosis; in diabetes mellitus, diffuse (Fig. 5.25B) or occasionally nodular hyaline deposits (Kimmelstiel–Wilson nodules) may be seen in glomeruli.

Thickening of Bowman's capsule may occur due to various combinations of hyperplasia of parietal epithelial cells in crescents, invasion by monocytes, thickening of the basement membrane, and periglomerular fibrosis. These changes may be particularly marked in glomerular ischemia due to vascular occlusion.

Glomerular tuft atrophy may occur subsequent to scarring, which causes tubular constriction, inhibits or stops tubular fluid flow, and causes dilation of Bowman's capsule and secondary atrophy of the glomerular tuft (glomerulocystic change).

Nonglomerular histologic changes in GN include tubular proteinuria, which is prominent in membranous GN but is most marked in glomerular amyloidosis. Other histologic changes include those of ischemic origin due to decreased glomerular, and hence efferent arteriolar and peritubular blood flow and acute and chronic interstitial inflammation. Hence, tubular atrophy, interstitial fibrosis, and scarring occur in advanced lesions, eventually producing the nonspecific histologic picture of end-stage kidney. Tubulointerstitial and glomerular damage may be coincident and due to the same mechanism rather than either one's being primary.

B. Pathogenesis of Generalized Glomerulonephritis

Glomerulonephritis may result from the deposition in glomeruli of circulating immune complexes unrelated to glomerular components, from *in situ* formation of antibodies against GBM, or from activation of the alternative pathway of complement. Some types of GN are of unknown pathogenesis. By far the most commonly identified pathogenesis of GN in domestic animals is immune-complex deposition.

In **immune-complex glomerulonephritis,** circulating nonglomerular antigen–antibody complexes localize in glomeruli and are visible by immunofluorescence or electron microscopy as granules within, or on either side of, the GBM. Causative antigens may be exogenous, e.g., serum sickness, or endogenous, e.g., nucleic acid in systemic lupus erythematosus. Immune-complex deposition may cause acute or chronic, membranous or proliferative lesions. The classical example of immune-complex GN is acute, or single-shot, serum sickness. When a large quantity of foreign protein is injected intravenously into an experimental animal, immune complexes occur in glomeruli in a characteristic lumpy-bumpy pattern as seen by

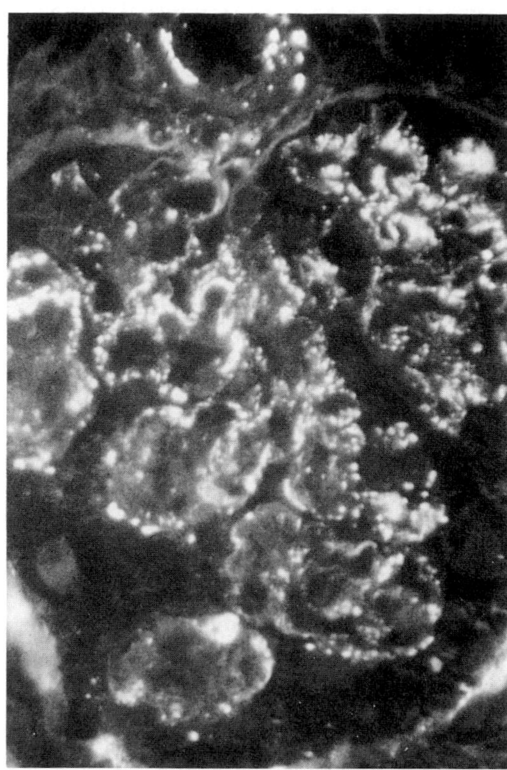

Fig. 5.26 C3 granular (lumpy-bumpy) immunofluorescence. Post-infectious glomerulonephritis. (Courtesy of B. N. Wilkie.)

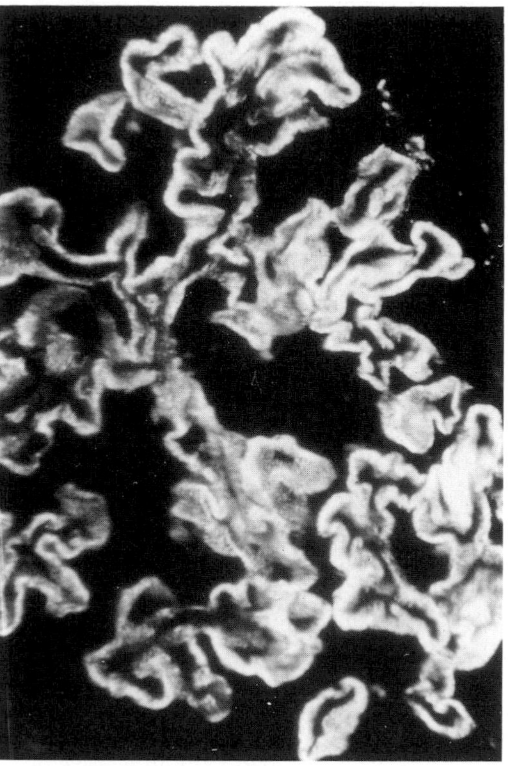

Fig. 5.27 IgG linear immunofluorescence in membranous glomerulonephritis. (Courtesy of B. N. Wilkie.)

immunofluorescence (Fig. 5.26). By electron microscopy, the complexes are seen as irregular electron-dense deposits in a subendothelial or subepithelial location or within the mesangium. The immune complexes usually contain complement as well as antigen and antibody. In general, it has been believed that immune-complex deposition, and hence glomerular damage, occurs during the period of equivalence of antigen and antibody concentrations or during slight antigen excess. An alternative view is that antigens capable of penetrating the basement membrane localize, or are planted, in a subepithelial position, and then bind antibody of low avidity. This antigen localization may be charge dependent. As well as taking part in the usual immune-complex GN, dirofilarial antigens, for example, can apparently be deposited directly in basement membrane, inducing *in situ* formation of immune complexes, and producing linear fluorescence, which is usually a characteristic of anti-GBM disease (Fig. 5.27). Candidates for planted antigens that may localize in glomeruli and result in *in situ* formation of immune complexes include viral, bacterial, and parasitic products, drugs, DNA, and large aggregated proteins, e.g., aggregated immunoglobulin G (IgG). The relative importance of circulating soluble immune complexes versus *in situ* formation of complexes in causing immune-complex GN is not resolved. Another modification of the classical soluble immune-complex disease model is that insoluble or poorly soluble complexes play a major role in subendothelial and mesangial deposit diseases.

Chronic serum sickness occurs when repeated small doses of foreign protein are given to an animal, and circulating immune complexes are continually present. This condition of continued antigenemia occurs during various microbial and parasitic infections, such as feline leukemia virus infection and canine dirofilariasis, as well as during continued release of endogenous antigens, such as nucleoprotein in systemic lupus erythematosus or tumor-specific or tumor-associated antigens.

It is not completely straightforward to ascribe the cause of GN to immune complexes since the presence of immunoglobulins and complement in a lesion does not necessarily indicate that they are responsible for the lesion; C3, C1q, and IgM are sticky molecules that may adhere to previously injured tissue. As well, the significance of circulating soluble immune complexes is controversial, since they may be present in the absence of GN and, even if present, they may be more markers for the disease than actual causative agents, since glomerular damage may be caused by various combinations of insoluble, soluble, and *in situ*-formed immune complexes. To go one step further, some investigators dispute the primary role of immune complexes in the pathogenesis of glomerulonephritis and suggest that glomeruli that have suffered primary damage by other agents, such as hydrocarbons, are then susceptible to secondary immunologic damage.

The reasons for localization of immune complexes in various glomerular sites, namely subendothelial, intramembranous, subepithelial, or mesangial, are not clear. Localization may be affected by the size, shape, charge, and chemical composition of the complexes. Thus, large complexes tend to localize in the mesangium and cause mesangiopathic GN, whereas small complexes (or antigens) penetrate the glomerular loop to produce the membranous or proliferative form. Antibody avidity may affect localization; complexes containing high-avidity antibody localize in the mesangium, whereas those with low-avidity antibody may localize subepithelially. Penetration of the basement membrane by complexes may be aided by products of inflammation, such as IgE-mediated release of histamine and serotonin from platelets and basophils, which is induced by antigen. The location of deposits may change with time; subepithelial deposits (humps) separated by spikes of GBM may become surrounded by GBM and hence become intramembranous deposits.

Modification of glomerular immune complexes occurs; they may be eliminated or may enlarge. Complexes may be eliminated by solubilization by excess antigen, phagocytosis by neutrophils, macrophages, or mesangial cells, passage through mesangial channels and egress at the vascular pole, excretion by mesangial cells through epithelial cells into the urinary space, degradation within the mesangial matrix, extracellular degradation by proteases, or by solubilization by complement. Thus, for example, removal of the source of persistent antigenemia in pyometra of dogs by ovariohysterectomy results in resolution of GN and cessation of proteinuria. Conversely, complexes may enlarge due to combination with various blood-borne reactants, such as small amounts of antigen, free antibody, immune complexes of the same or different specificity, complement components, or antibodies against immunoglobulins or complement components (immunoconglutinin or C3 nephritic factor).

In **anti-GBM glomerulonephritis,** antibodies are formed against intrinsic GBM antigens, resulting in a linear pattern of immunofluorescence reflecting the uniform distribution of immunoglobulins and complement along the GBM. There is a notable lack of dense or other deposits on electron-microscopic examination. This lesion was the first recognized immune-mediated nephritis, and was induced in rats by injection of anti-rat-kidney antibodies obtained from rabbits or ducks immunized with rat kidney tissue; this experimental model is also referred to as Masugi or nephrotoxic nephritis. Although arbitrarily separated, anti-GBM GN and immune-complex GN are not separate conditions but are actually two poles of a spectrum of immune-mediated glomerular disease. In fact, the typical linear immunofluorescence pattern of anti-GBM GN is gradually converted to the granular pattern typical of immune-complex GN with time, as linearly arrayed immune complexes become reorganized into dense aggregates in subepithelial and subendothelial locations.

Anti-GBM GN occurs as a component of Goodpasture's syndrome in humans, but occurs much less frequently than does immune-complex GN. In domestic animals, anti-GBM disease is apparently rare, having been reported in a horse and suspected, but not proved, in several dogs.

Although these descriptions of immune-complex GN and anti-GBM disease are conceptually useful, the mechanisms operative in clinical cases are often less well defined and more complex. Thus, in the well-recognized acute poststreptococcal disease in humans, factors implicated in glomerular injury include immune-complex deposition, damage by antibodies that cross-react with streptococci and GBM, activation of the alternative complement pathway, and cell-mediated reactivity to altered GBM.

C. Mechanisms of Immunologic Glomerular Injury

Several mechanisms result in glomerular injury once immune complexes are formed or deposited in glomeruli in either immune-complex GN or in anti-GBM disease. The best-established mechanism is that of complement fixation with resultant chemotaxis of neutrophils. Complement components C3a, C5a, and C567 attract neutrophils which, in the process of ingesting complexes, release lysosomal enzymes, arachidonic acid metabolites, and oxygen-derived free radicals, and hence cause GBM damage. This is the complement–leukocyte-dependent mechanism. The terminal membrane attack complex of complement, C5b-9, can damage glomeruli independent of neutrophils. Complement fragments cause release of histamine from mast cells, and hence caused increased capillary permeability, which may be important in allowing deposition of further immune complexes in the capillary wall. Since damage also occurs in the absence of complement or neutrophils, complement–neutrophil-independent mechanisms also exist, but have not been well understood. The rapidly evolving knowledge about cytokines may help to fill this void.

It is paradoxical that, although complement participates in glomerular injury, it also is capable of solubilizing immune complexes and accelerating their removal. Hence, hereditary hypocomplementemia, as occurs in Finnish Landrace lambs, may contribute to persistence of immune complexes and facilitate damage.

Interaction of complement fragments with platelets can initiate coagulation, thrombosis, and fibrinolysis; Hageman factor links the complement, coagulation, and kinin-forming systems. Fibrin and its degradation products are often present in glomeruli in GN, and fibrinogen that leaks into the urinary space is a stimulus to monocyte infiltration, proliferation of parietal epithelial cells, and crescent formation.

Monocytes play a role in glomerular damage also, especially through their interaction with mesangial cells. Monocytes may be beneficial in removing immune complexes, but may cause enzymatic damage, as do neutrophils. There is evidence that they transform to cells of fibroblastic type in glomerular crescents.

The central role of mesangial cells in production of the cellular lesions of GN is increasingly being recognized.

Mesangial cells can be stimulated to produce inflammatory mediators, including oxygen free radicals, interleukin-1, arachidonic acid metabolites, and a variety of growth factors, and may initiate GN in the absence of inflammatory cells. Macrophages and other immune cells can also release a variety of mediators, such as interleukin-1, beta-endorphin, tumor necrosis factor, and platelet-derived growth factor (PDGF), which promote growth of mesangial cells and hence increased production of mesangial matrix. Proliferating mesangial cells release autocoids, such as interleukin-1 and PDGF, producing an amplifying loop of inflammation. The growth-promoting factors are antagonized by suppressive factors such as transforming growth factor-beta. Immunomodulatory peptides released by proliferating mesangial cells stimulate replication and activation of macrophages. These activated macrophages amplify the inflammatory lesion and also phagocytize immune complexes.

Cell-mediated hypersensitivity reactions occur in some humans with progressive GN, and may help cause glomerular damage.

Cytotoxic antibodies directed against glomerular antigens may cause direct cell injury without formation of deposits. These antibodies may be directed against mesangial cell antigens, endothelial cell-surface proteins, or visceral epithelial cell glycoproteins.

In addition to the immunologic causes of glomerulonephritis previously discussed, a number of nonimmunologic causes of glomerular injury have been invoked. These include increased glomerular capillary pressure, coagulation in response to endothelial injury, serum lipid abnormalities, and glomerular hypertrophy.

D. Prevalence of Glomerulonephritis

The frequency of diagnosis of GN in domestic animals has increased dramatically recently, mostly because of increased awareness and understanding of GN by clinicians and pathologists. There may also be a real increase in prevalence caused by poorly understood factors, such as the increased use of modified live virus vaccines, which may result in persistent antigenemia and predispose to immune-complex disease. Immune complexes commonly circulate throughout life, but few individuals develop significant lesions, so various factors such as genetic susceptibility or defective immune or other mechanisms may be operative in affected animals. Many associations of infectious and other diseases with GN have been identified (Table 5.1). In essence, any infection of low pathogenicity which is able to produce persistent antigenemia has the potential to cause immune-complex disease. Most of the animal glomerulonephritides characterized to date are of immune-complex origin and of the membranoproliferative type. The morphology of the glomerular lesion is of little assistance in identifying its cause, however, since many agents cause the same type of lesion, and conversely one agent can produce a spectrum of glomerular changes. Most cases in animals are idiopathic, and hence may be referred to as primary; those occurring in association with other diseases or in which glomerular lesions contain known antigens are referred to as secondary.

TABLE 5.1

Causes of Immune-Mediated Glomerulonephritis in Domestic Animals

Viral	Canine adenovirus 1 (infectious canine hepatitis)
	Feline leukemia virus
	Feline infectious peritonitis
	Feline progressive polyarthritis
	Equine infectious anemia
	Hog cholera
	African swine fever
	Bovine virus diarrhea
	Aleutian mink disease
Bacterial	*Borrelia burgdorferi*
	Canine pyometra
	Campylobacter fetus
	Chronic pancreatitis
	Subacute valvular endocarditis
Protozoal	African trypanosomiasis
	Canine leishmaniasis
	Coccidiosis
Helminths	*Dirofilaria immitis*
Neoplasms	Various
Autoimmune	Antiglomerular basement membrane disease
	Immune-mediated hemolytic anemia
	Systemic lupus erythematosus
	Polyarteritis
Hereditary	Hypocomplementemia in Finnish Landrace lambs
	Canine familial renal disease

Associations of particular types of GN with specific clinical presentations, clinical course, and outcome are rare in veterinary medicine but common in human medicine. An exception is membranous GN, which is often associated with the nephrotic syndrome. Most other forms of GN are associated with chronic renal failure.

The prevalence and importance of GN varies with species. In general, mild glomerular lesions (hypercellularity and occasional glomerular adhesions) are common, chronic lesions leading to renal failure are less common, and the acute disease is rare.

Glomerulonephritis is a common finding in **dogs** and is a leading cause of renal failure; it is usually membranoproliferative. In canine pyometra, tubulointerstitial lesions appear to be of more significance than GN, which may be present as an age-related change rather than as a product of pyometra.

In **cats,** GN is common, is predominantly membranous, and is a major cause of the nephrotic syndrome and/or renal failure.

In **horses,** GN is fairly common, but renal failure is rare. Glomerulonephritis often occurs in horses with equine infectious anemia (Fig. 5.22A), and the renal lesions may be important. *Streptococcus equi* and herpesvirus infections are suggested as causes of GN in horses.

Acute fatal GN occurs sporadically in **swine,** but is of little economic importance. Mesangial hyaline droplet formation and mesangiolysis are common in the glomeruli of pigs with mastocytosis. Deposition of immune complexes containing IgG and C3 is common in the mesangium of normal slaughter swine, but the mesangioproliferative GN is not of clinical significance.

In **ruminants,** immunologic evidence of GN is common, but clinical disease is not. Glomeruli of sheep and goats are often hypercellular and have membranous changes, but the changes appear to have little clinical significance. An interesting exception is the membranoproliferative GN of **Finnish Landrace sheep,** which is present at birth, and is characterized by recessive inheritance of a deficiency of the complement component C3; in affected lambs, blood levels of C3 are about 5% of normal. This congenital deficiency contributes to the development of membranoproliferative (mesangiocapillary) GN, probably owing to impaired complement-mediated solubilization of immune complexes in glomeruli. Affected lambs are clinically normal at birth, but die between 1 and 3 months of age because of renal failure. At autopsy, the kidneys are enlarged, have pale cortices and glomeruli, which are grossly visible as red spots. The glomerular lesion is characterized by mesangial proliferation, capillary wall thickening, and often by the formation of glomerular crescents. Subendothelial electron-dense deposits are present and consist of C3, smaller amounts of IgM and IgA and, with prolonged survival, progressively larger amounts of IgG; this pattern resembles type I membranoproliferative GN of humans. Glomerular changes begin in the lambs *in utero* and develop progressively after birth. Choroid plexus lesions also occur due to immune-complex deposition, and lead to encephalopathy.

E. Morphology of Glomerulonephritis

Acute GN may not significantly alter the gross appearance of the kidney, which may be slightly or markedly enlarged, pale, soft, and edematous. The glomeruli may be visible as fine red dots. Petechial hemorrhages may be visible if bleeding has occurred from the inflamed glomeruli. In **subacute GN,** the kidney is enlarged, perhaps greatly, and pale with a smooth surface and nonadherent capsule (there may be numerous cortical petechiae indicating recurrent acute episodes). The capsule is tense, and the cut surface bulges; the cortex is wide and yellow-gray, which demarcates it from a normal-colored medulla. This subacute phase is anatomically and developmentally arbitrary and grades into the **chronic** phase, in which the kidney is shrunken and contracted with a generalized fine granularity of the capsular surface (Fig. 5.28). The capsule may be adherent. On the cut surface, the cortex is rather uniformly narrowed, and corticomedullary markings are obscured. Fine cysts may be present, developed from obstructed tubules. This stage when contraction is severe is grossly indistinguishable from chronic interstitial nephritis. It can usually be distinguished from the end result of pyelonephritis, which tends to produce more irregular contraction and scarring, often with intervening areas of normal parenchyma.

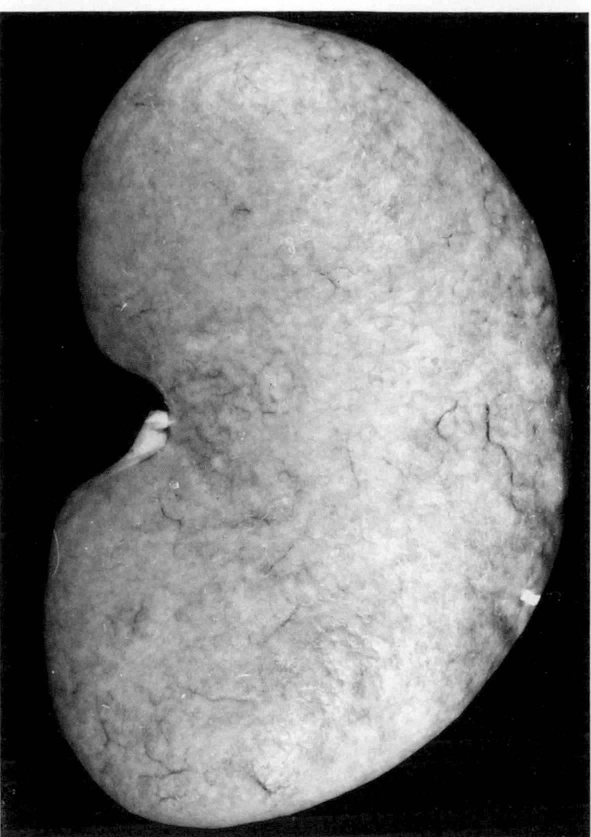

Fig. 5.28 Pale granular kidney of subacute–chronic glomerulonephritis. Dog.

The **histologic features of the acute phase** are those of exudative inflammation. Initially hyperemic, the glomeruli soon become ischemic as a result of edematous thickening of the capillary walls and swelling of endothelial and epithelial cells. Neutrophils marginate in the capillaries and, with the swollen and proliferated native cells of the glomerulus, give a distinct impression of hypercellularity. The tuft swells and occupies most of the capsular space; any remaining space may contain migrated leukocytes, precipitated protein, or extravasated erythrocytes. Occasionally, fibrin thrombi form in the capillaries and cause focal necrosis and hemorrhage into the capsular space (Fig. 5.29A,B). This form of hemorrhagic GN with the formation of fibrin thrombi is the usual picture seen in swine with petechial hemorrhages as a gross manifestation. Concomitantly, interstitial edema develops. The tubular epithelium may contain hyaline droplets; casts of protein, erythrocytes, and leukocytes form in the urine.

Although functional changes vary greatly, some can be anticipated. The swelling and resultant ischemia of the glomeruli reduce filtration so that there is oliguria. The concentrating capacity of the tubules is unimpaired, as

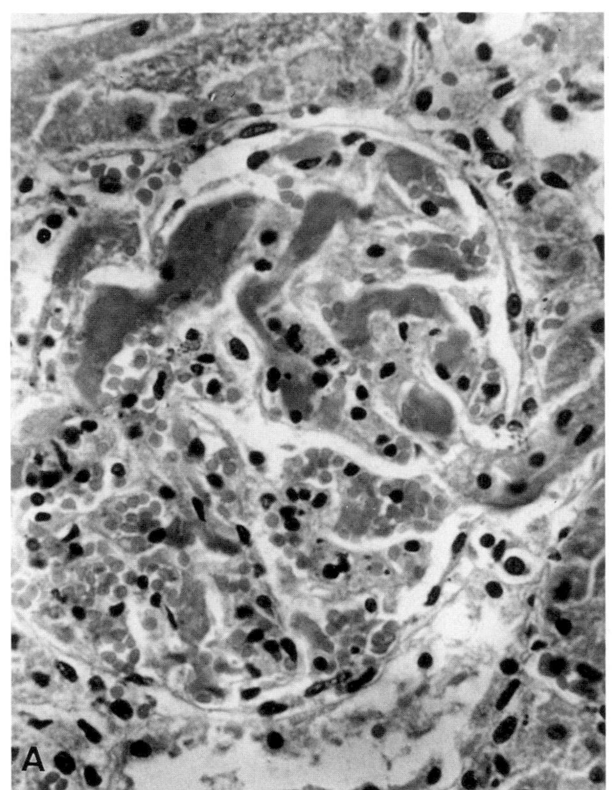

Fig. 5.29A Fibrinoid thrombi in glomerular capillaries. Calf. Colisepticemia.

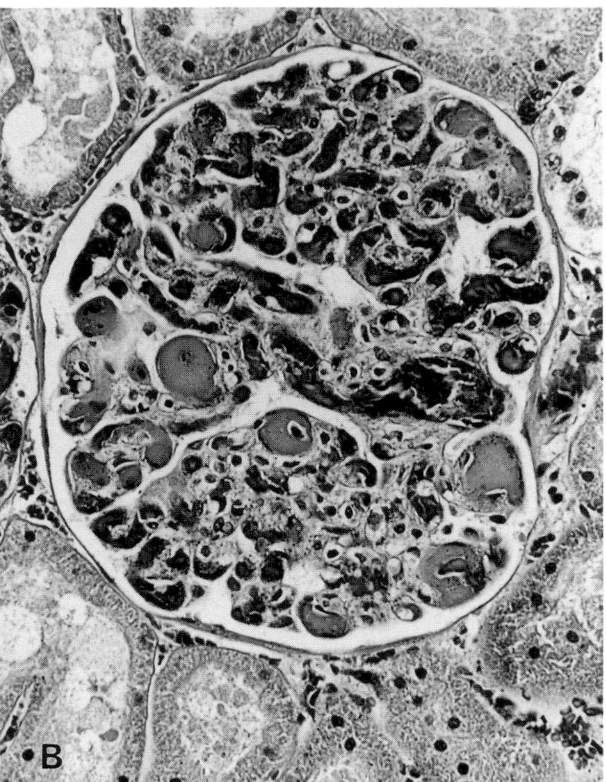

Fig. 5.29B Fallow deer, adult male. Pale-staining glomerular hyaline thrombi. Disseminated intravascular coagulation (epizootic hemorrhagic disease). (Slide courtesy of F. Leighton.)

yet, so the urine is of high specific gravity. It also contains protein, and hyaline, granular, and red-cell casts.

In the **subacute phase,** either mesangial hyperplasia or glomerular crescent formation may predominate. Fatty degeneration of the tubular epithelium may occur in this stage, as may hyaline droplet formation or necrosis. Casts of protein, leukocytes, and necrotic epithelial cells are present in the tubules.

In the **chronic** phase, fibrous scarring of glomeruli occurs. There may be a reduction in the apparent number of glomeruli as sclerotic glomeruli blend with surrounding scar tissue. If the original proliferative phase was mesangial, scarification may obliterate the tufts, transforming them to large or small masses of collagen and preserving the capsular space. If the proliferation was initially epithelial, fibrosis may completely obliterate the capsular space but, since the two forms usually coexist, obliteration of both glomerulus and capsule is usual. Although all glomeruli are usually involved, the degree varies somewhat, so that many retain some function. The interstitial reaction initiated during the edematous exudative phase develops prominently with fibrosis and lymphocytic infiltration. Large numbers of tubules undergo disuse, ischemic, or pressure atrophy and are replaced by scar tissue, and the fibrosis becomes slowly self-perpetuating. Tubules that remain connected to functioning glomeruli may become dilated and develop epithelial hypertrophy and hyperplasia; these are in part responsible for the fine granularity of the surface and streakiness of the cut surface.

In chronic GN at the stage of decompensated renal failure, there is an increased volume of urine with a fixed, low specific gravity. Albuminuria may be only slight, and casts may be absent. Death occurs in uremia. Acute GN does not inevitably lead to fatal chronic GN. In fact, healed mild glomerular lesions with full renal function are much more common than debilitating or fatal chronic generalized GN. The only evidence of previous injury may be mild mesangial sclerosis and the presence of occasional small adhesions between peripheral capillary loops and the parietal epithelium.

Once the glomerular filtration rate has decreased to 30–50% of normal, progression to end-stage renal failure tends to be inexorable. This sequence is thought to occur partly because of continuation of the primary glomerular condition, partly because of addition of complicating factors such as hypertension, and perhaps partly because of adaptive changes in glomeruli in a failing kidney. These adaptive changes include hypertrophy and glomerular capillary hypertension, with resulting epithelial and endothelial injury and proteinuria. Mesangial cells respond by hyperplasia and by production of extracellular matrix; combined with intraglomerular coagulation, this response leads to glomerulosclerosis. A proposed common determinant of glomerulosclerosis is a sustained increase in glomerular permeability to macromolecules. In any case, these further reductions of renal mass contribute to a vicious cycle of continuing glomerulosclerosis.

Bibliography

Arthur, J. E. *et al.* The long-term prognosis of feline idiopathic membranous glomerulonephropathy. *J Am Anim Hosp Assoc* **22:** 731–737, 1986.

August, J. R., and Leib, M. S. Primary renal diseases of the cat. *Vet Clin North Am: Small Anim Pract* **14:** 1247–1260, 1984.

Benderitter, T. *et al.* Glomerulonephritis in dogs with canine leishmaniasis. *Ann Trop Med Parasitol* **82:** 335–341, 1988.

Bruijn, J. A., Hoedemaeker, P. J., and Fleuren, G. J. Pathogenesis of anti-basement membrane glomerulopathy and immune-complex glomerulonephritis: Dichotomy dissolved. *Lab Invest* **61:** 480–488, 1989.

Cohen, A. H. Morphology of renal tubular hyaline casts. *Lab Invest* **44:** 280–287, 1981.

Couser, W. G. Mechanisms of glomerular injury in immune-complex disease. *Kidney Int* **28:** 569–583, 1985.

Crowell, W. A., Duncan, J. R., and Finco, D. R. Canine glomeruli: Light- and electron-microscopic change in biopsy, perfused, and *in situ* autolysed kidneys from normal dogs. *Am J Vet Res* **35:** 889–896, 1974.

Dore, M., Morin, M., and Gagnon, H. Proliferative glomerulonephritis leading to nephrotic syndrome in a cow. *Can Vet J* **28:** 40–41, 1987.

Emancipator, S. N., and Lamm, M. E. IgA nephropathy: Pathogenesis of the most common form of glomerulonephritis. *Lab Invest* **60:** 168–183, 1989.

Frelier, P. F., Armstrong, D. L., and Pritchard, J. Ovine mesangiocapillary glomerulonephritis type I and crescent formation. *Vet Pathol* **27:** 26–34, 1990.

Grauer, G. F. *et al.* Renal lesions associated with *Borrelia burgdorferi* infection in a dog. *J Am Vet Med Assoc* **193:** 237–239, 1988.

Grauer, G. F. *et al.* Experimental *Dirofilaria immitis*-associated glomerulonephritis induced in part by *in situ* formation of immune complexes in the glomerular capillary wall. *J Parasitol* **75:** 585–593, 1989.

Hayashi, T., Ishida, T., and Fujiwara, K. Glomerulonephritis associated with feline infectious peritonitis. *Jpn J Vet Sci* **44:** 909–916, 1982.

Jaenke, R. S., and Allen, T. A. Membranous nephropathy in the dog. *Vet Pathol* **23:** 718–733, 1986.

Jeraj, K. P. *et al.* Immune complex glomerulonephritis in a cat with renal lymphosarcoma. *Vet Pathol* **22:** 287–290, 1985.

Jergens, A. E. Glomerulonephritis in dogs and cats. *Compend Cont Ed Pract Vet* **9:** 903–911, 1987.

Kashgarian, M., Hayslett, J. P., and Spargo, B. H. Renal disease. *Am J Pathol* **89:** 187–272, 1977.

Koeman, J. P., Biewenga, W. J., and Gruys, E. Proteinuria in the dog: A pathomorphological study of 51 proteinuric dogs. *Res Vet Sci* **43:** 367–378, 1987.

Kurtz, J. M. *et al.* Naturally occurring canine glomerulonephritis. *Am J Pathol* **67:** 471–482, 1972.

Leifer, C. E. *et al.* Proliferative glomerulonephritis and chronic active hepatitis with cirrhosis associated with *Corynebacterium parvum* immunotherapy in a dog. *J Am Vet Med Assoc* **190:** 78–80, 1986.

MacDougall, D. F. *et al.* Canine chronic renal disease: Prevalence and types of glomerulonephritis in the dog. *Kidney Int* **29:** 1144–1151, 1986.

MacIver, A. G. Diagnosis and classification of primary glomerulonephritis: A review. *Diagn Histopathol* **5:** 231–281, 1982.

Magil, A. B. Histogenesis of glomerular crescents. Immunohistochemical demonstration of cytokeratin in crescent cells. *Am J Pathol* **120:** 222–229, 1985.

Majid, H. N., and Winter, H. Glomerulonephritis in lambs with coccidiosis. *Aust Vet J* **63:** 314–316, 1986.

McCluskey, R. T. Modification of glomerular immune complex deposits. *Lab Invest* **48:** 241–244, 1983.

Nash, A. S., Mohammed, N. A., and Wright, N. G. Experimental immune complex glomerulonephritis and the nephrotic syndrome in cats immunised with cationised bovine serum albumin. *Res Vet Sci* **49:** 370–372, 1990.

Olson, J. L., and Heptinstall, R. H. Nonimmunologic mechanisms of glomerular injury. *Lab Invest* **59:** 564–578, 1988.

Ravnskov, U. Nonsystemic glomerulonephritis: Exposure to nephro- and immunotoxic chemicals predispose to immunologic harassment. *Med Hypotheses* **30:** 115–122, 1989.

Remuzzi, G., and Bertani, T. Is glomerulosclerosis a consequence of altered glomerular permeability to macromolecules? *Kidney Int* **38:** 384–394, 1990.

Shirota, K., and Nomura, Y. Ultrastructure of glomerulopathy in swine. *Jpn J Vet Sci* **50:** 1–8, 1988.

Shirota, K. *et al.* Glomerulopathy in a cat with cyanotic congenital heart disease. *Vet Pathol* **24:** 280–282, 1987.

Stone, E. A. *et al.* Renal dysfunction in dogs with pyometra. *J Am Vet Med Assoc* **193:** 457–464, 1988.

Stuart, B. P., Phemister, R. D., and Thomassen, R. W. Glomerular lesions associated with proteinuria in clinically healthy dogs. *Vet Pathol* **12:** 125–144, 1975.

Taboada, J., and Palmer, G. H. Renal failure associated with bacterial endocarditis in the dog. *J Am Anim Hosp Assoc* **25:** 243–251, 1989.

Tamura, T. *et al.* Mesangial hyaline droplet formation and mesangiolysis in the renal glomeruli seen in pigs with mastocytosis. *Jpn J Vet Sci* **48:** 1183–1189,1986.

Tornroth, T., and Skrifvars, B. The development and resolution of glomerular basement membrane changes associated with subepithelial immune deposits. *Am J Pathol* **79:** 219–236, 1975.

Veis, J. H. *et al.* The biology of mesangial cells in glomerulonephritis. *Proc Soc Exp Biol Med* **195:** 160–167, 1990.

Wardle, E. N. Cytokine growth factors and glomerulonephritis. *Nephron* **57:** 257–261, 1991.

White, M. R., Crowell, W. A., and Blue, J. L. A nephrotic-like syndrome with an associated mesangioproliferative glomerulopathy in a cow. *Vet Pathol* **23:** 439–442, 1986.

Wilkinson, J. E. *et al.* Fibrillary deposits in glomerulonephritis in a horse. *Vet Pathol* **22:** 647–649, 1985.

F. Amyloidosis

Amyloidosis is a systemic disease in which amyloid, an eosinophilic, homogeneous, hyaline material, is deposited in the walls of small blood vessels and extracellularly in a variety of sites, particularly in renal glomeruli. Amyloidosis has been referred to as a final common pathway for protein deposition in various tissues in a variety of conditions. The most common forms of amyloidosis are **immunocytic** (primary), in which case **amyloid AL** is produced from immunoglobulin light chains in plasma cell dyscrasias, or **reactive systemic** (secondary), in which **amyloid AA** is derived from serum amyloid A (SAA) protein, an acute-phase immunoregulant product of hepatic and other cells that is produced in excess as a result of chronic antigenic stimulation. In addition, various **hereditary** forms exist in humans. Commonly associated with amyloid is amyloid P component, a member of the family of proteins known as pentraxins.

Most cases of amyloidosis in domestic animals are idiopathic, but appear to be of the reactive systemic type. The deposits of amyloid may be found in many organs and may be concentrated in one or other of them, such as the liver or spleen, but the kidney is the organ most commonly involved in amyloidosis. Localization of amyloid is usually glomerular, but medullary localization predominates often in Shar-Pei dogs, in cats, in Dorcas gazelles, and occasionally in cattle.

Amyloidosis is most common in older **dogs** and is usually idiopathic, although some cases do occur in association with chronic suppurative and granulomatous lesions in other tissues; affected dogs develop progressive renal insufficiency and proteinuria, which may be sufficiently severe to cause the nephrotic syndrome. Dogs with medullary amyloidosis without glomerular involvement may have little or no proteinuria. Amyloidosis is less common in **cats** than in dogs, and marked proteinuria is a less prominent finding. In **cattle,** glomerular amyloidosis can cause severe proteinuria; medullary amyloidosis is reported as a common subclinical disease. A chronic suppurative or tissue-destructive process is occasionally demonstrable in affected cattle. Amyloidosis occurs in **horses** used for antiserum production; **pigs** rarely develop amyloidosis.

With small deposits of amyloid, the gross appearance of the kidney may be normal except for a slight increase in size and a peculiar translucence of the glomeruli. The characteristic renal change is one of paleness, enlargement, and increase in consistency. In cattle, the kidneys may be very large. The capsule strips smoothly to reveal a cortical surface with a finely stippled appearance due to numerous fine yellow spots, which are glomeruli, and gray points of translucence, which are dilated tubules. On cut surface, the cortex is widened and presents the same appearance as the capsular surface, rather like pumice stone. Affected glomeruli stain brown-red when exposed to an iodine solution; subsequent exposure to dilute sulfuric acid changes the color to purple (Fig. 5.30).

Histologically, amyloid is first deposited in the mesangial area and in the subendothelium of glomerular capillaries. Nodules of amyloid gradually develop until the glomeruli, when uniformly involved, are enlarged and converted to homogeneous spheres with loss of endothelial and epithelial nuclei (Fig. 5.31A). Similarly, amyloid is deposited in tubular basement membranes, and eventually broad cuffs of amyloid appear around the tubules. The physical presence of amyloid causes ischemia and pressure atrophy of nephrons, and resultant scarring. The tubules contain a striking number of pink hyaline casts of protein and are dilated, sometimes to such an extent that normal renal structure is not recognized (thyroidization) (Fig. 5.31B). Urinalysis reveals a high level of protein, and the loss of protein from this source may cause hypoproteinemic edema. The amyloidotic kidney, especially when medullary amyloidosis predominates, may have various of the features of end-stage renal disease, including interstitial fibrosis and lymphoplasmacytic infiltration, tu-

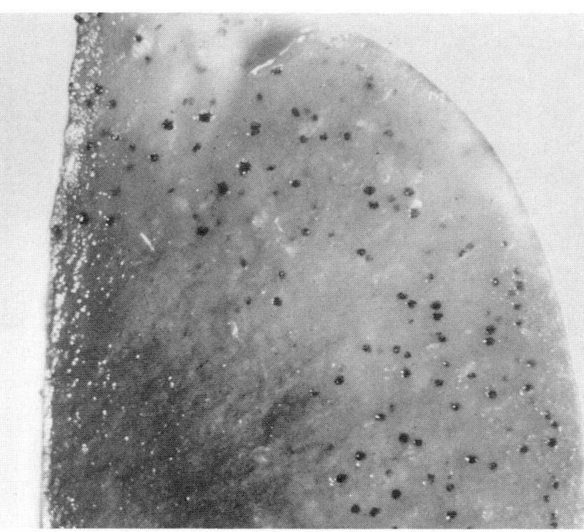

Fig. 5.30 Amyloidosis. Cow. Glomeruli are prominent after exposure to iodine, then dilute sulfuric acid.

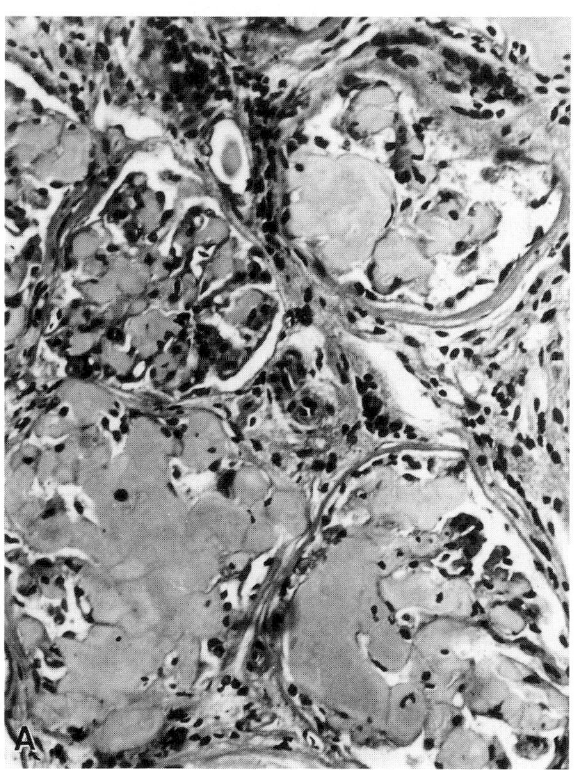

Fig. 5.31A Amyloidosis. Dog. Severe lesions in glomeruli have caused atrophy of tubules and aggregation of tufts.

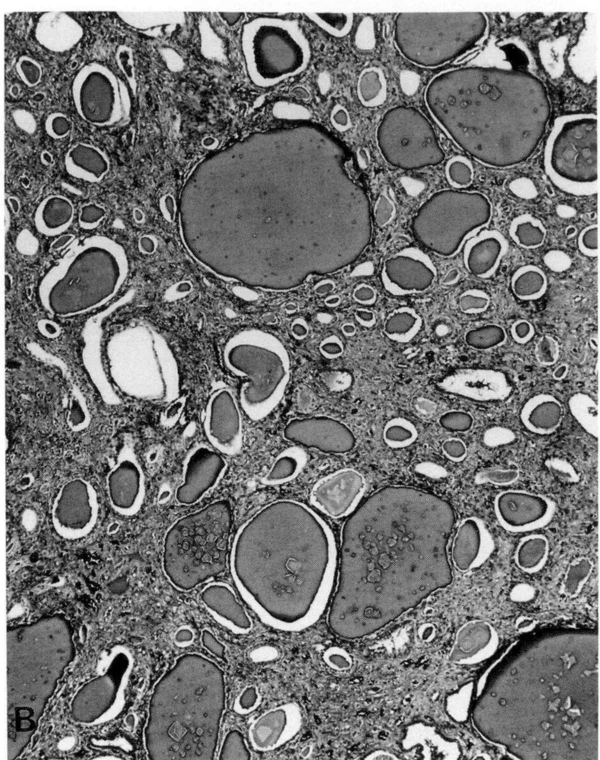

Fig. 5.31B Sow. Marked proteinuria thyroidization in medulla. Glomerulosclerosis. (Slide courtesy of D. Johnson.)

bular atrophy, tubular dilation, mineralization, intratubular deposition of oxalate crystals, glomerular atrophy, and glomerulosclerosis.

Thrombosis of the pulmonary arteries or renal veins is occasionally a prominent finding in dogs with the nephrotic syndrome due to amyloidosis; they are in a hypercoagulable state due to stimulation of production of acute-phase proteins, such as fibrinogen, while simultaneously losing low-molecular-weight anticoagulants, such as antithrombin III, because of increased glomerular permeability.

The **cat** differs somewhat from other species, in that amyloid is deposited mainly in the papilla and outer medulla, with relative sparing of the glomeruli. The kidneys are very firm, shrunken, and coarsely nodular. The papilla, in cats dying in renal failure, is necrotic, or excavated in some that survive. The nodularity is due to scarring extending from medulla to capsular surface. The capillary and tubular basement membranes in the medulla are thick and hyaline, and this is presumed to produce capillary occlusion with papillary necrosis on the one hand, and occlusion of collecting ducts with obstructive atrophy and fibrosis in the medullary rays on the other. The prevalence of amyloidosis in cats is much increased on diets providing excess vitamin A (see Bones and Joints, Volume 1, Chapter 1).

Amyloid is nonspecifically eosinophilic in routine sections and weakly birefringent in polarized light. The diagnosis is thus usually confirmed with special stains. Amyloid is stained a light orange-red with Congo red, and then exhibits green birefringence in polarized light; elimination of the Congo red staining affinity of amyloid by oxidation of tissue sections in potassium permanganate indicates that the amyloid is of the AA type. Amyloid exhibits a bright yellow fluorescence after staining with thioflavine-T, which may be required in cats because of poor staining of amyloid with Congo red in this species. These staining patterns of amyloid are due to its characteristic beta-pleated pattern, which also confers on it resistance to proteolysis and insolubility, and hence its resistance to removal from tissues. The characteristic nonbranching 10–15 nm diameter fibrils of amyloid may be seen by electron microscopy. Because all amyloid fibrils have a β-pleated sheet structure, the term β-fibrilloses has been proposed as a more appropriate description of amyloid deposits and amyloidosis.

Bibliography

DiBartola, S. P., and Benson, M. D. The pathogenesis of reactive systemic amyloidosis. *J Vet Intern Med* **3:** 31–41, 1989. (review)

DiBartola, S. P. *et al.* Familial renal amyloidosis in Chinese Shar-Pei dogs. *J Am Vet Med Assoc* **197:** 483–487, 1990.

Kim, D. H. *et al.* Light- and electron-microscopic observations on bovine amyloid-laden kidneys. *Jpn J Vet Sci* **46:** 633–639, 1984.

Rideout, B. A. *et al.* Renal medullary amyloidosis in Dorcas gazelles. *Vet Pathol* **26:** 129–135, 1989.

Stone, M. J. Amyloidosis: A final common pathway for protein deposition in tissues. *Blood* **75:** 531–545, 1990. (review)

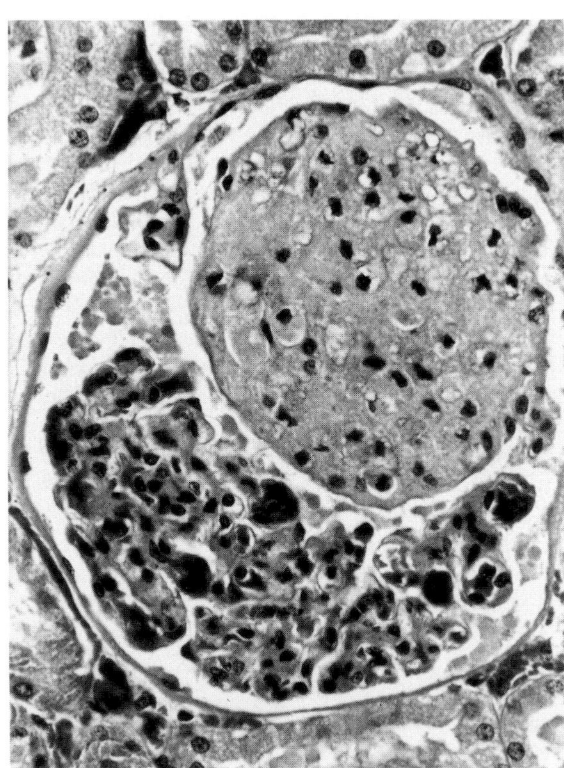

Fig. 5.32 Glomerular lipidosis. Dog.

G. Glomerular Lipidosis

Large foam cells, which by appropriate techniques are seen to contain sudanophilic droplets, may be found in one or more lobules of glomerular tufts in many dogs (Fig. 5.32). In paraffin preparations, the cells are closely packed and finely vacuolated, and the cell boundaries are distinct. These large cells appear to arise from mesangial cells. This lesion is not associated with glomerulonephritis and has no functional significance.

Lipid embolization of renal arterioles and glomerular capillaries occurs occasionally in dogs with diabetes mellitus or following trauma. The lipid in these cases is intravascular rather than within foam cells.

Bibliography

Brown, T. P., and Fitzpatrick, R. K. Glomerular lipid emboli in a diabetic dog. *Vet Pathol* **23:** 209–211, 1986.

Zayed, I. *et al.* A light and electron microscopical study of glomerular lipoidosis in beagle dogs. *J Comp Pathol* **86:** 509–517, 1976.

V. Diseases of Tubules

Diseases of tubules are primarily reflected in morphologic changes in lining epithelial cells, although specific defects of function due to enzyme deletions may not have a morphologic representation. Degenerations are best regarded as homeostatic disturbances of intracellular functions which may become balanced at new levels or be sufficiently severe that the cell or part of it dies. As previously noted, the tubules and interstitium are intimately associated, and damage to one affects the other; thus, many disorders are termed tubulointerstitial diseases and are discussed later. Regeneration of tubular epithelium can occur (Fig. 5.33A,B), but postnatal development of new nephrons is limited to a short period, depending on species. The response of the kidney to destruction of tubules is limited to compensatory hypertrophy of remaining nephrons. Thus, the tubules remaining in damaged kidneys are often large and dilated.

Degeneration and swelling of tubular cells cause the kidney to enlarge and bulge on cut surface. Hydropic degeneration occurs due to damage to mitochondrial membranes and formation of vacuoles, and is potentially reversible. Necrotic tubular cells are eosinophilic, have pyknotic nuclei, and slough into the tubular lumen where they are seen as cellular or coarsely granular casts (Figs. 5.33A, 5.34A,B). Tubules filled with proteinaceous fluid usually indicate that there is increased glomerular permeability in that nephron; extreme proteinuria may indicate the presence of the nephrotic syndrome clinically. Tamm–Horsfall mucoprotein, which is produced in the ascending limb of the loop of Henle and the distal tubules, and/or autolytic tubular epithelial cytoplasm may appear as a granular pink substance in many cortical tubules, but this is not a lesion. Hyaline droplets, which are pink homogeneous globules

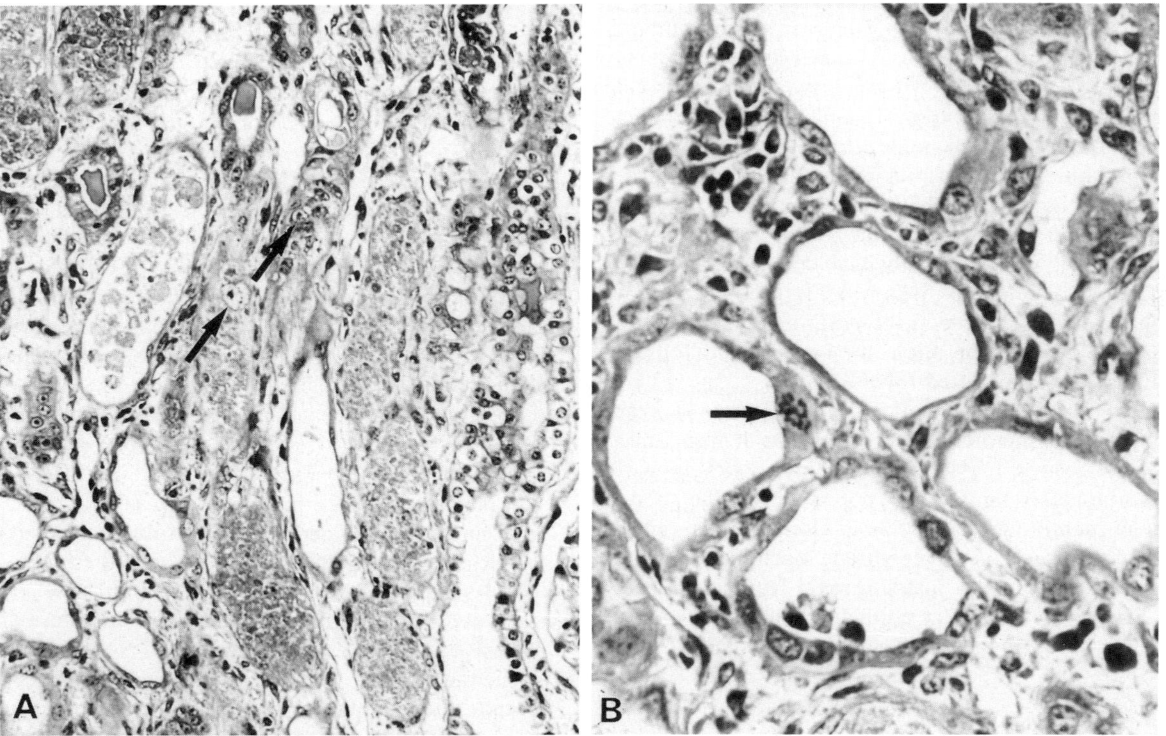

Fig. 5.33 Nephrosis. *Amaranthus retroflexus*. Calf. (A) Granular and hyaline casts. Tubules lined by flattened epithelium. Regenerating epithelial cells in tubules (arrows). (B) Mitotic figure in regenerating tubule (arrow).

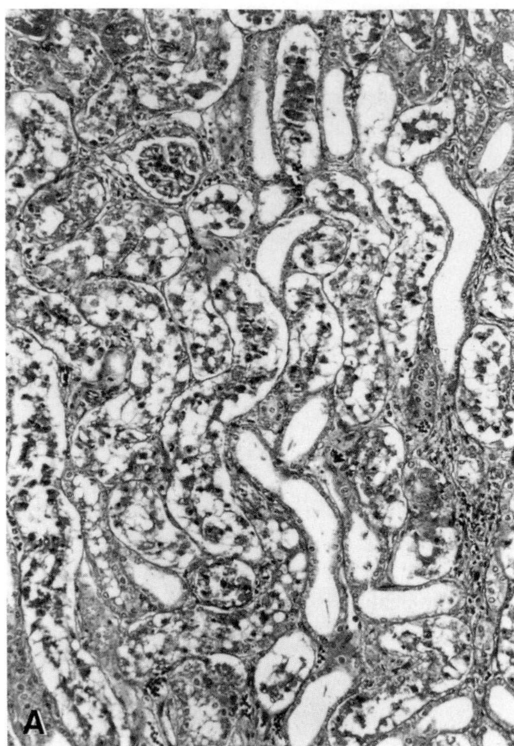

Fig. 5.34A Acute tubular necrosis due to mercuric chloride poisoning. Necrosis, fragmentation, and shedding of tubular epithelium.

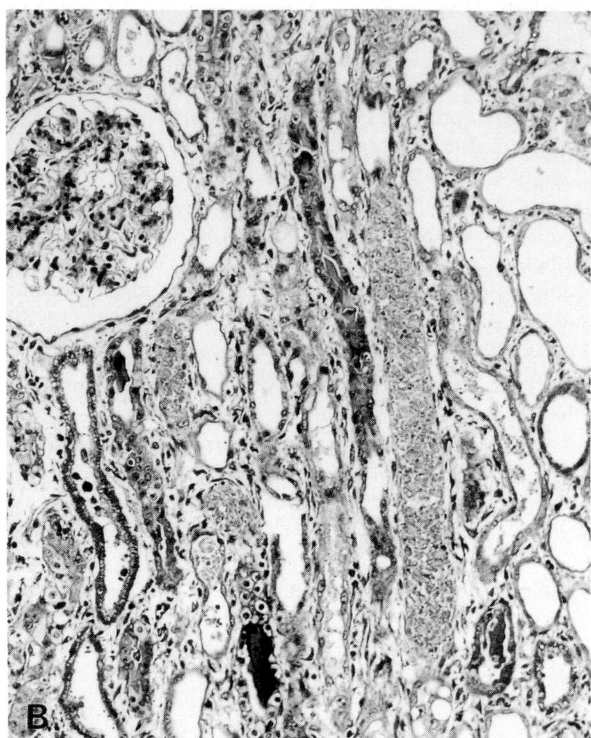

Fig. 5.34B Subacute nephrosis. Calf. *Amaranthus retroflexus*. Granular and hyaline casts, dilation of Bowman's spaces, interstitial edema, and tubules lined by flattened epithelium.

of protein, appear in the cytoplasm of proximal tubular cells in nephrons with increased glomerular permeability. The hyaline droplets are lysosomes swollen with protein which is undergoing proteolysis and will be returned to the circulation as amino acids. Protein reabsorption by proximal tubules is a physiological process; hyaline droplets indicate that this mechanism is saturated.

Fatty degeneration is difficult to evaluate in swine, dogs, and cats, which normally have considerable quantities of fat in the renal epithelium; infiltration fat accumulates in the loop of Henle in the outer medulla in starved animals. In fatty degeneration, the fat is usually found in the cells of the convoluted tubules.

Thickening of the basement membrane is seen in a variety of situations involving chronic tubule damage and is usually associated with atrophic tubular epithelium. In renal amyloidosis, amyloid is deposited on the tubular basement membrane, as well as in glomeruli. Disruption of the tubular basement membrane occurs in ischemic necrosis and frequently in focal renal lesions, and may allow herniation of tubular epithelial cells, with some of these cells persisting as interstitial foam cells.

A. Acute Tubular Necrosis

Acute tubular necrosis, or nephrosis, is a condition in which tubular degeneration is the primary process, and it is an important cause of **acute renal failure.** Nephrosis is an imprecise term applied to noninflammatory renal disease, particularly tubular degeneration; acute tubular necrosis (ATN) is a more accurate descriptor of the changes to be discussed here. Affected animals are oliguric or anuric and die within a few days unless given appropriate therapy. The principal causes of ATN are ischemia and nephrotoxins. Another major cause of acute renal failure is postrenal, namely, complete urinary outflow obstruction. Severe acute glomerulonephritis can also cause acute renal failure, but is uncommon in domestic animals. The renal tubules, and particularly the proximal straight tubule and the medullary thick ascending limb, are metabolically very active and are hence the renal components most susceptible to ischemia or nephrotoxins. Lower nephron nephrosis was a term applied in the past to ATN but is inaccurate and no longer in use.

Ischemic or **tubulorrhectic acute tubular necrosis** follows a period of hypotension (shock) which causes marked renal ischemia. Prolonged renal ischemia causes renal cortical necrosis; that is, all cortical structures are affected. Massive hemolysis is a cause of ATN and produces an ischemic pattern known as hemoglobinuric nephrosis. Neither hemoglobin nor myoglobin is a primary nephrotoxin, but they contribute to renal failure produced by other causes, such as hypotension. Ischemic ATN is characterized histologically by focal necrosis along nephrons, particularly of the proximal tubules, and distal tubules to some extent, plus disruption of tubular basement membranes (tubulorrhexis) and occlusion of lumina by casts. Eosinophilic hyaline and granular casts occur commonly in the distal tubules and collecting ducts and consist of Tamm–Horsfall mucoproteins, degenerate epithelial cells, hemoglobin, myoglobin, and other plasma proteins. Interstitial edema and accumulation of leukocytes in dilated vasa recta are common findings, and they may predate the occurrence of overt ATN. Glomeruli are usually normal. After about 1 week, epithelial regeneration may be seen as tubules lined by flattened epithelium with hyperchromatic nuclei and mitoses (Fig. 5.33A,B). The renewed cells are smaller than normal initially and may appear close-packed on the basement membrane. Their relationship with each other is also abnormal, and they tend frequently to pile up in small clusters which eventually disappear. If the initial injury is mild and/or supportive therapy is adequate, recovery of architecture may be complete within about 2–3 weeks.

Nephrotoxic acute tubular necrosis, or exogenous toxic nephrosis, is contrasted here with ischemic ATN, and specific examples are given. Renal tubules, and especially proximal tubules, are particularly susceptible to a wide variety of toxic agents as a consequence of their great metabolic activity and their exposure to agents in the large volume of ultrafiltrate they resorb in the process of urine formation. Their enzyme systems are thus exposed to, and inactivated by, agents such as heavy metals, which bind to sulfhydryl groups. Nephrotoxic ATN is usually characterized histologically by extensive necrosis of predominantly proximal tubules, but with preservation of tubular basement membranes (Fig. 5.34A). These two features distinguish toxic from ischemic ATN, in which necrosis is patchy and disrupts basement membranes. Preservation of tubular basement membrane is necessary to provide the framework for epithelial regeneration, and hence ischemic damage to tubules often has a worse prognosis for the kidney and the animal than does toxic damage. Ischemia often complicates toxic ATN because the swelling of tubular epithelial cells caused by the toxin impairs intrarenal blood flow.

The pathogenesis of acute renal failure and oliguria in either ischemic or toxic ATN remains controversial. Obstruction of tubular flow by cellular debris and casts and by interstitial edema appears to be an important factor (Fig. 5.34B). Other mechanisms proposed include preglomerular vasoconstriction, possibly due to activation of the renin–angiotensin system; leakage of tubular fluid into the interstitium (tubular backleak); and impaired glomerular permeability or vascular reactivity. Oliguria is probably the result of various combinations of these factors. At the oliguric stage of acute renal failure, hyperkalemia is a life-threatening event. If the animal survives the oliguric phase, diuresis occurs, and electrolyte imbalances, such as hypokalemia, may contribute to death. As tubular regeneration proceeds, azotemia resolves, and tubular function slowly returns.

TABLE 5.2

Nephrotoxic Agents in Domestic Animals

Exogenous	Antimicrobials
	Aminoglycosides (neomycin, kanamycin, gentamicin, streptomycin, tobramycin, amikacin)
	Cephalosporins
	Polymixins
	Tetracyclines
	Sulfonamides (sulfapyridine, sulfathiazole, sulfadiazine)
	Amphotericin B
	Metals (arsenic, bismuth, cadmium, lead, mercury, thallium)
	Paraquat
	Monensin
	Antineoplastic agents (doxorubicin, methotrexate)
	Ethylene glycol
	Chlorinated hydrocarbons
	Contrast media
	Methoxyflurane
	Sodium fluoride (superphosphate fertilizer)
	Oxalates (various plants)
	Mycotoxins (ochratoxin A, citrinin)
	Amaranthus retroflexus (pigweed)
	Tannins [*Quercus* spp. (oak)]
	Terminalia oblongata (yellow-wood)
	Isotropis
	Lantana camara
	Animal venoms
	Menadione (vitamin K_3)
	Cantharidin (blister beetle)
Endogenous	Bile
	Hemoglobin
	Myoglobin

B. Nephrotoxic Tubular Necrosis

Numerous toxic substances can cause ATN in domestic animals (Table 5.2). Some of these agents are no longer important as nephrotoxins; for example, organomercurials were commonly used as fungicides on seed grains, which were occasionally fed inadvertently to animals and humans with disastrous results. This use of mercury has been banned. Similarly, highly chlorinated naphthalenes, which cause hyperkeratosis and nephrosis in cattle, have been excluded from the farm environment. Sulfonamides were formerly important as nephrotoxins, but newer formulations are more soluble and less toxic. Some newly introduced agents have nephrotoxicity as a side effect, e.g., aminoglycosides. Numerous additional antibiotics which are toxic to humans, e.g., penicillin, semisynthetic penicillins, and polymixins, may also prove to be toxic to domestic animals. The toxicity of many of the exogenous agents is exacerbated by various systemic states, such as dehydration or shock, which concomitantly impair renal function in the affected animal. Discussion of specific examples of nephrotoxins follows.

Bibliography

Abuelo, J. G. Renal failure caused by chemicals, foods, plants, animal venoms, and the misuse of drugs. An overview. *Arch Intern Med* **150:** 505–510, 1990.

Angus, K. W., and Hodgson, J. C. Renal ultrastructure in lamb nephrosis. *J Comp Pathol* **103:** 241–251, 1990.

Bach, P. H., and Lock, E. A. (eds.). "Nephrotoxicity *In Vitro* to *In Vivo* Animals to Man." New York, Plenum Press, 1989.

Baker, S. B. de C., and Davies, R. L. F. Experimental haemoglobinuric nephrosis. *J Pathol Bacteriol* **87:** 49–56, 1964.

Bennett, W. M. Lead nephropathy. *Kidney Int* **28:** 212–220, 1985.

Berns, A. S. Nephrotoxicity of contrast media. *Kidney Int* **36:** 730–740, 1989.

Bratton, G. R., and Zmudzki, J. Laboratory diagnosis of Pb poisoning in cattle: A reassessment and review. *Vet Hum Toxicol* **26:** 387–392, 1984.

Brown, S. A., and Engelhardt, J. A. Drug-related nephropathies. Part I. Mechanisms, diagnosis, and management. Part II. Commonly used drugs. *Compend Cont Ed Pract Vet* **9:** 148–160, 281–288, 1987.

Commandeur, J. N. M., and Vermeulen, N. P. E. Molecular and biochemical mechanisms of chemically induced nephrotoxicity: A review. *Chem Res Toxicol* **3:** 171–315, 1990.

Cotter, S. M., Kanki, P. J., and Simon, M. Renal disease in five tumor-bearing cats treated with Adriamycin. *J Am Anim Hosp Assoc* **21:** 405–409, 1985.

Davis, J. W. *et al.* Experimentally induced lead poisoning in goats: Clinical observations and pathologic changes. *Cornell Vet* **66:** 489–496, 1976.

Diamond, J. R., and Yoburn, D. C. Nonoliguric acute renal failure. *Arch Int Med* **142:** 1882–1884, 1982.

DiBartola, S. P. Acute renal failure: Pathophysiology and management. *Compend Cont Ed Pract Vet* **2:** 952–958, 1980.

Divers, T. J. *et al.* Acute renal disorders in cattle: A retrospective study of 22 cases. *J Am Vet Med Assoc* **181:** 694–699, 1982.

Dobyan, D. C., Nagle, R. B., and Bulger, R. E. Acute tubular necrosis in the rat kidney following sustained hypotension. Physiologic and morphologic observations. *Lab Invest* **4:** 411–422, 1977.

Finn, W. F. Nephron heterogeneity in polyuric acute renal failure. *J Lab Clin Med* **98:** 21–29, 1981.

Goldberg, I. D., Garnick, M. B., and Bloomer, W. D. Urinary tract toxic effects of cancer therapy. *J Urol* **132:** 1–6, 1984.

Hamir, A. N., Sullivan, N. D., and Handson, P. D. Acid-fast inclusions in tissues of dogs dosed with lead. *J Comp Pathol* **93:** 307–317, 1983.

Honda, N. Acute renal failure and rhabdomyolysis. *Kidney Int* **23:** 888–898, 1983.

Humes, H. D. Role of calcium in pathogenesis of acute renal failure. *Am J Physiol* **250:** F579–F589, 1986.

Kelly, D. F., Amand, W. B., and Fein, D. A. Acute nephrosis in a cat. *J Am Vet Med Assoc* **159:** 413–416, 1971. (Bismuth)

Kennedy, S., and Rice, D. A. Renal lesions in cattle fed sodium hydroxide-treated barley. *Vet Pathol* **24:** 265–271, 1987.

Mason, J., and Thiel, G.(eds.). Workshop on the role of renal medullary circulation in the pathogenesis of acute renal failure. *Nephron* **31:** 289–323, 1982.

Matthews, K. A. *et al.* Nephrotoxicity in dogs associated with methoxyflurane anesthesia and flunixin meglumine analgesia. *Can Vet J* **31:** 766–771, 1990.

Schmitz, D. G. Toxic nephropathy in horses. *Compend Cont Ed Pract Vet* **10:** 104–111, 1988.

Schuh, J. C. L, Ross, C., and Meschter, C. Concurrent mercuric blister and dimethylsulfoxide (DMSO) application as a cause of mercury toxicity in two horses. *Equine Vet J* **20:** 68–71, 1988.

Spangler, W. L., and Muggli, F. M. Seizure-induced rhabdomyolysis accompanied by acute renal failure in a dog. *J Am Vet Med Assoc* **172:** 1190–1194, 1978.

Tsukamoto, H. *et al.* Nephrotoxicity of sodium arsenate in dogs. *Am J Vet Res* **44:** 2324–2330, 1983.

1. Aminoglycosides

These antibiotics are widely used against Gram-negative infections, and include, in decreasing order of nephrotoxicity, **neomycin, kanamycin, gentamicin, streptomycin, tobramycin,** and **amikacin.** Aminoglycosides are obligate nephrotoxins; in cats, aminoglycosides are ototoxic as well as nephrotoxic. Foals are particularly prone to nephrotoxicosis. Aminoglycosides are not metabolized but are eliminated from the body primarily by glomerular filtration; they selectively accumulate in, and cause damage to, proximal tubules. The changes in tubular cells include damage and loss of the brush border, and formation of cytosegrosomes and myeloid bodies; this overloading of lysosomes with phospholipids (lysosomal phospholipidosis) results from aminoglycoside-induced inhibition of phospholipases. Lysosomal dysfunction and/or leakage may lead to tubular cell necrosis. Damage is dose related and is enhanced by pre existing renal impairment. Toxicity is manifest clinically by inability to concentrate urine, polyuria, enzymuria, proteinuria, hematuria, cylindruria, and azotemia. Acute renal failure may ensue. Aminoglycoside nephrotoxicity is reversible; recovery from the nephrosis may occur even in the face of continued therapy because the regenerating cells have increased resistance to aminoglycoside toxicity.

2. Tetracyclines

Tetracyclines cause several syndromes of renal disease in humans: progressive azotemia due to their antianabolic effect, a reversible Fanconi syndrome due to the use of outdated tetracycline containing degradation products, and reversible nephrogenic diabetes insipidus. An overdose of oxytetracycline can produce acute tubular necrosis and renal failure in dogs. Tetracycline administration has been reported to cause acute nephrosis and death in calves due to the presence of tetracycline degradation products; high doses of oxytetracycline can cause acute nephrosis in treated cattle. Use of tetracyclines is contraindicated in animals in renal failure; tetracyclines are excreted from the body primarily by the kidneys; thus, renal dysfunction leads to increased serum drug concentrations and enhanced nephrotoxic potential. Doxycycline, a newer semisynthetic tetracycline, is not reported to be nephrotoxic.

3. Sulfonamides

Severe nephropathy may follow the ingestion of excessive doses of sulfonamides, especially if treated animals

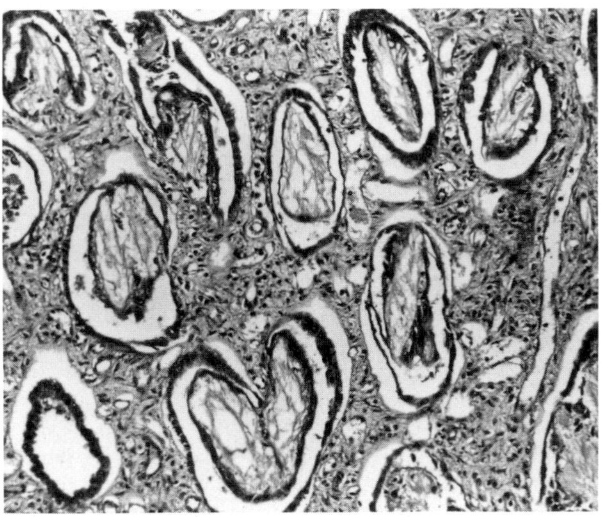

Fig. 5.35 Sulfonamide nephrosis. Calf. Sulfa crystals (removed in processing) have been covered by epithelium from collecting tubules.

are dehydrated. Toxicity was much more common previously when only less-soluble forms of the drug were available, e.g., sulfapyridine, sulfathiazole, and sulfadiazine. Crystalline nephropathy is now rare as the newer shorter-acting sulfonamides have greater solubility. Affected kidneys are slightly enlarged and congested, and the sulfonamide crystals are grossly visible in the medulla, pelvis, and in some cases, even in heavy deposits in the bladder. The deposits are yellow, and form pale radial lines in the medulla. Crystals are not observed in section as they are dissolved during processing. The epithelium of the proximal convoluted tubules and of Bowman's capsule undergoes severe hydropic degeneration. There is little evidence of necrosis in the distal and collecting tubules, but epithelial proliferation and swelling are prominent, and the tubules become densely populated with large dark-staining cells. Some papillary formations into the lumen may even be present, and commonly in the collecting tubules, there is more or less complete duplication of the epithelium, the inner epithelium enclosing a faintly basophilic hyaline precipitate (Fig. 5.35). There is a diffuse but mild interstitial reaction about the corticomedullary junction. It appears that the renal lesions are due to both local toxic and mechanical effects and that hypersensitivity does not play a role in animals as it apparently does in humans.

4. *Amphotericin*

Amphotericin B is an antifungal agent, a polyene antibiotic, whose most important toxic effect is renal dysfunction. It causes decreased renal blood flow and glomerular filtration due to renal vasoconstriction. Necrosis of proximal and distal tubules occurs, and there is mineralization of intratubular casts.

Bibliography

Garry, F., Chew, D. J., and Hoffsis, G. F. Enzymuria as an index of renal damage in sheep with induced aminoglycoside nephrotoxicosis. *Am J Vet Res* **50:** 428–432, 1990.

Hinchcliff, K. W. *et al.* Phenolsulfonphthalein pharmacokinetics and renal morphologic changes in adult pony mares with gentamicin-induced nephrotoxicosis. *Am J Vet Res* **50:** 1848–1853, 1989.

Kacew, S., and Bergeron, M. G. Pathogenic factors in aminoglycoside-induced nephropathy. *Toxicol Lett* **51:** 241–259, 1990.

Laurent, G., Kishore, B. K., and Tulkens, P. M. Aminoglycoside-induced renal phospholipidosis and nephrotoxicity. *Biochem Pharmacol* **40:** 2383–2392, 1990.

Riond, J. L., and Riviere, J. E. Pharmacology and toxicology of doxycycline. *Vet Hum Toxicol* **30:** 431–443, 1988.

Rubin, S. I. *et al.* Nephrotoxicity of amphotericin B in dogs: A comparison of two methods of administration. *Can J Vet Res* **53:** 23–28, 1989.

TerHune, T. N., and Upson, D. W. Oxytetracycline pharmacokinetics, tissue depletion, and toxicity after administration of a long-acting preparation at double the label dosage. *J Am Vet Med Assoc* **194:** 911–917, 1989.

Ziv, G. Clinical pharmacology of polymixins. *J Am Vet Med Assoc* **179:** 711–713, 1981.

5. *Ethylene Glycol*

Dogs and cats are commonly poisoned by ingestion of ethylene glycol. The seasonal incidence of this poisoning coincides with the changing of engine antifreeze solutions in the spring and autumn. Cattle are also occasionally poisoned. Ethylene glycol, which is present in a 95% concentration in antifreeze solutions, has a sweet taste and is usually voluntarily ingested, especially by young male dogs. Cats are more susceptible, but less commonly affected, than dogs; the minimum lethal dose is 1.5 ml/kg for cats and 6.6 ml/kg for dogs.

Ethylene glycol, which itself is of low toxicity, is rapidly absorbed from the gastrointestinal tract, and most is excreted unchanged in the urine. A small percentage is oxidized by alcohol dehydrogenase in the liver to glycoaldehyde, which is in turn oxidized to glycolic acid, glyoxylate, and finally oxalate. Glycolic acid (glycolate) is the primary toxic metabolite of ethylene glycol. Other end-products of metabolism are lactic acid, hippuric acid, and carbon dioxide.

Depression, ataxia, and osmotic diuresis develop within a few hours after ingestion of ethylene glycol. Although oxalate crystals are deposited around cerebral vessels and in perivascular spaces (Fig. 5.36A), nervous signs are due to the effect of aldehydes and possibly to the severe metabolic acidosis which develops as a result of accumulation of lactic acid, glycolate, and glyoxylate. Over the next 12 hr, pulmonary edema, tachypnea, and tachycardia occur. If the animal survives for 1–3 days after ingestion, acute renal failure develops, primarily due to renal tubular damage caused by glycoaldehyde, glycolic acid, glyoxylic acid, and oxalate. Severe renal edema impairs intrarenal blood flow and contributes to nephrosis and renal failure. Soluble calcium oxalates in the blood precipitate in the

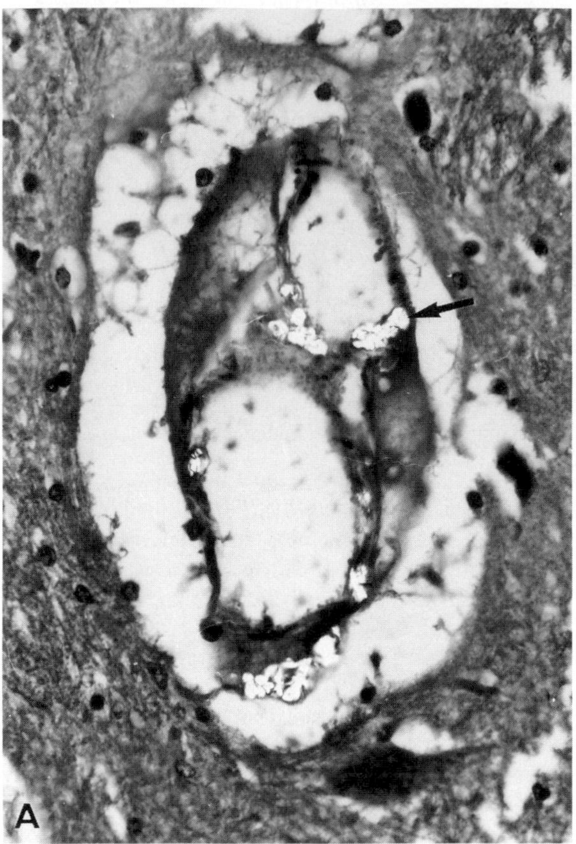

Fig. 5.36A Oxalate encephalitis. Dog. Ethylene glycol poisoning. Oxalate crystal (arrow). Partially crossed polarization filters. (Slide courtesy of R. W. Wilson.)

ultrafiltrate of the renal tubules as the pH of the fluid decreases. Calcium oxalate crystals may be found in tubular lumina (Fig. 5.36B), in tubular cells, and in the interstitium; they are light yellow, arranged in sheaves, rosettes, or prisms, and are birefringent with polarized light. Tubular lesions, which are most severe in proximal tubules, range from hydropic degeneration to necrosis to regeneration.

In animals surviving the acute toxic insult, calcium oxalate crystals are thought to be of importance in causing renal failure. Large numbers of crystals in tubules are virtually pathognomonic of ethylene glycol poisoning; a few crystals may be seen with chronic tubular obstruction. Occasional calcium oxalate crystals are normally seen in urine sediment of dogs; large numbers of these crystals are highly suggestive of poisoning. Hypocalcemia due to the formation of crystals is usually mild in dogs. Animals which survive the acute exposure toxicity may have renal interstitial fibrosis. Few crystals may be left in the tubules; they tend to be removed in the weeks following their deposition. The diagnosis may be confirmed by detection of ethylene glycol in stomach content or blood by gas chromatography early in the toxicosis, or by detection

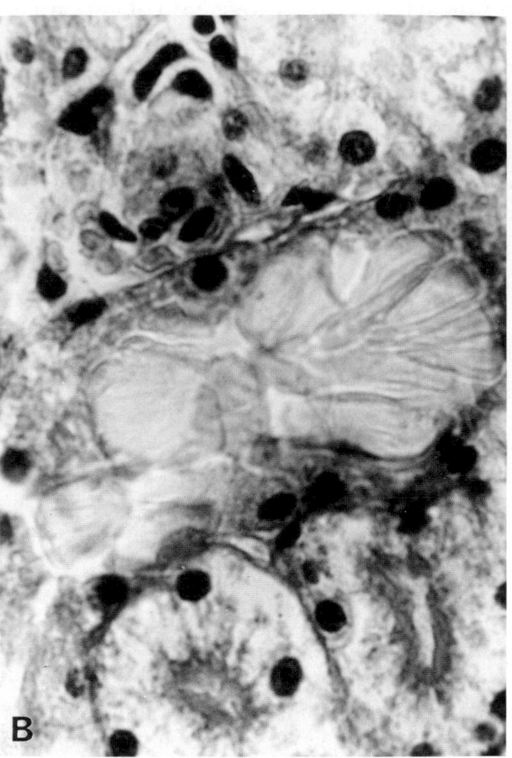

Fig. 5.36B Oxalate crystals in proximal tubule. Dog.

of glycolic acid in urine, serum, or ocular fluid by mass spectrometry later in the toxicosis.

6. Oxalate

Plants are the usual source of oxalate poisoning in sheep and cattle. **Plants** which may contain toxic amounts of oxalate are *Halogeton glomeratus,* halogeton; *Sarcobatus vermiculatus,* greasewood; *Rheum rhaponticum,* the common garden rhubarb; *Oxalis cernua,* soursob; *Rumex* spp., sorrel, dock. Plants of lesser importance are *Portulacca oleracea, Trianthema portulacastrum,* and *Threlkeldia proceriflora,* as well as some cultivated species such as mangels and sugar beet. Young plants may contain the equivalent of 7% or more of potassium oxalate; the amount decreases with maturity and drying of the plant. These plants are eaten only in unusual circumstances and not readily. Species of **grasses** in the genera *Cenchrus, Panicum,* and *Setaria,* which are widely cultivated in tropical and subtropical areas and which accumulate large amounts of oxalate, have been associated with renal oxalosis in cattle and sheep and with skeletal disease in horses, the latter due to conditioned calcium deficiency (see Bones and Joints, Volume 1, Chapter 1).

The **fungi** *Aspergillus niger* and *A. flavus* can produce large quantities of oxalates on feedstuffs. Large doses of **ascorbic acid** (vitamin C) have caused oxalate nephrotoxicosis in humans and in a goat; ascorbic acid is a metabolic precursor of oxalate. **Primary hyperoxaluria,** a rare inherited metabolic condition, occurs in humans, cats, and perhaps dogs (Tibetan spaniels). **Pyridoxine (vitamin B_6) deficiency** and **methoxyflurane** anesthesia can also cause renal oxalosis.

Mortality rates of 10% may occur in sheep when, as frequently happens in some areas, these animals graze on almost pure stands of halogeton or of soursob. It is more usual, however, for fatalities to be sporadic. Under natural conditions, sheep may ingest as much as 75 g of oxalate a day; thus, the ovine rumen must degrade the salt efficiently. Depending on the diet before exposure to oxalate-containing plants and, therefore, on the microbial composition of the rumen, some variation is to be expected in the ability of ruminal contents to degrade the salt. Cattle are less commonly affected under range conditions than are sheep, but cattle and sheep are equally susceptible to experimental poisoning. Horses are resistant to oxalate-induced nephrosis and succumb to acute gastroenteritis only after receiving unnaturally large amounts of the chemical; they may develop osteodystrophia fibrosa with prolonged exposure.

Chelation of calcium by unmetabolized oxalate in the ingesta contributes to hypocalcemia. Following absorption, oxalates combine with calcium to form insoluble calcium oxalate; hypocalcemic tetany may result. Calcium oxalate may crystallize in vessel lumens or walls, causing vascular necrosis and hemorrhage, or in renal tubules, causing tubular obstruction and acute renal failure. The nephrotoxicity of oxalates involves more than mechanical obstruction, and may be due in part to intracellular chelation of calcium and magnesium and hence interference with oxidative phosphorylation. Clinically, weakness, prostration, and death may follow within 12 hr of ingestion of oxalate-containing plants.

Oxalates are produced endogenously in the degradation of glycine, an important constituent amino acid of collagen and elastin. Uptake of normal dietary oxalate may increase in a variety of enteric diseases (enteric oxalosis). Oxalosis can be prominent in the kidneys of aborted bovine fetuses, and may reflect maternal intake of oxalate-containing plants or moldy feed. A few oxalate crystals can frequently be found in scarred tubules in any species; these crystals are usually without significance.

Bibliography

Boermans, H. J., Ruegg, P. L., and Leach, M. Ethylene glycol toxicosis in a pygmy goat. *J Am Vet Med Assoc* **193:** 694–696, 1988.

Chaplin, A. J. Histopathological occurrence and characterization of calcium oxalate: A review. *J Clin Pathol* **30:** 800–811, 1977.

Collier, M. A., Brown, C. M., and Stick, J. A. Renal disease and oxalosis in horses. *Mod Vet Pract* **66:** 631–634, 735–739, 1985.

Jansen, J. H., and Arnesen, K. Oxalate nephropathy in a Tibetan spaniel litter. A probable case of primary hyperoxaluria. *J Comp Pathol* **103:** 79–84, 1990.

McKenzie, R. A. *et al.* Acute oxalate poisoning of sheep by buffel grass. *Aust Vet J* **65:** 26, 1988.

Mueller, D. H. Epidemiologic considerations of ethylene glycol intoxication in small animals. *Vet Hum Toxicol* **24:** 21–24, 1982.

Panciera, R. J. *et al.* Acute oxalate poisoning attributable to ingestion of curly dock (*Rumex crispus*) in sheep. *J Am Vet Med Assoc* **196:** 1981–1984, 1990.

Proia, A. D., and Brinn, N. T. Identification of calcium oxalate crystals using alizarin red S stain. *Arch Pathol Lab Med* **109:** 186–189, 1985.

Sanford, S. E. Oxalate nephropathy associated with seizures in mink. *Can Vet J* **29:** 1005–1006, 1988.

Schiefer, B., Hewitt, M. P., and Milligan, J. D. Fetal renal oxalosis due to feeding oxalic acid to pregnant ewes. *Zbl Vet Med (A)* **23:** 226–233, 1976.

Smith, B. J. *et al.* Early effects of ethylene glycol on the ultrastructure of the renal cortex in dogs. *Am J Vet Res* **51:** 89–96, 1990.

Thrall, M. A., Dial, S. M., and Winder, D. R. Identification of calcium oxalate monohydrate crystals by x-ray diffraction in urine of ethylene glycol-intoxicated dogs. *Vet Pathol* **22:** 625–628, 1985.

7. Mycotoxins

Aspergillus and *Penicillium* spp. produce a number of nephrotoxic mycotoxins, namely **ochratoxins, citrinin, oxalate,** and **viridicatum toxin,** which can contaminate feed grains. Ochratoxin A is the only member of the group that is significant in disease. In pigs, ochratoxin A and citrinin produce proximal tubular degeneration and atrophy, cortical interstitial fibrosis, and glomerular hyalinosis; the renal insufficiency produced is usually subclinical. Acute renal disease occurs very rarely, and is manifested by severe perirenal edema resembling that produced by redroot pigweed (*Amaranthus retroflexus,* see Section V,C,5 of The Kidney in this chapter). Ochratoxin A has been suggested as the cause of endemic (Balkan) nephropathy in humans.

Moldy feed also produces mycotoxic nephropathy in horses. Citrinin produces tubular degeneration in swine, horses, and sheep. Ochratoxins normally are degraded in the rumen; thus, toxicity is unlikely to occur in ruminants.

Bibliography

Elling, F. *et al.* Ochratoxin A-induced porcine nephropathy: Enzyme and ultrastructure changes after short-term exposure. *Toxicology* **23:** 247–254, 1985.

Hanika, C. *et al.* Citrinin mycotoxicosis in the rabbit: Ultrastructural alterations. *Vet Pathol* **23:** 245–253, 1986.

Krogh, P. *et al.* Renal enzyme activities in experimental ochratoxin A-induced porcine nephropathy: Diagnostic potential of phosphoenolpyruvate carboxykinase and gamma-glutamyl transpeptidase activity. *J Toxicol Environ Health* **23:** 1–14, 1988.

Thornton, R. H., Shirley, G., and Salisbury, R. M. A nephrotoxin from *Aspergillus fumigatus* and its possible relationship with New Zealand mucosal disease-like syndrome in cattle. *N Z J Agric Res* **11:** 1–14, 1968.

8. Amaranthus

Ingestion of redroot pigweed, *Amaranthus retroflexus,* causes perirenal edema and acute renal failure due to toxic nephrosis in swine and cattle, and uncommonly in horses. The nephrotoxic principle of *A. retroflexus* has not yet been identified; the plants often contain high levels of

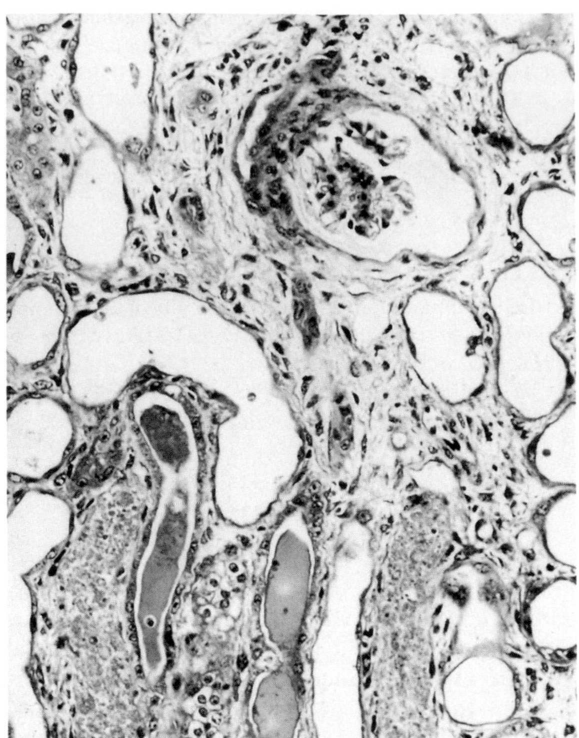

Fig. 5.37 Fibrosis beginning around glomeruli and between tubules following tubular necrosis due to *Amaranthus retroflexus*.

nitrate and oxalate, but neither nitrate nor oxalate poisoning usually occurs and perirenal edema is not produced. Phenolic compounds have been identified in the leaves of *Amaranthus,* and may be of similar importance to those in *Quercus* spp. (see Section V,C,9 of The Kidney in this chapter). Lush growth of pigweed occurs in early summer, and this plant often dominates the weed growth in disused lots and yards to which animals are moved when other pasture is depleted. Weakness, recumbency, and often death follow 5–10 days after grazing begins.

Grossly, there is marked perirenal edema, which may be bloodstained and may be accompanied by edema of mesenteries, bowel wall, and ventral abdominal wall, with moderate ascites and hydrothorax. The kidneys are pale but not usually enlarged. Histologically, there is degeneration and coagulation necrosis of both proximal and distal tubules (Figs. 5.33A,B, 5.34B); there may also be mild glomerular epithelial injury and hypercellularity. Tubules contain granular casts. Animals which survive have cortical interstitial fibrosis and tubular dilation. The perirenal edema seen in acute cases is apparently due to tubular backleak, with subsequent lymphatic drainage and leakage into perirenal connective tissue. The probable cause of death is heart failure due to hyperkalemia. Survivors may develop interstitial fibrosis (Fig. 5.37).

Bibliography

Sizelove, W. *et al*. Perirenal edema in a calf. *Vet Hum Toxicol* **30:** 265–266, 1988.

9. Other Plant Toxicoses

Poisoning of ruminants and occasionally of horses by acorns, leaves, and buds of **oak shrubs and trees (*Quercus* spp.)** occurs wherever these grow and in areas where the acorns are accepted as a dietary staple in late autumn and early winter. There are many species and varieties of oaks, but not all are palatable. They are all potentially poisonous by virtue of the tannins they contain, but, in small quantities, they are eaten with impunity. Ingestion of large amounts of the material can cause hydrothorax, ascites, marked perirenal edema, alimentary tract ulceration, and acute tubular necrosis, and can result in large death losses. The toxic substances are gallotannins; they are hydrolyzed to tannic acid, gallic acid, and pyrogallol, which appear to be the active toxic metabolites. Binding of tannins to endothelial cells results in endothelial damage and accounts for perirenal edema and fluid leakage into body cavities. The alimentary lesions are due to the strong ability of oak tannins to bind to peptide linkages and precipitate protein; this astringent effect of tannins is used in leather tanning. The gastrointestinal and mesenteric edema and ulcerative enterocolitis that develop in poisoned horses are also partly the product of disseminated intravascular coagulation.

In acute oak poisoning, there is marked perirenal edema and hemorrhage, the kidneys are swollen and pale and, in cattle, are rather uniformly sprinkled with cortical hemorrhages of 2–3 mm diameter. The glomeruli are ischemic but otherwise normal except for dilation of the urinary space after several days. There may be microscopic hematuria. Necrosis of the epithelium of the proximal tubules can be complete, to produce within the basement membranes dense homogeneous casts. In less severe injury, adjacent groups of tubules may vary considerably in the extent of degeneration (Fig. 5.38). Some animals may recover but, in others, the renal lesion progresses with shrinkage and diffuse fibrosis and scattered collections of mononuclear cells. The completeness of the necrosis in groups of tubules with intratubular hemorrhage distinguishes the nephrosis of acute oak poisoning from that of most other causes.

Poisoning by the **yellow-wood tree, *Terminalia oblongata,*** in Australia is reputed to produce lesions similar to those of oak poisoning. Yellow-wood produces at least two toxic factors: punicalagin, a hepatotoxic tannin, and an unidentified nephrotoxin. In acute yellow-wood poisoning of cattle and sheep, coagulative periacinar hepatic necrosis predominates; subacute and chronic intoxications are characterized by renal fibrosis and atrophy.

Several species of the genus ***Isotropis*** are toxic to ruminants. In both cattle and sheep, reference is made to abomasitis and enteritis, petechial hemorrhages throughout the gastrointestinal tract, and accumulation of fluid in the body cavities and subcutis. The renal lesions are dominated by necrosis of proximal tubular epithelium. In many acute poisonings, there is abundant proteinaceous fluid in Bowman's space.

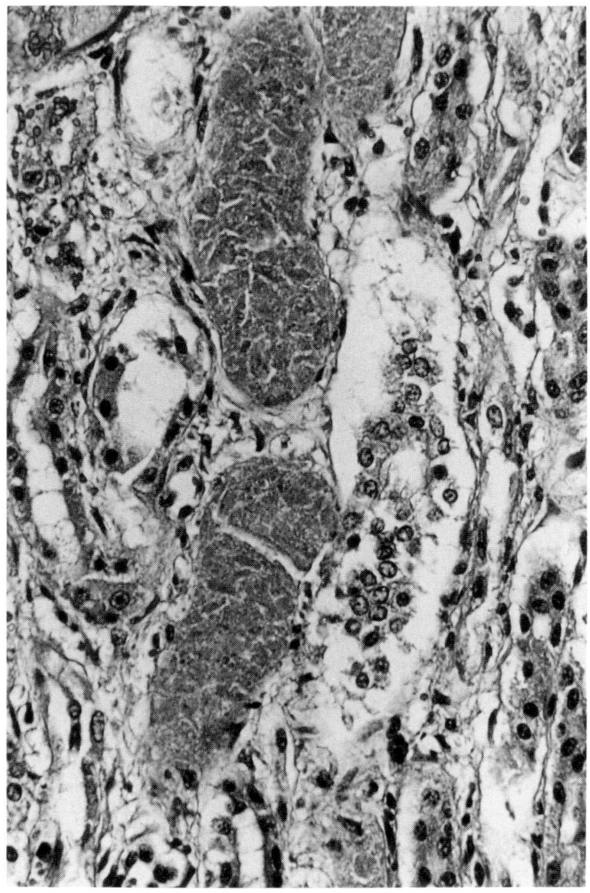

Fig. 5.38 Hereford calf. Six months. Oak poisoning. Necrotic tubule adjacent to more normal tubules. (Slide courtesy of R. Werdin.)

Bibliography

Anderson, G. A. *et al.* Fatal acorn poisoning in a horse: Pathologic findings and diagnostic considerations. *J Am Vet Med Assoc* **182:** 1105–1110, 1983.

Filippich, L. J. *et al.* Hepatotoxic and nephrotoxic principles in *Terminalia oblongata*. *Res Vet Sci* **50:** 170–177, 1991.

Gardiner, M. R., and Royce, R. D. Poisoning of sheep and cattle in western Australia due to species of *Isotropis* (Papilionaceae). *Aust J Agric Res* **18:** 505–513, 1967.

Kasari, T. R., Pearson, E. G., and Hultgren, B. D. Oak (*Quercus garryana*) poisoning of range cattle in southern Oregon. *Compend Cont Ed Pract Vet* **8:** F17–F29, 1986.

Spier, S. J. *et al.* Oak toxicosis in cattle in northern California: Clinical and pathological findings. *J Am Vet Med Assoc* **191:** 958–964, 1987.

C. Specific Tubular Dysfunctions

Renal tubular dysfunction may occur secondary to other conditions; for example, glucosuria occurs when the tubular transport maximum for glucose is exceeded in diabetes mellitus and acute enterotoxemia, and heavy-metal toxicity causes glucosuria and aminoaciduria due to tubular degeneration. The primary tubular transport defects identified in domestic animals are hyperuricosuria in Dalmatian dogs, essential cystinuria, the syndrome of multiple resorptive defects in basenji dogs, renal tubular acidosis, and primary renal glucosuria. Hyperuricosuria and cystinuria are of importance because they predispose to urolithiasis, and are discussed in Section IV, of The Lower Urinary Tract in this chapter.

Basenjis and several other breeds of dogs may develop a proximal tubular disorder similar to the **Fanconi syndrome** in humans; the condition is hereditary in basenjis. The syndrome in dogs is characterized by polyuria, polydipsia, hyposthenuria, glucosuria, normoglycemia, hyperphosphaturia, proteinuria, and aminoaciduria. The aminoaciduria may be generalized or limited to cystinuria. Affected dogs have impaired renal tubular reabsorption of glucose, phosphate, sodium, potassium, uric acid, and amino acids. Polyuria results from the glucosuria and natriuresis. The syndrome develops in adult dogs and is usually slowly progressive. Dehydration and acidosis result in renal papillary necrosis and death due to renal failure. Histologic renal changes are nonspecific, and include interstitial fibrosis and tubular atrophy. Affected dogs often have marked karyomegaly in occasional tubular cells. Ultrastructural abnormalities have not been noted in tubular cells.

The renal tubular acidosis that occurs as part of the Fanconi syndrome is the most common example in dogs of **proximal** or **type II renal tubular acidosis,** in which proximal tubules fail to reabsorb filtered bicarbonate. Proximal renal tubular acidosis is usually a self-limiting

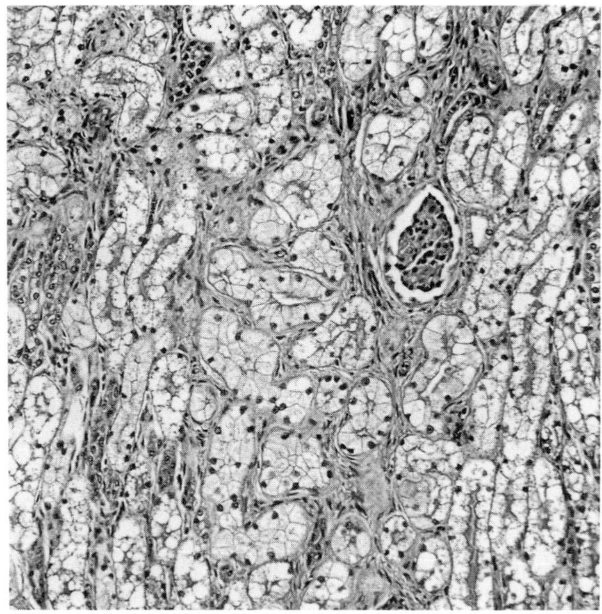

Fig. 5.39 Salers calf, newborn, term. Beta-mannosidosis. Marked vacuolation of renal tubular epithelial cells. (Slide courtesy of L. Bryan.)

disease that is not evident clinically. **Distal renal tubular acidosis (type I)** occurs in dogs, cats, and horses, is caused by defective excretion of hydrogen ions by distal tubules, and produces hyperchloremic metabolic acidosis that is more severe than that in the proximal form.

Primary renal glucosuria may occur as a singular transport abnormality without other defects. This defect is an inherited disorder in Norwegian elkhounds.

Salers calves affected with **β-mannosidosis** primarily have a variety of neurologic deficits but also have greatly enlarged kidneys that are characterized by marked vacuolation of the cytoplasm of proximal tubular epithelial cells (Fig. 5.39); this lysosomal storage disease is inherited as an autosomal recessive trait. Although the renal lesion is histologically dramatic, renal dysfunction is not reported (see the Nervous System, Volume 1, Chapter 3).

Bibliography

Abbitt, B. *et al.* β-Mannosidosis in twelve Salers calves. *J Am Vet Med Assoc* **198:** 109–113, 1991.

DiBartola, S. P., Chew, D. J., and Horton, M. L. Cystinuria in a cat. *J Am Vet Med Assoc* **198:** 102–104, 1991.

Mueller, D. L., and Jergens, A. E. Renal tubular acidosis. *Compend Cont Ed Pract Vet* **13:** 435–444, 1991.

Rothstein, M., Obialo, C., and Hruska, K. A. Renal tubular acidosis. *Endocrinol Metabol Clin North Am* **19:** 869–887, 1990.

Ziemer, E. L. *et al.* Renal tubular acidosis in two horses: Diagnostic studies. *J Am Vet Med Assoc* **190:** 289–293, 1987.

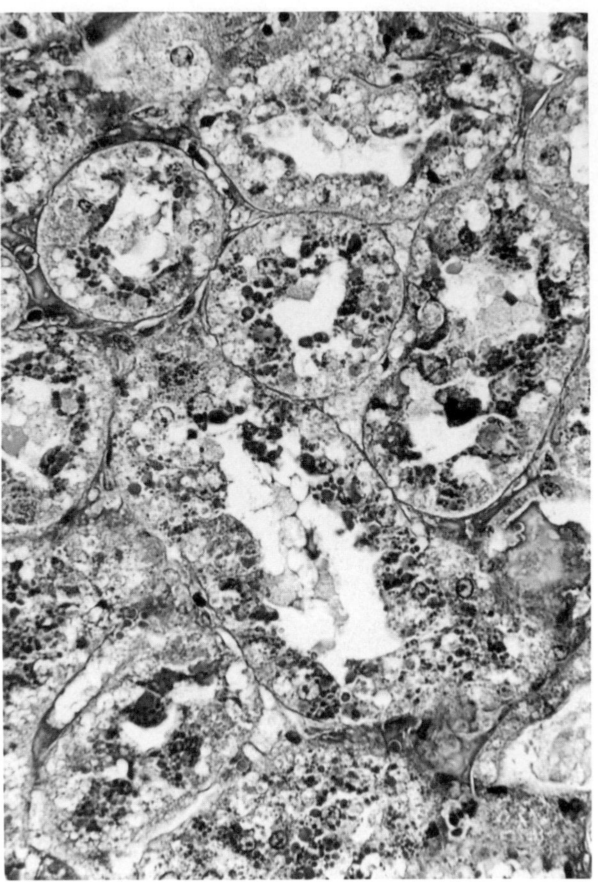

Fig. 5.40 Sheep. Renal tubular hyaline droplets. Hemolysis caused by chronic copper poisoning. (Slide courtesy of L. Bryan.)

D. Pigmentary Changes

Following acute hemolytic crises of any cause, the kidneys may be very dark, almost black, as a consequence of concentrated **hemoglobin.** Initially, the discoloration is uniform, but shortly most of the hemoglobin is dispersed except from scattered clusters of nephrons, in which it persists for many days to produce a diffuse brown speckling of the cortices. The color alone provides a good distinction between this pigmentary change and the red or blue speckling that occurs in acute hemorrhagic glomerulitis. It is particularly characteristic of the hemolytic crisis of chronic copper poisoning in sheep. Microscopically, the hemoglobin appears as fine red granules in the epithelial cells of the tubules (Fig. 5.40) and as red casts in the lower reaches of the nephron, especially Henle's loop and the collecting tubules. The same histologic picture occurs following incompatible blood transfusions and in paralytic myoglobinuria of horses, in which disease the pigment is **myoglobin.** Nutritional myopathy of young animals does not produce this renal lesion because the myoglobin content of their muscle is very low. Hemoglobin and myoglobin pigmentation persists after hemoglobin or myoglobin are no longer detectable grossly in urine samples.

Hemosiderosis occurs in the course of chronic hemolytic anemia and as residue from acute hemoglobinuric episodes. The pigment is found in epithelial cells of proximal tubules, where it is produced by the degradation of resorbed hemoglobin, and it may be sufficient to produce a distinctive brown coloration of the cortex.

Lipofuscinosis of the kidneys of adult cattle, also referred to as hemochromatosis and xanthomatosis, consists of the deposition of brown iron-free pigments with staining characteristics of lipofuscin (Fig. 5.41A). The pigmentation also affects striated muscles, giving them a dark brown appearance. On the cut surface of the kidney, the pigmentation occurs in radial dark lines in the cortex but spares the medulla. Microscopically, it is present as fine, brown granules in the epithelial cells of the convoluted tubules. An environmental lipofuscinosis of the liver, kidney, and other organs is discussed with the Liver and Biliary System (Chapter 2 of this volume).

Cloisonné kidney is a nonclinical pigmentary condition in goats. The renal cortices are uniformly brown or black, due to thickening and brown pigmentation of basement membranes restricted to the convoluted portions of the proximal tubules (Fig. 5.41B). The basement membrane thickening is due to the deposition of ferritin and hemosiderin, which is presumably the result of repeated episodes of intravascular hemolysis. A similar renal discoloration

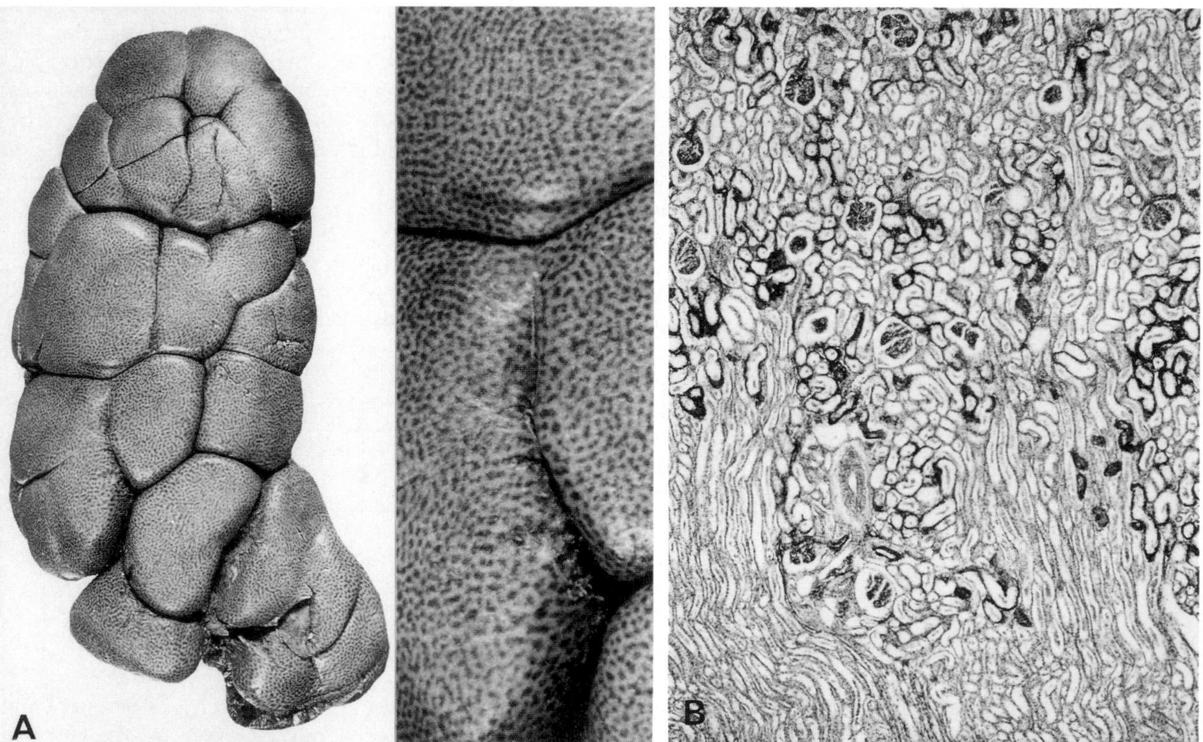

Fig. 5.41 (A) Lipofuscinosis. Kidney. Ox. (Inset) Close-up of subcapsular surface. (B) Cloisonné kidney. Goat. (Slide courtesy of A. Zubaidy.)

and basement membrane thickening has been reported in a horse, but was found to be due to lipofuscinosis.

In congenital **porphyria** of cattle, swine, and cats, brown pigmentation affects the cortex. Histologically, the pigment is present in the tubular epithelium and the interstitial tissue. The pigment is excreted in the urine, which, if allowed to stand in light, develops a port-wine color due to photic activation of porphyrins. The urine and tissues fluoresce blue-green in ultraviolet light.

A green-yellow pigmentation of swollen kidneys is common in **icterus** of hepatic origin and less notable in hemolytic icterus unless there is concomitant hepatic injury. It is described in Section V,E, of The Kidney in this chapter with hepatorenal syndromes. Olive-green coloration of the renal cortex is common in newborn lambs, calves, and foals. The pigment is bilirubin, and its presence is probably due to immaturity of hepatic conjugating mechanisms.

Light green to green-yellow discoloration of liver, and hepatic, renal, and other lymph nodes is occasionally observed in cattle at slaughter. Histologically, numerous brown acicular crystals are present in the cytoplasm of hepatocytes, macrophages, and renal tubular epithelial cells. Crystals may be present in renal tubules, and renal calculi are rarely present. The crystals are **2,8-dihydroxyadenine,** a metabolite of the purine adenine. The crystal deposition and pigmentation are of little significance, and the cause of this condition is unknown.

Bibliography

Giddens, W. E. *et al.* Feline congenital erythropoietic porphyria associated with severe anemia and renal disease. *Am J Pathol* **80:** 367–386, 1975.

Grossman, I. W., and Altman, N. H. Caprine cloisonné renal lesion. Ultrastructure of the thickened proximal convoluted tubular basement membrane. *Arch Pathol Lab Med* **88:** 609–612, 1969.

Marcato, P. S., and Simoni, P. Pigmentation of renal cortical tubules in horses. *Vet Pathol* **19:** 572–573, 1982.

McCaskey, P. C. *et al.* Accumulation of 2,8-dihydroxyadenine in bovine liver, kidneys, and lymph nodes. *Vet Pathol* **28:** 99–109, 1991.

Plumlee, K. H. Red maple toxicity in a horse. *Vet Hum Toxicol* **33:** 66–67, 1991.

Sutton, R. H., and Atwell, R. B. Renal haemosiderosis in association with canine heartworm disease. *J Small Anim Pract* **23:** 773–777, 1982.

Tremblay, R. R. M., and Baird, J. D. Chronic copper poisoning in two Holstein cows. *Cornell Vet* **81:** 205–213, 1991.

Winter, H. "Black kidneys" in cattle—a lipofuscinosis. *J Pathol Bacteriol* **86:** 253–258, 1963.

E. Hepatorenal Syndromes

The term hepatorenal syndrome is vague, and more specific diagnoses should be sought, but a number of more or less distinct associations of renal disease can occur secondarily in animals with hepatic disease. They may be the result of hypovolemia, failure of clearance of gastrointestinal bacteria and endotoxins from the portal blood with development of disseminated intravascular coagulation, or be due to various hepatic metabolites. Hypotension may result from the vasodepressor, cardiodepressor, and diuretic effects of cholemia; thus, the uremia in jaundiced patients may be of prerenal origin. Concentrations of bilirubin and bile acids may be greatly elevated in the blood, especially in obstructive jaundice, and the pigment accumulates in tubular epithelium, which is frequently swollen and hydropic (**cholemic nephrosis**); the actual toxicity of bilirubin and bile salts is still under debate. Some nephrotoxins are also (or mainly) hepatotoxic, e.g., carbon tetrachloride and *Lantana camara*. **Pseudohepatorenal syndromes** include conditions in which liver and kidneys are both affected, but in which renal disease is not secondary to hepatic disease; included are a wide variety of infectious, circulatory, genetic, and other systemic disorders.

F. Glycogen Nephrosis

In diabetes mellitus in dogs and cats, glycogen is deposited in the tubular epithelium producing marked vacuolation of the epithelium in the outer medulla and innermost cortex. Glycogen can be readily demonstrated by appropriate techniques. The deposition occurs in the ascending limb, disappears following insulin administration, and has no effect on renal function. Often in diabetes mellitus of long duration, there is hyaline thickening of the afferent arteriole, which may extend to the capillary basement membranes of the glomerulus.

G. Nephrogenic Diabetes Insipidus

This condition has been reported in several dogs with polyuria, polydipsia, and hyposthenuria. Affected dogs are unresponsive to water deprivation, to exogenous administration of antidiuretic hormone, and to infusion of hypertonic saline. The basis of the defect is a lack of responsiveness of the cells of the distal tubules and collecting ducts to the hormone. The defect may be congenital, or acquired as the result of tubulointerstitial diseases such as pyelonephritis or hypercalcemic nephropathy, or due to the effect of drugs such as tetracycline.

H. Hypokalemic Nephropathy

Chronic potassium depletion in humans, caused by diarrhea, adrenal overactivity, and some renal diseases, can result in impaired urine concentration and polyuria. Coarse vacuolation of the proximal convoluted tubules is due to reversible dilation of intercellular spaces. A vacuolar degeneration of proximal tubular cells has been reported in ewes deliberately given 11–17 times the recommended dose of thiabendazole. Many of the ewes developed hypokalemia, hypoproteinemia, and uremia before death; potassium loss was thought to occur through the kidneys. In a proposed case of hypokalemic nephropathy in a dog, chronic vomition due to a gastric foreign body was thought to be the cause of potassium depletion. Corticosteroids produce hypokalemia and reversible vacuolar degeneration of tubular cells. Hypokalemia may be related to the tubular dilation commonly seen in baby pigs with diarrhea, and is related to experimental production of renal cysts.

Bibliography

Alpern, R. J., and Toto, R. D. Hypokalemic nephropathy—a clue to cystogenesis? *N Engl J Med* **322:** 398–399, 1990.

Breitschwerdt, E. B., Verlander, J. W., and Hribernik, T. N. Nephrogenic diabetes insipidus in three dogs. *J Am Vet Med Assoc* **179:** 235–238, 1981.

Clark, R. G., and Lewis, K. H. C. Deaths in sheep after overdosage with thiabendazole. *N Z Vet J* **25:** 187–190, 1977.

Fioretti, A. *et al.* Cholemic nephrosis in equine fetuses. *Equine Pract* **8:** 11–14, 1986.

Green, J. *et al.* Jaundice, the circulation and the kidney. *Nephron* **37:** 145–152, 1984.

Punukollu, R. C., and Gopalswamy, N. The hepatorenal syndrome. *Med Clin North Am* **74:** 933–943, 1990.

I. Miscellaneous Tubular Conditions

In addition to the standard patterns of parenchymal cell degeneration, several miscellaneous histologic changes may be found in renal epithelium. Some of the **pyrrolizidine alkaloids** cause megalocytosis in the proximal tubules. The lesion is similar in type to that in hepatocytes but much less conspicuous and not observed to cause functional disturbance. Some pyrrolizidine alkaloid-containing plants, particularly *Crotalaria* spp., cause significant glomerular megalocytosis and sclerosis in pigs (see Liver and Biliary System, Chapter 2 of this volume.).

Occasional nuclei in tubules of old dogs may be polyploid. In the proximal tubules, eosinophilic, crystalline, intranuclear inclusions (**brick inclusions**) are commonly encountered in old dogs. Similar inclusions occur in the liver, their source is unknown and, although they resemble the inclusions produced in experimental animals by heavy metals such as bismuth, they do not contain heavy metals. In cells in the same location, subacute **lead poisoning** produces amorphous acid-fast inclusion material in nuclei, which are large, pale, and vesicular.

Large, eosinophilic, intranuclear inclusions occur in hepatocytes and renal collecting duct epithelial cells in goats. The pathogenesis of this **nuclear glycogenosis** is unknown, and it does not appear to be of functional significance.

Eosinophilic intracytoplasmic inclusion bodies have been reported in the renal collecting duct epithelial cells of dogs. The inclusions consisted of **iridovirus** particles, and the infection appeared not to be significant.

Bibliography

Betton, G. R. Identification of viral inclusions in the papillary collecting duct epithelium of the dog. *Vet Pathol* **19:** 716–718, 1982.

Fenwick, B. W., Muir, S., and East, N. Hepatic and renal tubular cell nuclear glycogenosis in goats. *J Comp Pathol* **96:** 399–405, 1986.

Thompson, S. W. *et al*. The protein nature of acidophilic crystalline intranuclear inclusions in the liver and kidney of dogs. *Am J Pathol* **35:** 1105–1115, 1959.

VI. Tubulointerstitial Diseases

This term comprises diseases which involve primarily the interstitium and tubules, and acknowledges that inflammatory and degenerative diseases of the interstitium almost always impair tubular function. Hence, **interstitial nephritis,** which may be acute or chronic, focal or generalized, suppurative or nonsuppurative, and **pyelonephritis** are classified as tubulointerstitial diseases. There is obviously overlap with the previous category of acute tubular necrosis, since animals which survive acute tubular necrosis often develop interstitial inflammation and fibrosis. Also included as tubulointerstitial disease may be nephropathy due to any of hypercalcemia, hypokalemia, analgesics, and oxalates, as well as immunologically mediated tubulointerstitial disease. In humans, and probably also in domestic animals, tubulointerstitial nephritis can be caused by a vast array of agents, including infections, toxins, immunologic disorders, chemicals, and therapeutic drugs (Fig. 5.42A,B).

Interstitial inflammation and fibrosis and tubular atrophy and degeneration are predominant histologic features of these diseases. Interstitial nephritis is usually hematogenous and part of systemic disease, whereas pyelonephritis is usually urogenous; both are usually due to infectious agents, although agents are often not identified, especially in chronic cases. Injury to glomeruli and vessels is usually secondary in tubulointerstitial disease, although they are eventually involved because of the interdependence of renal structures. There is experimental evidence that glomerular disease may lead to tubular cell damage; some low-molecular-weight proteins are directly toxic to tubular cells and will hence contribute to tubulointerstitial nephritis.

The hallmark of glomerular disease is persistent proteinuria, whereas tubulointerstitial diseases are more likely to demonstrate defects of concentrating ability or specific tubular defects of resorption or secretion. However, the end point of both classes of renal disease and the usual clinical presentation is decompensated renal failure with isosthenuria and uremia.

Immunologically mediated tubulointerstitial disease has been identified in humans, and rarely in domestic animals. Hypersensitivity reactions occur to a variety of drugs, e.g., methicillin. Tubular immune-complex disease occurs in some patients with lupus nephritis and glomerulonephritis, indicating that autoantibodies may cross-react with glomerular and tubular basement membranes; antitubular

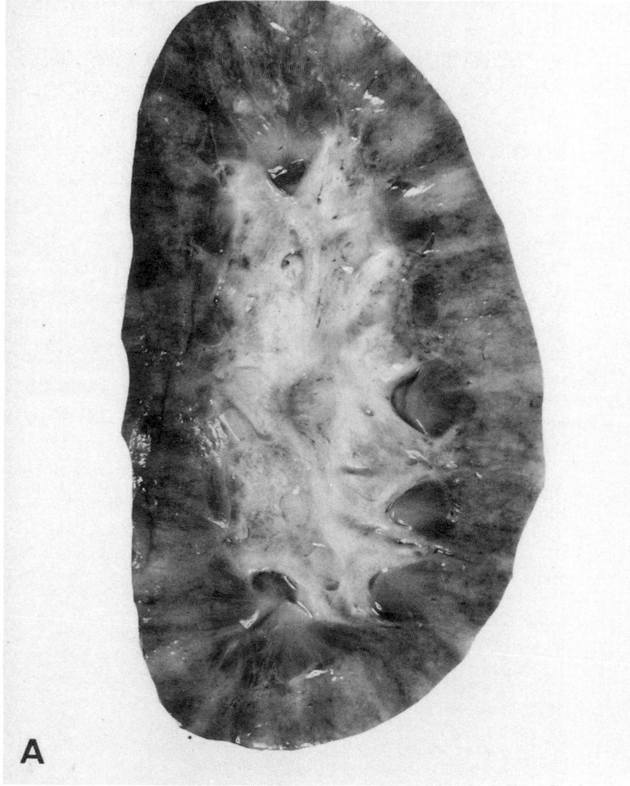

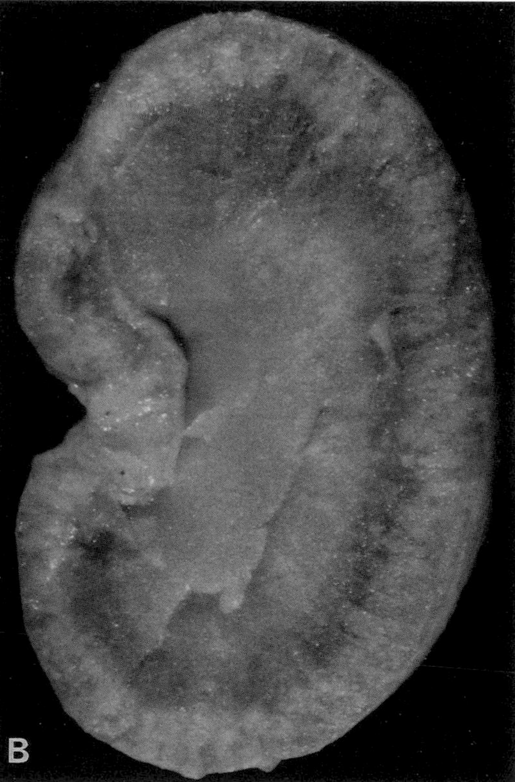

Fig. 5.42 (A) Acute interstitial nephritis. Pig. (B) Chronic renal fibrosis and mineralization (end-stage kidney) in Shih Tzu dog.

basement membrane autoantibody has been identified in a dog.

A. Nonsuppurative Interstitial Nephritis

Focal inflammation with slight scarring and some lymphohistiocytic cells is common in kidneys. The causes are seldom known and probably not specific; some lesions may be primarily inflammatory, and some may be foci of antigen persistence in scars of other origins.

As a form of nephritis, this may be acute or chronic, and multifocal or generalized, probably depending on the intensity of the insult and the efficiency of the host's responses. **Acute** interstitial nephritis is characterized by acute clinical onset, and histologically by interstitial edema, leukocytic infiltration, and focal tubular necrosis. In **chronic** interstitial nephritis, there is mononuclear cell infiltration, interstitial fibrosis, and generalized tubular atrophy. Many infectious agents are capable of causing nonsuppurative interstitial nephritis, and some are discussed here, but agents are often not identified in naturally occurring cases, especially in the chronic stages.

Interstitial nephritis is common in dogs and cats, both as a primary disease and secondary to glomerular diseases. Acute generalized interstitial nephritis can be caused by *Leptospira canicola* infection in dogs. *Leptospira canicola* is commonly associated with interstitial nephritis in the United Kingdom, although its importance is declining because of the efficacy of vaccination; *L. icterohaemorrhagiae* and canine adenovirus 1 (infectious canine hepatitis) are also commonly involved. According to serologic evidence, leptospirosis is common in domestic animals and, in severe cases, interstitial nephritis often occurs. The most severe infections are usually caused by *L. pomona* in cattle and swine, and *L. canicola* and *L. icterohaemorrhagiae* in dogs. Inflammatory cells gradually disappear, marked interstitial fibrosis and loss of nephrons cause contracture of the kidney, and chronic interstitial nephritis results. Diffuse interstitial nephritis is less common in large domestic animals than in dogs; the usual end result of leptospirosis in cattle and swine is multifocal interstitial nephritis. Leptospirosis is discussed in detail in Section VI,D of The Kidney in this chapter.

Encephalitozoon cuniculi, an obligate intracellular microsporidian parasite, causes diffuse nonsuppurative to granulomatous interstitial nephritis and granulomatous encephalitis in dogs. The renal lesion is characterized by heavy, almost pure, interstitial infiltrates of plasma cells. The Gram-positive organisms occur in tubular epithelial cells, tubular lumina, and in vessel walls. The disease is discussed with The Nervous System (Volume 1, Chapter 3).

The best-known form of multifocal nonsuppurative interstitial nephritis is the white-spotted kidney of calves.

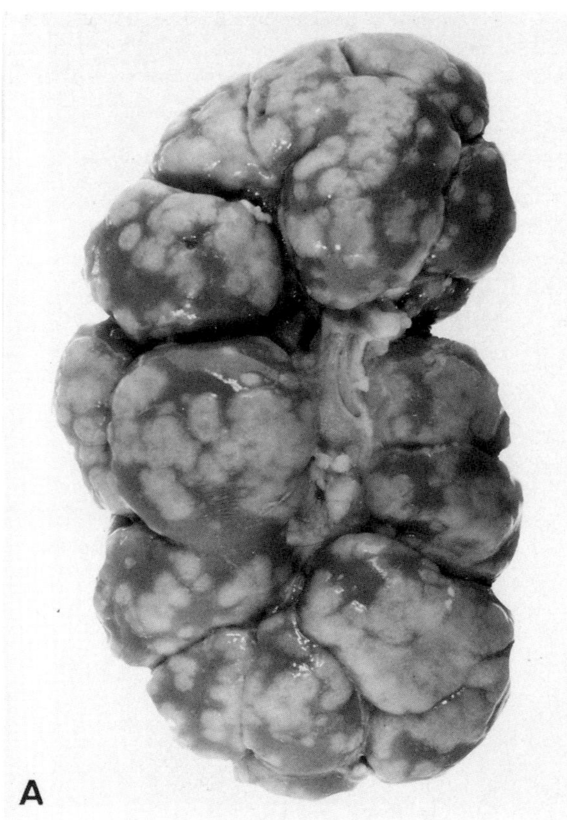

Fig. 5.43A White-spotted kidney. Calf.

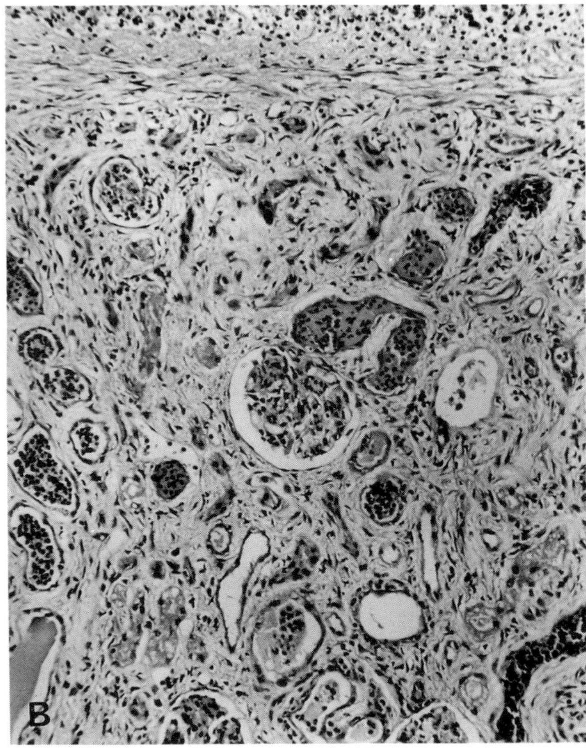

Fig. 5.43B Section of cortex in 5.43A showing interstitial reaction.

This is common and appears to be of little significance because it is largely an incidental finding in young calves and is probably obliterated with advancing age. The cause is usually undetermined but is most likely the result of bacteremia; *Escherichia coli* can occasionally be recovered from the lesions. *Salmonella* and *Brucella* are other suggested causes. Affected kidneys contain multiple small white nodules as large as 1 cm diameter throughout the cortex. The larger nodules may bulge from the capsular surface of the kidney and adhere to the capsule (Fig. 5.43A). Histologically, the initial lesion is a microabscess, which is soon replaced by numerous lymphocytes and occasional plasma cells and macrophages. Progressive fibrosis results in healing by scar tissue. The inflammation and scarring may cause tubular obstruction and/or atrophy (Fig. 5.43B).

Multifocal interstitial nephritis also occurs in cattle in the course of malignant catarrhal fever, theileriosis, and lumpy-skin disease; in sheep, in sheep pox; and in the horse, in equine infectious anemia. The renal lesions do not contribute significantly to the course of these diseases but are of some diagnostic importance; their gross and histologic features are given elsewhere. Multifocal pyogranulomatous lesions are a rather consistent finding in the kidneys of cats with feline infectious peritonitis. Canine herpesvirus produces severe necrotizing nephritis as part of the systemic disease in puppies (see The Female Genital System. Volume 3, Chapter 4).

B. Suppurative Interstitial Nephritis

Bacterial infection of the kidneys may be either **hematogenous** (Fig. 5.44A,B), and cause embolic suppurative nephritis, or **urogenous,** and cause pyelonephritis. Pyelonephritis means inflammation of both the pelvis and renal parenchyma, and, whereas pelvic inflammation may result from septic renal foci (Fig. 5.45), most cases of pyelonephritis arise from ascending urinary infections.

Adenoviral infection of sheep is most significant as a cause of pneumonia, but also causes mild, multifocal, suppurative interstitial nephritis, with characteristic large, basophilic, intranuclear inclusion bodies in endothelial and/or interstitial cells.

C. Embolic Suppurative Nephritis

This is analogous to abscess formation in any organ, and occurs when any of a wide variety of bacteria is seeded in the kidneys in the course of bacteremia or septic thromboembolism. Bacteria alone or in small clumps, and small septic emboli, lodge mainly in glomerular and peritubular capillaries (Figs. 5.24A, 5.46), and may produce multiple small abscesses or fewer large ones. Larger emboli lodge in afferent vessels and produce septic infarcts, which may be unilateral. Many bacteria undoubtedly pass through the glomerular capillary walls into the tubules, where they are probably harmless unless there is stasis of urine. Developed abscesses are generally cortical rather than medullary but in bacteremia caused by Gram-negative enterobacteria, microscopic suppurative foci may be scattered in the medulla. If healing of the suppurative lesions occurs, it is by scar formation. The healed lesions of isolated abscesses are occasionally seen, but extensive renal scarring as a sequel to multiple abscessation is rare, as the

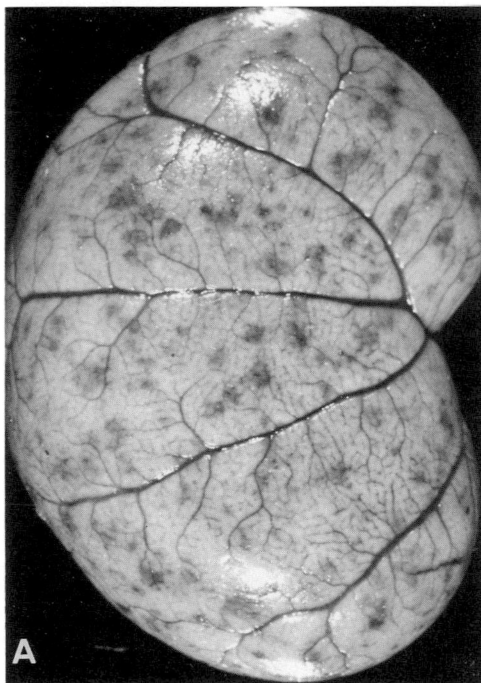

Fig. 5.44A Multifocal embolic nephritis. Cat. *Pasteurella multocida*.

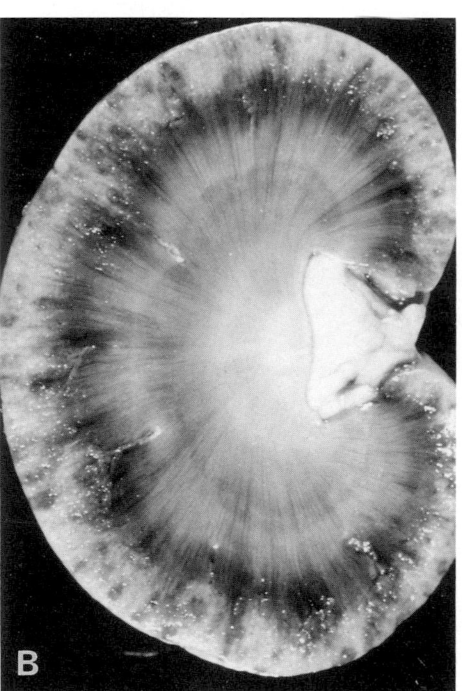

Fig. 5.44B Cut surface of kidney in (A).

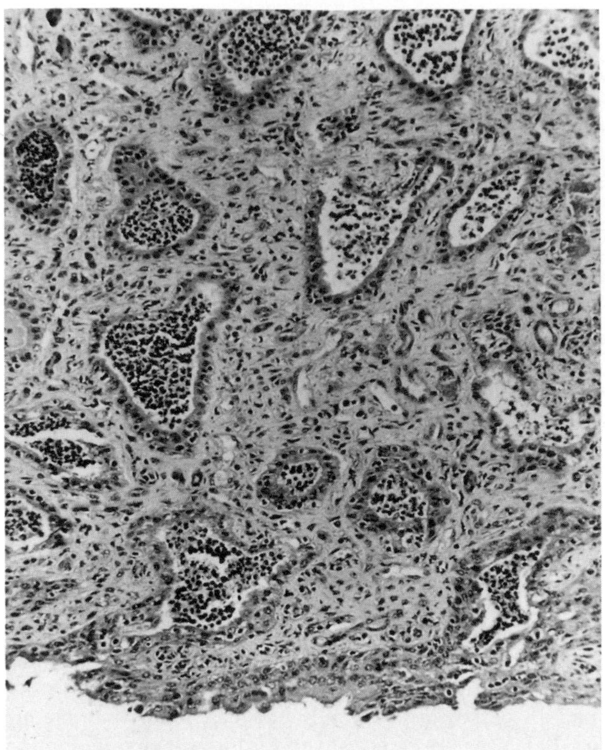

Fig. 5.45 Descending pyelonephritis in white-spotted kidney. Calf.

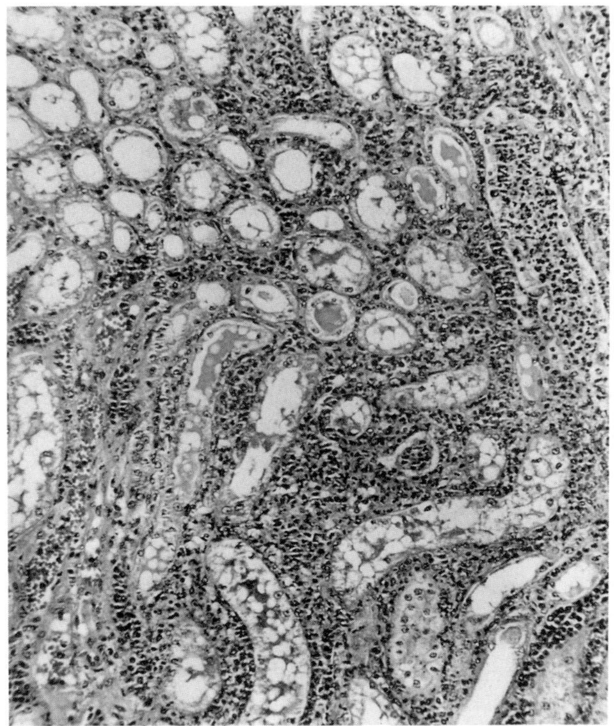

Fig. 5.46 Hematogenous interstitial nephritis. Dog. *Klebsiella pneumoniae*.

animal is likely to die of the primary disease or from renal insufficiency early in the course of the disease.

In horses, the most common cause of embolic suppurative nephritis is *Actinobacillus equuli,* which is acquired *in utero,* during parturition, or shortly after birth; it is probably an umbilical infection. Death may occur due to fulminating septicemia. In foals which survive for several days, typical microabscessation is seen in the kidneys and other organs, and polyarthritis is present. The abscesses are usually green-yellow foci of as large as 3 mm diameter, which contain a small droplet of pus. The most common cause of embolic nephritis in swine is probably *Erysipelothrix rhusiopathiae*. Embolic glomerulonephritis may be seen grossly as glomerular hemorrhages; microabscesses form in the interstitium. In adult cattle, most cases are caused by *Actinomyces pyogenes* from valvular endocarditis, the septic emboli often producing large, randomly distributed abscesses and infarcts. In sheep and goats, renal abscessation caused by *Corynebacterium pseudotuberculosis* is common.

Bibliography

Bush, B. M., and Evans, J. M. Infectious canine hepatitis and chronic renal failure. *Vet Rec* **90:** 33–34, 1972.

Cole, J. R. *et al.* Infections with *Encephalitozoon cuniculi* and *Leptospira interrogans,* serovars *grippotyphosa* and *ballum,* in a kennel of foxhounds. *J Am Vet Med Assoc* **180:** 435–437, 1982.

DiBartola, S. P. *et al.* Clinicopathologic findings associated with chronic renal disease in cats: 74 cases (1973–1984). *J Am Vet Med Assoc* **190:** 1196–1202, 1987.

Eddy, A. A. *et al.* A relationship between proteinuria and acute tubulointerstitial diseases in rats with experimental nephrotic syndrome. *Am J Pathol* **138:** 1111–1123, 1991.

Finnie, J. W., and Swift, J. G. Adenovirus infection in ovine kidney and liver. *Aust Vet J* **68:** 184, 1991.

Hartley, W. J., and Done, J. T. Cytomegalic inclusion-body disease in sheep. A report of two cases. *J Comp Pathol* **73:** 84–87, 1963.

Mezza, L. E. *et al.* Antitubular basement membrane autoantibody in a dog with chronic tubulointerstitial nephritis. *Vet Pathol* **21:** 178–181, 1984.

Morrison, W. I., Wright, N. G., and Cornwell, H. J. C. An immunopathologic study of interstitial nephritis associated with experimental canine adenovirus infection. *J Pathol* **120:** 221–228, 1976.

Shirota, K., and Fujiwara, K. Nephropathy in dogs induced by treatment with antiserum against renal basement membrane. *Jpn J Vet Sci* **44:** 767–776, 1982.

Smyth, J. A. *et al.* Adenoviral infection of the renal interstitium of a lamb. *Vet Pathol* **27:** 290–292, 1990.

Szabo, J. R., and Shadduck, J. A. Experimental encephalitozoonosis in neonatal dogs. *Vet Pathol* **24:** 99–108, 1987.

Timoney, J. F., Sheahan, B. J., and Timoney, P. J. *Leptospira* and infectious canine hepatitis (ICH) virus antibodies and nephritis in Dublin dogs. *Vet Rec* **94:** 316–319, 1974.

Toto, R. D. Review: Acute tubulointerstitial nephritis. *Am J Med Sci* **299:** 392–410, 1990.

Wright, N. G. *et al.* Chronic renal failure in dogs: A comparative clinical and morphological study of chronic glomerulonephritis and chronic interstitial nephritis. *Vet Rec* **98:** 288–293, 1976.

TABLE 5.3

Common Leptospiral Serovars of Disease Significance in Domestic Animals

Serovar	Maintenance host	Distribution	Species disease significance
autumnalis	Rodents	Global, tropics especially	+ ? Dogs
bratislava	Pigs, horses, (dogs?)	Global	+ + + + Pigs + Horses, dogs
canicola	Dogs	Global	+ + + Dogs + All species
grippotyphosa	Raccoon, skunk, small rodents	Global	+
hardjo type hardjo-bovis	Cattle	Global	+ Cattle, all species
type hardjoprajitno	Cattle	Europe	+ + + Cattle
icterohaemorrhagiae	Rats	Global	+ + + + Dogs, humans
pomona type kennewicki	Pigs	Global? (some exceptions)	+ + + + Pigs
	Wildlife, cattle	Global? (some exceptions)	+ + + Cattle, all species
tarassovi	Pigs	Europe, Australasia	+ + + Pigs

*D. Leptospirosis**

Leptospirosis is an important, largely hidden, complex, neglected, and intriguing spirochetal infection of animals and humans caused by serovars of *Leptospira interrogans*. It is particularly important as a cause of abortion and stillbirth in farm animals but also causes loss through acute disease (septicemia, hepatitis, nephritis, meningitis) in these and other animals. Many aspects of leptospirosis are poorly understood because of difficulties in diagnosis, the changing pattern of disease because of vaccination and antibiotic use, and the complexities of host–leptospiral relationships. Although some generalizations are helpful, leptospirosis is best understood in terms of the individual relationship between specific serovars and particular host species rather than as a single disease with a common epidemiology, host response, and approach to control.

Leptospirosis can be caused by any of the 180 serovars belonging to the 19 serogroups of *Leptospira interrogans*. The use of serotyping to distinguish isolates into serovars is increasingly being replaced by restriction enzyme analysis of chromosomal DNA to identify genotypes. This is a simpler and more informative process. For example, genotyping has divided serovar *hardjo* into two distinct types, hardjo-bovis and hardjoprajitno, which differ both in geographic distribution and in virulence. Recent studies further suggest that these two genotypes belong to two separate species, as *L. borgpetersoni* serovar *hardjo* strain bovis and *L. interrogans* serovar *hardjoprajitno*. Thus, genetically unrelated leptospires, belonging to one of the probably six species of what used to be described as *L. interrogans,* may be antigenically identical. Restriction enzyme analysis has also assigned most North American serovar *pomona* isolates to serovar *kennewicki,* and further identified pig-associated and cattle-associated subtypes.

Although many serovars are recognized globally, only a limited number are usually endemic to a particular region (Table 5.3). Geographic differences in the distribution of serovars are marked, but the true incidence and prevalence of leptospirosis are largely undetermined for most countries and regions. Serologic surveys tend to be flawed because antigens chosen may not represent serovars present in the country, because serologic prevalence does not necessarily indicate disease significance, because sampling is often done on the basis of convenience rather than in a carefully designed, epidemiologically valid manner, and because titers designated as significant [usually $\geq$ 1:100 in the microscopic agglutination test (MAT)] may underestimate the true seroprevalence of some host-adapted serovars.

Each serovar is adapted to and may cause disease in particular maintenance hosts although they may cause disease in any other species, the incidental hosts. The general distinctions between these types of hosts are shown in Table 5.4, which also shows reactions of serovars with an intermediate type of host–parasite relation.

The natural reservoir of pathogenic leptospires is the proximal convoluted tubules of the kidney, and in certain maintenance hosts, the genital tract. In maintenance hosts particularly, transmission may be direct, through urine splashing, in postabortion discharges, venereally, through milk, or transplacentally in congenitally affected animals. Infection of incidental hosts is more commonly indirect, through environmental contamination by the urine of carrier animals. Close contact of maintenance hosts aids spread but, especially for incidental hosts, environmental conditions determine the success of indirect transmission. Optimal conditions for survival of leptospires are moist, warm (optimal 28°C), and neutral or mildly alkaline conditions (flood fever, swamp fever). Under ideal conditions, leptospires may survive weeks or months in waterlogged soil (mud fever) or stagnant water. Under adverse conditions, survival is measured in minutes. Leptospirosis thus occurs especially in the autumn in temperate climates (fall fever), and in the winter in tropical climates, seasons which may also coincide with the greater population sizes of wildlife shedders.

*Contributed by John F. Prescott

TABLE 5.4

General Distinctions between Maintenance and Incidental Hosts in Leptospiral Infection

Characteristic	Maintenance host	"Intermediate" host	Incidental host
Susceptibility to infection by the serovar	+ + + +[a]	+ + +	+ +
Endemic transmission within host species	+ + + +	+ + + +	+
Pathogenicity for the host	+ +	+ + +	+ + +
Type of disease caused	Chronic, reproductive loss especially	Acute or chronic	Acute or chronic
Persistence in kidney	+ + + +	+ + + +	+
Persistence in genital tract	+ + + +	−	−
Microscopic agglutinating antibody response	Low titer, sometimes nil	High titer	High titer
Efficacy of vaccination in controlling losses	± to + + + +	+ + + +	+ + + +
Examples	Pig, *bratislava* Cattle, *hardjo*	Pig, *pomona* Dog, *canicola*	Pigs and cattle, *canicola, grippotyphosa* Cattle, *pomona*

[a] Arbitrary scale for comparison.

Leptospires penetrate exposed mucosal surfaces or water-softened skin and disseminate throughout the body, in a leptospiremic phase lasting as long as 7 days, but especially to the liver, kidneys, lungs, placenta, udder, and cerebrospinal fluid. The development of agglutinating and opsonizing antibody ~6 days after infection clears the organisms from sites other than those which immunoglobulins penetrate poorly (proximal convoluted tubules of the kidney, cerebrospinal fluid, vitreous humor of the eye), and, for certain serovars, the genital tract (oviducts, uterus, vagina in females; testes, epididymes, prostate, and seminal vesicles in males) of maintenance hosts.

Most leptospiral infections are supposedly subclinical, particularly in nonpregnant and nonlactating animals, detected only by the presence of antibody or of minor lesions of interstitial nephritis at slaughter. Infection may also cause acute or subacute systemic disease during the leptospiremic phase or, after leptospiremia has ceased, chronic disease in the form of abortion or stillbirth, infertility, or recurrent uveitis.

Acute and often severe disease may occur in the leptospiremic phase, particularly in young animals. Jaundice is a common manifestation of acute disease and occurs because of hemolysis due to hemolysin production and because of hepatocellular injury of both toxic and ischemic origin. The clinical disease is characterized by fever, jaundice, hemolytic anemia, hemoglobinuria, pulmonary congestion, and occasionally meningitis. Capillary injury of unknown cause occurs in acute disease. Anemia is initially the result of hemolysins but may later be due to antibodies causing an intravascular hemolytic anemia by reaction with leptospiral products coating red blood cells. Postsepticemic localization of leptospires in the kidneys is associated with focal or diffuse interstitial nephritis and with acute, transient tubular degeneration.

Renal failure is a recognized consequence of infection with *canicola* and other serovars in dogs but is not often described in other animals, even though interstitial nephritis, especially in pigs, can be extensive. Leptospires reach the kidney hematogenously and migrate randomly, persist briefly in the interstitial spaces, and enter tubules at all levels of the nephron. Once antibody develops, the leptospires localize to the proximal convoluted tubules where they may multiply. The physiological changes to glomerular filtrate lower in the nephron, and formed urine, damage leptospires. The interstitial phase is accompanied by marked vascular alterations that produce hyperemia, edema, and endothelial swelling. Tubular epithelial degeneration is likely to be the combined result of hypoxia due to hypovolemia and red cell loss, of poorly described bacterial toxins including lipooligosaccharides and sphingomyelinases, of free hemoglobin, and of the interstitial inflammatory reaction to leptospires. Leptospiral antigen is demonstrable by immunoperoxidase staining in epithelial cell phagosomes, and is the counterpart of minute, round, black spherical bodies seen with silver stains. Tubular degeneration is well established by 2 weeks and is accompanied by interstitial infiltration of plasma cells and lymphocytes, which may be focal or diffuse. Leptospiral antigen is present in peritubular macrophages. The renal lesions may be insignificant, or may cause chronic debility or death in uremia.

Abortion, stillbirth, or the birth of congenitally infected young may follow weeks or months after maternal leptospiremia and is the most important form of the disease in ruminants and pigs. Serovar *bratislava* may also cause infertility in swine, as possibly may serovar *hardjo* infection in cattle. Horses are particularly likely to develop recurrent uveitis (periodic ophthalmia) following serovar *pomona* infection.

Leptospires are delicate, slender spirochetes (6–20 $\mu m \times 0.1\ \mu m$), with hooked ends like question marks, which led to the name *L. interrogans*. They do not stain with the usual aniline bacterial dyes but may be stained by Giemsa or, in tissue, by silver-impregnation techniques of Levaditi or Warthin–Starry. Dark-field microscopy is generally used in routine laboratory study. Demonstration of leptospires by dark-field microscopy of fluids, or silver staining of tissue sections, are insensitive methods which give both false-negative and false-positive results. Immunofluorescence of urine, or of homogenates of tissues such as fetal lung and kidney or of placenta, is an excellent diagnostic technique, almost equivalent in sensitivity to isolation in experienced laboratories. It is a method of choice in the diagnosis of leptospirosis. Difficulties may be experienced with serovar *bratislava*. Leptospires die readily in tissues or body fluids unless kept at 4°C. Results may be improved if tissues are submitted to laboratories in leptospiral transport medium.

1. Cattle

Serovars of major importance are *hardjo* and *pomona* type kennewicki in North America and *hardjo* in Europe. There is serologic evidence of infection with other serovars including *canicola, grippotyphosa,* and *icterohaemorrhagiae,* among others, but these serovars are not often implicated in disease, although geographic variations will occur. Serovar *hardjo* has become increasingly recognized with a concomitant, apparent decline in importance of serovar *pomona*. Cattle are reservoir hosts for *hardjo*. Serovar *hardjo* type hardjoprajitno, which is recognized in Europe but not in North America or Australia and New Zealand, appears to be more virulent than type hardjo-bovis. In Northern Ireland, where type hardjoprajitno occurs, *hardjo* was recognized in one study as responsible for nearly half of all abortions. This type was isolated from most aborted or stillborn fetuses, whereas type hardjo-bovis was isolated mainly from the kidney and genital tract of carrier cows. In one large study in Ontario, Canada, where only hardjo-bovis rather than hardjoprajitno is thought to occur, serovar *hardjo* was identified in about 6% of abortions; no serovar *pomona* was recognized.

The most severe (but uncommon) manifestation of acute infection occurs in calves infected with incidental serovars, especially *pomona*. Hemoglobinuria is usually the first sign noticed and may be transient or last 2–3 days. In fatal cases, it gives the urine a port-wine color. Hematuria from hemorrhage into renal tubules may give rise to blood clots in the urinary tract. There is fever, anemia, icterus, dyspnea because of pulmonary congestion, and occasionally meningitis. High levels of albumin and bilirubin are present in the urine. In cows, agalactia with small quantities of blood-tinged milk, which may be stained yellow and thickened like colostrum, is also typical. Abortion may occur during the acute phase or several weeks later during convalescence. The fetus is frequently decomposed, indicating death some time before abortion.

The most common form of the disease is a less severe, subacute form characterized in dairy cows by a 2- to 10-day drop in milk production with transient pyrexia. In this milk drop syndrome or flabby udder mastitis form, the milk has the consistency of colostrum, with thick clots, yellow staining, and the udder has a soft texture. This form is commonly associated with serovar *hardjo* type hardjoprajitno, but may be caused by all serovars.

The chronic form of the disease, most commonly associated with serovars *hardjo* and *pomona,* is fetal infection in pregnant cows, presenting as abortion, stillbirth, or the birth of premature and weak infected calves. Abortion and stillbirth is often the only manifestation of infection, but may be related to an episode of illness up to 6 weeks (*pomona*) or 12 weeks (*hardjo*) earlier. Serovar *hardjo* type hardjoprajitno appears to be more virulent than, and to cause more abortion than, *hardjo* type hardjo-bovis.

The hematologic changes are mild in cases not characterized by hemoglobinuria and severe in those that are. Animals with acute intravascular hemolysis will have moderate to marked anemia, but hemoglobin levels may be erroneously high because of the measurement of free hemoglobin associated with hemoglobinemia.

The postmortem appearance of an animal that dies of acute leptospirosis is characterized by mild icterus and severe anemia. Hemorrhages may be absent, or ecchymoses may be numerous on serous membranes and in the subcutis. The lungs are pale, edematous, and expanded, and the fluid, stained by bilirubin, widens the septa. The liver is enlarged, friable, anemic, and bile stained. It may contain hemorrhages and small zones of necrosis about the central veins, but necrotic foci are not usually seen grossly. Hemoglobinuria is to be expected but may not be present. The kidneys are swollen; during a hemolytic crisis they are dark, but later the pigmented foci become restricted to small groups of tubules and have an appearance suggestive of numerous small hemorrhages. Still later, the kidneys show more or less numerous small grayish foci of interstitial reaction that are rather indistinct and more numerous in the cortex than in the medulla (Fig. 5.47). It is doubtful whether cattle die of chronic interstitial nephritis caused by leptospires, but in animals that have recovered from the acute diseases, foci of renal inflammation are the only morphologic traces remaining.

The histologic changes in bovine leptospirosis are neither prominent nor specific. Edema of the lungs is apparent, and in scattered groups of alveoli and septal lymphatics, there are thin laces of fibrin. Zonal necrosis occurs in the liver; it is usually periacinar and typically a change of severe anemic anoxia. The Kupffer cells are hyperplastic and contain excessive amounts of hemosiderin, and there is a diffuse but mild cellular infiltration in the portal triads. In the uncommon infections caused by *L. icterohaemorrhagiae,* necrosis in the liver and dissociation of the cords of hepatic cells are more likely to occur than in infections caused by the other serovars. If the survival period in the acute hemolytic disease is sufficiently long, the biliary canaliculi become distended with bile.

In the acutely fatal disease, there are often marked degenerative changes in the epithelium of the cortical renal tubules, the changes varying in severity from hydropic swelling to necrosis and desquamation. The desquamated

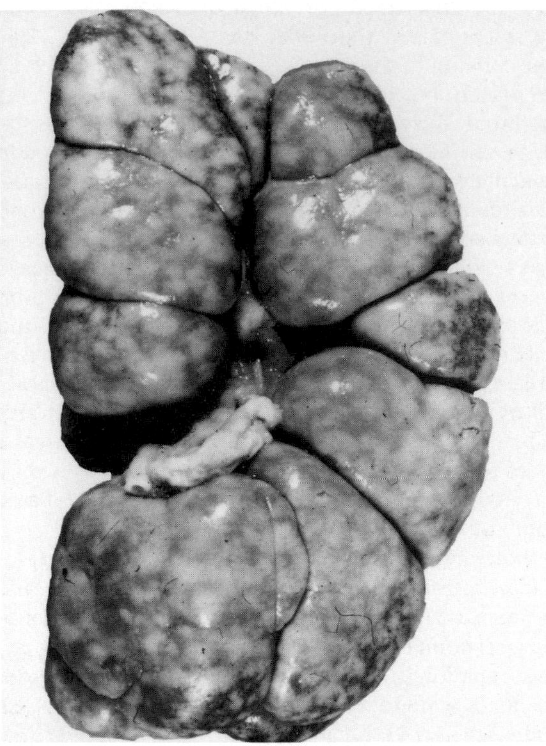

Fig. 5.47 Leptospirosis. Interstitial nephritis caused by serovar *pomona*. Ox.

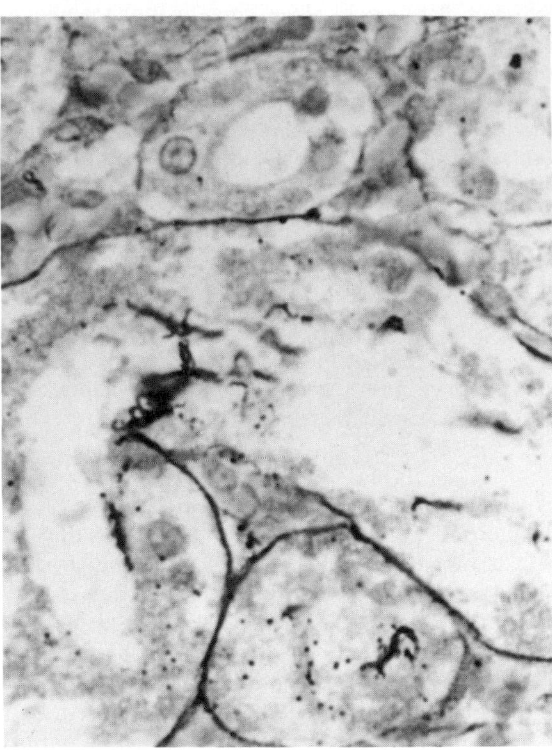

Fig. 5.48 Intratubular leptospires in kidney. Ox. Silver stain.

epithelium produces, in the tubules, granular and cellular casts in addition to the hyaline ones of albuminuria and hemoglobinuria and those due to direct bleeding into the tubules. Pigmentation by intracellular hemoglobin and biliary pigments does not become fully evident until 2 days, and the tubules, which then are strikingly involved, occur in clusters. There is also edema of the kidneys, with distension of the interstitial tissues with fluid, and in this there is a mild but diffuse infiltration of plasma cells and lymphocytes. In the acute disease, the organisms can often be demonstrated by appropriate stains in the liver, in which they are partly intracellular, and in the kidneys, in which they occur in the tubular epithelium and frequently as clusters in the tubular lumen (Fig. 5.48).

In recovery from the acute disease and in due course in subclinical illness, the organisms localize in microcolonies in the kidneys. The microcolonies are in intratubular clumps; it is exceptional to find organisms in the interstitial tissue. The organisms are shed in the urine. Renal localization is associated with more or less widespread focal interstitial nephritis (Fig. 5.49A,B). The inflammatory reaction is virtually confined to the cortex. The focal nephritis is of conventional type, the principal participants in the cellular reaction being lymphocytes and plasma cells. The reaction subsides very slowly, and the inflammatory cells decrease in number as the focal lesions scarify. An odd feature of the active lesions is the atypical regenerative pattern of tubular epithelium within the areas of inflamma-

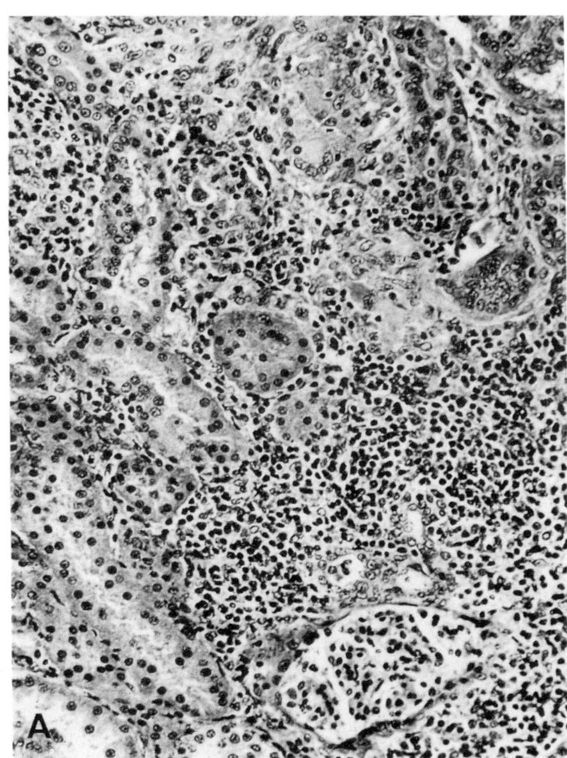

Fig. 5.49A Interstitial nephritis. Leptospirosis. Ox. Scattered giant cells and focal hyperplasia of tubular epithelium.

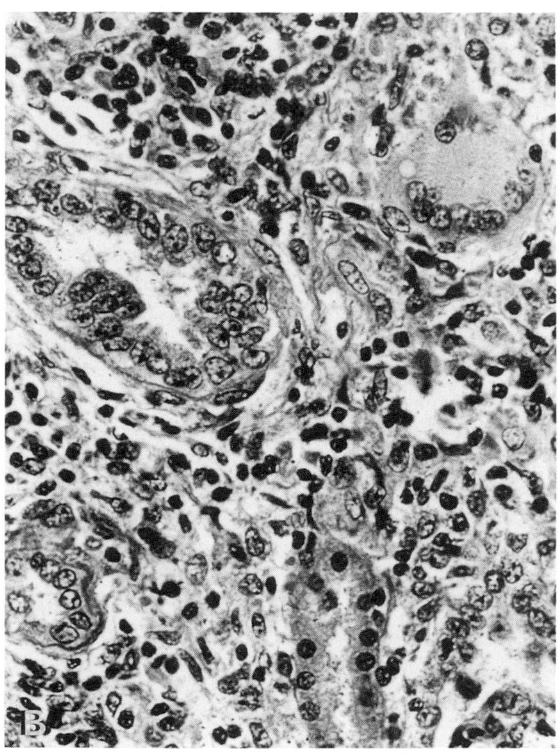

Fig. 5.49B Interstitial nephritis. Leptospirosis. Ox. Detail of (A).

tion; the regenerating cells produce a few bizarre syncytia as well as a few giant cells morphologically similar to those of a foreign-body reaction (Fig. 5.49B).

The aborted fetuses show no specific changes, although the organism can often be demonstrated in the fetal tissues (see The Female Genital System, Volume 3, Chapter 4). The fetuses are sometimes edematous, but the edema is not specific, and in many cases there is advanced autolysis or putrefaction by the time the fetus is aborted. The placenta may show mild microscopic changes of placentitis; there is a tendency for it to be unduly retained.

2. Sheep, Goats, and Deer

Sheep, goats, and deer may be less susceptible than cattle to clinical leptospirosis. The major serovar in sheep is *hardjo,* which is maintained in a maintenance cycle independent of cattle. Other serovars may also cause disease. Acute disease in lambs resembles that described in calves. *Hardjo* infection of ewes may cause late-term abortion, stillbirth, and weak lambs, and agalactia in recently lambed ewes. Other serovars may sometimes cause abortion. Leptospirosis in goats is not often described, but clinical and pathologic changes are similar to those described for cattle. Fatal nephritis of farmed young red deer due to serovar *pomona* has been described in New Zealand. Kidneys were two to three times normal size and showed histologic changes of severe chronic active nephritis, characterized by extensive, segmental inflammation of cortical interstitial tissue.

3. Dogs

Dogs are susceptible to infection with a number of serovars, but those best recognized to cause severe disease are *canicola* and *icterohaemorrhagiae*. *Canicola* is host-maintained in the dog, but widespread use of vaccination has virtually eradicated this infection from dogs in many countries. *Icterohaemorrhagiae* is generally acquired from rats, and other serovars (*autumnalis, bratislava, pomona*) from their respective hosts (Table 5.3). Serologic evidence of infection with serovar *bratislava* is increasingly recognized, and this organism may cause nephritis and abortion in dogs. Clinical infections with serovars other than *canicola* and *icterohaemorrhagiae* may be under-reported.

It is not possible to separate, on the basis of clinical evidence, acute infections caused by different serovars, although, as a generalization, *icterohaemorrhagiae* exerts its effect more specifically on the liver; *canicola,* on the kidney; and other serovars in a less severe way on both organs. *Icterohaemorrhagiae* is associated with severe icterus, and *canicola,* with severe renal injury, but the syndromes shown by these and other serovars may overlap.

The hyperacute infection, which is usually one of puppies and usually caused by *icterohaemorrhagiae,* is acute in onset, with the course of a fulminating septicemia; death occurs in a few hours to 2–3 days. There is fever, dehydration, hypersensitivity, and a marked tendency to hemorrhage, providing for hematemesis, melena, epistaxis, and petechiae on the mucous membranes. In the acute disease, in which icterus is a prominent feature, the onset may be sudden, with the development of icterus delayed, or the onset may be insidious, with icterus as the first abnormality observed. There is frequently an oculonasal discharge, which may suggest distemper, especially in younger animals. The temperature is usually only mildly elevated at the time of clinical evaluation.

Widespread hemorrhages characterize both the hyperacute and the acute disease, although icterus is usually absent in the former case. The most consistent gross lesions occur in the kidneys, and in acute cases consist of subcapsular hemorrhages with multifocal ecchymotic and petechial hemorrhages throughout cortical areas but most prominent in subcapsular regions. With chronicity, these foci become pale, and the capsule is increasingly adherent. Residual lesions in dogs given viable *canicola* and killed 100 days later consisted of symmetrically enlarged kidneys with nodular and wedge-shaped lesions 4–8 mm in diameter at the corticomedullary junction. Lesions have been described in the liver of dogs with spontaneous infections of *grippotyphosa* that vary from gross enlargement, with focal lesions, sclerosis, ascites, and atrophy, to fibrosis and nodular hyperplasia.

In animals dying acutely, focal necrosis is frequent in the liver but may not be present. The characteristic change, but not a specific one, is dissociation of the cells of the parenchymal cords. The dissociated cells become discrete and rounded, the cytoplasm becomes eosinophilic and coarsely granular, and the nuclei become shrunken and dark. Regeneration is sometimes prominent and evidenced by cytomegaly, binucleation, and mitoses. The Kupffer cells contain excess hemosiderin, and many biliary canaliculi are plugged. The organisms can be demonstrated by appropriate techniques in the sinusoids and in the hepatic epithelial cells. Serovar *grippotyphosa* may cause chronic active hepatitis, with peribiliary fibrosis, and lobular disarray, with irregular fibrosis.

In dogs that survive the acute septicemic, icteric type of disease, or fail to manifest a septicemic phase at all, the clinical and pathologic emphasis shifts from the liver to the kidneys; the resultant syndrome is the usual way in which infections by *canicola* are manifest. The signs are those of renal insufficiency and vary in their severity and rapidity of progression; death may supervene rather rapidly from the renal failure of acute diffuse nephritis, but it also appears that initially inapparent infections may set in motion a train of events in the kidneys that after a long time, possibly many years, results in the renal failure of chronic interstitial nephritis. In these, the renal syndromes, the lesion caused directly by the leptospires is acute diffuse interstitial nephritis, from which recovery may occur to a focal pattern, or which may progress to subacute and chronic interstitial nephritis.

In the acute phase, the renal changes are severe but largely characterized by degeneration rather than by reaction. The brunt of the injury is borne by the convoluted tubules, the epithelium of which manifests changes varying from hydropic degeneration to necrosis. The latter may be extensive enough to denude considerable areas of tubular basement membrane. In the course of a couple of days, regeneration begins, during which, as described in cattle, atypical syncytial giant cells may form. These acute changes in the kidney are accompanied by interstitial edema and a diffuse but sparse infiltration by leukocytes, principally lymphocytes and plasma cells. The leptospires are demonstrable in the tubular epithelium and in the lumina of tubules, frequently in clusters. Early in the renal phase, the organisms may be found in any part of the cortex, but later they are more restricted in their distribution and are then mainly to be found in the more superficial, subcapsular areas. With chronicity, the interstitial cellular exudate is decreased, and fibrosis increases, with mild diffuse and moderate focal interstitial sclerosis and thickened Bowman's capsule and basement membranes with focal periglomerular fibrosis. There is increased cellularity of the renal pelvis, and the fibrosis extends into the papillae. The lymph nodes and spleen may be enlarged and edematous or hemorrhagic, and microscopically there is depletion of lymphocytes and increase of sinusoidal reticular cells. Erythrophagocytosis is prominent.

4. *Swine*

Although any leptospiral serovar may cause disease in pigs, until recently the most important serovar recognized in North America was *pomona* (type kennewicki), a subtype of which is host-adapted to swine. In Australia and some European countries, *tarassovi* (formerly *hyos*), another pig-adapted serovar, causes losses as serious as those of *pomona*. Understanding of leptospirosis in swine is rapidly changing with the recognition of the widespread and dominant prevalence of antibodies to the Australis serogroup (serovars *bratislava, lora, muenchen*) and the isolation particularly of *bratislava* and *muenchen* from aborted and stillborn pigs. The role and importance of Australis serogroup leptospires is only partially understood, in part because of the difficulty of isolating these leptospires. Incidental infections with serovars *canicola, grippotyphosa, hardjo,* and other serovars have been locally important. Antibody to *icterohaemorrhagiae* is widespread, but the serovar is of rare disease significance.

Only a small proportion of infected animals develop clinical illness, usually an unrecognized transient episode of mild fever, anorexia, and depression. Hemoglobinuria and icterus may occur rarely in piglets.

The principal aspect of the disease in pigs, apart from transmissibility to other species, is abortion and the birth of weak piglets, which may reach outbreak proportions. This is particularly likely to occur if pregnant sows with no acquired immunity are exposed during the second month of pregnancy. Abortion is associated with heavy leptospiral infection of the fetus.

The usual pattern of leptospirosis in pregnant sows, caused by serovars other than those of the Australis serogroup, is for the litter to be delivered 1–3 weeks prematurely, with some of the fetuses mummified, some more recently dead, and some born alive, only to die shortly afterward. The mummified fetuses are unrevealing, but the organism can usually be recovered from the fresher ones, some of which in each litter are expected to have lesions. Not all aborted fetuses in the litter will yield leptospires. A straw-colored pleural effusion, somewhat viscid, may be accompanied by effusion of lesser volumes in the other serous cavities. Petechial hemorrhages may be present in the pulmonary pleura, epicardium, renal cortex, and peripelvic tissue, and occasionally elsewhere. The liver and spleen are swollen and dark, and tan foci of necrosis, 2–5 mm in size, in the liver, especially near the margins, are characteristic when present.

Histologic changes are also inconstant, but part or all of the picture is usually seen in one or more of the piglets, especially in those dying at or very soon after birth. The hepatitis is acute, with infiltrated neutrophils and lymphocytes in portal areas and surrounding the foci of coagulation necrosis (Fig. 5.50A). Focal myocarditis with coagulation necrosis and mononuclear infiltration is less frequent than infiltration beneath epicardium and endocardium (Fig. 5.50B). These latter infiltrations, also of mononuclear cells, are light but quite diffuse. In addition to many minor foci of interstitial reaction in the kidney, large, fairly circumscribed infiltrates of mononuclear cells are present in the peripelvic parenchyma, and sometimes involving the papilla (Fig. 5.51A) and encroaching on the

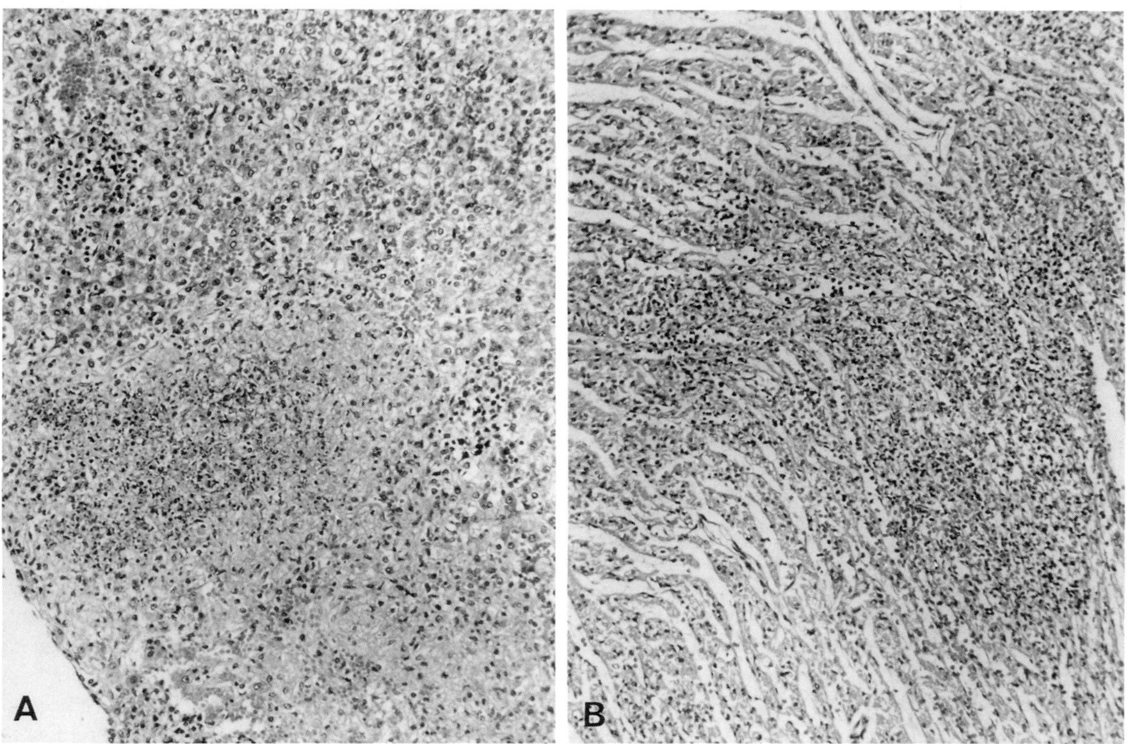

Fig. 5.50 Leptospirosis. Porcine neonate. (A) Hepatitis with subcapsular necrosis. (B) Interstitial lymphocytic myocarditis.

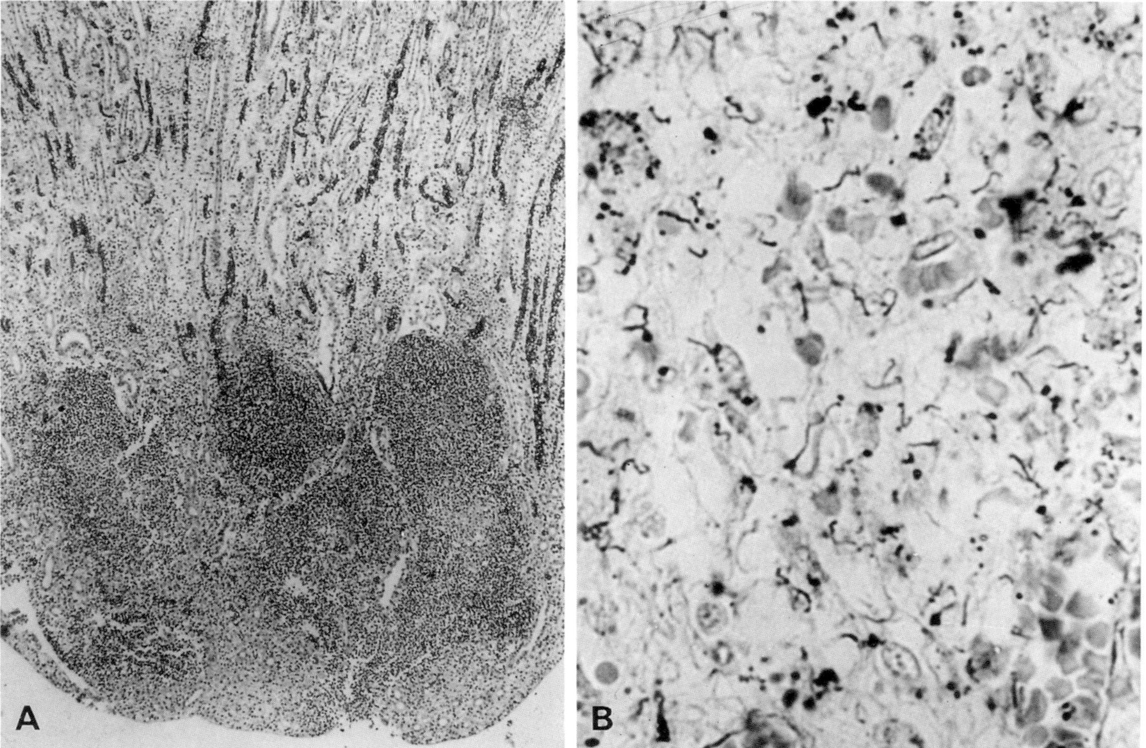

Fig. 5.51 Leptospirosis. Porcine neonate. (A) Renal papillitis. (B) Organisms in foci of papillitis.

parahilar cortex. The medullary tissues swarm with organisms (Fig. 5.51B).

The lesions as described are not specific for *pomona* infections. They have been observed also in *tarassovi* and can be anticipated with some other serovars.

Infection with serovars belonging to the Australis serogroup produce subtler losses than those described for *pomona* or other serovars. The lesions have not been described. In Northern Ireland and the United States of America late-term abortion and stillbirth have been reported, characterized by the birth of live, dying, and dead piglets within a litter. Late-term abortion is less characteristic than production of small litters of viable piglets, accompanied by stillborn piglets and by piglets which die shortly after birth. Diagnosis is problematic because of the extreme difficulty of isolation of serovars *bratislava* and *muenchen*.

A distinct infertility (repeat breeder) syndrome associated with Australis serogroup infection has been described in Northern Ireland. Disease is most noticeable in sows bred to infected boars for the first time or when susceptible animals are introduced into infected herds. Serovars *bratislava* and *muenchen* are commonly isolated from the genital tracts of sows and boars in infected herds. Venereal transmission is thought to be common.

The majority of instances of chronic interstitial nephritis in pigs, lesions of which are often observed at slaughter, are leptospiral in origin, associated particularly with serovar *pomona*.

5. *Horses*

There is widespread serologic evidence of leptospiral infection in horses, but acute disease is apparently rare. Clinical features include fever, anorexia, depression, and icterus in the acute disease and abortion, premature foaling, and chronic uveitis (periodic ophthalmia) in the chronic disease. Improved diagnostic techniques have confirmed the importance of leptospirosis in horses. It is now recognized that horses are maintenance hosts for *bratislava,* that leptospires are involved in fatal hepatic and renal disease in foals, that leptospires may be more important in abortion than previously thought, and that leptospirosis continues to cause chronic uveitis in horses.

Leptospires of a variety of serovars have been isolated or identified by immunofluorescence in Northern Ireland in neonatal foals or adults with fatal icterus. Different serovars, including *bratislava, canicola, grippotyphosa, hardjo, icterohaemorrhagiae,* but particularly *pomona,* may also cause subacute disease characterized by fever, but inconstantly by icterus, in adults. Although of generally minor significance *per se,* these infections have important chronic sequelae in the form of abortion or chronic uveitis. In North America, serovars in leptospiral abortion are, in order of importance, *pomona, grippotyphosa,* and *bratislava,* the first two being incidental infections. Abortion therefore tends to be seasonal (late fall and early winter). Giant-cell hepatitis in aborted fetuses has been associated with leptospiral infection; the lesions were characterized by dissociation of hepatocytes, disruption of hepatic cords, and numerous large, multinucleated hepatocytes. Recurrent uveitis may develop several months after leptospiral infection, particularly with serovar *pomona.* Antibody in the aqueous humor of the eye may considerably exceed serum antibody and assist in diagnosis in such cases.

Bibliography

Amatredjo, A., and Campbell, R. S. F. Bovine leptospirosis. *Vet Bull* **43:** 875–891, 1975.

Baker, T. F. *et al.* The prevalence of leptospirosis and its association with multifocal interstitial nephritis in swine at slaughter. *Can J Vet Res* **53:** 290–294, 1989.

Baldwin, C. J., and Atkins, C. F. Leptospirosis in dogs. *Compend Cont Ed Pract Vet* **9:** 499–508, 1987.

Bishop, L. *et al.* Chronic active hepatitis in dogs associated with leptospires. *Am J Vet Res* **40:** 839–844, 1979.

Bolin, C. A. *et al.* Reproductive failure associated with *Leptospira interrogans* serovar *bratislava* infection of swine. *J Vet Lab Diagn Invest* **3:** 152–154, 1991.

Champagne, M. J. *et al.* Detection and characterization of leptospiral antigens using a biotin/avidin double-antibody sandwich enzyme-linked immunosorbent assay and immunoblot. *Can J Vet Res* **55:** 239–245, 1991.

Donahue, J. M. *et al.* Diagnosis and prevalence of leptospira infection in aborted and stillborn horses. *J Vet Diagn Invest* **3:** 148–151, 1991.

Ellis, W. A. The diagnosis of leptospirosis in farm animals. *In* "The Present State of Leptospirosis Diagnosis and Control," W. A. Ellis, and T. W. A. Little (eds.), pp. 13–24. Dordrecht, Netherlands, Martinus Nijhoft, 1986.

Ellis, W. A. Effects of leptospirosis on bovine reproduction. *In* "Current Therapy in Theriogenology," 2nd Ed., D. W. Morrow (ed.), pp. 267–271. Philadelphia, Pennsylvania, W.B. Saunders, 1986.

Ellis, W. A. *Leptospira australis* infection in pigs. *Pig Vet J* **22:** 83–92, 1989.

Fairley, R. A. *et al.* Leptospirosis associated with serovars *hardjo* and *pomona* in red deer calves (*Cervus elephus*). *N Z Vet J* **32:** 76–78, 1984.

Hanson, L. E. *et al.* Current status of leptospirosis immunization in swine and cattle. *J Am Vet Med Assoc* **161:** 1235–1243, 1972.

Hathaway, S. C., and Little, T. W. A. Epidemiological study of *Leptospira hardjo* infection in second-calf dairy cows. *Vet Rec* **112:** 215, 1983.

Hathaway, S. C. *et al.* Serological survey of leptospiral antibodies in sheep from England and Wales. *Vet Rec* **110:** 99–101, 1982.

Prescott, J. F. *et al.* Seroprevalence and association with abortion of leptospirosis in cattle in Ontario. *Can J Vet Res* **52:** 210–215, 1988.

Scanziani, E., Sironi, G., and Mandelli, G. Immunoperoxidase studies on leptospiral nephritis of swine. *Vet Pathol* **26:** 442–444, 1989.

Sillerud, C. L. *et al.* Serologic correlation of suspected *Leptospira interrogans* serovar *pomona*-induced uveitis in a group of horses. *J Am Vet Med Assoc* **191:** 1576–1578, 1987.

Songer, J. G., and Thiermann, A. B. Leptospirosis. Zoonosis update. *J Am Vet Med Assoc* **193:** 1250–1254, 1988.

Thompson, J. C., and Manktelow, B. W. Pathogenesis of renal lesions in haemoglobinaemic and nonhaemoglobinaemic leptospirosis. *J Comp Pathol* **101:** 201–214, 1989.

Williams, R. D. *et al.* Experimental chronic uveitis. Ophthalmic signs following equine leptospirosis. *Invest Ophthalmol* **10:** 948–954, 1973.

E. Pyelonephritis

Pyelonephritis is inflammation of the pelvis and renal parenchyma, usually resulting from infection ascending from the lower urinary tract. It is characterized by inflammation, necrosis, and eventually deformity of the calyces, in association with areas of tubulointerstitial inflammation and necrosis, and is hence distinguishable from other forms of nephritis. It is usually accompanied by ureteritis and cystitis. In acute pyelonephritis, cellular infiltration and necrosis predominate, with pelvic and medullary involvement more severe and advanced than involvement of the cortex. In chronic pyelonephritis, fibrosis replaces inflammation. In both cases, the disease process is asymmetrical within the kidney, and chronic pyelonephritis may produce very irregular contracture of the kidneys with pelvic deformities. **Pyonephrosis** is the term applied to severe suppuration of the kidney in the presence of complete or nearly complete ureteral obstruction; the infected hydronephrotic kidney is converted to a sac of pus. Suppuration may extend through the renal capsule during the course of pyelonephritis to produce a **perinephric abscess.**

The pathogenesis of pyelonephritis begins with establishment of infection in the lower urinary tract; urinary tract infection in general is dealt with under cystitis. Organisms involved in urinary tract infection are usually endogenous bacteria of the bowel and skin, such as *Escherichia coli,* staphylococci, streptococci, *Enterobacter, Proteus,* and *Pseudomonas,* and more specific urinary pathogens, such as *Corynebacterium renale, C. cystitidis,* and *C. pilosum* in cattle, and *Eubacterium suis* in pigs. Mycoplasmas are rarely involved in cattle. Infection is often mixed, and whereas *C. renale* may be present in bovine pyelonephritis, and is an obligate parasite of urinary mucosae, various enteric pathogens may be of more pathogenetic importance. Virulence of bacteria in the urinary tract, as elsewhere, is enhanced by the presence of pili on their surface. Pili assist adhesion of *C. renale* to urinary epithelium; this process is pH dependent. The type of pili expressed by the bacteria may also be important later in the course of pyelonephritis; type 1 fimbriate *E. coli* induce greater activation of neutrophils and hence more renal scarring than do nonfimbriate or P-fimbriate *E. coli.*

One of the urinary tract defenses against bacterial infection and colonization is shedding of mature epithelial cells with attached bacteria. Normal voiding of urine, plus immune and other mechanisms, usually maintains sterility of the bladder, but once bacteria enter the bladder, e.g., via catheterization, they grow well in urine of low osmolality or alkaline pH. Stasis of urine is an important predisposing factor in the pathogenesis of cystitis and of pyelonephritis. Urinary obstruction may be caused by ureteral anomalies in young animals, kinked ureters in pigs, pregnancy, urolithiasis, and prostatic hypertrophy. Females are predisposed to urinary tract infection because of their short urethras, urethral trauma, and possibly hormonal effects. Clinically, infection is indicated by bloody or cloudy urine, with pyuria and bacteriuria. The presence of antibody-coated bacteria in urine, as detected by the fluorescent antibody technique, indicates that the bacteria are of renal rather than bladder origin, and is indicative of pyelonephritis.

Once infection is established in the bladder, probably the most significant mechanism in causing renal infection is **vesicoureteral reflux.** This retrograde flow of urine up the ureters during micturition may carry bacteria as far as the urinary space of glomeruli (intrarenal reflux). Reflux may occur during micturition, especially if there is urinary obstruction, or as a result of external compression of the bladder, as occurs during manual compression of the bladder in dogs and cats for collection of urine samples. Vesicoureteral reflux is very common in puppies, and is a function of the short intravesical length of the ureters and hence an easily overcome vesicoureteral valve; reflux decreases with age and the development of greater intravesical length of the ureter and its more oblique entry through the bladder wall. Vesicoureteral reflux of sterile urine does little renal damage; the ureteral muscular layers may hypertrophy. Cystitis may alter normal ureteral peristalsis, perhaps causing reversed peristaltic waves.

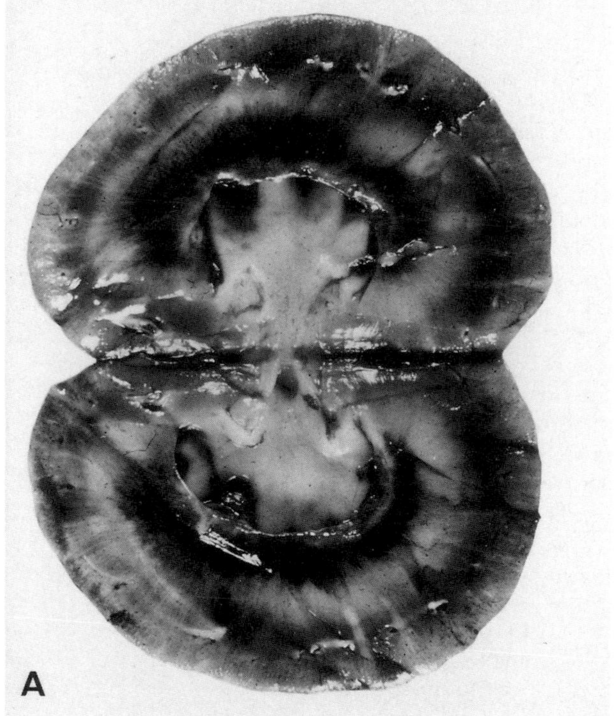

Fig. 5.52A Acute pyelonephritis. Dog. There is ulceration of the renal crest and hemorrhage in medulla. Pale streaks extend to cortical surface.

Hence, persistent renal infection may result from vesicoureteral reflux, and possibly from reversed peristalsis, in animals with bladder infection and thus contribute to chronic active pyelonephritis. Progression of pyelonephritis probably depends on persistence of bacterial infection, or at least of bacterial antigens. Protoplasts (L-forms) may be produced after antibacterial therapy and persist in the medulla; their significance is unknown.

For a number of reasons, the medulla is the part of the kidney most susceptible to infection. It is relatively hypoxic because of the low hematocrit in vasa recta; hypertonicity depresses the phagocytic activity of leukocytes; and ammonia may interfere with activation of complement. In pigs, the renal poles are more susceptible to infection because the collecting ducts of their compound papillae do not collapse as readily as do those of the simple papillae of the central lobes, when exposed to the increased pelvic pressure of vesicoureteral reflux; hence, intrarenal reflux is more common at the poles. Invasion of the kidney from the pelvis probably progresses by way of the collecting ducts, as is suggested by the early development of lines of suppuration along the straight tubules and the presence of bacterial colonies in the tubules, and by direct invasion across the degenerate eroded pelvic epithelium.

Pyelonephritis is often bilateral, but not necessarily symmetrical. Acute disease is seen most commonly in sows, and chronic pyelonephritis, in cows and dogs. A

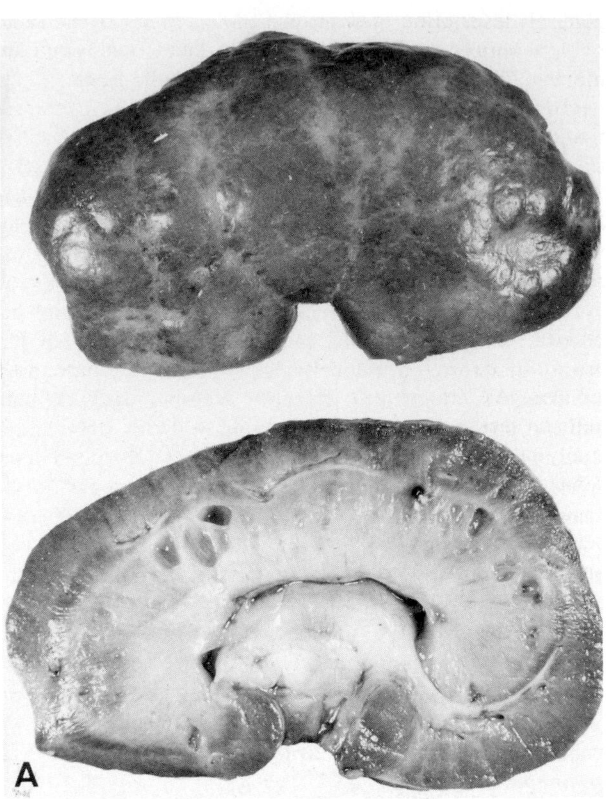

Fig. 5.53A Chronic pyelonephritis. Dog. Ulceration of renal crest and deep irregular scars, which are most prominent at the poles.

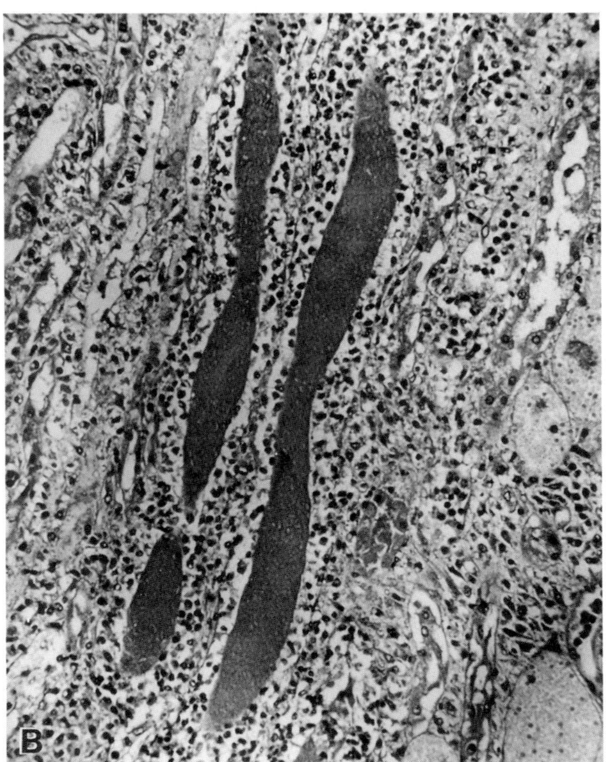

Fig. 5.52B Acute ascending pyelonephritis. Ox. Bacterial colonies in collecting tubules with suppuration.

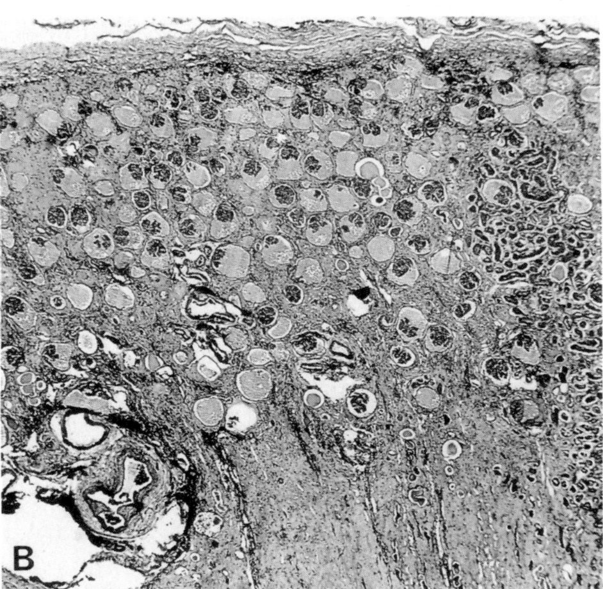

Fig. 5.53B Cortical and medullary scarring in pyelonephritis. Dog. Note inflammatory cells at corticomedullary junction and beneath capsule.

general description will be given of acute and chronic pyelonephritis before species differences are noted in more detail. Acute disease characteristically begins with necrosis and inflammation of papilla or renal crest (necrotizing papillitis) in an irregular pattern (Fig. 5.52A). Bacteria may be abundant in the collecting tubules (Fig. 5.52B). Associated wedge-shaped areas of parenchyma are swollen, dark red, and firm. Hyperemia subsides, and suppurative tubulointerstitial nephritis and tubular necrosis then predominate in these radially distributed wedges. Tubules are obliterated by the inflammation, tubular obstruction and dilation occur, and glomeruli, although initially resistant, may be obliterated. Leukocytic casts are present in tubules. As the process becomes chronic, mononuclear cells replace neutrophils, and fibrosis proceeds and eventually predominates. Contraction of the scars and loss of renal substance results in a wide variety of patterns of renal scarring, usually with deep cortical depressions. The scars in pyelonephritis extend from capsule to pelvis and are distinguished from those of other nephritides and infarcts by the associated fibrosis and deformities of the renal papilla and dilation of calyces and pelvis. The pelvis often contains exudate and debris. The papillary defects may be small and difficult to detect in mild cases. More or less total involvement of the kidney may produce a firm pale shrunken kidney with an irregular surface (Fig. 5.53A) which may be difficult to differentiate from other end-stage kidneys resulting from ischemic lesions.

In **dogs** and **cats,** acute pyelonephritis is not often detected, but scars attributed to chronic pyelonephritis are common. In dogs, accumulation of colloidlike material in tubules and glomerular capsules dilated due to scarring may produce a thyroidlike histologic appearance (thyroidization) (Fig. 5.53B). Calculi may form in the pelvis on the nidi provided by cellular debris.

In **swine,** acute pyelonephritis is seen occasionally, but the chronic disease is rare. Acute pyelonephritis occurs in sows postpartum or 3–4 weeks postbreeding; young males are occasionally affected, and some of these have urinary tract anomalies. Bloodstained urine or discharge may be seen, but it is not unusual for prostration and death to occur in 12 hr or so. Severe cystitis and ureteritis are usually present with yellow-brown or bloody mucoid exudate. The renal poles are preferentially involved, and the infection may be fulminant and erupt through the renal capsule to produce retrorenal hemorrhage and inflammation. Less severe examples of tubulointerstitial nephritis

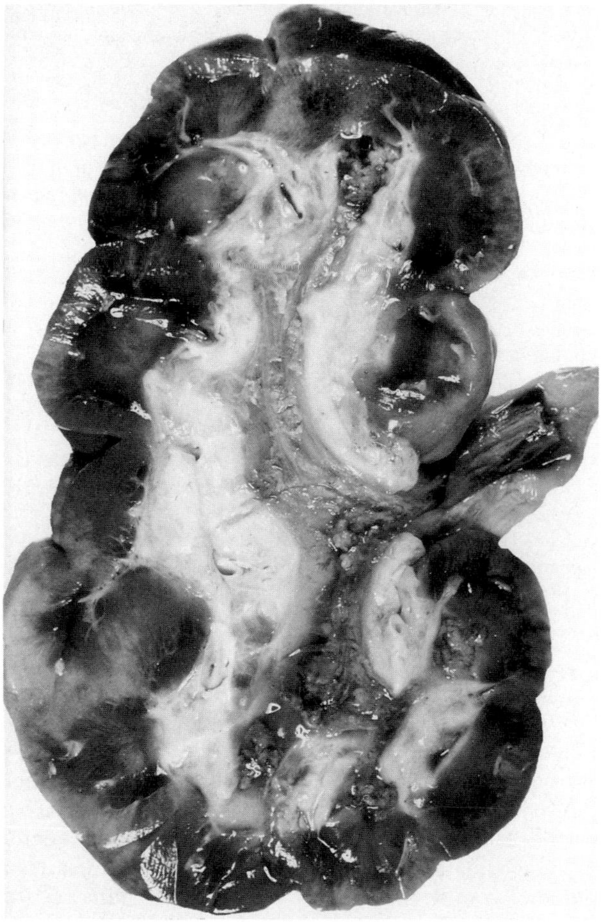

Fig. 5.54 Acute pyelonephritis. Ox. Casts and detritus in calyces and ureters, erosion of papillae, and irregular interstitial inflammation of parenchyma.

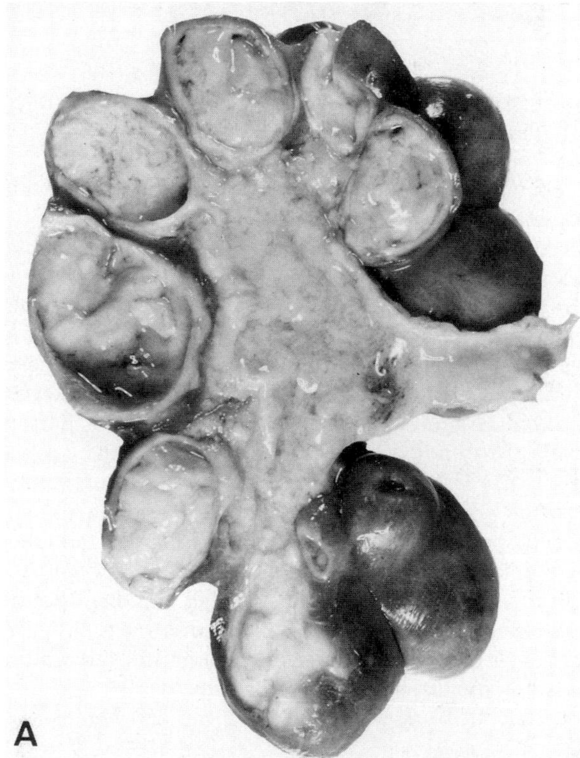

Fig. 5.55A Chronic pyelonephritis. Ox. Renal parenchyma is scarred and atrophic. Exudate fills the distended, thickened calyces.

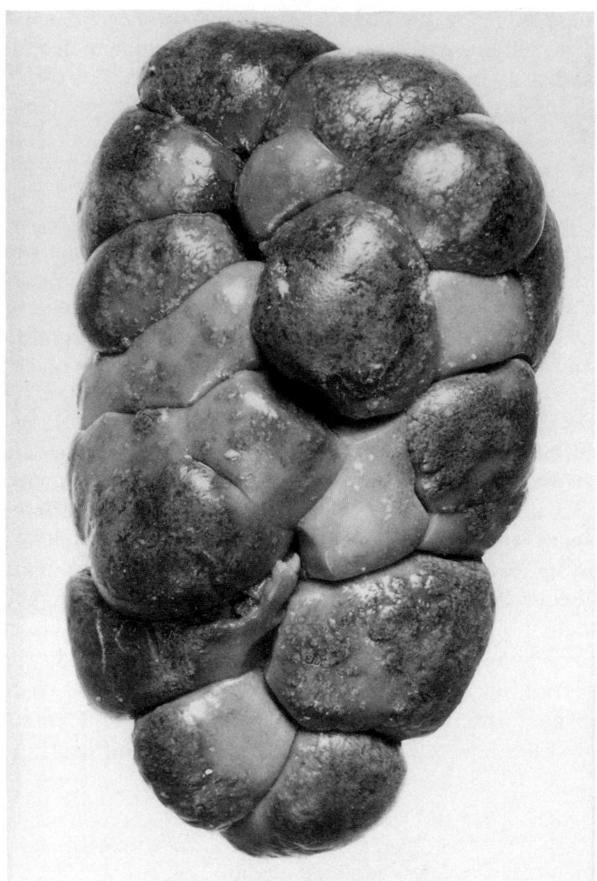

Fig. 5.55B Chronic pyelonephritis. Ox. Scarred lobes alternate with lobes showing multifocal suppuration.

also occur, and are seen as pale areas of cellular infiltration involving wedges or entire lobes.

In **cattle,** chronic pyelonephritis is a significant sporadic disease in cows, but acute pyelonephritis (Fig. 5.54) is usually only an incidental finding. Tubulointerstitial nephritis in affected cows may be minimal, and a slowly progressive, suppurative destructive papillitis may predominate. The medulla of each lobe is fairly uniformly destroyed. Eventually the cortex remains as a narrow capsule surrounding large amounts of pus in the calyces (Fig. 5.55A). Alternatively, and perhaps more commonly, the pattern of radially distributed tubulointerstitial nephritis develops as previously described. Enlarged tan lobes are granular due to interstitial inflammation, and interstitial fibrosis may become extensive (Fig. 5.55B). Rupture of the kidney occurs in males with obstructive urolithiasis after development of fulminant pyelonephritis, but rupture is less common in cattle than in swine.

Pyelonephritis is uncommon in sheep and horses.

Bibliography

Appleton, J. A., Munnell, J. F., and DeBuysscher, E. V. Scanning electron microscopy of experimentally induced pyelonephritis in the rat. *Am J Vet Res* **42:** 351–355, 1981.

Biertuempfel, P. H., Ling, G. V., and Ling, G. A. Urinary tract infection resulting from catheterization in healthy adult dogs. *J Am Vet Med Assoc* **178:** 989–991, 1981.

Crow, S. E., Lauerman, L. H., and Smith, K. W. Pyonephrosis associated with *Salmonella* infection in a dog. *J Am Vet Med Assoc* **169:** 1324–1326, 1976.

Feeney, D. A., Osborne, C. A., and Johnston, G. R. Vesicoureteral reflux induced by manual compression of the urinary bladder of dogs and cats. *J Am Vet Med Assoc* **182:** 795–797, 1983.

Fukuoka. T., and Yanagawa, R. Comparison of experimental infection in mice of *Corynebacterium renale* piliated and nonpiliated clones. *Jpn J Vet Res* **35:** 79–86, 1987.

Jergens, A. E., Miles, K. G., and Turk, M. Bilateral pyelonephritis and hydroureter associated with metastatic adenocarcinoma in a dog. *J Am Vet Med Assoc* **193:** 961–963, 1988.

Laberke, H. G., Klingebiel, T., and Quack, G. A contribution to the morphology and pathogenesis of thyroid-like lesions in the kidney. *Path Res Pract* **176:** 284–296, 1983.

McCullagh, K. G. *et al.* Experimental pyelonephritis in the cat. 3. Collagen alterations in renal fibrosis. *J Comp Pathol* **93:** 9–25, 1983.

Nicolet, J., and Fey, H. Antibody-coated bacteria in urine sediment from cattle infected with *Corynebacterium renale. Vet Rec* **105:** 301–303, 1979.

Panangala, V. S. *et al.* Isolation of *Mycoplasma bovirhinis* from the kidneys of a bull with urinary obstruction and subacute nephritis. *J Am Vet Med Assoc* **197:** 381–382, 1990.

Ransley, P. G., and Risdon, R. A. Renal papillae and intrarenal reflux in the pig. *Lancet* **ii:** 1114, 1974.

Sato, H., Yanagawa, R., and Fukuyama, H. Adhesion of *Corynebacterium renale, Corynebacterium pilosum,* and *Corynebacterium cystitidis* to bovine urinary bladder epithelial cells of various ages and levels of differentiation. *Infect Immun* **36:** 1242–1245, 1982.

Sloet van Oldruitenborgh-Oosterbaan, M. M., and Kalsbeek, H. C. Ureteropyelonephritis in a Friesian mare. *Vet Rec* **122:** 609–610, 1988.

Steinhardt, G. F. Reflux nephropathy. *J Urol* **134:** 855–859, 1985.

Thomas, J. E. Urinary tract infection induced by intermittent urethral catheterization in dogs. *J Am Vet Med Assoc* **174:** 705–707, 1979.

Topley, N. *et al.* Type 1 fimbriate strains of *Escherichia coli* initiate renal parenchymal scarring. *Kidney Int* **36:** 609–616, 1989.

Wallace, L. L. M. *et al.* Polypoid cystitis, pyelonephritis, and obstructive uropathy in a cow. *J Am Vet Med Assoc* **197:** 1181–1183, 1990.

F. Hypercalcemic Nephropathy

Hypercalcemia occurs often in dogs, and may be sufficiently severe to cause renal failure (hypercalcemic nephropathy). The leading cause is pseudohyperparathyroidism, a paraneoplastic syndrome, in which a nonendocrine tumor, usually lymphosarcoma or adenocarcinoma of the apocrine glands of the anal sac, is a source of ectopic substances that stimulate bone resorption (see The Endocrine Glands and The Hematopoietic System, Volume 3, Chapters 3 and 2). Other less common causes of hypercalcemia are primary hyperparathyroidism, hypervitaminosis D and like diseases, osteolytic neoplasms, acute or chronic renal failure, and hypoadrenocorticism. Hypercalcemia results in inactivation of adenyl cyclase, and hence decreased cyclic adenosine monophosphate formation; sodium transport is impaired in the ascending limb of the loop of Henle, the distal tubule, and collecting ducts. Natriuresis results. As well, hypercalcemia interferes with antidiuretic hormone receptors in the collecting ducts, resulting in renal diabetes insipidus. The resultant polyuria and compensatory polydipsia are reversible if the primary cause of the hypercalcemia is removed. If hypercalcemia persists, progressive renal mineralization occurs beginning with tubular basement membranes and epithelium, particularly in the outer zone of the medulla (Fig. 5.56) and eventually involving glomeruli. Tubular epithelial mineralization and cast formation causes tubular obstruction, and eventually loss of nephrons.

Other less significant examples of renal mineralization also occur. The deposition of calcium salts in the form of clumps of granules in the lumen and lining of collecting tubules and in the adjacent interstitium is rather common. They are associated with hypomagnesemia in some species; they are not significant.

Mineralization is very common in dogs, most unusual in other species, and occurs very quickly in casts, in dead and degenerate epithelium, and in injured basement membranes. In uremia, it may also involve the glomeruli and small blood vessels. Mineralization is a frequent result of secondary hyperparathyroidism induced by chronic renal insufficiency and coexists with similar deposits in the lungs, gastric mucosa, and other organs (see Uremia, Section I,D of The Kidney in this chapter). Dogs fed a high-phosphorus diet similarly develop diffuse renal mineralization.

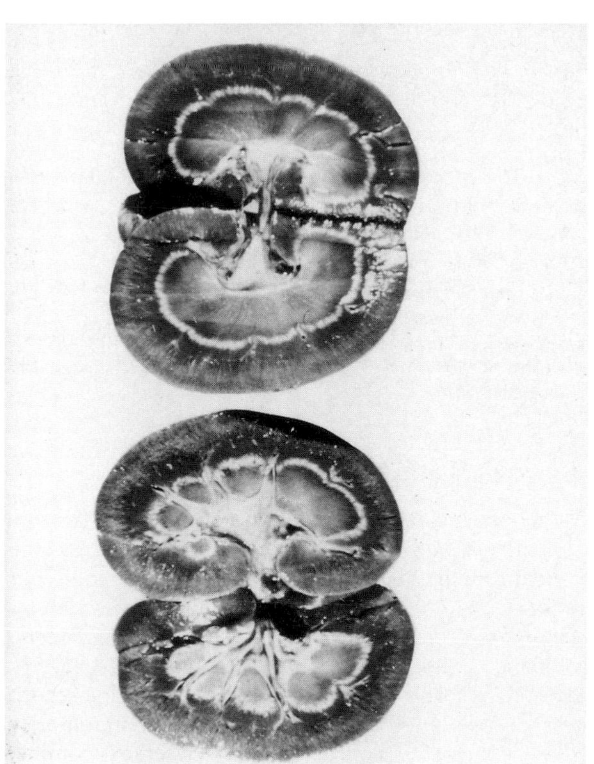

Fig. 5.56 Hypercalcemic nephropathy. Dog.

G. Miscellaneous Interstitial Lesions

Extramedullary hematopoiesis occurs in the kidneys of dogs under a variety of circumstances, all of which probably have a common denominator of bone-marrow depression or injury. When the kidneys are the site of hematopoiesis, it is usual that the liver, lymph nodes, spleen, adrenals, and lungs are also. The most pronounced hematopoiesis occurs in canine pyometra.

Bone occasionally develops in association with urinary tract tissue, for example, following urinary tract surgery or in hydronephrotic kidneys. Transitional epithelium stimulates transformation of mesenchymal cells to osteoblasts.

Renal **telangiectasis** is a rare cause of hematuria in dogs.

Bibliography

Adams, J. S. Vitamin D metabolite-mediated hypercalcemia. *Endocrinol Metabol Clin North Am* **18:** 765–778, 1989.

Boland, R. L. Plants as a source of vitamin D_3 metabolites. *Nutr Rev* **44:** 1–8, 1986.

Bundza, A. Osseous metaplasia of the renal pelvis in slaughter swine. *Can Vet J* **31:** 529, 1990.

Ganote, C. *et al.* Acute calcium nephrotoxicity. An electron microscopical and semiquantitative light microscopical study. *Arch Pathol Lab Med* **99:** 650–657, 1975.

Gunson, D. E. *et al.* Environmental zinc and cadmium pollution associated with generalized osteochondrosis, osteoporosis, and nephrocalcinosis in horses. *J Am Vet Med Assoc* **180:** 295–299, 1982.

Holt, P. E., Lucke, V. M., and Pearson, H. Idiopathic renal hemorrhage in the dog. *J Small Anim Pract* **28:** 253–263, 1987.

Levi, M., Peterson, L., and Berl, T. Mechanism of concentrating defect in hypercalcemia. Role of polydipsia and prostaglandins. *Kidney Int* **23:** 489–497, 1983.

Lucke, V. M., and Hunt, A. C. Renal calcification in the domestic cat. A morphological and x-ray diffraction study. *Pathol Vet* **4:** 120–136, 1967.

Majeed, S. K. Mineralisation in kidney and stomach of beagle dogs. *Vet Q* **7:** 162–164, 1985.

Meuten, D. J. *et al.* Hypercalcemia in dogs with adenocarcinoma derived from apocrine glands of the anal sacs. *Lab Invest* **48:** 428–435, 1983.

Mundy, G. R. The hypercalcemia of malignancy. *Kidney Int* **31:** 142–155, 1987.

Peterson, M. E., and Feinman, J. M. Hypercalcemia associated with hypoadrenocorticism in sixteen dogs. *J Am Vet Med Assoc* **181:** 802–804, 1982.

Talcott, P. A., Mather, G. G., and Kowitz, E. H. Accidental ingestion of a cholecalciferol-containing rodent bait in a dog. *Vet Hum Toxicol* **33:** 252–256, 1991.

H. Parasitic Lesions in the Kidneys

The most common parasitic lesion in the kidneys is the focal scar of reaction to the larvae of *Toxocara canis* in dog kidneys (Fig. 5.57A). These small granulomas, 2–3 mm in diameter, are found on the surface and cross section of the cortex. In the early stages of development, the lesions are gray-yellow and have soft centers; later they become firm and white, and the superficial ones cause dimpling of the cortex. Each granuloma surrounds an entrapped larva (Fig. 5.57B), which usually is hard to find in sections. The granuloma is composed largely of epithelioid cells and lymphocytes with an occasional eosinophil. Healing of the lesions occurs after the death and removal of the larvae; the residual scars are typical and consist of dense concentrically arranged fibrous tissue. Similar lesions are produced in calves by the migratory larvae of *T. cati* and *T. canis* acquired by fecal contamination of feed, and by *T. (Neoascaris) vitulorum* especially in buffaloes. In cats, *T. canis* can produce disseminated granulomatous disease marked by the presence of large numbers of eosinophils in granulomas. Occasionally ascarid larvae are found in other sites occupying granulomas similar to those in the canine kidney (Fig. 5.58).

Stephanurus dentatus is the kidney worm of swine. It is widely distributed in tropical and subtropical countries, and the prevalence in grazing swine in such areas can be very high. The worms encyst in perirenal fat and adjacent tissues, the cysts communicating with the renal pelvis.

The life cycle of *Stephanurus dentatus* can be direct or, experimentally, involve earthworms as transport hosts. The latter mechanism has not been shown to occur naturally. Eggs are passed in the urine of the pig, sometimes in immense numbers, and the larvae hatch in 2–3 days. The infective stages are vulnerable to sunlight and drying. Infection may occur by penetration through the skin or by ingestion, and prenatal infections occur. Following oral infection, third-stage larvae migrate from the small and large intestine via the portal circulation and mesenteric lymphatics to the liver. A few migrate across the peritoneal cavity. After skin infection, most larvae migrate to the lungs and reach the intestines following tracheal migration. Deaths due to peritonitis and intestinal intussusception occur in some pigs 20–30 days after heavy infections and are associated with larval migration from the mesenteric nodes to the liver. The infective larvae migrate in the tissues of the pig, especially in the liver where they may stay for several months. The hepatic migrations provoke considerable injury and severe interstitial hepatitis with lesions of the same character but much more severe than those produced by the larvae of *Ascaris suum*. *Stephanurus dentatus* also produces portal phlebitis with thrombosis in some pigs (see the Liver and Biliary System, Chapter 2 of this volume). The liver is usually enlarged and may be very hard. It is pale, and the lobulation is remarkably emphasized by the perilobular fibrosis which develops. Many lobules are obliterated by contracting and proliferating scar tissue in the portal areas, and all lobules are more or less reduced in size in the diffuse hepatitis of heavy or prolonged larval infestation.

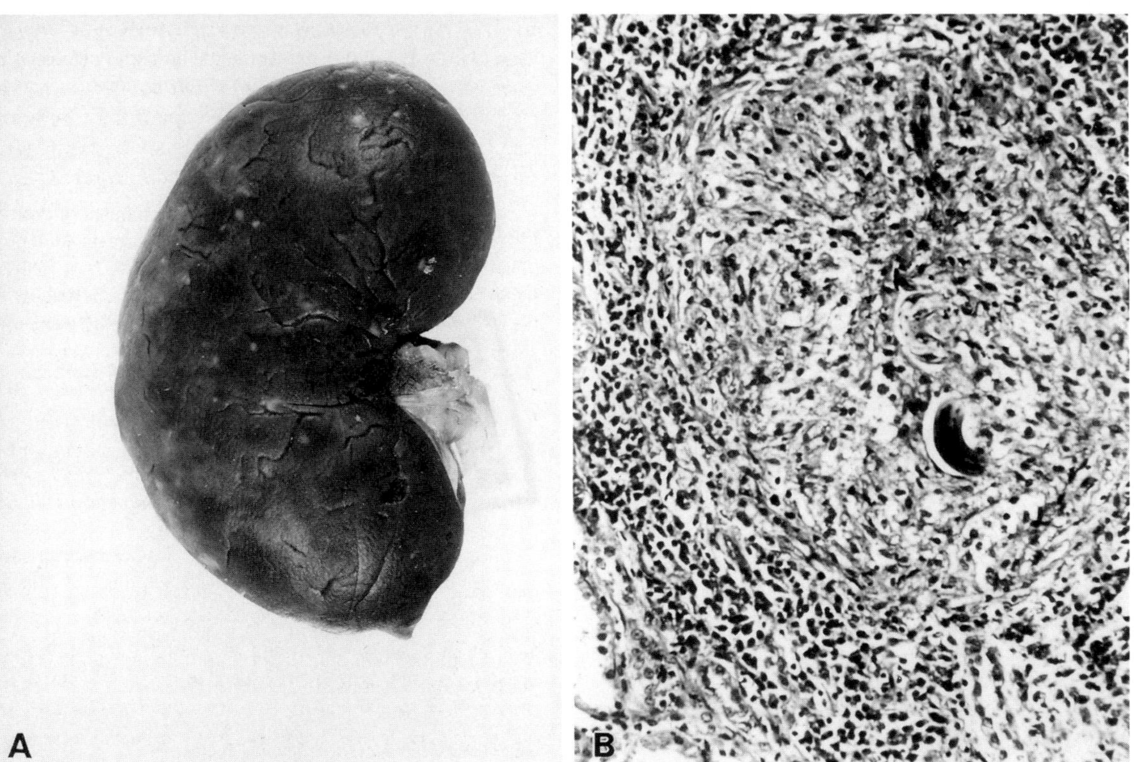

Fig. 5.57 (A) Cortical granulomas caused by *Toxocara canis*. Kidney. Dog. (B) Section from (A) showing larva in granuloma.

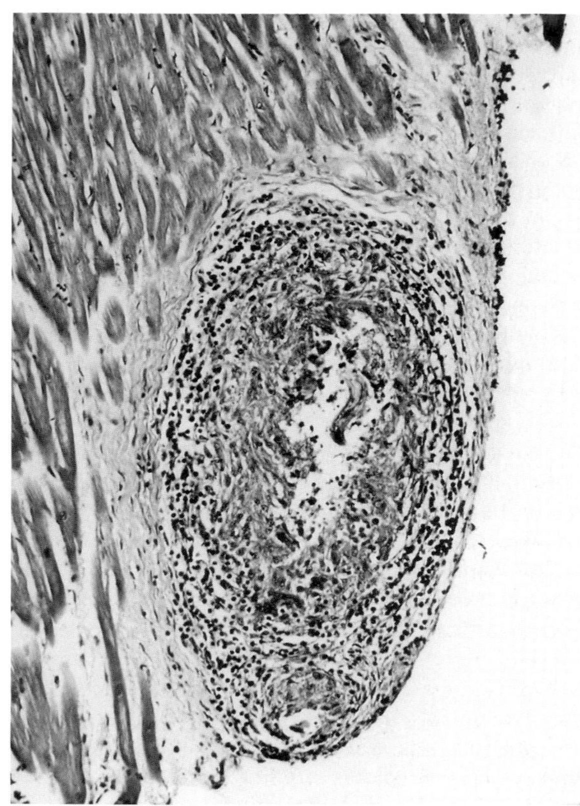

Fig. 5.58 Dog. Myocardial granuloma containing an ascarid larva. (Courtesy of G. W. Thomson.)

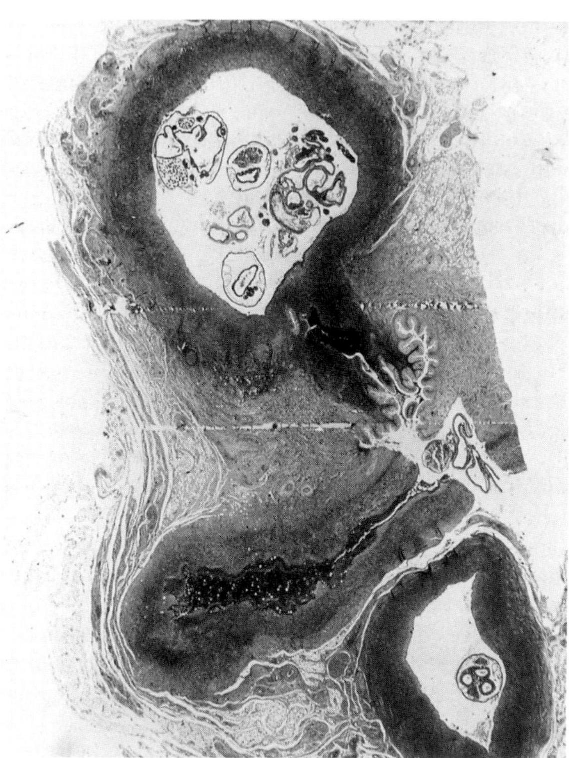

Fig. 5.59 Encysted *Stephanurus dentatus* in hilus of kidney. Pig.

Many larvae are destroyed in the liver, being encapsulated in small abscesses that are eventually obliterated. From the liver, the larvae migrate across the peritoneal cavity to the perirenal region. Many become encysted in abscesses in adjacent tissue, especially the pancreas, and it is not unusual for some to invade the vertebral canal and cause posterior paralysis. The definitive site is the tissue around the renal pelvis and ureter wherein the adults encyst (Fig. 5.59). Occasionally, the cysts may be found in the kidney itself. The cysts communicate with the lumen of the ureter, allowing escape of eggs. Developmental stages in the definitive host take a long time, and patency may not be established for 9 months or more. Once patency is established, the mature females may lay eggs for 3 years or longer.

Dioctophyma renale is the giant kidney-worm, the largest of parasitic nematodes. The worm is red and cylindrical, and in dogs the females measure 20–100 cm long and 4–12 mm in diameter. Males are 14–45 cm long and 4–6 mm in diameter. *Dioctophyma renale* is usually found in dogs, mink, cats, and other fish-eating mammals but is recorded in the pig, ox, and horse. It has a world-wide distribution, but its incidence is unknown.

The life cycle involves one intermediate and often one paratenic host. Eggs passed in the urine are very resistant to the external environment and may survive for 2–5 years. Embryonation requires 1–7 months, depending on the climatic conditions. The embryonated eggs are ingested by the intermediate hosts, which are aquatic oligochaetes (mud-worms) (*Lumbriculus variegatus*), and encyst in their body cavities. The paratenic hosts are fish and frogs, of which the northern black bullhead (*Ictalurus melas*) and the green frog (*Rana clamitans*) are known to serve in North America. Other fish and frogs may also act as paratenic hosts, but *L. variegatus* is the only known intermediate host. Following ingestion of infective larvae, they penetrate the gut wall and migrate across the peritoneal cavity to the kidney. The life cycle from egg to adult requires 3.5–6 months, but may take 2 years.

The adult worms live in the renal pelvis but may encyst in a body cavity, the uterus, mammary gland, or bladder. The adults are very destructive, causing initially a hemorrhagic pyelitis, which shortly becomes suppurative, and the parenchyma is progressively destroyed until the tunic contains only the worm and exudate.

Dogs, the domestic species usually affected by *D. renale,* are regarded as abnormal hosts because usually only one or a very small number of worms is present, and worms of both sexes are found in only about one third of infections. Intrarenal parasites in dogs are more common in the right kidney than the left, but in ~60% of infected dogs, parasites are in the peritoneal cavity only. Simultaneous renal and peritoneal infections occur in ~15% of dogs. Thus, most canine infections are not patent.

In the peritoneal cavity, *D. renale* often entwines a lobe

of the liver and may cause erosion of the hepatic capsule with hemoperitoneum, or produce infarction and rupture. On occasion they rear up to startle surgeons engaged in exploratory laparotomy.

The definitive hosts are wild fish-eating carnivores, mink in particular, in which the worms are smaller and usually located in the kidney.

Capillaria plica may be found in the lumen of the renal pelvis, ureter, or urinary bladder of dogs, foxes, and smaller carnivores. Although widely distributed, it is not a common parasite. The life cycle is not clearly known but is probably indirect, earthworms being intermediate hosts. Ingestion of earthworms from infected premises causes patent infections in 61–68 days. Pathologic effects usually are not attributed to *C. plica* infection, but hematuria and dysuria are produced occasionally; worms embedded in bladder, ureter, or pelvis may invoke mild submucosal inflammation.

Other species of *Capillaria* occur in the urinary bladder of other animals: *C. micronata* in mink and *C. feliscati* in the cat; the latter may be the same as *C. plica*. Light infestations are common but harmless, the anterior end of the worm embedded in the surface layer of epithelium provoking at most a light cellular infiltration of the lamina propria.

Klossiella equi is a sporozoan parasite of the kidney of the horse and its relatives, including the zebra, donkey, and burro. It is apparently quite rare and harmless. The life cycle is not fully known. It is thought that, following infection with sporocysts from the environment, sporozoites are released and enter the circulation. One schizont generation develops in glomerular endothelium and another in proximal tubular epithelium. Sporogony occurs in the epithelium of the thick limb of Henle's loop, and sporocysts are passed in the urine (Fig. 5.60). Heavy infections can result in rupture of tubules and lymphoplasmacytic interstitial nephritis.

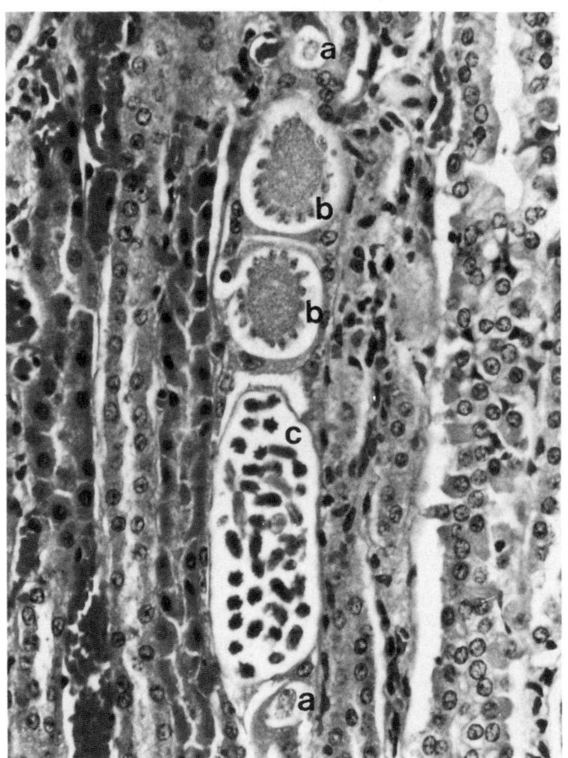

Fig. 5.60 *Klossiella equi*. Horse. Within tubular epithelial cells are gamonts (a), sporonts (b), and sporocysts (c).

Granulomas may be found in the renal pelvis in schistosomiasis of cattle and sheep (see The Cardiovascular System, Volume 3, Chapter 1), and larvae of *Setaria digitata* may produce granulomas in the bladder of cattle in Asia (see The Peritoneum and Retroperitoneum, Chapter 4 of this volume).

Micronema deletrix, a saprophagous nematode that may produce granulomatous masses in the nasal cavity of horses and occasionally is responsible for cerebral vasculitis and hemorrhagic necrosis, also localizes in the kidney. Renal infections are characterized by granulomatous inflammation with production of cream-colored masses, which resemble neoplasms macroscopically.

Bibliography

Anderson, W. I., Picut, C. A., and Georgi, M. E. *Klossiella equi* induced tubular nephrosis and interstitial nephritis in a pony. *J Comp Pathol* **98:** 363–366, 1988.

Bartsch, R. C., and Van Wyk, J. A. Studies on schistosomiasis. 9. Pathology of the bovine urinary tract. *Onderstepoort J Vet Res* **44:** 73–94, 1977.

Celerin, A. J., and McMullen, M. E. Giant kidney worm in a dog. *J Am Vet Med Assoc* **179:** 245–246, 1981.

Chalmers, G. A. *et al. Micronema deletrix* in the kidney of a horse. *Can Vet J* **31:** 451–452, 1990.

Mace, T. F., and Anderson, R. C. Development of the giant kidney worm, *Dioctophyma renale* (Goeze, 1782) (Nematoda: Dioctophymatoidea). *Can J Zool* **53:** 1552–1568, 1975.

Osborne, C. A. *et al. Dioctophyma renale* in the dog. *J Am Vet Med Assoc* **155:** 605–620, 1969.

Parsons, J. C. *et al.* Disseminated granulomatous disease in a cat caused by larvae of *Toxocara canis*. *J Comp Pathol* **99:** 343–346, 1988.

Senior, D. F. *et al. Capillaria plica* infection in dogs. *J Am Vet Med Assoc* **176:** 901–905, 1980.

Smith, H. J., and Hawkes, A. B. Kidney worm infection in feral pigs in Canada with transmission to domestic swine. *Can Vet J* **19:** 40–43, 1978.

Taylor, J. L. *et al. Klossiella* parasites of animals: A literature review. *Vet Parasitol* **5:** 137–144, 1979.

Wilson-Hanson, S., and Prescott, C. W. *Capillaria* in the bladder of the domestic cat. *Aust Vet J* **59:** 190–191, 1982.

VII. Renal Neoplasia

Primary renal tumors are uncommon. One abattoir survey in the United Kingdom found 8.5, 0.9, and 4.3 cases per million animals in cattle, sheep, and pigs, respectively. Renal tumors were found in ~0.15% of horses in two large surveys. Primary renal tumors compose about 1% of all canine neoplasms and probably about 0.5% of feline neoplasms.

A. Renal Adenoma

Renal adenomas are rare; they are said to occur more often in cattle and horses than in other species. In dogs, they compose about 15% of primary renal epithelial tumors. Renal adenomas, and carcinomas also, arise from epithelium of the proximal convoluted tubules. Adenomas usually are incidental autopsy findings. Grossly, they tend to be solitary nodules less than 2 cm across but occasionally are huge. They grow expansively. Microscopically, the tumor cells usually are cuboidal with moderate to abundant acidophilic cytoplasm. They form solid sheets, or papilliform or tubular structures, and stromal tissue is scant. Tumors with mixed architectural patterns occur. Histologic differentiation of adenoma and renal carcinoma sometimes is impossible; a few "adenomas" may be small, well-differentiated carcinomas.

B. Renal Carcinoma

Carcinomas are the most common primary renal tumors of dogs, cattle, and sheep. They occur in mature and old animals; thus, their incidence is relatively low in some species. The average age of affected dogs is ~8 years. Males are affected about twice as often as bitches. Common presenting signs are hematuria, palpable abdominal mass, and weight loss. Polycythemia associated with erythropoietin production is very rarely seen; polycythemia typically resolves after removal of the tumor. Hypertrophic osteoarthropathy may be seen in cases of renal carcinoma with pulmonary metastases.

Grossly, renal carcinomas are spherical or ovoid masses, usually located in one pole of the kidney (Fig. 5.61A). Usually they are well demarcated from the remainder of the kidney, which is atrophic and compressed. Often the tumor is much larger than the original size of the host kidney but still has a discrete border. The tumor is usually gray or light yellow, often with darker areas of necrosis and hemorrhage. Invasion of the renal pelvis, ureter, renal vein, and hilar lymphatics may be visible (Fig. 5.61B).

Histologically, there is a variety of cell types and architectures, but if examined carefully, small or large areas composed of renal clear cells are often found. These cells have vacuolated cytoplasm, and only the basal nucleus and cytoplasmic outline are visible. The vacuoles contain fat. The presence of clear cells, even in metastases, should suggest renal carcinoma but is not pathognomonic—similar cells occur in certain endocrine tumors and other carcinomas. In other areas, the cells are cuboidal with denser acidophilic or basophilic cytoplasm. They may be arranged in sheets, papillary, or tubular structures, and occasionally they line small cystic spaces. All of these patterns may occur in a single tumor, and apparently there is no prognostic value associated with any pattern. The

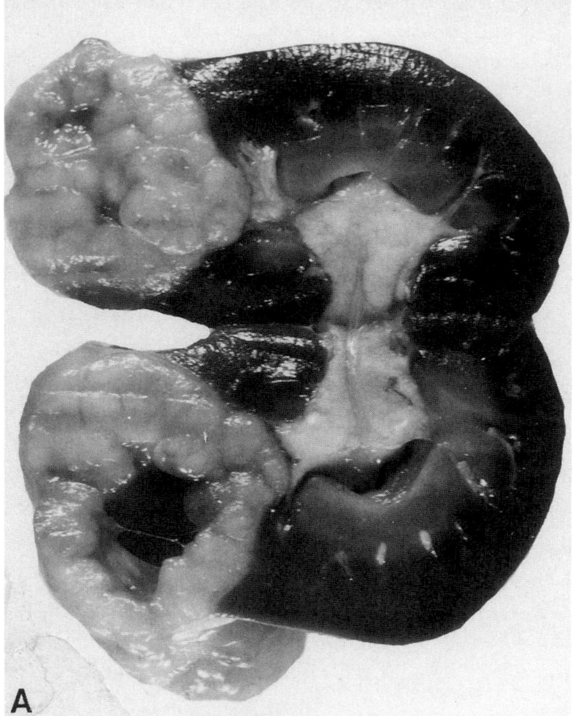

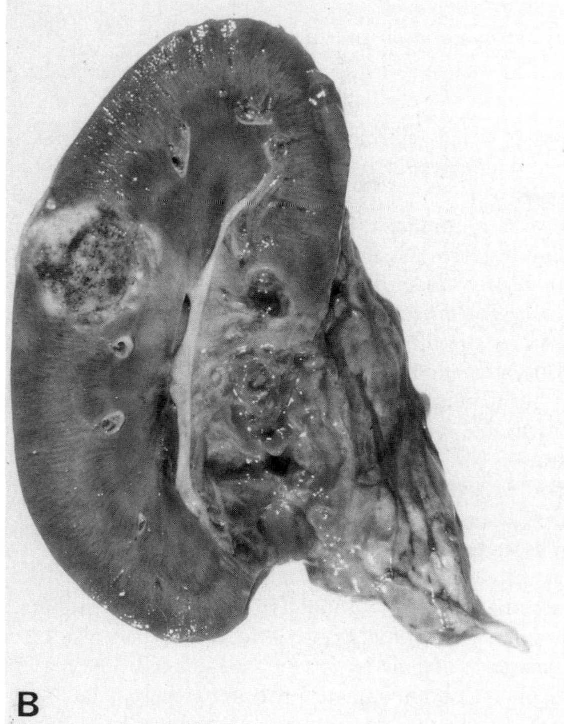

Fig. 5.61 (A) Renal carcinoma showing cystic degeneration. Sheep. (B) Renal carcinoma. Dog. There is extension to pelvis and pelvic structures.

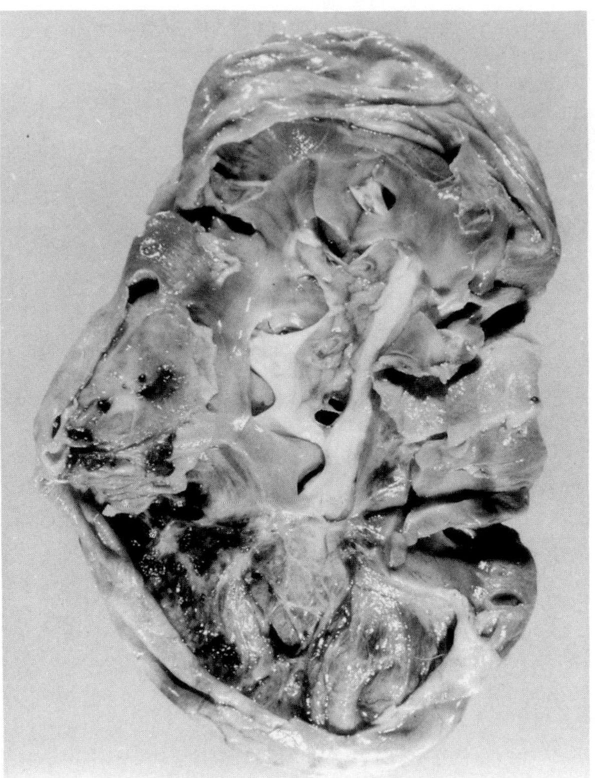

Fig. 5.62 Renal cystadenocarcinoma. German shepherd dog.

stroma of renal carcinomas is scant but highly vascularized, which predisposes to the extensive necrosis often seen grossly.

Renal carcinomas tend to grow expansively, but satellite nodules often develop from local permeation. Invasion of the renal vein is always likely but may not result in metastases. Peritoneal implantation sometimes occurs. Usually by the time a dog is presented for examination, widespread metastases are present, especially in lungs and liver, but also in brain, heart, and skin. Such behavior is not invariable, and in some cases unilateral nephrectomy is curative.

Middle-aged and older German shepherd dogs with generalized nodular dermatofibrosis concurrently also have **renal cystadenocarcinomas** or cystadenomas, which are usually bilateral (Fig. 5.62); the carcinomas will occasionally metastasize to regional lymph nodes, peritoneum, liver, spleen, lung, and bone. Affected bitches also often have multiple uterine leiomyomas; the syndrome may be the result of a paraneoplastic process in which renal tumor-derived growth factors stimulate accumulation of fibrous tissue in various sites. The syndrome is apparently inherited in an autosomal dominant mode.

C. Nephroblastoma

Nephroblastoma (embryonal nephroma, Wilms' tumor) is the most common primary renal tumor of pigs and chickens. Abattoir surveys of pigs in the United Kingdom found 3.5 per million swine slaughtered, and in the United States 43.5 per million, with a frequency of 197 cases per million in one area. Nephroblastomas occur far less often in calves and in dogs, and are very uncommon in other species. They are seen usually in young animals and sometimes in fetuses, but also in mature sows, and are more common in adult dogs than in pups. In rats, various carcinogens, including dimethylnitrosamine, can induce formation of nephroblastomas and other tumors.

Nephroblastomas are true embryonal tumors which arise in primitive nephrogenic blastema and in foci of renal dysplasia. The presence in them of tissues such as cartilage and skeletal muscle, which normally are not associated with the kidney, indicates an origin in pluripotential mesenchyme before it becomes metanephrogenic. These tumors establish the important principle that all component tissues of the kidney arise from a common blastema.

Grossly, nephroblastomas may attain a huge size and cause abdominal enlargement. They are often multiple in the affected kidney, growing expansively and compressing the adjacent parenchyma, and they are encapsulated. They are usually unilateral, but a few are bilateral (Fig. 5.63A), and these sometimes unite across the midline to form a single large mass. Widespread metastases to lung and liver occur in over half the canine cases, but are rare in pigs and calves. The cut surface of nephroblastomas is variegated or lobulated, and the larger ones have extensive areas of hemorrhagic necrosis. The characteristic cut surface reveals a myxomatous soft, gray-white, or tan tissue, which feels spongy. Histologically, the characteristic features are primitive glomeruli with primitive Bowman's spaces, abortive tubules, and a loose spindle cell stroma (Fig. 5.63B), which may show some differentiation to a variety of mesenchymal tissues, including striated muscle, collagen, cartilage, bone, and adipose tissue. The mesenchymal components may predominate over epithelial elements in certain tumors, especially in ruminants. Tubular and glomerular differentiation indicate a good prognosis; anaplasia and a sarcomatous stroma are associated with metastasis and a poor prognosis.

D. Other Tumors

Transitional cell papilloma and **carcinoma** of the renal pelvis are very rare tumors which occur in the dog, cow, pig, and horse. Squamous and glandular metaplasia develop in the carcinomas. Transitional cell tumors are discussed with the urinary bladder, Section II,B of The Lower Urinary Tract, in this chapter.

Primary mesenchymal tumors of the kidney occur but may be diagnosed only after very careful examination to exclude a primary focus in some other tissue. Fibrous and vascular tumors are the most common types; **benign cortical fibromas** occur in older dogs. Renal **interstitial cell tumors** occur in the cortex and medulla of old dogs and arise from cells distinct from interstitial fibroblasts. A vimentin-positive tumor termed a **congenital mesoblastic**

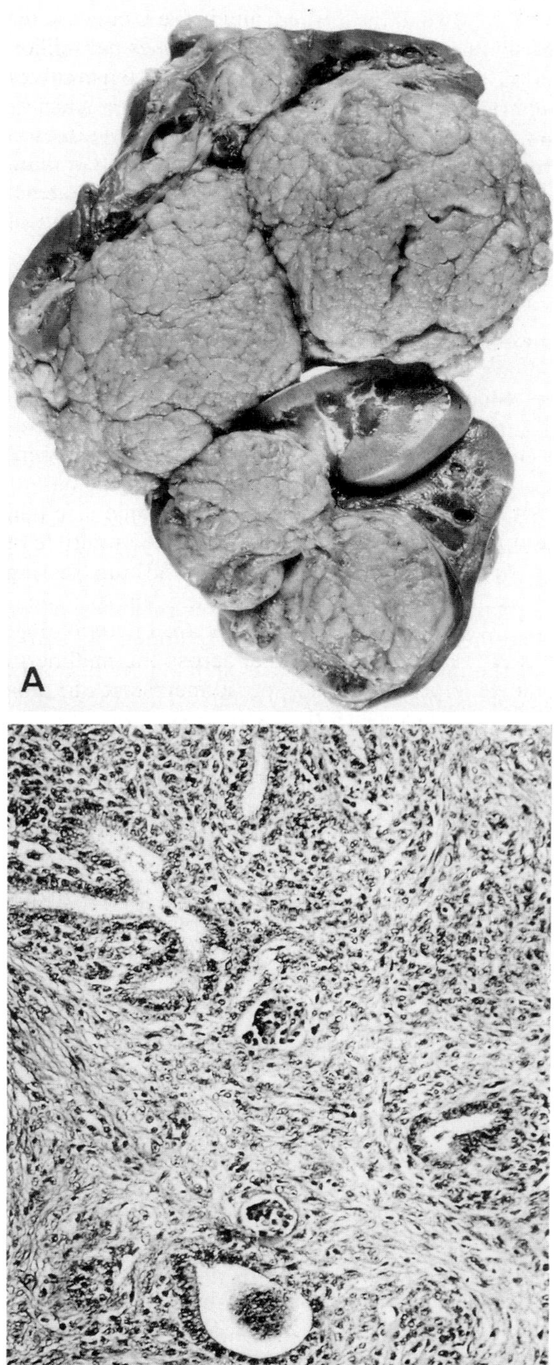

Fig. 5.63 (A) Bilateral nephroblastomas. Pig. Lobulated tumors distort and replace renal parenchyma. (B) Nephroblastoma. Pig. Note tubular and glomerular structures.

nephroma has been reported in a dog; the tumor was composed of fibromatous and myxomatous areas.

Metastatic tumors are common in the kidneys, and disseminated neoplasms of any type are likely to localize there, especially in the cortices, and to be bilateral. Many such metastases are of microscopic size, and they are of hematogenous origin. Retrograde lymphatic invasion along the renal lymphatics may occur from carcinomas in adjacent organs.

Renal involvement in **lymphosarcoma** is common in those species in which the neoplasm is common. The involvement may be diffuse or nodular. When the nodular lesions are grossly visible, they are numerous, poorly defined, fatty in appearance, and project hemispherically above the surface. The capsule is not adherent. When lymphomatous involvement is diffuse, the organ is enlarged and has a uniform white fatty appearance. The differentiation of lymphomatous metastases from interstitial nephritis often requires microscopic examination and, indeed, metastases may sometimes be discovered, especially in cats, only by microscopic examination. Peripelvic and periureteral infiltrates which cause hydronephrosis are common in cattle.

In dogs, primary **pulmonary adenocarcinoma** with renal metastases may be difficult or impossible to distinguish from primary renal carcinoma with pulmonary metastases since their microscopic appearance is quite similar.

Bibliography

Britt, J. O., Ryan, C. P., and Howard, E. B. Sarcomatoid renal adenocarcinoma in a cat. *Vet Pathol* **22:** 514–515, 1985.

Clark, W. R., and Wilson, R. B. Renal adenoma in a cat. *J Am Vet Med Assoc* **193:** 1557–1559, 1988.

Eble, J. N., and Hull, M. T. Morphologic features of renal oncocytoma: A light- and electron-microscopic study. *Hum Pathol* **15:** 1054–1061, 1984.

Gilbert, P. A., Griffin, C. E., and Walder, E. J. Nodular dermatofibrosis and renal cystadenoma in a German shepherd dog. *J Am Anim Hosp Assoc* **26:** 253–256, 1990.

Gorse, M. J. Polycythemia associated with renal fibrosarcoma in a dog. *J Am Vet Med Assoc* **192:** 793–794, 1988.

Hayashi, M. *et al.* Histopathological classification of nephroblastomas in slaughtered swine. *J Comp Pathol* **96:** 35–46, 1986.

Hodgin, E. C. Meningeal hemangioma and renal hamartoma in a heifer. *Vet Pathol* **22:** 420–421, 1985.

Lappin, M. R., and Latimer, K. S. Hematuria and extreme neutrophilic leukocytosis in a dog with renal tubular carcinoma. *J Am Vet Med Assoc* **192:** 1289–1292, 1988.

Marsden, H. B., and Lawler, W. Wilms' tumour and renal dysplasia: An hypothesis. *J Clin Pathol* **35:** 1069–1073, 1982.

Mooney, S. C. *et al.* Renal lymphoma in cats: 28 cases (1977–1984). *J Am Vet Med Assoc* **191:** 1473–1477, 1987.

Sandison, A. T., and Anderson, L. J. Tumors of the kidney in cattle, sheep, and pigs. *Cancer* **21:** 727–742, 1968.

Splitter, G. A., Rawlings, C. A., and Casey, H. W. Renal hamartoma in a dog. *Am J Vet Res* **33:** 273–275, 1972.

Srivastava, A. K., Sharma, D. N., and Dwivedi, J. N. Nephroblastoma in a calf. *Vet Rec* **125:** 245–246, 1989.

Stenzl, A., and deKernion, J. B. Pathology, biology, and clinical staging of renal cell carcinoma. *Sem Oncol* **16** (Suppl. 1, Feb): 3–11, 1989.

Takeda, T. *et al.* Congenital mesoblastic nephroma in a dog: A benign variant of nephroblastoma. *Vet Pathol* **26:** 281–282, 1989.

Vitovec, J. Carcinomas of the renal pelvis in slaughter animals. *J Comp Pathol* **87:** 129–134, 1977.

Watson, A. D. J. *et al.* Nephroblastoma in two dogs. *Aust Vet J* **64:** 94–96, 1987.

West, H. J., Kelly, D. F., and Ritchie, H. E. Renal carcinomatosis in a horse. *Equine Vet J* **19:** 548–551, 1987.

THE LOWER URINARY TRACT

I. General Considerations

The lower urinary tract consists of **ureters, urinary bladder, and urethra.** The ureters and bladder, and also the renal pelvis, are lined by transitional stratified epithelium, the urothelium. The ureters are of uniform diameter throughout, and usually course directly to the bladder, although they may be tortuous and dilated distally in baby pigs. The ureters enter the bladder wall obliquely and are covered by a mucosal flap. Histologically, the ureteral mucosa is present in longitudinal folds; there are poorly defined internal and external longitudinal muscle layers and a prominent middle circular layer, and either adventitia or peritoneal serosa. Peritonitis may involve the ureters and interfere with their peristalsis. Ureters of horses have simple branched tubuloalveolar mucous glands in the propria–submucosa. The male urethra has a thin lining of transitional epithelium; that of the female is similar but has stratified squamous epithelium at its termination. Histologically, the bladder is an expanded ureter. Lymphoid nodules are commonly found in the lamina propria of all domestic animals. The transitional epithelium varies from 3 to 14 cells thick, depending on species and degree of distension. Theliolymphocytes are common in ruminants. Eosinophilic intracytoplasmic inclusion bodies of canine distemper seen in urinary bladder epithelial cells must be differentiated from similar nonspecific inclusions.

The urothelium of the renal pelvis, ureter, and perhaps the trigone of the bladder originates from mesoderm, whereas in the rest of the bladder, it has an endodermal origin. This urothelium responds to chronic irritation from infections, calculi, excreted chemicals, etc., by proliferation and metaplasia, and metaplasia of squamous or mucous types often is superimposed on predominantly proliferative lesions. Both proliferative and metaplastic lesions of the urothelium are regarded as premalignant changes; thus, papillary growths may give rise to transitional, squamous or adenocarcinoma, and squamous, or adenocarcinoma may develop in metaplastic lesions of the corresponding type. Downward proliferation of urothelium, a common reactive change, results in the formation of von Brunn's nests when groups of proliferating cells are isolated in the submucosa. If the center of the nest undergoes liquefaction, cystitis cystica, ureteritis cystica, or pyelitis cystica results. Pyelitis, ureteritis, or cystitis glandularis develops if the epithelium lining the cyst undergoes mucous metaplasia. (Mucous glands are normal in the horse renal pelvis.) Most of the adenomas and adenocarcinomas of the lower urinary tract develop in these areas of mucous metaplasia. A few may arise in submucosal glands or mesonephric and urachal remnants. Urothelium which is not exposed to urine has a tendency to undergo metaplasia to an intestinal type epithelium—such is the fate of some cystic urachal remnants, which normally are lined by transitional epithelium.

The function of the ureter is to propel urine from the kidney to the bladder by peristalsis. In this it is assisted by the renal pelvis. Ureteral peristalsis is controlled by one or more pacemakers, which are located in the recesses of the renal pelvis, and by the activity of the ureteropelvic junction, which determines whether a pacemaker stimulus initiates a peristaltic wave. At low urine-production rates, peristalsis may occur with every fifth pacemaker stimulus, but during diuresis, every stimulus initiates a peristaltic wave. The ureters pass obliquely through the muscular wall of the bladder at the ureterovesical junction. The segment of ureter in the bladder wall, the intravesical ureter, forms the basis of the **vesicoureteral valve,** which prevents reflux of urine from bladder to ureter. When the length of the intravesical ureter is short, as is often the case in puppies, reflux frequently occurs. Thus the competence of the valve is influenced by the angle of the ureteral entry and the thickness of the bladder wall. The urinary bladder stores urine and, in concert with the urethra, expels it. During continence, the bladder is relatively flaccid, and the urethra acts as a valve. During micturition, contraction of the detrusor muscle—the urinary bladder musculature—pumps urine through the relaxed urethra. Sphincter mechanism incompetence or detrusor instability can lead to incontinence, seen most commonly in bitches.

Embryologically the ureters are formed by buds from the mesonephric ducts, which develop craniad to their entrance into the cloaca. The cloaca is divided into a dorsal rectum and ventral urogenital sinus by the urorectal fold in such a way that the urogenital sinus is continuous with the allantois. (The allantois originates as an evagination of the hindgut.) At this stage of development, the mesonephric duct and ureteral bud form a Y shape—one arm of the Y is the ureteral bud, and the other arm plus the stem of the Y are formed by the mesonephric duct. As the allantois and urogenital sinus develop, the stem of the Y is absorbed, and the mesonephric duct and ureteral bud enter the urogenital sinus independently. In females the entire urethra, plus the vaginal vestibule, is derived from the urogenital sinus, but in males only the prostatic urethra is so derived. The penile urethra forms by closure of a groove, the urethral groove, on the caudal face of the penis. The bladder, which is formed from the cranial part of the urogenital sinus and the caudal part of the allantoic diverticulum, communicates with the allantois via the urachus, which forms from the cranial part of the intraembryonic allantoic diverticulum. The communication is severed at birth, and the urachus closes but remains as the umbilical ligament of the bladder.

Most ailments of the lower urinary tract are associated with obstruction and infection, which often are concomitant. Unlike the gastrointestinal tract, which has a normal microbial flora through its length, only the most distal part of the male urethra, and the female vagina, normally host micro-organisms. The operation of sphincterlike mechanisms in the urethra and vesicoureteral valves, and the intermittent pulsatile flow of urine from the kidneys and bladder, normally prevent the movement of organisms higher up the tract. The susceptibility of the urinary bladder of the female to severe infections is undoubtedly related to its short distensible urethra and its proximity to the external environment and especially the rectal flora. On the other hand, the anatomy of male urethras, with their flexures, ossa, and appendages, make them prone to obstruction, particularly by calculi. Specific factors concerned in the establishment and maintenance of infections in the urinary bladder and their spread to the kidney are discussed with cystitis and pyelonephritis. The causes and effects of obstruction are considered with urolithiasis (Section IV of The Lower Urinary Tract) and hydronephrosis (Section III,F of The Kidney).

Urine may be obtained for urinalysis or culture by cystocentesis at autopsy. The bladder may be dilated in downer animals, even in states of dehydration, due either to the absence of the correct posture needed for urination or to decreased medullary tonicity due to hypoproteinemia (low urea production), which has led to polyuria. Dog bladders are often constricted at necropsy and hence have a thick wall. If the bladder can be dilated by pulling it between the fingers, the thickening is not pathologic. Horse urine normally contains mucus and crystals.

Bibliography

Constantinou, C. E., Silvert, M. A., and Gosling, J. Pacemaker system in the control of ureteral peristaltic rate in the multicalyceal kidney of the pig. *Invest Urol* **14:** 440–441, 1977.

Dagle, G. E. *et al.* Cytoplasmic inclusions in urinary bladder epithelium of dogs. *Vet Pathol* **16:** 258–259, 1979.

Djurhuus, J. C. Dynamics of upper urinary tract. III. The activity of renal pelvis during pressure variations. *Invest Urol* **14:** 475–477, 1977.

Gleason, D. M., Bottaccini, M. R., and Drach, G. W. Urodynamics. *J Urol* **115:** 356–361, 1976.

Goss, R. J. *et al.* The physiological basis of urinary bladder hypertrophy. *Proc Soc Exp Biol Med* **142:** 1332–1335, 1973.

Holt, P. E. Urinary incontinence in the bitch due to sphincter mechanism incompetence: Prevalence in referred dogs and retrospective analysis of sixty cases. *J Small Anim Pract* **26:** 181–190, 1985.

Krawiec, D. R. Urinary incontinence in dogs and cats. *Mod Vet Pract* **69:** 17–24, 1988.

Lappin, M. R., and Barsanti, J. A. Urinary incontinence secondary to idiopathic detrusor instability: Cystometrographic diagnosis and pharmacologic management in two dogs and a cat. *J Am Vet Med Assoc* **191:** 1439–1442, 1987.

Michell, A. R. Ins and outs of bladder function. *J Small Anim Pract* **25:** 237–247, 1984.

II. Anomalies of the Lower Urinary Tract

A. Ureters

Agenesis of the ureters is due to failure of the ureteral bud to form, and may be unilateral or bilateral. It occurs in dogs accompanied by renal agenesis (see Anomalies of Development, Section II of The Kidney). **Duplication** of a ureter is caused by formation of two ureteral diverticula from the mesonephric duct. The caudal ureter drains the caudal part of the kidney, and the cranial one drains the cranial part. Usually the caudal ureter empties normally, whereas the other is ectopic. Duplication is rare but occurs in dogs and pigs. Ureteral **dysplasia** occurs in association with renal dysplasia. Ureteral **valves** are seen occasionally in dogs.

Ectopic ureter is the most important ureteral anomaly. Rather than terminating at the trigone of the bladder, the affected ureter may empty into the vas deferens, vesicular gland, or urethra of the male or the bladder neck, urethra, or vagina of the female. In bitches, the ectopic ureter usually terminates in the vagina or urethra. There are two possible causes: either the ureteral bud arises too far craniad to be incorporated into the urogenital sinus, or the differential growth of the sinus is abnormal, and the ureter fails to migrate to its usual location. Ectopic ureters occasionally empty into the rectum because of anomalous cloacal division by the urorectal fold. Very rarely they empty into the cervix, uterus, or uterine tube, possibly as a result of aberrant origin from the paramesonephric (müllerian) duct.

Ectopic ureter is most common in dogs and is diagnosed as much as 20 times more frequently in females than in males. However, this sex difference may be apparent or exaggerated since affected females are usually incontinent from birth, whereas affected males may not be. Termination of the ectopic ureter proximal to the external urethral sphincter in males leads to retrograde filling of the bladder rather than to incontinence. Ectopia can be unilateral or bilateral and is often associated with other urinary tract abnormalities, including bladder agenesis or hypoplasia, renal agenesis or hypoplasia, ureteral or bladder duplication, and branching of the terminal ureter. Certain dog breeds have a high risk for the defect, including the Siberian husky, Newfoundland, Labrador retrievers, West Highland white terrier, fox terrier, and miniature and toy poodles; the defect is familial in Siberian huskies and Labrador retrievers. Ectopic ureter also occurs in White Shorthorn bulls and tends to involve the region of the seminal vesicles.

Ureteral anomalies often predispose to hydronephrosis and urinary tract infection that may culminate in pyelonephritis.

B. Urinary Bladder

Duplication of the urinary bladder occurs in dogs and causes dysuria, incontinence, and sometimes abdominal distension and cryptorchidism. The extra bladder originates dorsally between the urinary tract and uterus or rectum. Cystic remnants of the urorectal fold may be responsible for the defect.

Patent or **pervious urachus** is the most common malformation of the urinary bladder and is seen more often in foals than in other animals. Animals with this defect dribble urine from the umbilicus because the urachal lumen fails to close and remains as an open channel between the apex of the bladder and the umbilicus; a patent urachus is susceptible to infection and abscessation. Rupture of the urachus causes uroperitoneum. The condition must be differentiated from perinatal rupture of the bladder. Occasionally, urachal obliteration is partial, and rests of epithelium remain intact to develop into cysts at any point between the umbilicus and the bladder. These cysts may become quite large but usually are small and multiple and are attached to the midline of the bladder. Occasionally they adhere to the intestinal serosa. The urachus is normally lined by transitional epithelium, but metaplasia is common in urachal cysts and sinuses, which are then lined by squamous or mucus-secreting columnar epithelium. Urachal remnants in the bladder wall may give origin to neoplasms.

Diverticula of the bladder may be acquired secondary to partial obstruction to the outflow of urine, or they may result at an abnormally weak area of the wall from the pressure of normal contractions. Diverticula are usually seen at the vertex, where they represent incomplete closure of the urachus with an area of discontinuity in the muscle. Contraction of the bladder tends to distend the diverticulum, but rupture does not occur. Stasis of urine in the diverticulum eventually leads to persistent infection and inflammation. Calculi may form in the diverticulum.

C. Urethra

Urethral agenesis, duplicated urethra, ectopic urethra, and imperforate urethra occur rarely in dogs. Hypospadias is described with male genitalia. The most common urethral anomaly is **urethrorectal** or **rectovaginal fistula,** which is caused by incomplete division of the cloaca into rectum and urogenital sinus by the urorectal fold. In males, the communication involves the pelvic urethra, and affected dogs urinate from the rectum. In females, the opening is in the vagina and may be associated with imperforate anus. These defects occur in dogs, pigs, and horses, and usually predispose to urogenital tract infections but sometimes are incidental autopsy findings.

In male goats, a urethral diverticulum is normally present and is not anomalous, but is an impediment to catheterization.

Bibliography

Benko, L. Cases of bilateral and unilateral duplication of ureters in the pig. *Vet Rec* **84:** 139–140, 1969.

Dean, P. W., and Robertson, J. T. Urachal remnant as a cause of pollakiuria and dysuria in a filly. *J Am Vet Med Assoc* **192:** 375–376, 1988.

Dean, P. W., Bojrab, M. J., and Constantinescu, G. M. Canine ectopic ureter. *Compend Cont Ed Pract Vet* **10:** 146–157, 1988.

Divers, T. J., Byars, D., and Spirito, M. Correction of bilateral ureteral defects in a foal. *J Am Vet Med Assoc* **192:** 384–386, 1988.

Hinkle, R. F., Howard, J. L., and Stowater, J. L. An anatomic barrier to urethral catheterization in the male goat. *J Am Vet Med Assoc* **173:** 1584–1586, 1978.

Holt, P. E., Long, S. E., and Gibbs, C. Disorders of urination associated with canine intersexuality. *J Small Anim Pract* **24:** 475–487, 1983.

Hoskins, J. D., Abdelbaki, Y. Z., and Root, C. D. Urinary bladder duplication in a dog. *J Am Vet Med Assoc* **181:** 603–604, 1982.

Kuzma, A. B., and Holmberg, D. L. Ectopic ureter in a cat. *Can Vet J* **29:** 59–61, 1988.

Osuna, D. J., Stone, E. A., and Metcalf, M. R. A urethrorectal fistula with concurrent urolithiasis in a dog. *J Am Anim Hosp Assoc* **25:** 35–39, 1989.

Perlman, M., Williams, J., and Ornoy, A. Familial ureteric bud anomalies. *J Med Genet* **13:** 161–163, 1976.

Pollock, S., and Schoen, S. S. Urinary incontinence associated with congenital ureteral valves in a bitch. *J Am Vet Med Assoc* **159:** 332–335, 1971.

Pringle, J. K., Ducharme, N. G., and Baird, J. D. Ectopic ureter in the horse: Three cases and a review of the literature. *Can Vet J* **31:** 26–30, 1990.

Rawlings, C. A., and Capps, W. F. Rectovaginal fistula and imperforate anus in a dog. *J Am Vet Med Assoc* **159:** 320–326, 1971.

Weaver, M. E. Persistent urachus—an observation in miniature swine. *Anat Rec* **154:** 701–704, 1966.

D. Acquired Anatomic Variations

Displacements of ureters and urethra are sometimes caused by local inflammatory and neoplastic swelling. Their main significance to the urinary system is related to obstruction of urine flow. Ureteral and urethral displacements may also occur with variations of position of the bladder. Torsion of the bladder is uncommon; it may be partial or complete about the long axis of the organ. Presence of part of the bladder within the pelvis in dogs, so-called pelvic bladder, is thought to be normal variation dependent on the degree of distension of the bladder and is not a cause of incontinence.

Dorsal **retroflexion** occurs in male dogs with tenesmus in response to prostatic enlargement or constipation. The normal position is assumed following emptying. A more serious type occurs in prolapse of the vagina in cows and sows and occasionally in perineal hernia of older male dogs. In these cases, the bladder may be present in the hernial sac and, because of the retroflexion, there is obstructive kinking of the neck of the bladder and sometimes of the urethra and ureters. If the ureters are patent, the accumulation of urine in the bladder contributes to the size of the hernia. Hydronephrosis or rupture of the bladder may occur if the condition is not corrected.

Eversion of the bladder (invagination into and through the urethra) occurs in females and is permitted by the short, wide urethra in this sex. The bladder may arrive in the vagina. It can occur in any of the larger species and is perhaps most common in mares. Eversion is predisposed to by circumstances in which straining occurs, often after parturition. The everted bladder may contain intestines. Eversion of the bladder is to be distinguished from **prolapse** of the bladder; in eversion, the mucosal surface protrudes from the vulva, whereas in prolapse the bladder has been displaced through a rent in the vagina, and the serosal surface appears.

Hydroureter, or dilation of a ureter, may be due to obstruction by calculi, neoplasms, or inflammatory debris, or due to accidental ligation, and will lead to hydronephrosis. Dilation without physical obstruction occurs in association with peritonitis and may be due to loss of muscle tone. Dilation of ureters is often present in neonatal pigs with enteric infections. Congenital hydroureter and hydronephrosis often occur in piglets in association with epitheliogenesis imperfecta.

Ureters may **rupture** as a consequence of physical trauma or may be accidentally **transected** during surgery, e.g., ovariohysterectomy. Leakage of urine from the ureter may result in formation of a urinoma—a retroperitoneal accumulation of urine sometimes referred to as a pseudocyst.

Dilation of the bladder may be of local obstructive or neuroparalytic origin. The wall is thin and almost transparent, and the distended organ may extend almost to the liver. Brief periods of distension may allow quick return of normal contractibility, but severe or prolonged distension may result in loss of tone, which is not restored before bacterial complications terminate the condition. The causes of obstruction include calculi, prostatic enlargement in dogs, accumulated inflammatory detritus or blood clots in the urethra, urethral strictures, and tumors of the neck of the bladder or urethra.

Neurogenic distension follows spinal injury with loss of tonic parasympathetic outflow from the sacral plexus. Spinal myelitis, as in canine distemper and rabies, may also cause paralysis of the bladder. Perhaps it most commonly follows herniation of intervertebral disks in the dog. Cystitis is the usual complication. In horses in particular, bladder paralysis and distension can lead to sabulous urolithiasis.

Distension of the bladder occurs when calves fed indigestible milk-replacer starve to death. They are usually recumbent for several hours before death, but this is probably due to weakness rather than nervous disease. Renal concentrating ability is depressed by starvation because of lack of urea and a partial insensitivity to antidiuretic hormone and mineralocorticoids. Possibly the bladder distension is caused by overproduction of dilute urine.

Hypertrophy of the bladder is fairly common in dogs and less so in other species. It is a response to long-standing partial obstruction to the outflow of urine.

Rupture of the bladder (cystorrhexis) often occurs following urethral obstruction, such as occurs in urolithiasis, but rarely following pelvic trauma. The interval between obstruction and rupture depends somewhat on the competence of the vesicoureteral valve and whether hydronephrosis develops. Rupture of the bladder occurs in newborn foals, affecting either the dorsal or ventral aspect of the viscus. Males are most often affected. Some ruptures are congenital, and most are probably caused by birth trauma. Twists in the amniotic portion of the umbilical cord may compress the urachus, causing distension of both bladder and urachus and predisposing to rupture.

Bibliography

Bertone, A. L., and Smith, D. F. Ruptured urinary bladder in a yearling heifer. *J Am Vet Med Assoc* **184:** 981–982, 1984.

Holt, P. E., and Mair, T. S. Ten cases of bladder paralysis associated with sabulous urolithiasis in horses. *Vet Rec* **127:** 108–110, 1990.

Kritchevsky, J. E. *et al.* Peritoneal dialysis for presurgical management of ruptured bladder in a foal. *J Am Vet Med Assoc* **185:** 81–82, 1984.

Mahaffey, M. B. *et al.* Pelvic bladder in dogs without urinary incontinence. *J Am Vet Med Assoc* **184:** 1477–1479, 1984.

O'Brien, D. P. Disorders of the urogenital system. *Sem Vet Med Surg (Small Anim)* **5:** 57–66, 1990.

Peter, A. T., Arighi, M., and Gaines, J. D. Herniation of distal jejunum into the partially everted urinary bladder of a cow. *Can Vet J* **30:** 830–831, 1989.

Richardson, D. W., and Kohn, C. W. Uroperitoneum in the foal. *J Am Vet Med Assoc* **182:** 267–271, 1983.

Tidwell, A. S., Ullman, S. L., and Schelling, S. H. Urinoma (paraureteral pseudocyst) in a dog. *Vet Radiol* **31:** 203–206, 1990.

Wegmann, E. Urinary bladder eversion in a mare with colic. *Mod Vet Pract* **68:** 174, 1987.

White, R. A. S., and Herrtage, M. E. Bladder retroflexion in the dog. *J Small Anim Pract* **27:** 735–746, 1986.

III. Circulatory Disturbances

Hemorrhages are the most important and common of circulatory disturbances. In the ureters and urethra, they are associated with obstructive calculi, and ureteral hemorrhage is part of acute ascending infections. In the bladder, they are located in the propria mucosa and may occur in any septicemia. Small hemorrhages with the shape of tiny hematomas are common and considered diagnostically significant in hog cholera, African swine fever, porcine salmonellosis, and equine purpura hemorrhagica. Larger hemorrhages are present in bracken fern poisoning of cattle. Hemorrhage occurs with acute cystitis and neoplastic diseases, and hemorrhage with hematoma formation is seen with rupture of the bladder.

Bibliography

Lloyd, K. C. K. *et al.* Ulceration in the proximal portion of the urethra as a cause of hematuria in horses: Four cases (1978–1985). *J Am Vet Med Assoc* **194:** 1324–1326, 1989.

IV. Urolithiasis

Urolithiasis is the presence of calculi, or uroliths, in the urinary passages. Calculi are grossly visible aggregations of precipitated urinary solutes, urinary proteins, and proteinaceous debris; minerals predominate in **calculi,** and matrix usually predominates in **urethral plugs.** Many calculi have a laminated structure and are hard spheres or ovoids with a small amount of organic matrix impregnated with inorganic salts. Urethral plugs are masses of sandy sludge with a much higher organic component whose form is largely determined by the shape of the cavity they fill. Even densely mineralized calculi of the same type may have quite a different appearance, depending on whether they are located in renal pelvis or urinary bladder. Many calculi contain significant quantities of contaminants such as calcium oxalates in silica calculi; a few are relatively pure.

The diseases caused by uroliths are among the most important urinary tract problems of domesticated animals. Several factors are important in predisposing to calculus formation, and several are important in precipitating disease. These are not the same for all diseases. Obviously, calculogenic material must occur in urine in quantities sufficient to be precipitated. Sometimes this concentration is achieved because a substance is metabolized in an unusual way, as is uric acid in Dalmatian dogs; or it may be processed abnormally by the kidney, as is cystine in cystine stone formers; or abnormally high levels of a substance in the diet, such as silicic acid in native pastures, may produce potentially dangerous urinary levels. Regardless of the type of calculus, certain factors are more or less important; these are **urinary pH,** in terms of its optimum for solute precipitation, and **reduced water intake,** in relation to the degree of urine concentration. Deficiency of vitamin A is frequently suggested as a predisposing factor, but the evidence is equivocal; it may contribute in exceptional circumstances by producing metaplastic changes in the urinary epithelium.

Urine is often supersaturated with respect to the components of stone-forming salts, and this **supersaturation** is the essential precursor to initiation of urolith formation (nucleation). Supersaturation may be in the **unstable** region where spontaneous precipitation occurs (homogeneous nucleation, the precipitation-crystallization theory of urolith initiation), or in the **metastable** range where precipitation occurs by epitaxy or heterogeneous nucleation (one type of crystal grows on the surface of another type). Although formerly it was thought that urinary proteins such as uromucoid, which make up 5–20% or more of most calculi, were preeminent initiators of crystal formation in the metastable range (the matrix-nucleation theory of urolith initiation), it is now believed that in many cases either coprecipitation of proteins and minerals occurs or proteins are adsorbed onto formed crystals. It is possible that crystals of one salt, for which urine is supersaturated in the unstable range, cause epitactic induction of crystals of another salt for which supersaturation is metastable. A foreign body, such as a suture or a grass awn, can act as a nidus for urolith formation.

Crystals are much more common in urine than are calculi. Even though equine urine, for example, is normally supersaturated with calcium carbonate, and crystalluria is normal, horses experience a low prevalence of calculi. The factors which promote crystal growth and crystal aggregation or, more important, prevent them in some animals, are poorly understood. Experimentally, high levels of urinary inorganic pyrophosphate and magnesium are important inhibitors of calcium phosphate and calcium oxalate crystallization, and pyrophosphate also inhibits aggregation of calcium phosphate crystals. Certain urinary macromolecules, probably glycosaminoglycans, are also strong inhibitors of crystal aggregation in experimental systems. Deficiency of inhibitors of crystallization may be important in calcium oxalate and calcium phosphate calculogenesis (crystallization-inhibition theory of urolith initiation). Nothing of substance is known about why calculi stay in the renal pelvis and urinary bladder until they are large enough to cause disease.

The important and less important types of urinary calculi are given according to species (Table 5.5). Brief discussions of some of these follow a discussion of their pathologic effects.

The division indicated in the table is arbitrary. Obviously silica calculi are important only where ruminants are pastured, and clover stones are important only where subterranean clover grows. In general, calculi are important in cattle, sheep, dogs, and cats, less important in horses, and unimportant in pigs. In pigs, uroliths are found occasionally in the renal pelvis of old animals and, more often, in the pelvis of dehydrated sucklings (Fig. 5.1) (see Uremia, Section I,D of The Kidney, in this chapter). In horses, they occur sometimes as single or several, spherical, or faceted carbonate stones in the bladder; urethral obstructions are rare. In dogs, several breeds are predisposed to formation of calculi, namely dachshunds, Dalmatians, cocker spaniels, Pekingese, basset hounds, poodles, schnauzers, and small terriers.

TABLE 5.5

Composition and Importance of Calculi

Species	Common Types	Uncommon Types
Dog	Struvite Cystine Urate Oxalate	Xanthine Silica
Cat	Struvite	Oxalate Urate Cystine
Ox	Silica Struvite Carbonate	Xanthine
Sheep	Silica Struvite Oxalate "Clover stones" Carbonate	Xanthine
Horse	Carbonate	—
Pig	—	Urate

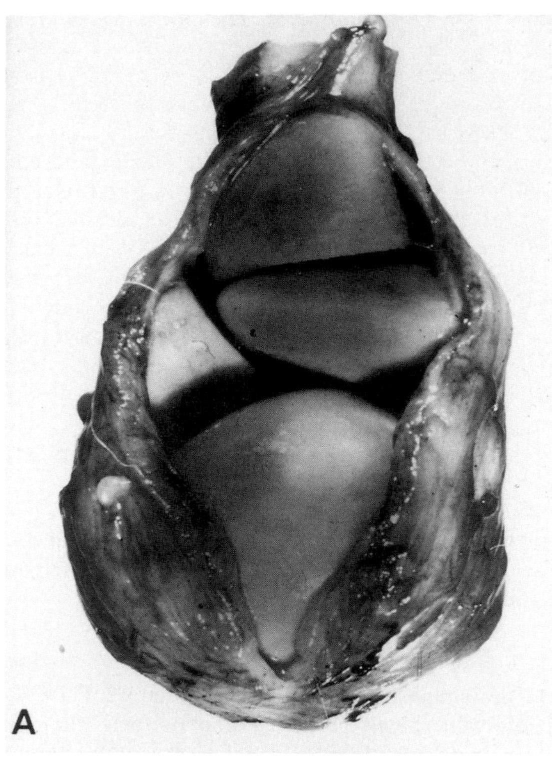

Fig. 5.64A Faceted calculi filling bladder. Dog.

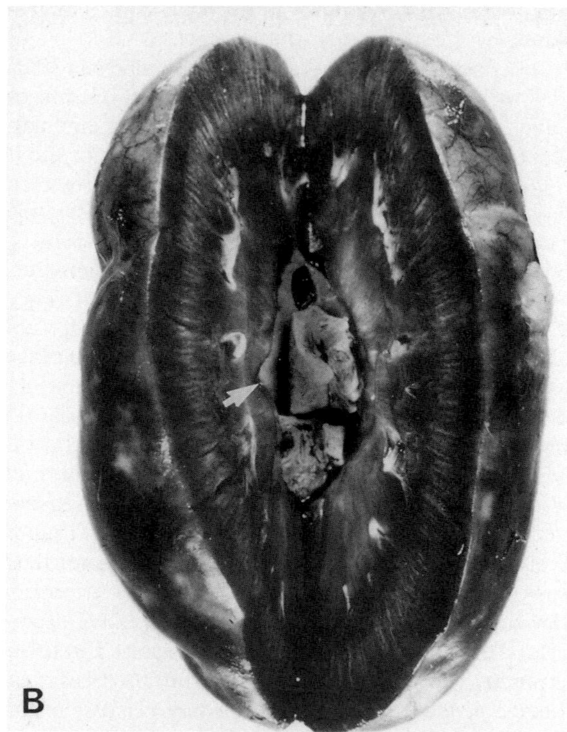

Fig. 5.64B Calculus, renal pelvis. Dog. Renal crest is ulcerated (arrow). Cortex is irregularly scarred.

Calculi may form in any part of the urinary duct system, from the renal pelvis to the urethra. Some uroliths clearly originate in the lower urinary tract, but the point for embryogenesis of most is not known (Fig. 5.64A). In experimental urolithiasis produced by oxalates or calcium phosphate in laboratory animals, the calculi, initially microscopic, form in the collecting tubules and encrust on the renal papilla. They may grow large enough to make voidance impossible (Fig. 5.64B). It is not known whether this is a general phenomenon. The tubular microlithiasis may simply represent crystallization in the highly concentrated urine of the medulla, or, alternatively, it may indicate the production there of an abnormal or excessive matricial substance. Obstructive nephroliths and ureteroliths occasionally develop in horses and cause secondary chronic tubulointerstitial nephritis; the suggested pathogenesis is renal medullary crest necrosis resulting from the use of non-steroidal antiinflammatory drugs in dehydrated horses, with subsequent mineralization of the sloughed necrotic renal crest material.

Small calculi may be voided in the urine, but impaction in the urethra is common in males. The common sites of urethral impaction are the ischial arch, the sigmoid flexure of ruminants, the vermiform appendage of rams (Fig. 5.65), the proximal end of the os penis in dogs, and anywhere along the urethra of male cats. At the point of impaction, there is local pressure necrosis with ulceration of the mucosa and, because the urinary stasis favors bacterial growth, acute hemorrhagic urethritis develops and often ascends to the bladder and even to the kidney. Hydronephrosis is not a prominent development with urethral calculi, and rupture of the urethra with leakage of urine into the surrounding tissues, often associated with infection and acute cellulitis, terminates the condition fairly quickly.

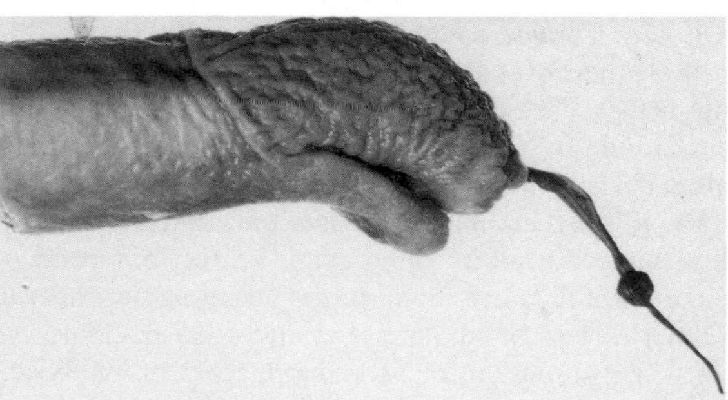

Fig. 5.65 Calculus impacted in vermiform appendage. Ram.

A. Silica Calculi

In ruminants these calculi are hard, white to dark brown, radiopaque, often laminated, and as much as 1 cm across. In the bladder of ruminants they are spherical, ovoid, or mulberry-shaped and have smooth surfaces, but in the kidney they are angular and irregular, having the shape of the minor calyces where they are located almost exclusively.

"Pure" silica stones contain about 75% silica as silica dioxide. Mixed calculi contain some calcium oxalate or carbonate. Silica calculi contain about 20% organic matter. Most have a friable core, which is high in amorphous silica and low in organic matter. The core is surrounded by a layer of organic matter, which separates it from the outer concentric laminations, which are high in silica.

Silica calculi are very common in pastured ruminants and are a major cause of urinary tract obstruction. They occur rarely in horses and dogs. Silica calculi are present in more than 50% of steers on native (unimproved) range in western Canada; fewer than 5% develop urethral obstruction. The singularity of adjacent laminae in the calculi is consistent with intermittent deposition as urine composition changes. Certain grasses contain 4–5% or more of silica; the level increases through the growing season. Most of it is relatively insoluble, but that in the cell sap is relatively soluble, unpolymerized silicic acid. Rumen fluid becomes saturated with respect to silicic acid. After absorption, some is returned to the gut in digestive secretions; less than 1% of dietary silica is excreted in urine and as much as 60% is resorbed from the filtrate. However, when urine production is very low, either because of the nature of the diet or because of high insensible fluid losses in hot climates, the concentration of silicic acid in urine may reach five times the saturation level. Even so, precipitation from solution requires other substances, probably proteins of renal or serum origin, in the urine. Calculus formation is reduced to subclinical levels by adding salt to the ration, thereby ensuring high water consumption.

Silica calculi are reported in dogs from Kenya and the United States. In Kenya they occur in both sexes, and are mainly renal and asymptomatic. In the United States, male dogs are affected in most cases, and the stones, located in the bladder and urethra, often cause urinary obstruction. Unlike cystic silica calculi in ruminants, bladder stones in dogs have very irregular shapes; many silica uroliths have a jack-stone configuration. Dietary factors probably are involved in calculus formation in dogs as they are in ruminants. Urine pH does not appear to be important.

B. Struvite Calculi

Struvite stones are white or gray, radiopaque, chalky, usually smooth, and easily broken. They may be pure struvite but usually contain other compounds such as calcium phosphate, and ammonium urate, oxalate or carbonate. They may be single and large, or numerous and sandlike. Struvite is magnesium ammonium phosphate hexahydrate; formerly it was called triple phosphate, a misnomer.

Struvite calculi are important in dogs, cats, and ruminants (Fig. 5.66). In **dogs,** they are the most common type; females are particularly susceptible perhaps because they develop bladder infections more often than males. Struvite calculi are often single, rapidly forming masses which

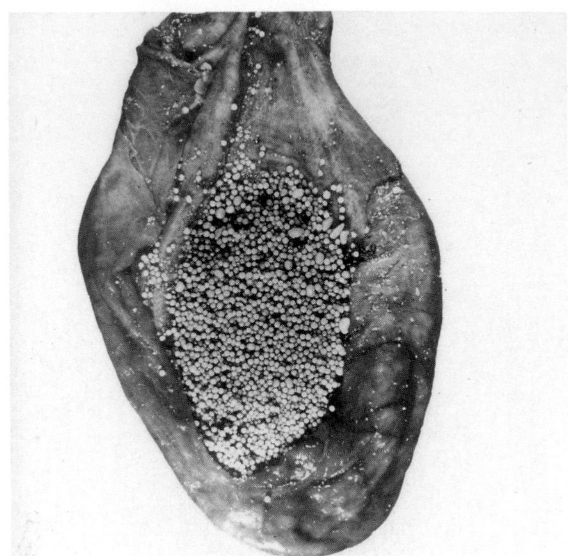

Fig. 5.66 Struvite calculi in urinary bladder. Cow.

mold to the shape of the cavity they occupy. They are called **infection calculi** in recognition of their common association with infection. Bacterial ureases from staphylococci and *Proteus* induce supersaturation of urine with struvite by increasing urine pH and ammonium ions. Alkaline urine decreases struvite solubility and increases ionization of trivalent phosphate, both of which favor calculus formation. Factors other than urease production which are associated with infection probably are important in the genesis of struvite stones. A high incidence of struvite calculi in miniature schnauzers may be related to a familial susceptibility to urinary tract infections.

In **cats,** discrete struvite calculi often develop in the urinary bladder of both sexes, but are more common in middle-aged, spayed female cats. Struvite crystalluria is seen often in cats with and without calculi; the reasons for aggregation of crystals into sterile calculi are obscure. Formation of uroliths can be induced in previously normal cats fed calculogenic diets containing 0.15–1.0% dry weight magnesium. Coagulase-positive staphylococci and other bacteria are commonly cultured from the urine or calculi of some affected cats, and the formation of infection-induced struvite calculi is similar to that mentioned for dogs; these calculi are much less common than are sterile struvite uroliths.

Of considerably more importance than discrete calculi are the amorphous accumulations of protein, cellular debris, and struvite crystals that form sabulous urethral plugs in male cats. This condition is variously known as the **feline urologic syndrome** (FUS) and as lower urinary tract disease (LUTD), and is probably the most common and important urinary tract disease of cats. It is characterized by dysuria, hematuria, and urethral obstruction. If unrelieved, the obstruction can lead to bladder distension, hemorrhagic cystitis, azotemia, and death (Fig. 5.67). The obstructive material, which becomes molded to the shape of the urethra in male cats, may be either struvite sand or rubberlike protein matrix, or a mixture of the two; the protein apparently is unique to feline calculi but is not characterized.

The pathogenesis of FUS is multifactorial. Various viruses, including feline cell-associated herpesvirus (FCAHV) (a close relative of bovine herpesvirus 4) and calicivirus, have been implicated as potential urinary pathogens in cats. Other suggested predisposing factors include inhibition of urethral growth by early castration, and exclusive use of dry food. Addition of magnesium and phosphate to the diet causes disease in some, presumably predisposed, cats and, conversely, reduction of dietary magnesium reduces the incidence. Alkaline urine pH may be of more significance in formation of struvite crystals than is magnesium intake. The apparent increased incidence during cold winter months may be due to decreased fluid consumption or increased intervals between urinations. The incidence of FUS has decreased as more cats have been fed low-ash cat foods [total mineral <6%, Mg 0.05–0.10%, Mg <20 mg/100 kcal dose equivalent (DE)].

In **ruminants,** struvite calculi usually occur in feedlot cattle on high-grain rations, and obstruction may develop in as many as 10% of steers. As in cats, calculi usually form a gritty sludge with a high proportion of matrix.

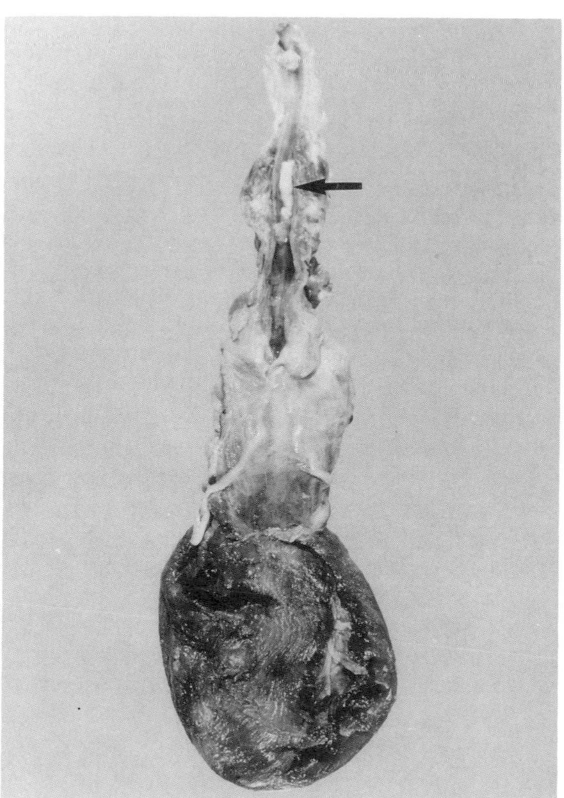

Fig. 5.67 Feline urologic syndrome. Plug of struvite crystals in urethra (arrow) with hemorrhagic cystitis.

Inhibition of urethral growth by early castration predisposes to obstruction, and increased water consumption tends to prevent obstruction. Animals with crystalluria often have crystals adhering to preputial hairs. Diets high in phosphate can cause a very high incidence of calculi in sheep; a calcium-to-phosphorus ratio of 1:2 or wider appears to be the critical factor, but the form in which they are fed and the balance of other constituents such as magnesium, sodium, and potassium are probably also important. Additional potassium tends to promote phosphate urolithiasis. Magnesium deficiency leads to renal mineralization and tubular microlithiasis, at least in laboratory species, and both sodium and magnesium are competitive with calcium, and increase the solubility of calcium salts in urine. There may also be a genetic effect on urolithiasis in sheep; urolithiasis is more likely to develop in sheep that excrete phosphorus mainly in urine than in those that excrete phosphorus mainly in feces.

C. Oxalate Calculi

Oxalate calculi are hard, heavy, white or yellow, and typically covered with jagged spines, though some are smooth. They tend to be large and solitary in the bladder.

Oxalate calculi occur as the calcium oxalates, whewellite (calcium oxalate monohydrate) and weddellite (calcium oxalate dihydrate). Their development is not well understood but obviously hypercalciuria and hyperoxaluria are involved. There are several causes of hypercalciuria (see Hypercalcemic Nephropathy, Section VI,F of The Kidney, in this chapter). Oxalic acid is synthesized from glyoxylic and ascorbic acid and may be ingested in certain foods—the relevance of these facts is obscure. Hyperuricosuria may be involved in oxalate precipitation, since sodium hydrogen urate may act as a heterogeneous nucleator.

Oxalate (and silica) calculi may be important in sheep grazing grain stubble, but the source of the oxalate is not known. Oxalate-containing plants apparently are not a source since oxalate is metabolized in the rumen; nonetheless occasional exceptions to this general rule do seem to occur. Feeding a low-calcium diet (0.3% Ca) has produced oxalate urolithiasis in steers, possibly because of increased bone resorption resulting in increased plasma concentrations of hydroxyproline, an oxalate precursor. High magnesium intakes inhibit formation of oxalate calculi, whereas low levels induce formation in some species.

In dogs, oxalate calculi are of some importance, but little is known of their origins. Calcium oxalate and calcium phosphate (hydroxyapatite or calcium apatite) calculi occur in dogs with primary hyperparathyroidism and hypercalcemia.

D. Uric Acid and Urate Calculi

These calculi are usually multiple, hard, concentrically laminated, yellow to brown, and moderately radiodense. In the bladder, they are frequently spherical and less than

5 mm across. Most contain ammonium urate with some uric acid and phosphate; in others, sodium urate is the predominant salt.

Urate stones are most common in dogs, especially Dalmatians, but also occur in pigs (see Uremia, Section I,D of The Kidney, in this chapter) and rarely in cats. Dalmatians excrete high levels of uric acid in their urine. This is due to defective hepatocellular uptake of uric acid, which results in incomplete conversion of uric acid to allantoin, a more soluble product of purine metabolism; this defect is an inherited autosomal recessive trait. Hepatic uricase levels are normal. It is not clear whether the defective transport system also involves renal tubules and prevents reabsorption of uric acid from glomerular filtrate. Dogs with portosystemic shunts have ammonium biurate crystals in their urine, and may have urate-containing calculi in kidneys and bladder.

Urates exist in supersaturated urine as lyophobic colloids which are flocculated by high levels of ammonium ion and, to a lesser extent, by low pH. Urea-splitting organisms may be important in the development of urate calculi since production of ammonium ion favors calculus formation. Also, although higher pH inhibits precipitation of uric acid, it favors precipitation of ammonium urate, as well as phosphates, which are often found in urate calculi.

E. Cystine Calculi

Cystine calculi are small and irregular, soft and friable, waxy, and yellow turning to green on exposure to daylight. Many cystine calculi consist of pure cystine; others may also contain calcium oxalate, struvite, brushite (calcium hydrogen phosphate dihydrate), and complex urates.

Cystine stones occur in dogs, especially dachshunds, and rarely in cats. They compose about 10% of canine calculi, and as much as 30% in Europe, being second to struvite calculi in incidence. Cystine calculi occur in males only, but cystinuria is recorded in females. Many dogs have high levels of urinary cystine because of defective tubular reabsorption from glomerular filtrate. Blood cystine levels are normal, demonstrating that this is a transport defect rather than an inborn error of metabolism. Many dogs with cystinuria also have high levels of other amino acids in their urine, but these are more soluble than cystine. Cystine precipitates in acid urine, but factors other than urinary pH probably are important in the genesis of cystine stones, since dogs with crystalluria do not always form them. The genetics of cystinuria is poorly understood; a familial tendency is suggested in Irish terriers, and inheritance as an autosomal recessive trait with sex-modified expression is postulated.

F. Clover Stones

Sheep grazing estrogenic pastures, particularly subterranean clover, or injected or implanted with estrogens, may have an incidence of fatal urinary obstruction as high as 10%. There are probably three separate developmental patterns and, in each, the obstructing material is soft or pulpy and scantily mineralized. Probably the most common pattern is urethral obstruction by desquamated cells and secretions of accessory glands originating in the pelvic urethra under the influence of estrogen. The second type, the so-called clover stone, is usually found in the renal pelvis as a yellow, soft material which leads eventually to fibrosis and shrinkage of the kidney. It affects both sexes equally. These calculi contain benzocoumarins, which may be metabolites of phytoestrogens. Third, sudden and serious mortalities may occur in male sheep grazing subterranean clover during its period of rapid maturation. The urethral process becomes impacted with a soft white paste consisting mainly of calcium carbonate and an unidentified organic material probably related to isoflavones.

G. Xanthine Calculi

Xanthine stones are yellow to brown-red, often concentrically laminated, friable, and irregularly shaped. They are radiolucent. Xanthine is a metabolite of purines and seldom appears in urine because normally it is degraded by xanthine oxidase to uric acid.

Xanthine calculi occur occasionally in sheep and calves and are reported in a dog. A high incidence in sheep was circumstantially related to deficiency of molybdenum in unimproved pasture; molybdenum is a component of xanthine oxidase. Several cases in calves in Japan were also associated with deficiency of xanthine oxidase. Xanthine precipitates in acid urine. Calculi usually form in the collecting ducts and calyces of the kidney, and may cause hydronephrosis.

H. Other Types of Calculi

Several other types of calculi develop in animals; they may be important locally or simply be curiosities. **Tetracycline** and **barium** stones, iatrogenic and rare, fall into the latter category. Other chemical compounds are more common but often constitute a minor part of certain uroliths. Stones with a high **carbonate** content are associated with very alkaline urines and are seen in ruminants consuming high-oxalate plants or clover-dominated pastures.

In horses, calculi most commonly consist of **calcium carbonate,** usually in the crystalline form of calcite, and substituted vaterite (the Ca of $CaCO_3$ is replaced in various amounts by Mg and Mn); weddellite (calcium oxalate dihydrate) may also be present. These crystal types are the same as those present in normal equine urine.

Bibliography

Briggs, O. M., Rodgers, A. L., and Harley, E. H. Uric acid urolithiasis in a Dalmatian coach hound. *J S Afr Vet Assoc* **53:** 205–208, 1982.

Brown, R. G. Low-ash cat foods: The role of magnesium in feline nutrition. *Can Vet J* **30:** 73–76, 1989.

Cuddeford, D. Role of magnesium in the aetiology of ovine uro-

lithiasis in fattening store lambs and intensively fattened lambs. *Vet Rec* **121:** 194–197, 1987.
da Silva Curiel, J. M. A. *et al.* Ammonium urate urolith resulting in hydronephrosis and hydroureter in a dog with a congenital portosystemic shunt. *Can Vet J* **31:** 116–117, 1990.
DiBartola, S. P., Chew, D. J., and Horton, M. L. Cystinuria in a cat. *J Am Vet Med Assoc* **198:** 102–104, 1991.
Divers, T. J., Reef, V. B., and Roby, K. A. Nephrolithiasis resulting in intermittent ureteral obstruction in a cow. *Cornell Vet* **79:** 143–149, 1989.
Dutt, B., Majumbar, B. N., and Kehar, N. D. Vitamin A deficiency and urinary calculi in goats. *Br Vet J* **115:** 63–66, 1959.
Ehnen, S. J. *et al.* Obstructive nephrolithiasis and ureterolithiasis associated with chronic renal failure in horses: Eight cases (1981–1987). *J Am Vet Med Assoc* **197:** 249–253, 1990.
Escolar, E., Bellanto, J., and Rodriquez, M. Study of cystine urinary calculi in dogs. *Can J Vet Res* **55:** 67–70, 1991.
Gaskell, C. J. Feline urologic syndrome (FUS)—theory and practice. *J Small Anim Pract* **31:** 519–522, 1990.
Hesse, A. Canine urolithiasis: Epidemiology and analysis of urinary calculi. *J Small Anim Pract* **31:** 599–604, 1990.
Huntington, G. B., and Emerick, R. J. Oxalate urinary calculi in beef steers. *Am J Vet Res* **45:** 180–182, 1984.
Klausner, J. S., O'Leary, T. P., and Osborne, C. A. Calcium urolithiasis in two dogs with parathyroid adenomas. *J Am Vet Med Assoc* **191:** 1423–1426, 1987.
Kruger, J. M., and Osborne, C. A. The role of viruses in feline lower urinary tract disease. *J Vet Intern Med* **4:** 71–78, 1990.
Ling, G. V. *et al.* Epizootiologic evaluation and quantitative analysis of urinary calculi from 150 cats. *J Am Vet Med Assoc* **196:** 1459–1462, 1990.
Mair, T. S., and Osborn, R. S. The crystalline composition of normal equine urine deposits. *Equine Vet J* **22:** 364–365, 1990.
Momotani, E. *et al.* Pathological changes of xanthinurolithiasis in calves. *Nat Inst Anim Health Q* **19:** 65–71, 1979.
Muldoon, L. D., and Resnick, M. I. Secondary urolithiasis. *Endocrinol Metabol Clin North Am* **19:** 909–918, 1990.
Osborne, C. A., Hammer, R. F., and Klausner, J. S. Canine silica urolithiasis. *J Am Vet Med Assoc* **178:** 809–813, 1981.
Osborne, C. A. *et al.* Struvite urolithiasis in animals and man: Formation, detection, and dissolution. *Adv Vet Sci Comp Med* **29:** 1–101, 1985.
Osborne, C. A. *et al.* Relationship of nutritional factors to the cause, dissolution, and prevention of feline uroliths and urethral plugs. *Vet Clin North Am: Small Anim Pract* **19:** 561–581, 1989.
Poole, D. B. R. Observations on the role of magnesium and phosphorus in the aetiology of urolithiasis in male sheep. *Irish Vet J* **42:** 60–63, 1989.
Pope, G. S. Isolation of two benzocoumarins from "clover stone," a type of renal calculus found in sheep. *Biochem J* **93:** 474–477, 1964.
Roch-Ramel, F. Renal excretion of uric acid in mammals. *Clin Nephrol* **12:** 1–6, 1979.
Schneeberger, E. E., and Morrison, A. B. Increased susceptibility of magnesium-deficient rats to a phosphate-induced nephropathy. *Am J Pathol* **50:** 549–558, 1967.
Smith, L. H. Solutions and solute. *Endocrinol Metabol Clin North Am* **19:** 767–772, 1990.
Smyth, J. A. *et al.* Urolithiasis in weaned pigs. *Vet Rec* **119:** 158–159, 1986.
Udall, R. H., and Chow, F. H. C. The etiology and control of urolithiasis. *Adv Vet Sci Comp Med* **13:** 29–57, 1969.
Waltner-Toews, D., and Meadows, D. H. Urolithiasis in a herd of beef cattle associated with oxalate ingestion. *Can Vet J* **21:** 61–62, 1980.

V. Inflammation of the Lower Urinary Tract

Inflammation of the lower urinary tract revolves around inflammation of the bladder. Ureteritis is rare in the absence of cystitis, and clinical urethritis in animals usually is associated with obstruction by a calculus from the bladder. Under normal circumstances, the bladder is resistant to infection, and bacteria are quickly eliminated by the normal flow of normal urine. Predisposition to urinary tract infection (UTI) occurs when there is stagnation of urine due to obstruction, incomplete voiding at micturition, or urothelial trauma. Other risk factors for UTI include catheterization, vaginoscopy, urinary incontinence, vaginitis, and administration of antibiotics or corticosteroids within the last 60 days. Of itself, normal voiding is not sufficient to prevent and eliminate bladder infection. Indeed, complete voidance does not occur, but residual urine is rapidly diluted or added to by continuing excretion. Defense mechanisms in the bladder and urethra which prevent bacterial adhesion to mucosal surfaces are essential if bacteria are to be removed by urine flow. Local production of IgA and surface mucins probably are important in preventing attachment of organisms to the normal urothelium, and IgG may have similar activity in specific UTIs. Urinary oligosaccharides may be able to detach adherent bacteria. Voiding of sloughed urothelial cells with attached bacteria aids clearance of bacteria. Incomplete voiding at micturition may be a result of diverticula of the urinary bladder or vesicoureteral reflux. The presence of residual urine can maintain a bladder infection, allowing organisms to take advantage of any opportunity to invade the urothelium.

Unlike human urine, which tends to be a good medium for bacterial growth, animal urines, especially those of dogs and cats, usually have antibacterial activity. This activity is related to urine pH and particularly to urine osmolality. In general, the farther the pH is from the optimal range of 6–7, the less likely it is to support bacterial growth. The antibacterial effect of acid urines is related to their concentration of undissociated organic acids. High concentrations of urea and other solutes increase urine osmolality and contribute significantly to its bacteriostatic effect.

The usual causes of cystitis are **bacteria** from the urethra, which are almost always from the rectal flora. When bacteria breach the surface defenses of the urothelium and attach to or penetrate the epithelial cells, the cells are desquamated and shed in the urine. When the urothelium is penetrated, neutrophils and macrophages in the submucosa respond in the usual way. Leukocytes in urine usually are not phagocytic. A variety of bacteria may be involved in bladder infections (see Pyelonephritis, Section VI,E of The Kidney, in this chapter) and these include in all hosts *Escherichia coli, Proteus vulgaris,* streptococci, and staphylococci. The *Corynebacterium renale* group (*C. renale, C. pilosum, C. cystitidis*) is important in cows, and less so in other species, and is usually mixed with other organisms. *Eubacterium suis* is the primary cause of cystitis and pyelonephritis in swine and a leading cause of death in sows. Cystitis is common in young animals with patent urachus, and the bacterial flora is mixed. **Mycoplasmas** are uncommon causes of UTI in dogs and cattle. Urogenital infections causing prostatitis, orchitis, nephritis, and cystitis may occur in canine **blastomycosis.** *Aspergillus* and *Candida* are unusual causes of cystitis in dogs and cats.

Bacterial pathogens of the urinary tract, such as *E. coli,* can express a formidable array of virulence factors, including P fimbriae (pili), non-fimbrial adhesins, type 1 fimbriae, aerobactin (an iron chelator), hemolysin, capsular polysaccharide (K antigen), and anticomplementary serum resistance. The most urovirulent strains often express multiple virulence factors simultaneously. Bacterial adhesins bind to glycolipid receptors on urothelial cells. In humans, *E. coli* with P fimbriae bind to renal pelvic urothelium and are thought to be responsible for pyelonephritis. Type 1 fimbriae are of most importance in bladder colonization. In order to infect the urinary tract, uropathogens must compete with the normal bacterial flora of the distal urethra, vulva, or prepuce.

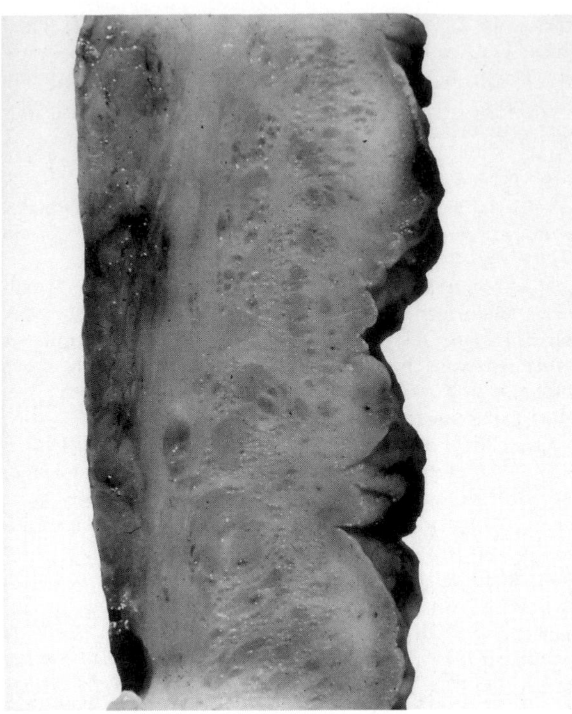

Fig. 5.68 Emphysematous cystitis. Dog. Not associated with diabetes mellitus.

A. Cystitis

Cystitis does occur without obvious predispositions of the types described. There is a higher incidence in females, which is probably associated with the short urethra. Pathological urine may be a better medium for bacterial growth than normal urine and, although the glucosuria of diabetes mellitus promotes bacterial growth, the influence of other reducing substances and of even slight levels of proteinuria may be significant in the development of cystitis with this disease. Decreased leukocyte efficiency may also be involved. Emphysematous cystitis develops in some dogs and cats with diabetes mellitus, and is thought to be caused by fermentation of sugar by glucose-fermenting bacteria. Emphysematous cystitis occurs less commonly in nondiabetic animals (Fig. 5.68). Hormone-induced changes as occur in hyperestrogenism may also affect the functional integrity of the urethral and vesical epithelium, and the role of hormones in the production of glycosaminoglycans in the urogenital tract may also change the susceptibility to UTIs. During estrus in sows, estrogen causes the urine pH to rise, producing an alkaline environment suitable for the growth of *E. suis*.

As well as the opportunistic bacterial UTIs which develop in all species, there are a few diseases of which inflammation of the lower urinary tract is often a part. Hemorrhagic cystitis sometimes occurs in **malignant catarrhal fever** in cattle and deer, and occasionally is the dominant gross feature in the disease. Linear granulomas occur in the renal pelvis, ureter, and bladder of cattle with ***Schistosoma mattheei*** infections. Cystitis in horses and cattle grazing ***Sorghum*** spp. is associated with ataxia caused by degenerative encephalomyelopathy; the bladder lesions are almost certainly neurogenic in origin. The cause of a similar **epizootic cystitis of horses** in Australia is not known.

Sterile hemorrhagic cystitis may occur in dogs and cats treated for neoplastic or immunologic diseases with **cyclophosphamide.** Activated metabolites of the drug cause mucosal ulceration, hemorrhage, and edema. Signs of cystitis may follow an 8-week course of therapy. Concurrent treatment with other drugs, degree of diuresis, and preexisting cystitis may influence the prevalence of cyclophosphamide-induced lesions. Fibrosis and mineralization of the bladder may result in persistent hematuria and incontinence. Transitional cell carcinoma may develop in the bladder of dogs in association with prolonged cyclophosphamide therapy.

Cystitis is differentiated into acute and chronic forms, but there is considerable overlap in both the lesions and the causes. In simple acute catarrhal inflammation, there is moderate hyperemia and submucosal edema, and the surface is covered with a layer of tenacious catarrhal exudate. The urine is cloudy. Histologically, there is degeneration and desquamation of the epithelium and a prominent leukocytic infiltration. The submucosal vessels are dilated and cuffed by leukocytes. In somewhat more severe grades of inflammation, leukocytes may infiltrate all layers of the bladder wall, and hemorrhage from the dilated vessels may be severe enough to produce large clots in the bladder. These hemorrhagic complications are common in cystitis (Fig. 5.69A) following urethral obstruction, especially in cats and cattle. When the inflammatory process is severe, the cystitis may be of superficial fibrinous or deep diphtheritic type (Fig. 5.69B). In both, there is a thick, dirty yellow friable encrustation, which may peel with difficulty. A large portion of the mucosa may become necrotic in addition to deep layers of the bladder wall. Ulcerations may penetrate the wall to the serosa or predispose to rupture.

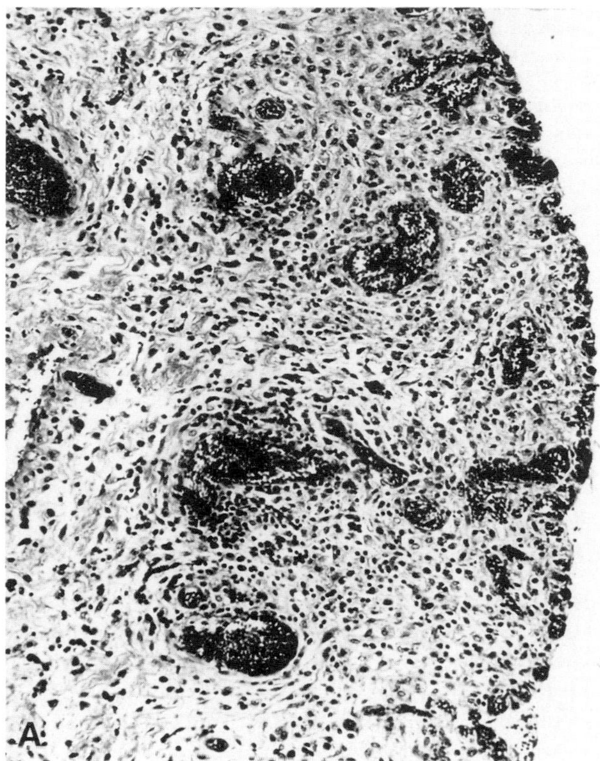

Fig. 5.69A Acute hemorrhagic cystitis with complete loss of epithelium. Ox.

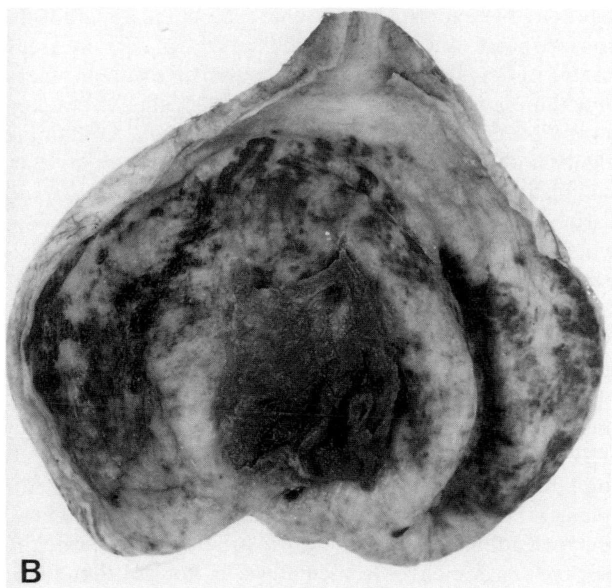

Fig. 5.69B Acute fibrinous cystitis. Dog.

Chronic cystitis may also take a number of anatomic forms. The simplest occurs in association with vesical calculi. The mucosa is irregularly reddened and usually thickened. There is some epithelial desquamation, and the submucosa is heavily infiltrated with inflammatory cells of mononuclear type. There are few neutrophils. In addition, there is often connective tissue thickening of the submucosa and hypertrophy of the muscularis.

There are also some special anatomic forms of chronic cystitis. In **follicular cystitis,** which is common in dogs, the mucosa is studded with gray-white nodules about 1 mm across (Fig. 5.70A), which may be confluent or surrounded by a zone of hyperemia. Histologically, the nodules are aggregations of proliferating lymphocytic cells. These are immediately beneath the epithelium, which may be normal or ulcerated.

Chronic polypoid cystitis is common in any species (Fig. 5.70B). In this, the mucosa is thrown into many folds or villus-like sessile projections. The polyps are covered by epithelium over a core of proliferated connective tissue densely infiltrated with mononuclear leukocytes. The polyps often undergo mucoid degeneration in cattle, or the epithelium may undergo metaplasia to a mucus-secreting, glandular type. Such polyps may break down and cause

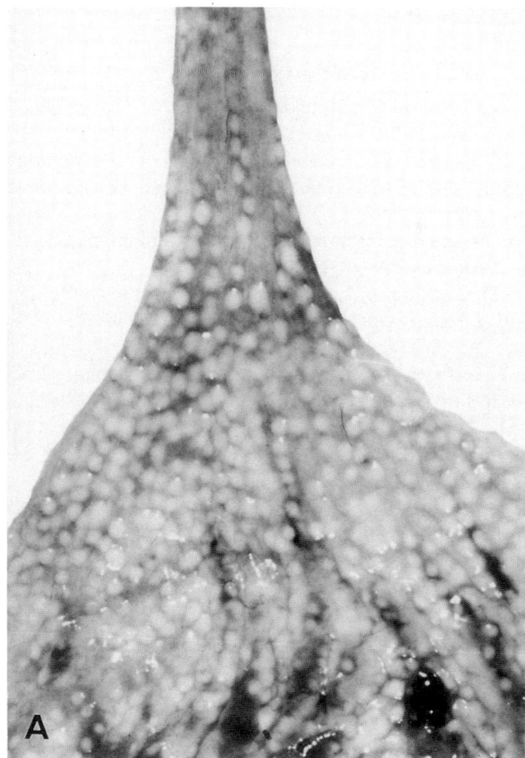

Fig. 5.70A Follicular cystitis. Dog.

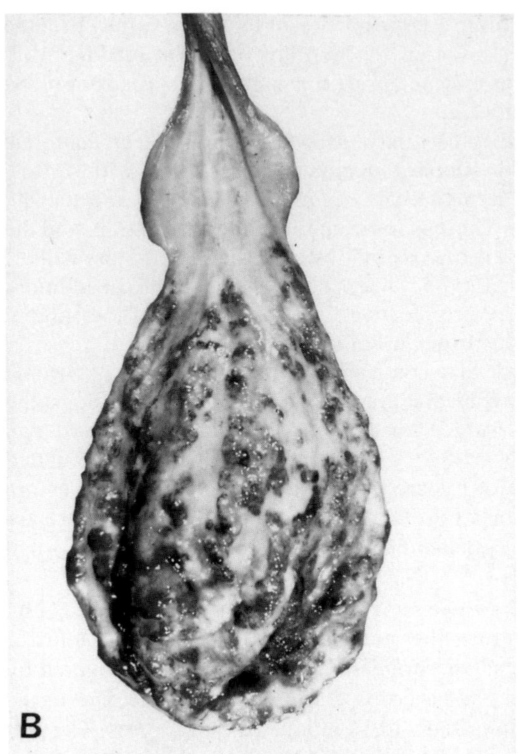

Fig. 5.70B Polypoid cystitis. Dog.

intermittent hematuria. Biopsy is required to differentiate them from neoplasms.

Bibliography

Anderson, B. C. Emphysematous cystitis in a cow. An incidental lesion. *Vet Med Small Anim Clin* **78:** 406–407, 1983.

Brobst, D. F., Cottrell, R., and Delez, A. Mucinous degeneration of the epithelium of the urinary tract of swine. *Vet Pathol* **8:** 485–489, 1972.

Brumfitt, W. Progress in understanding urinary infections. *J Antimicrob Chemother* **27:** 9–22, 1991.

Dee, S. A. Diagnosing and controlling urinary tract infections caused by *Eubacterium suis* in swine. *Vet Med* **86:** 231–238, 1991.

Freshman, J. L. *et al.* Risk factors associated with urinary tract infection in female dogs. *Prevent Vet Med* **7:** 59–67, 1989.

Herenda, D., Dukes, T. W., and Feltmate, T. E. An abattoir survey of urinary bladder lesions in cattle. *Can Vet J* **31:** 515–518, 1990.

Jang, S. S. *et al. Mycoplasma* as a cause of canine urinary tract infection. *J Am Vet Med Assoc* **185:** 45–47, 1984.

Johnson, J. R. Virulence factors in *Escherichia coli* urinary tract infection. *Clin Microbiol Rev* **4:** 80–128, 1991.

Johnston, S. D., Osborne, C. A., and Stevens, J. B. Canine polypoid cystitis. *J Am Vet Med Assoc* **166:** 1155–1160, 1975.

Kirkpatrick, R. M. Mycotic cystitis in a male cat. *Vet Med Small Anim Clin* **77:** 1365–1371, 1982.

Laing, E. J., Miller, C. W., and Cochrane, S. M. Treatment of cyclophosphamide-induced hemorrhagic cystitis in five dogs. *J Am Vet Med Assoc* **193:** 233–236, 1988.

McKenzie, R. A., and McMicking, L. I. Ataxia and urinary incontinence in cattle grazing sorghum. *Aust Vet J* **53:** 496–497, 1977.

Middleton, D. J., and Lomas, G. R. Emphysematous cystitis due to *Clostridium perfringens* in a nondiabetic dog. *J Small Anim Pract* **20:** 433–438, 1979.

Mulholland, S. G. Lower urinary tract antibacterial defense mechanisms. *Invest Urol* **17:** 93–97, 1979.

Richardson, D. W., and Kohn, C. W. Uroperitoneum in the foal. *J Am Vet Med Assoc* **182:** 267–271, 1983.

Root, C. R., and Scott, R. C. Emphysematous cystitis and other radiographic manifestations of diabetes mellitus in dogs and cats. *J Am Vet Med Assoc* **158:** 721–728, 1971.

Shaw, D. H. Lower urinary tract infections: How they arise and how the body combats them. *Vet Med* **85:** 344–349, 1990.

Sherding, R. G., and Chew, D. J. Nondiabetic emphysematous cystitis in two dogs. *J Am Vet Med Assoc* **174:** 1105–1109, 1979.

Yang, W. H., and Shen, N. C. Gas-forming infection of the urinary tract: An investigation of fermentation as a mechanism. *J Urol* **143:** 960–964, 1990.

Zachary, J. F. Cystitis cystica, cystitis glandularis, and Brunn's nests in a feline urinary bladder. *Vet Pathol* **18:** 113–116, 1981.

Zanotti, S. *et al.* Endocarditis associated with a urinary bladder foreign body in a dog. *J Am Anim Hosp Assoc* **25:** 557–561, 1989.

B. Enzootic Hematuria

Enzootic hematuria is a syndrome in mature cattle characterized by persistent hematuria and anemia, and associated with hemorrhages or neoplasms in the lower urinary tract. In more than 90% of cases, the hematuria originates from tumors of the urinary bladder. Outbreaks of the disease are reported in sheep.

Enzootic hematuria occurs on all continents but is restricted to particular locations. In endemic areas, as many as 90% of adult cattle may be affected. The syndrome is attributed to chronic ingestion of **bracken fern** and is reproducible experimentally; there are some apparent inconsistencies since enzootic hematuria occurs in areas devoid of bracken and does not occur in many areas where bracken is present. There are two subspecies of bracken fern: *Pteridium aquilinum* subsp. *aquilinum,* containing eight varieties, and *P. aquilinum* subsp. *caudatum,* containing four varieties, and it is not known whether all varieties are toxic. Also, the extent and persistence with which toxic ferns are grazed probably influence the incidence of bladder lesions. In areas where bracken does not grow, other ferns, such as *Cheilanthes sieberi* (mulga or rock fern from Australia), appear to be capable of producing enzootic hematuria. In Kenya, a high incidence of bladder tumors in Zebu cattle is associated neither with ingestion of bracken nor with enzootic hematuria.

Bracken fern contains several toxic substances including a thiaminase, a variety of carcinogens (quercetin, shikimic acid, prunasin, ptaquiloside, aquilide A, and others), and a bleeding factor of unknown structure. The principle responsible for enzootic hematuria is not yet identified. There appears to be a link between bracken fern and bovine papilloma virus in the development of bladder neo-

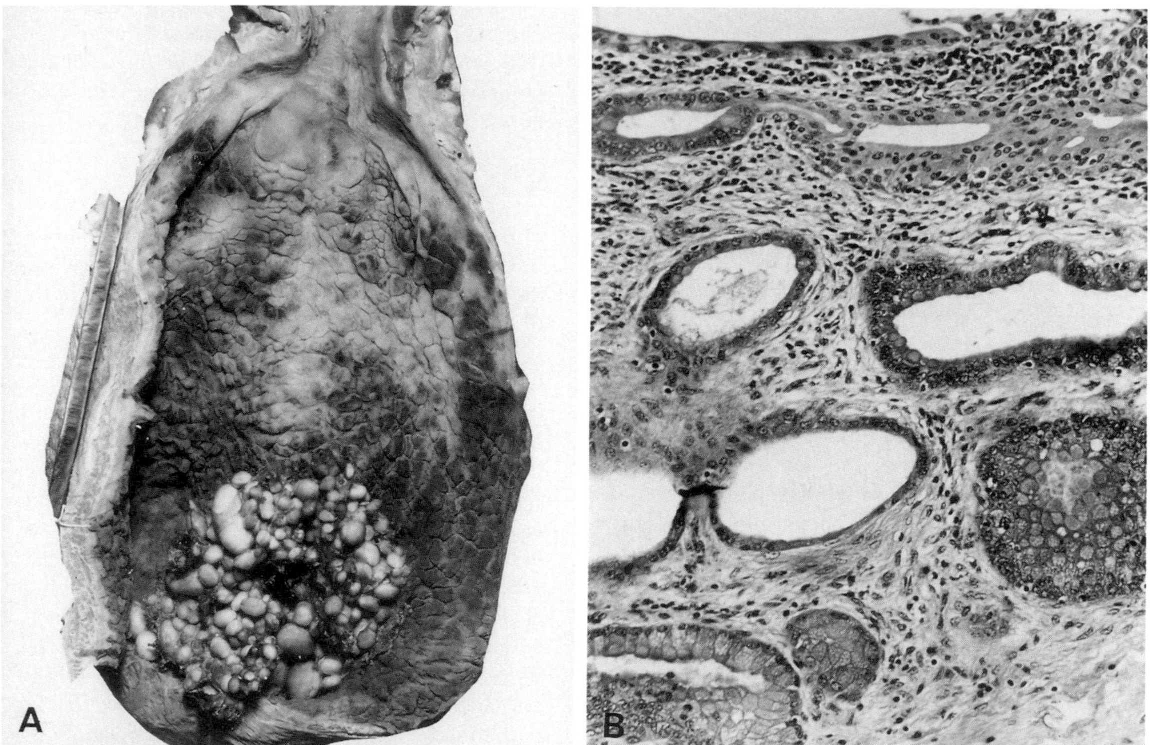

Fig. 5.71 (A) Enzootic hematuria. Cow. Dark angiomatoid lesions and confluent nodular tumors involving most of the bladder mucosa. (B) Mucous adenocarcinoma of urinary bladder in enzootic hematuria. Cow. There is ulceration and inflammation of the bladder surface (above, right).

plasms in animals with enzootic hematuria; the relationship of oncogenic viruses to bracken is discussed with The Alimentary System, Chapter 1 of this volume.

Cattle fed low levels of bracken fern develop microscopic, followed by macroscopic, hematuria. Microhematuria usually is associated with petechial, ecchymotic, or suffusive hemorrhages in the urothelium of the renal calyces, pelvis, ureter, and bladder. These lesions appear to be a manifestation of the hemorrhagic syndrome characteristic of acute bracken fern poisoning (see The Hematopoietic System, Volume 3, Chapter 2). In some cases, microscopic hematuria occurs before gross lesions are visible. Diffuse or patchy areas of pink discoloration develop in the bladder mucosa and, microscopically, ectasia and engorgement of capillaries are present. These altered vessels are prone to hemorrhage into the bladder wall or lumen, and nodular hemangiomatous lesions develop in affected areas. In a few animals, macroscopic hematuria is associated solely with these non-neoplastic changes, but usually it is caused by development of tumors which ulcerate and bleed into the lumen (Fig. 5.71A,B). Occasionally tumors also develop in the renal pelvis and ureter, and hepatic hemangiomas accompany bladder tumors in a few animals.

Several types of epithelial and mesenchymal neoplasms may develop, including transitional and squamous cell carcinoma, papilloma, adenoma, hemangioma, hemangiosarcoma, leiomyosarcoma, fibroma, and fibrosarcoma. Multiple tumors of more than one type may be present, and in more than 50% of affected cattle, mixed epithelial-mesenchymal neoplasms develop. Papillomas, fibromas, and hemangiomas with carcinomas are the most common types. Malignant types may invade locally, and about 10% of epithelial malignancies metastasize to iliac nodes or lungs. Chronic cystitis usually accompanies the neoplastic changes. The gross and microscopic appearance of the inflammatory and neoplastic lesions is conventional; Brunn's nests may develop in the mucosa. Epithelial neoplasms appear to develop from the hyperplastic and metaplastic (squamous and mucous) changes in the urothelium which often accompany the vascular lesions described.

Bibliography

Evans, I. A. *et al.* The carcinogenic, mutagenic, and teratogenic toxicity of bracken. *Proc R Soc Edin* **81B:** 65–77, 1982.

Fenwick, G. R. Bracken (*Pteridium aquilinum*)—Toxic effects and toxic constituents. *J Sci Food Agric* **46:** 147–173, 1988.

Hopkins, N. C. G. Aetiology of enzootic haematuria. *Vet Rec* **118:** 715–717, 1986.

Hopkins, N. C. G. Enzootic haematuria in Nepal. *Trop Anim Hlth Prod* **19:** 159–164, 1987.

Page, C. N. The taxonomy and phytogeography of bracken—a review. *Botanical J Linnean Soc* **73:** 1–34, 1976.

Pamukcu, A. M., Price, J. M., and Bryan, G. T. Naturally occurring and bracken-fern-induced bovine urinary bladder tumors. Clinical and morphological characteristics. *Vet Pathol* **13:** 110–122, 1976.

Yoshikawa, T. *et al.* Histopathogenesis of bracken fern-induced experimental tumor of urinary bladder. *Jpn J Vet Sci* **43:** 875–885, 1981.

VI. Neoplasms of the Lower Urinary Tract

Neoplasia of the lower urinary tract is uncommon but most often occurs in cattle (Figs. 5.71A, 5.72) (see Enzootic Hematuria, Section V,B of The Lower Urinary Tract, in this chapter), dogs, and cats. There are few data for other animals; thus, the following discussion concerns mainly these species; almost all bovine tumors are part of enzootic hematuria. Tumors of the **urinary bladder** account for only 0.5% of all canine neoplasms, and there is a similar prevalence in cats. They occur somewhat more often in female than in male dogs in some studies, but are more frequent in male dogs in other studies and in human males. The Scottish terrier, Shetland sheepdog, beagle, and collie seem to be at greater risk than other breeds. The greater susceptibility of the urinary bladder than of other parts of the tract to neoplasia may be due to more prolonged exposure of the bladder mucosa to urinary carcinogens. With the exception of rhabdomyosarcoma, neoplasia of the lower urinary tract usually occurs in old animals.

Bladder neoplasia may be caused by a variety of industrial chemicals (2-naphthylamine, benzidine), tryptophan metabolites (*ortho*-aminophenol), chronic irritation, foreign bodies (sutures), viruses, bracken fern, and cyclophosphamide. Grading of urinary tract neoplasms according to tumor invasiveness, node involvement, and presence of metastases may assist with prognostication and selection of therapy; the use of biological markers (antigens, tumor products) shows promise of improving clinical staging of urinary tumors in human medicine.

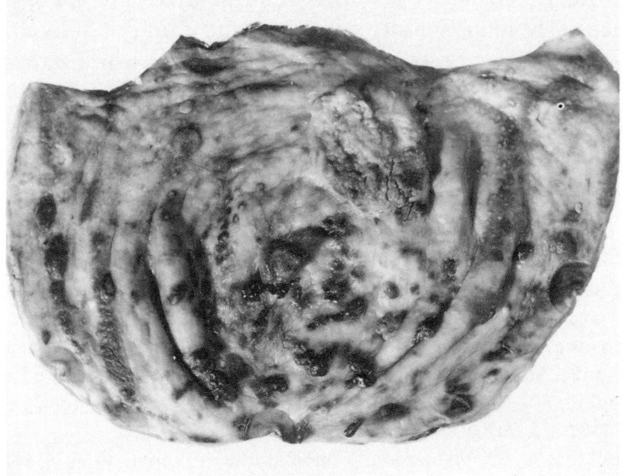

Fig. 5.72 Chronic polypoid cystitis with multiple sessile and papillary areas of carcinoma.

Secondary tumors are rare, but those of the bladder compose ~5% of tumors of this organ. These originate in pelvic organs or as peritoneal implants.

A. *Epithelial Tumors*

Epithelial tumors compose ~80% of the lower urinary tract neoplasms. They occur as adenomas, papillomas, and carcinomas, and most of them develop in the bladder of old animals.

Adenomas are rare in all species; they originate from areas of mucous metaplasia of the urothelium and may be single or multiple with a papilliform or pedunculated appearance. Microscopically, they form glandular structures, some of which contain mucin. **Papillomas** constitute ~17% of primary tumors of the urinary bladder. They tend to be multiple and may be pedunculated or sessile, occasionally involving most of the mucosa. They are covered by well-differentiated transitional epithelium, which is demarcated by basement membrane from a delicate supporting stroma. Squamous metaplasia of the epithelium may develop. Papillomas are susceptible to superficial necrosis, which results in hematuria. In dogs, some papillomas undergo malignant transformation to form transitional-cell or adenocarcinomas. Papillary hyperplasia, to be differentiated from papilloma, occurs in the urinary bladder of cattle and can cause urinary obstruction and hydronephrosis.

Carcinomas of the lower urinary tract are of four histologic types, namely transitional-cell, squamous cell, adeno-, and undifferentiated carcinoma. Together they make up ~60% of primary bladder tumors in dogs and cats; the majority of these are transitional-cell carcinomas. Carcinomas may be solitary or multiple and usually do not reach a large size before they cause hematuria or death from urinary complications. Epithelial metaplasia and squamous and glandular hyperplasia are often present in the urothelium adjacent to epithelial neoplasms; von Brunn's nests are found most often in association with adenocarcinomas.

Transitional-cell carcinomas may be papillary, polypoid, or sessile. Occasionally they are not visible on the vesical mucosa, even though the bladder wall is infiltrated diffusely; the tumors may be present in any part of the bladder, but are often in the bladder neck or trigone. Tumors originating in the prostatic urethra are easily overlooked at gross necropsy. Although there is some variation in structure, the papillary tumors, or parts of them, often are clearly transitional in type, whereas the nonpapillary tumors are usually more anaplastic and invasive. Both patterns, however, may be repeated in the metastases. A few transitional-cell carcinomas contain areas of squamous metaplasia. About 50% of them metastasize, sometimes in a rampant or unpredictable manner. The usual pattern is for late metastasis to regional lymph nodes and lungs, but peritoneal implantation or retrograde lymphatic spread to the soft tissue and bones of the hindlimbs is common. Occasionally solitary metastasis to bone occurs. Transitional-cell carcinoma sometimes develops in association with cyclophosphamide therapy in dogs.

Squamous cell carcinomas and **adenocarcinomas** usually are nonpapillary infiltrative growths, which grossly are nodular or sessile and often ulcerated. They develop in areas of squamous or mucous metaplasia. Histologically they are pure, without transitional-cell areas (Fig. 5.71B). Squamous cell carcinomas and adenocarcinomas occur in dogs and cattle, and also in cats. Squamous cell carcinomas occur most often in bitches in the urethra, the distal two thirds of which is lined by stratified squamous epithelium. Apparently these are less likely to metastasize than are transitional-cell tumors. **Undifferentiated carcinomas** are those very rare primary neoplasms which do not conform to one of the histologic types previously mentioned.

B. Mesenchymal Tumors

Mesenchymal tumors compose less than 20% of tumors of the lower urinary tract. Neoplasms causing enzootic hematuria in cattle are about 10% mesenchymal and 55% mixed, with most of the nonepithelial tumors in these mixtures being hemangiomas. A few vascular tumors also occur in the bladder and about the urethra of dogs, but most mesenchymal tumors in dogs are leiomyomas or fibromas. **Leiomyomas** originate in the muscular coats of the urinary bladder and form well-defined projecting spherical white nodules. The nodules may be multiple and seem to have a predilection for the neck of the bladder, where they may interfere with urinary outflow. Histologically, they are typical of smooth-muscle tumors. **Leiomyosarcomas** are very rare and generally do not metastasize. **Fibromas** probably arise from subepithelial connective tissue, are usually solitary, and have a typical gross and microscopic appearance. **Fibrosarcomas** are rare; they are likely to metastasize, often widely. Rhabdomyosarcoma is a rare tumor in any location (see Diseases of Muscle, Volume 1, Chapter 3). **Botryoid** (shaped like a bunch of grapes) **rhabdomyosarcoma** occurs in the urinary bladder and occasionally the urethra of young dogs; large breeds, particularly the St. Bernard, seem to be over-represented. The youthfulness of the victims (younger than 18 months in most cases) raises the possibility that these tumors arise in rests of embryonic myoblasts. Grossly the tumors usually occur at the trigone and project into the bladder near the neck as botryoid masses. They infiltrate the wall and may metastasize, but usually draw attention to themselves through urinary obstruction before this occurs. Microscopically, there is usually a mixture of fusiform and pleomorphic cells with some strap cells and multinucleated cells. Cytoplasmic cross striations are sometimes present (Fig. 5.73). Immunoperoxidase staining of the intermediate filament desmin may aid in the diagnosis of this tumor.

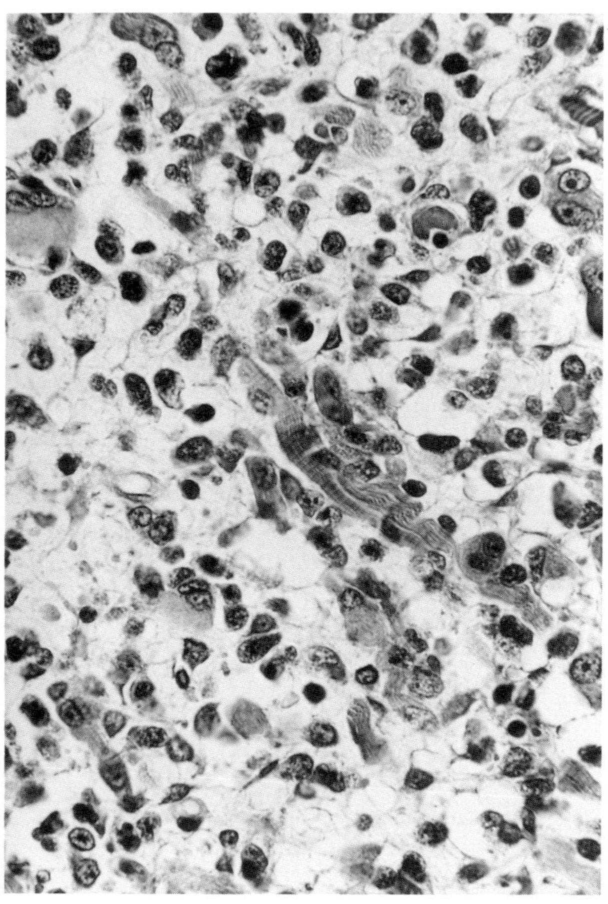

Fig. 5.73 English setter, 2 years old. Urinary bladder. Botryoid rhabdomyosarcoma, with a striated strap cell. (Slide, courtesy of M. Ayroud.)

Bibliography

Bourne, C. W., and May, J. E. Urachal remnants: benign or malignant. *J Urol* **118:** 743–747, 1977.

Brearley, M. J., Thatcher, C., and Cooper, J. E. Three cases of transitional cell carcinoma in the cat and a review of the literature. *Vet Rec* **118:** 91–94, 1986.

Bryan, G. T. The pathogenesis of experimental bladder cancer. *Cancer Res* **37:** 2813–2816, 1977.

Davies, J. V., and Read, H. M. Urethral tumours in dogs. *J Small Anim Pract* **31:** 131–136, 1990.

Esplin, D. G. Urinary bladder fibromas in dogs: 51 cases (1981–1985). *J Am Vet Med Assoc* **190:** 440–444, 1987.

Fradet, Y. Biological markers of prognosis in invasive bladder cancer. *Sem Oncol* **17:** 533–543, 1990.

Friedell, G. H. Carcinoma, carcinoma *in situ*, and "early lesions" of the uterine cervix and the urinary bladder: Introduction and definitions. *Cancer Res* **36:** 2482–2484, 1976.

Hall, R. R., and Prout, G. R. Staging of bladder cancer: Is the tumor, node, metastasis system adequate? *Sem Oncol* **17:** 517–523, 1990.

Hicks, R. M., and Chowaniec, J. Experimental induction, histology, and ultrastructure of hyperplasia and neoplasia of the urinary bladder epithelium. *Int Rev Exp Pathol* **18:** 199–280, 1978.

Krawiec, D. R. Canine bladder tumors: The incidence, diagnosis, therapy, and prognosis. *Vet Med* **86:** 47–54, 1991.

Magne, M. L. *et al.* Urinary tract carcinomas involving the canine vagina and vestibule. *J Am Anim Hosp Assoc* **21:** 767–772, 1985.

McCaw, D. L., Hogan, P. M., and Shaw, D. P. Canine urinary bladder transitional cell carcinoma with skull metastases and unusual pulmonary metastases. *Can Vet J* **29:** 386–388, 1988.

McKenzie, R. A. An abattoir survey of bovine urinary bladder pathology. *Aust Vet J* **54:** 41, 1978.

Murphy, W. M., and Soloway, M. S. Urothelial dysplasia. *J Urol* **127:** 849–854, 1982.

Nikula, K. J. *et al.* Transitional cell carcinomas of the urinary tract in a colony of beagle dogs. *Vet Pathol* **26:** 455–461, 1989.

Patnaik, A. K., Schwarz, P. D., and Greene, R. W. A histopathologic study of twenty urinary bladder neoplasms in the cat. *J Small Anim Pract* **27:** 433–445, 1986.

Schwarz, P. D., and Willer, R. L. Urinary bladder neoplasia in the dog and cat. *Prob Vet Med* **1:** 128–140, 1989.

Skye, D. V. Hydronephrosis secondary to focal papillary hyperplasia of the urinary bladder of cattle. *J Am Vet Med Assoc* **166:** 596–598, 1975.

Van Vechten, M., Goldschmidt, M. H., and Wortman, J. A. Embryonal rhabdomyosarcoma of the urinary bladder in dogs. *Compend Cont Ed Pract Vet* **12:** 783–793, 1990.

Vitovec, J. Carcinomas of the renal pelvis in slaughter animals. *J Comp Pathol* **87:** 129–134, 1977.

Ward, A. M. Glandular neoplasia within the urinary tract. The aetiology of adenocarcinoma of the urothelium with a review of the literature. I. Introduction: The origin of glandular epithelium in the renal pelvis, ureter and bladder. *Virchows Arch Pathol Anat* **352:** 296–311, 1971.

Wimberley, H. C., and Lewis, R. M. Transitional cell carcinoma in the domestic cat. *Vet Pathol* **16:** 223–228, 1979.

Acknowledgments

I thank Jo Boyle and Pat Wallace for histologic sections, Tim Sullivan for gross photography, Ted Eaton for photographic processing, and the pathologists of the Veterinary Laboratory Services Branch and the Ontario Veterinary College for case material.

CHAPTER 6 The Respiratory System

D. L. DUNGWORTH
University of California, Davis

I. General Considerations

The responses of the respiratory tract to injury, and the resulting patterns of disease, are determined largely by the structural and functional complexity of the system. Most of the diseases of the respiratory system are caused by damaging agents arriving by either the airborne (aerogenous) or blood-borne (hematogenous) routes, each with its own special pathogenetic considerations.

The respiratory system is constantly under assault from potentially injurious agents, which include airborne microorganisms, oropharyngeal flora, toxic particulates and gases in ambient air, and a wide array of infectious agents and extrinsic or intrinsic toxins delivered via the pulmonary circulation. Pulmonary defense mechanisms are remarkably effective under most circumstances in preventing disease agents from entering or remaining in the lung and in neutralizing these agents if they penetrate initial barriers.

A brief overview of general structural and functional features of the respiratory system is presented to provide a framework for understanding its responses to injury.

The **nasal airways,** in contrast to most respiratory conducting passages, are noncollapsible structures, which are encased in bone and contain osseous and cartilaginous turbinates (conchae) and are divided by a cartilaginous nasal septum. The mucosa of the nasal cavity has at least four distinct epithelial types: stratified squamous, transitional, ciliated respiratory, and olfactory epithelium. The submucosa has a richly supplied vascular plexus and abundant submucosal glands. The nasal airways contribute ~50% of total respiratory resistance, and hyperemia of nasal plexuses plays an important regulatory role in modulating nasal airway caliber and resistance to airflow.

Most of the epithelial lining of nasal mucosa is composed of ciliated respiratory epithelium which is pseudostratified and shares many similarities in structure and response to injury with tracheal and bronchial epithelium. Ciliated respiratory epithelium of the nasal mucosa includes ciliated, mucous, nonciliated columnar, cuboidal, and basal cells. Olfactory epithelium forms a large percentage of total nasal epithelium in some species and is composed of olfactory sensory cells, sustentacular cells, and basal cells. Olfactory epithelium is rich in cytochrome P-450–dependent monooxygenase enzyme activity and is susceptible to many of the respiratory toxins that are also metabolized in the lung, and which can damage bronchiolar epithelium and components of alveolar septa.

The **nasopharynx** is lined by ciliated pseudostratified epithelium with zones of stratified squamous epithelium. Abundant lymphoid nodules are present throughout the submucosa. The auditory (Eustachian) tubes extend from the nasopharynx to the middle ears and have ventral diverticula in horses forming the guttural pouches, which are subject to ascending bacterial and fungal infections.

The **larynx** is supported by cartilages which resist deformation and obstruction of the lumen, and the mucosa is lined by stratified squamous epithelium as well as ciliated respiratory epithelium.

Trachea and bronchi in most domestic animals are lined by pseudostratified epithelium composed of ciliated, mucous, and nonciliated cells. Major varieties of nonciliated cells are serous, basal, and neuroendocrine. Also within the epithelium are resident inflammatory cells such as lymphocytes and globule leukocytes, and intraepithelial nerve fibers. Tracheal and bronchial epithelium consists of a stable cell population with continual low-level turnover and differentiation of new epithelial cells. Following injury to tracheobronchial epithelium, a stereotypic pattern of repair usually follows. Ciliated cells are terminally differentiated and have little or no regenerative capacity. Sloughing of these cells with replacement of the epithelial lining with nonciliated cell types is a frequent early event following mucosal injury. Mucous cells and nonciliated cells are the primary cells that effect epithelial repair, with a lesser contribution by basal cells. Basal cells may play a more important role in attachment of columnar cells to the basement membrane than they do in epithelial regeneration. Mucous cells and nonciliated cells have the capacity to regenerate themselves as well as to undergo differentiation into ciliated cells and other epithelial types of the trachea and bronchi.

Normal mucociliary clearance of particulates that interact with the mucosa requires coordinated ciliary function and a normal lining of the gel–sol liquid layer of mucus, which is derived from surface mucous cells and submucosal glands. Submucosal glands include both mucous cells and serous secretory cells. In addition to its barrier function, mucous secretory capacity, and mucociliary transport function, tracheobronchial epithelium synthesizes and secretes neutral endopeptidase. This is an important enzymatic regulator of airway neuropeptides such as substance P and neurokinin A, which in turn can stimulate increased vascular permeability and airway smooth muscle contraction. Nonciliated epithelial cells (Clara cells), which are components of tracheobronchial epithelium of some animal species, have high cytochrome P-450 monooxygenase activity and can activate many xenobiotic compounds to toxins that can cause pulmonary injury. Furthermore, tracheobronchial epithelial cells actively metabolize arachidonic acid to eicosanoids such as prostaglandin E_2 and 12-HETE (hydroxyeicosatetraenoic acid), which may regulate local smooth-muscle tone and vascular flow. Bronchial epithelial cells also can up-regulate expression of intercellular adhesion molecule-1 (ICAM-1) following injury and interaction with cytokines; ICAM-1 promotes adhesion and migration of circulating neutrophils and monocytes into airways during an inflammatory reaction.

Trachea, bronchi, and bronchioles contain lymphoid tissue (bronchus-associated lymphoid tissue or BALT) in the lamina propria and submucosa, analogous to gut-associated lymphoid tissue (GALT) in function. In addition, there can be a more diffuse distribution of lymphocytes and plasma cells. Other cells such as macrophages, dendritic cells, neutrophils, and mast cells at low density within the lamina propria participate in normal baseline immune and inflammatory processes. Both B cells and T cells have been demonstrated in BALT, with B cells the predominant component. B cells have been demonstrated to be positive for immunoglobulin A (IgA), IgG, IgM, and IgE antibodies. Immunoglobulin A cells are distributed throughout the lamina propria and in association with BALT; BALT and GALT IgA cells are the principal source of IgA in serum. Viral-specific and bacterial-specific secretory IgA antibody on the respiratory mucosa is recognized as one of the most important components of host immunity to respiratory pathogens. In respiratory secretions, IgA can prevent binding of bacteria and adsorption of virus to respiratory epithelial cells, and block infection. High viral-specific IgA in upper respiratory tract secretions is recognized as being associated with the most effective form of immunity to respiratory viral reinfection. Concentrations of IgA are highest in the airways, but IgG and IgM predominate in the alveoli. An important feature of the distribution of lymphocytes in the respiratory tract is the existence of localized traffic. Antigen-reactive cells are generated mainly in local lymph nodes (e.g., mediastinal and bronchial), and activated lymphocytes (memory cells) migrate preferentially back to BALT and other pulmonary sites.

Trachea and bronchi contain hyaline cartilage rings, and intrapulmonary bronchi are surrounded by abundant peribronchial connective tissue which compartmentalizes the largest conducting airways from the surrounding alveolar tissue. Airway patency in trachea and bronchi is maintained by the minimally deformable cartilage rings. The abundant peribronchial connective tissue insulates bronchi from lung-volume-induced changes in airway diameter and acts under most circumstances to prevent suppurative inflammatory processes from spreading from the bronchial wall directly into surrounding alveolar tissue. Although bronchi have large individual cross-sectional areas, it is estimated that ~80% of resistance to airflow in pulmonary conducting airways is present in the first 4–7 divisions of the bronchial tree. Airflow is rapid in these airways, and even minimal bronchoconstriction or airwall edema and inflammatory cell infiltration can result in profound increases in overall respiratory resistance and auscultable airway sounds.

Bronchioles, in contrast to bronchi, have no cartilage in their walls to prevent airway collapse. Instead, airway patency is dependent on the close attachment of interalveolar septa to a thin connective tissue layer in the bronchiolar wall. As the lung increases in volume during inspiration, the radially arranged interalveolar septa pull on the bronchiolar wall in a radial tethering fashion to result in maximal luminal diameter during maximal lung volume. During expiration, the radial tethering forces of the interalveolar septa decrease, and the bronchiolar lumen decreases in diameter. Small bronchioles may collapse normally toward the end of the expiratory cycle, and airflow out of the pulmonary acini supplied by the bronchioles ceases unless there is sufficient collateral ventilation. Because of their smaller diameter, collapsibility, and thin-walled structure, bronchioles are much more susceptible to pathologic processes occurring in the surrounding alveolar parenchyma than are bronchi. Their small luminal size makes them much more likely to become obstructed by inflammatory exudate during an acute inflammatory reaction. Inflammatory processes centered on bronchioles are highly likely to extend into adjacent alveoli. Although the resistance to airflow in individual bronchioles is high, the total cross-sectional area of all generations of bronchioles is much greater than that of bronchi. Therefore, pathologic processes affecting small numbers of bronchioles might not result in clinical signs of airway obstruction. A large percentage of bronchioles must be affected before clinical evidence of disease is detected (e.g., hypoxemia due to ventilation/perfusion abnormalities or dyspnea due to small airway obstruction).

Bronchioles in proximal generations are often lined by epithelium which is indistinguishable from that in distal bronchi. More distally, small-caliber bronchioles are lined by a simple columnar to cuboidal epithelial lining almost entirely composed of ciliated cells and nonciliated bronchiolar (Clara) cells. The nonciliated cells function as stem cells for repair in the bronchiole and have the capacity to divide and differentiate into ciliated cells or other nonciliated cells. The nonciliated cells lining bronchioles in some animal species have abundant agranular endoplasmic reticulum in their apical cytoplasmic projections and are the pulmonary cells with the greatest concentration of cytochrome P-450-monooxygenase enzyme systems. The latter places them among the most exquisitely sensitive pulmonary cells to toxic injury by xenobiotic compounds.

Alveolar parenchyma is divided into structural and functional units called **acini.** An acinus is the gas-exchange unit of the lung supplied by a single terminal bronchiole. An acinus includes all of the branches of respiratory bronchioles, alveolar ducts, alveolar sacs, alveoli, and associated blood vessels supplied by branching of one terminal bronchiole. Many acini (equivalent to primary lobules) are grouped together and surrounded by connective tissue septa in some species such as cattle, sheep, and horses to form grossly visible lobules. An earlier convention of dividing alveolar parenchyma into primary and secondary lobules has been dropped because of the confusion it caused. Patterns of respiratory disease often follow these grossly and histologically detectable structural units, and the lesion distributions are frequently referred to as being panacinar, centriacinar, or lobular.

The most important cells of the alveolar parenchyma are type I and type II alveolar epithelial cells (pneumonocytes or pneumocytes), alveolar capillary endothelial cells, fibroblasts and other interstitial cells, and alveolar macrophages.

Type II alveolar epithelial cells (granular pneumocytes) are cuboidal cells, lining interalveolar septa, and contain characteristic osmiophilic lamellar inclusions in their cytoplasm. The primary recognized functions of type II cells are to synthesize pulmonary surfactant and to serve as progenitor cells for replacement and turnover of alveolar epithelium. Pulmonary surfactant is a complex mixture of phospholipids and small amounts of protein synthesized by type II epithelial cells. Its main function is to decrease surface tension in the alveolar space during expiration. Type II alveolar cells divide during alveolar development and postnatal lung growth and serve as stem cells following normal turnover and loss of alveolar epithelial cells. Type II cells can proliferate rapidly to repopulate denuded basement membrane following injury to type I alveolar epithelial cells. Following division and migration to cover the bare basement membrane, type II cells can differentiate into type I alveolar epithelial cells. Type II cells synthesize a variety of matrix components including fibronectin, type IV collagen, and proteoglycans. Type II cells also metabolize arachidonic acid to form eicosanoids, such as prostaglandin E_2, which may modulate function of other alveolar cells, and there is evidence that they can express major histocompatibility complex (MHC) class II molecules and function as antigen-presenting cells.

Type I alveolar epithelial cells are squamous cells which line ~93% of the alveolar surface. They have limited capacity to adapt to injury, in part because of their large membrane surface area and minimal enzymatic defense mechanisms. Injury to type I cells is usually quickly followed by sloughing of these cells from the alveolar basement membrane.

Alveolar capillary endothelial cells are part of the largest capillary bed of any tissue in the body. They function as the initial permeability barrier between the capillary lumen and pulmonary interstitium and have important transport functions for solutes, water, and gases. They have numerous metabolic functions including the uptake or clearance of serotonin, norepinephrine, prostaglandins E and F, bradykinin, hormones, and drugs. Endothelial cells have angiotensin-converting enzyme activity, which converts angiotensin I to angiotensin II. Cytochrome P-450 monooxygenase activity has been identified with immunocytochemical techniques in alveolar endothelium, and this may in part explain the sensitivity of endothelial cells in some species to toxic damage by xenobiotic compounds. Endothelial cell exposure to mediators such as leukotriene B_4 and cytokines such as tumor necrosis factor and interleukins 1–8 can up-regulate expression of endothelial cell adhesion molecules to facilitate attachment and migration of neutrophils and other leukocytes into interstitium and alveoli.

Alveolar fibroblasts include a morphologically heterogenous group of connective tissue cells (e.g., interstitial cells) that may have varying protein synthetic activity, contractile function, and cell and matrix interactions. They are responsible for synthesis of interstitial matrix and collagen types I, III, IV, V, and VI, as well as elastin. Collagen types I and III predominate. Pulmonary fibroblasts also synthesize laminin, fibronectin, glycosaminoglycans, and proteoglycans which, together with the other synthesized components, contribute to the mechanical properties of lung.

Macrophage populations in the lung include alveolar macrophages, interstitial macrophages, pulmonary intravascular macrophages, and dendritic cells.

Alveolar macrophages form the first line of pulmonary defense against infectious agents and particles that are able to penetrate defense mechanisms of the upper respiratory tract and intrapulmonary airways. In normal lung, alveolar macrophages are derived from blood monocytes that migrate into the lung after undergoing a maturation step in the interstitial space. During inflammatory states, alveolar macrophages are derived directly from infiltrating blood monocytes. Macrophages can also be derived from division of local macrophages, although this probably contributes little to the expansion of pulmonary macrophage populations that occur in most inflammatory lung diseases.

Alveolar macrophages have a wide array of functions in addition to their capacity to phagocytose and kill infectious agents and to degrade other phagocytosed particles. They function as regulatory cells controlling inflammatory, immune, and repair processes through release of a wide array of cytokines and other regulatory molecules. Inflammatory and immune functions are promoted by macrophage synthesis and release of cytokines such as interleukin-1, tumor necrosis factor, alpha and gamma interferon, and histamine release factor, as well as by release of inflammatory mediators that include leukotriene B_4 and C_4, platelet-activating factor, and thromboxane A_2. Repair processes are generally promoted or otherwise regulated by release of cytokines that include transforming growth factor-beta and -alpha, fibroblast growth factor, insulinlike growth factor, and platelet-derived growth factor (PDGF). Alveolar macrophages play a role in induction of cellular and humoral immune responses through antigen presentation and other accessory cell functions, but the dendritic cells in the lung may be much more effective at accessory cell function than macrophages.

Dendritic cells are bone marrow-derived motile leukocytes with enhanced antigen-presenting capacity in the interstitium of alveolar parenchyma and the lamina propria of airways. These cells have numerous, long, irregular dendritic processes, an extremely irregular and folded nucleus, and an absence of phagolysosomes. They constitutively express high levels of MHC class I and II molecules and common leukocyte antigen but are incapable of phagocytosing particles efficiently. The cells lack many of the cytoplasmic surface markers of mononuclear phagocytes.

Pulmonary intravascular macrophages (PIMs) are unique mononuclear phagocytes found in the lung. They are large, mature macrophages, present in the pulmonary alveolar capillaries, which form membrane adhesive complexes with the underlying endothelium. Species in which PIMs have been found include cattle, sheep, pigs, goat, cats, and humans. These cells are highly phagocytic and play a role in the clearance of circulating bacteria and particulates in the pulmonary circulation. They also release an array of inflammatory mediators following interaction with particulates, including leukotriene B_4, and hence can help recruit neutrophils and other inflammatory cells into the lung during an acute inflammatory reaction.

A. Pulmonary Defense

Pulmonary defenses serve principally to protect the delicate alveolar parenchyma of the lung from damage. This is accomplished by removing harmful agents as much as possible in the nasal passages and conducting airways. Alveolar mechanisms form a second level of defense. The upper respiratory tract functions to warm and humidify inspired air, and to remove larger particles and water-soluble gases by means of the mucous lining. Warming and humidifying occur principally during passage of air through the nose, and are facilitated by the extensive surface area and the rich, readily engorged vascular plexus in the submucosa, particularly of the turbinates and nasal septum. Many particles in inspired air are first deposited on the mucous lining of nasal passages and conducting airways and are then cleared by movement of the mucociliary blanket. The larger the particles, the more efficient is their removal in the upper airways. Deposition on surfaces is mainly by inertial impaction, gravitational sedimentation, diffusion, or a combination of these. Inertial impaction is chiefly in the nasal passages and pharynx and at points of branching of airways where the airstream changes its direction and where turbulence occurs. The efficiency of nasopharyngeal trapping depends on the anatomical complexity of the nasal passages, especially with regard to the turbinates, and on the pattern of respiration. The gravitational settlement of particles is directly proportional to their size and density, and is favored in the relatively still air of deeper parts of the respiratory system. Diffusion of particles is due to molecular collision and affects only the very smallest of them—particles of less than ~ 0.3 μm in size. Since displacement velocity by diffusion is low, deposition by this method is effective only in the alveoli where movement of gases is also by diffusion rather than linear flow.

Deposition of particles greater than ~ 10 μm aerodynamic diameter is virtually complete above the larynx. In addition, a large percentage of inhaled particulates smaller than 10 μm also interact initially with the mucosa of the nasal cavity and nasopharynx. As a result, many viral and bacterial diseases have initial stages of replication or multiplication in the epithelium and lymphoid tissue of the upper respiratory system before they either spread systemically or are nebulized during inspiration to be redistributed into the lower respiratory tract. With decreasing particle size less than 10 μm, an increasing proportion of inhaled particles pass into the deep lung, many being subsequently exhaled. The critical feature, from the point of view of pulmonary homeostasis, is that droplet nuclei and other irritant or infectious particles ~ 1–2 μm in diameter mostly deposit at the bronchiolar–alveolar junction. This is because the total cross-sectional area of airspaces increases suddenly, linear velocity of the airstream falls to zero, and there is time for the particles to deposit by gravitational settling. As will be discussed later, this is one of the reasons for the vulnerability of the bronchiolar–alveolar junction to damage by inhaled irritants.

Statements on relationship between particle size and deposition are relative rather than absolute. Sizes quoted for mathematical modeling of particle deposition are in terms of equivalent cross-sectional diameters of unit density spheres (aerodynamic diameter). The most obvious exception to the generalization that particles greater than 10 μm in diameter do not penetrate beyond the larynx is that fine fibers as long as 100 μm or longer, notably of asbestos, do reach alveolar parenchyma. Additionally, there might be opportunity for redistribution of particles deposited in the proximal respiratory tract by reflux of excess secretions or aspiration of fluid.

Once particles are deposited on the mucus of airways, clearance by normally functioning mucociliary transport is highly efficient. Most particles are removed from central airways within a few hours and even from distal airways within 24 hr. The mucociliary blanket consists of cilia bathed in a watery sol on top of which lies mucus with physical properties of a viscoelastic gel. Whether the mucus usually forms a patchy or continuous surface layer is still debated, but it appears to be mostly continuous in trachea and large bronchi of healthy individuals and perhaps patchy in smaller airways. In any event, the cilia beat mostly in the watery hypophase except during the active forward stroke when their tips contact the overlying mucus. The net effect of a ciliary frequency of ~1000 beats per minute is to propel the mucus toward the pharynx at a linear velocity in the order of 5–15 mm/min. The greater density of ciliated cells in proximal airways, the more rapid ciliary beat, and possibly absorption of a portion of the aqueous periciliary fluid are believed to prevent swamping of these airways, especially the trachea, by fluid collected from the large number of distal airways.

Most of the mucous secretions of the respiratory tract, and the particulate matter they carry, reach the pharynx and are swallowed. The concentration of material into the nasopharynx coincides with well-developed diffuse and focal lymphoid tissue of the tonsillar region and dorsal nasopharynx. This enhances the efficiency of development of immune responses, but also makes the region vulnerable to primary infections by organisms such as *Brucella* spp. and *Mycobacterium a. paratuberculosis*. Swallowing of material originating in the lungs also serves as a mode of spread of diseases such as tuberculosis and as part of the migratory pathway of helminth eggs and larvae.

The specific roles and controlling influences of mucous cells, serous cells, and other secretory cells in surface epithelium and submucosal glands, and the differences among species, are still poorly understood. In addition to the physical aspects of the sol and gel phases of the secretion, however, a variety of other components with defensive capabilities are recognized. As mentioned previously, the major immunoglobulin is locally synthesized IgA, although IgE, IgG, and other classes are present. Important nonspecific humoral components of the secretions are interferon, which helps limit viral infection in nonimmune hosts, and lysozyme (muramidase) and lactoferrin, which have selective antibacterial activity. Tracheal antibacterial peptides are secreted by bovine tracheal cells, but their relative importance in defense needs to be established. The normal bacterial flora of the nose and nasopharynx are important in that by specific adherence of their specialized surface structures (adhesins) to receptors on cilia and surfaces of epithelial cells, they prevent adherence and colonization by more virulent flora.

The physical and humoral defenses of the mucociliary blanket, which are constantly in operation, are boosted by cellular and humoral mechanisms recruited from blood at the onset of inflammation, and by sneezing, coughing, and bronchoconstriction provoked by irritation of airway receptors. Normal mucociliary function depends on structurally and functionally intact ciliated epithelium as well as normal viscous properties and quantity of secretions. Interference with one or more of these predisposes to infection, as will be considered under pathogenesis of bronchopneumonia.

Alveolar defense against small-sized particles depends heavily on phagocytosis by alveolar macrophages. Phagocytosis of readily ingested particles, for instance, opsonized bacteria, is largely complete by 4 hr after alveolar deposition. Actual physical removal of particulates from alveoli is inefficient, in contrast to their removal when deposited on the mucociliary blanket. Fifty percent clearance of particles deposited in alveoli takes from several days to months or longer, depending on their physical nature and irritant capability. Most particles are therefore phagocytosed by macrophages and either inactivated or sequestered. The alveolar macrophages move toward the bronchioles and hence eventually onto the mucociliary blanket. Reasons for their centripetal movement are not known, but the surface-lining liquid in alveoli is also believed to move centripetally, possibly because of its continual secretion and a "milking" action of respiratory movements. Alternative fates of particles in alveoli are clearance in the lining liquid without phagocytosis, or penetration into the pulmonary interstitium. The latter becomes of increasing importance as the particulate load increases. It appears that most particles reach the interstitium by endocytosis across the alveolar type I epithelial cells. Once in the interstitial space, particles move with the flow of lymph and are phagocytosed by interstitial macrophages. Particle-laden macrophages associated with lymphatics occur in peribronchiolar and perivascular clusters, and some eventually find their way to the local lymph nodes. Overloading the alveolar macrophage system favors accumulation of particles in the interstitium, as occurs in the pneumoconioses.

Sterility of alveoli is thus maintained largely by the ability of macrophages to kill ingested bacteria and to secrete cytokines and other regulatory molecules, as referred to earlier. These activities are enhanced by immunoglobulin, particularly through the opsonizing effect of IgG, which is the predominant immunoglobulin in the alveolar lining liquid. Surfactant also has important opsonizing functions.

Lysozyme, lactoferrin, and complement are also present in alveolar lining liquid. Humoral components capable of inhibiting inflammatory mediators or destructive enzymes are of great importance, particularly the glutathione peroxidase system and catalase, which help protect against injury by reactive oxygen radicals, and α_1-antitrypsin (α_1-antiprotease), which is important in protection against the development of alveolar emphysema and acute lung injury.

Just as factors interfering with mucociliary defense

mechanisms of airways predispose to bronchopneumonia, so will factors depressing alveolar defenses, especially the alveolar macrophage (see pathogenesis of bronchopneumonia in Section VI,F,1 of this chapter).

The entire output of the right ventricle flows through the low pressure pulmonary circulation. The densely anastomosing network of capillaries in alveolar septa provides the equivalent of sheet flow when they are all patent. This arrangement provides both for easy trapping of emboli in the pulmonary vascular bed and for minimizing the deleterious effects of blockage. Effects of blockage are minimized further by the dual pulmonary and bronchial arterial blood supplies to the lung. Nevertheless, emboli carry risks, and they are associated with a variety of lesions according to the nature of the emboli. The types of emboli vary greatly. Unusual ones are epidermal fragments and hair inadvertently introduced into the blood at the time of injection, or fragments of nucleus pulposus from intervertebral disks. More commonly, they are bacteria, fungi, protozoa, endogenous fat, normal cells (which may be represented by megakaryocytes), or abnormal cells (which are principally neoplastic). They can also be fragments of bland or septic thrombi, helminth parasites for which the respiratory system is a natural or accidental habitat, or even parasitic ova, as is required by *Parelaphostrongylus tenuis* of deer for the continuation of its life cycle. In general, the benefit of the lung's acting as a blood filter is the prevention of emboli reaching the systemic circulation and the protection of organs such as the brain, heart, and kidneys against infarction. The detriments are spread of infection, metastasis of tumors, and pulmonary thromboembolism causing shock. The last named is rare in animals.

Bibliography

Adamson, I. Y. R., and Bowden, D. H. Bleomycin-induced injury and metaplasia of alveolar type 2 cells. *Am J Pathol* **96:** 531–544, 1979.

Adrian, R. W. Segmental anatomy of the cat's lung. *Am J Vet Res* **25:** 1724–1733, 1964.

Ayers, M. M., and Jeffery, P. K. Proliferation and differentiation in mammalian airway epithelium. *Eur Respir J* **1:** 58–80, 1988.

Baron, J., and Voigt, J. M. Localization, distribution, and induction of xenobiotic-metabolizing enzymes and aryl hydrocarbon hydroxylase activity within lung. *Pharmacol Ther* **47:** 419–445, 1990.

Billups, L. H. *et al.* Pulmonary granulomas associated with PAS-positive bodies in brachycephalic dogs. *Vet Pathol* **9:** 294–300, 1972.

Brain, J. D., and Valberg, P. A. Deposition of aerosol in the respiratory tract. *Am Rev Respir Dis* **120:** 1325–1373, 1979.

Breeze, R. G., and Wheeldon, E. B. The cells of the pulmonary airways. *Am Rev Respir Dis* **116:** 705–777, 1977.

Dahl, A. R. *et al.* Cytochrome P-450-dependent monooxygenase in olfactory epithelium of dogs: Possible role in tumorigenicity. *Science* **216:** 57–59, 1982.

Evans, M. J., and Moller, P. C. Biology of airway basal cells. *Exp Lung Res* **17:** 513–531, 1991.

Green, G. M. *et al.* Defense mechanisms of the respiratory membrane. *Am Rev Respir Dis* **115:** 479–514, 1977.

Gross, P., Pfitzer, E. A., and Hatch, T. F. Alveolar clearance: Its relation to lesions of the respiratory bronchiole. *Am Rev Respir Dis* **94:** 10–19, 1966.

Hare, W. C. D. The bronchopulmonary segments in the sheep. *J Anat* **89:** 387–402, 1955.

Heffner, J. E., and Repine, J. E. Pulmonary strategies of antioxidant defense. *Am Rev Resp Dis* **140:** 531–554, 1989.

Heppleston, A. G., and Young, A. E. Alveolar lipoproteinosis: An ultra-structural comparison of the experimental and human forms. *J Pathol* **107:** 107–117, 1972.

Holtzman, M. J. Arachidonic acid metabolism. Implications of biological chemistry for lung function and disease. State of the art. *Am Rev Respir Dis* **143:** 188–203, 1991.

Kradin, R. L. *et al.* Accessory cells of the lung. I. Interferon-gamma increases Ia^+ dendritic cells in the lung without augmenting their accessory activities. *Am J Respir Cell Mol Biol* **4:** 210–218, 1991.

Laplante, C., and Lemaire, I. Interactions between alveolar macrophage subpopulations modulate their migratory funtion. *Am J Pathol* **136:** 199–206, 1990.

Lauweryns, J. M., and Baert, J. H. Alveolar clearance and the role of the pulmonary lymphatics. *Am Rev Respir Dis* **115:** 625–683, 1977.

Mauderly, J. L., and Hahn, F. F. The effects of age on lung function and structure of adult animals. *Adv Vet Sci Comp Med* **26:** 35–78, 1982.

McLaughlin, R. F., Tyler, W. S., and Canada, R. O. A study of the subgross pulmonary anatomy in various mammals. *Am J Anat* **108:** 149–166, 1961.

Miller, B. E., and Hook, G. E. R. Hypertrophy and hyperplasia of alveolar type II cells in response to silica and other pulmonary toxicants. *Environ Health Perspect* **85:** 15–23, 1990.

Newhouse, M., Sanchis, J., and Bienenstock, J. Lung defense mechanisms. *N Engl J Med* **295:** 990–998, 1045–1052, 1976.

Proctor, D. F. The upper airways. I. Nasal physiology and defense of the lungs. *Am Rev Respir Dis* **115:** 97–129, 1977.

Robinson, N. E. Some functional consequences of species differences in lung anatomy. *Adv Vet Sci Comp Med* **26:** 2–34, 1982.

Sorokin, S. P., and Brain, J. D. Pathways of clearance in mouse lungs exposed to iron oxide aerosols. *Anat Rec* **181:** 581–626, 1975.

Travis, J., and Fritz, H. Pulmonary perspective: Potential problems in designing elastase inhibitors for therapy. *Am Rev Respir Dis* **143:** 1412–1415, 1991.

Veit, H. P., Farrell, R. L., and Troutt, H. F. Pulmonary clearance of *Serratia marcescens* in calves. *Am J Vet Res* **39:** 1646–1650, 1978.

Warner, A. E., and Brain, J. D. The cell biology and pathogenic role of pulmonary intravascular macrophages. *Am J Physiol* **258:** L1–L12, 1990.

Warner, A. E., Barry, B. E., and Brain, J. D. Pulmonary intravascular macrophages in sheep. Morphology and function of a novel constituent of the mononuclear phagocyte system. *Lab Invest* **55:** 276–288, 1986.

B. Lung Development and Growth

The lungs begin to develop as a ventral groove in the endodermal tube, which evaginates to form the lung bud. Five stages of intrauterine lung development and growth are recognized. These are the embryonic, pseudoglandular, canalicular, saccular, and alveolar stages of growth.

During the **embryonic** stage of lung growth (30–50 days of gestation in a bovine fetus), the branches of the lung bud continue to grow and divide to form the segmental bronchi, which are surrounded by mesenchyme. Ciliated cells are developed in the airways at this period. During the **pseudoglandular** stage of lung growth (50–120 days of gestation in the bovine fetus), the remainder of the primary conducting airways develop by asymmetric dichotomous branching. Ciliated cells as well as mucous cells become differentiated within the airway epithelium, and bronchial glands and cartilage develop. At the end of the pseudoglandular period, all branches of conducting airways have developed and are embedded in mesenchymal stroma. Distal airway branches are lined by cuboidal to columnar epithelial cells, which contain abundant cytoplasmic glycogen. During the **canalicular** stage of growth (120–180 days of gestation), the vascular system becomes extensively developed, and capillaries become closely approximated with airway epithelium. The distal airways continue to give rise to more distal spaces, which will become respiratory exchange surfaces such as alveolar ducts and alveoli. The framework of the pulmonary acinus begins to form along with increased vascular density, and there is a proportionate reduction in the relative amount of mesenchyme to air spaces. Type I and type II alveolar epithelial cells begin to differentiate in the newly formed terminal air spaces. During the **saccular** stage of lung growth (180–240 days of gestation in the bovine fetus), lung volume and gas-exchange surface increase markedly, and there is further reduction in mesenchyme between air spaces. Small crests with two capillary layers protrude into the immature saccules to result in further subdivision of the air spaces. During the **alveolar** stage of lung growth (240–260 days), true alveoli form by further ingrowth of septa from the intersaccular crests. The ingrowth of the septa is associated with the simplification of the capillary structure so that there is a single capillary layer per interalveolar septum.

Further subdivision of alveolar septa results in continued increases in alveoli and alveolar surface area during the period of rapid postnatal growth. Airways increase in diameter and length through coordinated growth as overall lung volume and weight increase.

The rate and coordination of intrauterine lung growth are influenced by a number of complex factors. Compression of the thoracic cavity during development, such as occurs secondarily to chest wall abnormalities or diaphragmatic hernia, results in pulmonary hypoplasia with abnormally low numbers of alveoli. Decreased respiratory efforts of the fetus, and conditions associated with loss of volume of amniotic fluid (oligohydramnios), also result in pulmonary hypoplasia. Endogenous pulmonary growth factors such as gastrin-related peptide and transforming growth factor-beta, as well as hormonal factors such as thyroxine and glucocorticoids, regulate intrauterine lung development. Most of the congenital pulmonary anomalies described subsequently under this heading presumably are associated with localized or generalized disturbances of one or more of these regulating factors.

Bibliography

Boyden, E. A., and Thompsett, D. H. The postnatal growth of the lung in the dog. *Acta Anat* **47:** 185–215, 1961.

Castleman, W. L., and Lay, J. C. A morphometric and ultrastructural study of postnatal lung growth and development in calves. *Am J Vet Res* **51:** 789–795, 1990.

de Zabala, L. E., and Weinman, D. E. Prenatal development of the bovine lung. *Zblet Vet Med (C). Anat Histol Embryol* **13:** 1–14, 1984.

King, R. J., Jones, M. B., and Minoo, P. Regulation of lung cell proliferation by polypeptide growth factors. *Am J Physiol* **257:** L23–L38, 1989.

Reid, L. M. Lung growth in health and disease. *Br J Dis Chest* **78:** 113–134,1984.

Thurlbeck, W. M. Postnatal growth and development of the lung. *Am Rev Respir Dis* **111:** 803–844, 12975.

Thurlbeck, W. M. Lung growth. *In* "Pathology of the Lung," W. M. Thurlbeck (ed.), pp. 1–10. New York, Thieme Medical Publishers, 1988.

Winkler, G. C., and Cheville, N. F. Morphometry of postnatal development in the porcine lung. *Anat Rec* **211:** 427–433, 1985.

C. *Patterns of Respiratory Disease*

Respiratory diseases can be caused by a large variety of infectious or noninfectious agents. The site of damage in the respiratory tract is determined by the interplay of portal of entry of the agent, the nature and concentration of the agent, and the relative susceptibility of the tissues exposed to the agent. The portal of entry is the major determinant.

Aerogenous insult, as would be expected, usually leads to damage centered on airways. Nasal passages and upper airways are mostly affected by irritants contained in large particles, by highly soluble gases, or by infectious agents whose cell receptors are most numerous or more readily accessible in upper respiratory epithelium. Distal airways are more affected by fine particles, weakly soluble gases, and by infectious agents with affinity for bronchiolar or alveolar epithelium. The greater vulnerability of the bronchiolar–alveolar junction to damage is also an extremely important determinant at this level (see Bronchopneumonia, Section VI,F,1 of this chapter).

In instances in which viruses have tropism for both terminal bronchiolar epithelium and type II alveolar epithelial cells, viral replication occurring in these cells results in an inflammatory reaction centered on terminal airways as well as on surrounding interalveolar septa (i.e., proximal acinar areas) to result in a mixed pattern of damage (bronchointerstitial pneumonia.) The pattern of damage induced by viruses as well as other infectious agents can be greatly altered by variations in the efficiency of the systemic and pulmonary immune systems. For instance, when an immunosuppressive virus such as canine distemper virus infects dogs, it can induce a much more diffuse interstitial pneumonia with bronchiolitis than is typical for other less immunosuppressive paramyxoviridae, such as parainfluenza virus.

Hematogenous insult to the lungs is manifest, depending on the cause, as diffuse, patchy, or widely disseminated multifocal lesions without orientation on airways. An important exception to the generalization that blood-borne agents affect alveolar septa and pulmonary interstitium more than airways occurs when an ingested toxin specifically damages bronchiolar epithelium. An example of this is the necrosis of nonciliated bronchiolar epithelial (Clara) cells of the horse caused experimentally by 3-methylindole toxicosis. Localization of damage to nonciliated bronchiolar cells in the horse can be explained by cellular binding and then selective metabolism of 3-methylindole to toxic intermediates by the cytochrome P-450–monooxygenase system present in nonciliated cells of this species.

Other, less common types of injuries to the respiratory tract are traumatic, as by penetration of a foreign body, or by extension of lesions along fascial planes and lymphatics from adjacent tissues or cavities.

Differences in patterns of lesions among species of animals are well recognized, and some can be explained by species differences in anatomy or tissue distributions of metabolizing enzymes. One example is the complete lobular septation and absence of collateral ventilation (low interdependence) in the bovine lung, which predisposes it to poor resolution of bronchopneumonia and to the development of acute interstitial emphysema under conditions of greatly forced expiratory efforts with concurrent bronchoconstriction and increased airway resistance. Species-associated differences in distribution of metabolizing enzymes among pulmonary cells are presumably the explanation for differing patterns of damage of experimental 3-methylindole toxicosis in horses and cattle. In horses it induces necrosis of only bronchiolar epithelial cells, whereas in cattle it causes widespread damage to alveolar type I epithelium and alveolar capillary endothelium, as well as to bronchiolar epithelium.

II. Nasal Cavity and Sinuses

A. Congenital Anomalies

Congenital anomalies of the nasal region are rare but occur in all species. They are usually part of more extensive craniofacial defects in which they accompany various combinations of malformations of mouth and eyes. Animals with absent, underdeveloped, or severely distorted nasal regions are usually stillborn or die immediately after birth, often because of an imperforate buccopharyngeal membrane (choanal atresia). The milder defect of cleft palate is compatible with life, but affected animals generally die because of aspiration pneumonia.

A variety of localized, developmentally related defects that affect the nasal region can take time to become apparent. Defects of tooth-germ origin are especially likely to be of this type. Maxillary cysts in foals or young adult horses can distort the profile of the maxillary bone sufficiently to cause obstruction of the ipsilateral nasal passage, destruction of the nasal turbinates, and deviation of the nasal septum.

B. Metabolic Disturbances

Deposits of amyloid sometimes occur in the nasal submucosa of horses. The deposition is not part of a generalized amyloidosis, although there might be concurrent cutaneous amyloidosis, particularly of head, neck, and cranial thorax. The nasal vestibule and anterior portions of the septum and turbinates are mostly involved, but the deposits may extend to the larynx. The amyloid may be in nodules of various sizes or as a diffuse deposition. Resulting stenosis can be severe enough to cause signs of nasal obstruction. The amyloid deposits have a smooth surface and the usual waxy sheen of amyloid on the cut surface. The amyloid is deposited in the walls of submucosal vessels and the basement membrane of mucosal glands as well as in the connective tissues. Macrophages and lymphocytes are usually intermingled with the interstitial amyloid deposits, and giant cells are found adjacent to nodular deposits. There may be severe ulceration of the mucosa, especially overlying large nodular masses.

Nasal amyloidosis in horses appears to be analogous to AL amyloidosis in humans, in which the major amyloid protein is composed of light chains of immunoglobulin or of light chain fragments. Primary (AL) amyloidosis is idiopathic or associated with myelomatosis in humans. One case of nasal and cutaneous amyloidosis in a horse was associated with a malignant lymphoid tumor.

C. Circulatory Disturbances

The arteries, veins, and capillaries of the nasal mucosa are capable of remarkable adaptive changes in the content of blood. Vascular engorgement occurs by relaxation of the arteries and contraction of the thick tunica media of the veins. This lability of the vessels is responsible for the frequency of hyperemia and edema. Active hyperemia is part of the acute stage of inflammation. Passive congestion is the result of local or general circulatory failure.

Of more concern is nasal hemorrhage or **epistaxis.** The term epistaxis is used in a general sense to refer to hemorrhage from the nose, but this does not necessarily mean that the source of bleeding is within the nasal passages or sinuses. The hemorrhage might be from the nasopharynx or from deep within the respiratory tract. This distinction is particularly important in horses in which, in epistaxis associated with heavy exercise, the blood originates from the lung. The condition is more appropriately termed exercise-induced pulmonary hemorrhage and will be described under that heading. Bloodstained foam is frequently present in and issuing from the nose of cadavers, especially sheep. This is an indication of terminal pulmonary congestion, edema, and hemorrhage.

Hemorrhage originating within the nasal region is most commonly caused by traumatic, inflammatory, or neoplastic breakdown of vessels. It may also be part of any of the hemorrhagic diatheses (see The Hematopoietic System, Volume 3, Chapter 2). In some of the hemorrhagic diatheses, such as those of thrombocytopenic origin, the bleeding may be copious. Hemorrhage in rhinitis is associated with mucosal ulceration, a frequent feature of acute inflammation and some specific types of chronic inflammation. In most inflammatory hemorrhages, the extravasation is initially submucosal. Mycotic infections of the guttural pouches can cause epistaxis in horses. Rarely, nasal hemorrhage may be the result of hypertension or vascular aneurysms.

D. Inflammation of the Nasal Cavity

1. Rhinitis

The nasopharyngeal mucous membrane has a normal resident microbial flora established by specific adherence of bacteria via adhesins to sugar-containing surface binding sites on epithelial cells. An important role of the normal flora is to exclude adherence and subsequent colonization of the mucosa by more virulent organisms, particularly Gram-negative ones. Injury to the mucosal surface can lead to pathogenic activity by certain of the normal flora or, more importantly, affect surface binding sites so that adherence and colonization by pathogenic microorganisms can occur. Similar changes can occur because of systemic immunodeficiency states or nonspecific stress situations such as occur postoperatively. Fungal and other opportunistic infections which commonly follow prolonged antibiotic therapy are probably also attributable to removal of the normal blocking bacterial flora.

Primary injurious agents are usually viruses. Allergens are probably important in cattle and to a lesser extent in dogs, cats, and other species. Irritant volatile gases, dust, and excessive dryness of the atmosphere are occasional causes of injury to the nasal epithelium. Rhinitis usually results from the interaction between viruses, or other devitalizing influences, and bacteria or fungi.

Rhinitis can be differentiated, according to its course, as acute or chronic. It can be differentiated morphologically, according to the nature of the response, into serous, catarrhal, purulent, ulcerative, pseudomembranous, hemorrhagic, or granulomatous inflammation. Most cases of acute rhinitis begin with a serous exudation, which changes in the course of the disease to a catarrhal and then purulent inflammation. Pseudomembranous, ulcerative, or hemorrhagic rhinitis is a sign of very severe damage. Chronic rhinitis is most commonly manifested by proliferative changes, but sometimes it causes atrophy, which affects mainly the nasal conchae in large breeds of dogs.

During the initial **serous** stages of rhinitis, whether viral, allergic, or nonspecific, the mucosa is swollen and gray to red depending on the degree of hyperemia. Histologically, the epithelial cells show hydropic degeneration and loss of cilia. There is hyperactivity of the goblet cells and submucosal glands. The secretion is a thin, clear seromucin, which contains a few leukocytes and epithelial cells. The underlying lamina propria is edematous and sparsely infiltrated by inflammatory cells. The swelling of the mucous membrane tends to cause mild respiratory discomfort and the familiar sneezing and snuffling.

Within hours or a few days, serous rhinitis is modified partly by changes in glandular secretion and partly by bacterial infection. The hyperemia, edema, and swelling are then aggravated, and the discharge becomes **catarrhal** (mucous) or frankly purulent because of the emigration of large numbers of leukocytes and desquamation of epithelial cells. Regenerative hyperplasia of surviving epithelium can occur, but in purulent rhinitis, extensive ulcerations may be evident.

In subacute to chronic rhinitis, diffuse or localized polypoid thickenings of the mucosa develop (Fig. 6.1A). The **nasal polyps** are initially sessile but can, when larger, become pedunculated. The ease with which the nasal lamina propria becomes engorged and edematous, plus the tendency of protruberances into the nasal meatus to compromise venous and lymphatic drainage because of constriction in their basal regions, are probable factors in the persistence or progression of inflammatory polyps. They occur occasionally in horses and cats, and less commonly in other species. Polyps are soft, pink-gray, irregularly nodular, pedunculated, or sessile masses. They have a chronically inflamed edematous core resembling myxoma tissue, covered by variously hyperplastic, metaplastic, or ulcerated epithelium. Old polyps can become more fibrous.

Two special types of polyp deserve mention. One is the **hemorrhagic nasal polyp** (progressive hematoma) arising from the ethmoid region of the horse. This is a unilateral hemorrhagic mass, which can extend to the nostril or choanae. It tends to enlarge progressively and can recur after surgical excision. Histologically, it consists mostly of organizing hemorrhages of various ages with extensive siderosis and calcification of connective tissue fibers. The extent to which capillary angiomatous changes are the forerunners of hemorrhage and hematoma formation is uncertain. It has been suggested that equine paranasal sinus cysts have a common pathogenetic factor with hemorrhagic nasal polyps, namely repeated hemorrhages into submucosal tissues. The other special form of polyp affecting the nasal region is the **nasopharyngeal polyp of cats,** which arises in the middle ear or Eustachian tube.

Chronic catarrhal or **suppurative rhinitis** causes progressive fibrosis of the lamina propria with atrophy of the glands and atrophy with focal squamous metaplasia of nasal epithelium. The atrophic epithelium is dry and shiny. **Pseudomembranous rhinitis** may be fibrinous or fibrinonecrotic (diphtheritic), but it is usually the former, and the fibrinous membranes can be peeled off without leaving gross underlying defects. The deeper, fibrinonecrotic inflammations are associated with severe bacterial infections and frequently have a dry yellowish quality that indicates infection with *Fusobacterium necrophorum*. The fibrinonecrotic membrane is firmly adherent to the under-

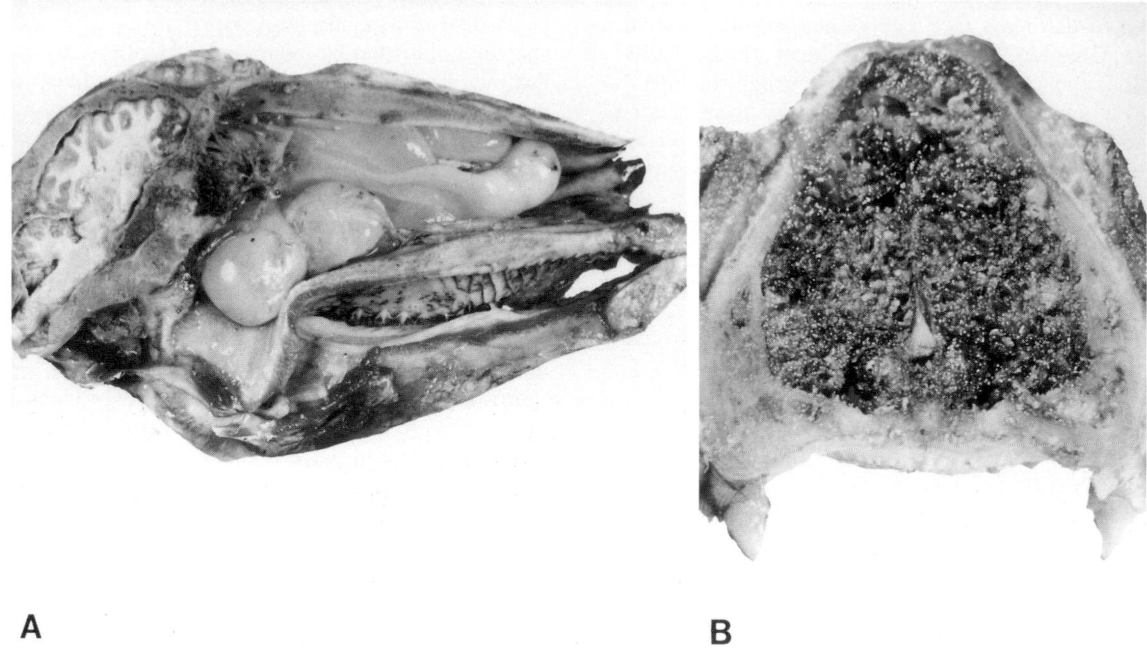

Fig. 6.1 (A) Myxomatous polyps in chronic rhinitis. Sheep. (B) Chronic diffuse, proliferative rhinitis. Cat.

lying tissue and when removed leaves a raw, ulcerated surface.

Granulomatous rhinitis is a typical lesion in some specific diseases. The lesions are nodular and polypoid or become large, space-occupying masses. The smaller ones are more firm, the larger ones, more friable or gelatinous. The histologic structure is specific for the disease.

Rhinitis occurs commonly as part of a more generalized disease process. Important specific entities in which rhinitis is the sole or a major lesion will be covered subsequently. A chronic, nonspecific rhinitis is an important condition in the dog, and to a lesser extent in the cat. The term lymphoplasmacytic is sometimes applied because lymphocytes and plasma cells are the predominant inflammatory cell components. There is a chronic unilateral or bilateral mucopurulent to hemorrhagic discharge, and the inflammatory proliferation leads to diffuse or polypoid thickening of the nasal mucosa and obstruction of nasal passages (Fig. 6.lB). The glandular elements are hyperplastic, the epithelium is variously ulcerated, hyperplastic, and metaplastic (squamous), and the edematous, fibrotic stroma is heavily infiltrated by lymphocytes and plasma cells. There is no sign of foreign bodies, at least in the chronic lesion, and bacterial cultures do not reveal significant organisms. The pathogenesis is unclear, but following initial damage, which is no longer detectable, there is probably a vicious cycle involving impaired local defenses, further infection, and damage by normally nonpathogenic flora and self-sustaining inflammation. The last named is presumably associated with release of cytokines and inflammatory mediators generated by interaction of lymphocytes, plasma cells, and other elements. Pooling of exudate in obstructed portions of the lumen and compromised venous and lymphatic drainage in the hyperplastic mucosa are also likely to be factors leading to progression of the lesion.

Rhinitis of itself can have unfortunate sequelae. Aspiration of nasal exudate can lead to bronchopneumonia. The potential for reflux flow in the valveless veins of the head explains the occurrence of intracranial thrombophlebitis, abscess, or meningitis; these are, however, rare. Sinusitis probably is the most common sequel to rhinitis.

2. *Sinusitis*

Inflammation of the paranasal sinuses often goes undetected unless it has caused facial deformity or a fistula in the overlying skin. Sinusitis is of most significance in the horse because of the size and complexity of its paranasal sinuses and the compounding effects of limited drainage and tendency for periodontitis to extend to sinusitis. Sinusitis is very common in sheep as a response to larvae of *Oestrus ovis*. It also follows penetration of infection in dehorning wounds, fractures, and periodontitis. Seromucinous sinusitis of little significance occurs in viral infections of the upper respiratory tract. In acute catarrhal or purulent rhinitis, the mucosal swelling tends to occlude the orifices of the sinuses. The secretions and exudates then accumulate and render chronic purulent sinusitis almost inevitable. The histologic features of sinusitis are the same as those of rhinitis. The accumulation of seromucinous secretion is referred to as **mucocele,** and the accumulation of purulent exudate is referred to as **empyema** of the sinus. Purulent inflammation of the sinuses is more significant than rhinitis because of proximity to the brain.

It is also less likely to spontaneously drain and resolve and therefore more likely to cause epithelial atrophy and metaplasia, and distortion of the bony walls of the sinuses by pressure or osteomyelitis.

Bibliography

Bedford, P. G. C. Origin of the nasopharyngeal polyp in the cat. *Vet Rec* **110:** 541–542, 1982.

Burgener, D. C., Slocombe, R. F., and Zerbe, C. A. Lymphoplasmacytic rhinitis in five dogs. *J Am Anim Hosp Assoc* **23:** 565–568, 1987.

Cook, W. R., and Littlewort, M. C. G. Progressive haematoma of the ethmoid region in the horse. *Equine Vet J* **6:** 101–108, 1974.

Delmage, D. A. Some conditions of the nasal chambers of the dog and cat. *Vet Rec* **92:** 437–442, 1973.

Gibbs, G., Lane, J. G., and Denny, H. R. Radiological features of intranasal lesions in the dog: A review of 100 cases. *J Small Anim Pract* **20:** 515–535, 1979.

Harvey, C. E. *et al.* Chronic nasal disease in the dog: Its radiographic diagnosis. *Vet Radiol* **20:** 91–98, 1979.

Lane, J. G. *et al.* Nasopharyngeal polyps arising in the middle ear of the cat. *J Small Anim Pract* **22:** 511–522, 1981.

Lane, J. G., Longstaffe, J. A., and Gibbs, C. Equine paranasal sinus cysts: A report of 15 cases. *Equine Vet J* **19:** 537–544, 1987.

Leyland, A., and Baker, J. R. Lesions of the nasal and paranasal sinuses of the horse causing dyspnoea. *Br Vet J* **131:** 339–346, 1975.

Negus, V. "The Comparative Anatomy and Physiology of the Nose and Paranasal Sinuses." Edinburgh and London, Livingstone, 1958.

Platt, H. Haemorrhagic nasal polyps of the horse. *J Pathol* **115:** 51–55, 1975.

van Andel, A. C. J., Gruys, E., and Kroneman, J. Amyloid in the horse: A report of nine cases. *Equine Vet J* **20:** 277–285, 1988.

3. Rhinitis in Specific Diseases

In addition to the specific diseases to be discussed, rhinitis is a prominent feature of a variety of respiratory or more generalized infectious diseases. The nature, cause, and specificity of the various forms of rhinitis differ according to species. Examples are canine distemper, the feline respiratory disease complex, the specific diseases of cattle described under ulcerative and erosive stomatitis, and equine influenza, equine rhinopneumonitis, and equine viral arteritis.

a. Inclusion-Body Rhinitis of Swine This disease is widespread in Europe. It also occurs in the United States and other major pig-raising areas of the world but appears to be relatively unimportant. The disease is caused by a cytomegalovirus (family Herpesviridae, subfamily Betaherpesvirinae) which characteristically produces large basophilic intranuclear inclusions in swollen glandular epithelia of the nasal cavity.

Inclusion-body rhinitis is most commonly an acute to subacute disease of suckling piglets of ~1–5 weeks of age. The signs are those usual for rhinitis with modest fever. The early discharge is seromucinous, but it may become catarrhal or purulent if the course is prolonged, probably owing to secondary bacterial infection. The morbidity is high, but the mortality in the absence of suppurative complications is low; the complications include sinusitis, otitis media, and pneumonia.

The uncomplicated histologic changes in the mucosa are those of a nonsuppurative rhinitis, with a tendency to squamous metaplasia, and the presence of specific basophilic inclusions in the epithelial cells of the glands and their ducts (Fig. 6.2). The inclusions are large and readily visible at low magnification. Affected glands occur in irregular clusters, and all their epithelial cells tend to contain inclusions. The inclusion bodies can persist for a month but become less numerous as the course of the disease advances.

As the inclusion develops, the nucleus and cytoplasm of the affected cell expand. The cytoplasm becomes clear and finely granular, and cell borders become indistinct. The inclusion body fills the nucleus except for small peripheral indentations, in which minute neutrophilic or acidophilic bodies may be found. The affected nuclei continue to swell, and the nuclear membrane loses its distinctiveness; by this time the inclusion bodies resemble bluish-gray smears among degenerating cytoplasm. Sloughing of the epithelium is followed by liquefaction and the accumulation of leukocytic debris. The necrotic glands are obliterated by collapse of the lamina propria and infiltration by lymphocytes. There is slight vascular reaction in this disease. The infiltrating cells are predomi-

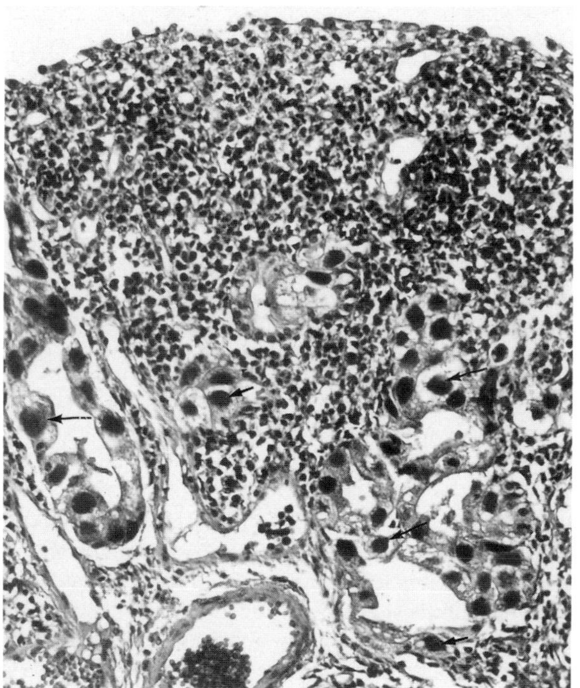

Fig. 6.2 Large, basophilic intranuclear inclusions (arrows) in inclusion-body rhinitis. Pig.

nantly lymphocytes and, although distributed diffusely, they tend to form more dense aggregates in the superficial layers of the lamina propria. Regeneration of glands may take place by downgrowth and differentiation from the superficial epithelium.

Although rhinitis is the main manifestation of the infection, and dissemination is probably via the nasal route, the systemic clinical signs and presence of inclusion bodies in other epithelial tissues are indicative of a viremic phase. In addition to the nasal location, typical inclusion bodies can be found in lacrimal and Harderian glands, in glomerular and renal tubular epithelium, and, sparsely, in hepatocytes, lining cells of sinusoids in liver, adrenal glands and lymph nodes, and other secretory epithelia. The viremic phase may last for 2–3 weeks and is followed by persistent infection in pulmonary macrophages.

Piglets which die of the disease do so in the period of generalization. Involvement of sinusoidal and endothelial cells produces petechial hemorrhages, and edema is present in the subcutis and thorax. Focal necrosis occurs in parenchymal tissues, and in the liver it may become massive. The piglets are anemic; the presence of inclusion bodies in intravascular and splenic mononuclear cells suggests that the anemia may be the result of bone marrow injury. Focal gliosis with intranuclear inclusions in scattered glial cells occurs throughout the central nervous system.

Infection in susceptible pregnant sows has been associated with fetal mummification, stillbirth, neonatal deaths, and failure of surviving piglets to thrive. Evidence for transplacental infection is, however, circumstantial.

Bibliography

Booth, J. C., Goodwin, R. F. W., and Whittlestone, P. Inclusion-body rhinitis of pigs: Attempts to grow the causal agent in tissue cultures. *Res Vet Sci* **8:** 338–345, 1967.

Corner, A. H. *et al.* A generalized disease in piglets associated with the presence of cytomegalic inclusions. *J Comp Pathol* **74:** 192–199, 1964.

Duncan, J. R., Ramsey, F. K., and Switzer, W. P. Electron microscopy of cytomegalic inclusion disease of swine (inclusion body rhinitis). *Am J Vet Res* **26:** 939–947, 1965.

Goodwin, R. F. W., and Whittlestone, P. Inclusion-body rhinitis of pigs: An experimental study of some factors that affect the incidence of inclusion bodies in the nasal mucosa. *Res Vet Sci* **8:** 346–352, 1967.

Plowright, W., Edington, N., and Watt, R. G. The behaviour of porcine cytomegalovirus in commercial pig herds. *J Hyg (Lond)* **76:** 125–135, 1976.

b. ATROPHIC RHINITIS OF SWINE Atrophic rhinitis of swine is characterized by moderate to severe atrophy of the nasal turbinates (conchae) associated with distortion or shortening of the snout in advanced cases. The turbinate atrophy is caused primarily by a protein toxin produced by toxigenic isolates of *Pasteurella multocida*. The toxin is lethal to mice on intraperitoneal inoculation and is dermonecrotic in guinea pigs following intradermal injection. Most toxigenic isolates of *P. multocida* are of capsular type D, but some are of capsular type A. Although the *P. multocida* toxin is the proximate cause of atrophy, colonization of respiratory mucosa by toxigenic *P. multocida* and its multiplication to produce damaging levels of toxin require the presence of additional factors. Foremost among these is prior or concurrent infection by *Bordetella bronchiseptica* which, mainly through the action of its cytotoxin, acts synergistically to increase colonization by the toxigenic *P. multocida*. *Bordetella bronchiseptica* alone can experimentally cause only mild, clinically insignificant atrophy.

Other factors known to be capable of enhancing the severity of the clinical disease, for instance cytomegalovirus infection (inclusion body rhinitis) or adverse environmental and nutritional circumstances, probably also act by facilitating colonization by toxigenic *P. multocida*. Nutritional defects, particularly those involving calcium and phosphorus, can also interfere with metabolism of bone at the time when rapid growth and remodeling of turbinates in young pigs make them most susceptible to the effects of *P. multocida* toxin. Nutritional deficiencies alone, however, do not cause atrophic rhinitis. Turbinate atrophy can be caused by intranasal or parenteral injection of purified *P. multocida* toxin or of toxin produced by recombinant techniques in *Escherichia coli*. Antibody to toxin is protective and is cross-protective between capsular types D and A. The molecular mode of action of the toxin is not known but, by what appears to be receptor-mediated activity, it is capable of experimentally inducing progressive degeneration of conchal cartilage and of osteoblasts and increased osteoclastic bone resorption of turbinates. These are the key features of the naturally occurring disease.

Atrophic rhinitis occurs with high incidence in most of the major pig-raising areas of the world. It is an important cause of economic loss because in young pigs, it causes decreased rate of growth and reduced efficiency of feed conversion. The endemic disease is insidious in onset and progression, but there can be acute episodes when a herd first becomes affected.

Acute signs are observed in young piglets and consist of rhinitis with sneezing, coughing, and a serous or mucopurulent nasal discharge. Large or small flecks of blood may be expelled by sneezing when damage is severe, and occasionally the hemorrhage is profuse. There is not a constant association between clinical signs of acute rhinitis and atrophic changes. Rhinitis occasionally is found not to have resulted in atrophy, at least of a permanent nature, and in some herds a high incidence of atrophy of the turbinates may be present in slaughtered pigs without there having been at any time clinical signs of rhinitis or facial deformity.

Facial deformity, which is an expression of severe disease in the rapidly growing young pig, is seldom evident before 5–6 weeks of age. It consists of shortening and distortion of the snout and facial bones (Fig. 6.3) As a result of the shortening, the overlying skin forms thick transverse folds. Asymmetry of the disease process causes deviation of the snout toward the more severely affected

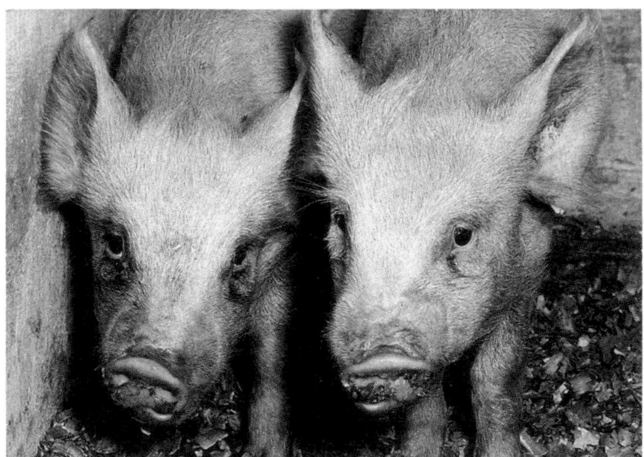

Fig. 6.3 Atrophic rhinitis with deviation of snout.

side; when the intranasal lesions are symmetric, the nose may be shortened and turned upward. Characteristically, there is often patchy encrustation of dried tears and dirt just below the medial canthus of the eye; this is usually attributed to lacrimal spillage caused by obstruction of the nasolacrimal duct, but increased lacrimation may also play a role.

The lesions of atrophic rhinitis range from indefinite to severe, and no clear dividing line separates the normal from the diseased. The lesions are most severe anterior to the nasofrontal suture. When mild, they may be detectable only in the ventral scroll of the ventral turbinate, but with increasing severity, gross changes become detectable in the entire ventral turbinate, in the dorsal turbinate, and farther back in the nasal cavity until even the ethmoids are involved. The nasal mucosa usually has fewer gross changes. It may be edematous and covered by a thin seromucinous exudate on the anterior portions and thick purulent exudate in posterior recesses and cells of the ethmoid, or it may be pale and dry.

The grossly detectable changes in the conformation of bones are always of the same type, but there are wide variations in the extent of the lesions. In the least-affected specimens, the ventral scrolls of the ventral turbinates are reduced in size, pliable, and soft. The width of the ventral meatus is increased. This is often accompanied by slight bulging of the nasal septum toward the less-affected side. With progression of the lesions in the turbinates, there is loss of scrolls of the ventral turbinate and then of the dorsal turbinate (Fig. 6.4). In extreme cases, nothing remains of the turbinates save for folds of mucosa on the lateral aspect of the empty nasal chamber. The bones surrounding the nasal cavity are often thinned. In some animals, especially those whose general health is not significantly affected by the disease and which continue to grow, hypertrophic changes frequently coexist with atrophic changes in the facial bones and rarely with hypertrophic changes in the turbinates. Combined hypertrophic and atrophic changes in the turbinates produce a series of longitudinal folds. Hypertrophy of the facial bones affects chiefly the

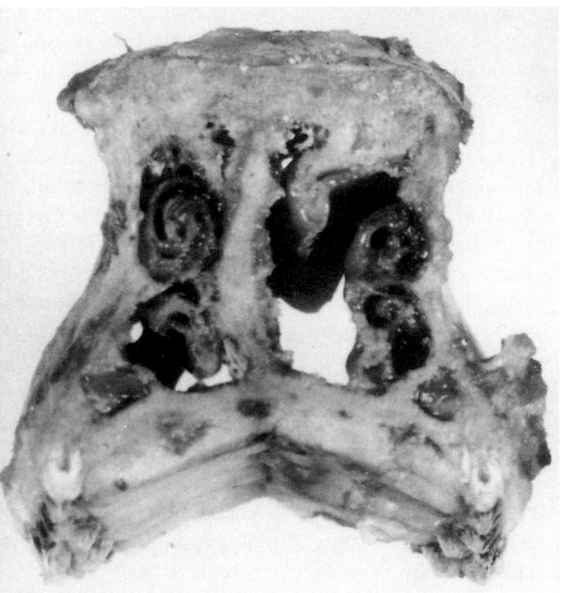

Fig. 6.4 Asymmetry of turbinates and facial skeleton with deviation of septum in atrophic rhinitis. Pig.

dorsal part of the nasal bones so that the conformation is broad and flat rather than narrow and convex. The alveolar processes may also be thickened, although the lateral plates of the maxillae tend to be attenuated.

Atrophy of turbinates in response to the toxin can occur at any age but is most severe when it begins in young animals. At this early age, the anterior parts of the conchae still have a core of hyaline cartilage; growth is by endochondral ossification on the inner or concentric side of the cartilage model and by membranous bone apposition forming radiating trabeculae on the outer or eccentric side. Lamellar bone is present in the more caudal, earlier-developed parts of the conchae. Each of these tissues is affected by the toxin after intramuscular injection. It is assumed that the evolution of changes in these hard tissues is the same in the natural disease and in the atrophy produced by injected toxin, although the rate of change may be different according to toxin levels.

The hyaline cartilage of the rostral extremity of the turbinates disappears quickly. Residual cartilage fails to undergo the hypertrophic sequence and is invaded by fibroblastlike cells and multinucleate cells. Endochondral ossification is suspended as both inner and outer surfaces of cartilage are eroded by chondroclasts. Trabecular bone on the outer surfaces is diminished or absent. The osteoblasts may be normal or show degenerative changes consisting of aggregated chromatin, irregular folding of nuclear and plasma membranes, and dilation of cisternae of the endoplasmic reticulum. Osteoclast numbers are increased, especially on the eccentric surface of the scroll.

The inflammatory lesions in the nasal mucous membranes are usually non-specific and vary according to the stage of the disease. In early stages, there is loss of ciliated and goblet cells and proliferation of cuboidal cells to form layers one to several cells deep. Submucosal glands become hyperactive and distended with mucus. Neutrophils infiltrate the superficial and glandular epithelium and occasionally form microabscesses. Subsequently, there is infiltration of the lamina propria by lymphocytes and plasma cells. The only indication of a specific acute infection occurs in piglets from herds where cytomegalovirus infection is prevalent. There is no direct correlation between severity of the acute rhinitis and the later development of permanent atrophy of the turbinates. In established cases of atrophic rhinitis, there is chronic nonspecific mucosal inflammation with variation from epithelial ulceration to squamous metaplasia, and atrophy or cystic dilation of the glands within a fibrotic lamina propria.

c. ATROPHIC RHINITIS IN OTHER SPECIES Chronic rhinitis with morphologic features similar to those of the porcine disease is occasionally observed in individuals of other species, mainly dogs, and as an endemic disease in some goat herds in Norway. Toxigenic strains of *Pasteurella multocida* do not readily colonize the normal nasal mucosa of pigs. The bacterial properties which allow colonization are not known, although apparently they do not include adhesins. Until these properties are known, the different susceptibilities of host species will not be explained.

The disease in goats closely resembles that in pigs, including a predominance of toxigenic strains in the nasal flora. All toxigenic strains were of capsular type D. Notably, there were no inflammatory lesions of significance in the nasal mucosa.

Bibliography

Baalsrud, K. F. Atrophic rhinitis in goats in Norway. *Vet Rec* **121:** 350–353, 1987.

Chanter, N. Molecular aspects of the virulence of *Pasteurella multocida. Can J Vet Res* **54:** S45–S47, 1990.

Chanter, N., and Rutter, J. M. Colonisation by *Pasteurella multocida* in atrophic rhinitis of pigs and immunity to the osteolytic toxin. *Vet Microbiol* **25:** 253–265, 1990.

Chanter, N., Magyar, T., and Rutter, J. M. Interactions between *Bordetella bronchiseptica* and toxigenic *Pasteurella multocida* in atrophic rhinitis of pigs. *Res Vet Sci* **47:** 48–53, 1989.

Drummond, J. G. *et al.* Effects of atmospheric ammonia on young pigs experimentally infected with *Bordetella bronchiseptica. Am J Vet Res* **42:** 963–968, 1981.

Foged, N. T., Pedersen, K. B., and Elling, F. Characterization and biological effects of the *Pasteurella multocida* toxin. *FEMS Microbiol Lett* **43:** 45–51, 1987.

Goodwin, R. F. W., Chanter, N., and Rutter, J. M. Detection and distribution of toxigenic *Pasteurella multocida* in pig herds with different degrees of atrophic rhinitis. *Vet Rec* **126:** 452–456, 1990.

Kimman, T. G. *et al.* Stimulation of bone resorption by inflamed nasal mucosa, dermonecrotic toxin-containing conditioned medium from *Pasteurella multocida,* and purified dermonecrotic toxin from *P. multocida. Infect Immun* **55:** 2110–2116, 1987.

Martineau-Doize, B., Frantz, J. C., and Martineau, G.-P. Effects of purified *Pasteurella multocida* dermonecrotoxin on cartilage and bone of the nasal ventral conchae of the piglet. *Anat Rec* **228:** 237–246, 1990.

Petersen, S. K. *et al.* Recombinant derivatives of *Pasteurella multocida* toxin: Candidates for a vaccine against progressive atrophic rhinitis. *Infect Immun* **59:** 1387–1393, 1991.

d. STRANGLES IN HORSES Strangles is an acute contagious disease of horses characterized by inflammation of the upper respiratory tract and abscessation in the regional lymph nodes. It is caused by *Streptococcus equi,* an obligate parasite on upper respiratory mucous membranes of Equidae. Other hemolytic streptococci of Lancefield group C are frequent commensals in the upper respiratory tract of horses. The main species (subspecies) are *Streptococcus zooepidemicus,* and *S. equisimilis.* The former is much more commonly pathogenic and can be isolated from a variety of suppurative processes such as wound infections, sinusitis, and pneumonia secondary to respiratory viral infection. It can cause endometritis and abortion in mares, and umbilical infection, septicemia, and polyarthritis in newborn foals. *Streptococcus zooepidemicus,* and rarely *S. equisimilis,* are causes of respiratory catarrh which may, on other than bacteriologic grounds, be indistinguishable from strangles. This is especially true for mild cases of the latter in which lymphadenitis is absent or is mild and nonsuppurative.

Streptococcus equi in exudates is very resistant to the external environment and can survive for many months in stables. The initial source of infection, however, is usually a carrier animal or one with active but not necessarily clinically obvious disease. Outbreaks of the disease occur mainly in young animals under crowded conditions. Carrier horses are difficult to detect because shedding of organisms is intermittent, and the site of recovery can shift between nasal and pharyngeal regions in a single animal.

The pathogenesis of the infection involves epithelial adherence, especially to soft palate and pharynx, and internalization of the organism into epithelial cells. There is intense chemotaxis of neutrophils to the mucosa and regional lymph nodes. Smears of pus show short chains of the organism, typically not in leukocytes. The intense chemotaxis is stimulated by factors derived from the alternative complement pathway, which is activated by peptidoglycan of the bacterial cell wall. Surface M protein and hyaluronic acid allow the organism to resist phagocytosis. Hemolysin production is not necessary for pathogenicity, but all strains produce a potent cytotoxin which allows the organism to resist intracellular digestion and to cause rapid degeneration of polymorphonuclear neutrophils.

Recovery from strangles confers immunity to a second attack in ~70% of horses, the acquired resistance apparently due to IgA and IgG subclasses produced locally in the nasopharynx. The serum of recovered cases, and of some vaccinated with bacterin-type preparations, contains complexes of IgA and bacterial M protein, which are probably responsible for the glomerulonephritis and the leukocytoclastic vasculitis which is the basis of complicating purpura hemorrhagica.

The incubation period of strangles is 3–4 days, although it may be as short as 2 or as long as 15 days. Onset is indicated by fever, slight cough, and nasal discharge. The nasal discharge is bilateral, and in a few days it changes from serous to catarrhal and then purulent. Catarrhal conjunctivitis occurs concurrently and, in cases which pursue a typical course, inflammatory swellings of the lymph nodes of the head and neck develop. The submandibular and retropharyngeal nodes are the first and usually the most severely affected. The acute inflammatory swelling is firm, but the nodes begin to fluctuate as liquefaction and suppuration develop. The typical and favorable outcome of the lymphadenitis is for the abscesses to rupture onto the skin 1–3 weeks after onset of infection. Rupture is preceded by depilation and oozing of serum. The discharged pus is copious, creamy, and yellow-white. Abscessation of lymph nodes is not an invariable feature of strangles, but clinical diagnosis is seldom made in its absence.

The nasal lesions are those of a purulent rhinitis but are otherwise nonspecific. Large amounts of creamy yellow pus collect in the folds of the turbinates and may produce temporary distortion. The mucosa is edematous, hyperemic, and occasionally ulcerated.

In the typical course of strangles previously described, the outcome is favorable. The course, however, may be either milder or more severe with an unfavorable outcome. In herds of mixed ages, ~20% of clinically affected animals will develop complications. In older horses, the course tends to be milder and confined to catarrhal rhinitis and pharyngitis without nodal abscessation, or the nodal abscesses may become sterile and encapsulated. When the course is severe, infection may spread to the paranasal sinuses and by way of the Eustachian tubes to the guttural pouches to cause chronic empyema of these cavities. Extensive cellulitis may develop in the connective tissues of nose, pharynx, or throat. Retropharyngeal abscesses may discharge into the pharynx, allowing pus to be aspirated into the lungs. Metastatic abscesses (bastard strangles) occasionally form in the liver, kidneys, synovial structures, and brain. The internal organs most frequently affected, however, are the mediastinal and mesenteric lymph nodes. Abscesses in mediastinal and mesenteric lymph nodes tend to be very large and, although frank rupture is unusual, the suppurative process can permeate to adjacent serous membranes and cause a purulent pleuritis or peritonitis. Two other important sequelae are purpura hemorrhagica and local damage to cranial nerves, resulting in laryngeal paralysis (roaring), facial nerve paralysis, or Horner's syndrome.

Bibliography

Bryans, J. T., Doll, E. R., and Shephard, B. P. The etiology of strangles. *Cornell Vet* **54:** 198–205, 1964.

Galan, J. E., and Timoney, J. F. Mucosal and nasopharyngeal responses of horses to protein antigens of *Streptococcus equi. Infect Immun* **47:** 623–628, 1985.

Galan, J. E., and Timoney, J. F. Immune complexes in purpura hemorrhagica of the horse contain IgA and M antigen of *Streptococcus equi. J Immunol* **135:** 3134–3137, 1985.

George, J. L. *et al.* Identification of carriers of *Streptococcus equi* in a naturally infected herd. *J Am Vet Med Assoc* **183:** 80–84, 1983.

Muhktar, M. M., and Timoney, J. F. Chemotactic response of equine polymorphonuclear leucocytes to *Streptococcus equi. Res Vet Sci* **45:** 225–229, 1988.

Sweeney, C. R. *et al.* Complications associated with *Streptococcus equi* infection on a horse farm. *J Am Vet Med Assoc* **191:** 1446–1448, 1987.

Sweeney, C. R. *et al.* Description of an epizootic and persistence of *Streptococcus equi* infections in horses. *J Am Vet Med Assoc* **194:** 1281–1286, 1989.

e. GLANDERS Glanders is an infectious disease caused by a Gram-negative bacillus, *Pseudomonas mallei*. It is mainly an equine infection, but it does occur occasionally in humans, and it can be acquired naturally by carnivorous animals which eat diseased flesh of horses. Goats and sheep are susceptible to contract infection, but cattle and pigs are not. A variety of other generic names have been used for the organism, most commonly *Loefflerella, Pfeifferella, Malleomyces,* and *Actinobacillus*. The disease in horses is characterized by nodular lesions in the lungs, and ulcerative and nodular lesions of the skin and respiratory mucosa. "Farcy" is the term often applied to the cutaneous lesions.

Glanders is, historically, a very old disease and flourished especially among cavalry horses. Since the advent of motorized vehicles and accurate serological diagnostic procedures, it has virtually or completely disappeared from many countries. It still exists, however, in some parts of eastern Europe and Asia.

Pseudomonas mallei is sensitive to the external environment, and infection is acquired directly or indirectly from excretions and discharges of affected animals. In horses, the disease is usually chronic, and the organisms are confined to the lesions and discharges, especially those of the skin and nasal mucosa. In the acute disease, which occurs in some horses and is the usual form in donkeys, the organism is distributed in most tissues and may be excreted in feces, urine, saliva, and tears. Although the most common form of the disease in horses is respiratory, the route of infection is probably oral, because this is the only experimental way to produce the typical chronic respiratory disease; intranasal or intratracheal inoculation reproduces the acute disease. Percutaneous infection can occur, but this is unusual.

In the absence of definitive information, it is assumed that the organisms traverse the pharyngeal mucosa, and perhaps the intestinal mucosa, and are conveyed to the lungs where lesions almost always occur. From there, hematogenous spread is believed to result in the nasal, cutaneous, and nodal lesions. This sequence of events is speculative, however, and not entirely satisfying. The chronic syndrome of glanders is frequently divided into nasal, pulmonary, and cutaneous varieties. The division is convenient for description, but the varieties are not distinct. Emphasis may at any time change from one variety to another, and the same animal may suffer the three varieties at the same time. Involvement of all three sites is common in the acute form of glanders in donkeys and in exacerbations of the chronic disease in horses.

Rhinitis in glanders usually commences as a unilateral nasal catarrh, but the inflammation may be bilateral and also involve the pharynx and larynx. The nasal excretion is copious, purulent, and greenish yellow. It is frequently flecked with blood and fragments of desquamated epithelium. The typical nasal lesions are multiple small nodules lying in the submucosa and surrounded by a narrow hyperemic halo. Each nodule consists of a focus of intense cellular infiltration with an inner core of neutrophils and a periphery of macrophages. The core liquefies, and the overlying mucosa may slough. The nodules may be isolated or semiconfluent with suppurative cores separated by granulation tissue. A discrete slough of the necrotic tissue over individual nodules can occur, leaving a crateriform ulcer which has a sharp margin and a smooth base. The ulcers sometimes perforate the septum in severe cases. New generations of nodules develop, ulcerate, and heal irregularly. It is usual to find nodules, ulcers, and white stellate scars mixed together in an affected horse. There is variation from case to case in the number of lesions which can be found. In milder cases, a few discrete foci are present in the posterior portions of the nasal cavity, and the anterior portions show only hyperemia and catarrh. Lymphadenitis of the submaxillary and retropharyngeal nodes is regularly present. Depending on the age and activity, nodules or scars may be found. When lesions occur on the larynx, they are of the same type as those occurring in the nose. Lesions in the tracheal mucosa are usually ulcerative but are occasionally pyogranulomatous nodules.

Lesions of glanders can be found in lungs in all but a very small percentage of cases. The typical lesion is the nodule, but in some acute cases, there may be a more diffuse pneumonia. The nodules have a miliary distribution throughout the lungs, but they are most visible beneath the pleura. They are basically pyogranulomatous lesions, but the relative proportion of exudative and proliferative components varies. The more exudative foci typically have necrotic centers composed of karyorrhectic neutrophils. In acute stages, there is hemorrhagic and fibrinous exudation. In more mature lesions, liquefied or caseonecrotic centers are surrounded by epithelioid cells, occasional giant cells, and lymphocytes, which blend with an outer layer of granulation tissue (Fig. 6.5A). The core may be gritty because of dystrophic calcification, but the salts are deposited irregularly and incompletely. In old lesions, the capsule is thin and fibrous (Fig. 6.5B). The more proliferative nodules develop a grayish semitranslucent core of granulomatous tissue consisting of epithelioid and giant cells with an admixture of leukocytes in a fibroblastic stroma. The more diffuse lobular pneumonia has

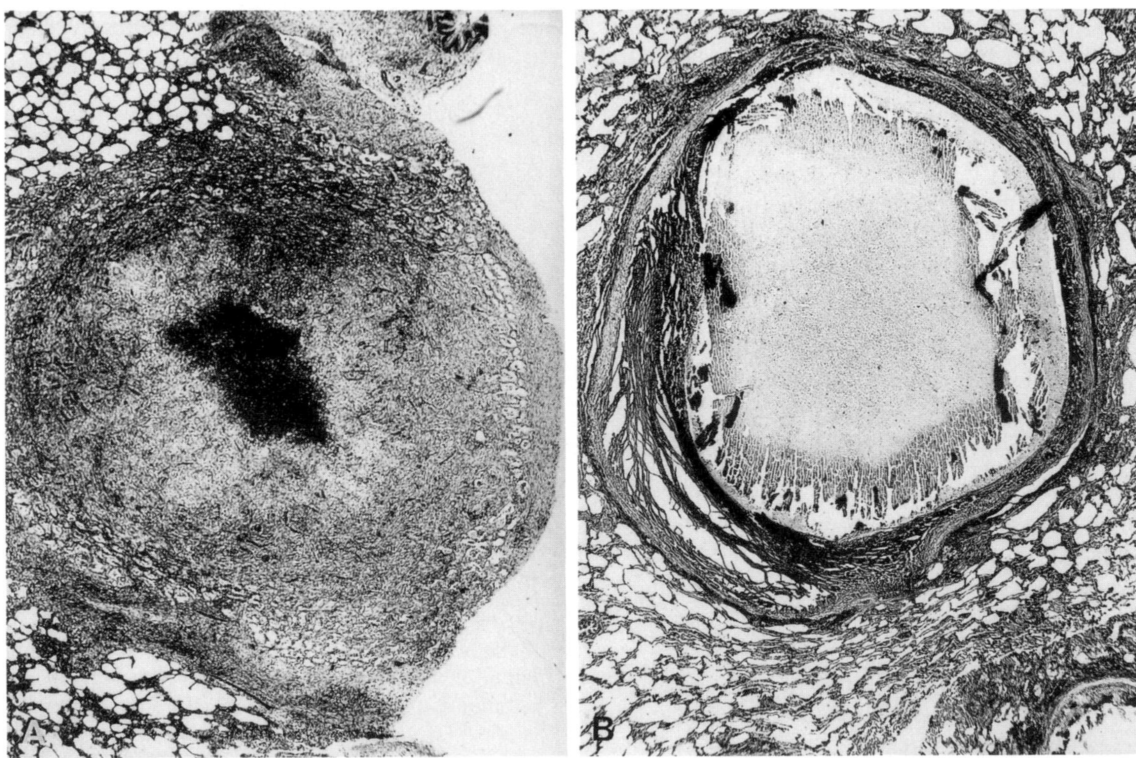

Fig. 6.5 Glanders. Horse. (A) Pyogranulomatous pulmonary nodule with central necrosis. (B) Chronic pulmonary nodules with irregular calcification and thin fibrous capsules.

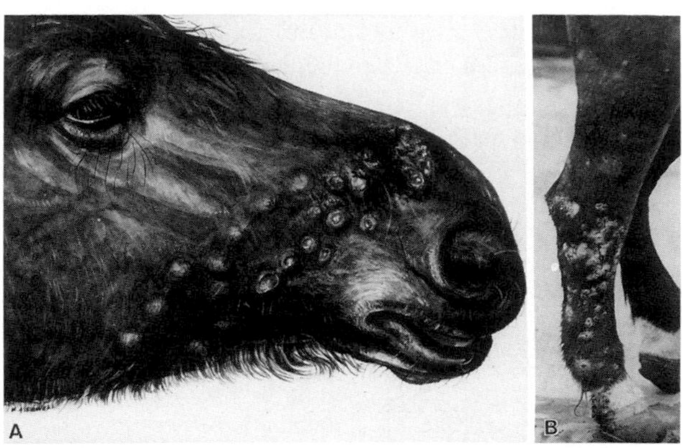

Fig. 6.6 (A) Glanders. Horse. Ulcers and farcy buds along facial lymphatics. (Reproduced from "Glanders," by W. Hunting, H. and W. Brown and Co., 1908, London.) (B) Cutaneous glanders with nonulcerated buds. Horse. (Reproduced from "Glanders," by W. Hunting, H. and W. Brown and Co., 1908, London.)

the same range of components as the nodules but extends without clear demarcations other than those provided by interlobular septa.

Lesions of glanders in the alimentary tract are rare, although they do occur in experimental infections in which large numbers of organisms are given by mouth. Hematogenous metastases are common in the spleen and less common in other viscera or in locomotor organs. Metastatic lesions are similar in structure to the pulmonary nodules.

In equine farcy, the cutaneous lesions of glanders, the cordlike thickening of the subcutaneous lymphatics has caused them to be referred to as farcy pipes. Chains of nodules (buds), which tend to ulcerate, are distributed along the corded lymphatics (Fig. 6.6A,B), and the regional nodes are enlarged. The lymphangitis is purulent, and remarkable only for the unusual degree of leukocytic necrosis.

Bibliography

Duval, C. W., and White, P. C. The histological lesions of experimental glanders. *J Exp Med* **9:** 352–380, 1907.

Hunting, W. "Glanders, a Clinical Treatise." London, H. & W. Brown, 1908.

McFadyean, J. Glanders. *J Comp Pathol* **17:** 295–317, 1904.

f. MELIOIDOSIS Melioidosis is occasionally known as pseudoglanders. The causative organism is *Pseudomonas (Malleomyces) pseudomallei,* which is closely related to *P. mallei*. Geographic strains may differ in virulence, and there are breed differences in susceptibility of sheep and goats. Melioidosis is primarily a disease of rodents, but is occasionally a highly fatal disease of humans. All domestic species are occasionally infected, sometimes in small outbreaks in regions where the infection is endemic. The principal occurrence has been in Southeast Asia, but it is also present in parts of western Europe, the Caribbean, and Australia. Rats have been regarded as the usual source of infection but, since the organism can persist for as long as 30 months in soil and water of endemic areas, it is probably an accidental pathogen. Infection can occur through cutaneous wounds, and it can be transmitted by insects. Ingestion is probably the most important natural route of infection. Although the high incidence of disease in confined and intensively managed piggeries suggests respiratory transmission, the sources of infection are likely to be circumstantial, such as a contaminated water supply.

The usual course following infection is pyemia followed by localization of the organism and abscessation in a wide variety of tissues, particularly lymph nodes, spleen, lung, liver, joints, and central nervous system. Depending on the severity of the process, there may be an acute disease associated with fulminating suppuration or a more indolent one associated with chronic abscessation. Melioidosis in horses can resemble glanders. Melioidosis in dogs may cause dermal abscesses and epididymitis in addition to other organ involvement. In cattle, acute fatal infection, pneumonia, arthritis, placentitis, and endometritis are important variants of the disease. Assuming variations in virulence of the organism and of susceptibility of animals, unless localization involves a vital organ, the disease is most likely to be met as an incidental finding at autopsy or at slaughter.

Outbreaks of melioidosis, as well as isolated cases, occur in sheep, goats, and pigs, and the infection can be transmitted to these species more regularly than to other domestic animals. Pneumonia and arthritis are common in the clinical course of the disease, which otherwise is nonspecific. Goats may develop a chronic infection or recover. The lesions are those of pyemia with multiple abscesses in the lungs, regional lymph nodes, and spleen and less often in other viscera and joints. The splenic abscesses are <1 cm in diameter, and they project from the surface of the organ (Fig 6.7A). Larger purulent cavities, as well as multiple small abscesses, occur in the lungs and are associated with focal adhesive pleuritis (Fig. 6.7B). The abscesses are encapsulated and contain a creamy or caseous, yellow-green pus. In some cases, there is purulent exudate in the bronchi. Except for the lamination which occurs in old lesions of caseous lymphadenitis caused by *Corynebacterium pseudotuberculosis,* there is nothing in the morphology of the lesions to distinguish the two diseases in sheep and goats. Experimental infections in sheep can produce, in addition to the lesions of the natural disease, microabscesses in the brain and lesions in the nasal mucosa similar to those of glanders.

Bibliography

Cottew, G. S. Melioidosis in sheep in Queensland. A description of the causal organism. *Aust J Exp Biol Med Sci* **28:** 677–683, 1950.

Cottew, G. S. Melioidosis. *Aust Vet J* **31:** 155–158, 1955.

Davie, J., and Wells, C. W. Equine melioidosis in Malaya. *Br Vet J* **108:** 161–166, 1952.

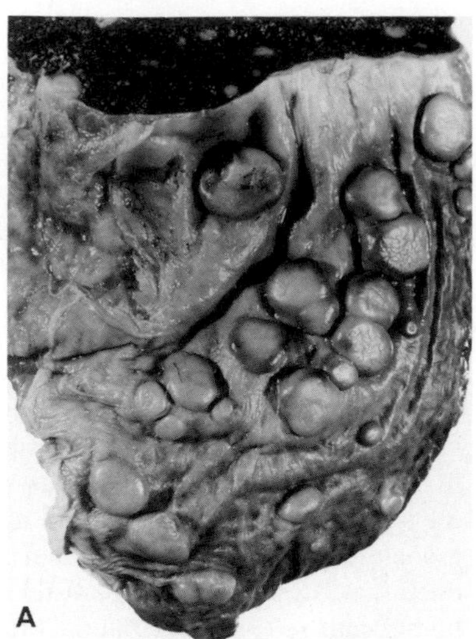

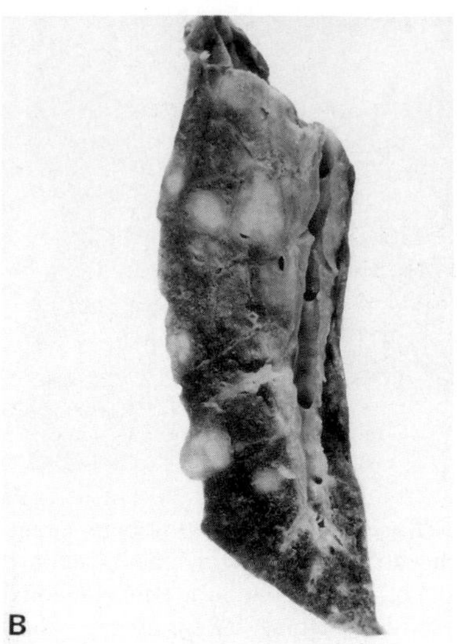

Fig. 6.7 (A) Splenic abscessation in meliodosis. Sheep. (Courtesy of W. T. Hall and Queensland Department of Agriculture.) (B) Chronic pulmonary abscessation in melioidosis. Sheep. (Courtesy of W. T. Hall and Queensland Department of Agriculture.)

Ketterer, P. J., Donald, B., and Rogers, R. J. Bovine melioidosis in south-eastern Queensland. *Aust Vet J* **51:** 395–398, 1975.

Olds, R. J., and Lewis, F. A. Melioidosis in goats. *Aust Vet J* **30:** 253–261, 1954.

Olds, R. J., and Lewis, F. A. Melioidosis in a pig. *Aust Vet J* **31:** 273–274, 1955.

Stedham, M. A. Histopathology of melioidosis in the dog. *Lab Invest* **36:** 358, 1977.

Sutmoller, P., Kraneveld, F. C., and van der Schaaf, A. Melioidosis (*Pseudomalleus*) in sheep, goats, and pigs on Aruba (Netherland Antilles). *J Am Vet Med Assoc* **130:** 415–417, 1957.

g. Infectious Bovine Rhinotracheitis This is an acute, contagious disease of cattle caused by bovine herpesvirus-1 (BHV-1) and is characterized by inflammatory lesions in the upper respiratory tract, trachea, and conjunctiva. Serologically identical virus causes infectious pustular vulvovaginitis (IPV) and balanoposthitis, but infectious bovine rhinotracheitis (IBR) isolates can be distinguished from those of IPV by molecular analysis. The standard method is by comparing DNA fragment patterns after restriction endonuclease digestion. On this basis, IBR isolates are classified as BHV-1.1 and IPV isolates, as BHV-1.2a or b. Both BHV-1.1 and BHV-2a have been shown capable of causing abortion. The herpesvirus isolates from meningoencephalitis and more generalized infections in young calves were also classified serologically as BHV-1. However, restriction endonuclease DNA analysis and DNA:DNA hybridization have revealed significant differences and led to the meningoencephalitis isolates being designated BHV-1.3 or as a separate virus, bovine encephalitis herpesvirus (BEHV). Bovine herpesvirus-1 has also been implicated as a cause of vaginitis and balanitis in swine.

On clinical and virologic evidence, IBR in cattle is widely distributed throughout the world, and on serologic evidence, the infection is more widespread than the disease. The disease occurs chiefly where cattle are crowded, and most outbreaks occur among animals kept in feedlots or indoor fattening pens. The disease in dairy cattle is usually milder. The onset in feedlots is usually preceded by introduction of animals from an outside source and, from there on, the pattern is typically that of an epidemic maintained by the continual movement of cattle into and out of the feedlots. The morbidity is high, but many cases are mild and unrecognized. The fatality rate is usually low, but it can exceed 30% in exceptional outbreaks.

The clinical course is characterized by fever, increased respiratory rate, coughing, and serous nasal discharge. Lacrimation is common. If the course is prolonged, the nasal discharge becomes mucopurulent, and inspiratory dyspnea develops. The lesions in typical and uncomplicated cases are those of seromucinous rhinotracheitis and possibly conjunctivitis. In cases of greater severity, which are usually associated with bacterial complications, there is a glairy or mucopurulent exudate with acute diffuse inflammation, and focal hemorrhages, erosions, and ulcerations. In the most severe cases, and especially in fatal ones, there are widespread fibrinopurulent or fibrinonecrotic membranes on nasopharyngeal, laryngeal, and tracheal surfaces (Fig. 6.8A). The region of most severe damage varies, but in field outbreaks the necrotizing and diphtheritic inflammation is often most dramatic in the larynx and adjacent pharynx and trachea (Fig. 6.8B). Bacteria contribute to the severity of these lesions, particularly *Pasteurella* spp., *Mycoplasma* spp., and *Fusobacterium necrophorum*.

The histologic changes can be anticipated from the gross

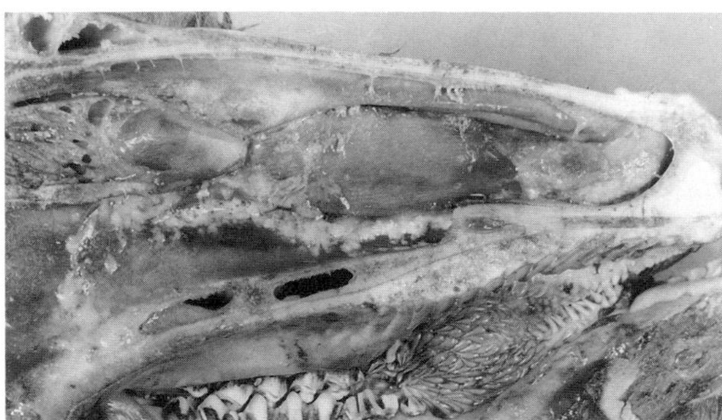

Fig. 6.8A Infectious bovine rhinotracheitis. Inflamed mucous membranes of nasal cavity partially covered by fibrinopurulent exudate.

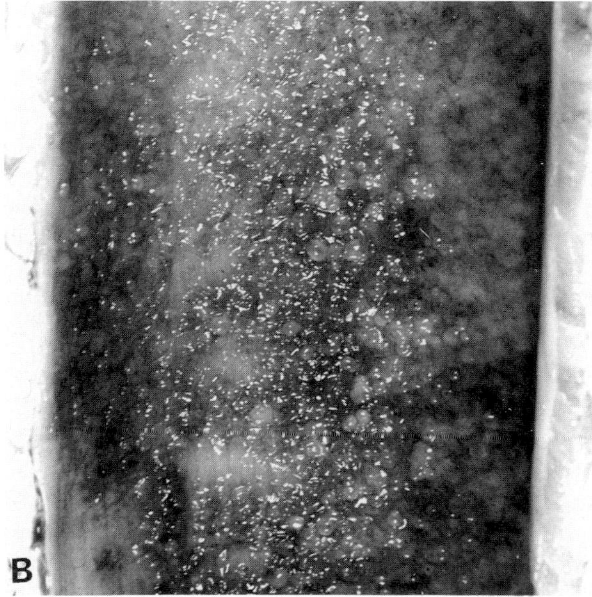

Fig. 6.8B Infectious bovine rhinotracheitis. Granular surface of ulcerated tracheal mucosa.

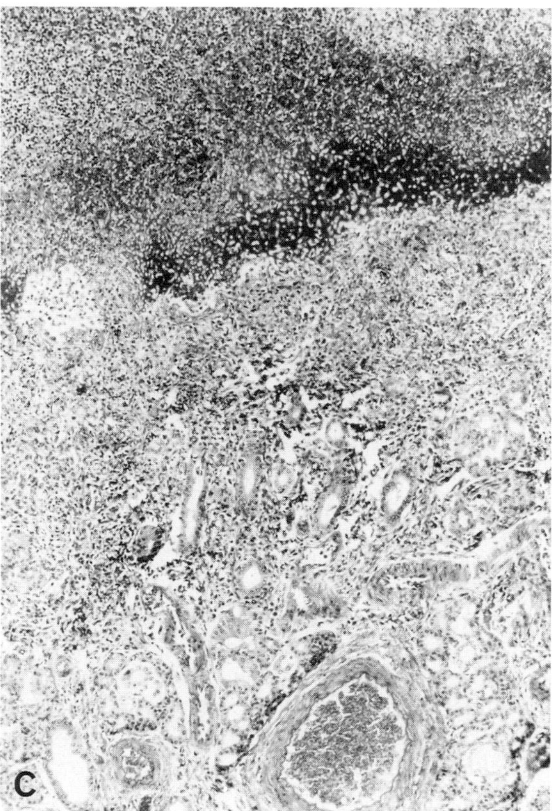

Fig. 6.8C Infectious bovine rhinotracheitis. Acute rhinitis with ulceration and fibrinonecrotic covering.

appearance of the lesions. In mild cases, there is serous to mucopurulent inflammation with little epithelial necrosis. In fatal cases, the emphasis is on extensive epithelial necrosis and formation of a surface layer of admixed fibrin and necrotic debris (Fig. 6.8C). There is an intense vascular, neutrophilic, and mononuclear response in the underlying viable tissue. Acidophilic intranuclear viral inclusion bodies, best demonstrated after use of acid fixatives, can sometimes be found in infected cells. Because they appear for only a transient period ~2–3 days after infection, they are mostly seen in experimental situations and are of little practical diagnostic value. They can rarely be detected in autopsy samples from field cases, although they occasionally persist long enough to be found in bronchial or alveolar epithelium.

Assessment of the role of BHV-1 in causing pneumonia is complicated because in most descriptions of both the experimental and naturally occurring respiratory form of the disease, it is impossible to distinguish the effect of the virus itself, its role in predisposing to severe secondary bacterial pneumonia, and the confounding effect of preexisting pneumonic lesions which are common in calves or feedlot animals. It seems fairly safe to conclude that the lung is not significantly affected in the mild viral disease. At the other end of the disease spectrum, severe viral infection seriously impairs pulmonary defenses and leads to the extensive secondary bacterial pneumonia usually present in fatal cases. The mechanisms by which viral damage and its amplification by various mediator cascades predispose to secondary bacterial infection are not known in detail. Some idea of the complexity of factors is given subsequently in Section VI,F,1 on bronchopneumonia. *Pasteurella* spp. are usually involved, and the lungs commonly show severe fibrinous pneumonia with or without pleuritis (see pneumonic pasteurellosis, in Section VI,H,2 of this chapter). An additional feature is interstitial emphysema, which frequently follows the labored respiration caused by upper and lower airway obstruction. The most severe viral lesion, in which secondary organisms may not play a significant role, is in fulminating infections. In these instances, there is a severe, necrotizing bronchitis and bronchiolitis, and there is extensive serofibrinous flooding of alveoli.

The pattern of generalized disease in newborn calves is spectacular. Affected calves are usually <1 month of age and are part of a herd in which infectious bovine rhinotracheitis affects all age groups. The calves are febrile and have serous ocular and nasal discharge, inspiratory difficulty, anorexia, depression, and sometimes a laryngeal stertor suggesting laryngeal necrobacillosis. There is acute rhinitis and erosive pharyngitis, with intense hyperemia under the eroded areas and yellowish pellicles of epithelium at the margin. The epiglottis may be similarly involved, but the more distal parts of the respiratory tract remain unaffected. The most prominent changes are in the epithelium of the esophagus and forestomachs, which appear as if plastered with clumps of curdled milk. This caseous material is adherent necrotic epithelial debris. The necrosis involves the epithelium to its full depth, with intense neutrophil infiltration. Surviving epithelial cells and those at the margins of the lesions contain inclusion bodies in their vesicular nuclei. Additional lesions of systemic viral action include acute lymphadenitis with focal cortical necrosis, especially in nodes draining the upper respiratory tract. Necrotic foci can also be seen in the kidney, spleen, and liver. Miliary white necrotic foci 1–2 mm in diameter are particularly prominent in the liver. They are either uniformly distributed or concentrated in the right lobe.

When abortion is caused by the virus, the fetuses are edematous, and advanced autolysis indicates death of the fetus perhaps 2 days before abortion. There are no characteristic gross lesions, but microscopic lesions occur in many parenchymatous organs and lymph nodes as well as in the placenta. They consist of foci of intense necrosis and leukocytic infiltration, and are most prominent and consistent in the liver, where they may be confused with lesions of listeriosis. Specific inclusion bodies often are not found in autolyzed fetuses. Vaccinal strains of virus produced in cell cultures are as effective as field virus in causing abortion, and the natural infections may not be preceded or accompanied by signs of rhinitis or other illness. It appears that cows pregnant <~5 months are less likely to abort following exposure to bovine herpesvirus-l.

Bibliography

Abinanti, F. R., and Plumer, G. J. The isolation of infectious bovine rhinotracheitis virus from cattle affected with conjunctivitis—observations on the experimental infection. *Am J Vet Res* **22:** 13–17, 1961.

Allan, E. M. *et al.* The pathological features of severe cases of infectious bovine rhinotracheitis. *Vet Rec* **107:** 441–445, 1980.

Bratanich, A. C. *et al.* Comparative studies of BHV-1 variants by *in vivo—in vitro* tests. *J Vet Med (B)* **38:** 41–48, 1991.

Crandell, R. A., Cheatham, W. J., and Maurer, F. D. Infectious bovine rhinotracheitis—the occurrence of intranuclear inclusions in experimentally infected animals. *Am J Vet Res* **20:** 505–509, 1959.

Evermann, J. F., and Henry, B. E. Herpetic infections of cattle: A comparison of bovine cytomegalovirus and infectious bovine rhinotracheitis. *Compend Cont Ed Pract Vet* **11:** 205–214, 1989.

McKercher, D. G., Wada, E. B., and Straub, O. C. Distribution and persistence of infectious bovine rhinotracheitis virus in experimentally infected cattle. *Am J Vet Res* **24:** 510–514, 1963.

Miller, J. M., Whetstone, C. A., and Van Der Maaten, M. J. Abortifacient property of bovine herpesvirus type 1 isolates that represent three subtypes determined by restriction endonuclease analysis of viral DNA. *Am J Vet Res* **52:** 458–461, 1991.

Ohmann, H. B., Babiuk, L. A., and Harland, R. Cytokine synergy with viral cytopathic effects and bacterial products during the pathogenesis of respiratory tract infection. *Clin Immunol Immunopathol* **60:** 153–170, 1991.

Studdert, M. J. Bovine encephalitis herpesvirus. *Vet Rec* **126:** 21–22, 1990.

Yates, W. D. G. A review of infectious bovine rhinotracheitis, shipping fever pneumonia, and viral–bacterial synergism in respiratory disease of cattle. *Can J Comp Med* **46:** 225–263, 1982.

h. Feline Viral Rhinotracheitis This is principally an upper respiratory disease caused by the serologically homogeneous feline herpesvirus-1 (FHV-1) and is one of the major components of the feline respiratory disease complex. The other major component is feline calicivirus infection, with feline reovirus and the feline-adapted strain of *Chlamydia psittaci* (feline pneumonitis agent) being minor causes. *Mycoplasma felis* is probably relegated to the role of an opportunist capable of causing mucopurulent conjunctivitis, usually in association with viral or chlamydial infection.

Feline viral rhinotracheitis is characterized by fever, sneezing, salivation, oral respiration, coughing, and serous to mucopurulent nasal and conjunctival discharges. Most cats recover in 7–14 days, but mortality can be high in young kittens or debilitated animals, including those whose immune system is depressed by feline immunodeficiency virus or feline leukemia virus infection.

The distribution of gross lesions corresponds to the predilection sites for viral replication, namely the epithelium of nasal passages, pharynx, soft palate, conjunctivae, tonsils, and, to a lesser extent, trachea. The initial serous inflammation becomes mucopurulent or fibrinous within a few days. Lethal cases usually have extensive fibrinous rhinotracheitis, possibly with extension to an acute viral or secondary bacterial pneumonia. Tonsils are enlarged and often petechiated. The regional lymph nodes are also usually enlarged, reddened, and edematous. Ulcerations of the tongue are seen rarely and only in severely affected cats. This contrasts with the frequent finding of vesicular to ulcerative lesions on tongue, hard palate, or nostrils of cats with calicivirus infection. The ocular involvement is usually limited to purulent conjunctivitis, but it can progress to ulcerative keratitis.

Microscopically, the respiratory and conjunctival lesions are associated with intranuclear viral replication causing epithelial cell death and the multifocal necrosis characteristic of active herpesvirus infection. The virus is virulent enough in its own right to cause extensive lesions, but mixed secondary bacterial infection by organisms such as *Pasteurella multocida, Bordetella bronchiseptica, Streptococcus* spp., and *Mycoplasma felis* enhance the suppurative response. Most active viral replication and cell necrosis occur from 2 to 7 days after infection, and during this period, herpesvirus inclusions are present in the nuclei of affected cells. They are typically large, acidophilic, and surrounded by a clear halo (Cowdry type A). Fixation in acid fixative such as Bouin's solution is best for their demonstration. They may be found in lesions from cats dying of the disease, but they are rarely detected beyond 7 days after infection and cannot be relied on for diagnosis. Cells bearing inclusion bodies become large and pale with a perinuclear clear zone, or ballooned and granular. There is loss of epithelial organization, and the disrupted epithelium is soon eroded or ulcerated. An acute inflammatory reaction develops with exudation of fibrin and many neutrophils. Focal necrosis accompanied by acute inflammation may be found in tonsils and local lymph nodes. Necrosis and resorption of turbinates have also been described.

Pulmonary involvement is uncommon except in fatal cases. In fulminating cases of viral infection, there is widespread multifocal necrotizing bronchitis, bronchiolitis, and interstitial pneumonia, with extensive serofibrinous flooding of airspaces. In other instances, there is a secondary bacterial bronchopneumonia.

Naturally occurring infection by feline herpesvirus-1 rarely causes manifestation of the wider tissue tropisms seen with other members of the family, such as BHV-1, but they occur occasionally. The virus is suspected of being a cause of abortion, but this has been difficult to prove in natural outbreaks. Experimentally, it has been possible to produce abortion and generalized neonatal infection by intravenous or intravaginal inoculation of the virus into pregnant cats. Necrosis accompanied by inclusion bodies has also been found in sites of osteogenesis in a wide variety of bones of kittens after intravenous inoculation. Degeneration of olfactory nerve fibers and focal lymphocytic infiltration of the olfactory bulbs have occurred in experimentally infected, germ-free cats, but the extent of lesions in the brain has not been properly documented.

Feline calicivirus infection is the other main component of the feline respiratory disease complex. Although clinical signs overlap with those of feline herpesvirus infection, and occasionally both viruses occur together, calcivirus has more affinity for epithelium of the mouth and lung than for that of the upper respiratory tract and conjunctiva. The tendency of virulent strains of calicivirus to affect lungs is discussed with pneumonia.

The cat-adapted strain of *Chlamydia psittaci* (*C. felis*) is mostly a cause of persistent conjunctivitis analogous to trachoma in humans. The disease is misleadingly called feline pneumonitis, since mild or inapparent bronchointerstitial pneumonia is the only manifestation of pulmonary infection.

Bibliography

Crandell, R. A. Feline viral rhinotracheitis (FVR). *Adv Vet Sci Comp Med* **17:** 201–224, 1973.

Gaskell, R. M., and Povey, R. C. Feline viral rhinotracheitis: Sites of viral replication and persistence in acutely and persistently infected cats. *Res Vet Sci* **27:** 167–174, 1979.

Kahn, D. E., and Hoover, E. A. Infectious respiratory diseases of cats. *Vet Clin North Am* [*Small Anim Pract*] **6:** 399–413, 1976.

Palmer, G. H. Feline upper respiratory disease: A review. *Vet Med Small Anim Clin* **75:** 1156–1158, 1980.

Povey, R. C. A review of feline viral rhinotracheitis (feline herpesvirus 1 infection). *Comp Immunol Microbiol Infect Dis* **2:** 373–387, 1979.

4. Allergic Rhinitis

Sporadic instances of what probably is an allergic rhinitis are observed occasionally in dogs, cats, and horses. Clinically and in its response to treatment, the disease resembles hay fever in humans. It is diagnosed on the basis of oculonasal discharge, sneezing, nose rubbing, head shaking, and perhaps epistaxis, and the presence of eosinophils in nasal exudate or lavage fluid. There is no definitive information on either the pathologic or immunologic basis of the condition.

Frequently in cattle, and occasionally in sheep, there is a seasonal rhinitis, which in its clinicopathologic features is consistent with an allergic pathogenesis. Some evidence has been provided that affected cattle are allergic to pollen antigens. The disease has been reported mainly from Australia, but it does occur elsewhere. It is more common in Channel Island breeds. A familial predisposition in crossbred cattle has also been reported. It occurs chiefly in the summertime when the pastures are in bloom and affects individuals or most of a herd or flock. Affected animals have nasal discharge, lacrimation, sneezing, and evidence of nasal itching. The nasal mucosa is pale and thick from edema fluid, and mucosal erosions may be visible in the anterior nares. The exudate is at first serous but later becomes mucopurulent or contains floccules of detritus and mucus. Eosinophils are a prominent component of the exudate.

Histologically, the surviving nasal epithelium is hyperplastic or eroded and is infiltrated by eosinophils. The glandular epithelium can be hypertrophied, and mucus is produced in excess; if the orifices of excretory ducts are occluded by the superficial reaction, the mucus accumulates in the ducts and eventually lifts off the debris on the surface. In more severe cases, in which there is extensive superficial diphtheresis, many of the small mucosal vessels show fibrinoid necrosis.

Nasal granuloma is generally considered to be a more chronic form of allergic rhinitis. The affected mucosa is mainly in the posterior portion of the nasal vestibule and the anterior region of the nasal septum and ventral meatus. In long-standing cases, the lesions extend further caudally

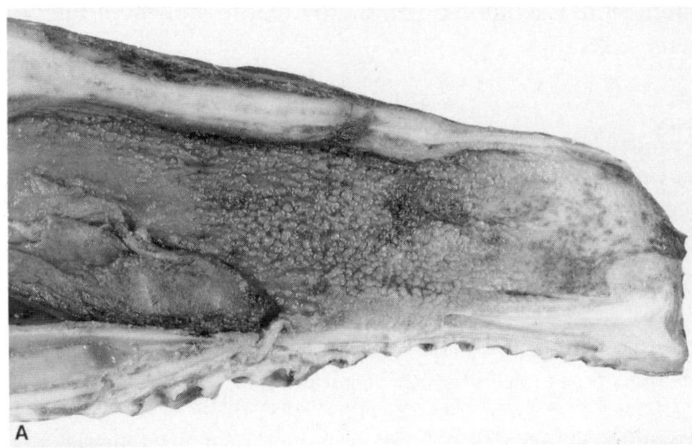

Fig. 6.9A Hyperplastic mucosa of anterior nasal septum in nasal granuloma. Ox.

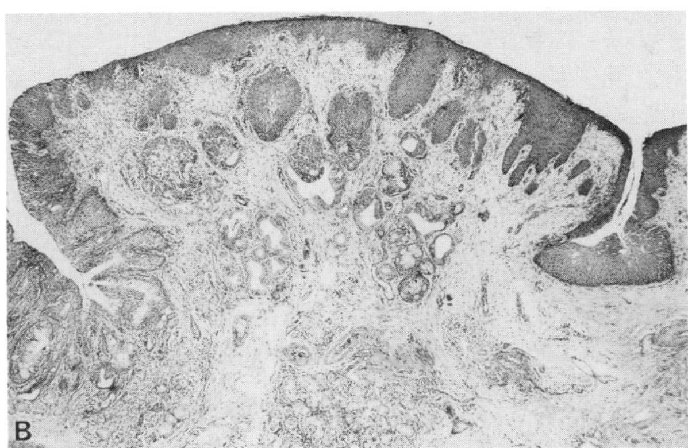

Fig. 6.9B Hyperplastic mucosa of anterior nasal septum in nasal granuloma. Ox.

to involve the posterior nasal cavity and even the larynx and proximal trachea. The hyperplastic epithelium is granular or has multiple nodular projections covered by intact epithelium (Fig. 6.9A). Histologically, the nodules typically consist of hyperplastic and metaplastic epithelium covering a superficial edematous lamina propria with a central core of inflammatory granulation tissue (Fig. 6.9B). Nonkeratinizing squamous epithelium usually covers the surface of the nodules. Goblet cell hyperplasia is more pronounced in the terminal portions of nasal gland ducts, which often form the lateral boundaries of the nodules. Active lesions have prominent eosinophil infiltration of the superficial lamina propria and epithelium. They are associated with increased numbers of submucosal mast cells. Vascular proliferation, fibroplasia, and accumulation of mostly lymphocytes and plasma cells in the cores of nodules are features of chronicity. Correlation of acute inflammatory events with degranulation of mast cells and accumulation of eosinophils is strong evidence that an immediate (type I) hypersensitivity is involved. Further support for this hypothesis has been provided by experimental production of closely similar lesions by repeated intranasal exposure of cattle to powdered ovalbumin. In view of the varied components of chronic lesions, however, it is probable that other classes of hypersensitivity (types III and IV) also play some role. It is believed that the condition is due to hypersensitivity to a variety of plant pollens or fungal spores. Because there appears to be a familial predisposition in Jersey cattle and to a limited extent in other cattle, the existence of susceptible atopic animals has been proposed. The condition is therefore sometimes referred to as atopic rhinitis.

Less commonly, nasal granulomas in cattle are attributable to fungal infection. They also occur mostly in the anterior portion of the nasal cavity but tend to be larger polypoid masses. They frequently have yellow-green cores associated with massive eosinophil accumulation. Histologically, components of the lesions are similar to those previously described for the chronic allergic granulomas, but hyphae and chlamydospores of fungi surrounded by macrophages, giant cells, and eosinophils are present. Various fungi normally saprophytic on plants have been isolated. It is tempting to speculate that the mycotic granulomas represent the small proportion of the more nonspecific allergic granulomas in which the causative allergen is able to vegetate.

Bibliography

Allan, E. M., Gibbs, H. A., and Wiseman, A. Pathological features of bovine nasal granuloma (atopic rhinitis). *Vet Rec* **112:** 222–223, 1983.

Carbonell, P. L. Bovine nasal granuloma: Gross and microscopic lesions. *Vet Pathol* **16:** 60–73, 1979.

Krahwinkel, D. J. *et al.* Familial allergic rhinitis in cattle. *J Am Vet Med Assoc* **192:** 1593–1596, 1988.

Pemberton, D. H., and White, W. E. Bovine nasal granuloma in Victoria. 2. Histopathology of nasal, ocular and oral lesions. *Aust Vet J* **50:** 89–97, 1974.

Pemberton, D. H., White, W. E., and Hore, D. E. Bovine nasal granuloma (atopic rhinitis) in Victoria, experimental reproduction by the production of immediate type hypersensitivity in the nasal mucosa. *Aust Vet J* **53:** 201–207, 1977.

5. *Granulomatous Rhinitis*

Local damage to nasal mucosa or reduced defenses because of impaired immune responses or other systemic influences make the nasal cavity prey to occasional opportunistic fungal or yeast infections. The range of fungi varies with species of animal affected.

Aspergillus fumigatus is the commonest cause in the dog, but it is rare in other species. The usual lesion is a chronic, necrotizing to granulomatous reaction producing large amounts of friable exudate, which often consists mainly of necrotic fungal hyphae. Viable surface hyphae can sometimes be seen grossly as a blue-green mat. The lesion is slowly aggressive and causes destruction of turbinates and sometimes the nasal septum, but it rarely erodes through the nasal, maxillary, or palatine bones. As with other fungal infections, there is usually suspicion of predisposition by localized or generalized impairment of immunity. Similar lesions can be caused by *Penicillium* spp.

Cryptococcus neoformans is the most frequent cause

of granulomatous rhinitis in cats and also occurs sporadically in horses and dogs and other species. The lesion in cats is more gelatinous than granulomatous, since it consists mainly of massed organisms with their abundant polysaccharide capsular material (Fig. 6.10A,B). Reaction by macrophages, epithelioid cells and lymphocytes is usually minor. Impaired immune responsiveness and ability of the capsular polysaccharide to cause antibody masking and immune paralysis are reasons for the lack of inflammatory response. The lesions are polypoid nodules or more widely space-occupying and slowly destructive masses. In cats, there is often facial swelling. Extension through the bony boundaries of the nasal cavity can involve skin and possibly oral mucosa. Local extension occurs to eyes or brain, and occasionally there is wider dissemination to local lymph nodes and lung or a variety of visceral organs (see Pulmonary Mycoses, Section VI,H,6 of this chapter).

Actinomycosis and actinobacillosis, the latter in sheep especially, sometimes involve or are limited to the nasal cavities. The incidence of nasal and facial actinobacillosis in sheep is highest in drought-feeding conditions, probably as a result of injury to the lips. Caseous fistulating tracts in the subcutis and nasal submucosa are the usual manifestations.

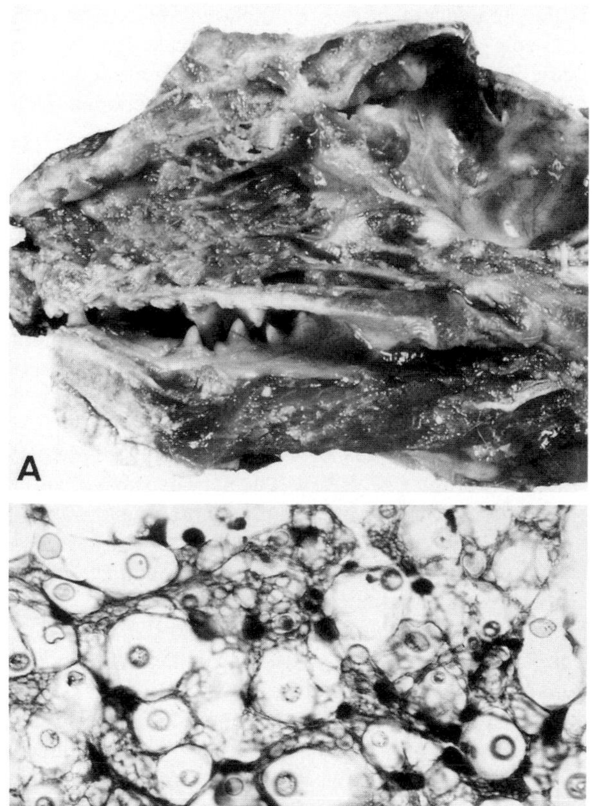

Fig. 6.10 Cryptococcosis. Cat. (A) Filling of nasal passages and obliteration of turbinates. (B) *Cryptococcus neoformans* surrounded by clear zones of unstained capsular material.

Zygomycotic infections of horses are uncommon ulcerative, granulomatous lesions of the nasal and facial regions, particularly the nostril. They are limited to warm climates and are caused by fungi in the *Conidiobolus* or *Basidiobolus* genera. *Conidiobolus incongruus,* a common soil saprophyte, is often responsible for destructive granulomatous rhinitis in Australian sheep in seasons of unseasonable summer rains. There is massive swelling and distortion, usually unilateral, of the maxillary region. There is extensive destruction of turbinates, palate, and facial bones by necrotizing and granulomatous inflammation in which the fungus is easily demonstrated.

Rhinosporidiosis in animals is a chronic polypous rhinitis caused by *Rhinosporidium seeberi*. The disease occurs in horses and cattle, and to a lesser extent in dogs, goats, and waterfowl. It also occurs in humans, sometimes in a more generalized form. The disease is endemic in India and Sri Lanka, and it is sporadic in some other tropical and subtropical countries.

Rhinosporidium seeberi grows *in vitro* only in cell cultures. Its mode of transmission is unknown, and knowledge of its life cycle is sketchy. The definitive stage is the sporangium, which has a diameter of 100–400 μm and is visible to the naked eye as a white spot in the lesions or squash preparations. The sporangia have thick, double-contoured, chitinous walls and contain numerous spherical sporangiospheres ~7 μm in diameter. The mature sporangium releases the sporangiospheres into tissue or into the nasal discharge, and these in turn form new sporangia to complete the cycle.

The source of the organism is unknown; the only recognized association of infection is with proximity to water. Initiation of the disease is thought to be influenced by local trauma to the nasal mucosa; an association has been observed between rhinosporidiosis and the nasal lesions produced by *Schistosoma nasalis,* as well as with punctures of the nasal septum for nose leads in draught oxen.

The lesion is a polyp, usually single and unilateral. The polyps range from sessile to pedunculated and cauliflowerlike. They vary in size up to a diameter of 2–3 cm. They are soft, pink, and bleed easily because of their insubstantial myxomatous nature. On section, the sporangia may be visible grossly. Histologically, the bulk of the polyp consists of a stroma of fibrous or fibromyxoid tissue covered by usually intact epithelium. The organisms are present in the stromal tissues as spherical bodies of various sizes. There is scant reaction to them except when sporangia rupture. Then there is a granulomatous and occasionally a neutrophilic response.

Bibliography

Bridges, C. H. Maduromycosis of bovine nasal mucosa (nasal granuloma of cattle). *Cornell Vet* **50:** 468–483, 1960.

Harvey, C. E. *et al.* Nasal penicilliosis in six dogs. *J Am Vet Med Assoc* **178:** 1084–1087, 1981.

Humber, R. A., Brown, C. C., and Kornegay, R. W. Equine

zygomycosis caused by *Conidiobolus lamprauges*. *J Clin Microbiol* **27:** 573–576, 1989.

Londero, A. T., Santos, M. N., and Freitas, C. J. B. Animal rhinosporidiosis in Brazil. Report of three additional cases. *Mycopathologia* **60:** 171–173, 1977.

McKenzie, R. A., and Connole, M. D. Mycotic nasal granuloma in cattle. *Aust Vet J* **53:** 268–270, 1977.

Roberts, E. D., McDaniel, H. A., and Carbrey, E. A. Maduromycosis of the bovine nasal mucosa. *J Am Vet Med Assoc* **142:** 42–48, 1963.

Roberts, M. C., Sutton, R. H., and Lovell, D. K. A protracted case of cryptococcal nasal granuloma in a stallion. *Aust Vet J* **57:** 287–291, 1981.

Wilkinson, G. T., Sutton, R. H., and Grono, L. R. *Aspergillus* spp. infection associated with orbital cellulitis and sinusitis in a cat. *J Small Anim Pract* **23:** 127–131, 1982.

Wysmann, E. Ueber Aspergillosen beim Rind. *Schweiz Arch Tierheilkd* **83:** 166–171, 1941.

E. Parasitic Diseases of the Nasal Cavity and Sinuses

1. Myiasis

The larvae of a number of flies of the family Oestridae are parasites of nasal cavities of domestic animals. *Cephalopina titillator* deposits its larvae in the nasal passages of camels. Species of the genus *Cephenomyia* are the head bots of deer. *Rhinoestrus purpureus,* the Russian gadfly, is parasitic in horses. Its larvae can also be found in the conjunctival sac. The life cycles and effects of each of these parasites are similar to those of their most ubiquitous relative, the nasal bot of sheep, *Oestrus ovis*.

The first-stage larvae of *Oestrus ovis* are deposited by the flies on the nares, and molt twice as they migrate through the nasal passages. Larvae which find their way through small openings into sinuses or recesses of turbinates are unable to leave after they have grown, so they remain and eventually die there. Development in the nasal passages can take as long as 10 months, although larvae deposited early in summer are able to mature in that season. Pupation occurs on the ground.

The larvae attach themselves to the mucous membrane by their mouth parts. They produce mucosal defects at the points of attachment and, since the cuticle is spinous, a more general irritation as they move about. Affected sheep develop a catarrhal rhinitis with a sometimes copious discharge. Irritation of the mucosa of the sinuses, especially the frontal, can cause a gelatinous hypertrophy of the mucous membrane, which may almost obliterate the sinus. Apart from persistent annoyance and the debility that this may cause, there are seldom untoward effects of the parasitism. Sometimes larvae penetrate the cranial cavity, and secondary bacterial infections spread from the olfactory mucosa to the meninges; such complications are rare. Mild infestations of *Oestrus ovis* occur in goats pastured with affected sheep.

2. Linguatulosis

The cause is *Linguatula serrata,* a tongue-shaped parasite considered by most to be a degenerate arthropod. Males are ~2 cm in length and females, 10–12 cm; the parasite has cosmopolitan distribution. The definitive hosts are carnivores, but in aberrant parasitisms, herbivores and humans may be host to the final stage. Herbivorous animals are the intermediate hosts, and the nymphs can be detected in their mesenteric lymph nodes. Carnivores are infected by eating the infected viscera of herbivores, and the nymphs migrate to the nasal passages and mature. The parasites may be found anywhere in the nasal cavity, and occasionally they find their way into the paranasal sinuses or pass via the Eustachian tube to the inner ear. They lie on the surface of the nasal mucosa and produce, at most, nasal irritation and a catarrhal to lightly bloodstained exudate.

The gravid females discharge a large number of eggs, which are removed by sneezing. The larvae develop in the alimentary tract of the intermediate host and migrate to the mesenteric nodes and other organs where they encyst and develop into the infective nymphs. The cysts are common in mesenteric nodes of cattle and sheep in some countries. They appear as small cysts containing brownish fluid; older lesions may calcify and resemble tubercles.

3. Miscellaneous Parasitisms

Schistosoma nasalis, a cause of granulomatous rhinitis in cattle, goats, and horses in India, is described with other species of the genus in The Cardiovascular System (Volume 3, Chapter 1). The only other trematode that is normally parasitic in the upper respiratory tract of animals is *Troglotrema acutum,* a European parasite of mink, skunks, and foxes. The first and second intermediate hosts are snails and frogs, respectively. The adult parasites occur in the paranasal sinuses. In foxes, they are attached to the mucous membrane. In mink and skunks, however, they lie in cysts beneath the mucosa. The cysts, which also contain the eggs, are formed by suppurative granulation tissue. The reaction extends to cause a local rarefying osteomyelitis which may eventually perforate and release purulent discharge into the cranial cavity, into the nasal cavity, or to the exterior.

The larvae of the genus *Habronema* may be deposited by flies in the anterior nares. The larvae subsequently burrow through the skin and produce granulomas similar to those of cutaneous habronemiasis. *Capillaria aerophila,* whose final habitat is the tracheobronchial system of carnivores, is found occasionally in the nasal passages and frontal sinuses. The leeches *Limnatis nilotica* and *L. africana* are taken in while drinking and attach to the mucosa of the pharynx and nasopharynx. They suck large quantities of blood, but the emergency caused by their presence depends on the development of large edematous swellings in the affected areas, which lead to dyspnea and, in severe cases, asphyxiation. The nematode *Syngamus nasicola* is found in the nasal passages of ruminants in tropical countries.

The mite *Pneumonyssoides* (*Pneumonyssus*) *caninum* is occasionally found in the nasal passages and sinuses of dogs. It is usually an incidental finding not associated with signs or development of lesions, but there are occasional reports of the mites causing catarrhal rhinitis and sinusitis with sneezing, and one in which they were associated with bronchitis.

Bibliography

Buckley, J. J. C. On *Syngamus nasicola* from sheep and cattle in the West Indies. *J Helminthol* **12:** 47–62, 1934.

Krishna, L., Charan, K., and Paliwal, D. P. Pathological study on the larval forms of *Linguatula serrata* infection in goats. *Ind Vet J* **50:** 317–318, 1973.

Patnaik, M. M. A note on bovine syngamosis *Ind Vet J* **40:** 272–274, 1963.

Sinclair, K. B. The incidence and life cycle of *Linguatula serrata* (Frohlich 1789) in Great Britain. *J Comp Pathol* **64:** 371–383, 1954.

F. Neoplastic Diseases of the Nasal Cavity and Sinuses

With the exception of endemic ethmoidal tumors to be described subsequently, primary sinonasal tumors are uncommon. They occur frequently enough, however, to be an important entity in dogs and, to a lesser extent, in cats and horses. There is no clear relationship between frequency of nasal tumors in various breeds of dogs and lengths of their noses. The breeds with significantly increased risk, such as collie and German shepherd, do have long noses, however, and this has led to the generalization that dolichocephalic breeds as a whole are at greater risk. Origin from the nasal cavity is usual in dogs and cats, but in horses tumors of the paranasal sinuses arise almost as frequently as those from the nasal cavity. Any of the tissues forming the lining or present in the boundaries of the nasal cavity and sinuses can give rise to either benign or malignant tumors. In general, most are carcinomas, followed in decreasing frequency by sarcomas of cartilage, fibrous tissue, or bone (Fig. 6.11). The precise mix of types varies according to species.

Epithelial tumors of the nasal cavity and sinuses are classified as follows:

- Papilloma
- Adenoma
- Carcinoma
  - Squamous cell (epidermoid) carcinoma
    - Spindle cell variant
  - Transitional carcinoma
  - Adenocarcinoma
  - Mucoepidermoid carcinoma
  - Adenoid cystic carcinoma
  - Undifferentiated (anaplastic) carcinoma
- Olfactory neuroblastoma

Squamous cell carcinomas predominate in the cat and horse. In the cat, a large proportion originate from the nasal vestibule, whereas in the horse the maxillary sinus is a common site (Fig. 6.11A). It is speculated that the latter may arise from epithelial remnants in dental alveoli. Transitional carcinomas are the most common in dogs, with lower numbers of squamous cell carcinomas (Fig. 6.11B), adenocarcinomas, and undifferentiated carcinomas occurring in about equal frequency.

Transitional carcinomas are so called because they assume the stratified cuboidal appearance of transitional epithelium (Fig. 6.11C). Because of their characteristic appearance they are sometimes referred to as respiratory epithelial carcinomas and, in the literature on human nasal tumors, they are often classified as nonkeratinizing squamous cell tumors. Transitional carcinomas typically consist of thick stratified layers of mostly cuboidal cells with rounded nuclei, indistinct cell borders, and a distinct basement membrane beneath the layer of neoplastic cells (Fig. 6.11D). Large transitional carcinomas have complex infolding or pleating of the thick epithelial bands separated by delicate fibrovascular septa. Small microcysts are sometimes present within the epithelial layers. Because the microcysts have a resemblance to glandular acini, their very obvious presence can lead to transitional carcinomas being classified as adenocarcinomas. Adenocarcinomas, however, have a predominance of papillary fronds and glandular acini formed by a single layer of cuboidal to tall columnar cells with a basement membrane, unlike the microcysts of the transitional tumor, which are within a thick layer of tumor cells. Mucin-filled acini are a fairly common feature of adenocarcinomas.

Adenoid cystic carcinomas are rare tumors with a multilobular organization and at least some lobules with a characteristic striking cribriform pattern. Possibly these tumors arise from salivary gland tissue in the soft palate rather than from nasal epithelial structures.

Undifferentiated carcinomas are mostly solid tumors in which there are large packets or nodules of round to polygonal cells with no discernible pattern. Unless multiple sampling reveals regions with a pattern resembling one of the more differentiated types of carcinoma, special methods are needed to separate these tumors from others such as olfactory neuroblastomas, amelanotic malignant melanomas, lymphoreticular tumors, and poorly differentiated mast cell tumors.

Carcinomas with mixed phenotypic expression are fairly common, especially if multiple sections are examined. Transitional carcinomas sometimes have scattered foci of squamous metaplasia or adenocarcinomatous regions. Mucoepidermoid carcinomas have mucin-filled acinar components and foci with usual features of squamous cell carcinoma. Both glandular and squamous elements must fulfill criteria for malignancy.

The olfactory neuroblastoma (esthesioneuroblastoma, esthesioneuroepithelioma) is a rare tumor which mostly arises in the ethmoturbinate region of the caudal nasal cavity. Penetration of the cribriform plate and into the cerebral cortex is commonly observed. Most of the reported tumors have occurred in cats. It is unclear whether they arise from one or more of olfactory neuroepithelial

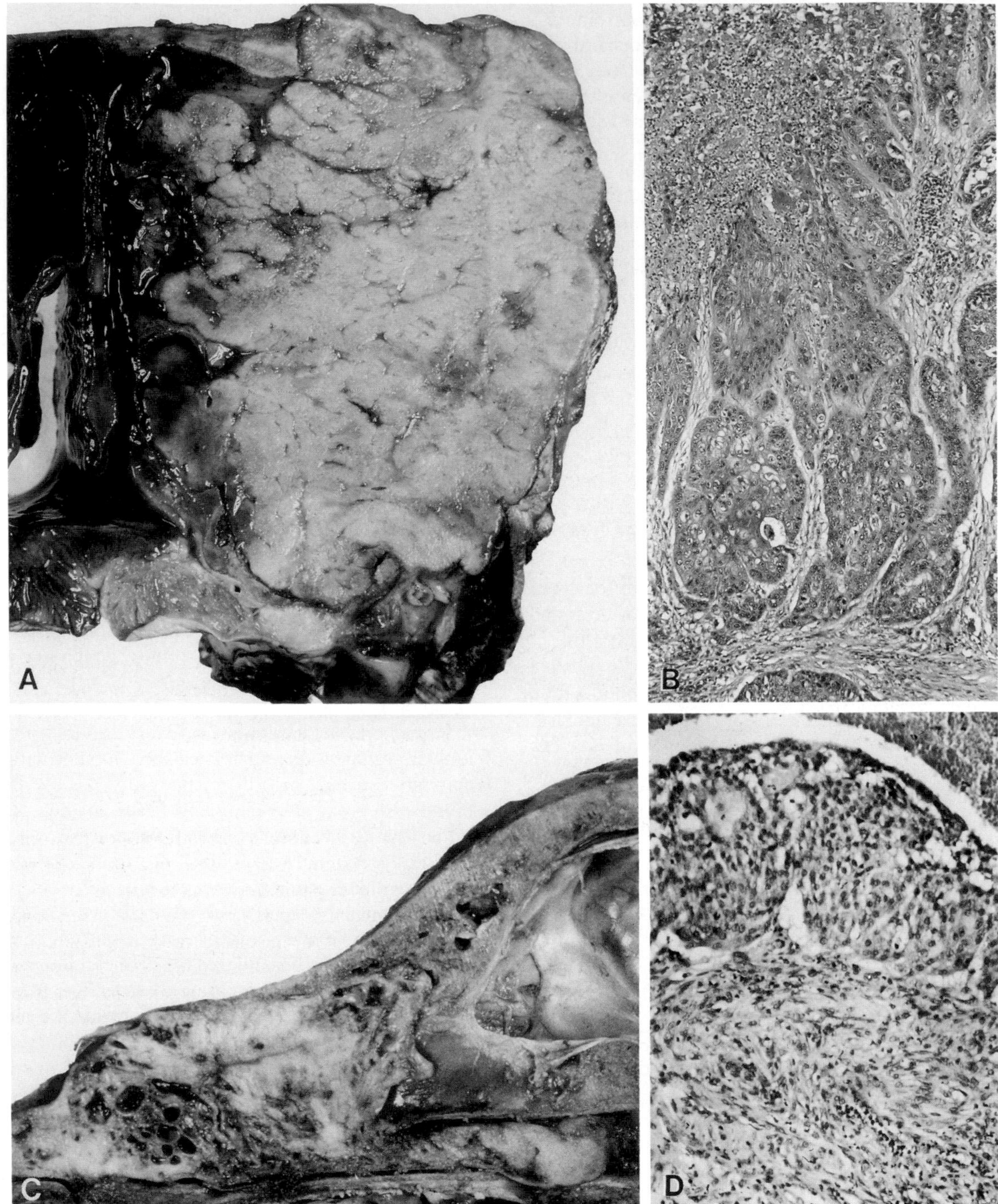

Fig. 6.11 (A) Squamous cell carcinoma of maxillary sinus. Horse. (B) Squamous cell carcinoma of nasal cavity. Dog. (C) Chondrosarcoma filling nasal cavity and extending into caudal nares. Dog. (D) Transitional carcinoma of nasal cavity with chronic inflammation and fibroplasia of lamina propria. Dog.

cells, remaining neural crest cells, or local components of the dispersed neuroendocrine system. Despite some morphologic variation, the tumors are typically highly cellular and consist of a uniform population of round to elongated cells with moderately dense nuclei and small amounts of cytoplasm. An important diagnostic feature is the presence of palisading around vessels and rosette formation. In the absence of these features, the olfactory neuroblastoma is not distinguishable on routine examination from lymphoreticular tumors or undifferentiated tumors of various origins. Definitive diagnosis, in any event, requires ultrastructural and immunocytochemical examinations. The presence of feline leukemia virus in feline olfactory neuroblastomas raises questions concerning the possible causative role of the virus. In dogs, paranasal meningiomas are uncommon tumors which develop as intranasal masses replacing ethmoturbinates and the cribriform plate and usually invading the olfactory region of the brain.

The tendency of the stroma of large, more rapidly growing sinonasal tumors to become edematous can result in difficulty in distinguishing the more undifferentiated carcinomas and sarcomas. Regardless of histogenetic type, malignant nasal tumors tend to be soft, pale, and fleshy to friable masses which slowly invade and destroy adjacent structures but rarely metastasize.

Endemic, or clustered, occurrence of tumors of the ethmoturbinate region in animals has been recognized in many countries for most of the century. Clustered cases have been reported in sheep from Germany, Spain, Canada, France, and the United States of America; goats from India, Spain, and France; cattle from Scandinavia, Brazil, India, and South Africa; pigs from Brazil, India, and China; and horses from Scandinavia. The endemicity depends on the observations that multiple cases occur in a few flocks and herds and may continue to occur over several years, and that more than one species can be affected on individual farms. The incidence patterns encourage the view that the neoplasms are caused by a virus, and success has been claimed for experimental transmission in sheep. Viral particles which structurally resemble retroviruses (type C particles) have been demonstrated electron-microscopically in the tumors from cattle, goats, and sheep, but a role for these viruses is not established. In view of the fact that jaagsiekte (pulmonary adenomatosis) in sheep is caused by a retrovirus, the virus must be considered a candidate.

The tumors in sheep are adenopapillomas or adenocarcinomas, and arise from the olfactory mucosa of the turbinate region. Ultrastructural evidence indicates their origin from sustentacular cells of olfactory mucosa or the dark cells of Bowman's glands. Histologic descriptions are consistent for the several species. The tumors are locally aggressive and destructive space-occupying lesions. Metastases to regional lymph nodes are reported in cattle.

Bibliography

Bradley, P. A., and Harvey, C. E. Intra-nasal tumours in the dog: An evaluation of prognosis. *J Small Anim Pract* **14:** 459–467, 1973.

Cohrs, P. Infektiose Adenopapillome der Riechschleimhaut beim Schaf. *Berl Muench Tieraerztl Wochenschr* **66:** 225–228, 1953.

Confer, A. W., and De Paoli, A. Primary neoplasms of the nasal cavity, paranasal sinuses and the nasopharynx in the dog: A report of 16 cases from the files of the AFIP. *Vet Pathol* **15:** 18–30, 1978.

Cox, N. R., and Powers, R. D. Olfactory neuroblastomas in two cats. *Vet Pathol* **26:** 341–343, 1989.

Hultgren, B. D. *et al.* Nasal–maxillary fibrosarcoma in young horses: A light and electron microscopic study. *Vet Pathol* **24:** 194–196, 1987.

Kuscher, A., Pommer, A., and Kment, A. Zur kasuistik bosartiger Neubildungen im Luftsack des Pferdes. *Berl Muench Tieraerztl Wochenschr/Wien Tieraerztl Mschr* **60**/31: 53–56, 1944.

Madewell, B. R. *et al.* Neoplasms of the nasal passages and paranasal sinuses in domesticated animals as reported by 13 veterinary colleges. *Am J Vet Res* **37:** 851–856, 1976.

McKinnon, A. O. *et al.* Enzootic nasal adenocarcinoma of sheep in Canada. *Can Vet J* **23:** 88–94, 1982.

Nair, M. K. *et al.* Viruslike particles in tumors of the mucosa of the ethmoid in Indian cattle. *Acta Vet Scand* **22:** 143–145, 1981.

Nieberle, K. Uber endemischen Krebs im Siebbein von Schafen. *Z Krebsforsch* **49:** 137–141, 1939.

Njoku, C. O. *et al.* Ovine nasal adenopapilloma: Incidence and clinicopathologic studies. *Am J Vet Res* **39:** 1850–1852, 1978.

Patnaik, A. K. *et al.* Paranasal meningioma in the dog: A clinicopathologic study of ten cases. *Vet Pathol* **23:** 362–368, 1986.

Pospischil, A., Haenichen, T., and Schaeffler, H. Histological and electron-microscopic studies of endemic ethmoidal carcinomas in cattle. *Vet Pathol* **16:** 180–190, 1979.

Pospischil, A. *et al.* Endemic ethmoidal tumour in cattle: Sarcoma and carcinosarcomas: A light- and electron-microscopic study. *Zentralblt Veterinaermed (A)* **29:** 628–636, 1982.

Schrenzel, M. D. *et al.* Type C retroviral expression in spontaneous feline olfactory neuroblastomas. *Acta Neuropathol* **80:** 547–553, 1990.

Stunzi, H., and Hauser, B. Tumours of the nasal cavity. *Bull WHO* **53:** 257–263, 1976.

Yonemichi, H. *et al.* Intranasal tumor of the ethmoid olfactory mucosa in sheep. *Am J Vet Res* **39:** 1599–1606, 1978.

Young, S. *et al.* Neoplasms of the olfactory mucous membrane of sheep. *Cornell Vet* **51:** 96–112, 1961.

III. Pharynx and Guttural Pouches

The pharynx, being common to upper respiratory and alimentary systems, shares the misfortunes of both. Because of the complicated organogenesis of the region, various congenital malformations are occasionally encountered. Most attention is drawn to defects in the dog and horse. In the dog, the excess of soft tissue over the skeletal framework, which occurs in brachycephalic breeds, leads to a variety of conditions of which excessive length of the soft palate, eversion of laryngeal saccules, and laryngeal collapse are most common. In the horse, complications are signaled by exercise intolerance and associated noisy respiration. Subepiglottic cysts, believed to arise from thyroglossal duct remnants, and entrapment of the epiglottis appear to be most frequent. Entrapment of the epiglottis below the aryepiglottic fold in horses is usually associated with congenital hypoplasia of the epiglottis or acquired shortening or distortion of the structure. A short epiglottis also predisposes to dorsal displacement of the soft palate, and sometimes epiglottic entrapment and dorsal displacement of the palate occur together.

A posterior diverticulum of the pharynx lies immediately dorsal to the esophagus in pigs. In young pigs, awns of barley and similar foreign materials occasionally lodge in the diverticulum and cause inflammation. The local reaction may cause dysphagia and death from starvation.

In some cases, the pharyngeal wall is perforated, and an ultimately fatal cellulitis spreads down the fascial planes of the neck. Perforation of the posterior dorsal wall of the pharynx by drenching guns occurs in sheep and is usually fatal.

Pharyngeal inflammation is a part of inflammatory diseases affecting the upper respiratory system, upper alimentary system, or both. These have been covered elsewhere. An entity deserving of brief mention here is **equine chronic pharyngitis with lymphoid hyperplasia.** It is detected mostly by endoscopy in Thoroughbred race horses <5 years of age. In its most severe manifestation, there are polypoid projections in the dorsolateral boundaries of the pharynx with prominent white plaques or nodules representing lymphoid aggregates. The extent of lymphoid hyperplasia found in biopsies sometimes raises the suspicion of neoplastic proliferation, but follicular structure is retained, and there is a predominance of mature lymphocytes. It is presumed to be due to continued lymphoproliferative stimulus by a combination of persistent bacterial agents, possibly aided by excessive drying or other factors, such as viral infections, leading to reduced local defenses. *Streptococcus zooepidemicus* and *Moraxella* spp. have been linked to severe grades of involvement. Equine lymphofollicular pharyngitis is the equine analog of adenoids in children.

The **guttural pouches** of Equidae are ventral diverticula of the Eustachian tubes. They tend to become involved in inflammatory processes in analogous fashion to the paranasal sinuses. Complications differ, however, because severe guttural pouch inflammation can extend to involve nearby cranial nerves (VII, IX, X, XI, XII), vessels, and the cranial sympathetic trunk, or even spread to adjacent bones, middle ear, brain, or atlanto–occipital joint. Suppurative inflammation leading to empyema occurs mostly after upper respiratory infections, particularly with *Streptococcus equi* or other streptococci. Fibrinous or fibrinonecrotic (diphtheritic) inflammation is usually associated with fungal infection, generally *Aspergillus* spp., particularly *Aspergillus nidulans,* and hence is commonly referred to as **guttural pouch mycosis.** Fibrinonecrotic inflammation is highly suggestive of, but not pathognomonic for, fungal infection unless there is visible evidence of mycelial growth. Because the fibrinonecrotic inflammation extends deeply, and fungi when present can frequently invade vessels and other structures, severe complications are much more likely to follow than from guttural pouch empyema. Examples are thrombosis, aneurysm formation, and rupture of the internal carotid artery with epistaxis, ischemic lesions, or osteitis, and fusion of stylohyoid and petrous temporal bones. A less common condition is **guttural pouch tympany.** This is seen mostly in young animals, and the accumulation of air is presumed to be due to valvular action of the nasopharyngeal orifice of the Eustachian tube. Tumors of the guttural pouches are rare, but when encountered are most likely to be squamous cell carcinomas. Pharyngeal tumors are discussed with neoplasia of the mouth (The Alimentary System, Chapter 1 of this volume).

Bibliography

Boles, C. L., Raker, C. W., and Wheat, J. D. Epiglottic entrapment by arytenoepiglottic folds in the horse. *J Am Vet Med Assoc* **172:** 338–342, 1978.

Cook, W. R., Campbell, R. S. F., and Dawson, C. O. The pathology and aetiology of guttural pouch mycosis in the horse. *Vet Rec* **83:** 422–428, 1968.

Haynes, P. F. Persistent dorsal displacement of the soft palate associated with epiglottic shortening in two horses. *J Am Vet Med Assoc* **179:** 677–681, 1981.

Hoquet, F. *et al.* Comparison of the bacterial and fungal flora in the pharynx of normal horses and horses affected with pharyngitis. *Can Vet J* **26:** 342–346, 1985.

Koch, D. B., and Tate, L. P. Pharyngeal cysts in horses. *J Am Vet Med Assoc* **173:** 860–863, 1978.

Raker, C. W., and Boles, E. L. Pharyngeal lymphoid hyperplasia in the horse. *J Equine Med Surg* **2:** 202–207, 1978.

Wheeldon, E. B., Suter, P. R., and Jenkins, T. Neoplasia of the larynx in the dog. *J Am Vet Med Assoc* **180:** 642–647, 1982.

IV. Larynx and Trachea

A. Congenital Anomalies

Congenital anomalies of the larynx are rare. Hypoplasia of the epiglottis has been observed in horses and swine. Partial or complete agenesis of the trachea is a rare finding. Tracheal hypoplasia characterized by reduction in the luminal diameter of the entire trachea, sometimes associated with bronchial hypoplasia, occurs in dogs. The higher frequency in English bulldogs indicates the possibility of an inherited basis. Malformations of the cross-sectional shape, mostly in the form of tracheal collapse, are important in the dog and occur in the horse, cow, and goat. Tracheal collapse in dogs occurs principally in miniature breeds. The trachea becomes flattened dorsoventrally. The cartilages form shallow arcs, and the dorsal tracheal membrane is widened and flaccid. The membrane is thin in uncomplicated cases but becomes thickened when there is chronic or periodic acute tracheitis. These are frequent complications of the mechanical obstruction. The nature of the basic defect is still unclear. It may be a manifestation of a more generalized chondrodysplasia in toy breeds. A major feature is focal hypocellularity of cartilage and areas of replacement by fibrous tissue. Reduction of chondroitin sulfate and calcium are associated with reduction in density of chondrocytes. Thus far, however, the basic defect has not been identified.

In horses, lateral compression of the trachea produces the so-called "scabbard" trachea. In this species also, a scroll-like curling may affect the ends of the cartilages.

Acquired malformations of the trachea are caused by external pressure, in most cases from enlarged thyroid glands or regional lymph nodes, or inflammatory or neoplastic lesions within the wall.

B. Laryngeal Paralysis

Unilateral or bilateral paralysis of the larynx is the most common cause of abnormal respiratory noise (roaring) in horses. The condition is almost always a left-sided hemiplegia and is due to degeneration of the left recurrent laryngeal nerve. Resulting denervation atrophy affects all intrinsic laryngeal muscles supplied by this nerve, but not all are affected equally. The most obvious atrophy occurs in the cricoarytenoid muscle, which may be reduced to fascial remnants. Atrophy of the other muscles is less severe and is indicated by pallor and a reduction in size. The cricothyroid muscle, which is supplied by the cranial laryngeal nerve, is the only intrinsic muscle not affected. The cricoarytenoid muscle is the main abductor of the larynx. As a result of its paresis and atrophy, the left arytenoid cartilage sags into the lumen, thus interfering with airflow, particularly during the inspiration associated with severe exercise.

In cases detected clinically, microscopic examination reveals severe loss of myelinated fibers in middle and distal portions of the left recurrent laryngeal nerve. Less obvious loss occurs in subclinical cases. Ultrastructural features indicate progressive loss of fibers in the left recurrent nerve accompanied by chronic demyelination, remyelination, and abortive regenerative attempts. Similar but milder changes can be detected electron-microscopically in the distal right recurrent nerve. The reasons for the axonal disease are still disputed. The axons in the left recurrent laryngeal nerve are much longer than those in the right recurrent nerve, and this presumably makes them more susceptible to damage. The extent to which damage is caused by traumatic interruption of axoplasmic flow, neuritis by extension from guttural pouch disease, vitamin deficiency, or neurotoxins has still to be established. It is unlikely that there is a single cause, as evidenced by the circumstantial implication of delayed neurotoxicity by oral haloxon administration as a cause in Arabian foals. Another organophosphate, trichlorfon, also is linked circumstantially with an incident of left recurrent laryngeal nerve degeneration in horses.

Denervation atrophy of laryngeal muscles occurs occasionally in dogs, mostly in old, large, or giant breeds, and particularly in males. It is usually bilateral. The causes are not clear, but it can be associated with lesions in the recurrent laryngeal nerves or be part of generalized neuromuscular disease. Occasionally it is secondary to hypothyroidism. The condition appears to follow a hereditary degeneration of the nucleus ambiguus in the Bouvier des Flandres. Laryngeal paralysis occurs rarely in the cat.

C. Circulatory Disturbances

Active hyperemia occurs in acute inflammation, which is common. Laryngeal hemorrhages particularly affect the mucous membrane on the dorsal surface of the epiglottis and occur in many septicemic diseases. They are of some diagnostic significance in salmonellosis of swine and hog cholera. The hemorrhagic speckling of the tracheal mucosa in slaughtered cattle is produced by small extravasations in the submucosal lymphoid follicles. In cattle that die with severe dyspnea, and to a lesser extent in sheep, these follicular hemorrhages spread in a linear form. In severe cases, the whole mucosa is red-black. The hemorrhages are reflected in the regional lymph nodes, which are also red-black, firm, and enlarged.

Edema of the larynx is usually inflammatory and part of acute respiratory infections, or caused by inhalation of irritant materials, local trauma, or inflammation (Fig. 6.12). Mild edema of the glottis is occasionally observed in edema disease of swine. Edema occurs in cattle with acute interstitial pneumonia. It is also observed in cattle as part of a rapidly developing edema of the face and throat; this latter syndrome is probably of allergic origin, and it responds well to antihistamines. If neglected, it leads to asphyxiation. Laryngeal edema can also be part of the localized anaphylactic response to insect stings in most species. Edema of the fauces and larynx occurs in equine purpura hemorrhagica and in the same species as a response to the leech *Limnatis nilotica* or to lead poisoning.

The amount of edema varies, but in any case is most severe in the region of the epiglottis, the aryepiglottic folds, and the ventricles. Severe cases are obvious; mild cases show a soft swelling of the mucosa. The edema fluid is usually bloodstained when associated with acute

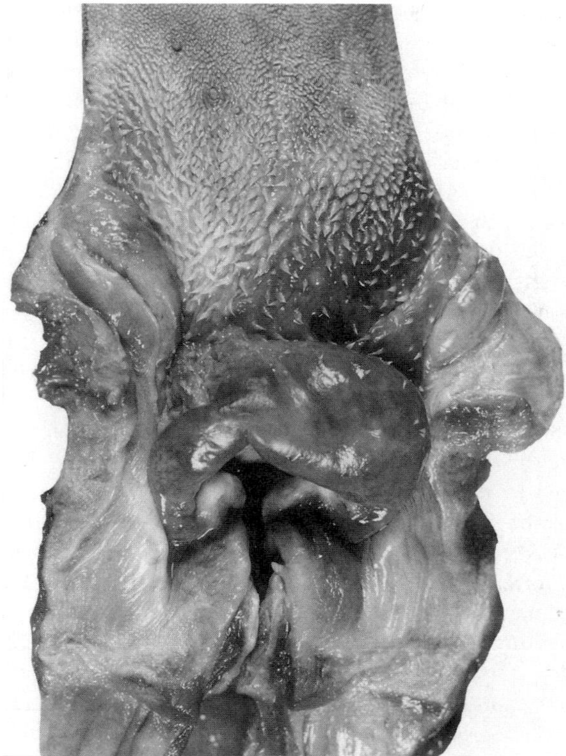

Fig. 6.12 Inflammatory edema of epiglottis associated with abscess in base of tongue. Dog.

inflammation and clear or pale yellow at other times. The fluid may disappear postmortem, but wrinkling of the mucous membrane remains to indicate the prior presence of fluid.

Severe mucosal and submucosal edema of the dorsal region of the distal half of the trachea occasionally causes death by asphyxiation in feedlot cattle. The loud inspiratory noise made by severely affected animals has given rise to the clinical term "honker syndrome." There is correlation with increased respiratory movements brought about by exercise or hot weather, usually in heavy cattle, but it is not known whether the condition is triggered by trauma, tracheal compression, inhalation of dusts, toxins in feed, or a combination of these.

D. Laryngitis and Tracheitis

The location of the larynx and trachea is such that frequently they become inflamed as part of inflammatory diseases of either the upper or lower parts of the respiratory tract. Their involvement in major upper respiratory tract diseases has already been covered. Tracheitis frequently accompanies bronchitis and is sometimes a minor component of pneumonias that do not arise by extension from severe upper respiratory disease. Laryngitis can, however, occur without wider involvement of the respiratory tract (Fig. 6.13). Laryngitis can occur as a part of oral necrobacillosis (calf diphtheria) caused by *Fusobacterium necrophorum* in calves and swine, or it may occur without lesions elsewhere. Laryngeal ulcers or scarred sites of previous ulceration are found in a small proportion of slaughtered feedlot cattle. They occur mainly at points of apposition of vocal processes and medial angles of arytenoid cartilages. It is speculated that mucosal damage by the repeated trauma of laryngeal closure is the main predisposing cause of ulceration. It has also been suggested that *Haemophilus somnus* infection is sometimes a factor. Lesions of acute or chronic diphtheria (*F. necrophorum*) and papillomatosis occur occasionally at the same sites and are believed to develop secondary to mucosal ulceration.

Laryngeal chondritis occurs in sheep, calves, and young horses. It is characterized by necrosis and ulceration of laryngeal mucosa over or just caudal to the vocal cord and the presence of a purulent tract leading to abscessation within the arytenoid cartilage. There is usually a more generalized laryngeal edema which is responsible for severe clinical signs and possibly death. The disease appears to occur most frequently in sheep, particularly in young rams of Texel or Southdown breeds. There is speculation that bulkiness of laryngeal and pharyngeal tissues in these animals predisposes to edema and ulceration of apposing surfaces of vocal cords, with subsequent activity of *Actinomyces pyogenes* and other bacteria leading to arytenoid abscessation.

Small foci of mineralization, often with accompanying granulomatous inflammation, occur in the lamina propria of the dorsal trachea and ventral turbinates of adult pigs, particularly males. A causal association with inhalation of dusty mineral-containing feed has been suggested, but this

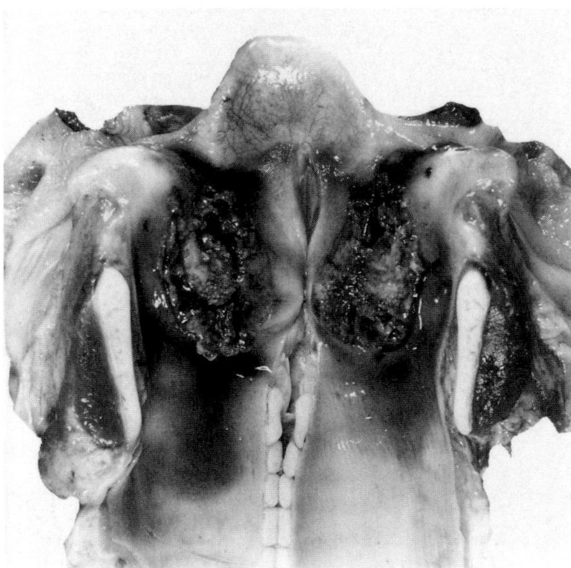

Fig. 6.13 Necrotic laryngitis. Calf.

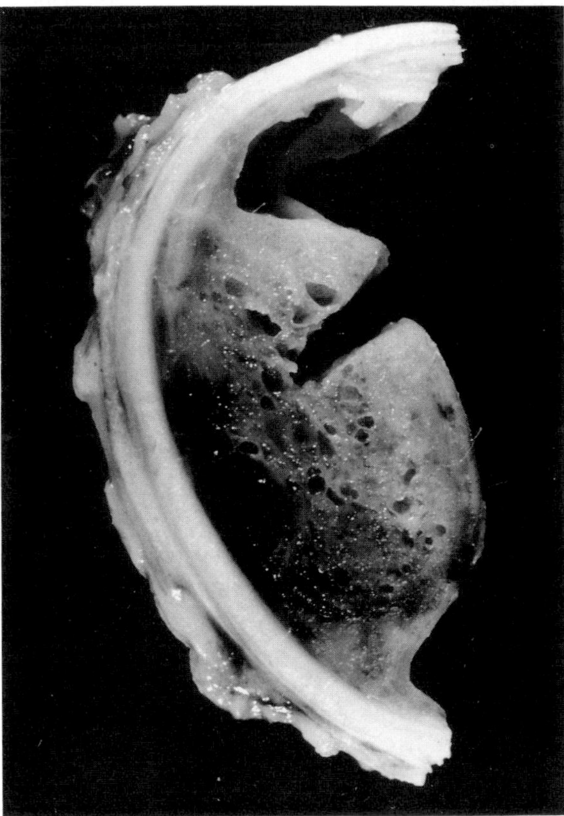

Fig. 6.14 Trachea. Sow. Acute fibrinohemorrhagic inflammation associated with *Streptococcus* sp. (Courtesy of I. W. Wilkie.)

is unlikely. More widespread mineralization is frequently also present in severely affected pigs. A diphtheritic laryngotracheitis caused by untyped streptococci is occasionally observed in pigs and may affect litters of piglets (Fig. 6.14).

A chronic and diffuse tracheitis can develop following tracheotomy. The reaction is most severe adjacent to the wound, the mucosa is swollen, and in the late stages, heavily scarred. Foci of chronic polypoid tracheitis are occasionally observed in dogs and cats. The thickening may be sufficient to cause significant stenosis and dyspnea. The cause is unknown, but the various pathogenetic factors involved are probably similar to those responsible for nasal polyps. Squamous metaplasia of tracheal epithelium is a feature of vitamin A deficiency and severe iodide toxicosis.

E. Parasitic Diseases of Larynx and Trachea

Syngamus laryngeus occurs in the larynx of cattle in tropical Asia and South America.

Capillaria aerophila (*Eucoleus aerophilus*), a relative of the genus *Trichuris,* parasitizes the trachea and bronchi of dogs, foxes, and occasionally, cats. The worms are slender and 2–3 cm long. The eggs are operculate and not easily distinguishable from those of *Trichuris vulpis* of the intestine or *Capillaria plica* of the urinary bladder. The eggs are laid in the airways, move with mucus to the pharynx, are swallowed, and passed in the feces. The larvae develop to the infective stage within the egg and remain there until the egg is swallowed by a suitable host. Hatching occurs in the intestine. The larvae reach the lungs in ~1 week and are mature in the trachea in ~6 weeks.

The effects of *C. aerophila* depend on the numbers present. Mild infestations are inapparent and provoke nothing more than a mild catarrhal inflammation. Heavy infestations cause more severe irritation as well as some obstruction to the lumen of the airways. Chronic coughing and intermittent dyspnea may then be observed, and secondary bacterial bronchopneumonia may occur.

Filaroides osleri is an ovoviviparous, filiform worm 5–15 mm in length. It is found in the dog and related species. The typical lesions are protruding submucosal nodules in the region of the tracheal bifurcation (Fig. 6.15A). The parasite has a wide geographic distribution, but is uncommon and seldom seen. The Filaroididae, unlike other metastrongyloids, do not require an intermediate host. The first-stage larvae of *F. osleri* are directly infective. The thin-walled eggs containing first-stage larvae are coughed up and swallowed and hatch before being passed as infective larvae in the feces. Pups are infected by larvae in the saliva or feces of their dams. *Filaroides osleri* represents a special hazard to wild canids because infection of pups can readily occur during regurgitative feeding. Larvae migrate from gut to lung through the blood.

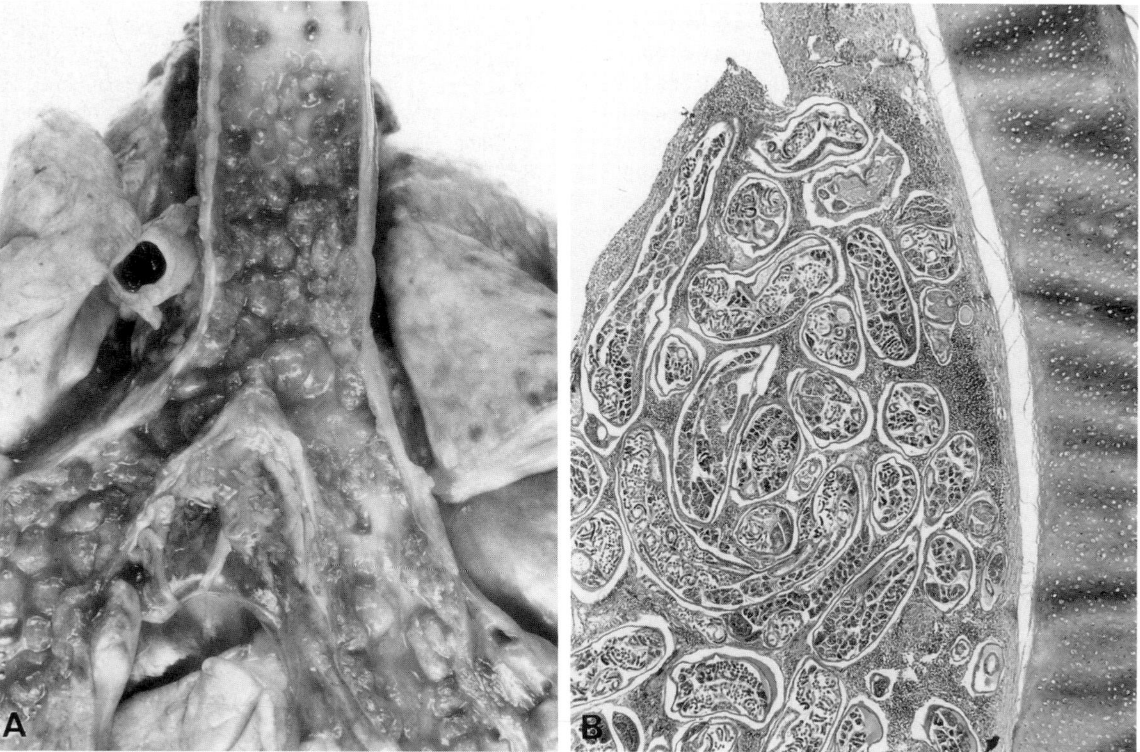

Fig. 6.15 (A) Parasitic tracheobronchitis. Nodules contain coiled *Filaroides osleri*. Dog. (B) Histologic section of nodule in (A) showing cross sections of worms and mononuclear cell reaction.

The lesions vary in size from nodules that are barely visible to larger nodules or plaques which project 1 cm or more into the lumen of the trachea (Fig. 6.15A). The larger masses are oval with the long axis parallel to that of the trachea. The parasites do not typically incite acute bronchitis or tracheitis although they can provoke paroxysmal coughing and dyspnea. The nodules and nodes are gray or whitish, and the worms are visible through the intact overlying mucosa.

The small nodules contain immature worms, and the larger ones contain a mass of tightly coiled adults (Fig. 6.15B). The worms lie in tissue spaces between the cartilage rings of the trachea and large bronchi and in the adventitia and lymphatics. The live worms provoke a minimal reaction consisting of a thin capsule and infiltration of the lamina propria by lymphocytes and plasma cells. Superficially the nodules are covered by intact epithelium except for small pores through which female worms protrude their tails to lay eggs. Dead worms provoke a foreign-body reaction with neutrophils and a few giant cells. Immature worms without significant tissue reaction may be found in the pulmonary lymphatics and occasionally in the alveoli. These immature worms are probably still migrating toward the trachea.

Spirocerca lupi occasionally forms nodules in the trachea or bronchi as an example of aberrant localization.

F. Neoplastic Diseases of Larynx and Trachea

Neoplasms of the larynx and trachea are rare, and information about them is fragmentary. Any tissue in or adjacent to the wall of these structures can give rise to tumors, so a variety of epithelial and mesenchymal tumors have been found. Epithelial tumors are most likely to be papillomas or squamous cell carcinomas. Adenocarcinomas are exceedingly rare. Leiomyomas and rhabdomyosarcomas can arise in or close to the wall. Chondromas or osteochondromas occasionally originate from the laryngeal or tracheal cartilages. The osteochondromas are usually cartilaginous nodules with central endochondral ossification. They are derived from perichondrial proliferation of developmental, inflammatory, or neoplastic basis. It is difficult or impossible to decide what the basic process is in any one tumor. Although it has been argued that the lesions should be classified as osteochondral dysplasias, the term osteochondroma is well established and can be understood to embrace the full range of pathogenetic possibilities. Chondrosarcomas and osteosarcomas are also rare findings. Mucosal involvement in lymphosarcoma or malignant mast cell tumor is an uncommon occurrence in cats and dogs, and deformation or invasion by adjacent neoplasms in the thyroid or lymph nodes has been mentioned.

Oncocytomas are rare benign tumors arising as solitary projecting nodules in or close to the lateral ventricle of the canine larynx, particularly in young dogs. They consist of lobular masses of pleomorphic cells with abundant, deeply eosinophilic, granular or foamy cytoplasm. Ultrastructurally there are numerous mitochondria and intermitochondrial glycogen granules. Oncocytes (oxyphil cells) occur in a variety of endocrine glands and epithelial tissues of humans, and occasionally give rise to tumors. Evidence indicates that they are atypical neuroendocrine cells; hence, oncocytomas are related to carcinoids and other tumors of the dispersed neuroendocrine system. Granular cell tumors and rhabdomyomas also arise in the laryngopharyngeal region of dogs with presentation similar to that of oncocytoma. The distinction between the three tumor types may not be possible by light microscopy; myotubes and cross-striations may not be demonstrable in the rhabdomyomas. Histochemical methods to demonstrate myoglobin and desmin and ultrastructural identification of myofibrils or Z lines distinguish the rhabdomyomas. The granular cell tumors are arranged in strands or clusters insinuated in stroma that may contain amyloid. The granules which are densely packed lysosomes stain with Schiff reagent and Sudan black.

Bibliography

Amis, T. C. Tracheal collapse in the dog. *Aust Vet J* **50:** 285–289, 1974.

Calderwood-Mays, M. B. Laryngeal oncocytoma in two dogs. *J Am Vet Med Assoc* **185:** 677–679, 1984.

Carb, A., and Halliwell, W. H. Osteochondral dysplasias of the canine trachea. *J Am Anim Hosp Assoc* **17:** 193–199, 1981.

Clayton, H. M., and Lindsay, F. E. F. *Filaroides osleri* infection in the dog. *J Small Anim Pract* **20:** 773–782, 1979.

Dallman, M. J., McClure, R. C., and Brown, E. M. Histochemical study of normal and collapsed tracheas in dogs. *Am J Vet Res* **49:** 2117–2125, 1988.

Done, S. H. Canine tracheal collapse—aetiology, pathology, diagnosis, and treatment. *Vet Ann* **18:** 255–260, 1978.

Duncan, I. D. *et al.* A correlation of the endoscopic and pathologic changes in subclinical pathology of the horse's larynx. *Equine Vet J* **9:** 220–225, 1977.

Duncan, I. D., Griffiths, I. R., and Madrid, R. E. A light- and electron-microscopic study of the neuropathy of equine idiopathic laryngeal hemiplegia. *Neuropathol Appl Neurobiol* **4:** 483–501, 1978.

Fau, D. Pathologie chirurgicale du tractus respiratoire superieur du chien. *Rev Med Vet* **132:** 651–660, 1981.

Gaber, C. E., Amis, T. C., and LeCouteur, R. A. Laryngeal paralysis in dogs: A review of 23 cases. *J Am Vet Med Assoc* **186:** 377–380, 1985.

Gilka, F., and Sugden, E. A. Focal mineralization and nonspecific granulomatous inflammation of respiratory mucous membranes in pigs. *Vet Pathol* **18:** 541–548, 1981.

Hardie, E. M. *et al.* Laryngeal paralysis in three cats. *J Am Vet Med Assoc* **179:** 879–882, 1981.

Jensen, R. *et al.* Laryngeal contact ulcers in feedlot cattle. *Vet Pathol* **17:** 667–671, 1980.

Jensen, R. *et al.* Laryngeal diphtheria and papillomatosis in feedlot cattle. *Vet Pathol* **18:** 143–150, 1981.

Lane, J. G. *et al.* Laryngeal chondritis in Texel sheep. *Vet Rec* **121:** 81–84, 1987.

Ligget, A. D., Weiss, R., and Thomas K. L. Canine laryngopharyngeal rhabdomyoma resembling an oncocytoma: Light-microscopic, ultrastructural and comparative studies. *Vet Pathol* **22:** 526–532, 1985.

Mangkoewidjojo, S., Sleight, S. D., and Convey, E. M. Pathologic features of iodide toxicosis in calves. *Am J Vet Res* **41:** 1057–1061, 1980.

O'Brien, J. A. *et al.* Neurogenic atrophy of the laryngeal muscles of the dog. *J Small Anim Pract* **14:** 521–532, 1973.

Pass, D. A. *et al.* Canine laryngeal oncocytomas. *Vet Pathol* **17:** 672–677, 1980.

Pommer, A., and Walzl, H. Die chronisch-polypose Tracheitis bei Katzen. *Wien Tierarztl Mschr* **44:** 129–135, 1957.

Raphel, C. F. Endoscopic findings in the upper respiratory tract of 479 horses. *J Am Vet Med Assoc* **181:** 470–473, 1982.

Rose, R. J., Hartley, W. J., and Baker, W. Laryngeal paralysis in Arabian foals associated with oral haloxon administration. *Equine Vet J* **13:** 171–176, 1981.

Suter, P. F., Colgrove, D. J., and Ewing, G. O. Congenital hypoplasia of the canine trachea. *J Am Anim Hosp Assoc* **8:** 120–127, 1982.

Thurlbeck, W. M. Chronic airflow obstruction. *In* "Pathology of the Lung." W. M. Thurlbeck (ed.), pp. 519–575. New York, Thieme Medical Publishers, 1988.

Urquhart, G. M., Harrett, W. F. H. , and O'Sullivan, J. G. Canine tracheo-bronchitis due to infection with *Filaroides osleri*. *Vet Rec* **66:** 143–144, 1954.

Venker-van Haagen, A. J. Larynxparalyse bij Bouviers en een fokadvies ter preventie. (Laryngeal paralysis in Bouviers Belge des Flandres and breeding advice to prevent this condition.) *Tijdschr Diergeneeskd* **107:** 21–22, 1982.

Venker-van Haagen, A. J. , Hartman, W., and Goedegebuure, S. A. Spontaneous laryngeal paralysis in young Bouviers. *J Am Anim Hosp Assoc* **14:** 714–720, 1978.

V. Bronchi and Bronchioles

Bronchi and bronchioles form the transitional zone between the upper and lower respiratory tract and therefore are often involved either as an extension of severe upper respiratory tract disease or as part of pulmonary disease. Congenital malformations are included with malformations of the lungs, and tumors arising in bronchi are considered with neoplasms of the lung.

A. Bronchitis

Agents inducing acute bronchitis and bronchiolitis usually do so by interacting initially with airway epithelial cells and inducing the stereotypic pattern of injury, sloughing, and epithelial repair (see General Considerations, Section I of this chapter). The most significant immediate pathophysiologic consequence of bronchial and bronchiolar inflammation is airway obstruction. This can result from one or more of intraluminal blockage by infiltration and accumulation of inflammatory exudate, bronchoconstrictive contraction of airway smooth muscle, and thickening of the wall by accumulation of cells and edema in the submucosa.

1. Acute Bronchitis

Morphologic manifestations of acute bronchitis include the same range of inflammation described for upper airways. The exudates may be catarrhal, mucopurulent, fibrinous, fibrinopurulent, or purulent. Epithelial necrosis is often a concurrent finding.

Catarrhal bronchitis is the simplest form of inflammation. Acute, mild irritation of the bronchial mucosa causes discharge of secretion from goblet and serous cells and from such seromucinous glands as are present. Since the types, relative numbers of epithelial secretory cells, and density of the glands differ from species to species, fine details of the response vary accordingly. Hyperemia and edema of the lamina propria accompany the secretory discharge. Ciliated epithelial cells are most sensitive to a wide array of injurious agents and are often the first to undergo necrosis and slough. The usual traffic of leukocytes through the epithelium becomes exaggerated. If the inflammation is transient, the integrity of the epithelium is restored rapidly by proliferation of nonciliated secretory cells and basal cells.

The course of bronchitis after the initial catarrhal phase depends on the nature of the irritant and the duration and severity of exposure. In common bacterial infections, **purulent** or suppurative **bronchitis** occurs, and the exudate in the bronchi becomes characteristically yellowish and viscid. The exuded dead and dying neutrophils collect in the lumen together with mucus and sloughed epithelial cells. **Ulcerative bronchitis** occurs in severe viral or bacterial infections during which large areas of epithelium are destroyed. In bacterial infections, there is often intercurrent purulent bronchitis. **Fibrinonecrotic bronchitis** is characterized by exudate forming a thick, yellow membrane which is firmly attached to many points. Reactions of this severity usually also involve the larynx, trachea, and cranioventral portions of the lungs and are typified by severe cases of infectious bovine rhinotracheitis, but can also be seen in mycotic bronchitis in cattle. Severe **necrotizing bronchitis** can occur in bronchiectasis or as a result of aspiration of foreign materials. In such lesions, the microflora is mixed, and the greenish or brown putrid debris is characteristic.

Severe bronchitis can resolve following removal or neutralization of the offending agent. Repair characterized by complete bronchial epithelial regeneration and only mild fibrosis of the bronchial lamina propria may often follow. In instances of severe or more prolonged injury to epithelium, fibrosis in the lamina propria becomes more prominent with time. Aggregates of lymphocytes, macrophages, and plasma cells in the lamina propria are common sequelae as acute bronchitis progresses through subacute to chronic duration. Prominent lymphofollicular hyperplasia of the bronchial and bronchiolar mucosa is a common feature of chronic mycoplasmal infections. Epithelial hyperplasia may also become prominent with prolonged mucosal injury of any cause. With more severe injury to the mucosa, especially in chronic suppurative reactions, bronchial wall destruction often results (see Bronchiectasis, Section V,B of this chapter). Fibrous polyps obstructing the bronchial lumen are an extremely rare response to severe bronchial mucosal injury.

Mild and limited bronchitis or tracheobronchitis rarely

causes death and is observed mainly as a clinical problem. **Infectious tracheobronchitis** (kennel cough) in dogs is an example of persistent, tracheobronchial inflammation that is characterized clinically by a hard, persistent, and usually nonproductive cough, which can become paroxysmal. Affected dogs usually recover, although signs can persist for 3 weeks or longer. Available evidence indicates that clinical signs are accompanied either by no significant gross lesions or, with about equal frequency, by catarrhal or mucopurulent tracheobronchitis. There is sometimes extension to a cranioventral bronchopneumonia and occasionally serous to mucopurulent rhinitis. Palatine tonsils and tracheobronchial and retropharyngeal lymph nodes are usually enlarged and reddened. Microscopically, various degrees of tracheobronchitis and bronchiolitis are usually present. These range from a focal, superficially necrotizing tracheobronchitis and bronchiolitis to a more severe process characterized by mucopurulent inflammation. There is epithelial degeneration and necrosis with disorganization of the normal pseudostratified pattern in the necrotizing lesions. The response in the underlying lamina propria is limited. The lesion is associated mainly with viral and bacterial infection. Viral infections contributing to this syndrome include parainfluenza type 2, canine adenovirus-2, and canine distemper virus. Extensive infiltration by neutrophils is characteristic of mucopurulent tracheobronchitis associated with *Bordetella bronchiseptica* infection. These bacteria attach to cilia and can induce ciliostasis within hours of attachment. Bacteria are often attached to cilia in sufficient numbers to be visible by light microscopy after staining for Gram-negative bacteria. *Mycoplasma cynos* has also been implicated in the complex etiology of infectious tracheobronchitis in dogs.

Severe bronchitis usually develops as a result of infection descending, usually aerogenously, from the upper respiratory system. Ascending infections can be important, particularly those involving verminous and granulomatous pneumonias. For instance, metastatic tubercles frequently erode into the airways to produce tuberculous bronchitis with subsequent spread as tuberculous bronchopneumonia. In a similar manner, pulmonary abscesses of caseous lymphadenitis can evacuate into bronchi, resulting in persistent caseous bronchitis.

The consequences of inflammation that are limited to larger bronchi are much less serious than the consequences of inflammation of small bronchi and especially of bronchioles. The larger bronchi lie in interstitial tissue outside the pulmonary lobules, and infectious processes are less likely to spread directly into surrounding parenchyma from bronchi than from bronchioles.

2. *Chronic Bronchitis*

Chronic bronchitis is usually of bacterial, parasitic, or presumed allergic cause. The relative importance of these causes varies according to species.

Chronic catarrhal or mucopurulent bronchitis is most important in **dogs,** where bronchial irritation and hypersecretion of mucus causes a chronic intractable cough. The condition is seen mostly in small breeds, particularly in obese animals. At postmortem, the major finding is excess mucus or mucopurulent exudate in the tracheobronchial tree. This ranges from pooling of turbid viscous fluid at the tracheobronchial junction to large amounts of tenacious, white or green to brown exudate in all airways. Sometimes the exudate is profuse enough to cause terminal foamy filling of the airways. The bronchial mucosa is thickened, often hyperemic, and edematous. Occasional polypoid projections into the lumen can be seen grossly in advanced cases, as can pale foci representing lymphoid nodules. Microscopically, the mucosal thickening and folding is caused mostly by increase in number and size of the mucosal glands and extensive infiltration of the lamina propria by lymphocytes, plasma cells, and occasional macrophages and neutrophils (Fig. 6.16). The superficial epithelium has prominent hyperplasia of goblet cells and usually has foci of ulceration or squamous metaplasia. Histochemical techniques reveal a shift in the character of secretions from sulfomucins to more viscous sialomucins. The intraluminal mucus is commonly mixed with abundant neutrophils. The amount of fibrosis, hyperemia, and edema in the bronchial wall depends on the age and severity of the lesion and whether there has been recent acute exacerbation. The airway involvement extends to involve bronchioles and, in ~25% of cases, there is a usually small area of associated bronchopneumonia. Hypertrophy of the smooth muscle in the wall of medium- and small-sized pulmonary arteries accompanies severe chronic bronchi-

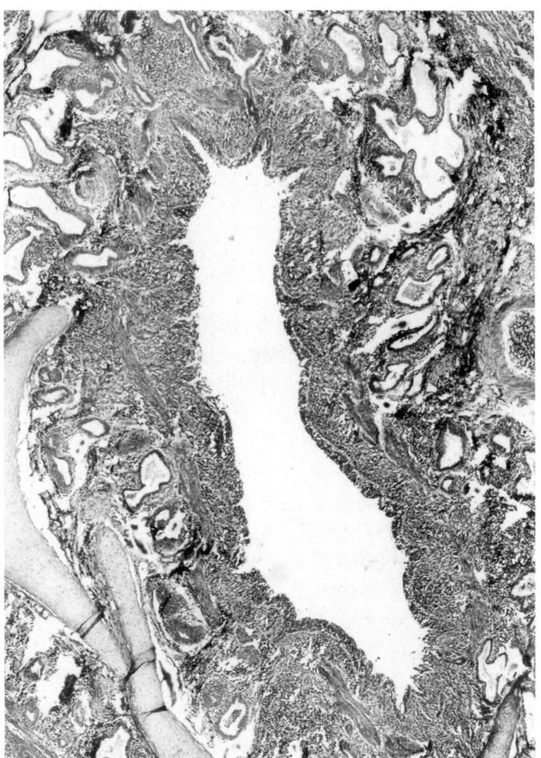

Fig. 6.16 Chronic bronchitis. Dog.

tis. The resulting pulmonary hypertension causes cor pulmonale that is occasionally detected clinically. Significant lesions of emphysema are not associated with chronic bronchitis in the dog, although there is often exaggeration of the marginal emphysema commonly found along the sharp ventral borders of the lungs in older dogs. A more common complication is alveolar atelectasis and bronchiectasis.

The pathogenesis of the chronic bronchitis in dogs is uncertain. It may occur in those dogs which fail to recover from a syndrome similar to infectious tracheobronchitis. Whatever the reasons for failure of the acute episode to resolve, eventually there occurs a vicious cycle of disruption of normal defense mechanisms and persistent interaction of bacteria and leukocytes capable of mediating continued inflammation. The most important infectious agent in dogs is *Bordetella bronchiseptica*.

Chronic suppurative bronchitis is a frequent sequel to bronchopneumonia in **cattle** and is usually associated with bronchiectasis. A variety of bacteria can be isolated from the suppurative lesions, with *Actinomyces (Corynebacterium) pyogenes* and *Pasteurella* spp. being the most important.

Although there is circumstantial evidence that allergens can be an important cause of bronchitis, rigorous proof is still lacking in most instances. The role of allergens in causing the chronic bronchiolitis–emphysema complex in the horse and the airway lesions associated with hypersensitivity pneumonitis are dealt with later. There remains a broad clinical syndrome, mostly in cats and dogs, which is commonly referred to as **asthma, allergic bronchitis,** or **allergic pneumonia.** Diagnosis is usually made on the basis of coughing, wheezing, respiratory distress, eosinophilia in blood or tracheobronchial lavage fluid, and alleviation of signs by sympathomimetic drugs and corticosteroids. There have been limited studies of the lesions associated with the clinical syndrome. Bronchial biopsies have demonstrated an edematous and hyperemic lamina propria with infiltration of eosinophils and fewer plasma cells and lymphocytes. The epithelium is highly susceptible to sloughing, which is exaggerated by sampling and processing artefacts. The lesions found postmortem usually are in an animal which has had repeated episodes or chronic involvement and therefore have features of a chronic bronchitis in which eosinophils are the predominant inflammatory cell. In the cat, there is narrowing of bronchial lumina because of extensive hyperplasia of the submucosal glands which are a prominent feature of normal cats in contrast to other species of domestic animals. The epithelial goblet cells are also hyperplastic. Numerous eosinophils infiltrate the epithelium and the edematous, hyperemic lamina propria. Plasma cells and lymphocytes are usually less conspicuous. Bronchial lumina are filled with mucus and sloughed cells mixed with many eosinophils. Eosinophils, plasma cells, and lymphocytes form an irregular collar in the adventitia of the bronchi, and small numbers of these cells infiltrate between the glandular acini. Hypertrophy of bronchial smooth muscle is common but not always present. Bronchioles are affected in severe cases (Fig. 6.17). Occasionally the lesion extends into peribronchiolar alveoli. Since lesions seen at postmortem are usually from an animal dying as a result of acute exacerbation, there is also a widespread patchy alveolar and interstitial edema. Sometimes, particularly in dogs, the numbers of eosinophils may be low relative to those of the other inflammatory cells.

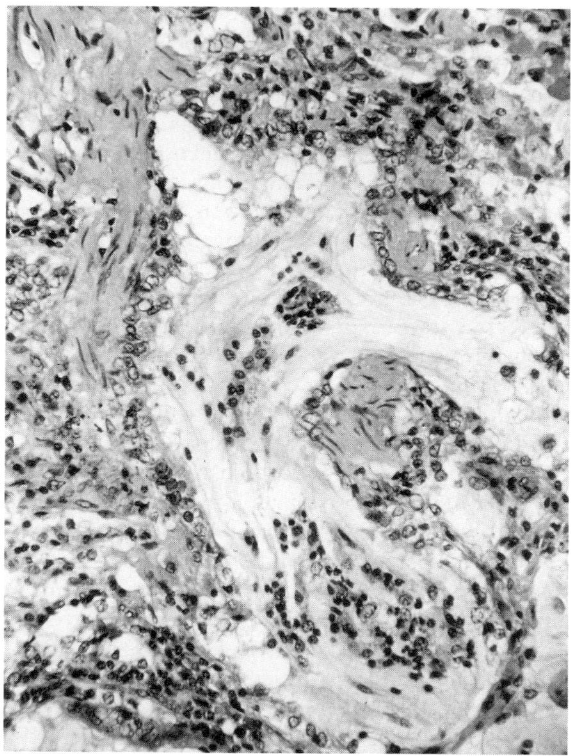

Fig. 6.17 Chronic bronchiolitis of presumed allergic origin with smooth muscle hypertrophy, mucus plugging, and eosinophils. Cat.

B. Bronchiectasis

Bronchiectasis is defined as permanent, abnormal dilation of bronchi. It most frequently occurs as an acquired lesion secondary to some form of bronchitis. The bronchitis may be of infective etiology or secondary to aspiration or another abnormality such as immotile cilia syndrome. It rarely occurs as a congenital malformation. There are two main anatomic varieties of bronchiectasis, saccular and cylindrical. **Saccular bronchiectasis** is less common and consists of thin-walled, circumscribed outpouchings of bronchial or bronchiolar walls. It is much more easily detected in lungs fixed by intratracheal infusion of fixative under pressure. This type of bronchiectasis can result from focal necrotizing bronchitis and bronchiolitis and occurs occasionally in sheep and cattle. It can also be found to a mild degree in the small airways of horses with the bronchiolitis–emphysema complex to be described later.

Cylindrical bronchiectasis affects bronchi partially or along their entire length (Fig. 6.18). In cattle, it is almost always a sequel to chronic suppurative bronchitis, which is in turn a frequent aftermath of bronchopneumonia. It therefore affects airways in cranioventral portions of the lung where bronchopneumonia occurs. Several pathogenetic events contribute to the development of bronchiectasis associated with bronchopneumonia. One is severe suppurative bronchitis with damage to and weakening of the bronchial wall by neutrophil lysosomal enzymes and associated oxygen radicals. This leads to pooling of exudate in the lumen. Secondly, inflammatory processes in more distal airways and alveolar parenchyma contribute to lower airway obstruction and atelectasis. The loss of alveolar tissue volume leads to traction on the walls of the airways during inspiration, which contributes to airway expansion over time. With lower airway obstruction and atelectasis, there is less-rapid airflow in the bronchial lumen, even during coughing efforts, to help maintain luminal patency. Mucociliary clearance is less effective because of damage to ciliated cells. This contributes further to mucus and inflammatory exudate accumulation in the bronchi. In **cattle,** the complete lobular septation and lack of collateral ventilation both lessen the effectiveness of resolution of bronchopneumonia and lead to more extensive atelectasis because of airway blockage. On both accounts, therefore, bronchiectasis is particularly likely to follow bronchopneumonia in this species.

Affected lungs have irregularly dilated bronchi in cranioventral regions. They are filled with viscous to caseous, yellow-green pus. The intervening parenchyma is atelectatic and sometimes fibrotic. In the cranial lobes the atelectasis tends to be complete, but in the caudal lobe there is often a mixture of areas of bronchopneumonia, hyperinflated lung, and atelectasis. In the bovine lung, in which the demarcation of lobules is distinct, dilation of the central bronchiole and alveolar collapse make a small hillock of each lobule, resembling the surface of a pineapple (Fig. 6.19A). The superficial appearance is often obscured by fibrous pleural adhesions, so the induration of the parenchyma and the dilated thin-walled bronchi filled with exudate are best appreciated when the lobe is sliced so that the bronchi are sectioned transversely. In severe cases, the dilated bronchi give a honeycombed or cystic appearance to the lobe (Fig. 6.19B).

Microscopically, depending on the severity and chronicity of the lesion, there are various degrees of reconstruction of the wall of the bronchus by granulation tissue. The lumen contains mucus, detritus, large collections of inflammatory cells, and frequently some blood. The mucosa may be destroyed by ulceration almost to the muscularis, or it may show a combination of ulcerative, atrophic, metaplastic, and hyperplastic changes. The bronchial walls are densely infiltrated with all types of leukocytes, and the lamina propria takes on the histologic properties of granulation tissue with progressive fibrosis. The necrotizing process can extend more deeply than the mucosa and destroy cartilage and submucosal glands. The destructive and suppurative process can involve the full width of

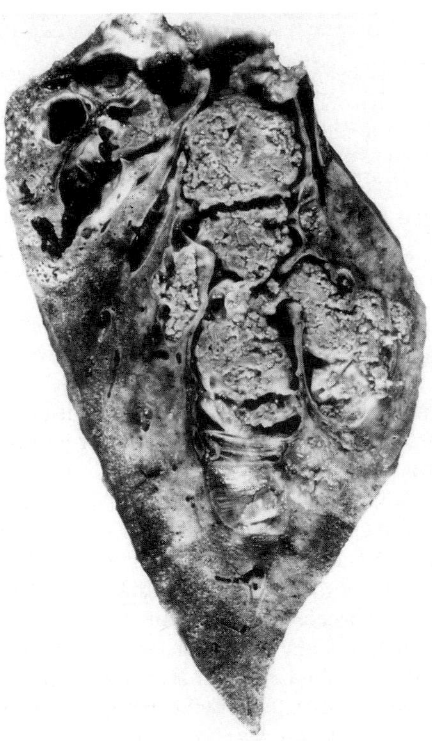

Fig. 6.18 Cylindrical bronchiectasis with inspissated exudate filling dilated airways. Dog.

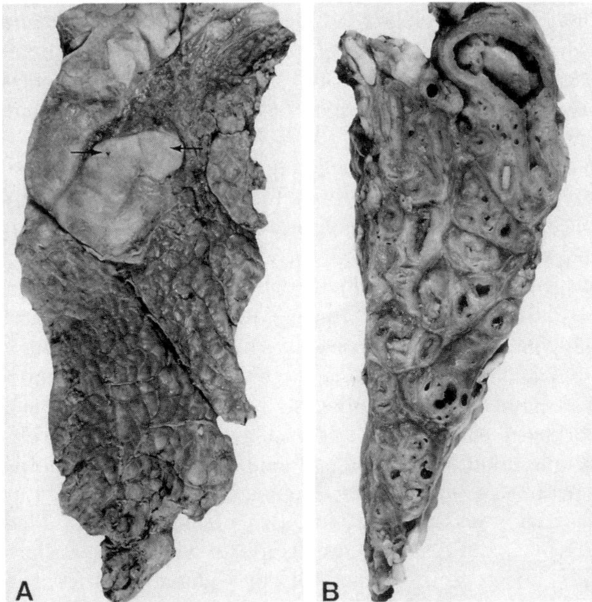

Fig. 6.19 (A) Bronchiectasis in cranial lobe. Air-trapping in lobules above (arrows). Ox. (B) Cut surface of (A).

the bronchial wall and some of the adjacent alveolar tissue and become equivalent to a lung abscess.

Cylindrical bronchiectasis in the **dog** (Fig. 6.18) arises against the background of severe chronic bronchitis but, in contrast to that in the cow, it is not so consistent a sequel. A major factor is probably the less frequent occurrence of alveolar atelectasis in the dog. Since there is very effective collateral ventilation in dogs, atelectasis is less likely to follow airway obstruction. This could be the reason bronchitis is less likely to cause bronchiectasis in this species. In addition to generalized bronchiectasis associated with severe, diffuse, chronic, mucopurulent bronchitis, the condition sometimes is limited to only one or two lobes, more often the middle lobes. Whether localized or generalized, the greatly dilated bronchi often contain casts of either crumbly or tenacious and rubbery, partially dehydrated exudate.

Chronic mucopurulent bronchitis with bronchiectasis and bronchiolectasis is rare in cats. Occasionally there is accompanying miliary broncholithiasis. In pigs, sheep, and goats, bronchiectasis is usually associated with severe parasitic bronchitis. Occasionally in all species, localized bronchiectasis follows obstruction by a foreign body, granuloma, or tumor.

The course of widespread bronchiectasis is chronic and unfavorable. Complications, other than bronchopneumonia, include bronchopleural fistula, septic thrombosis, and hemorrhage, or production of septic emboli with metastatic abscess formation, and secondary amyloidosis.

Although bronchiectasis occurs infrequently in dogs, dogs with **immotile cilia syndrome** usually develop bronchiectasis as part of a constellation of abnormalities associated with a basic ciliary defect. Kartagener's syndrome was the eponym applied to a congenital and often familial disorder in infants in which there was coexisting situs inversus, sinusitis, and bronchiectasis. The triad of Kartagener's syndrome is recognized in dogs. Only ~50% of the dogs with immotile cilia syndrome develop situs inversus. Abnormalities are referable to improper function of ciliated cells, particularly of respiratory and reproductive organs. The basic defect is usually associated with one of several ultrastructural abnormalities of cilia throughout the body, including absence of one or both of the inner and outer dynein arms, microtubular transposition, random microtubular orientation, and partial microtubular deficiency. Ciliary basal body abnormalities have also been described. Some dogs with the syndrome do not have ultrastructural changes in cilia. Littermates with the condition have been recognized in English pointers, English springer spaniels, and Old English sheepdogs. Breeding studies confirm the heritable nature of the disease in dogs and suggest that it is an autosomal recessive condition.

C. Bronchiolitis

Inflammation of bronchioles commonly occurs as an extension of bronchitis or concurrently with bronchitis and pneumonia. Bronchiolitis as a distinct pathologic entity occurs under several specific forms of pulmonary injury, with viral infection and pulmonary toxicity being the two most common forms in domestic animals. A notable example of viral bronchiolitis occurs with respiratory syncytial virus infection in cattle, where viral replication occurs in bronchiolar epithelial cells, in addition to bronchial and alveolar epithelial cells, to induce both airway inflammation and interstitial pneumonia. Bronchiolitis and bronchiolar obstruction can become a prominent feature of the disease, leading to severe hypoxemia due to ventilation/perfusion inequality, and forced expiratory efforts with obstructed airways leading to interstitial emphysema. Airway obstruction in viral bronchiolitis occurs by processes similar to those described for bronchitis, but hyperplasia of nonciliated bronchiolar epithelial cells often is much more pronounced in bronchiolitis. The epithelial hyperplasia and other viral cytopathic effects together cause severe narrowing or obstruction of the airway lumen.

Exposure to xenobiotic compounds, such as 4-ipomeanol, 3-methylindole and perilla ketone, can lead to severe bronchiolar injury as a result of necrosis of nonciliated bronchiolar epithelial cells, which possess high concentrations of cytochrome P-450-monooxygenase enzymes.

Relatively mild inflammatory lesions in bronchioles that result in thickening of the wall, if diffusely distributed, can lead to significant increases in respiratory resistance. According to Poiseuille's law, narrowing of the airway will increase resistance to the fourth power of the reduction in radius. Acute inflammatory conditions characterized by edema and infiltration or chronic conditions associated with fibrosis that reduce the bronchiolar lumen radius by half will increase resistance 16-fold.

Physical airway obstruction occurs more readily in bronchioles than in bronchi. This is partly explained by the ease with which bronchiolar walls collapse and by their small luminal size readily permitting occlusion by exudate. For these reasons, severe bronchiolitis characterized by accumulation of exudate and delayed epithelial repair is likely to lead to obliteration by organizing fibrous connective tissue.

Bronchiolitis fibrosa obliterans or organizing bronchiolitis is a nonspecific response to a variety of severe forms of damage to bronchioles and adjacent alveoli. It can follow viral infections such as influenza, inhalation of toxic gases (including 100% oxygen), or damage by lungworms or pneumotoxins such as those associated with acute interstitial pneumonia in cattle. Prerequisites are necrosis of epithelium at the bronchiolar–alveolar junction and the presence of an inflammatory exudate that may be rich in fibrin and chemotaxins for macrophages, fibroblasts, and endothelial cells. Fibroblast migration into the exudate and phagocytosis of debris and/or lysis of the fibrin are accompanied by collagen synthesis to lead to a permanently obstructive lesion in the bronchiolar lumen. The lesion is typically a polypoid projection of fibroblastic tissue partially or completely obliterating the bronchiolar lumen (Fig. 6.20A,B,C). In species with well-developed respiratory bronchioles (for instance, the dog), organiza-

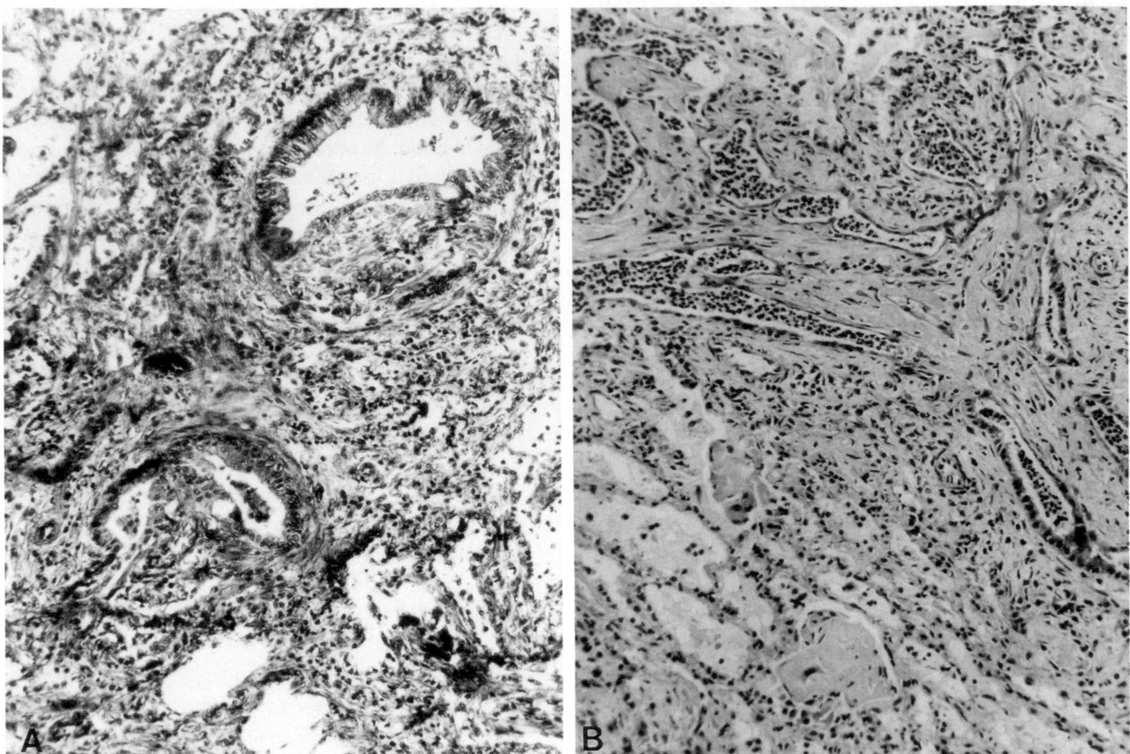

Fig. 6.20 (A & B) Patterns of obliterative bronchiolitis (bronchiolitis fibrosa obliterans). Calf.

tion of exudate often takes place from septa of alveoli situated at intervals along the length of the bronchioles. Organization of exudate into cellular granulation tissue can take place in as few as 7–10 days after onset of severe damage, and regeneration of epithelium over its surface can occur in the same period.

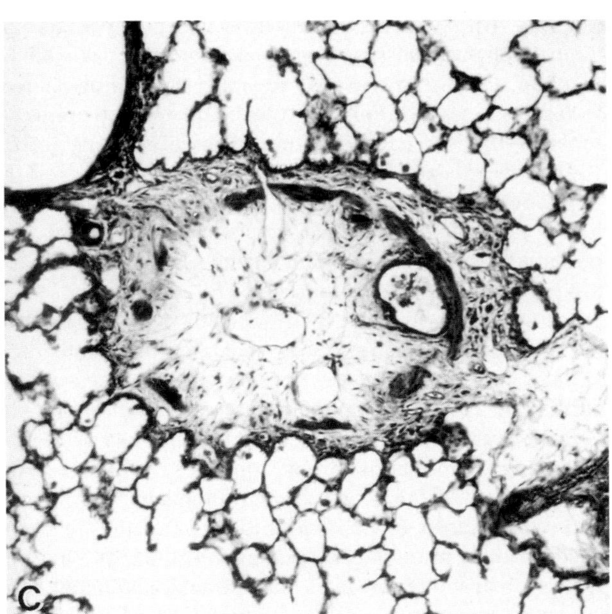

Fig. 6.20C Bronchiolitis obliterans. Dog. Experimental canine adenovirus-2 infection. (Reprinted from Castelman, W. L. *Am J Pathol* **119:** 495, 1985.)

Bibliography

Appel, M., and Bemis, D. A. The canine contagious respiratory disease complex (kennel cough). *Cornell Vet (Suppl.)* **68:** 70–75, 1978.

Carrig, C. B. *et al.* Primary dextrocardia with situs inversus, associated with sinusitis and bronchitis in a dog. *J Am Vet Med Assoc* **164:** 1127–1134, 1974.

Edwards, D. F. *et al.* Immotile cilia syndrome in three dogs from a litter. *J Am Vet Med Assoc* **183:** 667–672, 1983.

Edwards, D. F. *et al.* Kartagener's syndrome in a chow chow dog with normal ciliary ultrastructure. *Vet Pathol* **26:** 338–340, 1989.

Hamerslag, K. L., Evans, S. M., and Dubielzig, R. Acquired cystic bronchiectasis in the dog: A case history report. *Vet Radiol* **23:** 64–68, 1982.

Jensen, R. *et al.* Bronchiectasis in yearling feedlot cattle. *J Am Vet Med Assoc* **169:** 511–514, 1976.

Lettow, E. *et al.* Solitare Hohlraumbildung im Bronchialsystem bei einem Hund (angeborene Bronchialzyste?). *Tierarzl Umschau* **28:** 274–280, 282–283, 1973.

McCandlish, I. A. P. *et al.* A study of dogs with kennel cough. *Vet Rec* **102:** 298–301, 1978.

Pirie, H. M., and Wheeldon, E. B. Chronic bronchitis in the dog. *Adv Vet Sci Comp Med* **20:** 253–276, 1976.

Turk, M. A., Breeze, R. G., and Gallina, A. M. Pathologic changes in 3-methylindole-induced equine bronchiolitis. *Am J Pathol* **110:** 209–218, 1983.

VI. Lungs

A. Congenital Anomalies

Congenital anomalies of the lung are rare. Various forms have been recorded, in calves particularly. Major malformations such as pulmonary agenesis are incompatible with life and are often accompanied by other malformations. Accessory lungs are the most common finding. These are edematous, lobulated masses and can be found within the abdominal or thoracic cavities or subcutaneously. They may connect to the upper alimentary system (congenital bronchopulmonary foregut malformation). The main histologic features are dilated bronchiolar structures, hypoplastic bronchi, and various degrees of development of alveolar ducts and alveoli. Bronchial hypoplasia also appears to be the basic defect in what is usually referred to as congenital adenomatoid malformation or adenomatoid hamartoma. In this condition, one or more lobes of the normal lung are replaced by swollen, spongy or cystic, lobulated tissue. Histologically, as in accessory lungs, dilated bronchioles sometimes are large enough to be noted grossly as cystic spaces. Bronchi are hypoplastic and lack cartilage and smooth muscle in their walls. Alveolar structures may be more normal. However, if there is airway collapse and obstruction with secondary hyperinflation of the lung, enlarged alveoli may result (congenital lobar emphysema). Other anomalies include chondromatous hamartomas and pulmonary epidermoid cysts.

Pulmonary hypoplasia (Fig. 6.21) is particularly likely to accompany congenital diaphragmatic hernia. Congenital cysts and congenital bronchiectasis are localized variations on the same theme. Congenital alveolar dysplasia has been observed in pups. The gross form of the lungs is regular, but they retain a fetal appearance and become poorly aerated and poorly crepitant. The distribution, size, and shape of the alveoli are uneven. Alveoli are reduced in number, and there is excessive interstitial tissue that contains many dilated capillaries. The formed alveoli are lined by mature alveolar epithelium. In such cases, it is difficult or impossible to determine whether infection of the fetal lung played a pathogenetic role.

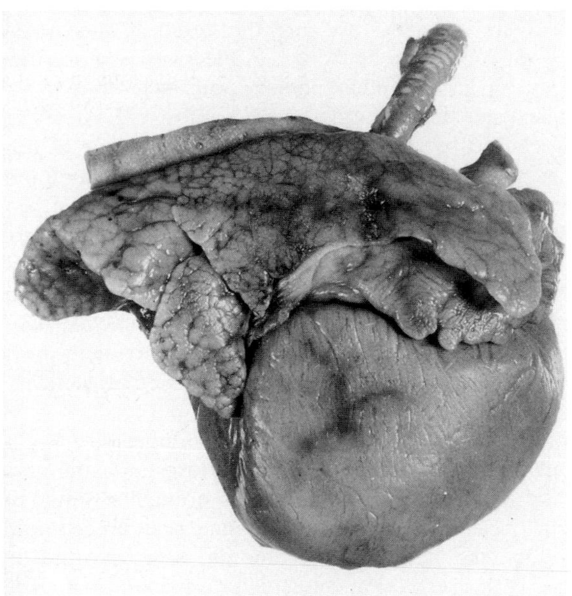

Fig. 6.21 Hypoplastic lung. Calf.

Abnormal lobulations and fissures are quite common and are found incidentally at postmortem examination.

Bibliography

Amis, T. C. *et al.* Congenital bronchial cartilage hypoplasia with lobar hyperinflation (congenital lobar emphysema) in an adult Pekingese. *J Am Anim Hosp Assoc* **23:** 321–329, 1987.

Ball, V., and Girard, H. Kystes aeriens congenitaux du poumon chez le chein. *Rec Med Vet* **118:** 5–12, 1942.

Brown, P. J. *et al.* Congenital bronchopulmonary foregut malformations in two young Friesian cattle. *Vet Rec* **122:** 208–209, 1988.

Dennis, S. M. Congenital respiratory tract defects in lambs. *Aust Vet J* **51:** 347–350, 1975.

Dieter, R. Ueber kongenitale Lungenveranderungen. *Arch Wiss Prakt Tierheilkd* **73:** 218–231, 1938.

Drolet, R., and Phaneuf, J. B. Pulmonary chondromatous hamartoma in a young cat. *Vet Rec* **113:** 541–542, 1983.

Joest, R. Intrathorakale Nebenlunge beim Pferde. *Tierarztl Arch* **3:** 329–333, 1923.

Milli, U. H., and Haziroglu, R. Pulmonary epidermoid cysts in a cat. *Vet Rec* **127:** 287, 1990.

Rubarth, S. On some congenital lung anomalies in animals. *Skand Vet Tidskr* **26:** 581–606, 1936.

Sjolte, I. P., and Christiansen, M. J. Zehn Falle von Nebenlungen bei Tieren. *Virchows Arch* **302:** 93–117, 1938.

Thomson, R. G. Congenital bronchial hypoplasia in calves. *Pathol Vet* **3:** 89–109, 1966.

van den Ingh, T. S. G. A. M., and van der Gaag, I. A congenital adenomatoid malformation of the lungs in a calf. *Vet Pathol* **11:** 297–300, 1974.

B. Atelectasis

Atelectasis means incomplete expansion of the lung and was originally applied to defective aeration of fetal lung at the time of birth. It is now also applied to collapse of previously air-filled pulmonary parenchyma. Atelectasis is therefore divided into congenital and acquired forms.

In **congenital (neonatal) atelectasis,** the lungs range from those of the stillborn animal which have never been aerated (**fetal atelectasis**) to minor degrees of incomplete expansion. In fetal atelectasis, the lungs appear as in the fetus but are dark reddish blue because of dilation of alveolar capillaries. They are of fleshy consistency and do not float. The alveoli are partially distended with fluid, and the epithelial cells are rounded. Sloughed epithelial cells (squames) from the oronasal regions and amniotic fluid are usually present in the alveolar fluid, possibly with bright yellow particles of meconium. Small numbers of squames can be present in the lungs of normal term fetuses but large numbers, especially if meconium is also present, indicate aspiration of amniotic fluid during the exaggerated respiratory movements of the asphyxiated fetus *in utero*. Patchy congenital atelectasis due to incomplete expansion is usually due to weak respiratory movements caused by general debilitation or damage to respiratory centers in the brainstem. Laryngeal dysfunction, obstruction of airways, and abnormalities of the lung or related thoracic structures are other possible causes. In the neonatal period, it is often not possible to distinguish atelectasis of incomplete expansion and acquired atelectasis of briefly aerated lung. The atelectasis is frequently seen affecting groups of lobules or occasionally more widespread regions during the first week of life. The larger zones are more likely to occur in weak, recumbent animals and mostly affect the lowermost region of the down side (Fig. 6.22). The atelectatic lobules are distinct because they are dark red, depressed below the surface of the surrounding aerated lung, and, in contrast to pneumonic lung, have a flabby consistency. The sectioned surface is homogeneous, dark red, and free blood is easily expressed from it. Microscopically, the alveolar walls are in close apposition. Only small amounts of fluid, epithelial debris (including squames from the upper oronasal regions or amniotic fluid), and alveolar macrophages are present.

Extensive neonatal atelectasis is a feature of **neonatal hyaline membrane disease (neonatal respiratory distress syndrome).** This is a common disease in human infants, particularly in premature babies and those born to diabetic mothers. A similar condition in animals is best recognized in foals, but has been reported in lambs, pigs, puppies, and a calf. Foals and pigs have been called barkers because of the doglike sound made during forced expiration. Foals which show evidence of presumed hypoxic brain damage are sometimes referred to as wanderers. Affected lungs are extensively atelectatic, although the borders of the lobes may be spared. They are heavy, fleshy, and often edematous. Cream-colored or bloodstained foam frequently exudes from cut surfaces and is present in large airways. The lungs sink or almost submerge in fixative. The main microscopic abnormalities are alveolar septal congestion, variably collapsed or edema-containing alveoli, and presence of acidophilic hyaline membranes lining alveolar ducts and distal portions of bronchioles. Focal hemorrhages and interstitial edema are common.

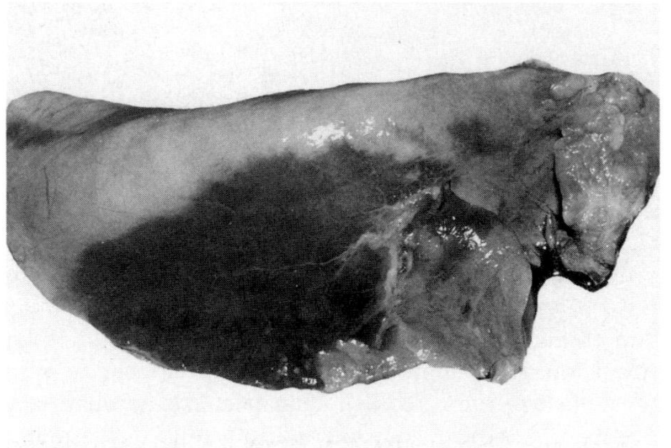

Fig. 6.22 Atelectasis of lateral aspect of right caudal lobe. Lamb.

There is general agreement that lack of normal surface-tension-reducing capacity of the alveolar lining liquid plays the central pathogenetic role. This in turn is linked to defective production by alveolar type II epithelial cells of the phospholipid surfactant material. There is still debate, however, as to the extent to which decreased surfactant activity is due to immaturity of type II cells or to a more specific metabolic derangement of their surfactant synthesis. Fetal hypothyroidism and possibly hypoadrenocorticism also play a role in the condition in piglets by being responsible for delayed maturation of type II cells. Other pathogenetic factors are fetal asphyxia, aspiration of amniotic fluid, reduction in pulmonary arteriolar blood flow, and inhibition of surfactant by fibrinogen, other serum constituents in edema fluid, or by components in aspirated amniotic fluid.

Acquired atelectasis and **alveolar collapse** are used synonymously. Acquired atelectasis is most commonly the **obstructive** type, which is caused by complete airway obstruction. Whether atelectasis follows obstruction depends on the size of airway obstructed and the degree of collateral ventilation. Complete blockage of lobar or segmental bronchi is necessary for atelectasis in the dog and cat, where collateral ventilation is extensive. Blockage of small bronchi or even bronchioles can result in atelectasis in bovine lungs where there is insignificant collateral ventilation. Lungs of sheep are also prone to atelectasis, pigs less so, and the horse is intermediate between ruminants and dogs. Atelectasis is more likely to develop in dependent lung regions where alveoli are smallest and airways, most easily compressed. Atelectatic lung caused by obstruction has the appearance of other forms of atelectasis. It is sunken relative to aerated lung, homogeneously dark red, and flabby. Evidence of bronchial obstruction by exudate, parasites, aspirated foreign material, granulomas, or tumors can often be seen grossly. Resorption of oxygen from nonventilated lung occurs quickly, but nitrogen is resorbed very slowly. Obstruction of airways by aspirated material or foamy exudate shortly before death does not, therefore, produce atelectasis in animals breathing air.

Microscopically, simple atelectasis appears as slightly congested alveolar walls lying in close apposition with slitlike residual lumina having sharp angular ends (Fig. 6.23). Atelectasis which is sometimes seen preceding the development of bronchopneumonia, or during the final phase of its resolution, is usually associated with small amounts of edema fluid and excess alveolar macrophages in the alveolar lumina. The edema accompanying large

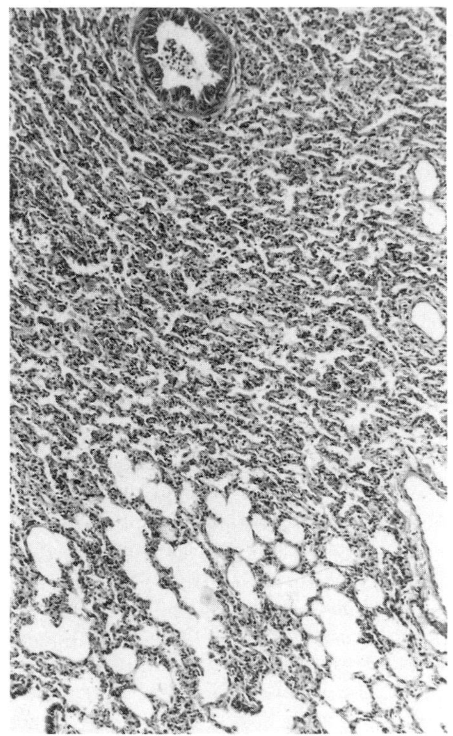

Fig. 6.23 Atelectasis. Lamb.

zones of atelectasis is due partly to leakage because of hypoxic damage and partly to the hypoxic vasoconstriction of vessels in the affected region. Reduced surfactant activity also plays a role. Microatelectasis of small groups of alveoli is often an artefact of immersion fixation, and the apparent blending of several alveolar septa is easily mistaken for interstitial pneumonia.

Acquired atelectasis of compression type is caused by pleural or intrapulmonary space-occupying lesions. Examples are hydrothorax, hemothorax, exudative pleuritis, and mediastinal and pulmonary tumors. In large animals, the atelectasis caused by pleural effusions often occurs below a sharply demarcated fluid line. Abdominal distension, as in severe ascites and ruminal tympany, may cause partial atelectasis, typically in the cranial regions where ventilatory movements are most easily compromised by intra-abdominal pressure.

What may be termed **hypostatic atelectasis** occurs in the lowermost zone of the lung of the down side in recumbent large animals. This is a hazard of prolonged anesthesia or of weakened animals, particularly if there is a condition causing chest pain. The contributing factors are shallow amplitude of respiration causing impaired ventilation of dependent lung, gradual loss of surfactant activity, and pooling of secretions in the lower airways.

Sharp-bordered, ribbon-shaped, or lobular zones of atelectasis are present to some extent in the cranioventral regions of the lungs of slaughtered sheep. Although many of these are associated with blockage of bronchioles and small bronchi with purulent exudate, some have no detectable blockage of airways, and the reason for the atelectasis is not known.

Massive atelectasis is seen mostly as a sequel to pneumothorax. What appears to be total atelectasis is seen in animals, usually dogs and cats, which die during the course of breathing 80–100% oxygen as part of intensive care. Because of the speed with which the oxygen is resorbed into the tissues, the lungs are usually completely devoid of gas by the time they are examined postmortem. They are uniformly shrunken, dark red, flabby, and ooze blood on cut section.

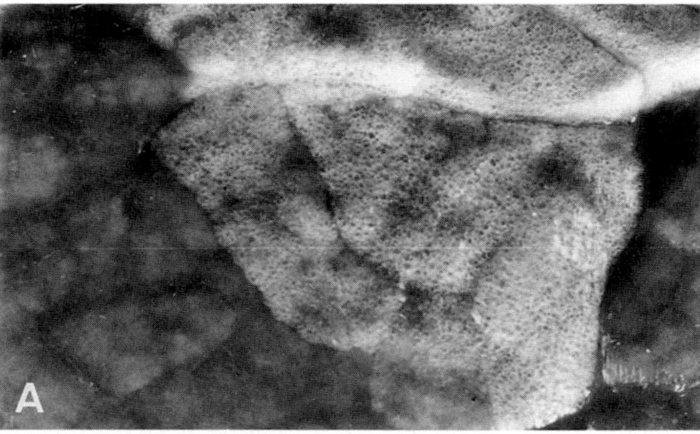

Fig. 6.24A Hyperinflation (compensatory emphysema) in lobules bordering areas of consolidation. Note the relative smallness of the consolidated lobules and mottling produced by peribronchial infiltrates.

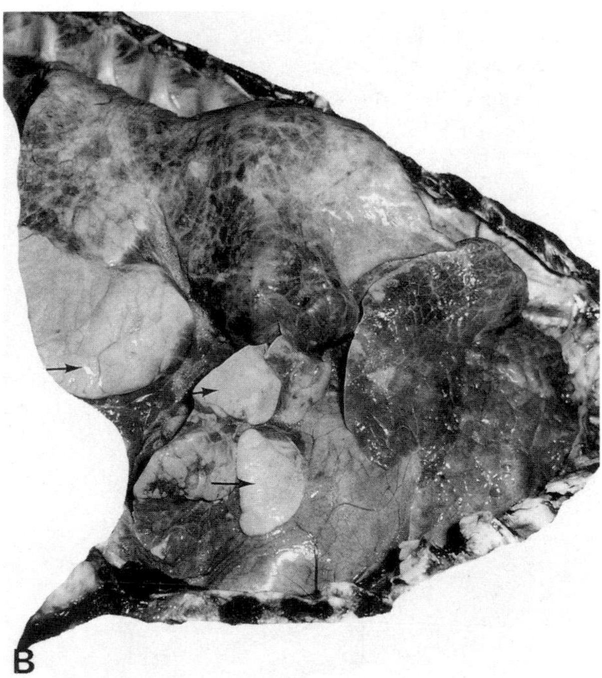

Fig. 6.24B Chronic bronchopneumonia. Cranial bronchiectasis, widespread lobular consolidation, interstitial bulla protruding in caudal lobe, and a few pale lobules caused by air trapping (arrows). Calf.

C. Emphysema of Lungs

Emphysema in its widest sense refers to tissue puffed up by air or other gas. In the lung there are two major forms. **Alveolar (vesicular) emphysema** is excessive amounts of air within airspaces of the lung. **Interstitial emphysema** is the presence of air within interlobular, subpleural, and other major interstitial zones of the lung. **Emphysema,** unless otherwise qualified, should be used only for alveolar emphysema. The most widely accepted current definition of human emphysema is abnormal enlargement of air spaces distal to the terminal bronchioles, accompanied by destruction of their walls and an absence of obvious fibrosis. Some broaden the definition to include abnormal enlargement of airspaces, with or without evidence of destruction. The advantage of requiring evidence of destruction of walls of the airspaces is that it enables more precise recognition of an irreversible, functionally significant lesion. Simple enlargement, or hyperinflation, can be a temporary and relatively insignificant lesion. An example of this is the so-called compensatory emphysema which occurs along the margin of a consolidated lung (Fig. 6.24A). What appear to be emphysematous lesions in lungs removed postmortem are often not significant antemortem changes but mostly result from failure of the lung to deflate normally (Figs. 6.19A, 6.24B). This is caused by air trapping, usually by blockage or spasm of airways. Accurate assessment of emphysema therefore can be obtained only in lungs inflated with fixative to a volume approximating the *in vivo* state. In the following discussion, emphysema will refer to abnormal enlargement of air spaces distal to terminal bronchioles with evidence of destruction of their walls.

Several morphologic types of emphysema are recognized in human lungs according to the distribution of the enlarged airspaces. **Centriacinar (centrilobular) emphysema** principally affects respiratory bronchioles and adjacent central portions of the respiratory acini, an acinus being defined as the terminal unit of lung supplied by a single terminal (nonrespiratory) bronchiole. **Panacinar (panlobular) emphysema** more uniformly involves all portions of acini. These two major anatomic types of emphysema in humans also differ with regard to other clinicopathologic features. Less important forms of emphysema are **paraseptal emphysema,** which affects distal alveoli bordering interlobular septa or pleura, and **irregular** or **paracicatricial emphysema,** which results from distortion of airspaces by adjacent contracted scar tissue.

Regardless of distribution, severely emphysematous lung is grossly voluminous, pale, and puffy. When the lesion is diffuse, the lungs fill the thoracic cavity even after the chest has been opened, and sometimes they bear imprints of the ribs. The enlarged air spaces are often visible as small vesicles, and in severe cases coalescence of air spaces can produce large air-filled bullae one to several centimeters in diameter. Histologically, enlarge-

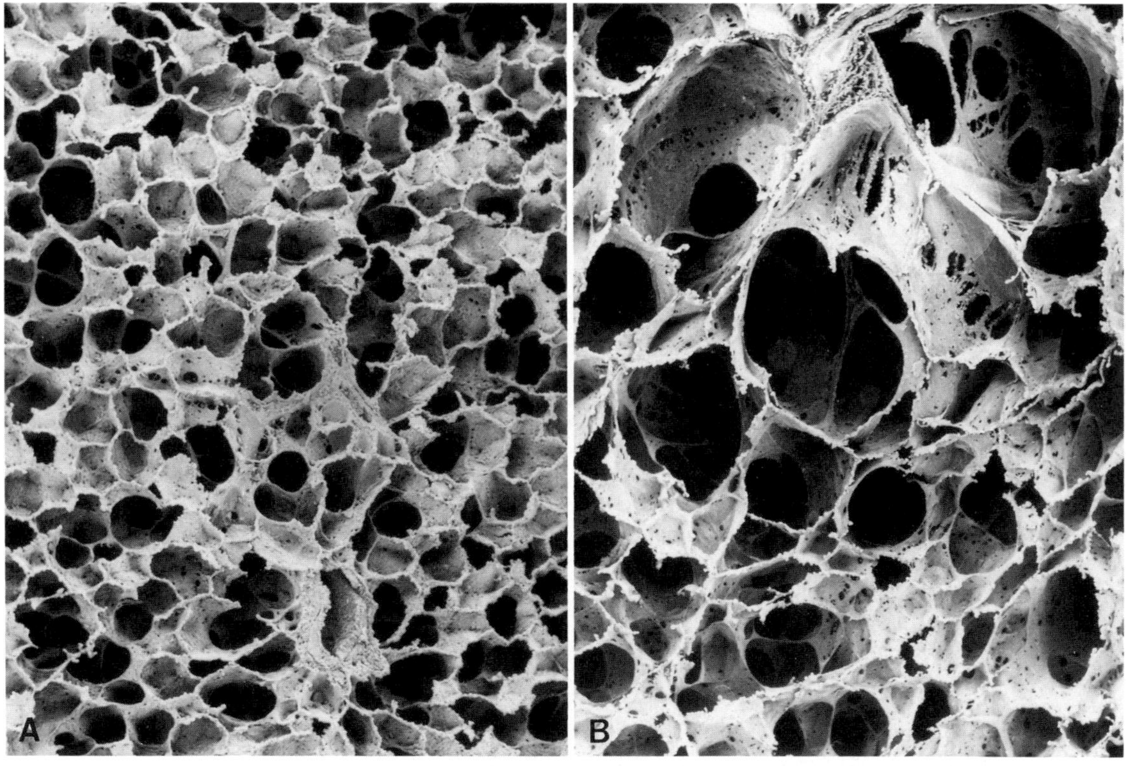

Fig. 6.25 (A) Scanning electron micrograph of normal lung. Horse. (B) Scanning electron micrograph of emphysematous lung. Same magnification as (A). Horse. Note alveolar enlargement and alveolar wall destruction.

ment and coalescence of air spaces in inflation-fixed lungs can readily be detected in moderate to severe cases. Scanning electron microscopy, which dramatically reveals the moth-eaten appearance (Fig. 6.25A,B), is best for visualization of early lesions.

With the exception of the chronic bronchiolitis–emphysema complex in the horse and congenital lobar or bullous emphysema in dogs (see the following paragraphs), naturally occurring emphysema is of little clinical significance in animals. It can be found postmortem in the apices and along the sharp ventral border of the lungs of old animals and is therefore seen mostly in dogs, (Fig. 6.26A,B) cats, and horses. Emphysematous bullae also occasionally occur in these regions and in rare instances rupture to cause fatal pneumothorax. Even when not noted grossly, subpleural air spaces, particularly along cranioventral margins of the lung, are often shown to be larger than more central ones at microscopic examination.

In contrast to that in animals, emphysema is an extremely important condition in humans, where it frequently coexists with chronic bronchitis and bronchiolitis in causing chronic obstructive pulmonary disease. Most of what is known about the pathogenesis of emphysema is therefore derived from the human condition or, more recently, from experimental animal models. With regard to pathogenetic factors in emphysema, there has been considerable speculation over the years concerning the relative importance of genetic factors, inflammatory alveolar destruction, atrophy of alveolar septa due to ischemic or unknown cause, and mechanical factors leading to widening and rupture of air spaces. Two important findings led to convergence of these ideas. One was the discovery that humans deficient in α_1-antitrypsin (now referred to commonly as α_1-protease inhibitor) have increased incidence and earlier onset of emphysema. The other was that intratracheal injection of papain in hamsters produced an emphysematous lesion. Further developments led to the current basic hypothesis that emphysema is caused by excessive proteolysis in the lung because of protease–antiprotease imbalance. The critical structural component undergoing lysis is elastin, because experimentally the development of emphysema is correlated well only with elastolytic activity and evidence of elastin breakdown. The neutrophil elastase (a serine protease) from lysosomal granules is believed to be the main source of elastolytic activity. In homozygous α_1-antitrypsin (α_1-antiprotease) inhibitor deficiency, the emphysema is panacinar in distribution and the protease–antiprotease imbalance is presumed to be due mainly to genetically controlled reduction in the antiprotease. In human centriacinar emphysema, such as associated with cigarette smoking, slowly smoldering inflammation at the bronchiolar–alveolar junctions (respiratory bronchiolitis) appears to be the forerunner of the emphysematous lesion. An important feature, however, is that although the respiratory bronchiolitis is generalized, the emphysema is mainly in the upper lobes. Currently, centriacinar emphysema in cigarette-smoking humans is considered to be basically due to an excess of

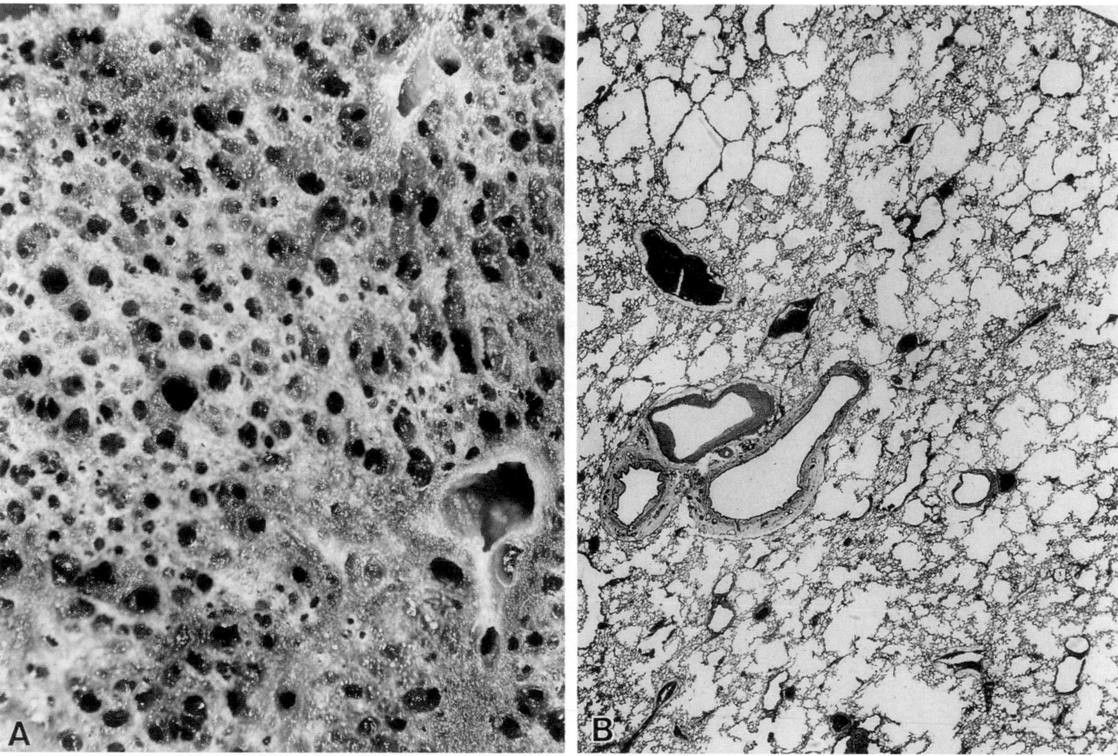

Fig. 6.26 (A & B) Emphysema. Lung. Dog.

elastase from neutrophils recruited to the inflamed sites. This is compounded by a lack of antiprotease activity caused by oxidative inactivation of antiproteases by components in cigarette smoke and by neutrophil-derived active oxygen species. It has been hypothesized that the preferential distribution of emphysema in upper lobes is associated with slower neutrophil traffic through capillaries in these regions of the lung.

Congenital lobar emphysema secondary to aplasia or hypoplasia of bronchial cartilage has been found in dogs. Pekingese are over-represented in the reports to date. Signs of respiratory difficulty have been associated with a single greatly emphysematous lung lobe compromising ventilation of the others. **Multifocal bullous emphysema** also occurs in dogs; in one report the emphysema was accompanied by bronchial hypoplasia.

Chronic bronchiolitis–emphysema complex in the horse has long been associated with the lay terms heaves or broken wind and more recently with the pathophysiological term chronic obstructive pulmonary disease. The term chronic bronchiolitis–emphysema complex is used here because it emphasizes the lesions which tend to coexist and the fact that the causes and pathogenesis are both complex and poorly understood. The most consistent finding in horses with clinical signs of chronic obstructive pulmonary disease is a generalized chronic bronchiolitis. Emphysema, as defined by enlargement and destruction of airspaces, is less common (Figs. 6.25B, 6.27), although in excised lungs the alveoli may appear hyperinflated because of air trapping. Rarely, emphysema is present without significant bronchiolitis. The emphysema is mostly in cranial regions, even when it accompanies a more generalized bronchiolitis.

Constant features of the chronic bronchiolitis are epithelial hyperplasia, goblet cell metaplasia, peribronchiolar fibrosis, and infiltration by lymphocytes and plasma cells. Lumina of bronchioles are narrowed by accumulation of exudate and peribronchiolar fibrosis. Mucus is usually a major component of the exudate and sometimes occurs in such large quantities that reflux into adjacent alveolar ducts and alveoli occurs (Fig. 6.28A,B). The major variable component of the bronchiolitis is the eosinophil. This is sometimes the most obvious feature, both of the intraluminal exudate and of the intraepithelial and peribronchiolar sites. At other times, relatively few eosinophils are scattered within the mucus and the bronchiolar wall. There often seems to be an inverse relationship between the amount of mucus and the number of eosinophils. There are usually increased numbers of mast cells surrounding the bronchioles. Neutrophils are less common than eosinophils, but sometimes the lesion has the characteristics of a mucopurulent bronchiolitis.

The relative importance of allergy, infection, and toxicity in causing the bronchiolitis is not established—it almost certainly can differ across a series of cases. The frequent presence of eosinophils, circumstantial evidence

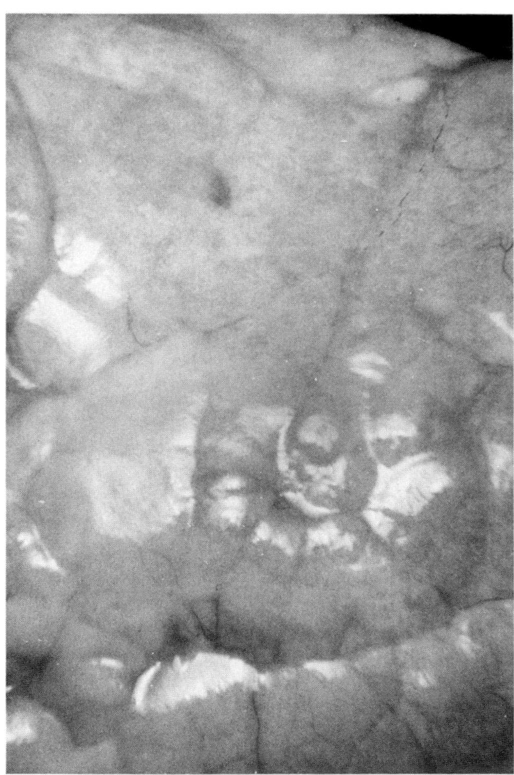

Fig. 6.27 Pale, puffy, emphysematous lung associated with chronic obstructive bronchiolitis. Horse.

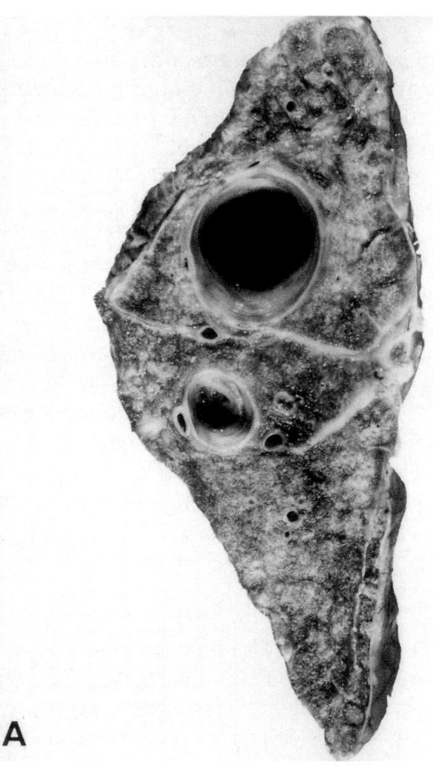

Fig. 6.28A Saccular bronchiectasis in chronic obstructive bronchiolitis. Horse.

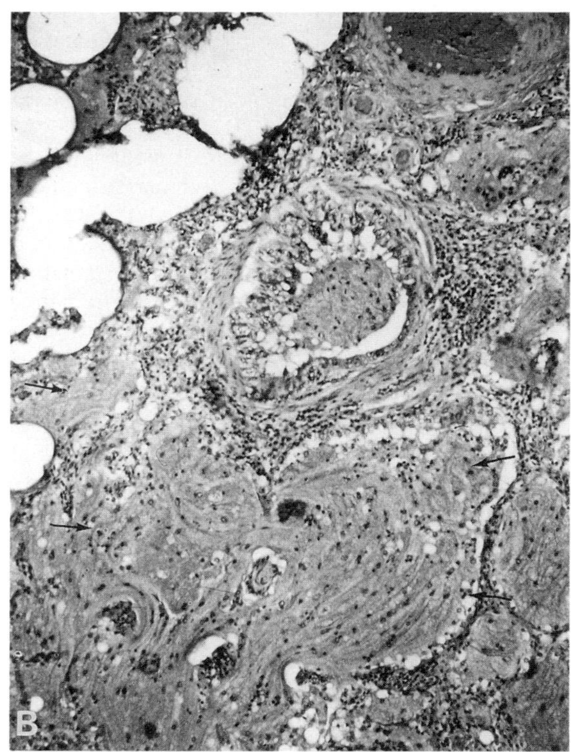

Fig. 6.28B Histologic detail of bronchiolitis in (A). Note mucus plugging of bronchiole and mucus reflux into adjacent alveoli (arrows).

of clinical exacerbation on exposure to moldy hay, bedding, or stable dust, and limited information from aerosol challenges using suspect fungal antigens all indicate that an allergic response to inhaled allergens (e.g., *Micropolyspora faeni, Aspergillus fumigatus,* and hay dust) is an important mechanism. Infection probably plays some part in a proportion of cases. Experimental evidence that blood-borne toxins, specifically 3-methylindole in the horse, can selectively damage bronchiolar epithelium introduces a further possible set of causes. From the point of view of the characteristic goblet cell metaplasia and mucus hypersecretion, there is evidence that histamine, prostaglandins, and leukotrienes released during type I allergic responses (anaphylaxis) have a stimulatory effect on mucus secretion. This could explain the association of goblet cell increases, mucus hypersecretion, eosinophils, and mast cells. As mentioned under allergic bronchitis, asthma and chronic allergic bronchitis and bronchiolitis are not clearly separable in animals.

Interstitial emphysema is distinguished from alveolar emphysema by the presence of air in the connective tissues and lymphatics of the lung, chiefly the interlobular septa but also beneath the pleura and around vessels and airways (Fig. 6.29A,B). Interstitial emphysema occurs mainly in lungs with well-developed interlobular septa. Lungs of the cow, sheep, and pig have this feature, but only the cow is readily susceptible to the lesion. Any condition causing forced expiratory maneuvers, even agonally, can cause the condition in the cow. It is common in slaughtered cattle. It occurs in most dramatic form as a prominent feature of acute interstitial pneumonia in cattle (acute bovine pulmonary emphysema and edema). A point to be emphasized is that there is no connection whatsoever between the pathogenesis of alveolar emphysema, as described previously, and interstitial emphysema in the cow. Although there is as yet no proof, it is presumed that air is forced into the complete but delicate interlobular septa because bronchioles are collapsed or otherwise blocked during forced expiration. For this to occur there has to be a lack of collateral ventilation and highly uneven deflation among neighboring lobules. In cows surviving a sufficient time with severe interstitial emphysema, the air can extend along lymphatics to the bronchial and mediastinal lymph nodes or along fascial planes of the mediastinum to beneath the skin of the back.

Bibliography

Anderson, W. I., King, J. M., and Flint, T. J. Multifocal bullous emphysema with concurrent bronchial hypoplasia in two aged Afghan hounds. *J Comp Pathol* **100:** 469–473, 1989.

Bradley, R., and Wrathall, A. E. Barker (neonatal respiratory distress) syndrome in the pig: The ultrastructural pathology of the lung. *J Pathol* **122:** 145–151, 1977.

Breeze, R. G. Heaves. *Vet Clin North Am [Large Anim Pract]* **1:** 219–230, 1979.

Cooper, J. E. Pulmonary cystic emphysema in piglets. *Vet Rec* **103:** 185–186, 1978.

Eriksson, S. Pulmonary emphysema and alpha-1-antitrypsin deficiency. *Acta Med Scand* **175:** 197–205, 1964.

Farrell, P. M., and Avery, M. E. Hyaline membrane disease. *Am Rev Respir Dis* **111:** 657–688, 1975.

Foley, F. D., and Lowell, F. C. Equine centrilobular emphysema. *Am Rev Respir Dis* **93:** 17–21, 1966.

Gillespie, J. R., and Tyler, W. S. Chronic alveolar emphysema in the horse. *Adv Vet Sci Comp Med* **13:** 59–99, 1969.

Gross, P. *et al.* Enzymatically produced pulmonary emphysema. A preliminary report. *J Occup Med* **6:** 481–484, 1964.

Herrtage, M. E., and Clarke, D. D. Congenital emphysema in two dogs. *J Small Anim Pract* **26:** 453–464, 1985.

Howard, E. B., and Ryan, C. P. Chronic obstructive pulmonary disease in the domestic cat. *Calif Vet* **36** (6): 7–11, 1982.

Mahaffey, L. W., and Rossdale, P. D. Convulsive and allied syndromes in new-born foals. *Vet Rec* **69:** 1277–1286, 1957.

Manktelow, B. W., and Baskerville, A. Respiratory distress syndrome in newborn puppies. *J Small Anim Pract* **13:** 329–332, 1972.

Perlmutter, D. H., and Pierce J. A. The α_1-antitrypsin gene and emphysema. *Am J Physiol* **257:** L147–L162, 1989.

Rossdale, P. D., Prattle, R. E., and Mahaffey, L. W. Respiratory distress in a newborn foal with failure to form lung-lining film. *Nature* **215:** 1498–1499, 1967.

Sartin, E. A., and Dubielzig, R. R. Congenital anomalies in the respiratory tree of a dog. *J Am Anim Hosp Assoc* **20:** 775–777, 1984.

Snider, G. L. The pathogenesis of emphysema—twenty years of progress. *Am Rev Respir Dis* **124:** 321–324, 1981.

Tennant, B. J., and Haywood, S. Congenital bullous emphysema in a dog: A case report. *J Small Anim Pract* **28:** 109–116, 1987.

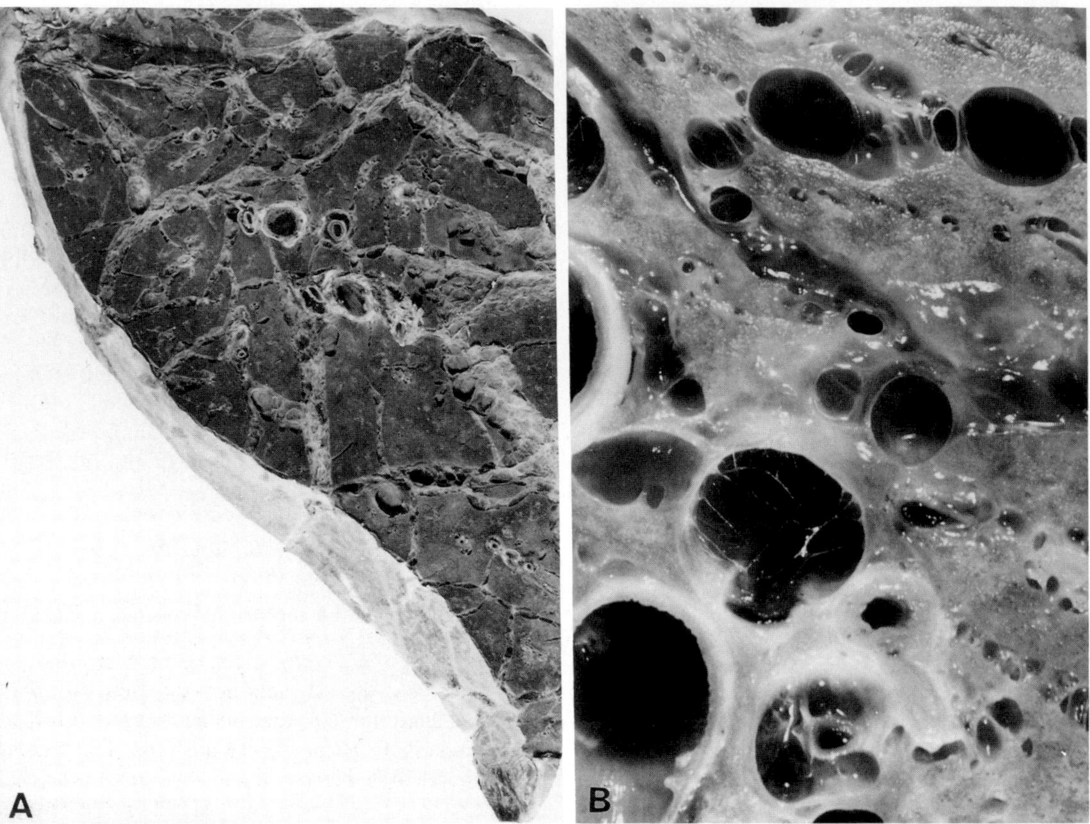

Fig. 6.29 (A & B) Interstitial emphysema secondary to acute interstitial pneumonia. Ox. Note bubbles of air in interstitial tissues and lymphatics of interlobular septa.

Wrathall, A. E. *et al.* Studies on the barker (neonatal respiratory distress) syndrome in the pig. *Cornell Vet* **67:** 543–598, 1977.

D. Circulatory Disturbances of Lungs

The lungs are affected by a large variety of circulatory disturbances. They are caused by abnormalities principally involving the pulmonary vessels and heart or by vascular changes secondary to pulmonary disease. The most important functional consequence is hypoxemia due to mismatching of ventilation and perfusion or shunting of blood through nonventilated regions of lung.

Pulmonary **ischemia** occurs following emphysematous or fibrotic attenuation of alveolar capillaries, and can be associated with severe reduction in blood volume. Because of the dual blood supply from pulmonary and bronchial arteries, and the extensive collateral circulation, congestion rather than ischemia is the usual sequel to arterial obstruction. Active **hyperemia** is part of the acute inflammatory response and is a feature of acute pulmonary injury of many types (see pneumonia, Section VI,F of this chapter). Pulmonary **congestion** is most commonly caused by left-sided or bilateral cardiac failure. It can also be due to changes in vascular tone causing redistribution of blood from the systemic to the pulmonary circulation. Such shifts commonly occur terminally or can be caused by autonomic disturbances, such as those produced by traumatic or other acutely damaging lesions in the hypothalamic region of the brain. The main importance of pulmonary congestion is that it leads to pulmonary edema.

1. Pulmonary Edema

Starling's equation for flow of liquid across a capillary membrane applies in general to pulmonary capillaries; that is, flow is dependent on the surface area and permeability characteristics of the vascular wall and on the balance of hydrostatic and osmotic pressures between the intravascular and interstitial compartments. The situation is more complicated in the lung, however, because the set of factors involved in the pathogenesis of alveolar edema also includes the permeability characteristics of the alveolar epithelium, air pressure, and surface tension acting on the alveolar surfaces, the role of alveolar oxygen in maintaining the permeability characteristics of alveolar capillaries, and preferential drainage of liquid through the pulmonary interstitium and possibly into the pleural space. Uncertainty exists about the exact magnitude of some of the factors and the routes by which water, solutes, and macromolecular substances cross endothelial and epithelial boundaries but the capacity of the pulmonary interstitium to act as a sink for excess fluid is critical to the maintenance of fluid balance.

Despite the low capillary hydrostatic pressure in the pulmonary circulation, there is a slow but steady flow of liquid from the alveolar interstitium into pulmonary lymphatics. Two factors are important in ensuring that alveoli do not become flooded under normal circumstances. One is that alveolar epithelium and its intercellular junctions are much less permeable than endothelial structures and therefore effectively seal off the alveolar lumen. The other is that the interstitial space is at lower pressure than intra-alveolar pressure. The interstitial pressure in the loose fascia surrounding vessels and airways where lymphatics are situated becomes increasingly subatmospheric (negative) toward the pulmonary hilus. The net effect is that liquid is drained from alveolar interstitium to lymphatics and to the loose connective tissue surrounding major vessels and airways, separating lobules, and in subpleural zones. The liquid then moves to the hilus of the lung and mediastinum. The bronchovascular interstitium and lymphatics therefore constitute a highly compliant sump. Provided the alveolar epithelium remains undamaged, alveolar edema does not occur until the capacity of the sump is overwhelmed. In slowly developing cardiogenic edema, the volume of interstitial liquid can be increased severalfold before alveolar flooding occurs. This explains why the first morphologic evidence of edema due to cardiac insufficiency is excess liquid in interstitium and lymphatics, particularly in the more compliant hilar regions. The increased capillary hydrostatic pressure and higher interstitial pressures caused by gravitational effects in dependent regions of the lungs predispose these sites to edema in large animals.

Physiological studies indicating different rates of movement of water and molecules of various size ranges and polarity have led to the development of mathematical models postulating the presence of pores of differing size ranges in the air–blood barrier. There is as yet no good correlation between the mathematical pore concept and ultrastructural evidence of sites of the pores. Probably water and small solutes pass through the endothelium by a transcellular route, and larger solutes, by way of intercellular junctions. Macromolecules appear to be largely transported by pinocytotic vesicles. Under some circumstances, water and protein are also actively transported across the alveolar epithelium. It is usually assumed that alveolar edema occurs by passage of edema fluid locally from interstitium to lumen. This is unquestionably the case for edema associated with increased capillary and type I epithelial permeability. It is not necessarily true for edema caused by increased capillary hydrostatic pressure (cardiogenic edema). There is the possibility that in this form of edema, excess fluid accumulates in the perivascular and peribronchiolar interstitium before overflowing into the alveoli through an as yet unidentified pathway close to the bronchiolar–alveolar junction. Although there is experimental evidence supporting this mechanism, its importance in naturally occurring, clinically significant cardiogenic edema remains to be established.

Pulmonary edema is a frequent complication of many diseases and is therefore one of the most commonly encountered pulmonary abnormalities. Most causes of edema act by increasing capillary hydrostatic (microvascular) pressure, by increasing permeability of the air–blood barrier, or by a combination of both factors. The total microvascular surface area is now recognized to be an important determinant, particularly in edema caused by increase in hydrostatic pressure. Decreased plasma oncotic pressure, such as occurs in hypoalbuminemia and lymphatic obstruction, caused for instance by widespread tumor infiltration of lymphatics and pulmonary lymph nodes, are less important.

Edema due to increased microvascular hydrostatic pressure is commonly the result of increased left atrial pressure in left-sided or bilateral cardiac failure and is commonly referred to as **cardiogenic edema.** The congestion and edema are important parts of the pulmonary complications of congestive heart failure (see The Cardiovascular System, Volume 3, Chapter 1). Increased capillary hydrostatic pressure is also the basis for the edema of hypervolemia developing in some cases of excessive fluid transfusion. Edema secondary to acute brain injury (neurogenic edema) appears to be due to both hemodynamic and capillary permeability changes. The immediate effect is increase in microvascular pressure associated with pulmonary hypertension, probably because of catecholamine release. Increase in capillary permeability occurs later.

Many agents cause pulmonary edema by damaging alveolar type I epithelium and capillary endothelium. The increase in permeability leads to edema of more rapid onset and of higher protein concentration than in cardiogenic forms. Inhaled corrosive gases (including 80–100% oxygen), systemic toxins, anaphylaxis in certain species such as the cow and horse, endotoxins, and shocklike states all can cause acute pulmonary edema. Reperfusion injury is now also recognized as a cause. As in edema elsewhere, there is no clear dividing line between these inflammatory edemas and serous exudates. Many of the toxic or shocklike states causing the edema accompanying acute pulmonary injury may be sufficiently severe to cause the set of abnormalities characterizing acute interstitial pneumonia. They will be considered further under that heading (Section VI,F,3 of this chapter). Loss or inhibition of phospholipid-rich surfactant in the alveolar lining layer can enhance edema formation because high surface tension at the air–liquid interface tends to draw fluid into the alveolus. This is probably not of primary importance except in neonatal hyaline membrane disease (respiratory distress syndrome) and perhaps in loss of surfactant activity accompanying prolonged shallow respiration.

Clinically evident pulmonary edema is a sign of serious underlying disturbance. Cardiogenic edema is not fatal if the cardiac insufficiency can be controlled, but pulmonary edema is often the cause of death from sudden cardiac decompensation. Whether other forms of pulmonary edema cause death depends on the severity and speed of onset of the underlying disease process and the edema it produces. Alveolar edema prevents ventilation of flooded alveoli. In the presence of surfactant material, it becomes stable foam by mixing with air in small airways, and the foam further compromises ventilation. As stated previously, clearance of interstitial edema fluid is through the compliant interstitial and lymphatic routes to the hilus of the lung and then into the mediastinum. Passage into the pleural space may also be important. Clearance of edema fluid from alveoli depends on protein content. Liquid (not protein) can be cleared rapidly by active metabolic transport of sodium across the alveolar epithelium into blood or interstitial spaces. Protein removal is slow, possibly by transcytosis (via pinocytotic vesicles) across the alveolar epithelium.

Edematous lungs are wet, heavy, and do not collapse completely when the thorax is opened. Frequently there is excess fluid in the thoracic cavity. Subpleural and interstitial tissues are edematous, and in lungs with well-developed interlobular septa, there is an accentuated pattern because the septa, become distended by edema fluid (Fig. 6.30A). Air can be mixed with edema in the bovine lung and distended, tortuous, and beaded lymphatics become visible grossly. Foam is discharged from the nostrils in severe cases, and foam variously mixed with fluid is often present in trachea (Fig. 6.30B) and intrapulmonary airways. Presence of foam indicates edema of at least moderate severity and the presence of alveolar surfactant not inhibited by fibrinogen or other high-molecular-weight constituents of serum. Fluid oozes from cut surfaces of edematous lungs.

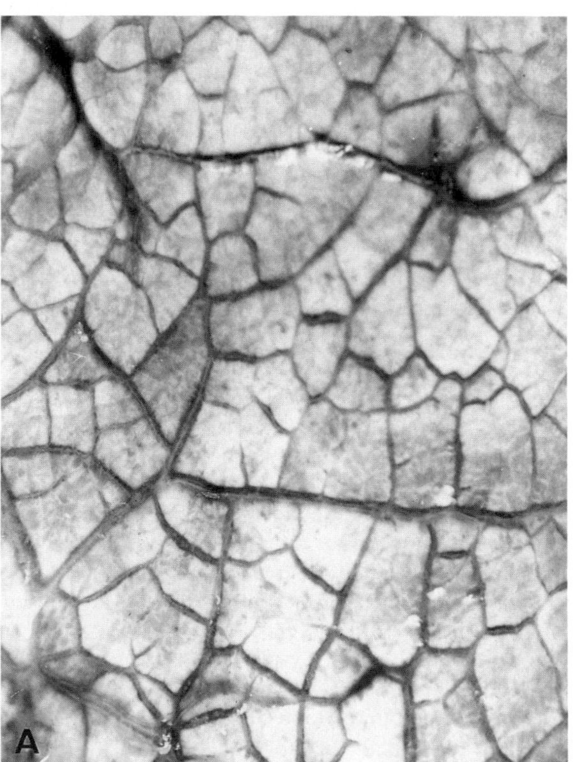

Fig. 6.30A Pulmonary edema. Ox. Interstitial accumulation of fluid accentuates the lobular pattern.

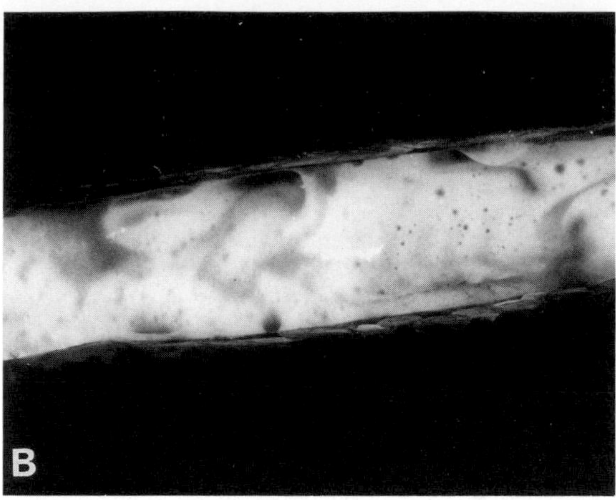

Fig. 6.30B Tracheal foam due to severe terminal pulmonary edema. Horse.

The color of edema fluid and foam depends on the amount of hemorrhage. If absent, the interstitial edema is clear, colorless to slightly yellow, and the foam is white. Various amounts of hemorrhage cause corresponding degrees of bloodstaining of fluid and foam. The pulmonary parenchyma varies from the dusky hue of cyanosis to reddish black according to the amount of congestion or hyperemia. When severe, the distinction between acute pulmonary edema and peracute pneumonia, especially interstitial pneumonia, is not possible grossly and can be blurred even on microscopic examination.

Histologically, edema fluid is acidophilic, homogeneous, or faintly granular material filling alveoli except for occasional discrete holes which represent trapped air bubbles. The same material is usually present in interstitial tissue and lymphatics around vessels and airways and in interlobular septa and subpleural zones in those species in which these are well developed. The amount of protein present in cardiogenic edema is small enough, particularly in dogs and cats, that it does not stain well after the leaching that occurs in formalin fixative. It can therefore easily be overlooked. Noting the presence of foam or fluid at gross examination, and distension of interstitial tissue and lymphatics microscopically, then takes on added importance. Coagulant fixatives containing mercury are best for demonstration of protein in edema fluid. Edema due to permeability defects is more acidophilic than cardiogenic edema, even after formalin fixation, and frequently contains strands or clumps of fibrin. The postmortem seepage of fluid into the alveoli of animals killed by barbiturate euthanasia solutions can easily be mistaken for edema. This artefact usually prevents detection of any antemortem edema unless the latter is revealed by dilation of interstitial lymphatics.

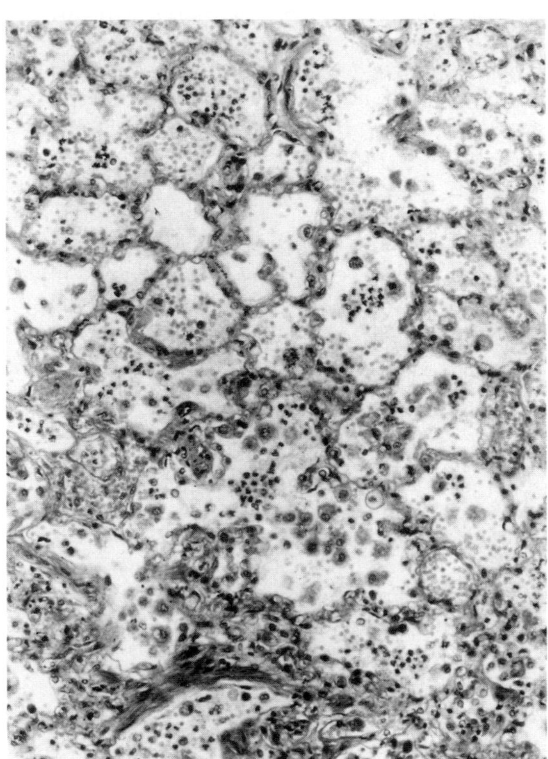

Fig. 6.31 Chronic pulmonary congestion due to heart failure. Dog.

When the lungs are congested, the capillaries are distended and intra-alveolar hemorrhages are common. Alveolar macrophages containing erythrocytes or hemosiderin are present and increase in number with duration of the congestion. These cells are known as heart failure cells (Fig. 6.31); they are not usually a prominent feature of congestive heart failure in animals, however. This is at least partly because of the shorter time animals with severe failure are kept alive compared to humans. A more usual feature accompanying the pulmonary hypertension of chronic cardiogenic edema in the dog and cat is hypertrophy of the muscular walls of small pulmonary vessels and thickening of pulmonary capillary walls by fibrous tissue, resulting in prominent circular profiles of capillaries with thickened walls within alveolar septa (Fig. 6.31). Occasionally, in terminal cardiac failure in the dog and cat, there is accumulation of leukocytes in pulmonary capillaries, severe damage to endothelium and alveolar type I epithelium, and filling of alveoli with fibrin-rich fluid. The cause is not established, but the morphologic evidence indicates acute pulmonary injury of shocklike antecedents (see acute interstitial pneumonia, in Section VI,F,3 of this chapter).

2. *Pulmonary Hemorrhage*

Hemorrhages occur frequently in the lung and beneath the pleura in the hemorrhagic diatheses, septicemias, disseminated intravascular coagulation (DIC), and severe congestion. They can also be caused by infarction, ruptured aneurysms, and trauma. Hemorrhages vary from petechiation to massive filling of large regions by blood. Aspiration of blood is frequent at slaughter. It has a characteristic pattern of multiple, small, bright red foci with feathery or indistinct borders. Massive hemorrhage sufficient to cause hemoptysis or exsanguination is occasionally observed in cattle. It is caused by erosion of a large vessel and rupture into a bronchus. It can be a complication of a bronchogenic abscess but is more often the sequel to septic thromboembolism and arteritis, usually caused by embolism from a septic thrombus in a large hepatic vein or the posterior vena cava. Clotted blood will be found in the forestomachs.

Exercise-induced pulmonary hemorrhage is the term currently used for hemorrhage occurring in horses during racing or training. It used to be referred to as epistaxis, but with endoscopic examination it has been shown that most horses (75% or more) examined soon after strenuous exertion have detectable hemorrhage, but only 1–10% have blood at the nostrils. The frequency of exercise-induced hemorrhage increases with age and severity of exertion. Bronchoscopic examinations reveal that the hemorrhage occurs in dorsocaudal lung regions. This is confirmed on postmortem examination of severely affected horses by finding grossly visible, patchy, bluish-brown discolored subpleural foci in the dorsocaudal portions of both caudal lobes. Histologically, the main features in affected regions are multifocal bronchiolitis, fibrosis, hemosiderophages in airspaces and interstitium, and extensive proliferation (neovascularization) of bronchial arteries. How these morphologic findings translate into pulmonary hemorrhage during exercise is debated. Current speculations favor increased microvascular pressure because of bronchopulmonary anastomoses and hemodynamic changes of severe exercise, and exaggerated forces acting on the alveolar septa because of uneven ventilation of neighboring lung lobules. The latter would be exaggerated during increased respiratory rate and amplitude in the presence of small airway disease and fibrosis.

3. *Embolism, Thrombosis, and Infarction*

The lungs are strategically situated to catch emboli carried in venous blood. In accordance with the general pathology of **embolism,** the outcome will depend on the nature of the embolic material and on the features of the pulmonary circulation. Because the lung is supplied by both pulmonary and bronchial arteries and has extensive collateral channels, infarction usually does not follow embolism and thrombosis unless the pulmonary circulation is already compromised. It is possible, for instance, to find a major pulmonary artery occluded by large, pale, friable thromboembolic material without gross abnormality of the pulmonary parenchyma. Bacterial emboli are associated with fulminating bacteremias and cause acute pulmonary edema or interstitial pneumonia. Septic emboli arising from infected thrombi cause thromboembolism, arteritis, usually multiple abscessation, and sometimes more extensive chronic suppurative pneumonia. In the cow, septic emboli arise mainly from thrombosis of the posterior vena cava due to local spread of a hepatic abscess. They can also originate in uterine and pelvic veins. Emboli arise mainly from mesenteric veins in horses, and they can originate from vegetative endocarditis in any species.

Tumor emboli vary in number from a few widely separated foci to extensive showering of capillaries and larger vessels with neoplastic cells. The latter is more common with highly invasive, anaplastic carcinomas such as some types of mammary carcinomas in bitches. An unusual form of embolism occurs where carcinoma cells lodge and proliferate within vessels to produce multiple discrete foci surrounded by smooth muscle and collagen. In some foci, there is thrombosis which stimulates organization by granulation tissue and frequently leads to death of the neoplastic cells and obliteration of the vascular lumen. Malignant cells usually proliferate more in perivascular lymphatics than in the vessels themselves.

Fat embolism is only occasionally important in animals. The fat can originate from bone marrow at sites of fracture and from severe hepatic lipidosis when the hepatocytes rupture. The emboli lodge in alveolar capillaries and produce sausage-shaped distensions, which are empty in routine paraffin sections. Megakaryocytes are frequently found in pulmonary capillaries, particularly in dogs. A small number of megakaryocytes derived from bone marrow are present in circulating blood and lodge in the lungs where they continue to produce platelets. This is a normal occurrence, but may be accentuated when there is compensatory extramedullary hematopoiesis in spleen and liver.

Pulmonary thrombosis can be triggered, as elsewhere, when there is hypercoagulability, stasis of blood, or vascular endothelial damage, as well as by embolism and endoarteritis. There is an association between pulmonary thrombosis and renal amyloidosis in dogs because of the loss of antithrombin III as part of the protein-losing nephropathy. The endoarteritis caused by *Dirofilaria immitis* or *Angiostrongylus vasorum* is also a cause of thrombosis in dogs; less commonly, thrombosis is secondary to ulceration of intimal atherosclerotic plaques. Disseminated intravascular coagulation in septicemic, toxic, and advanced neoplastic states is also an important cause (see The Cardiovascular System, Volume 3, Chapter 1). Pulmonary thrombosis of unexplained cause is found occasionally in all species.

Pulmonary infarction is an unlikely event unless the pulmonary circulation is already compromised. Thrombosis of large vessels is more likely to lead to congestion, edema, and atelectasis of the affected regions. Most infarcts occur in lungs which have generalized passive congestion. Thrombi occurring in conditions associated with general circulatory collapse, such as disseminated intravascular coagulation, are therefore particularly likely to cause infarction.

All recent infarcts are hemorrhagic. They occur most frequently in the caudal lobes (Fig. 6.32). They usually extend to the pleura and are particularly prone to affect the sharp costophrenic borders of the lung. At the costophrenic margin, they are wedge shaped with the broad base toward the hilus of the lung. When they involve only one pleural surface, they are cone shaped with the base at the pleura. The shape is difficult to appreciate when they are small because their margins blend laterally with adjacent congested parenchyma. Infarcted areas bulge on the pleural aspect and are red-blue to black. They are firm, and the overlying pleura becomes roughened, opaque, and covered by bloodstained exudate if the infarct is more than a few hours old. When the infarct is large, the occluded vessel can usually be detected at or near its apex. Histologically, an early infarct has extensive hemorrhage against a background of necrotic parenchyma. If the animal survives, there is lysis of red cells and a border of neutrophils and macrophages appears within 1–2 days. Organization by peripheral encroachment of granulation tissue occurs subsequently and eventually results in scar formation. The sequelae to septic infarction consist of the more severe changes described previously for septic thromboembolism.

4. Pulmonary Hypertension

Pulmonary hypertension can be initiated by high-pressure flow of blood in the pulmonary artery, as occurs in congenital left-to-right shunts, or by increased resistance in the pulmonary vascular system. The increased resistance to flow may be the result of left-sided heart failure, as occurs with mitral incompetence, luminal narrowing of vessels by arteriosclerotic changes, or by hypoxic vasoconstriction as seen in high-altitude disease of cattle (see The Cardiovascular System, Volume 3, Chapter 1). Regardless of initial cause, there occurs a vicious cycle of hypertension causing arteriosclerosis, which in turn leads to more hypertension. Probably the most common cause of hypertension is functional resistance to flow due to hypoxemia. The hypoxemia may reflect the low ambient oxygen tensions of high altitudes, the various forms of hypoventilation, or the various causes of abnormal ventilation/perfusion ratios. The histologic changes in the pulmonary vasculature may be minimal, consisting of muscularization and intimal thickening of small arteries, but in cattle, and to a lesser extent in sheep, muscular thickening in veins is prominent and develops rapidly.

Any subacute or chronic lesion causing narrowing or obliteration of pulmonary vessels can cause pulmonary hypertension. Thromboembolic situations may therefore produce hypertension and cor pulmonale. Widespread fibrosis in chronic interstitial pneumonias can also cause pulmonary hypertension by occluding small vessels. There is frequently hyperplasia of smooth muscle of bronchioles, alveolar ducts, and small vessels accompanying fibrosis, particularly in cattle. It is possibly caused by stimulation of smooth muscle cells by platelet-derived and other growth factors, which also stimulate the fibroblasts. The increase in smooth muscle tends to exacerbate the

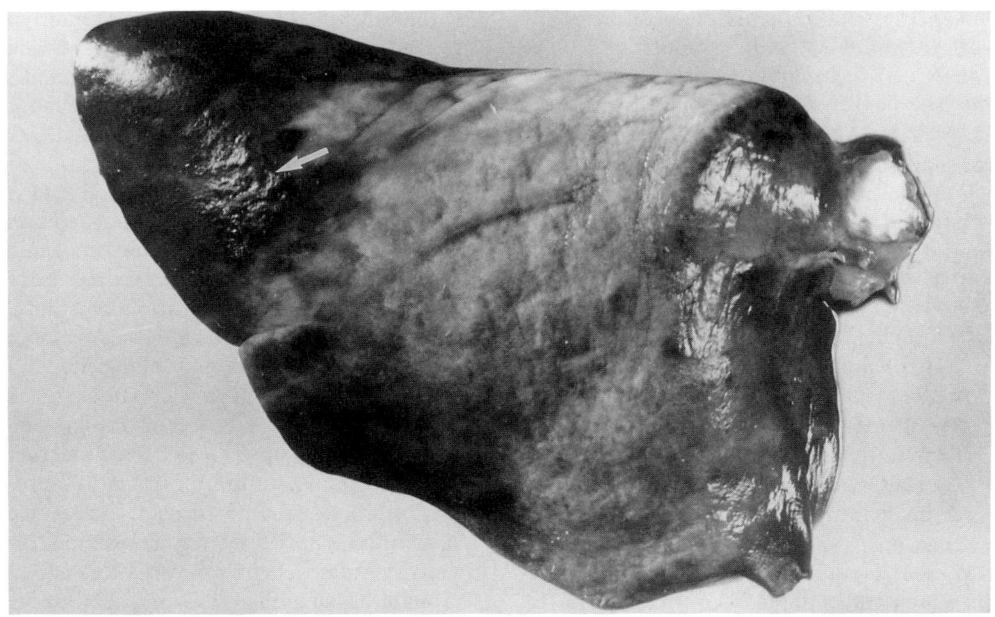

Fig. 6.32 Lung. Infarct. Dog. Note dark, swollen area in caudal part of caudal lobe and fibrin on pleura (arrow).

pulmonary hypertension. Chronic bronchitis and bronchiolitis stimulate muscular hypertrophy in the walls of small arteries, and this too can result in cor pulmonale. The effects of hypertension alone are mainly in the small muscular arteries where there is proliferation of myointimal and medial smooth muscle cells and in arterioles, which develop prominent muscle coats by proliferation of pericytes. Severe hypertension causes endothelial degeneration and intimal adventitial fibroplasia. Eventually leakage of plasma protein into the degenerating muscular and collagenous components of the wall can produce fibrinoid necrosis.

Bibliography

Breeze, R. G. *et al.* Thrombosis of the posterior vena cava in cattle. *Vet Annu* **16:** 52–59, 1976.

Cook, W. R. Epistaxis in the racehorse. *Equine Vet J* **6:** 45–58, 1974.

Donaldson, L. L. A review of the pathophysiology of exercise-induced pulmonary haemorrhage in the equine athlete. *Vet Res Comm* **15:** 211–216, 1991.

Drake, R. E., and Laine, G. A. Pulmonary microvascular permeability to fluid and macromolecules. *J Appl Physiol* **64:** 487–501, 1988.

Ell, S. R. Neurogenic pulmonary edema. *Invest Radiol* **26:** 499–506, 1991.

Lees, G. E., Suter, P. F., and Johnson, G. C. Pulmonary edema in a dog with acute pancreatitis and cardiac disease. *J Am Vet Med Assoc* **172:** 690–696, 1978.

Mansmann, R. A. *et al.* Chicken hypersensitivity pneumonitis in horses. *J Am Vet Med Assoc* **116:** 673–677, 1975.

Matthay, M. A. Resolution of pulmonary edema—New insights. *West J Med* **154:** 315–321, 1991.

Morgan, P. W., and Goodman, L. R. Pulmonary edema and adult respiratory distress syndrome. *Radiol Clin North Am* **29:** 943–963, 1991.

Nimmo-Wilkie, J. S., and Feldman, E. C. Pulmonary vascular lesions associated with congenital heart defects in three dogs. *J Am Anim Hosp Assoc* **17:** 485–490, 1981.

O'Callaghan, M. W., Pascoe, J. R., and Tyler, W. S. Exercise-induced pulmonary haemorrhage in the horse: Results of a detailed clinical, postmortem and imaging study. VIII. Conclusions and implications. *Equine Vet J* **19:** 428–434, 1987.

Raphel, C. F., and Soma, L. R. Exercise-induced pulmonary hemorrhage in thoroughbreds after racing and breezing. *Am J Vet Res* **43:** 1123–1127, 1982.

Robinson, N. E., and Derksen, F. J. Small-airway obstruction as a cause of exercise-associated pulmonary hemorrhage: An hypothesis. *Proc Am Assoc Equine Pract* **26:** 421–430, 1980.

Schneider, P., and Pappritz, G. Hairs causing pulmonary emboli. A rare complication in long-term intravenous studies in dogs. *Vet Pathol* **13:** 394–400, 1976.

Staub, N. C. New concepts about the pathophysiology of pulmonary edema. *J Thorac Imaging* **3:** 8–14, 1988.

Weir, E. K. *et al.* Vascular hypertrophy in cattle susceptible to hypoxic pulmonary hypertension. *J Appl Physiol* **46:** 517–521, 1979.

E. Inflammation of the Lungs

Pneumonia is the usual term for inflammation of the lungs involving alveolar parenchyma. There has been a tendency to use the term **pneumonia** for more acute and exudative inflammation and **pneumonitis** for more chronic, proliferative lesions. Since proliferative components are mostly within or become incorporated into the interstitium of the lung, pneumonitis and chronic interstitial pneumonia are largely synonymous terms. Alveolitis is another term used to describe acute exudative inflammation of alveolar tissue. Separate and sometimes conflicting use of pneumonia, pneumonitis, and alveolitis has more potential for confusion than clarification, however, so the term pneumonia will be used for pulmonary inflammation throughout this chapter. Salient morphologic and pathogenetic features of the various types of pneumonia are conveyed by additional descriptive terms.

The susceptibility of alveolar cells to injury and their capacity for regeneration have been briefly outlined in the first section of this chapter. When considering the response of alveolar tissue to injury, a brief review of alveolar cell responses and a few of the major regulatory molecules involved is warranted.

Type I alveolar epithelial cells are among the most sensitive cells to injury in the lung. The usual pattern of alveolar response to injury is for necrosis and sloughing of type I cells to occur during the acute exudative phase of inflammation. Provided the severity of the process is not sufficient to cause necrosis of type II cells and other components of the alveolar septa, the type II cells begin to proliferate within 24 hr and eventually completely line the previously denuded alveolar wall. Histologically, small clusters of alveolar cells can be detected 2–3 days after loss of type I cells, and by 6 days there can be complete lining of alveoli by cuboidal type II cells. Alveoli completely lined by type II cells give the appearance commonly referred to as epithelialization. In some instances, exaggerated proliferation of type II cells in dogs accompanied by variability of nuclear/cytoplasmic ratios is erroneously interpreted as a neoplastic process. The complete lining of alveoli by type II cells, which is a common response to injury, has also misleadingly been referred to as adenomatosis. Proliferation of type II cells marks the shift from the exudative to the proliferative stage of pneumonia and is usually accompanied by an alveolar exudate increasingly composed of macrophages and other mononuclear cells. Resolution of the epithelial lesion, once inflammation has subsided and provided there has not been scarring of the alveolar wall, is accomplished by transformation of type II cells into type I epithelium.

The character of alveolar exudate depends on its cause. In general, it changes with time from serous fluid (inflammatory edema) containing various quantities of fibrin, through a neutrophil phase that predominates in most bacterial infections, to an accumulation mostly consisting of alveolar macrophages. Both the dominant features and the rate of change vary according to cause of the inflammation. The degree of neutrophil infiltration into alveolar spaces and the amount of fibrin deposition and persistence are determined by a complex network of interactions at the alveolar level involving alveolar macrophages, capillary endothelial cells, circulating neutrophils, and serum components, as well as the nature and severity of the inciting agent.

Neutrophil movement and function in the alveolar space involve the classical processes of margination and adherence to endothelial cells, chemotaxis across the endothelial and epithelial barriers into the lung, and stimulation (up-regulation) of phagocytic and secretory functions. Depending on the nature of the inciting stimulus, various cell- and serum-derived inflammatory mediators are released to activate neutrophil adherence to capillary endothelial cells. Factors such as leukotriene B_4, platelet activating factor, and C5a can stimulate expression of integrin receptors on neutrophil surfaces. Interleukin-1 (IL-1) and tumor necrosis factor-α (TNF-α), which are also produced by activated macrophages, can act on endothelial cells to stimulate expression of endothelial leukocyte adhesion molecules and other adhesion molecules. These promote neutrophil–endothelial adherence prior to migration of the neutrophil into the alveolus along chemotactic concentration gradients. Chemotactic factors for neutrophil movement into the lung are well characterized and include IL-8, C5a, leukotriene B_4 and fibrin-degradation products. Interleukin-8 (neutrophil attractant/activation protein-1) is a 8400-dalton protein, which is released by many pulmonary cells including macrophages, type II cells, endothelial cells, and fibroblasts following exposure to a number of stimulants including IL-1 and TNF. Clearly, cytokines released from macrophages following a number of perturbations, including particulate and antigen exposure and stimulation by gamma interferon, play a major role in neutrophil recruitment into the lung.

The quantity of fibrin in alveolar exudate is an index of the amount of damage to the alveolar–capillary membrane because it reveals leakage of its precursor fibrinogen. Fibrin, together with other serum constituents and cell debris, forms the hyaline membranes found in conditions involving severe damage to the alveolar wall. The amount of fibrin deposited within and persisting in the alveolus is an important determinant of loss of alveolar function and repair by alveolar fibrosis. When alveolar epithelium is denuded, fibrinous membranes or plugs are infiltrated by macrophages, fibroblasts, and endothelial cells from the alveolar wall. Macrophages promote fibrosis by releasing fibronectin, which is chemotactic for fibroblasts, and by release of cytokines and growth factors including transforming growth factor-beta (TGFβ), platelet derived growth factor (PDGF), and insulinlike growth factors, all of which stimulate collagen synthesis and synthesis of glycosaminoglycans. Collagen-containing fibrous tissue can be detected as early as 7 days after initial fibrinous exudation.

Chronic inflammation of the alveolar septa is the major feature of chronic interstitial pneumonias and will be discussed more fully under that heading. Chronic bronchopneumonia, on the other hand, is much more likely to lead to destruction of alveolar walls and abscessation because of persistent suppuration caused by pyogenic bacteria. An aspect of the response of alveolar type II cells to chronic injury is their potential for undergoing metaplasia to squamous, ciliated, or fetal-type, glycogen-containing cells. One of the most important general features of the response of pulmonary epithelial cells to both acute and chronic injury is the extent to which transdifferentiation (metaplasia of one cell type to another) can occur in airways and alveoli. Persistent irritation or disruption of the normal epithelial interaction with basement membrane and alveolar stroma leads to persistence of atypical alveolar type II cells and the possibility that they will occasionally give rise to bronchioloalveolar tumors, as sometimes seems to occur in dogs and rodents.

Bibliography

Adamson, I. Y. R., Hedgecock, C., and Bowden, D. H. Epithelial cell–fibroblast interactions in lung injury and repair. *Am J Pathol* **137:** 385–392, 1990.

Albelda, S. M. Endothelial and epithelial cell adhesion molecules. *Am J Respir Cell Mol Biol* **4:** 195–203, 1991.

Berman, J. S. *et al.* Lymphocyte recruitment to the lung. *Am Rev Res Dis* **142:** 238–257, 1990.

Bertram, T. A. *et al.* Comparison of arachidonic acid metabolism by pulmonary intravascular and alveolar macrophages exposed to particulate and soluble stimuli. *Lab Invest* **61:** 457–66, 1989.

Car, B. D. *et al.* The role of leukocytes in the pathogenesis of fibrin deposition in bovine acute lung injury. *Am J Pathol* **138:** 1191–1198, 1991.

Crouch, E. Pathobiology of pulmonary fibrosis. *Am J Physiol* **259:** L159–184, 1990.

Goldstein, R. H. Control of type I collagen formation in the lung. *Am J Physiol* **261:** L29–40, 1991.

Hogg, J. C. Neutrophil kinetics and lung injury. *Physiol Rev* **67:** 1249–1295, 1987.

Kelley, J. Cytokines of the lung. *Am Rev Resp Dis* **141:** 765–788, 1990.

Kunkel, S. L. *et al.* Interleukin-8 (IL-8): The major neutrophil chemotactic factor in the lung. *Exp Lung Res* **17:** 17–23, 1991.

Leonard, E. J., and Yoshimura, T. Neutrophil attractant/activation protein-1 [NAP-1 (interleukin-8)]. *Am J Respir Cell Mol Biol* **2:** 479–86, 1990.

Said, S. I., and Foda, H. D.. Pharmacologic modulation of lung injury. *Am Rev Resp Dis* **139:** 1553–1564, 1989.

Sappino, A. P., Schürch, W., and Gabbiani, G. Biology of disease. Differentiation repertoire of fibroblastic cells: Expression of cytoskeletal proteins as marker of phenotypic modulations. *Lab Invest* **63:** 144–161, 1990.

Schleimer, R. P. *et al.* Do cytokines play a role in leukocyte recruitment and activation in the lungs? *Am Rev Respir Dis* **143:** 1169–74, 1991.

Serabjit-Singh, C. J. *et al.* The distribution of cytochrome P-450 monooxygenase in cells of the rabbit lung: An ultrastructural immunocytochemical characterization. *Mol Pharmacol* **33:** 279–289, 1988.

Sibille, Y., and Reynolds, H. Y. Macrophages and polymorphonuclear neutrophils in lung defense and injury. *Am Rev Resp Dis* **141:** 471–501, 1990.

Slauson, D. O. The mediation of pulmonary inflammatory injury. *Adv Vet Sci Comp Med* **26:** 99–144, 1982.

F. Anatomic Patterns of Pneumonia

The pulmonary inflammatory response varies according to the nature of the causative agents, their distribution (particularly the route by which they reach the lung), and their persistence. Pneumonia can be classified on a temporal basis as acute, subacute, or chronic, on an etiologic basis by major categories of causative agent, or according to morphologic features. Morphologically, there are two approaches. One approach is to classify according to the type of inflammation. Here there are two main subcategories: **exudative** pneumonias, in which the emphasis is on filling of alveoli by exudate with predominant **catarrhal, fibrinous, suppurative, hemorrhagic,** or **necrotizing** characteristics, and **proliferative** pneumonias in which the emphasis is on proliferation of alveolar type II cells, fibroblasts, macrophages, and possibly additional elements. The second, and more useful, morphologic approach is to classify pneumonias according to initial site of involvement and the pattern of spread of the lesion. On this basis, most pneumonias fall into three main categories: **bronchopneumonia, lobar pneumonia,** and **interstitial pneumonia.** The importance of this classification lies in the provision of clues regarding pathogenesis and possible causes.

There is often good linkage between the various classifications. For example, acute pneumonias are commonly of infectious cause, exudative in nature, and of bronchopneumonic pattern. Chronic pneumonias are of highly varied cause, proliferative in nature, and often of interstitial pattern. Other correlations, and exceptions to these generalizations, are identified in following sections.

1. Bronchopneumonia

The hallmark of bronchopneumonia is the origin of inflammation in the bronchioloalveolar junction, as an extension of bronchial inflammation. This is correlated with a predominantly aerogenous portal of entry of the causative agents, involvement usually of cranioventral regions of the lungs, and a patchy or variegated gross appearance. The irregular lobular involvement is reflected in the older term **lobular pneumonia.**

The defenses of the healthy lung are remarkably effective. Whether inflammation results from the constant bombardment of the lung by inhaled irritants depends on the balance between the intensity of the insult and the effectiveness of local defense mechanisms at each structural level of airways and parenchyma. In the distal respiratory tract, the bronchiolar–alveolar junctions are the sites of greatest vulnerability to damage by many types of inhaled particles and vapors, including droplet nuclei carrying infectious agents. There are three main reasons for the vulnerability of these regions. First, they are the major site of deposition of small particles (0.5–3.0 μm in diameter) capable of reaching deep lung. Second, the epithelium of bronchioles is probably susceptible to damage because it is not protected by the mucous blanket of larger airways or by an effective alveolar macrophage system. Third, the cellular (mostly macrophage) and noncellular material cleared from large volumes of alveolar parenchyma has to pass through the narrow lumen of its parent bronchiole, an easily plugged funnel or bottleneck, especially where lack of collateral ventilation hampers expulsion of exudate.

Epidemiologic and experimental evidence indicates that

the important infectious bronchopneumonias of animals usually develop only when the balance is tipped in favor of disease by an increase in numbers of pathogenic microorganisms reaching vulnerable bronchioloalveolar regions of the lung or when pulmonary defenses are underdeveloped or impaired. In most situations, both of these circumstances are present. Increased exposure to pathogenic microorganisms is particularly likely to occur when animals from a variety of sources are congregated. This is often associated with lack of immune experience with the organisms involved. An important aspect of increased exposure of pulmonary parenchyma to pathogenic microorganisms at times of environmental stress is the concurrent increased colonization of upper respiratory mucosa by agents such as *Pasteurella* spp. Reduced effectiveness of pulmonary defense mechanisms occurs in congenital and acquired immunodeficiency states and can also be caused by a variety of factors impairing the mucociliary blanket, alveolar macrophage defense systems, or both. Dehydration, extreme chilling, viral infection, inhalation of toxic gases and particles, certain anesthetics, and ciliary abnormalities inhibit mucociliary clearance and can predispose to bacterial colonization. Functions of alveolar macrophages and reinforcing activities of lymphoid cells are impaired by severe chilling, starvation, viral infection (including immunodeficiency viruses), toxic gases, metabolic disorders such as uremia and acidosis, and immunosuppressants such as corticosteroids. Chronic disease of heart or lungs also reduces pulmonary defensive capability.

Various combinations of these factors exist in circumstances recognized as predisposing to a high risk of bronchopneumonia and also the more aggressive lobar pneumonias. Most outbreaks are in young, intensively managed animals, especially soon after stresses associated with transport. Mixing of animals with different microbial floras and levels of acquired immunity is often involved as well. Sporadic cases of bronchopneumonia in individual animals are likely to be associated with interactive predisposing causes such as debility, immunodeficiency, preexisting cardiopulmonary disease, and prolonged anesthesia or recumbency of illness. Aspiration of foreign material can cause bronchopneumonia, but because of its severity, the inflammation more commonly has a lobar distribution.

The characteristic cranioventral distribution of infectious bronchopneumonias in animals indicates that in these regions the balance between insult and defense is most precarious. This is supported by the fact that pneumonia caused by inhalation of acutely irritant particles or gases does not have a cranioventral distribution. All the reasons for the cranioventral involvement have not been determined. It is reasonable to hypothesize that there is increased deposition of infectious particles in these regions, that defenses are more easily compromised, or both. There is slightly increased deposition of particles in cranial regions. This is believed to be due to the shorter and more abruptly branching airways. Gravitational influences impeding clearance of cranioventral regions, and possibly leading to pooling or reflux of secretions, are probably more important contributory factors. The smaller size of ventral airspaces and their greater vulnerability to collapse or blockage may also be involved. The possible roles of different rates of leukocyte traffic through the pulmonary capillary bed and different densities of intercellular adhesion molecules or other receptors have not been explored. There is evidence that *P. haemolytica* reaching the lungs in the blood also causes pneumonia in cranioventral regions. Since this is an unusual location for hematogenous injury, it supports the hypothesis that bacterial infection can become established and develop further in the cranioventral lung because local defense mechanisms are less effective there.

Bacteria are the main causes of clinically significant bronchopneumonia, most commonly after pulmonary defenses have been lowered by viral infection, severe stress, or other predisposing factors. Many species of bacteria are involved, the particular set of agents varying with animal species and sometimes geographic location. In sheep and cattle, *Pasteurella* spp. and *Actinomyces pyogenes* are common. In swine, *P. multocida, Actinobacillus pleuropneumoniae, Haemophilus* spp., *A. pyogenes, Bordetella bronchiseptica,* and *Salmonella choleraesuis* are often involved. In horses, the chief offenders are *Streptococcus* spp. and *Rhodococcus equi.* In dogs, *B. bronchiseptica, Klebsiella* spp., streptococci, staphylococci, and *Escherichia coli* are important. In cats, in which the disease is less common, *P. multocida* and a variety of other Gram-negative organisms are most often found. Bacteria tend to cause suppurative pneumonia. Exceptions, such as the fulminating fibrinonecrotic pneumonias that can be caused by *Pasteurella* and *Haemophilus* spp., will be addressed later. The involvement of viruses, mycoplasmas, and chlamydiae will also be considered further under specific pneumonias, as will their roles in causing the enzootic pneumonias of cattle, sheep, and swine.

The typical gross appearance of bronchopneumonia is of irregular consolidation in cranioventral regions. The cranial and middle lobes are most often affected in those species having well-defined lobation. Consolidated lung varies from dark red, through gray-pink to more gray, depending on the age and nature of the process. Palpable firmness (consolidation) of the tissue is the single most important gross criterion of pneumonia. The extent to which there is a lobular or sublobular mosaic of consolidated, atelectatic, congested, and more normal lung tissue depends partly on the severity and rate of spread of the pneumonia and partly on the degree of septation. It is most common in relatively slow-spreading bronchopneumonias of ruminants and swine which have well-developed septation (Fig. 6.33). The more uniform and rapidly spreading the pneumonia, the more homogeneous and extensive the consolidation. Even where complete lobes become involved, however, the bronchopneumonia pattern can often be detected on careful gross examination by the presence of multiple, small, evenly spaced, gray-white, bulging foci separated by narrow deep red zones. The bulging pale

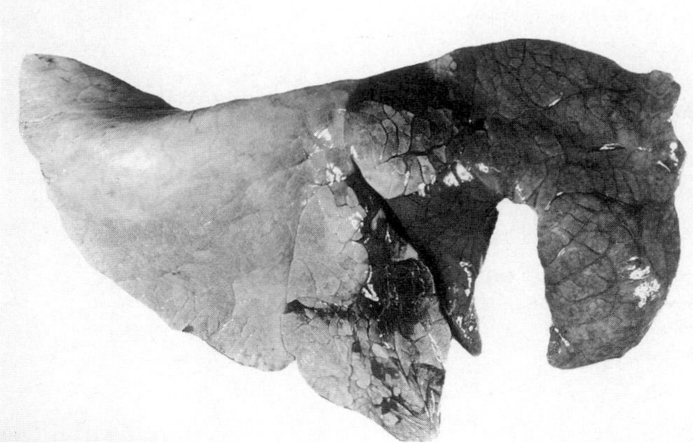

Fig. 6.33 Acute bronchopneumonia. Calf. Lobulation is emphasized in dark areas of consolidation by interlobular edema. Note focal pattern within affected lobules.

foci denote areas of exudation centered on bronchioles, and the deeper red zones represent more congested, edematous, and atelectatic alveolar parenchyma in peripheral acinar regions. This gross pattern is more usual in bronchopneumonia of dogs and cats, which have rudimentary interlobular septa, and in the enzootic bronchopneumonias of ruminants and swine. The pleura overlying mild to moderately inflamed pulmonary parenchyma usually has its normal smooth, glistening sheen. Where the inflammatory process is severe, however, it extends to the pleura to produce reddening, roughening, and superficial accumulation of yellow-gray fibrinous or fibrinopurulent exudate indicating pleuritis. The cut surface of affected lung reflects the variability of involvement seen on the pleural surface. In catarrhal or suppurative bronchopneumonias, consolidated lobules are moist on cut section; mucopurulent or purulent material can be expressed from small airways and can be seen in fluid or foamy state in the large airways. Frank abscesses can be present in severe suppurative inflammation (Fig. 6.34A). The cut surface of fibrinous inflammation, in contrast, has a dull, dryish appearance (Fig. 6.34B).

Histologically, the nidus of inflammation in bronchopneumonia is in the bronchioloalveolar junctions (Fig. 6.35A,B). In early bronchopneumonia, bronchioles and immediately adjacent alveoli are filled with neutrophils and sometimes an admixture of various amounts of cell debris, mucus, fibrin, and macrophages. The bronchiolar epithelium varies from necrotic to hyperplastic, depending on the nature and pathogenicity of causative agents, and there is mild acute inflammation of the peribronchiolar connective tissue. Bronchi often show similar but usually less severe changes. Necrotizing (Fig. 6.36) or proliferative lesions indicating the possibility of prior viral infection may be present (see specific viral infections), but pathognomonic inclusion bodies can be found only occasionally in clinical material. Adenovirus inclusion bodies are the exception and can usually be found in infection caused by this virus. Care must be taken not to interpret the apparently thickened epithelium of collapsed airways as evidence of epithelial hyperplasia. Alveoli peripheral to the severely inflamed bronchiolar regions are partially atelectatic and contain various amounts of edema or serofibrinous exudate, erythrocytes, macrophages, and a sprinkling of leukocytes. Vessels in the early acute stage are engorged and are responsible for the predominant red

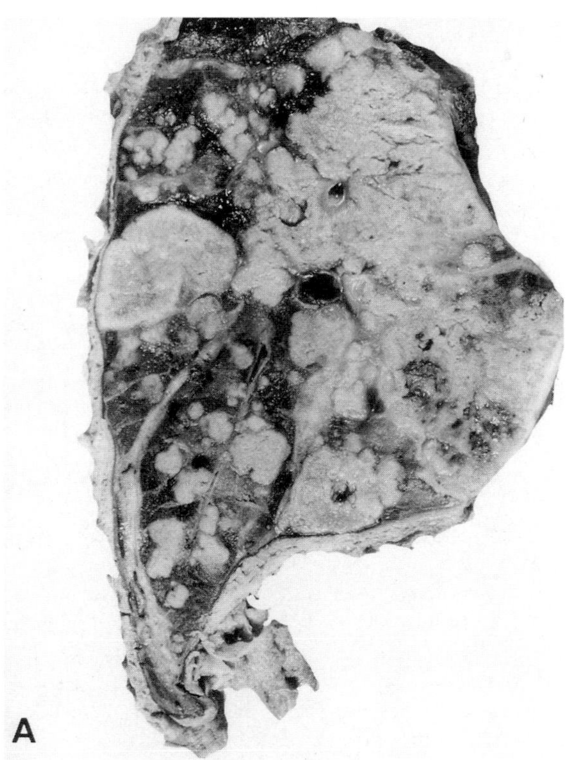

Fig. 6.34A Suppurative bronchopneumonia with abscessation and fibrinous pleuritis caused by streptococci. Horse.

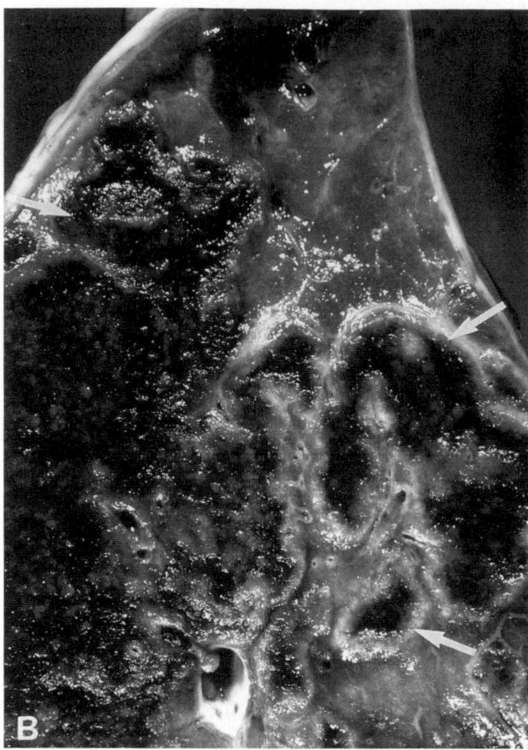

Fig. 6.34B Areas of necrosis (arrows) in lobar pneumonia. Cow.

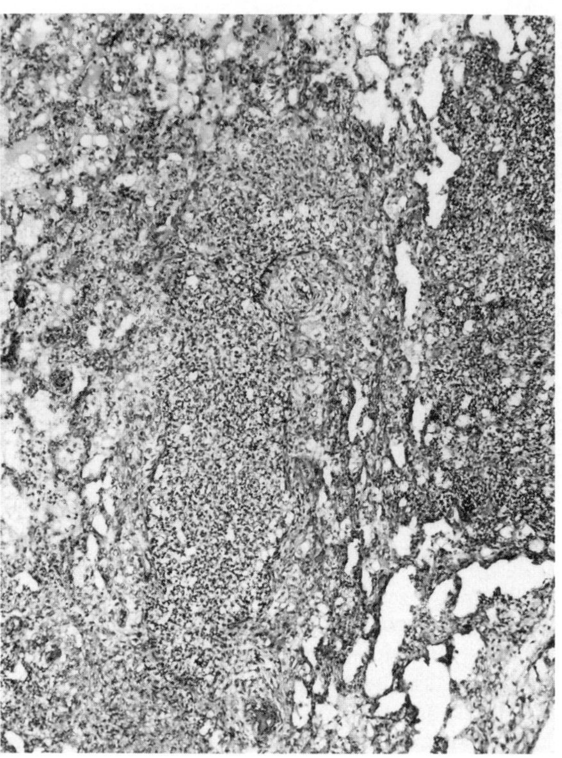

Fig. 6.36 Acute bronchopneumonia based on necrotizing bronchiolitis caused by adenovirus. Foal.

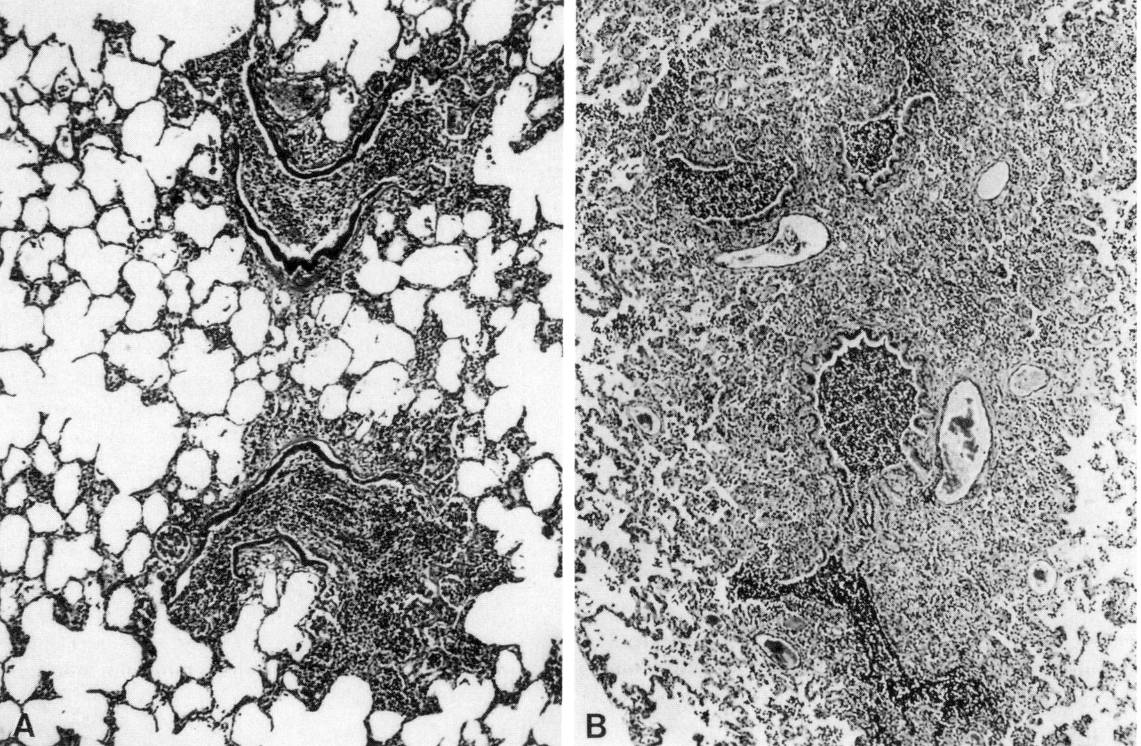

Fig. 6.35 (A) Initial lesion of bronchopneumonia at bronchioloalveolar junction. (B) Later stage of bronchopneumonia.

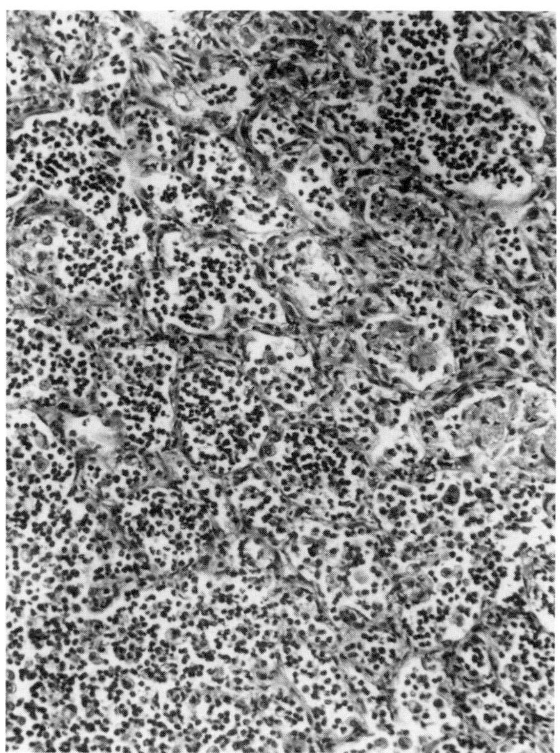

Fig. 6.37 Subacute suppurative bronchopneumonia. Pig.

color of the lung noted macroscopically. Edematous or serofibrinous fluid can be found in interstitial sites but is not an important feature of this early mild to moderate form of catarrhal bronchopneumonia.

The spread of infection after its initial foothold in the bronchiolo-alveolar regions is mostly by airways, both proximally through bronchioles and bronchi and distally through alveolar ducts and alveoli within a respiratory acinus (Fig. 6.37). The rate and extent of spread depends mainly on the balance between virulence of the causative agent and host defense. Rapid bacterial proliferation leads to severe suppurative pneumonia if pyogenic bacteria are involved, and fibrinous through hemorrhagic and necrotizing pneumonia if highly toxigenic bacteria such as *P. haemolytica* and *A. pleuropneumoniae* are the cause. In the latter instances, the pneumonia is likely to take on lobar characteristics, and spread of infection across edematous interlobular septa can become important.

The time sequence of inflammatory events varies with the severity and speed of onset, which in turn depend on the balance between the virulence of the agent and host defense. The red stage of consolidation is present for only 2–3 days in a typical bacterial pneumonia. The increasing amount of leukocytic or fibrinous exudation reduces capillary volume and results in a gray appearance within 5–7 days. Proliferation of alveolar type II cells can also occur during this period unless there is severe purulent or fibrinonecrotic inflammation. Variations on this theme will be dealt with under the heading of the special types of pneumonia or under specific etiologic agents.

Just as the rate at which bronchopneumonia reaches maturity and the type of inflammation vary greatly, so the rate and degree of resolution vary. A catarrhal or mild purulent bronchopneumonia can begin to resolve within 7–10 days and the lung return to normal within 3–4 weeks. Once the agent has been overcome by the cellular and humoral defenses, macrophages become the predominant cell and phagocytose debris and aid in lysis of fibrin. The macrophages and extracellular debris are mostly cleared through the airways with the aid of coughing and collateral ventilation. This milder inflammation is not associated with significant damage to alveolar basement membranes or capillaries, and resolution can occur without recognizable trace. In these cases, there is a stage as the inflammation begins to wane when the alveoli are lined by alveolar type II cells. Transformation to type I cells occurs as the inflammatory exudate is cleared. A transitory stage of partial atelectasis is usually present between clearance of exudate and regeneration of the pulmonary parenchyma. If there is a residual bronchiolitis or bronchitis, however, and especially if the lack of collateral ventilation impedes expulsion of exudate from small airways, the atelectasis, bronchiolitis, and bronchitis persist. This probably explains why resolution of bronchopneumonia is frequently incomplete in ruminants and swine, and why cattle in particular tend to develop chronic suppurative bronchiectasis and bronchopneumonia.

Severe bronchopneumonia causes death mostly by a combination of hypoxemia and toxemia. Complete resolution can occur, but requires integrity of alveolar basement membranes, readily cleared exudate, and rapid killing of the infectious agent. Necrosis of alveolar septa, intractable exudate, or persistence of the agent therefore preclude complete resolution, even if the animal survives. Often all three conditions occur together. The resulting complications range from healing with scarring, through atelectasis, chronic bronchopneumonia, and bronchiectasis, to abscessation or necrosis with sequestration.

Atelectasis is both a prelude and a sequel to bronchopneumonia. As a complication of bronchopneumonia, it follows resolution of parenchymal inflammation with persistence of obstructive bronchiolitis and bronchitis. Obstructive bronchiolitis can occur in three ways. In the simplest form, there is a chronic bronchiolitis with persistent plugging of the lumen by exudate. The second form occurs when there is necrosis of bronchiolar epithelium, presence of fibrin-rich exudate, and development of plugs or polypoid projections of granulation tissue (Fig. 6.20A). These can cause complete obliteration of the bronchiole if epithelial necrosis is total. An alternative finding is that re-epithelialization of incompletely obliterating granulation tissue can occur to produce multiple, small, rudimentary lumina analogous to a recanalized thrombus (Fig. 6.20B). These bronchiolar lesions are referred to as bronchiolitis fibrosa obliterans. The third form of bronchiolar obstruction is by compression or constriction of peribron-

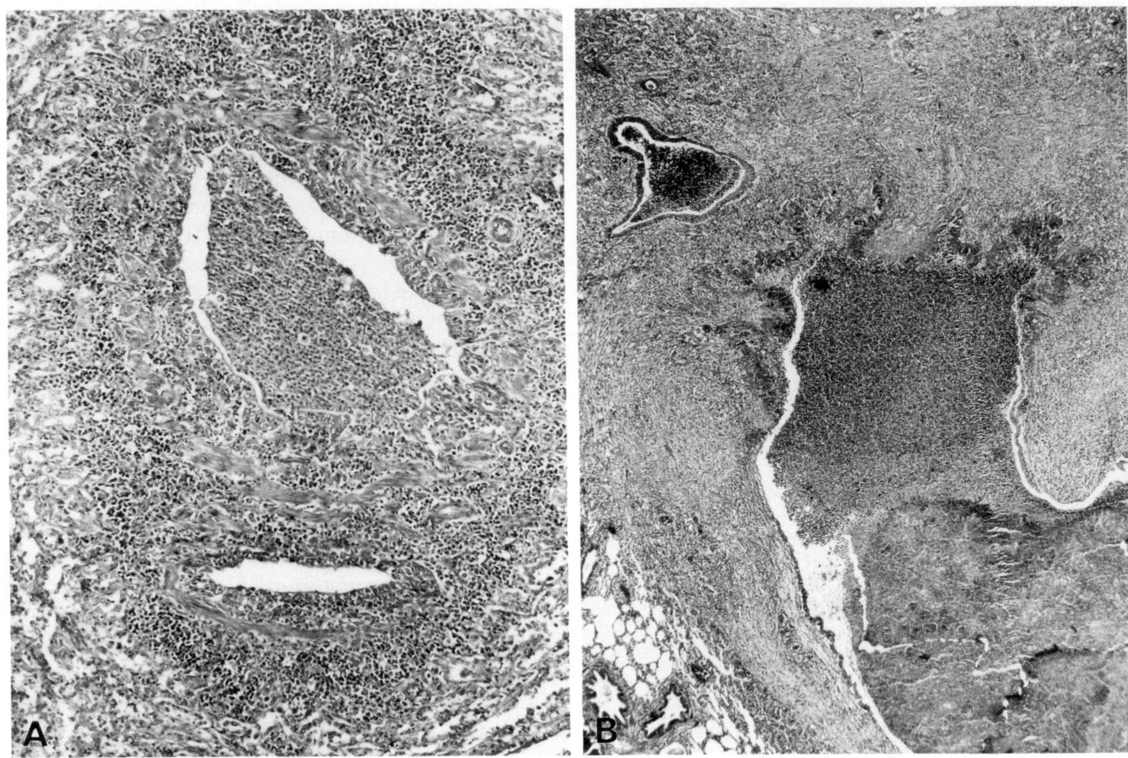

Fig. 6.38 (A & B) Development of bronchogenic abscess in chronic suppurative bronchopneumonia. Sheep.

chiolar origin. This can be caused by constricting fibrous tissue, in which case it denotes a preceding severe acute inflammation and usually occurs with obliterative bronchiolitis, or by lymphoid proliferations such as occur in mycoplasmal pneumonias.

Bronchopneumonia may become chronic. This is seen most commonly in cattle and to a lesser extent in sheep and swine. It is reasonable to associate the tendency for poor resolution of bronchopneumonia with complete lobular septation and lack of collateral ventilation. The virulence of the bacteria involved also undoubtedly plays some part. The lesions of chronic bronchopneumonia are those of chronic suppuration with fibrosis. The suppurative lesions in ruminants and swine tend to involve mostly the airways (Fig. 6.38A,B) and, in cattle especially, there is bronchiectasis and abscessation. Alveolar parenchyma is mainly atelectatic and fibrotic. Severe acute exudative pneumonias cause prominent widening of interlobular, subpleural, and peribronchial zones by accumulation of serofibrinous or fibrinopurulent exudate in the loose fascia and lymphatics. The exudate becomes organized and visible as broad seams of moist fibrous tissues, most frequently seen as an aftermath of lobar pneumonia in ruminants and swine. Similar changes occur in subpleural regions and as irregular interlobular septa in the horse as a sequel to severe exudative pneumonia. Organization of fibrin-containing pleural exudate often produces pleural adhesions.

Severe suppuration and abscessation of pulmonary parenchyma can be caused by pyogenic organisms. Suppuration is common in dogs when pneumonia is caused by *Bordetella bronchiseptica* and in foals when it is part of the pyogranulomatous response to *Rhodococcus equi*. In both cases, the exudate has a grayish-yellow slimy quality. Bronchopneumonia in the horse commonly causes abscessation because the organisms are usually pyogenic streptococci (Figs. 6.34A, 6.39). The suppuration usually begins deep in the consolidated areas. The alveolar tissues undergo necrosis in volumes large enough to be visible as many gray nodules, around each of which is a narrow hyperemic zone. These nodules coalesce, and most of the lobe may be converted to a fragile mass of dull gray detritus. Some of this can liquefy and be discharged into a bronchus so that a cavity remains. *Actinomyces pyogenes* causes pulmonary abscesses in sheep, cattle, and swine. The abscesses sometimes develop in the alveolar tissue, or they may be associated with chronic suppurative bronchitis, bronchiolitis, and bronchiectasis. The abscesses vary in size and number, and the purulent reaction usually extends to the pleura to produce dense adhesive pleuritis, or an abscess may fistulate to produce pleural empyema. Metastatic abscessation can occur in other organs. Erosion of a blood vessel occasionally leads to fatal pulmonary hemorrhage. A variety of other bacteria occasionally cause abscesses, the set of possible agents varying according to species of animal affected.

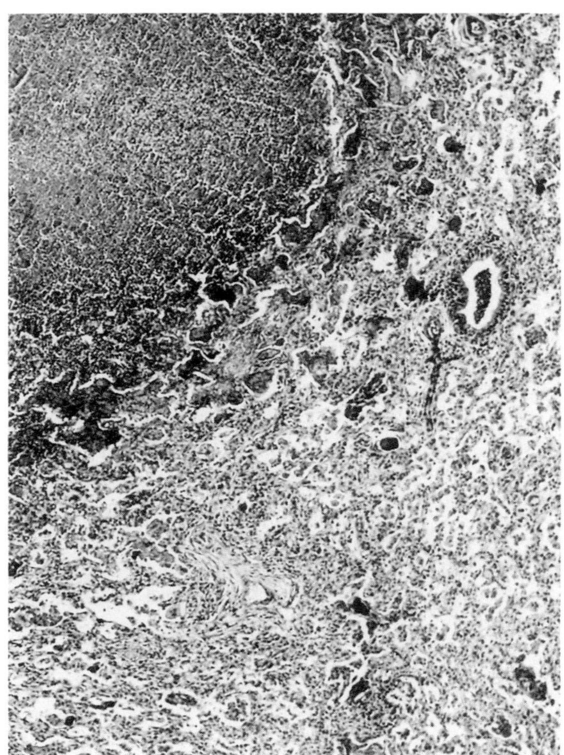

Fig. 6.39 Suppurative bronchopneumonia. Horse. Abscessation and fibrinous pleuritis caused by streptococci. Periphery of abscess.

2. *Lobar Pneumonia*

Lobar pneumonia, as the term implies, is one in which entire pulmonary lobes, or major portions of lobes, are diffusely and uniformly consolidated. Pathogenetically, lobar pneumonias are rapidly confluent, fulminating bronchopneumonias in which gross evidence of bronchiolar orientation and spread is not evident. Since lobar pneumonias have this close relationship to bronchopneumonias, it is not surprising that separation of the two is difficult and often arbitrary. This is further complicated by the fact that even though large areas of uniform consolidation may be seen on gross examination, microscopic evidence often reveals orientation of the inflammation about bronchioles and hence basically a bronchopneumonic pathogenesis. The term lobar is entrenched, however, and is useful to indicate a fulminating or highly aggressive bronchopneumonia. To use this term with as little confusion as possible, it is best applied as a gross designation of extensive pneumonic consolidation in which the parenchymal involvement appears uniform (Fig. 6.40). Exceptions to the uniform appearance are the necrotic foci which develop, for example, in pneumonic pasteurellosis of cattle or contagious bovine pleuropneumonia (Fig. 6.34B) and the exudative distension of interlobular septa in ruminants and swine.

Since lobar pneumonia can be regarded as a fulminating bronchopneumonia, it follows that similar pathogenetic factors are involved. Lobar pneumonia is the result of overwhelming spread of the inflammatory process, and is usually caused by the action of a virulent organism in an animal with severely impaired pulmonary defense. The prototype in animals is lobar pneumonia caused by *P. haemolytica* in cattle that have recently been stressed by transportation and frequently have a predisposing respiratory viral infection. A strong correlation exists between a fulminating pulmonary inflammation and production of profuse fibrinous exudate, as exemplified by the condition in cattle. Therefore a tendency has arisen to use the terms lobar and **fibrinous** interchangeably. This is unwarranted, however, because, although there is considerable overlap, not all lobar pneumonias are fibrinous and vice versa. Because of the predominance of pneumonic pasteurellosis as a cause of lobar pneumonia in cattle and other animals, details of the typical lesions will be presented under that heading. Other than by overwhelming *Pasteurella* infection, lobar pneumonia is sometimes caused by *Haemophilus somnus* in ruminants and *Haemophilus* spp. and *Actinobacillus pleuropneumoniae* in swine. *Mycoplasma mycoides* is incriminated in cattle and goats. Lobar pneumonia can occasionally be caused by *P. multocida* in cats and pigs. In horses, massive proliferation of streptococci or occasionally *Rhodococcus equi* can be responsible. Another cause in all species is the aspiration of foreign fluids or gastric contents.

Infectious lobar pneumonias diffusely affect large portions of cranioventral lung (Fig. 6.40). Those caused by aspiration affect portions of lung lowermost at the time of aspiration and therefore, in a recumbent animal, may involve the lateral zones of the caudal lobe of one side or the dorsal zones of both sides. As would be expected from their peracute or acute nature, lobar pneumonias are hemorrhagic, fibrinous, fibrinopurulent, or necrotizing and sometimes gangrenous (the latter usually caused by aspiration). The gross appearance varies with the age of the lesion from reddish black through deep red, to reddish brown or gray. In all but the peracute hemorrhagic cases,

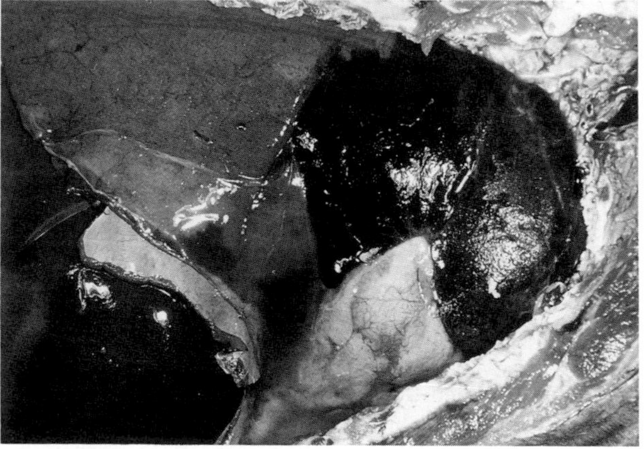

Fig. 6.40 Acute, fibrinous, lobar pneumonia and serofibrinous pleuritis of pneumonic pasteurellosis. Lamb.

there is usually roughening of the overlying pleura and a coating of fibrin. Two additional features are often seen in ruminants and swine and less often in horses. One is the prominent distension of interlobular septa by serofibrinous exudate, and the other is the development of irregular, discrete zones of necrosis with swollen, pale margins (Fig. 6.34B). The cut surface in early cases exudes bloody fluid and later, in the fibrinous lobar pneumonias, becomes grayish brown, finely granular, dry, and friable. Necrotic areas sometimes become crumbly and cavitated.

The initial stage of red consolidation (hepatization) is characterized by hyperemia of alveolar capillaries and flooding of alveoli with serofibrinous exudate admixed with various amounts of hemorrhage, small numbers of alveolar macrophages, and neutrophils (Fig. 6.41A). The amount of fibrin precipitated in alveoli as dense pink fibrillar or more homogeneous clumps rapidly increases. It is accompanied by neutrophils, which predominate in some regions. The capillaries are compressed by pressure of exudate, and many become occluded by thrombi. This is the stage of red-brown or gray consolidation, depending on the degree of ischemia and extent of hemorrhage and lysis of extravasated red cells. During this time, the interlobular septa (when present) and perivascular, peribronchiolar, and subpleural sheaths become widely distended by serofibrinous or fibrinous exudate within the loose connective tissue and especially in the lymphatics. The latter often become greatly distended by fibrin thrombi (Fig. 6.41B). Small airways in affected regions are filled with either a purulent exudate or a more fibrinous exudate similar to that filling alveoli. Arteries, and especially veins, passing through severely inflamed regions can develop vasculitis by local extension across their walls, and occasional thrombi are formed. There is a tendency for leukocytic aggregates in alveoli to become condensed or spindle shaped (oat shaped) under the influence of toxins from Gram-negative bacteria such as *Pasteurella* spp. (Fig. 6.41C); necrotic foci can also develop (Fig. 6.41D). A feature common to most lobar pneumonias is massive proliferation of bacteria, which can be readily detected even in sections stained by hematoxylin and eosin. They are especially prominent within developing necrotic foci and tend to be concentrated close to the leukocytic boundary zones.

This description of lobar pneumonia has drawn heavily on the fibrinous lobar pneumonias best exemplified by pneumonic pasteurellosis in cattle. However, the features of predominantly fibrinous pneumonia in a series of affected cattle are often a mix of lobar and bronchopneumonic patterns.

The **complications of lobar pneumonia** are more frequent and serious than those of the less severe bronchopneumonias. Death is frequent, usually with accompanying pleuritis and sometimes with pericarditis. If the animal survives, resolution without some degree of scarring is virtually impossible. Extensive organization by granulation tissue leading to fleshy fibrous tissue (carnification) is likely, as is chronic abscessation. Peritonitis may arise by hematogenous spread of the infection or direct extension from the pleura through the diaphragmatic lymphatics. Additional complications include toxemic degeneration of parenchymatous organs, endocarditis, fibrinous polyarthritis, meningitis, and hemolytic icterus. A late complication may be empyema of the pleural cavity following rupture of a subpleural abscess. Erosion and rupture of an abscess into a bronchus can cause a rapid onset of purulent bronchopneumonia or fatal hemorrhage if an artery is affected.

3. Interstitial Pneumonia

Diffuse or patchy damage to alveolar septa is the essential feature of interstitial pneumonia. It can be caused by many forms of pulmonary injury. The lack of a completely satisfactory morphologic designation embracing the variants of interstitial pulmonary disease has led to a confusing array of terms. Two terms are most commonly used: **interstitial pneumonia** and **diffuse fibrosing alveolitis.** The former is preferred because it more appropriately covers the broad range of morphologic, etiologic, and pathogenetic aspects. Other relevant terms, with emphasis on more chronic diseases, are chronic diffuse infiltrative lung disease and diffuse interstitial pulmonary fibrosis.

Interstitial pneumonias are inflammatory conditions in which there are predominantly exudative and proliferative responses involving alveolar walls. A variety of agents produce acute, diffuse damage to alveolar walls, causing an early intra-alveolar exudative phase that is quickly followed by proliferative and fibrotic responses. The acute pulmonary injury can be caused by, or associated with, conditions such as severe viral pneumonia, chemical lung injury, acute pancreatitis, shock, and septicemia. Often there is superimposed toxicity caused by the high concentrations of oxygen used therapeutically. Terms which refer to the various circumstances under which such acute damage occurs in humans include shock lung, respirator lung, and traumatic wet lung. Clinically, however, the common feature is acute respiratory distress and the collective term **adult respiratory distress syndrome** is generally used. The syndrome was originally called acute respiratory distress syndrome in adults to distinguish it from neonatal respiratory distress syndrome in human infants. For veterinary medicine, it is sufficient to refer to **acute respiratory distress syndrome** because there is no need to distinguish the adult and the less common neonatal forms. The clinician evaluating a patient with acute respiratory distress and the pathologist interpreting an acute interstitial pneumonia (alveolitis) are both dealing with acute pulmonary injury and therefore need to consider the same differential diagnoses.

Pathogenetically, interstitial pneumonia results from diffuse or patchy damage to alveolar septa. The absence of obvious orientation of the lesions in and around small airways differentiates interstitial pneumonia from bronchopneumonia. Grossly, the lesions are distributed widely throughout the lungs, often with greater involvement of dorsocaudal regions (Fig. 6.42A,B). This pattern is in

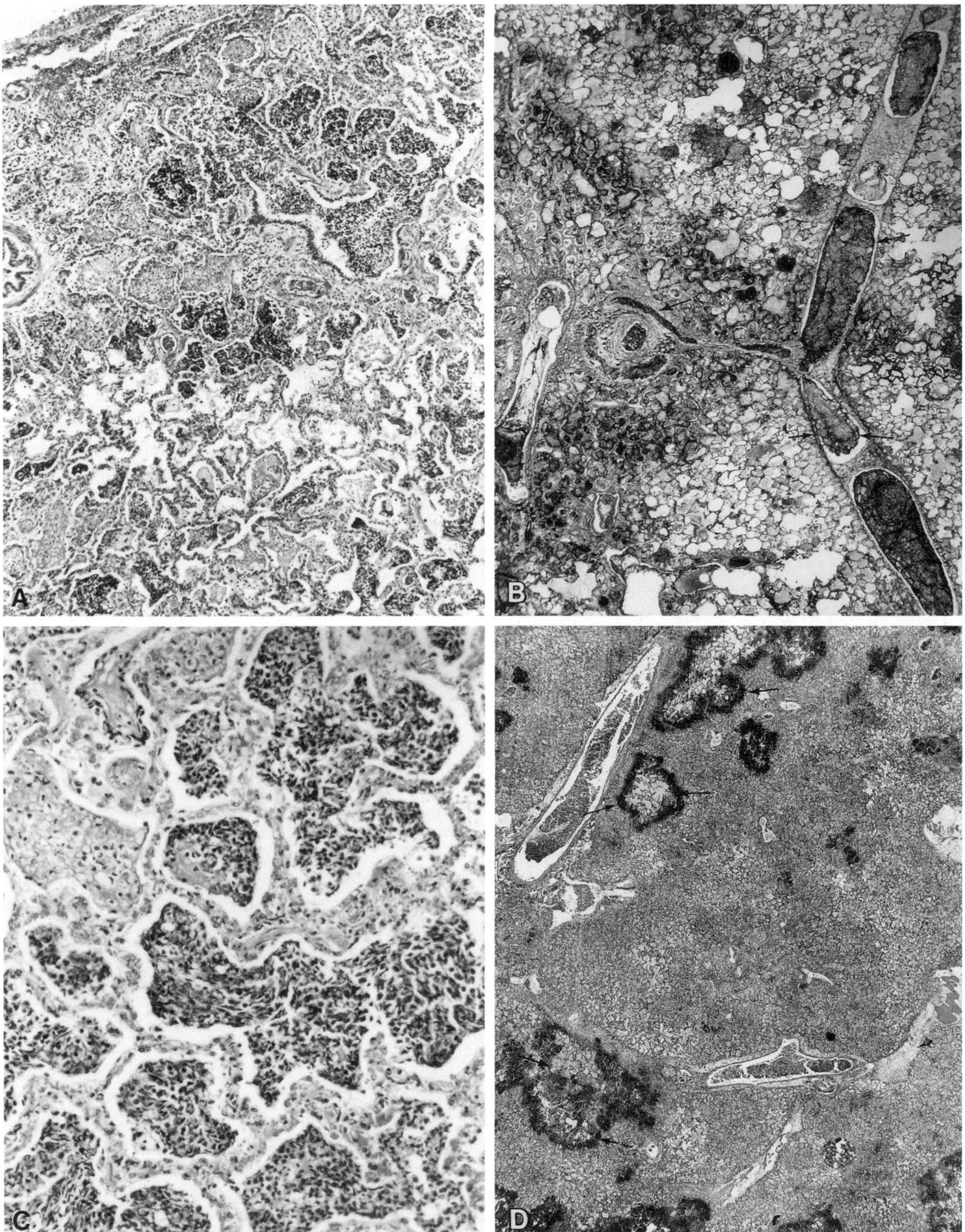

Fig. 6.41 (A) Acute lobar pneumonia with bronchiolar orientation. Ox. Alveoli filled with fibrin and leukocytes. (B) Acute fibrinous lobar pneumonia. Ox. Fibrin clots in septal and perivascular lymphatics (arrows). (C) Streaming oat-shaped leukocytes. Pneumonic pasteurellosis. Ox. (D) Necrotic foci (arrows) in acute fibrinous pneumonia of pasteurellosis. Pig. Necrotic tissue surrounded by dark-staining zones of leukocytes.

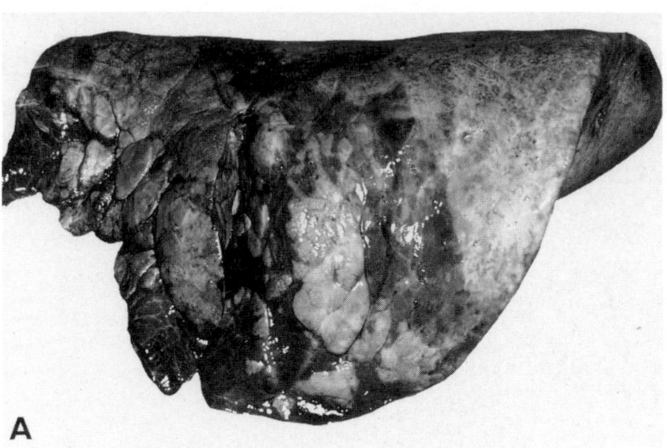

Fig. 6.42A Acute interstitial pneumonia. Ox. The lung has failed to collapse. Subpleural and interstitial emphysema is present.

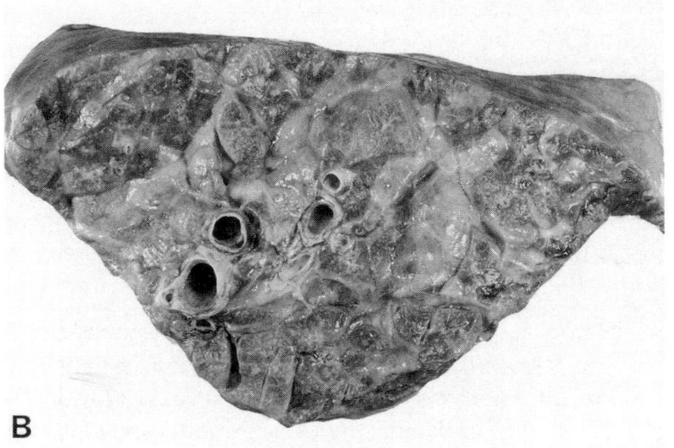

Fig. 6.42B Acute interstitial pneumonia. Ox. Cross section of caudal lobe. Emphysema and edema in interlobular septa and around vessels and airways.

sharp contrast to the cranioventral distribution of lesions in the common infectious lobar and bronchopneumonias.

The alveolar septal damage is caused by a blood-borne insult in most instances. This accounts for the widespread or random distribution of lesions within affected acini as opposed to the centriacinar localization of damage caused by most inhaled irritants. There are two notable exceptions to the generalization that deeply penetrating airborne lung irritants cause mainly centriacinar damage, and blood-borne irritants cause diffuse or random damage. One is that some blood-borne chemicals exert their toxic effect only after they are metabolized to reactive intermediates by microsomal enzyme systems, particularly monooxygenases. Depending on the chemical and the species of animal affected, damage can be limited to nonciliated bronchiolar epithelial (Clara) cells and the pulmonary alveolar parenchyma, spared, even through the parent chemical is in the blood. Necrosis of equine Clara cells by 3-methylindole is the best known example in domestic animals. The second exception to the generalization is that inhalation of irritants which become widely distributed in the lung causes sufficiently diffuse damage to present as interstitial pneumonias. Severe, acute, diffuse damage is associated with inhalation of very high concentrations of toxic gases or fumes because there is not an appreciable concentration gradient of the toxic substance between small airways and distal portions of the pulmonary acini. Inhalation of 100% oxygen is the best example. The pneumoconioses, on the other hand, are chronic progressive lesions caused by inhalation of inorganic dusts. Here, although there may initially be a greater tendency for the granulomatous or fibrotic foci to be located close to terminal airways, this often becomes obscured by the time the lesions progress to the point of causing clinical pulmonary dysfunction. There is no explanation for the tendency of interstitial pneumonias, whether of hematogenous or aerogenous origin, to be more severe in dorsocaudal regions of the lung.

Histologically, the interstitial pneumonias as defined here can range from acute to chronic. Although the term implies that the inflammatory response takes place predominantly within the alveolar walls and the interstitial tissues of the lung, interstitial pneumonias of acute onset have an initial phase in which the most obvious feature is exudation into alveolar lumina. The interstitial components soon predominate, however, if the animal survives. The apparent paradox that some interstitial pneumonias have an acute exudative phase is the principal reason for the alternative term of diffuse alveolitis. It is also the reason that acute interstitial pneumonia in cattle was initially called atypical interstitial pneumonia.

As in other organs, the morphologic responses of the lung following damage by a large variety of agents have many features in common, and the lesions often lack etiologic specificity. Acute injury, whether of toxic, metabolic, or infectious origin, causes damage principally to alveolar capillary endothelial cells and type I epithelial cells. Whether the endothelium or epithelium is damaged first depends on the nature, portal of entry, and intensity of the insult and, to some extent, the species affected. Usually, however, the alveolar type I epithelial cells eventually suffer most damage because of their poor reparative capacity and inability to regenerate. During this acute phase, the most dramatic features of the lesion are flooding of alveoli with serofibrinous exudate and congestion and edema of alveolar walls. Fibrin, other serum proteins, and cell debris frequently condense to form hyaline membranes lining airspaces or aggregates plugging their lumina (Fig. 6.42C). There is usually some admixture of leukocytes and erythrocytes in the alveolar exudate and an initial accumulation of mixed leukocytes within the alveolar interstitium. Mononuclear cells predominate if the inflammation persists.

Replacement of degenerate type I epithelium takes place on intact basement membranes by proliferation of type II epithelium, as described under patterns of alveolar response to injury. The resulting lining of alveoli by cuboidal cells (epithelialization) is a common feature of sub-

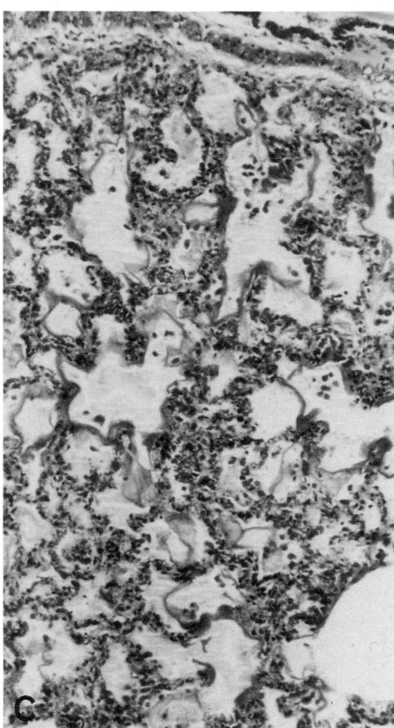

Fig. 6.42C Acute interstitial pneumonia caused by *Zieria arborescens* poisoning. Ox. Diffuse alveolar wall damage with edema and hyaline membrane formation.

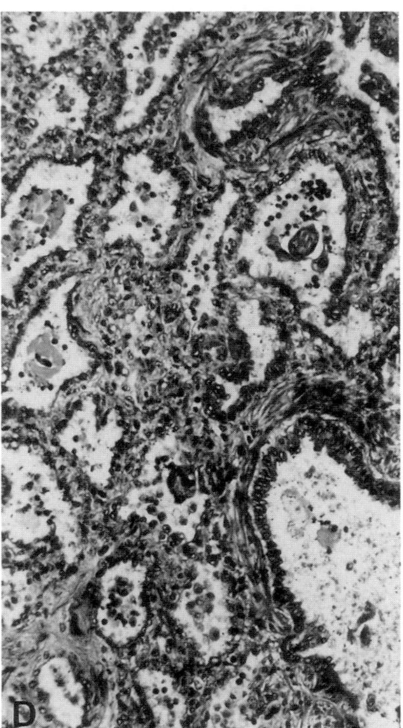

Fig. 6.42D Acute interstitial pneumonia. Ox. Note prominent epithelialization of thickened alveolar walls.

acute to chronic interstitial pneumonias (Figs. 6.42D, 6.43A,B). Once the inflammation has subsided, and if there is not severe scarring of the alveolar wall, complete resolution can be effected by differentiation of type II cells into type I epithelium.

Proliferation of alveolar type II cells marks the shift from the exudative to the proliferative stage of interstitial pneumonia. Onset of fibrosis is a critical feature of the proliferative phase because it is irreversible, at least in its mature form. Fibroblast proliferation can occur as early as 72 hr after severe alveolar damage. It is most evident when alveoli are filled with fibrinous exudate. Immature or profibroblasts can appear within alveoli in the lungs by 3 days after severe fibrinous exudation such as that caused by paraquat toxicity. Mature fibroblasts can be seen by 4 days, and collagen fibers can be detected histologically by 5–7 days. Interstitial fibrosis also occurs in such instances, though not to such a dramatic degree. It occurs more rapidly when there is considerable interstitial edema or serofibrinous exudation. Both intra-alveolar and interalveolar (interstitial) fibrosis, therefore, are sequelae to severe exudative lesions and can be a striking feature by 14 days after initial onset. If the animal survives and residual scarring is present, it is no longer possible to determine the relative contributions of intra- and interalveolar fibrosis (Fig. 6.44). Chronic, smoldering lesions in which there are prominent interstitial cellular accumulations, mostly of mononuclear cells, cause fibrosis within the alveolar walls.

The rate of fibrosis is therefore heavily dependent on the intensity of inflammation. Studies on mechanisms underlying fibrosis focus on two major areas. One is the biochemistry of collagen; the other, the nature of factors influencing collagen synthesis and degradation. A relative increase of type I collagen (dense fibers of high tensile strength) over type III (reticulin-type fibers) occurs wherever active fibroplasia can be recognized histologically or where there is extensive scarring. There may be an early, transient increase in type III collagen in conditions where the rate of accumulation of fibrous tissue is slow.

Factors influencing the balance of synthesis and degradation of collagen are extremely complex. Potentially any of the cellular and biochemical alterations in an inflammatory site can have an influence, and presumably most of them do. Stimulation (up-regulation) of fibroblast proliferation and synthesis of collagen are believed to be induced by macrophage-derived cytokines. Important among these are alveolar-macrophage-derived and platelet-derived growth factors (AMDGF and PDGF), interleukin-1, transforming growth factor-α, fibroblast growth factor, and granulocyte/macrophage colony stimulating factor (GM-CSF). Collagen synthesis can also be stimulated by factors such as fibronectin and laminin. Inhibition of fibroblasts and collagen synthesis (down-regulation) is even less well understood, but collagen can be degraded, before becoming heavily cross-linked to form scar tissue, by plasminogen activation, cysteine protease, and collagenase.

Cell–cell and cell–matrix interactions are also im-

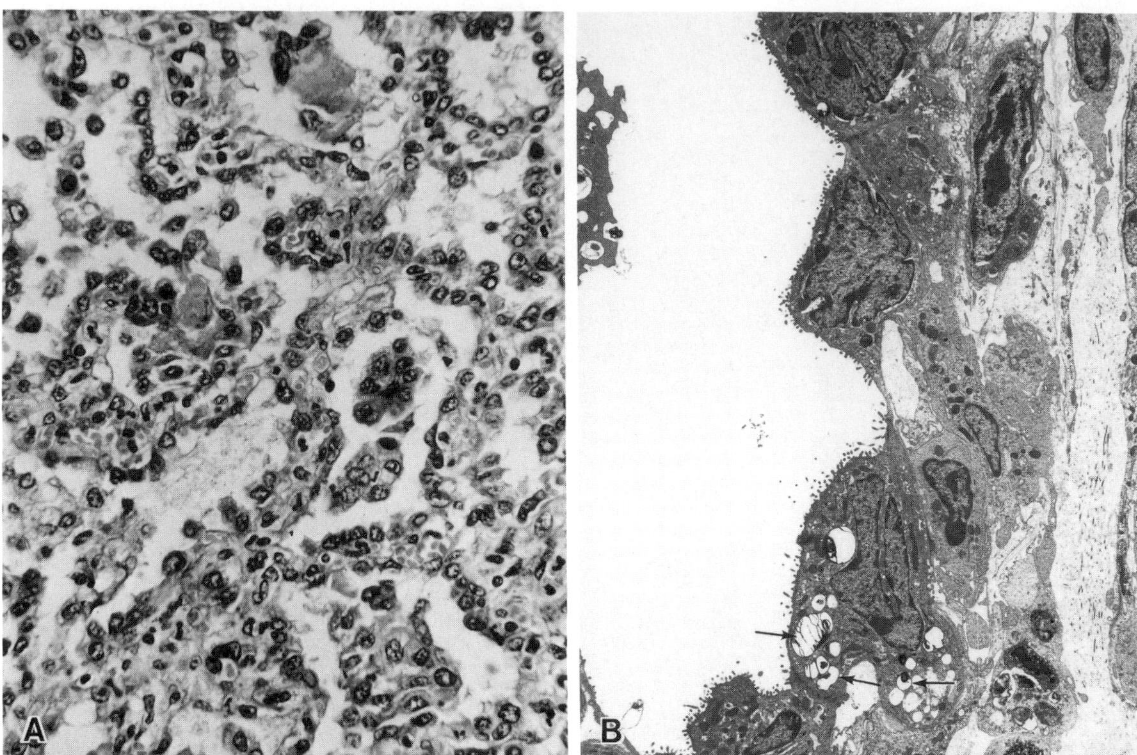

Fig. 6.43 (A) Acute interstitial pneumonia. Ox. Proliferation of alveolar type II epithelial cells forming partial cuboidal lining to alveoli 4–5 days after onset of damage. (B) Ultrastructure of (A) showing lining of alveolus by type II cells, some of which contain characteristic lamellar inclusions (arrows).

portant in maintenance of normal structure and prevention of fibroplasia. Ultrastructurally, alveolar type II epithelial cells can be seen to be in contact with plasma membranes of fibroblasts by means of foot processes, which pass through gaps in basement membrane. It is thought that the type II cells inhibit fibroblasts through these contacts, possibly with the aid of local production of factors such as prostaglandin E_2 (PGE_2). The type of collagen present in basement membrane is also important because there is evidence that type IV collagen promotes spreading of type II cells and conversion to type I epithelium. The presence of types I and III collagen leads to the persistence of type II cells. This could account, at least in part, for the presence of cuboidal type II cells lining airspaces with fibrotic walls.

If the animal survives, most acute interstitial pneumonias resolve with various amounts of residual scarring (Fig. 6.44). Chronic, progressive inflammation is not often encountered but, where a specific cause can be identified, is usually associated with persistence of, or repeated exposure to, the causative agent (e.g., dusts, drugs, or infectious agents). Often immunologic processes are known or suspected to be at least partly involved in the pathogenesis, even where a specific cause cannot be identified.

The central features of **chronic interstitial pneumonia** are intra-alveolar accumulation of various mononuclear cells (mostly macrophages), proliferation and persistence of alveolar type II cells, and interstitial thickening by accumulations of lymphoid cells and fibrous tissue. Granulomatous interstitial pneumonia is probably the most common chronic form (Fig. 6.45A,B,C). Hyperplasia of smooth muscle and distortion of airspaces (honeycombing) are sometimes present in more advanced cases, not necessarily in proportion to one another. Hyperplasia of smooth muscle, for instance, is a prominent feature of chronic progressive pneumonia (maedi) in sheep.

A large variety of agents representing all major etiologic categories of disease can cause interstitial pneumonia. The list of recognized causes or associations is much larger for humans than for animals. Most of the recognized spontaneous interstitial pneumonias in animals are caused by infectious or parasitic agents or by toxins entering via the digestive tract. Hypersensitivity pneumonitis (extrinsic allergic alveolitis) and pneumoconiosis occur occasionally. Occupational exposure to dusts, gases, fumes, and vapors, which compose the largest group of causative agents in humans, is essentially lacking in animals. Other important categories of interstitial pneumonia in humans for which there is little or no definitive information concerning analogous spontaneous conditions in animals are those caused by adverse drug reactions and those associated with collagen–vascular disorders such as systemic lupus erythematosus and rheumatoid arthritis.

Most interstitial pneumonias in animals are infectious

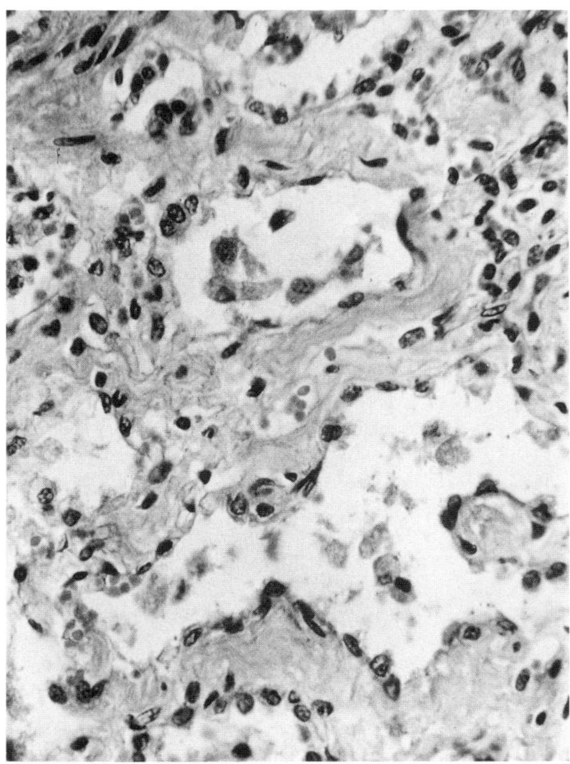

Fig. 6.44 Aftermath of acute interstitial pneumonia. Ox. Fibrosis of alveolar walls and persistence of type II cells.

in origin and are caused by **viral, bacterial, fungal,** or **parasitic diseases** (Table 6.1). Many agents are involved; most produce pulmonary lesions as the result of systemic or blood-borne infection, for example, toxoplasmosis (Fig. 6.46A,B).

Most **inhaled viruses,** particularly myxoviruses, can infect both airway and alveolar epithelium. When uncomplicated viral pneumonia occurs, the lesion is centered on bronchioles and adjacent alveolar parenchyma and is therefore a bronchopneumonia by pathogenetic pattern. Because interstitial accumulation of leukocytes rapidly becomes the dominant feature of the lesions, these viral pneumonias are often termed interstitial. Since the interstitial response in most instances is clearly associated with bronchioles and adjacent alveoli, such cases can be distinguished from the more characteristic interstitial pneumonias not associated with bronchioles. For these viral bronchopneumonias, a combined morphologic designation of **bronchointerstitial pneumonia** is preferable.

The pattern of viral pneumonia resulting from aerogenous exposure is affected by the extent to which viral proliferation is limited by the immune system and by the cell tropism of the virus. With influenza virus infection in mice, limitation of viral proliferation to airways is an important determinant in minimizing the severity of the disease. Cell tropism is important in pneumonia such as that caused by certain virulent strains of feline calicivirus in which type I alveolar epithelial cells are principally affected following aerosol infection. Although early lesions are in regions adjacent to bronchioles, this orientation becomes obscured by 4 days postinfection when the damage is more widespread.

Severe, diffuse pulmonary parenchymal damage caused by inhaled gases, fumes, or vapors is rarely encountered in animals because they do not have the occupational exposures that are usually responsible in humans. Occasional poisoning of cattle, pigs, and chickens by nitrogen dioxide generated in corn silos has been suspected but never proven. Acute pulmonary injury is occasionally seen in animals trapped in burning buildings. When asphyxiation is not immediate, the combined chemical and heat effects of smoke can cause widespread epithelial necrosis and exudation, and death within a few days.

With the advent of increased attention to intensive care units in veterinary hospitals, oxygen toxicity is emerging as an important form of inhaled chemical injury in animals. Most cases of oxygen toxicity are superimposed on the preexisting pulmonary abnormality which necessitated oxygen therapy. Susceptibility to oxygen toxicity varies with species, previous exposure history, metabolic state, and whether there is preexisting pulmonary damage. Concentrations over 50%, particularly in the 80–100% range, can produce damage in already compromised lungs after 2–3 days of exposure. The lesion is nonspecific, consisting of damage to alveolar–capillary endothelium, necrosis of bronchiolar epithelium and of alveolar type I cells, and serofibrinous exudation. The relative proportion of these changes also varies with species. Reactive oxygen species (superoxide, hydroxyl radicals, and hydrogen peroxide) are currently favored as the active metabolites. These are believed, in turn, to damage cell membranes by lipid peroxidation, to inactivate sulfhydryl-containing enzymes, and to damage a variety of macromolecules including DNA. The enhanced toxic effect of oxygen in the period shortly after acute pulmonary injury of some other cause suggests that alveolar epithelial cells exert some controlling influence on proliferating fibroblasts and has important implications for therapeutic use of high oxygen concentrations.

Ingested toxins or precursors are second in importance to infections as causes of interstitial pneumonia in animals generally. In cattle, they are probably the most important cause. Several plant- or feed-related substances can cause a nonspecific **acute interstitial pneumonia in cattle.** L-Tryptophan and 3-methylindole are implicated in causing the pasture-related form in cattle (commonly referred to as acute bovine pulmonary emphysema and edema, or fog fever). Similar pulmonary damage in cattle is caused by perilla mint ketone, toxin from moldy sweet potato (4-ipomeanol), stinkwood poisoning, and toxin from moldy garden beans. Pulmonary lesions are also produced in horses, pigs, sheep, and cattle by pyrrolizidine alkaloids from a variety of plants (mostly genera *Crotalaria, Trichodesma,* and *Senecio*). Crofton weed (*Eupatorium adenophorum*) is another poisonous plant that produces chronic interstitial pneumonia in horses. Toxicity is asso-

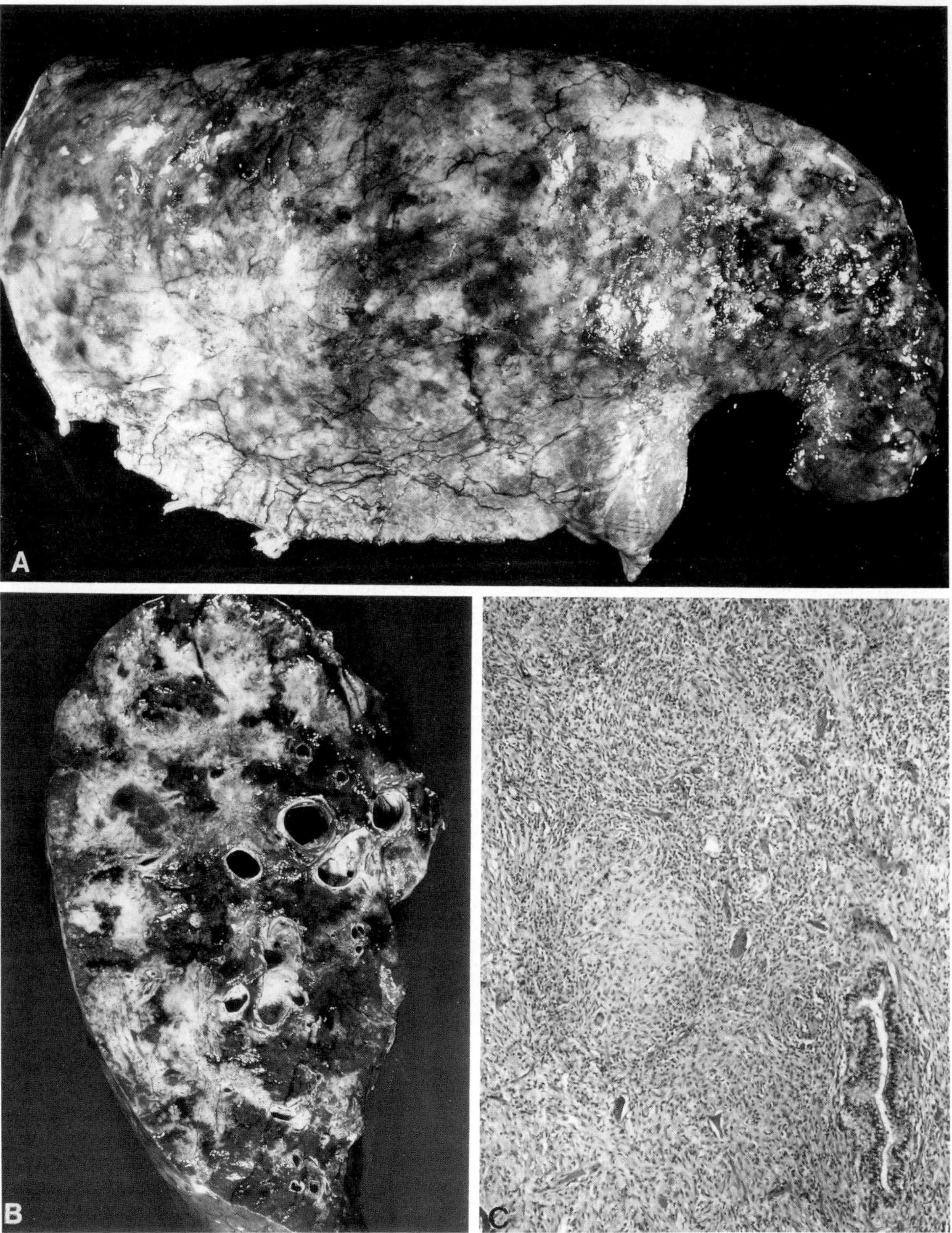

Fig. 6.45 (A) Chronic granulomatous interstitial pneumonia. Pulmonary coccidioidomycosis. Horse. (Courtesy of T. E. Dorr.) (B) Section of caudal lobe of (A) showing multiple, confluent foci of consolidation. (Courtesy of T. E. Dorr.) (C) Effacement of pulmonary parenchyma by granulomatous inflammation.

TABLE 6.1

Causes of Interstitial Pneumonia in Animals

Acute
- Infections
  - Principally systemic viral, bacterial, or parasitic involvement, e.g., canine distemper, feline infectious peritonitis, septicemic salmonellosis in calves and pigs, toxoplasmosis, and acute parasitism by lungworm or migrating ascarid larvae
- Inhaled chemicals
  - Oxygen (>50% concentration)
  - Smoke
- Ingested toxins or precursors
  - L-Tryptophan, perilla mint ketone, and furanoterpenoid from moldy sweet potatoes in cattle; paraquat and kerosene in dogs
- Adverse drug reactions
  - Uncertain
- Hypersensitivity
  - Acute hypersensitivity pneumonitis
- Endogenous metabolic/toxic conditions
  - Shock (particularly endotoxic)
  - Disseminated intravascular coagulation
  - Uremia, pancreatitis
- Unknown
  - Acute/subacute interstitial pneumonia in a variety of species, particularly horses and dogs

Chronic
- Infections
  - Principally systemic viral, bacterial, fungal, or parasitic involvement, e.g., ovine progressive pneumonia, chronic African swine fever, tuberculosis, pneumocystosis, histoplasmosis, and some verminous pneumonias
- Inhaled inorganic dusts (pneumoconioses)
  - Silicosis in horses
- Hypersensitivity
  - Hypersensitivity pneumonitis in cattle and horses; microfilariae of *Dirofilaria immitis* in dogs
- Ingested toxins or precursors
  - Pyrrolizidine alkaloids in horses, pigs, cattle, and sheep; Crofton weed toxicity in horses
- Irradiation
  - Experimental studies in dogs and other laboratory animals
- Collagen–vascular disorders
  - Uncertain
  - Possibly canine systemic lupus erythematosus
- Unknown
  - Occasionally in all species
  - Diffuse fibrosing alveolitis in cattle

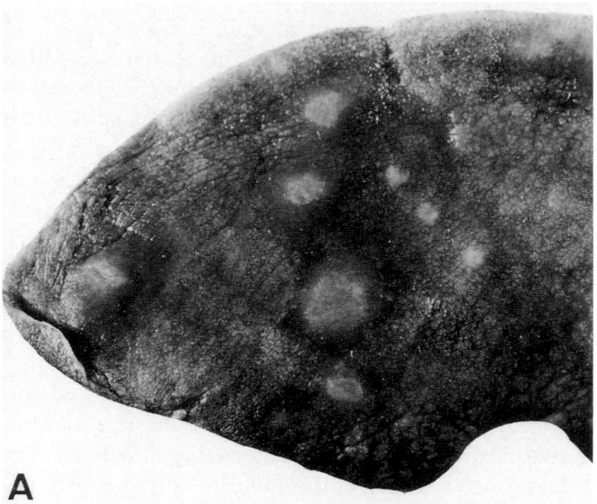

Fig. 6.46A Multifocal necrotizing interstitial pneumonia. Toxoplasmosis. Cat.

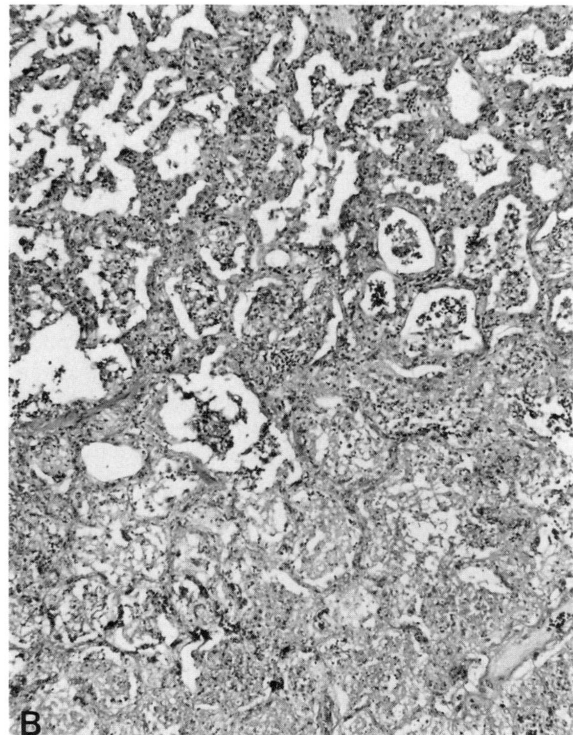

Fig. 6.46B Histology of periphery of a necrotic focus in (A).

ciated with ingestion of the flowering plant, but the nature of the toxin is not known. The lungs have a multifocal chronic interstitial pneumonia in which proliferation and metaplasia of alveolar epithelial cells and fibroplasia are the prominent features.

Pneumotoxins produce different patterns of pulmonary response according to the specific toxin and the species of animal affected. This appears to be due at least in part to the distribution of monooxygenase enzymes among pulmonary cells potentially at risk, because the actual damage often requires production of reactive metabolites from parent toxins by the action of the monooxygenase system.

Poisoning of dogs and cats by the herbicide paraquat is another common cause of acute interstitial pneumonia in animals. As with most other pneumotoxins, paraquat produces a nonspecific, acute-to-subacute lesion. Cases of malicious poisoning are more likely to cause fulminating pulmonary edema and hemorrhage because of the high dosage, whereas in accidental poisonings, there is more often time for hyperplasia of alveolar type II cells and fibroplasia to be superimposed on the earlier exudative changes. In the acute intoxication with survival as long as 2–3 days, the lungs are heavy, dark, and rubbery, and the alveolar spaces are filled with fluid and blood, with much fluid in the hilar connective tissue. Thin hyaline membranes are present in alveolar ducts. With longer survival, profuse fibroplasia thickens the alveolar septa. The alveolar lining cells which are destroyed in the acute phase are replaced from the peribronchial region by the epithelialization of type II cells. The extrapulmonary lesions which are almost consistent include patchy necrosis of the adrenal glomerulosa and of renal tubular epithelium. Affected animals are often placed on oxygen therapy, but it is difficult or impossible to determine whether oxygen has exacerbated the lesions because of the severity of the preexisting damage caused by paraquat. Poisoning by the rodenticide α-naphthylthiourea (ANTU) also causes respiratory distress, but it causes pulmonary edema and pleural effusion without the tendency to epithelial hyperplasia and fibroplasia if the animal survives. There is insufficient damage to components of the alveolar wall for it to be included as a cause of interstitial pneumonia as defined here.

Little is known concerning pulmonary damage caused by therapeutic use of drugs in animals. Development of acute pulmonary edema as part of the anaphylactic or anaphylactoid shock caused by drugs such as penicillin is widely recognized but not well documented.

Inhaled inorganic dusts (pneumoconioses) are uncommon in animals because they lack occupational exposures to dusts, which are the basis for pneumoconioses in humans. There are old reports of asbestosis in animals with industrially related exposure. A very mild form of pneumoconiosis was found in ponies used in coal mines. There were multiple compact aggregates of coal dust, particularly around small vessels adjacent to terminal and respiratory bronchioles. The amount of fibrosis was minimal. There have been reports of silicate pneumoconiosis or diatomaceous pneumoconiosis in animals kept in zoos. The minimal to mild, clinically insignificant lesions mostly consist of focal dust granulomas associated with lymphatics in perivascular, peribronchiolar, and other interstitial sites. Similar foci can be seen in the lungs of many animals living in a dusty environment, but the amount of dust retention appears to be greater in birds.

Silicate pneumoconiosis in horses is the only reported clinically important pneumoconiosis in animals. Multifocal granulomatous interstitial pneumonia with interstitial fibrosis (Fig. 6.47A) is associated with exercise intolerance of various degrees. Necrosis and mineralization are frequently present in the centers of granulomas in the most severely affected lungs (Fig. 6.47B). Small crystalline particles are difficult to detect in the macrophages by light microscopy but are plentiful when examined electron microscopically. The type of silicate responsible is cristobalite, one of the highly fibrogenic species.

In its most specific sense, **hypersensitivity pneumonitis (extrinsic allergic alveolitis)** refers to pulmonary disease caused by inhalation of organic antigens. Naturally occurring hypersensitivity pneumonitis in animals occurs in cattle and to a lesser extent in horses. Lesions are those of a lymphocytic interstitial pneumonia. Noncaseating granulomas can be found in the farmer's lung analog in cattle caused by spores of thermophilic actinomycetes (especially *Micropolyspora faeni*) from moldy hay. A lymphocytic and plasmacytic bronchitis and bronchiolitis is frequently a prominent feature of the disease in cattle and horses.

There is probably some degree of mixed immediate and delayed-type hypersensitivity in many infectious and parasitic conditions. An example of the latter is the interstitial pneumonia associated with microfilaria of *Dirofilaria immitis* in dogs with both occult and nonoccult heartworm disease. Immunologic mechanisms will undoubtedly be found to play some part in the pathogenesis of virtually all chronic interstitial pneumonias.

This is a convenient place to consider **eosinophilic syndromes** involving the lung. As would be expected of any set of diseases grouped on the basis of the presence of a particular inflammatory cell, these represent an ill-defined, poorly understood mixture. Little is known of the range of eosinophilic involvement of animal lungs, though their presence in helminth infections and presumed allergic bronchitis is well recognized. The term pulmonary infiltrates with eosinophilia has come into use to include all cases in which, as the name implies, there is radiologic evidence of interstitial pulmonary infiltrates together with a blood eosinophilia. Eosinophils may be present in bronchoalveolar lavage fluid with or without the blood eosinophilia. Since affected animals usually recover with corticosteroid treatment, the precise nature of the pulmonary lesion and the etiology often remain uncertain. The best known causes of pulmonary infiltrates with eosinophilia are dirofilariasis in dogs and migrating helminth larvae in many species. Involvement in hypersensitivity pneumonitis, allergic bronchitis and asthmatic states is more often suggested than clearly proven. Whether pulmonary infiltrates with eosinophilia can be part of adverse drug responses or immune-mediated disorders can be determined only by extensive, careful studies. Pulmonary infiltrates with eosinophilia is not a diagnosis, and there should be concerted efforts to make the term redundant by identification of the specific disease responsible in each case.

A variety of **endogenous metabolic and toxic conditions** can cause acute pulmonary injury leading to inflammatory edema or more severe alveolar wall damage and serofibrinous exudation as described for an acute interstitial pneumonia. Acute uremia frequently causes severe pulmonary edema. Acute pancreatitis in dogs is occasionally associated with radiologic evidence of pulmonary edema. Shock-like states, massive burns and trauma, and prolonged surgery can also produce acute pulmonary injury, and these are also a major cause of the acute respiratory distress syndrome in humans. Endotoxin is suspected to play an important role in many instances, for example, shock asso-

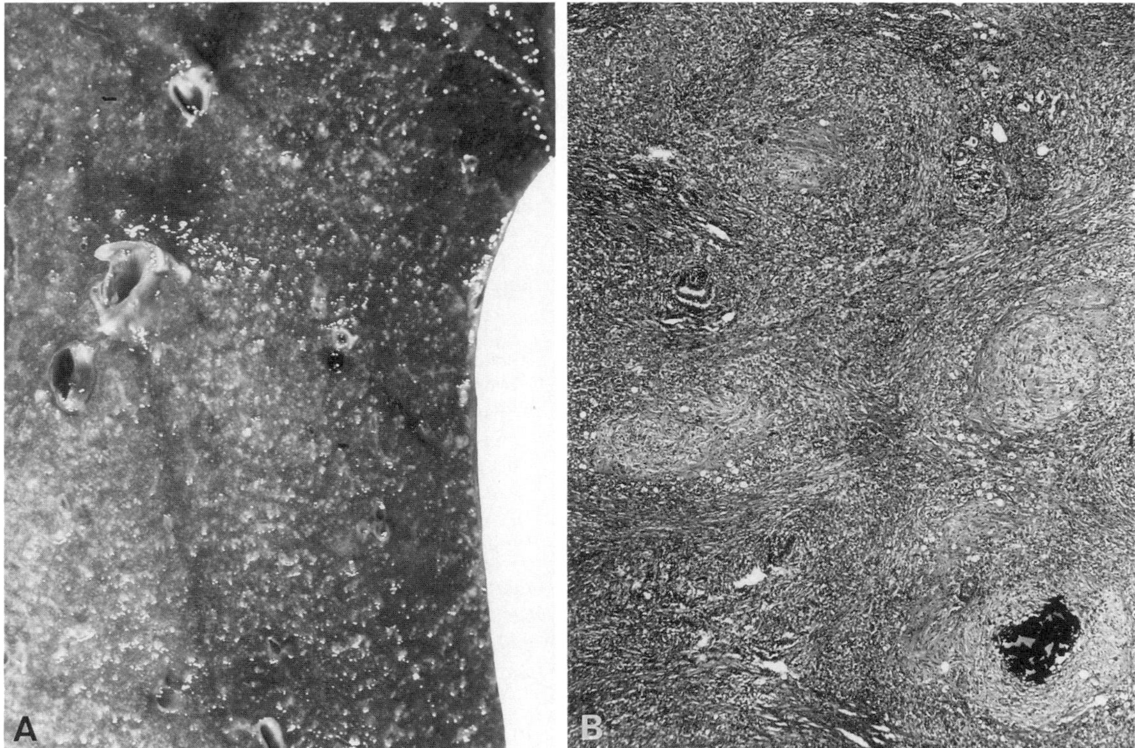

Fig. 6.47 (A) Multifocal granulomatous pneumonia of silicate pneumoconiosis. Horse. (B) Details of granulomas in (A). Some have central necrosis or mineralization.

ciated with severe enteric diseases in horses. But the situation is extremely complex because essentially all mediators implicated in any form of acute inflammation have to be considered. The complete range of possible factors involves the clotting cascade starting with activation of Hageman factor, the alternate pathway of complement activation, the arachidonic acid cascade, platelet-activating factor, interactive cytokines, lysosomal proteases, reactive oxygen species, and cationic proteins from neutrophil or eosinophil granules. The roles of tumor necrosis factor-α (TNFα) and lysosomal elastase are a particular focus of attention at the moment.

Acute and chronic interstitial pneumonias of unknown cause are encountered in all species, but the sporadic reports do not enable assessment of their prevalence. Since the clinicopathologic picture of interstitial pneumonias is often nonspecific, many are not identified by a specific cause, and go unreported. In cattle, acute interstitial pneumonia occurs in calves and feedlot cattle. Chronic interstitial pneumonia (diffuse fibrosing alveolitis) of adult cattle has been described. In pet animals, particularly dogs, acute interstitial pneumonia is occasionally seen where there is no evidence of access to a pneumotoxin such as paraquat. There seems sometimes to be an association with cardiac insufficiency. An acute shocklike pulmonary injury occurs in terminal cardiovascular collapse. Similar lesions, often with superimposed oxygen toxicity, are seen in animals which have been treated in intensive care units. Acute to subacute interstitial pneumonia occurs in horses of various ages, and thus far the causes are not known.

Bibliography

Ashbaugh, D. G. *et al.* Acute respiratory distress in adults. *Lancet* **2:** 319–323, 1967.

Bedrossian, C. W. M. Pathology of drug-induced lung diseases. *Semin Respir Med* **4:** 98–106, 1983.

Berkwitt L., Chew, D. J., and Rojko, J. Pulmonary granulomatosis associated with immune phenomena in a dog. *J Am Anim Hosp Assoc* **14:** 111–114, 1978.

Boyd, M. R. Role of metabolic activation in the pathogenesis of chemically induced pulmonary disease: Mechanism of action of the lung-toxic furan, 4-ipomeanol. *Environ Health Perspect* **16:** 127–138, 1976.

Brambilla, C. *et al.* Comparative pathology of silicate pneumoconiosis. *Am J Pathol* **96:** 149–170, 1979.

Breeze, R. G. *et al.* The pathology of respiratory diseases of adult cattle in Britain. *Folia Veterinaria Latina* **5:** 95–128, 1975.

Breeze, R. G., and Wheeldon, E. B. Fibrosing alveolitis. *In* "Spontaneous Animal Models of Human Disease," E. J. Andrews, B. C. Ward, and N. H. Altman (eds.), pp. 187–188. New York, Academic Press, 1979.

Breeze, R. G., and Carlson, J. R. Chemical-induced lung injury in domestic animals. *Adv Vet Sci Comp Med* **26:** 201–232, 1982.

Castleman, W. L., and Wong, M. M. Pulmonary ultrastructural lesions associated with retained microfilariae in canine occult dirofilariasis. *Vet Pathol* **19:** 355–364, 1982.

Collis, C. H. Lung damage from cytotoxic drugs. *Cancer Chemother Pharmacol* **4:** 17–27, 1980.

Confer, A. W. *et al.* Four cases of pulmonary nodular eosinophilic granulomatosis in dogs. *Cornell Vet* **73:** 41–51, 1983.

Dagle, G. E. *et al.* Pulmonary hyalinosis in dogs (from uranium ore dust). *Vet Pathol* **13:** 138–142, 1976.

Darke, P. G. G. *et al.* Acute respiratory distress in the dog associated with paraquat poisoning. *Vet Rec* **100:** 275–277, 1977.

Deneke, S. M., and Fanburg, B. L. Normobaric oxygen toxicity of the lung. *N Engl J Med* **303:** 76–86, 1980.

Dungworth, D. L. Interstitial pulmonary disease. *Adv Vet Sci Comp Med* **26:** 173–200, 1982.

Frank, L., and Massaro, D. Oxygen toxicity. *Am J Med* **69:** 117–126, 1980.

Gershwin, M. E., and Steinberg, A. D. The pathogenctic basis of animal and human autoimmune disease. *Semin Arthritis Rheum* **6:** 125–164, 1976.

Harding, J. D. J. *et al.* Experimental poisoning by *Senecio jacobaea* in pigs. *Pathol Vet* **1:** 204–220, 1964.

Heppleston, A. G. Changes in the lungs of rabbits and ponies inhaling coal dust underground. *J Pathol Bacteriol* **67:** 349–359, 1954.

Hunningshake, G. W., and Fauci, A. S. Pulmonary involvement in the collagen vascular diseases. *Am Rev Respir Dis* **119:** 471–503, 1979.

Johnson, R. P., and Huxtable, C. R. Paraquat poisoning in a dog and cat. *Vet Rec* **98:** 189–191, 1976.

Katzenstein, A. A., Bloor, C. M. and Liebow, A. A. Diffuse alveolar damage—the role of oxygen, shock, and related factors. *Am J Pathol* **85:** 210–228, 1976.

Kelly, D. F. *et al.* Pathology of acute respiratory distress in the dog associated with paraquat poisoning. *J Comp Pathol* **88:** 275–294, 1978.

Lazary, S. *et al.* Hypersensitivity in the horse with special reference to reaction in the lung. *In* "Allergology, Proceedings of the VIII International Congress of Allergology, Tokyo, 1973." pp 501–508 Amsterdam, Excerpta Medica; New York, American Elsevier Publishing Co. Inc., 1974.

Lewis, R. M., Shwartz, R., and Henry, W. B. Canine systemic lupus erythematosus. *Blood* **25:** 143–160, 1965.

Liebow, A. A. Definition and classification of interstitial pneumonias in human pathology. *Prog Respir Res* **8:** 1–33, 1975.

Liebow, A. A., and Carrington, C. B. Hypersensitivity reaction involving the lung. *Trans Stud Coll Physicians Phila* **34:** 47–70, 1966.

Liebow, A. A., and Carrington, C. B. The eosinophilic pneumonias. *Medicine (Baltimore)* **48:** 251, 285, 1969.

Longstaffe, J. A. *et al.* Paraquat poisoning in dogs and cats—differences between accidental and malicious poisoning. *J Small Anim Pract* **22:** 153–156, 1981.

Lord, P. F., Schaer, M., and Tilley, L. Pulmonary infiltrates with eosinophilia in the dog. *J Am Vet Radiol Soc* **16:** 115–120, 1975.

Main, D. C., and Vass, D. E. Cambendazole toxicity in calves. *Aust Vet J* **56:** 237–238, 1980.

Mansmann, R. A. *et al.* Chicken hypersensitivity pneumonitis in horses. *J Am Vet Med Assoc* **116:** 673–677, 1975.

O'Sullivan, B. M. Crofton weed (*Eupatorium adenophorum*) toxicity in horses. *Aust Vet J* **55:** 19–21, 1979.

Pauli, B., Gerber, H., and Schatzmann, U. "Farmer's Lung" beim Pferd. *Pathol Microbiol* **38:** 200–214, 1972.

Pratt, P. C. Pathology of adult respiratory distress syndrome. *In* "The Lung: Structure, Function and Disease," W. M. Thurlbeck and M. R. Abell (eds.), pp. 43–57. Baltimore, Maryland, Williams & Wilkins, 1978.

Scadding, J. G., and Hinson, K. F. W. Diffuse fibrosing alveolitis (diffuse interstitial fibrosis of the lungs). *Thorax* **22:** 291–304, 1967.

Schuster, N. H. J. Pulmonary asbestosis in a dog. *J Pathol Bacteriol* **34:** 751–757, 1931.

Schwartz, L. W. *et al.* Silicate pneumoconiosis and pulmonary fibrosis in horses from the Monterey–Carmel Penninsula. *Chest* **80:** S82–S85, 1981.

Smith, B. L., Poole, W. S. H., and Martinovich, D. Pneumoconiosis in the captive New Zealand kiwi. *Vet Pathol* **10:** 94–101, 1973.

Theiler, A. Jagziekte in horses (*Crotalariosis equorum*). *In* "7th and 8th Reports of the Director of Veterinary Research, Department of Agriculture, Union of South Africa." Capetown, South Africa Government Printers, 1920.

Turk, J. R., Brown, C. M., and Johnson, G. C. Diffuse alveolar damage with fibrosing alveolitis in a horse. *Vet Pathol* **18:** 560–562, 1981.

Wilkie, B. N. Allergic respiratory disease. *Adv Vet Sci Comp Med* **26:** 233–266, 1982.

Wiseman, A. *et al.* Bovine farmer's lung: A clinical syndrome in a herd of cattle. *Vet Rec* **93:** 410–417, 1973.

4. Bronchointerstitial Pneumonia

The most important attribute of a classification scheme in pathology is that it provides an effective framework for diagnosing, interpreting, and conveying information about disease processes. From this point of view, the designation of certain pneumonias as bronchointerstitial is justified. Bronchointerstitial pneumonia is commonly caused by aerogenous viral infections, particularly by myxoviruses. The essential features of the lesion are that it is centered on bronchioles, and interstitial accumulation of lymphocytes is a prominent feature. Sequential studies reveal that the early lesion is one of bronchiolar epithelial necrosis and accumulation of acute inflammatory components in the bronchioles and adjacent alveoli. Pathogenetically, the lesion is therefore a bronchopneumonia. Because of the mainly cell-mediated immune responses which develop, however, accumulation of lymphocytes in the peribronchiolar and adjacent alveolar interstitium become the dominant feature (Fig. 6.48A). This has resulted in the lesions' being referred to as interstitial pneumonia. From the standpoint of pattern recognition and interpretation, however, it is important to differentiate this type of response which is associated with bronchioles from the interstitial pneumonias that do not have a bronchiolar orientation. Hence the special designation of bronchointerstitial pneumonia. This is not merely an academic exercise, because careful analysis of whether parenchymal abnormalities are centered on bronchioles is one of the most important criteria in the histologic diagnosis and interpretation of pneumonias. In ruminants and swine, mycoplasma infection is the most common cause of bronchointerstitial pneumonia (Fig. 6.48B).

5. Abscesses of the Lung and Embolic Pneumonia

Pulmonary abscesses usually arise either from focal residues of severe, suppurative lobar or bronchopneumo-

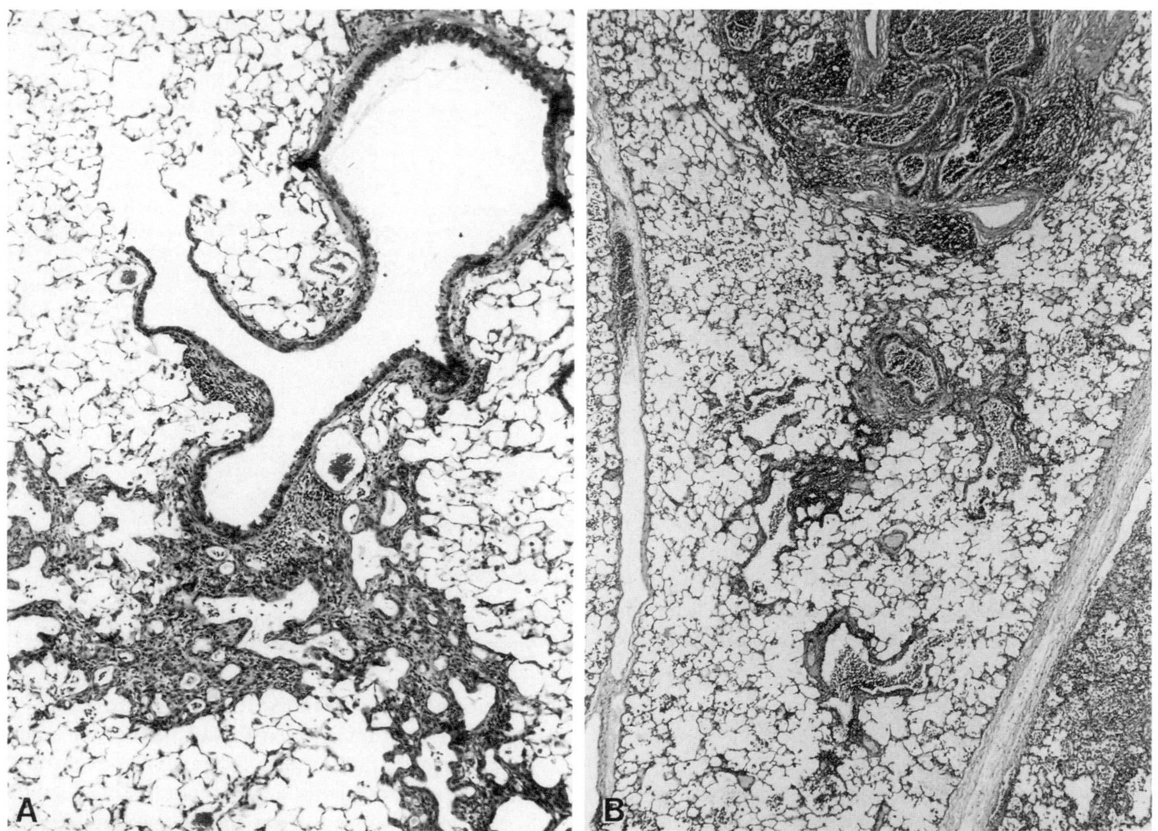

Fig. 6.48 (A) Bronchointerstitial pneumonia caused by myxoviruses. Parainfluenza-1 (Sendai virus). Mouse. (Courtesy of D. G. Brownstein.) (B) Bronchointerstitial pneumonia of mycoplasmosis. Calf.

nia or from septic emboli lodging in the pulmonary vascular bed (Fig. 6.49). Cranioventral location and associated scarring or bronchiectasis are evidence of origin from a suppurative pneumonia. Multiple, widely distributed abscesses indicate hematogenous origin and are usually associated with an obvious source of septic emboli elsewhere in the body, for example, septic thrombosis of the posterior vena cava in cattle. Isolated abscesses in dorsocaudal regions are more likely to have arisen from septic emboli, but in the absence of a pattern of abscesses in other organs, the origin remains uncertain. Difficulty is encountered in interpreting the pathogenesis of pulmonary abscesses in horses; they are relatively frequent and can arise by either major route. It is often impossible to determine the pathogenesis of isolated old abscesses.

Two less-common causes of pulmonary abscesses are aspirated foreign bodies, such as a plant awn, or direct traumatic penetration of the lung. Complications of abscessation include pleural fistulation and empyema, hemorrhage from a ruptured blood vessel, and fulminating suppurative bronchopneumonia subsequent to rupture into a bronchus.

The term embolic pneumonia could be extended to include pneumonias caused by any circulating particulates, including bacteria and parasites, but it is preferable to

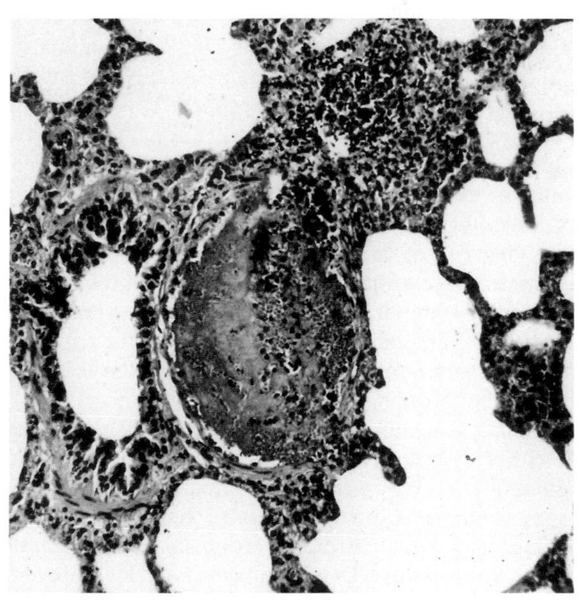

Fig. 6.49 Thromboembolic suppurative pneumonia. Ox. Early lesion associated with septic thrombus.

consider pneumonia caused by hematogenous infectious agents under the general heading of interstitial pneumonia, as was discussed earlier. Embolic pneumonias can be considered as a special category of interstitial pneumonia in which there are focally discrete lesions with clear relationship to the vascular bed. In addition to the abscesses caused by septic emboli mentioned previously, other examples are the hematogenous abscesses which are an integral part of specific diseases such as caseous lymphadenitis and melioidosis.

G. *Special Forms of Pneumonia*

1. Gangrenous Pneumonia

Gangrene can be a complication of other forms of pneumonia in which there is extensive necrosis of pulmonary parenchyma. It is occasionally seen in cattle as a result of penetration of a foreign body from the reticulum, but mostly it is a result of aspiration of foreign material and associated saprophytic, putrefactive bacteria. The yellowish- to greenish-black color and foul odor are characteristic. Extensive ragged cavitation rapidly develops. If a gangrenous cavity extends to the pleura, a foul empyema results with putrefactive pneumothorax.

2. Aspiration Pneumonia

Aspiration pneumonia refers to pneumonia caused by aspiration of foreign material, often in liquid form, reaching the lungs through the airways. This distinguishes it from pneumonias caused by inhalation of small respirable particles, which includes the bulk of aerogenous pneumonias. The response to the aspirated material depends on three factors: the nature of the material, the bacteria which are carried with it, and the distribution of the material in the lungs.

Widespread distribution of inhaled milk or combination of milk and gruel is observed occasionally in pail-fed calves. The course of the disease in these cases can be as short as 1 day. The gross appearance is not characteristic. The lungs remain inflated; they are hyperemic, and small amounts of exudate can be expressed from the small airways. Histologically, there is an acute bronchiolitis with various degrees of acute alveolar inflammation. Lipids, and sometimes plant material, can be seen in the lesions. Aspiration of ruminal contents can produce a similar picture in recumbent cattle, but in these cases the aspirated material is usually obvious, and there is often a hemorrhagic tracheobronchitis.

When the distribution of foreign material is more localized, either discrete foreign-body granulomas, bronchopneumonia (Fig. 6.50), lobar pneumonia, or gangrene of the lungs occurs. Cattle and lambs frequently aspirate inflammatory exudate from necrotic laryngitis. Lambs with nutritional myopathy affecting the muscles of deglutition aspirate milk and plant material, including whole grain. Pigs in dry, dusty environments and fed on dry, finely particulate food can aspirate starch granules and particles of plants from the feed. Any cause of dysphagia, pharyngeal paralysis in particular, is likely to lead to aspiration pneumonia. It is also a hazard of anesthesia. Aspiration of vomitus and medications occurs in all species. The aspiration of vomitus in a simple stomached animal is often rapidly disastrous, and death can occur from laryngeal spasm or acute pulmonary edema before there is time for much inflammation to develop. The possibility of aspirated material's being responsible must always be considered in any case of fulminating lobar or bronchopneumonia, especially one with a history of one of the predisposing conditions just mentioned. Careful search will usually reveal evidence of foreign material, but this is not the case when the material is largely or entirely liquid.

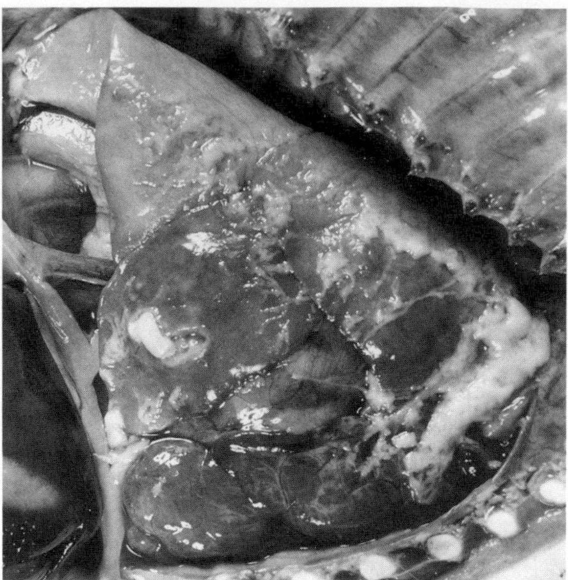

Fig. 6.50 Aspiration pneumonia. Cat. There is confluent bronchopneumonia and fibrinopurulent pleuritis.

3. Lipid Pneumonia

This is a special form of aspiration pneumonia in which droplets of oil are inhaled. It used to be fairly common in cats and other species given mineral oil (liquid paraffin) as a laxative, or cod-liver oil for its antirachitic properties. The reaction is typically macrophagic and proliferative, with some qualitative differences depending on the nature of the oil. In general, vegetable oils, such as olive oil, are not irritating, and they are eventually resorbed with little reaction or fibrosis. Oils of animal origin are irritants and provoke an early exudation of serofibrinous fluid and leukocytes. This is replaced later principally by macrophages, among which giant cells can be numerous. Foamy macrophages fill the alveoli, and the alveolar walls are thickened by infiltrated mononuclear cells and fibrosis. The oil is ultimately resorbed. The purest cellular response occurs to mineral oil, which is the usual offender in animals. The nature of the oil can be distinguished by its permanence and by its failure to stain with osmic acid.

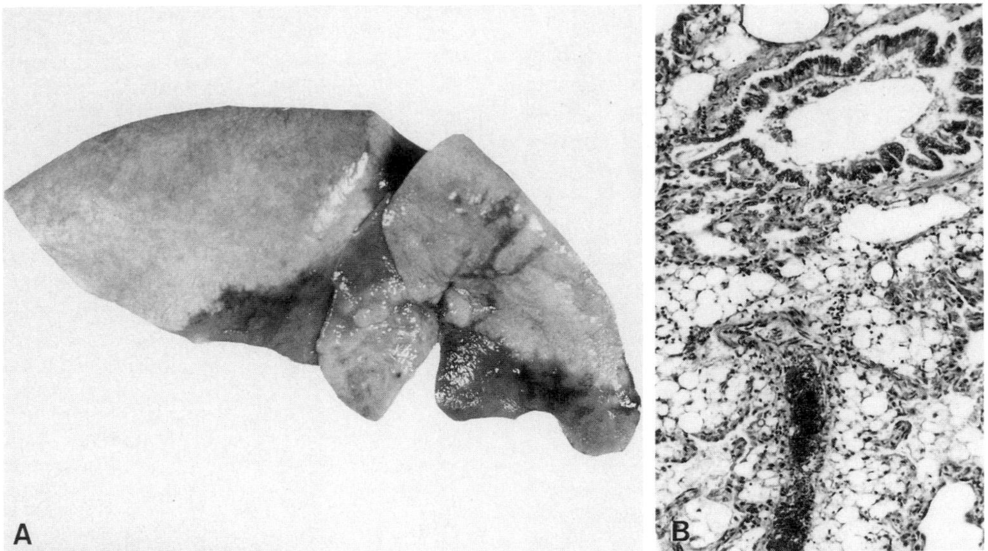

Fig. 6.51 (A) Lipid pneumonia. Cat. Bronchopneumonia with atelectasis in darker areas. (B) Lipid-laden macrophages in alveoli and perivascular lymphatics of (A).

The lipid is both extracellular and intracellular. Lipid-laden macrophages tend to fill the alveoli, and in time, they accumulate in the lymphatics which surround the bronchi and blood vessels (Fig. 6.51B). Fibrosis of alveolar walls and proliferation of alveolar type II epithelial cells are conspicuous, and the foamy macrophages tend to be incorporated into the alveolar septa by extension of the fibroplasia. Unless complicated by secondary bacterial infection, the lesions have a characteristic yellowish, homogeneous, or finely mottled appearance (Fig. 6.51A). They vary from multiple small nodules to complete consolidation of a lobe. Involvement is usually bilateral and tends to be in ventral regions. The bronchial lymph nodes are grossly normal, but histologically often contain droplets of oil.

Pneumonias caused by aspiration of foreign (exogenous) lipid must be differentiated from the so-called endogenous lipid pneumonias. Accumulation of lipid-filled macrophages and various amounts of interstitial response are common to both conditions. The most important distinguishing feature is that in lipid aspiration pneumonias there are large discrete extracellular globules of lipid. In paraffin-embedded sections these appear as clear spherical spaces with distinct borders formed by the compressed cytoplasm of macrophages and giant cells.

4. *Uremic Pneumonia*

Severe uremia causes increased permeability of the alveolar air–blood barrier and is therefore a cause of pulmonary edema. The usual form of uremic pneumonopathy occurs in dogs with chronic uremia in which, in addition to edema, the principal lesion is degeneration and calcification of smooth muscle and connective tissue fibers (see The Urinary System, Chapter 5 of this volume). This occurs mainly in the walls of respiratory bronchioles and alveolar ducts in mild cases. Severe involvement results in extensive mineralization of alveolar septa, which can be recognized grossly by the gritty, porous texture of the lung. Inflammatory cell components are not usually a significant feature of uremic pneumonopathy in dogs.

5. *Alveolar Filling Disorders*

This is a convenient term for lumping together an ill-defined group of conditions with overlapping morphologic features. They are usually found as incidental lesions in which alveoli are filled by one or more of (1) collections of large, foamy, lipid-filled macrophages with lipofuscin pigment and possibly cholesterol crystals (alveolar histiocytosis and endogenous lipid pneumonia); (2) amorphous acidophilic material (alveolar lipoproteinosis and phospholipidosis); or (3) clusters of macrophages and giant cells containing hyaline or faintly laminated material (pulmonary hyalinosis). The amount of inflammation varies from minimal to mild, depending on the variety of the disorder. The early feature in these conditions is accumulation of lipid-filled macrophages. Accumulation of macrophages can be caused by one or more of three factors: (1) their clearance is impeded by obstructed airways; (2) they are produced in excess; or (3) their mobility is impaired by increased adhesiveness or metabolic abnormality. These conditions are included here because some have obvious inflammatory components, especially the so-called endogenous lipid pneumonia, and inflammation plays a part in the pathogenesis of most of the conditions.

Alveolar histiocytosis and **endogenous lipid pneumonia** (foam cell pneumonia, cholesterol pneumonia) are opposite ends of a spectrum characterized by large focal accumulations of foamy macrophages. The condition is en-

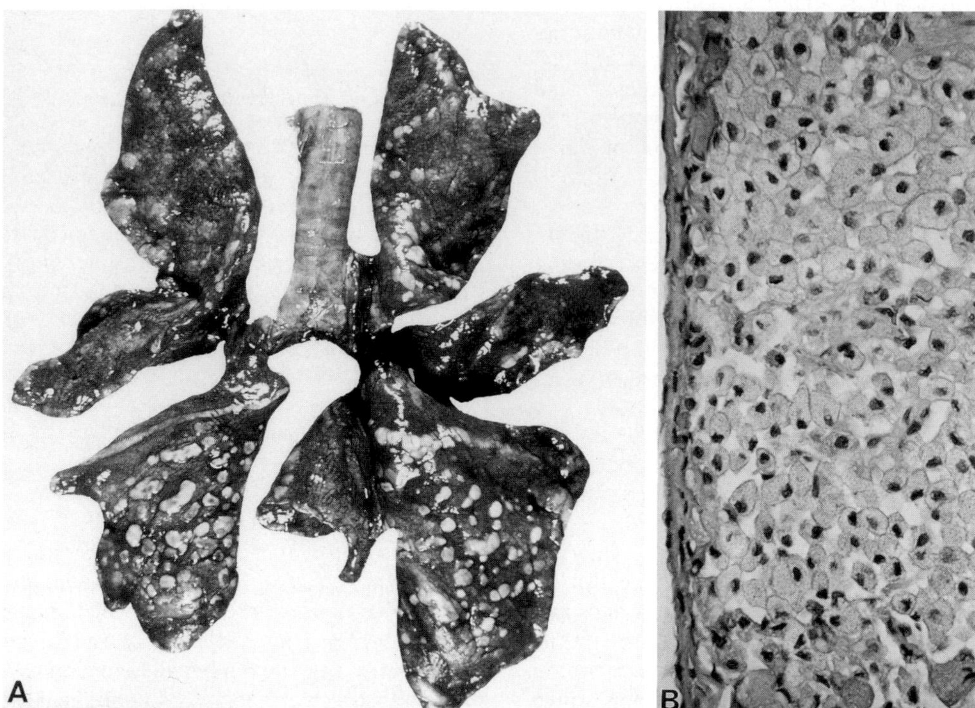

Fig. 6.52 (A) Endogenous lipid pneumonia. Cat. Multiple, discrete, pale subpleural nodules. (B) Histology of (A) showing accumulations of foamy macrophages.

countered mostly in laboratory rodents and fur-bearing animals. It is seen occasionally in cats and rarely in dogs. Grossly, the lungs have irregularly distributed, yellowish-white, firm foci. Most of foci are subpleural and appear as sharply defined small flecks or bulging nodules as much as a centimeter or more in width (Fig. 6.52A). The overlying pleura is often thickened, and the adjacent lymphatics may be prominent because of accumulations of macrophages and lipid.

Histologically, the bulk of the lesion in many instances is composed of distended alveoli filled with foamy macrophages (Fig. 6.52B), and the term **alveolar histiocytosis** is commonly applied. There is a small amount of interstitial fibrosis and accumulation of lymphocytes and plasma cells. In more severe cases, there are intracellular and extracellular cholesterol crystals, more severe interstitial fibrosis, accumulation of small numbers of neutrophils and mononuclear cells, and regions of alveolar type II cell proliferation. The large cholesterol crystals stimulate development of giant cells and intra-alveolar fibroplasia. The term **endogenous lipid pneumonia** (cholesterol pneumonia) is sometimes applied to these more severe mixed inflammatory and fibrotic lesions.

The causes of alveolar histiocytosis and endogenous lipid pneumonia are not clearly defined. In some instances, the accumulation of alveolar macrophages is associated with localized bronchitis and bronchiolitis and is therefore attributed to obstruction of alveolar clearance. In other instances there is no evident obstruction of clearance pathways, although initial sites of accumulation are in subpleural or paraseptal locations where clearance deficits are more likely to result in stasis of macrophages. It is probable that alveolar histiocytosis and endogenous lipid pneumonia are nonspecific responses to mild injury compounded by as yet unknown inherent species-dependent factors. The transition from histiocytosis to endogenous lipid pneumonia is gradual. Admixtures of neutrophils and small mononuclear cells, and evidence of macrophage breakdown, accompany the cholesterol formation and fibrosis of endogenous lipid pneumonia. The latter is therefore probably initiated by breakdown of macrophages, which sets in train a sequence of proinflammatory events involving neutrophils and lymphocytes.

Alveolar lipoproteinosis and **alveolar phospholipidosis** are characterized by accumulation of acellular acidophilic material within alveoli. Knowledge about the pathogenesis of these conditions is derived mostly from two types of experimental models, one induced by crystalline silica and the other by amphophilic drugs. The condition caused by high concentrations of inhaled silica or similar irritants is conventionally called lipoproteinosis, whereas the drug-induced condition is referred to as phospholipidosis because it is part of a more generalized phospholipid disturbance. In both instances, however, the main abnormality is intra-alveolar accumulation of large amounts of phospholipid derived from alveolar surfactant, together with small amounts of surfactant protein and other proteins. The material is strongly periodic acid–Schiff (PAS) positive and ultrastructurally is found to consist mostly of lamellar and tubular arrays of phospholipid and fragmented lamellar bodies derived from alveolar type II cells. Alveoli are lined by type II cells, but inflammatory and fibrotic changes are usually minimal. Evidence to date indicates that production and accumulation of large amounts of surfactant phospholipid in alveoli suppress inflammation.

Alveolar lipoproteinosis (phospholipidosis) is an important condition in rats and mice, but it is not a significant naturally occurring entity in domestic animals other than the goat, in which it appears in association with chronic interstitial pneumonia such as that caused by the caprine arthritis–encephalitis virus and possibly lungworm infestation.

Pulmonary hyalinosis, which consists of multifocal accumulations of macrophages and giant cells containing hyaline or laminated material, is seen in the lungs of dogs. Grossly detectable foci occur mainly subpleurally, especially at the narrow ventral margins of the lungs. They are grayish white to tan, nodular or confluent, and firm to gritty. Histologically, the cytoplasm of macrophages and giant cells is greatly distended and disrupted by amorphous or sometimes laminated material. The material is amphophilic, often staining with a pronounced bluish tinge with hematoxylin and eosin. It is strongly PAS positive, and limited ultrastructural observations have shown that it consists of packed segments of cytoplasmic membranes. Plasma cells, lymphocytes, and small amounts of fibrous tissue usually surround individual or clustered giant cells and macrophages.

The lesions can be found occasionally as incidental findings in the lungs of old dogs. They have been referred to as pulmonary granulomas with PAS-positive bodies and are reported mostly in brachycephalic breeds, particularly boxers. They are usually found accompanying chronic pulmonary injury such as pneumoconiosis or experimental radiation pneumonitis. The lesions of pulmonary hyalinosis in dogs are somewhat similar to those of pulmonary corpora amylacea of humans, but the two conditions are not clearly defined.

6. *Granulomatous Pneumonia*

Granulomatous or pyogranulomatous pneumonia may occasionally be caused by *Actinobacillus, Actinomyces,* or *Nocardia* spp. In these cases there is usually local damage to pulmonary tissue, such as by trauma or aspirated foreign body, or suspicion of systemic immunodeficiency. An example of the latter is the occasional finding of systemic nocardiosis, including multifocal pulmonary pyogranulomas, in dogs with distemper or in Arabian foals with combined immunodeficiency. More important granulomatous pneumonias are tuberculosis and fungal infections of the lung (pneumonomycoses), which are described under these specific headings. Another category of granulomatous pneumonias consists of those caused by inhaled or aspirated insoluble particles. These include the multifocal granulomas caused by inhaled silicious dusts in horses and foreign-body granulomas enclosing inhaled feed particles.

H. The Specific Infectious Pneumonias

Naturally occurring infectious pneumonias of clinical significance usually have complex causes. Interaction of two or more organisms is commonly involved, and often there are predisposing environmental factors. The relatively nonspecific nature of many pneumonic lesions compounds the difficulty of attributing them to specific causes. In the following discussion, features of pneumonias caused by, or strongly associated with, individual infectious agents will be presented first. The variety of agents implicated in causing conditions grouped under epidemiologic terms such as enzootic pneumonia will be summarized afterward.

1. *Viral Diseases*

Generalizations about the complex interactions of viral pathogens, pulmonary cells, and the immune and inflammatory responses are inevitably accompanied by significant exceptions. Nevertheless, most of the important viral pathogens of the lung have an aerogenous portal of entry, replicate in airway and alveolar epithelial cells, and induce a characteristic pattern of pulmonary inflammation in airways and proximal acinar alveolar tissue (bronchointerstitial pneumonia). If the virus also replicates in macrophages and/or is immunosuppressive or can evade host defense mechanisms, more diffuse interstitial pneumonia may result as well as dissemination to other tissues.

a. Paramyxovirus Infections

i. *Parainfluenza Virus* **Parainfluenza type 3 virus** induces acute respiratory disease in a wide variety of species including cattle, sheep, goats, and horses. Parainfluenza virus is best described in the veterinary literature as a cause of pneumonia in cattle. It can cause pneumonia alone, but more commonly is part of the etiologic complex of enzootic pneumonia in calves or more acute episodes of shipping-fever pneumonia. Uncomplicated **parainfluenza virus type 3** infection in **cattle** has been studied mainly in natural or experimental infections of calves. The disease is either clinically inapparent or causes coughing, moderate fever, tachypnea, and slight mucoid or mucopurulent nasal discharge. Signs are most evident from ~4 to 12 days after infection. Disease caused by the virus alone is more likely to be encountered in calves from 2 weeks to a few months of age depending on management practices. Uncomplicated infection does not appear to be an important cause of death.

The virus causes a bronchointerstitial pattern of pneumonia. Grossly there is usually evidence of mild mucopurulent inflammation of nasal passages and upper airways. Early macroscopic lung lesions are limited to irregular lobular foci of atelectasis or slightly consolidated purple-red foci in cranioventral regions (Fig. 6.53A). In more developed lesions, ~4–12 days after experimental infec-

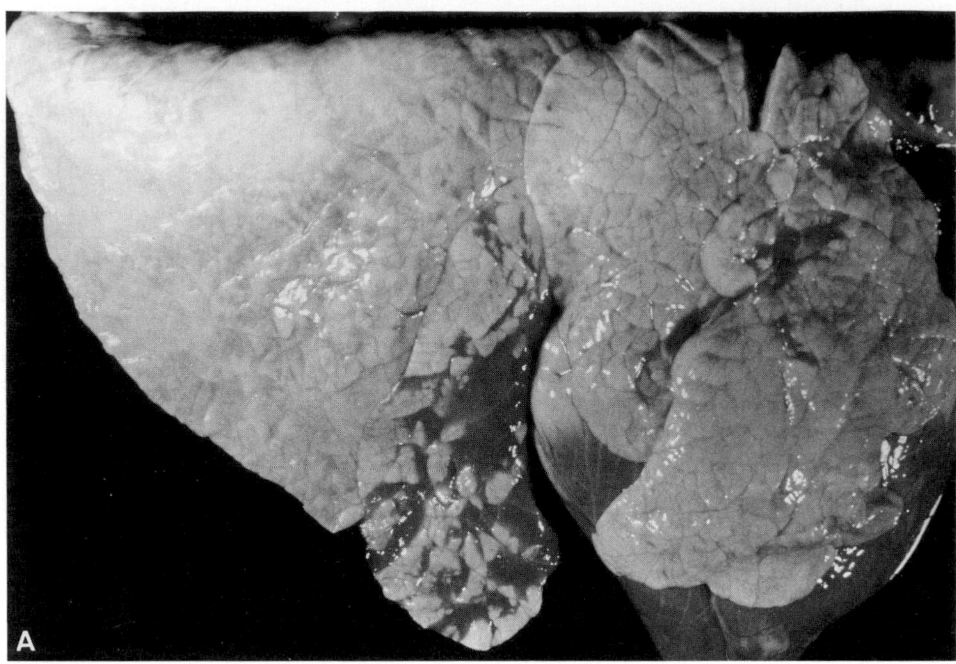

Fig. 6.53A Bronchointerstitial pneumonia. Calf. Experimental parainfluenza-3 virus infection.

tion, there is more confluent consolidation. Therefore, affected regions are less frequent and more atelectatic as they undergo resolution.

In the airways, parainfluenza virus replicates in ciliated, nonciliated, and mucous epithelial cells. In alveolar tissue, replication is largely confined to type II alveolar epithelial cells and macrophages. However, in other hosts such as rodents, parainfluenza virus also replicates in type I alveolar epithelial cells.

Histologically, in the more severe viral infections, there is initially an acute bronchitis and a more obvious bronchiolitis, with extension to adjacent alveoli. The bronchiolar and alveolar exudate is predominantly neutrophilic, although edema and hemorrhage may be present in the alveoli. From ~2 to 4 days after infection, bronchiolar epithelium is variously hyperplastic or vacuolated and necrotic. Acidophilic intracytoplasmic inclusions can be found at this stage in vacuolated bronchiolar epithelium and to a lesser extent in bronchial epithelium. Intracytoplasmic inclusions are present infrequently in type II alveolar epithelial cells. Occasional binucleate or multinucleate forms of type II cells are present. Multinucleated cells are rarely found in bronchioles. The F-glycoprotein in the envelope of parainfluenza virus has a fusion protein function which mediates viral entry into cells through fusion of the viral envelope and the host cell plasma membrane. During viral assembly, viral glycoproteins are inserted into the membrane of the infected cell, and this results in cell fusion and the formation of occasional multinucleated cells.

The exudate in bronchioles and alveoli contains macrophages and lymphocytes mixed with neutrophils and serofibrinous material. Many alveoli are atelectatic because of bronchiolar obstruction. Lymphocytes and plasma cells also accumulate around vessels, bronchioles, and within alveolar septa. Lesions are of maximal cellularity ~6–12 days after infection and are dominated by hyperplasia of bronchiolar epithelium and alveolar type II epithelial cells. Squamous metaplasia may be present.

Intracytoplasmic inclusions are seldom found after 7 days, the time of maximal epithelial proliferative response. Early bronchiolitis fibrosa obliterans can be seen in severely affected bronchioles at the peak of the pneumonic involvement, but it is more likely when secondary bacterial infections cause more severe exudative airway and alveolar inflammatory responses.

The severity of alveolar damage and the range of lesions produced depend on the extent to which virus reaches the alveolar epithelium and replicates, thus causing necrosis. This in turn is governed by the virulence of the strain of virus, the method of inoculation, and the viral immunity and innate susceptibility of the calf. Also, intercurrent immunosuppression as well as other forms of lung injury induced by pulmonary toxins such as 4-ipomeanol can exacerbate the severity of virus-induced lesions.

In general, experimental infections deliver more virus to deep regions of the lung and hence cause more alveolar damage. In natural infection, viral replication seems usually to be more limited to airways and hence is characterized more by bronchiolitis than by pneumonia. In severe experimental infections, the amount of alveolar epithelial damage can be pronounced. The degree of alveolar exudation and subsequent proliferation of alveolar type II epithelial cells (epithelialization) is correspondingly more

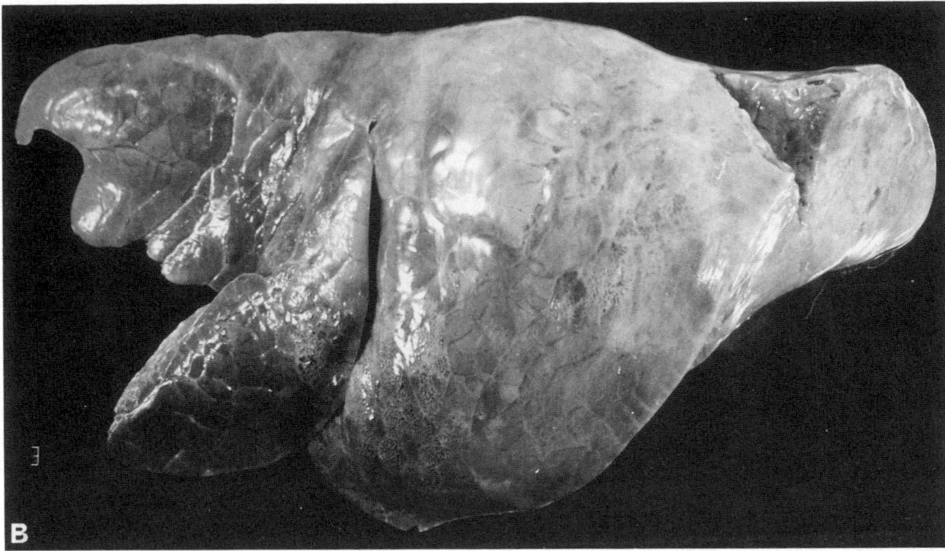

Fig. 6.53B Lung. Ox. Bovine respiratory syncytial virus (BRSV) infection. Note red consolidation in cranioventral lung and extensive interstitial emphysema in caudal lobe.

dramatic. The extent to which syncytial or multinucleated giant cells are seen on the alveolar walls or in the bronchiolar epithelium varies. Although intracytoplasmic inclusion bodies are present as the virus-induced lesions approach their peak, they are rarely encountered in calves that die with respiratory disease, because secondary bacterial damage usually obscures possible earlier viral lesions or causes death after the stage at which inclusion bodies are detectable.

One of the most important pathogenetic attributes of bovine parainfluenza type 3 virus is its ability to inhibit pulmonary bactericidal defense mechanisms, most notably at the level of alveolar macrophage function. Virus replicates in macrophages and can induce decreased phagocytosis and killing of bacteria.

The role of parainfluenza type 3 virus infection in **sheep** is similar to its role in cattle in that it acts mostly to pave the way for severe *Pasteurella* pneumonia. The experimental lesions in lambs are essentially the same as those produced in calves.

Parainfluenza type 2 virus infection in **dogs,** which was formerly referred to as parainfluenza SV-5, has been mentioned in its role as one of the causative agents of infectious tracheobronchitis. Lesions are those of a mild tracheobronchitis and bronchiolitis. The acute viral-induced airway lesions are characterized by mild epithelial necrosis with intercurrent mixed cellular inflammatory infiltrates and submucosal edema. The virus does not replicate in macrophages and does not induce significant bronchointerstitial pneumonia in immunocompetent dogs.

Bibliography

Allan, E. M. *et al.* Some characteristics of a natural infection by parainfluenza-3 virus in a group of calves. *Res Vet Sci* **24:** 339–346, 1978.

Betts, A. O. *et al.* Pneumonia in calves caused by parainfluenza virus type 3. *Vet Rec* **76:** 382–384, 1964.

Bryson, D. G. *et al.* The experimental production of pneumonia in calves by intranasal inoculation of parainfluenza type III virus. *Vet Rec* **105:** 566–573, 1979.

Bryson, D. G. *et al.* Ultrastructural features of experimental parainfluenza type 3 virus pneumonia in calves. *J Comp Pathol* **93:** 397–414, 1983.

Cutlip, R. C., and Lehmkuhl, H. D. Experimentally induced parainfluenza type 3 virus infection in young lambs: Pathologic response. *Am J Vet Res* **43:** 2101–2107, 1982.

Dawson, P. S., Darbyshire, J. H., and Lamont, P. H. The inoculation of calves with parainfluenza 3 virus. *Res Vet Sci* **6:** 108–113, 1965.

Ditchfield, J., Zbitnew, A., and Macpherson, L. W. Association of myxovirus parainfluenzae 3 (RE55) with upper respiratory infection of horses. *Can Vet J* **4:** 175–180, 1963.

Lemen, R. J. *et al.* Canine parainfluenza type 2 bronchiolitis increases histamine responsiveness in beagle puppies. *Am Rev Respir Dis* **141:** 199–207, 1990.

Li, X., and Castleman, W. L. Effects of 4-ipomeanol on bovine parainfluenza type 3 virus-induced pneumonia in calves. *Vet Pathol* **28:** 428–437, 1991.

Liggitt, D. *et al.* Impaired function of bovine alveolar macrophages infected with parainfluenza-3 virus. *Am J Vet Res* **46:** 1740–1744, 1985.

Omar, A. R., Jennings, A. R., and Betts, A. O. The experimental disease produced in calves by the J121 strain of parainfluenza virus type 3. *Res Vet Sci* **7:** 379–388, 1966.

Wagener, J. S. *et al.* Parainfluenza type II infection in dogs: A model for viral lower respiratory tract infection in humans. *Am Rev Repir Dis* **127:** 771–775, 1983.

ii. *Respiratory Syncytial Virus* Bovine respiratory syncytial virus belongs to the *Pneumovirus* genus of paramyxoviruses. Virulent strains of the virus are some of the synergistic agents involved in bovine respiratory disease but are also capable of causing outbreaks of respiratory disease and occasional deaths independently, most often in animals <1 year of age. Outbreaks usually occur in fall or early winter, generally within a few weeks of the animals' being housed. Late-weaned calves seem to be most prone to the disease. Prominent clinical signs are coughing and tachypnea, and in the most severely affected animals, there is respiratory distress with open-mouthed breathing and forced, grunting expiration.

Gross lesions in animals dying of the naturally occurring disease are irregular lobular or confluent regions of atelectasis and consolidation in cranioventral portions of the lungs (Fig. 6.53B). Interstitial emphysema is frequently present and is particularly evident in more caudal regions where there sometimes are large bullae within interlobular septa. There is often mucopurulent exudate within bronchi of pneumonic and atelectatic regions. The exudate may be foamy in major bronchi. Histologically, inflammation of trachea, bronchi, bronchioles, and proximal acinar areas, especially in cranioventral areas, is a major component of the disease. A special characteristic of the bronchiolar response is the frequent prominence of syncytial giant cells formed by proliferating nonciliated bronchiolar epithelial cells, some of which may contain acidophilic intracytoplasmic inclusion bodies. Alveoli are either atelectatic, because of bronchiolar obstruction, or contain a mixed cellular exudate in their lumina with mononuclear thickening of their septa. When alveoli are directly involved, alveolar epithelial proliferation with tendency to form large syncytial giant cells is as prominent as in bronchioles, and here also acidophilic intracytoplasmic inclusion bodies are sometimes seen. There is moderate accumulation of lymphocytes and plasma cells in the peribronchiolar and associated connective tissues.

Experimental infections with virulent strains of the virus produce a bronchointerstitial pneumonia with peak involvement ~5 to 8 days after infection. Syncytial giant cells of bronchiolar and alveolar epithelium are an outstanding feature during this period, and many contain intracytoplasmic inclusions (Fig. 6.53C). Both natural and experimental infections can lead to prominent bronchiolitis fibrosa obliterans in surviving animals. The virus has been shown to replicate in ciliated and nonciliated epithelial cells in bronchioles (Fig. 6.53D) and in type I and type II alveolar epithelial cells. Only limited viral replication occurs in macrophages.

Bronchoconstriction is a prominent feature of the disease, resulting in extensive airway obstruction and terminal interstitial emphysema. Although viral antigen can be readily demonstrated in cranioventral areas of the lung where severe bronchiolitis and pneumonia are present, it is not readily demonstrable in caudodorsal areas where evidence of bronchoconstriction is present. Respiratory syncytial virus-infected cells are capable of activating complement. There is evidence suggesting that mast cell degranulation occurs in airways throughout the lung during infection, possibly as a function of activated complement components, and that mast cell mediators such as histamine are responsible for the bronchoconstriction away from areas of viral replication. Other evidence indicates that the level of viral-specific IgE antibody in cattle predicts severity of disease signs during acute infection.

Research on human respiratory syncytial virus provides the greatest insight into hypersensitivity mechanisms that may modulate disease expression. Children making high IgE responses to the virus have the most severe disease.

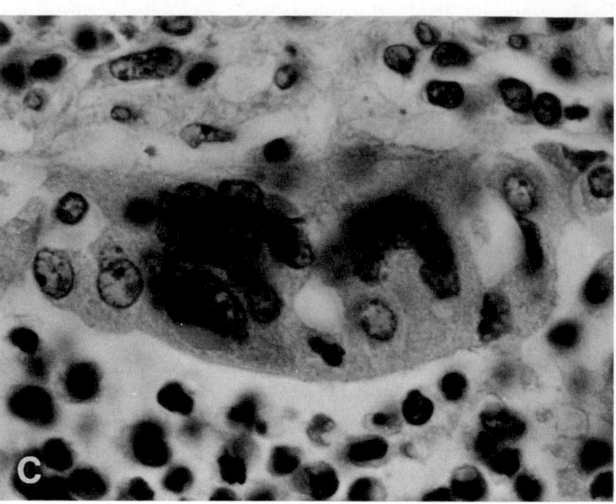

Fig. 6.53C BRSV infection. Cow. Bronchiolar syncytial epithelial cell containing eosinophilic intracytoplasmic inclusions (arrowheads). (Reprinted from Castleman, W. L. *et al., Cornell Vet* **75:** 473, 1985.)

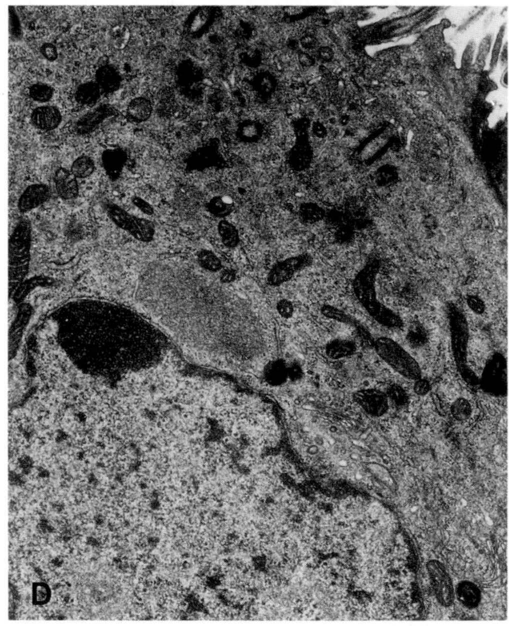

Fig. 6.53D BRSV infection. Calf. Trachea ciliated cell. Note fibrogranular nucleoprotein inclusions (arrowhead) and basal bodies in cytoplasm. (Reprinted from Castleman, W. L. *et al., Am J Vet Res* **46:** 554, 1985.)

Early vaccine trials demonstrated that alum-containing vaccines that stimulated IgE and poor neutralizing antibody actually potentiated disease symptoms when a spontaneous infection occurred. Secretory immunity following infection is not long-lived, and it is possible under spontaneous infection conditions that initial exposure to the virus in some cattle may actually sensitize them to the virus through genetically controlled IgE responses and that subsequent exposure to the virus may precipitate exaggerated viral airway disease.

There is evidence from studies on acute interstitial pneumonia in feedlot cattle that bovine respiratory syncytial virus may contribute to the development of the disease, but the situation is far from clear.

Sheep are also susceptible to respiratory syncytial virus and spontaneous infections in sheep have been detected. The pulmonary lesions induced by the sheep virus are similar to those induced by the bovine virus.

A respiratory syncytial virus has been isolated from cats, but its significance is not established.

Bibliography

Bryson, D. G. *et al.* Observations on outbreaks of respiratory disease in calves associated with parainfluenza type 3 virus and respiratory syncytial virus infection. *Vet Rec* **104:** 45–49, 1979.

Bryson, D. G. *et al.* Respiratory syncytial virus pneumonia in young calves: Clinical and pathologic findings. *Am J Vet Res* **44:** 1648–1655, 1983.

Bryson, D. G. *et al.* Ultrastructural features of alveolar lesions in induced respiratory syncytial virus pneumonia in calves. *Vet Pathol* **28:** 286–292, 1991.

Bryson, D. G. *et al.* Ultrastructural features of lesions in bronchiolar epithelium in induced respiratory syncytial virus pneumonia in calves. *Vet Pathol* **28:** 293–299, 1991.

Chanock, R. M. *et al.* Influence of immunological factors in respiratory syncytial virus disease. *Arch Environ Health* **21:** 347–355, 1970.

Kimman, T. G. *et al.* Pathogenesis of naturally acquired bovine respiratory syncytial virus infection in calves: Evidence for the involvement of complement and mast cell mediators. *Am J Vet Res* **50:** 694–700, 1989.

Lehmkuhl, H. D., and Cutlip, R. C. Experimentally induced respiratory syncytial viral infection in lambs. *Am J Vet Res* **40:** 512–514, 1979.

Lehmkuhl, H. D., and Cutlip, R. C. Experimentally induced respiratory syncytial viral infection in feeder-age lambs. *Am J Vet Res* **40:** 1729–1730, 1979.

Pirie, H. M. *et al.* Acute fatal pneumonia in calves due to respiratory syncytial virus. *Vet Rec* **108:** 411–416, 1981.

Stewart, R. S., and Gershwin, L. J. Role of IgE in the pathogenesis of bovine respiratory syncytial virus in sequential infections in vaccinated and nonvaccinated calves. *Am J Vet Res* **50:** 349–355, 1989.

van den Ingh, T. S. G. A. M., Verhoeff, J., and van Nieuwstadt, A. P. K. M.I. Clinical and pathological observations on spontaneous bovine respiratory syncytial virus infections in calves. *Res Vet Sci* **33:** 152–158, 1982.

iii. *Canine Distemper Virus* Canine distemper remains one of the most ubiquitous and serious of the diseases of dogs. In spite of the development of effective vaccines, the disease remains endemic in most parts of the world. All members in the Canidae (e.g., dog, dingo, fox, coyote, wolf, jackal), Procyonidae (e.g., raccoon, coati, kinkajou, panda), and Mustelidae (e.g., ferret, mink, badger, weasel, otter) families are thought to be susceptible, but cases have not been proven in some species of these families. Clearly the canine distemper virus is a remarkable pathogen that can cause infection and disease in a wide variety of domestic and wild animals. This variety has been apparently extended to include seals, porpoises, and dolphins, which have sustained substantial mortalities as the result of canine distemper or a canine distemperlike infection. In seals, two agents appear to be involved—canine distemper virus and phocid distemper virus, possibly a mutant of the classic virus. Investigators have also discovered the distemper virus causing a fatal central nervous system disease in javelinas (collared peccaries), a feral animal of the United States Southwest not previously thought to be susceptible. The ferret is remarkably susceptible to distemper virus and for this reason was used extensively in investigation of the disease.

Carré first demonstrated that the causative agent is a filterable virus. This virus is a paramyxovirus, subgroup Morbillivirus, a large RNA virus closely related to measles virus of humans and to rinderpest virus of cattle. Various isolates of the virus cannot be distinguished serologically, but they differ in the type and severity of the disease they produce.

Infection by canine distemper virus is pantropic, and the manifestations protean. The disease is described here because respiratory signs and lesions, although variable in severity, are relatively constant in occurrence. Effective antibacterial therapy has greatly reduced the incidence of secondary bronchopneumonia, but it is still frequently seen in neglected cases. Intestinal disease is also common in dogs with distemper.

The disease is a summation of the effects of the virus and of secondary infections with other organisms. These secondary infections are particularly important in this disease because one of the primary sites of action of the virus is the lymphoid tissue, causing suppression of immune function. Secondary bacterial infections in the alimentary tract are nonspecific, but in the respiratory tract *Bordetella bronchiseptica* is frequently associated with suppurative bronchopneumonia. Activated toxoplasmosis develops in dogs whose immune systems have been damaged by the distemper virus, and in fact toxoplasmosis as a clinical disease seldom occurs in dogs other than in association with canine distemper or other diseases that cause immunodeficiency.

The virus is shed in all the excretions from infected animals during the systemic phase of the infection, and natural transmission is usually by inhalation. The pathogenesis of the infection has been followed in dogs, the distribution of the virus having been monitored by the use of immunofluorescence. After aerosol exposure, the virus appears in macrophages of the bronchial lymph nodes and tonsils during the first 24 hr. The virus proliferates in the bronchial lymph nodes and 2–5 days after exposure is distributed throughout the lymphatic tissue, including bone marrow, thymus, and spleen. The animals become febrile and viremic at this stage, and cells of the buffy coat contain virus. The infection is primarily confined to the lymphoid tissues until 8–9 days after exposure. In some infections, the virus spreads no further, and the disease is mild or inapparent. The control of the infection at this stage is correlated with the development of neutralizing antibody. If protective titers develop within the first 2 weeks of infection, spread of virus does not occur, and virus disappears from lymphoid tissues. If protective levels of antibody are not reached, the infection persists in lymphoid tissues and spreads to the epithelium of the alimentary, respiratory, and urogenital tracts, and the skin and endocrine glands, and may reach the brain. In the central nervous system, the virus appears first in perivascular and meningeal macrophages, but infection of the choroid plexus epithelium occurs early, and the cerebrospinal fluid contains large amounts of virus. The critical timing involved in the rise of neutralizing antibody titer, and its role in influencing the pattern of disease, appears to offer a partial explanation for the variability in the severity of the disease produced by the canine distemper virus. The disease is more severe in young animals in which the immune system is less well developed but, even among littermates infected by the same strain of virus, the disease is unpredictable in severity.

The incubation period of canine distemper, as indicated by the onset of acute fever, is rather constant at ~5 days. The febrile reaction is typically diphasic with a second peak occurring at ~11 days, but this diphasic response is seldom observed clinically. The fever is continuous for the course of the systemic infection, which may last some weeks. The clinical signs are variable in their severity and in their emphasis on particular systems. A syndrome consisting of catarrhal oculonasal discharge, pharyngitis, and bronchitis is common but may be so mild as to be missed. Signs of pulmonary involvement accompany moderate to severe damage, whether purely viral with edema and interstitial inflammation or mainly bacterial with bronchopneumonia. The alimentary disturbance is usually expressed as diarrhea, which becomes more severe as the disease advances. The feces become semifluid, slimy, foul, and occasionally streaked with blood. The animals lose weight, and dehydration results. Vesicles and pustules develop in the skin in some cases. These cutaneous lesions are confined to the epidermis beginning in the deeper layers, and are particularly to be found on the thin skin of the abdomen and inner aspects of the thighs. They are bacterial complications usually produced by staphylococci and streptococci. Cutaneous hyperkeratosis and parakeratosis also occur, but these never reach the degree of development that is seen in ferrets and mink except on the footpads (Fig. 6.54A) and nose. In dogs, there is at most a generalized scurfiness of the skin. Small zones of moist alopecia are common on the palpebral margins and oral commissures.

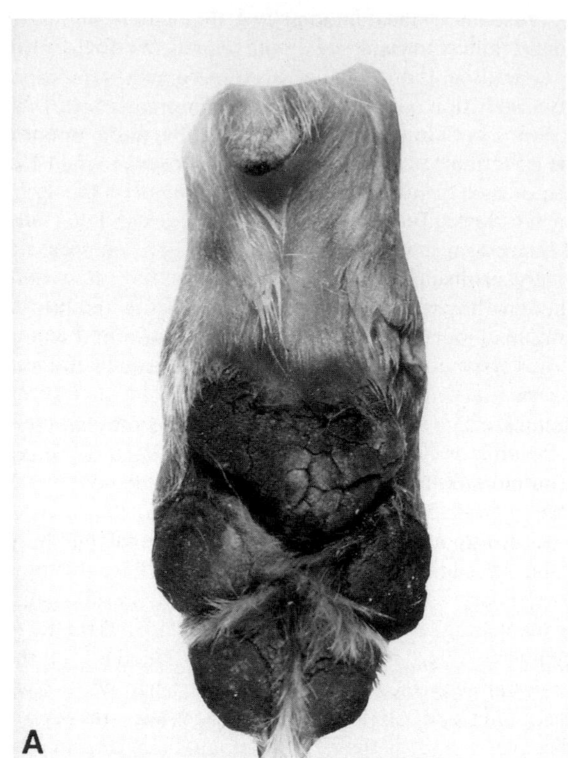

Fig. 6.54A Canine distemper. Hyperkeratosis of footpads.

Blindness, or some loss of vision, is common. Keratitis developing as an extension of conjunctivitis is rare. Few if any dogs, however, escape completely from a retinitis if the disease becomes generalized, and in many there are degenerative and inflammatory changes in the optic nerves and pathways. There may be complete or focal retinal degeneration, patchy edema of the retina with focal detachments, and retinal ischemia with pallor and contraction of the papilla that can be recognized ophthalmoscopically. Pigmented proliferations of the pigment epithelium are visible in the tapetal fundus.

The onset of neurologic signs is usually sudden and follows the systemic signs by 1–5 weeks, but it can be longer, and in some cases only neurologic signs are recognized. Certain patterns of signs can be identified: generalized convulsions of cerebral cortical origin; ataxia, the result of cerebellar or vestibular dysfunction; posterior paralysis due to cord damage. However, the neurologic signs of distemper are usually progressive and the result of multifocal damage. Convulsions, depression, paralysis, and rhythmic motor movements (myoclonus) are the most common. Myoclonus may persist as a residual sign of the disease in animals that recover from the infection.

The gross lesions seen in canine distemper will depend on the phase of the disease when the animal dies or is killed. When death occurs early in the course of the disease and systemic effects are still prominent, as is usual in pups, gross lesions can be expected. In most cases which die or are killed because of the encephalitic effect of the virus, however, there may be little to be seen grossly.

Visceral lesions of canine distemper are common in the respiratory system, but they may be subtle. Inflammation of the nasopharynx is serous in initial stages and in the course of 3 or more weeks becomes catarrhal and sometimes purulent. The mucosal vessels of the larynx and trachea are congested. The bronchi contain a small amount of foamy serous fluid which has come from the edematous lungs, and they may contain a mucopurulent exudate in complicating bacterial pneumonia. The lungs are edematous, and when this is severe, there is also serous effusion in the pleural sacs. The specific lesion is an interstitial pneumonia. To a variable extent, the lungs may reveal the smooth liverlike appearance associated with extensive serofibrinous filling of alveoli, but the more usual lesions are reddish-tan patches immediately beneath the pleura, and grayish zones of firmer consistency along the sharp margins of the lobes. Deflation is incomplete in such lungs.

Lesions are regularly present in the lymphoid organs, but except for the thymus, these changes are difficult to recognize grossly. If the animal dies or is killed during the acute systemic phase of the disease, the lymph nodes may be variable in size. Some are large and edematous; others, small and atrophic. In the large, edematous nodes, cortical and medullary distinction may be lost. The thymuses of affected animals at this stage are greatly reduced and in some cases are difficult to identify. Later in the course of the disease, lymphoid tissue of lymph nodes and thymuses can regenerate and may be of normal size in animals dying in the chronic neurologic phase of the disease.

Many animals dying of canine distemper are severely emaciated and their muscles, wasted. The lobular pattern of the liver is sometimes prominent because of mild fatty change and centrilobular congestion. Large irregular whitish areas of necrosis and mineralization are often seen in the myocardium of very young suckling pups, which are most apt to die during the acute early phase of the disease.

The histologic changes in canine distemper, when present, are fairly specific; specificity depends on the demonstration of the viral inclusion bodies or, better yet, detection of viral antigen by immunofluorescence.

The number and distribution of inclusion bodies vary from case to case and with the phase of the disease. Their appearance coincides with, or follows shortly after, the appearance of systemic signs of illness, from ~10 to 14 days after infection. By about the fifth or sixth weeks, their numbers diminish rapidly in most tissues and disappear. Of the non-neural tissues, they persist longest in the lung. Inclusion bodies can be found in the central nervous system before changes of encephalomyelitis are present, and they persist in the neural tissue when they have disappeared from all extraneural sites, provided that infection of the brain has occurred.

The inclusion bodies are acidophilic and occur in either the nucleus or cytoplasm or both, depending on the tissue. They are usually easier to find and recognize with confidence in brain and epithelial tissues. In lymph nodes, they can be very easily confused with eosinophilic debris unless their specificity can be proven by fluorescent antibody.

The earliest lesions of canine distemper are those affecting the lymphoid tissues. These are rarely seen in clinical cases, as dogs only rarely die during this period, but in experimental series it has been shown that as early as the sixth day after exposure there is a depletion of lymphocytes in the cortical zone of the lymph nodes. By the ninth day, the lymph nodes are largely depleted of lymphocytes, and the cortical zones are reduced to thin rims. Individual lymphocytes undergo necrosis, and the sinusoids and cords are infiltrated by neutrophils. Similar lesions develop in the spleen, and small foci of necrosis may be scattered throughout the white pulp (Fig. 6.54B). Large multinucleated syncytial cells form in the nodes; often these cells contain acidophilic inclusion bodies. Approximately 2 weeks after exposure, hyperplasia of the reticulum cells develops, focally at first and later as diffuse sheets of cells. In some fatally infected animals, the nodes are not repopulated by lymphocytes. The nodes are of normal size, but filled with only proliferating large mononuclear cells when the animal dies 25–35 days after infection. Repopulation of the node by both B and T cells can occur in convalescent dogs. The recovery is not complete in some of these dogs, and some die with neurologic signs. The thymus also undergoes a severe lymphocytic depletion in parallel with the lymph nodes. The thymic atrophy is due to both loss of cortical thymocytes as well as great

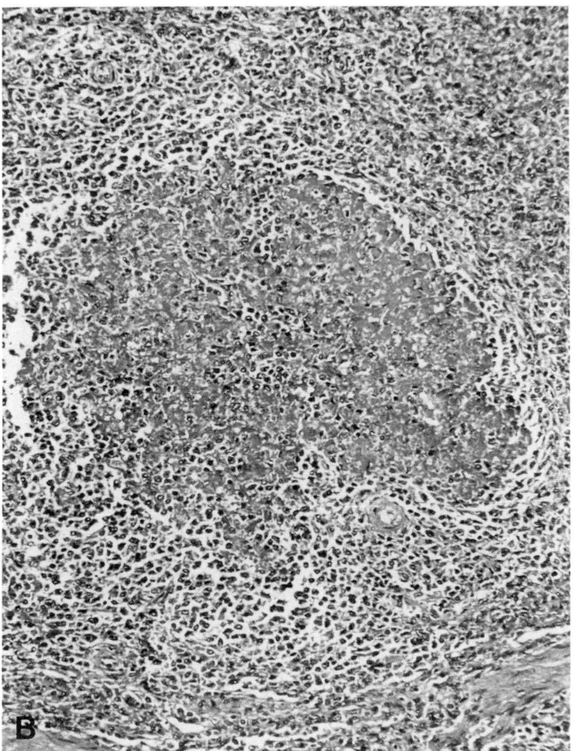

Fig. 6.54B Canine distemper. Necrotic focus. Spleen.

reduction in the medulla. In some animals which die, the thymuses show no tendency to regenerate, but regeneration, if it is to occur, commences at the same time as it does in the nodes.

Severe leukopenia is a characteristic feature of canine distemper. It is due chiefly to a lymphopenia. The lymphopenia develops at the time the initial necrosis of lymphatic tissue occurs and is most likely the result of viral multiplication and destruction of the lymphoid tissues. The lymphopenia persists in the acute disease until death or recovery, but some animals die of encephalitis after the circulating lymphocyte levels have returned to normal. Lymphopenia coincides with the onset of the leukocyte-associated viremia, but persists long after viral antigen can no longer be demonstrated in the buffy coat.

The characteristic changes in the lung produced by the virus of canine distemper are those of interstitial pneumonia (Fig. 6.55), but the lesion found at autopsy may be complicated by secondary bacterial bronchopneumonia. The change is diffuse in the lungs, although more severe in some areas than in others. Syncytial giant cells formed by alveolar type II epithelial cells are a characteristic feature of the interstitial pneumonia caused by the virus. Many contain the acidophilic intracytoplasmic viral inclusions (Fig. 6.56). As the systemic phase is overcome in the chronic disease, residual changes tend to persist in patches beneath the pleura and about venules and small bronchioles as areas of thickened alveolar septa with epithelialization and accumulation of alveolar macrophages. Specific inclusion bodies can sometimes still be found in the cytoplasm of altered alveolar epithelium and in the bronchial mucosa. Among non-neural tissues, they are most likely to be found in the alveolar epithelium because they persist longest in these cells in terms of the disease process, and these cells are not so subject to postmortem lysis and sloughing as most epithelial cells.

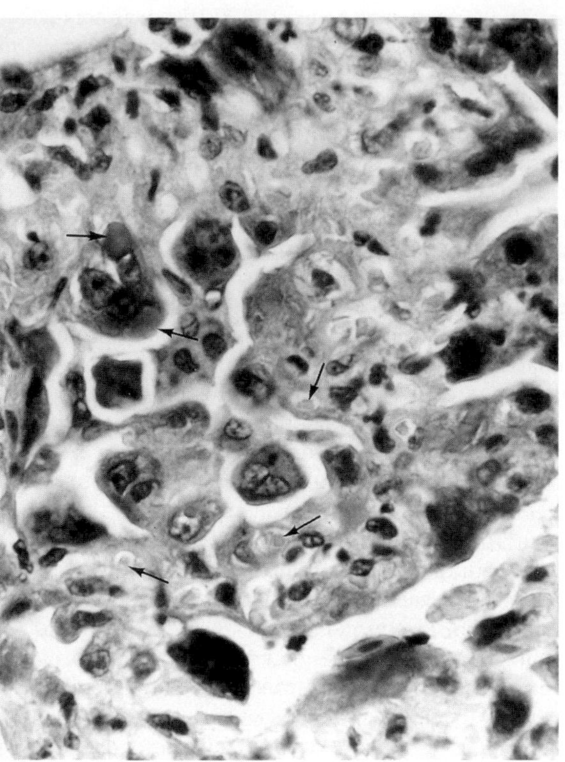

Fig. 6.56 Canine distemper. Giant cells in alveoli with intracytoplasmic inclusions (arrows).

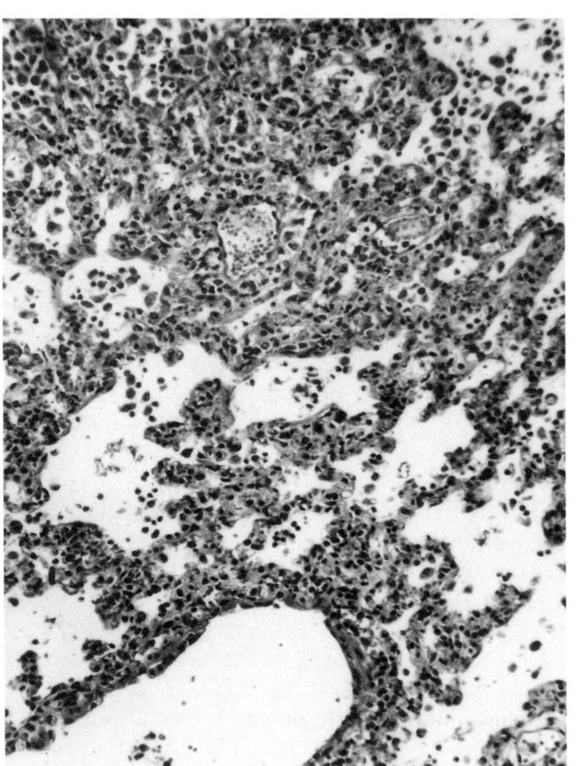

Fig. 6.55 Canine distemper. Acute interstitial pneumonia with predominance of mononuclear cells in alveolar walls.

Intracytoplasmic inclusion bodies are regularly found in the transitional epithelium of the urinary tract in the acute systemic disease. Intranuclear inclusions are less common. In some cases, inclusions are found in the epithelium of the collecting tubules. The epithelial cells are often swollen and hydropic, and in the absence of these degenerative changes, inclusion bodies are unlikely to be found. Mild interstitial epididymitis and orchitis are common in canine distemper; inclusion bodies are found in the epididymal epithelium, and the interstitium is mildly infiltrated with mononuclear cells. Inclusion bodies can occasionally be found in the epithelium of the biliary and pancreatic ducts and in the pancreatic exocrine tissue. Inclusions are common in the gastric epithelium but uncommon in the intestine. In the stomach, they are found in superficial epithelium as well as in chief and parietal cells; the latter frequently show acute degenerative changes.

Necrosis and cystic degeneration of ameloblastic epithelium of the developing tooth give rise to the defective enamel seen in animals which have recovered from infection. The defects may consist of small focal depressions to large areas lacking enamel. The boundaries of the defects are discrete.

Intraocular lesions occur in most cases of canine distemper. Ulcerative keratitis may complicate a purulent conjunctivitis, but this is uncommon. More commonly, the anterior segment is not significantly changed except for leukocytic infiltrations in the ciliary body. Distinctive retinal lesions of variable severity and extent are present, and nuclear and cytoplasmic inclusions may be found in the retinal ganglion cells and glia, as well as in glia of the optic nerve. The retinal changes may be predominantly exudative in the acute cases, but in those of longer duration, they are predominantly degenerative (Fig. 6.57); in all cases, there is prominent proliferation of the pigmented epithelium. The earliest changes include severe degeneration of the retinal ganglion cells revealed as dispersion of the Nissl substance and migration of the nucleus to the margin of the cell. The degenerative changes in the ganglion cells are diffuse, but these cells tend to persist until the layered organization of the retina is lost. In acute retinitis, there is congestion and cuffing of the blood vessels in the optic nerve and ganglion cell layers. Patchy edema often separates the fibers of the optic nerve layer and the reticular layers and produces focal retinal detachments. Atrophy of the retina may be patchy or complete. In some cases, the atrophy is limited to the layer of rods and cones, the outer limbs of which shorten and disappear concurrent with pyknosis of the nuclei. In other foci or cases, the atrophy results in disorganization of the layers and, when the ganglion cell layer disappears also, the retina in such areas consists of disorganized remnants of the layer of bipolar cells. Swelling and proliferation of the cells of the pigment epithelium is common, more marked in the ventral than in the tapetal fundus, and is also common in the pars ciliaris retinae. Associated with the reactive changes in the pigmented epithelium is a migration of pigment into the retina. Pigmentation of the retina is rather common in old dogs, but in these it tends to be restricted to the periphery of the retina and is not obviously associated with reactive changes in the epithelium; in canine distemper, the pigmentation occurs centrally as well as peripherally, and activity of the epithelium may be sufficient to cause focal detachments of the retina. Changes in the optic nerve are inconstant, but papilledema may be observed in acute cases, and gliosis of the nerve head or demyelinating neuritis in chronic ones.

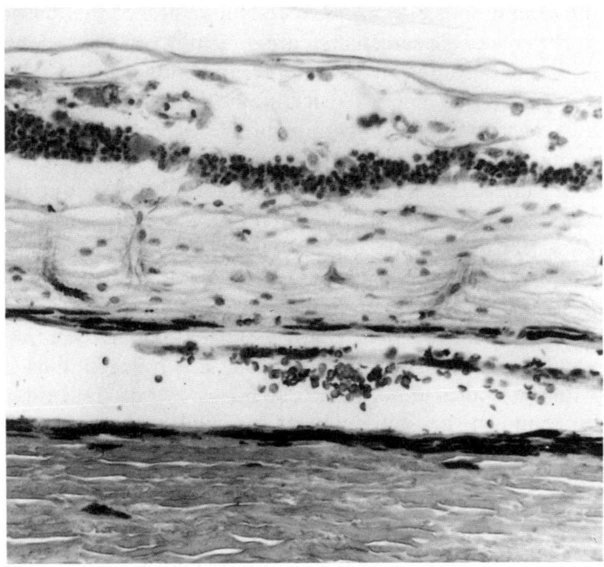

Fig. 6.57 Canine distemper. Severe retinal degeneration. Only a few ganglion cells and remnants of outer nuclear layer persist.

Demyelination is the salient feature of the encephalomyelitis of distemper. The lesions are widespread, but correlation with the clinical signs is often not apparent. The lesions have a pattern of development with regional differences in quality and severity. They are most severe and obvious in the cerebellum (Fig. 6.58A,B), surrounding the fourth ventricle, and in the optic tracts. Meningitis is always present, but usually mild and consists of accumulation of mononuclear cells, mainly lymphocytes, most obvious on the ventral surface of the brain. Inclusion bodies can be demonstrated in meningeal macrophages in both nuclei and cytoplasm.

Acute degenerative changes in the neurons occur extensively in the brain, but are modest in the cord. Experimental studies, both immunofluorescent and ultrastructural, associate this degeneration with viral infection of the neurons. The cells most susceptible to this virus-induced injury are the small pyramidal cells of the motor cortex and Purkinje cells of the cerebellum. More widespread neuronal degeneration occurs in subacute or chronic cases, particularly in the pyriform cortex, Ammon's horn, and deep structures in the temporal lobes. The degenerating neurons have eosinophilic granular cytoplasm and are often shrunken. The nuclei are pyknotic and may be eccentric. The surrounding neuropil is edematous, and the endothelial cells of the capillaries are swollen and proliferating. The malacic lesion remains virus associated in these cases, and inclusion bodies can be seen in the neurons and astrocytes, but the neuronal injury may be indirect and caused by immune mechanisms, ischemia, or anoxia.

Patchy demyelination is very common in dogs that come to autopsy. Early in the course of the cerebral involvement (this may be difficult to judge in clinical material because of the great variation in the onset in neurologic signs), there is vacuolation of the white matter. This vacuolation may be widely spaced or focal, giving the lesion a spongy appearance. In some foci, there is a reduction only in the intensity of myelin staining, which can be best demonstrated by myelin stains. At this stage, there is no perivascular infiltration and little or no astrocytic reaction, although viral inclusion bodies can be frequently seen in their nuclei. There appears to be no special affinity of the demyelinating process for particular tracts, but it is usually more severe in some locations than others. The commonly

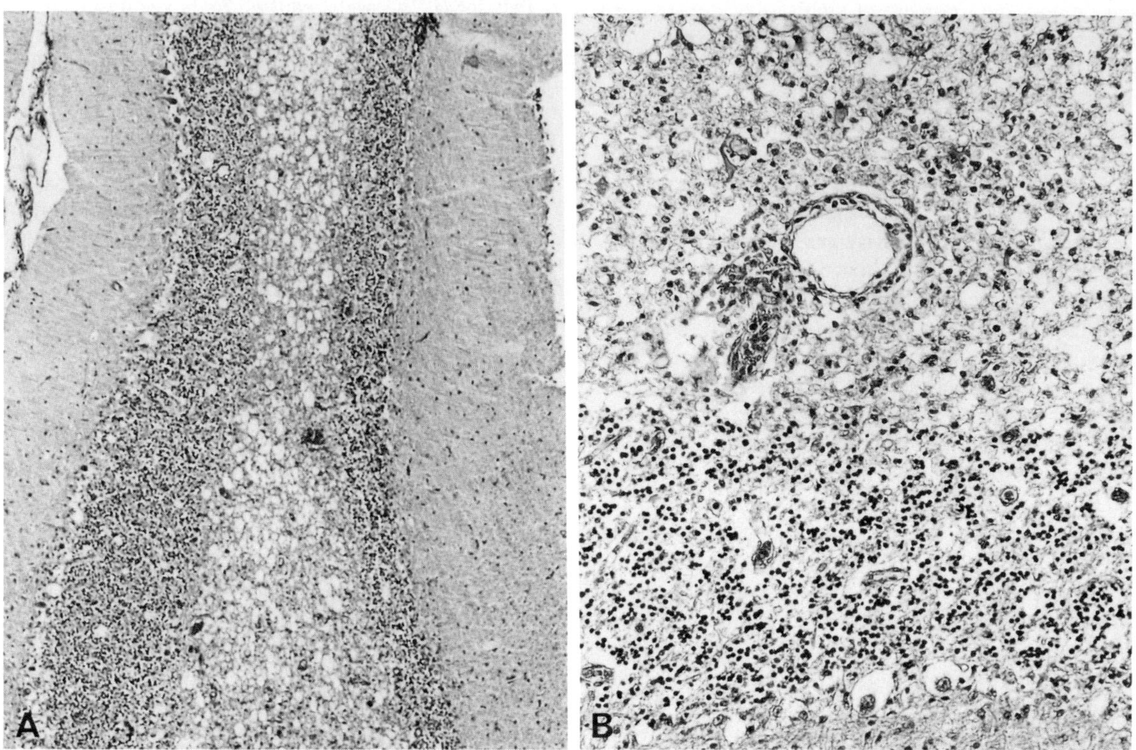

Fig. 6.58 (A) Canine distemper. Demyelination in cerebellar folium. (B) Canine distemper. Perivascular cuffing and demyelination in cerebellar folium.

involved sites are the anterior medullary velum, the cerebellar peduncles and arbor vitae, and the periphery of the optic chiasm and tracts. Demyelination is also common in subpial areas of the brainstem, either patchily or encircling it completely. Large foci of acute demyelination are uncommon in other parts of the brain.

Later stages of demyelination are characterized by reactive changes of astrocytes, consisting of diffuse proliferations of astrocytes and some microglia. Occasionally proliferating astrocytes form multinucleated syncytial cells. Inclusion bodies can be found in both types of astrocytes. The demyelination becomes more obvious, but it is usual for the original framework of the tissue to remain and to produce a lacelike appearance. Occasionally, especially in the folia of the cerebellum, there are foci of colliquative necrosis in which nothing remains except a few vessels and cells surrounded by fluid. These colliquative foci in the cerebellum may involve the granular layer but, as is usual for the lesions of canine distemper, spare the molecular layer. The demyelination reaction can progress to this stage with only very minor perivascular cuffing developing.

In canine distemper, perivascular cuffing is a late development and follows the demyelination. At the margins of larger foci in the chronic stage of the demyelination, thick perivascular cuffs of mononuclear cells form. At this stage, the lesions have a distinctly motheaten appearance. Macrophages are prominent in the lesion, and astrocytic proliferation and fusion continue. The astroglia have abundant, glassy cytoplasm and plump processes. Viral inclusion bodies in the astrocytic nuclei may be common (Fig. 6.59). Animals which survive the encephalomyelitis of canine distemper may be left with sclerotic astrocytic foci and myelin loss.

The role of the canine distemper virus in old dog encephalitis remains unclear. **Old dog encephalitis** (see The Nervous System, Volume 1, Chapter 3) is a disease of mature dogs characterized clinically by progressive motor and mental deterioration and pathologically by encephalitis with widely scattered perivascular infiltrations of lymphocytes and plasma cells and by intranuclear inclusions in the astrocytes and neurons. The inclusion bodies have been shown to contain paramyxovirus nucleocapsids and the viral antigen of canine distemper, but most investigators have been unable to recover the distemper virus from affected dogs or transmit the disease to either dogs or distemper-susceptible ferrets. The nature of the lesions and the localization are distinct between old dog encephalitis and the demyelinating encephalitis of canine distemper. The cerebellum, which is regularly involved in canine distemper encephalitis, is usually spared in old dog encephalitis, and clinical signs of the two entities are different. If the canine distemper virus can be a cause of old dog encephalitis, the pathogenetic mechanisms must differ from those that operate to produce the conventional disease.

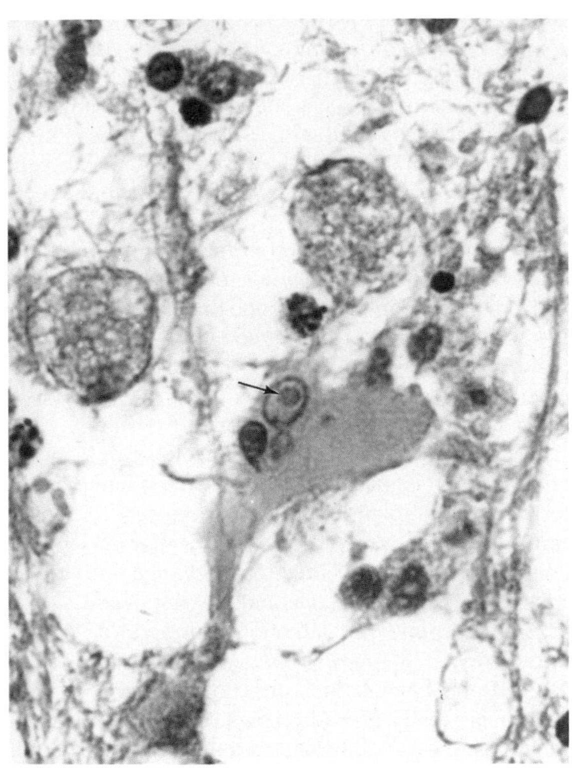

Fig. 6.59 Canine distemper. Myelin vacuoles, gitter cells, and one swollen astrocyte containing an intranuclear inclusion body (arrow).

Bibliography

Appel, M. J. G. Pathogenesis of canine distemper. *Am J Vet Res* **30:** 1167–1182, 1969.

Appel, M. J. G. Distemper pathogenesis in dogs. *J Am Vet Med Assoc* **156:** 1681–1684, 1970.

Appel, M. J. G., and Gillespie, J. H. Canine distemper virus. *Virol Monogr* **11:** 1–96, 1972.

Appel, M. *et al.* Canine distemper virus infection and encephalitis in javelinas (collared peccaries). *Arch Virol* **119:** 147–152, 1991.

Appel, M. *et al.* Where next for canine virus? *Nature* **353:** 508, 1991.

Axthelm, M. K., and Krakowka, S. Canine distemper virus: the early blood–brain barrier lesion. *Acta Neuropathol (Berl)* **75:** 27–33, 1987.

Blakemore, W. F., Summers, B. A., and Appel, M. G. J. Evidence of oligodendrocyte infection and degeneration in canine distemper encephalomyelitis. *Acta Neuropathol* **77:** 550–553, 1989.

Carre, H. Sur la maladie des jeunes chiens. *C R Acad Sci Paris* **140:** 689–690, 1489–1491, 1905.

Confer, A. W. *et al.* Biological properties of a canine distemper virus isolate associated with demyelinating encephalomyelitis. *Infect Immun* **11:** 835–844, 1975.

Cordy, D. R. Interstitial pneumonia with giant cells and inclusions. *J Am Vet Med Assoc* **114:** 21–26, 1949.

Dubielzig, R. R. The effect of canine distemper virus on the ameloblastic layer of the developing tooth. *Vet Pathol* **16:** 268–270, 1979.

Dunkin, G. W., and Laidlaw, P. P. Studies in dog distemper. *J Comp Pathol* **39:** 201–221, 1926.

Hall, W. W., Imagawa, D. T., and Choppin, P. W. Immunological evidence for the synthesis of all canine distemper virus polypeptides in chronic neurological diseases in dogs. Chronic distemper and old dog encephalitis differ from SSPE in man. *Virology* **98:** 283–287, 1979.

Higgins, R. J. *et al.* Canine distemper virus-associated cardiac necrosis in the dog. *Vet Pathol* **18:** 472–486, 1981.

Higgins, R. J. *et al.* Experimental canine distemper encephalomyelitis in neonatal gnotobiotic dogs. *Acta Neuropathol (Berl)* **57:** 287–295, 1982.

Higgins, R. J., Child, G., and Vandevelde, M. Chronic relapsing demyelinating encephalomyelitis associated with persistent spontaneous canine distemper virus infection. *Acta Neuropathol* **77:** 441–444, 1989.

Johnson, G. C., Krakowka, S., and Axthelm, M. K. Prolonged viral antigen retention in the brain of a gnotobiotic dog experimentally infected with canine distemper virus. *Vet Pathol* **24:** 87–89, 1987.

Jubb, K. V., Saunders, L. Z., and Coates, H. V. The intraocular lesions of canine distemper. *J Comp Pathol* **67:** 21–29, 1957.

Kennedy, S. *et al.* Histopathologic and immunocytochemical studies of distemper in seals. *Vet Pathol* **26:** 97–103, 1989.

Krakowka, S., and Koestner, A. Age-related susceptibility to infection with canine distemper virus in gnotobiotic dogs. *J Infect Dis* **134:** 629–632, 1976.

Krakowka, S., Axthelm, M. K., and Gorham, J. R. Effects of induced thrombocytopenia on viral invasion of the central nervous system in canine distemper virus infection. *J Comp Pathol* **97:** 441–450, 1987.

Krakowka, S., Confer, A., and Koestner, A. Evidence for transplacental transmission of canine distemper virus: Two case reports. *Am J Vet Res* **35:** 1251–1253, 1974.

Krakowka, S., Higgins, R. J., and Koestner, A. Canine distemper virus: Review of structural and functional modulations in lymphoid tissues. *Am J Vet Res* **41:** 284–292, 1980.

Lauder, I. M. *et al.* A survey of canine distemper. 2. Pathology. *Vet Rec* **66:** 623–631, 1954.

Lincoln, S. D. *et al.* Etiologic studies of old dog encephalitis. 1. Demonstration of canine distemper viral antigen in the brain of two cases. *Vet Pathol* **8:** 1–8, 1971.

Lincoln, S. D. *et al.* Studies of old dog encephalitis. 2. Electron microscopic and immunohistologic findings. *Vet Pathol* **10:** 124–129, 1973.

Lisiak, J. A., and Vandevelde, M. Polioencephalomalacia associated with canine distemper virus infection. *Vet Pathol* **16:** 650–660, 1979.

McCullough, B., Krakowka, S., and Koestner, A. Experimental canine distemper virus-induced lymphoid depletion. *Am J Pathol* **74:** 155–166, 1974.

Mitchell, W. J., Summers, B. A., and Appel, M. J. G. Viral expression in experimental canine distemper demyelinating encephalitis. *J Comp Pathol* **104:** 77–87, 1991.

Summers, B. A., Greisen, H. A., and Appel, M. J. G. Early events in canine distemper demyelinating encephalomyelitis. *Acta Neuropathol (Berl)* **46:** 1–10, 1979.

Vandevelde, M., and Kristensen, B. Observations on the distribution of canine distemper virus in the central nervous system of dogs with demyelinating encephalitis. *Acta Neuropathol* **40:** 233–236, 1977.

Vandevelde, M. *et al.* Chronic canine distemper virus encephalitis in mature dogs. *Vet Pathol* **17:** 17–29, 1980.

Vandevelde, M. *et al.* Immunoglobulins in demyelinating lesions in canine distemper encephalitis. *Acta Neuropathol (Berl)* **54:** 31–41, 1981.

Vandevelde, M. et al. Immunological and pathological findings in demyelinating encephalitis associated with canine distemper virus infection. *Acta Neuropathol (Berl)* **56:** 1–8, 1982.

Vandevelde, M. *et al.* Demyelination in experimental canine distemper virus infection: Immunological, pathological, and immunohistological studies. *Acta Neuropathol (Berl)* **56:** 285–293, 1982.

Vandevelde, M. *et al.* Glial proteins in canine distemper virus-induced demyelination. *Acta Neuropathol (Berl)* **59:** 269–276, 1983.

b. ORTHOMYXOVIRUS INFECTIONS Orthomyxoviruses typically cause inapparent to mild infections, mainly of the upper respiratory tract, unless they are unusually virulent or the affected animals are unduly susceptible. This is the pattern of human influenza. Where severe disease does occur, it is mostly due to the viral infection predisposing to secondary bacterial involvement. Virus particles are transmitted in aerosolized droplets, which are deposited, generally in accordance with their size, on the mucosa at different levels of the respiratory tract. In susceptible animals, viral neuraminidase causes destruction of surface glycoprotein, thus exposing the cell to viral attachment. Invasion of a few cells is sufficient to initiate focal lesions and progressive damage to the protective mucus layer. Attachment is the property of viral hemagglutinin. The virus enters the cell by endocytosis, and replication within the cell leads to the release of virions into the airways and to spread of the infection. Virtually every epithelial cell may become infected, and the protective mucociliary blanket is stopped as the epithelial cells are destroyed. The degenerative changes occur very rapidly but are also halted rapidly by production of new epithelium, which is resistant to infection.

The severity of these infections is often governed by the complications of compromised respiratory defenses, as discussed earlier in this chapter. Although the influenza viruses also involve the intestine and are viremic in birds, the viruses usually remain confined to the respiratory epithelium in animals, although viremia and infection of fetuses may occur with virulent infections.

The influenza viruses of pigs and horses belong to the A type, which is notable for the antigenic changes which can occur spontaneously in the hemagglutin and neuraminidase glycoproteins of the envelope. The changes may be the result of minor mutations which produce slight antigenic differences between viral strains, or they may be the result of gene acquisition producing a completely new type of envelope glycoprotein, and the potential for new pandemics. Several subtypes are identified, based on antigenic differences in the hemagglutin (H) or neuraminidase (N) proteins.

i. *Swine Influenza* Swine influenza is an acute contagious disease caused by type A viruses. The classic disease is caused by the subtype H_1N_1, which contains distinct antigenic variants which may circulate concurrently in pig populations in different parts of the world. Subtype H1N1 is the main agent of swine influenza in North America, is present in the pig population throughout the year, and produces disease of seasonal occurrence. The same subtype circulates widely in other parts of the northern hemisphere. Subtype H3N2 is prevalent in Europe; on serologic evidence, ~30% of pigs in England have been infected.

The swine viruses are zoonotic. There is circumstantial evidence that the classical swine subtype, H_1N_1, was acquired from humans in the 1918 pandemic, and the subtype H_3N_2 was also acquired from humans after its emergence in 1968 as Hong Kong flu. The traffic of infection can, however, be two-way, with humans acquiring infection by antigenic variants currently circulating in swine.

In surveyed pig populations, the serologic evidence of infection is much higher than the clinical evidence, which suggests that additional factors are necessary to convert the initial infections into disease. These factors are not understood, but the stress of climatic change and of management procedures is circumstantially important. So too may be concurrent viral infections such as by porcine coronaviruses.

Affected pigs have sudden onset of coughing and high fever, which rapidly spread to pigs of all ages. There is stiffness, weakness, and serous oculonasal discharge. The virus itself causes a mild illness lasting no more than a week; more severe illness and deaths are usually because of secondary bacterial pneumonia.

Uncomplicated viral infection rarely causes death, and the lesions have been studied mostly in experimental situations. Grossly, there is evidence of acute tracheobronchitis with reddened, swollen mucosa and filling of the airways by tenacious mucus, particularly in cranioventral regions. Because of the airway obstruction, there is alveolar atelectasis. This is seen as groups of clearly defined, plum-colored lobules in the cranioventral lung regions. The overall extent of the atelectasis depends on the severity of the viral bronchitis and bronchiolitis. In fatal cases, in addition to atelectasis, there is diffuse hyperemia and edema of the lungs, and the interlobular septa are widened by edema fluid. The airways contain bloodstained foam as well as thick mucus, and as a result, there can be terminal air trapping in non-atelectatic regions of the lung. The pleura is normal or covered by a small amount of serous or serofibrinous exudate, and there is excess fluid in the pleural cavity. The pulmonary lymph nodes are enlarged by hyperemia and edema. There is usually a nonspecific, severe congestion of the gastric mucosa along the greater curvature. In the more common instances where pigs die of secondary bacterial pneumonia, usually involving *Haemophilus* spp., *Pasteurella multocida*, or both, the lesions are characteristic of an acute bacterial bronchopneumonia.

Microscopically, there is patchy, acute inflammation of oculonasal membranes and mucosa of the tracheobronchial tree. The severity of infection is correlated with the extent of involvement of the respiratory tract. In mild cases, viral replication and the lesions it causes are limited to the upper respiratory tract. In severe infection, viral involvement extends to the bronchioles and alveolar parenchyma. Viral replication begins in epithelial cells by 2 hr after infection, and by 8 hr there is loss of cilia, extrusion of mucus, and vacuolar degeneration of epithelial cells. Within 24 hr, there is epithelial necrosis and sloughing with emigration of leukocytes, chiefly neutrophils, into the airway lumen. The net effect in severe infections is an acute bronchiolitis and bronchitis in which plugs of neutrophilic exudate are responsible for alveolar atelectasis. Extension of virus infection to alveolar epithelial cells causes alveolar flooding by serofibrinous exudate and neutrophils. The response after the first 24–48 hr becomes increasingly mononuclear. There is extensive infiltration of lymphocytes and smaller numbers of other leukocytes into the walls of airways and into the peribronchiolar and adjacent alveolar interstitium. Macrophages become the predominant cell in alveolar lumina. Epithelial proliferation and repair are easily detected histologically by the third to fourth days and lead to hyperplastic cells, which by light microscopy have an undifferentiated appearance. Return to ciliated and secretory cells occurs more slowly. The bronchial and bronchiolar epithelia frequently consist of several layers of stratified cells with the superficial ones degenerating and desquamating into the residual luminal exudate.

The lesion likely to be seen in the few animals dying primarily of the pure viral infection is one in which there is severe involvement of the bronchiolar–alveolar regions. The acute inflammatory exudate and associated interstitial accumulation of mononuclear cells give the characteristic bronchointerstitial pattern of pneumonia defined earlier. In pigs dying because of secondary bacterial infection, the exudative bacterial pneumonia obscures the earlier viral lesion.

Bibliography

Andrewes, C. H., Laidlaw, P. P., and Smith, W. The susceptibility of mice to the viruses of human and swine influenza. *Lancet* **ii:** 859–862, 1934.

Francis, T., and Shope, R. E. Neutralization tests with sera of convalescent or immunized animals and the viruses of swine and human influenza. *J Exp Med* **63:** 645–653, 1936.

Hjarre, A., Dinter, Z., and Bakos, K. Vergleichende Untersuchungen uber eine influenzaahnliche Schweinekrankheit in Schweden und Shopes Schweineinfluenza. *Nord Vet Med* **4:** 1025–1043, 1952.

Kammer, H., and Hanson, R. P. Studies on the transmission of swine influenza virus with *Metastrongylus* species in specific-pathogen-free swine. *J Infect Dis* **110:** 99–102, 1962.

Kammer, H., and Hanson, R. P. The *in vitro* association of swine influenza virus with *Metastrongylus* species. *J Infect Dis* **110:** 103–106, 1962.

Lewis, P. A., and Shope, R. E. Swine influenza. 2. A haemophilic bacillus from the respiratory tract of infected swine. *J Exp Med* **54:** 361–371, 1931.

Madec, F. *et al.* Pathological consequences of a severe outbreak of swine influenza (H_1N_1 virus) in the nonimmune sow at the beginning of pregnancy under natural conditions. *Comp Immun Microbiol Infect Dis* **12:** 17–27, 1989.

Nayak, D. P., Kelley, G. W., and Underdahl, N. R. The enhancing effect of swine lungworms on swine influenza infections. *Cornell Vet* **54:** 548, 1987.

Nayak, D. P. *et al.* Immunocytologic and histopathologic development of experimental swine influenza infection in pigs. *Am J Vet Res* **26:** 1271–1283, 1965.

Pritchard, G. C. *et al.* Porcine influenza outbreak in East Anglia due to influenza A virus (H_3N_2). *Vet Rec* **121:** 548, 1987.

Shope, R. E. Swine influenza. 1. Experimental transmission and pathology. *J Exp Med* **54:** 349–359, 1931.

Shope, R. E. The swine lungworm as a reservoir and intermediate host for swine influenza virus. 4. The demonstration of masked swine influenza virus in lungworm larvae and swine under natural conditions. *J Exp Med* **77:** 127–138, 1943.

Shope, R. E. The swine lungworm as a reservoir and intermediate host for swine influenza virus. 5. Provocation of swine influenza by exposure of prepared swine to adverse weather. *J Exp Med* **102:** 567–572, 1955.

Wibberley, G., Swallow, C., and Roberts, D. H. Characterization of an influenza A (H_3N_2) virus isolated from pigs in England in 1987. *Br Vet J* **144:** 196–201, 1988.

ii. *Equine Influenza* Equine influenza is caused by either of two subtypes of type A virus (A/equi 1, H_7N_7 and A/equi 2, H_3N_8). A role for type B virus is unconfirmed. The clinical syndrome caused by the influenza viruses overlaps those caused by equine herpesvirus 4 (rhinopneumonitis), equine arteritis virus (see The Cardiovascular System, Volume 3, Chapter 1), and perhaps equine parainfluenza type 3, rhinovirus, and reovirus. The subtypes of equine influenza virus have remained relatively stable with only antigenic drift in H_3N_8.

In common with other influenza infections, the disease spreads rapidly among susceptible horses. All ages in a previously unexposed population are susceptible, but the disease is seen most often in young animals brought together or mixed with older animals. Main clinical signs are coughing, serous to purulent oculonasal discharge, fever, and weakness. Most horses have a mild illness which resolves within 1–2 weeks, but death can occur either from secondary bacterial bronchopneumonia or from severe viral infection involving damage to brain, heart, gastrointestinal tract, kidney, and other parenchymal organs, as well as severe ocular and pulmonary lesions. Edematous swelling of subcutaneous tissues of legs and, less commonly, ventral trunk may also be present.

Respiratory lesions are those of hyperemia, edema, exudation, desquamation, and focal erosions in the upper respiratory tract. In severe cases, there is an acute bronchointerstitial pneumonia accompanied by more widespread pulmonary edema, as described for swine influenza, and a tendency for secondary bronchopneumonia caused mostly by streptococci but occasionally by *Escherichia coli, Pasteurella multocida,* or various other organisms normally resident on the nasopharyngeal mucosa.

Bibliography

Ahmed, M. T. Cases of purpura haemorrhagica as sequelae to equine influenza. *Ind Vet J* **15:** 213–215, 1938.

Bryans, J. T. *et al.* Epizootiologic features of disease caused by *Myxovirus* influenza A equine. *Am J Vet Res* **28:** 9–17, 1967.

Gerber, H., and Lohrer, J. Influenza A/equi-2 in der Schweiz 1965: III. Symptomatologie: 1. Reine Virusinfection. *Zentralblt Veterinarmed* **13:** 438–450, 1966.

Gerber, H. *et al.* Influenza A/equi-2 in der Schweiz 1965: II. Epizootologie. *Zentralblt Veterinarmed* **13:** 427–437, 1966.

Jones, T. C., and Maurer, F. D. The pathology of equine influenza. *Am J Vet Res* **4:** 15–31, 1943.

Wilson, J. C., Bryans, J. T., and Doll, E. R. Recovery of influenza virus from horses in the equine influenza epizootic of 1963. *Am J Vet Res* **26:** 1466–1468, 1965.

c. Rhinovirus Infections Rhinoviruses are one of the four genera of the family Picornaviridae. Two serotypes of rhinovirus are widespread among cattle populations. **Bovine rhinovirus** is generally believed to be of minor importance as a cause of respiratory disease in cattle. Viral isolation and serologic responses occasionally provide circumstantial evidence that it is involved in causing upper respiratory disease. Experimental production of disease is inconsistent, but there have not been attempts to confirm indications that the virus may produce a bronchointerstitial pneumonia. It seems most probable that viral replication and damage are limited to the upper respiratory tract in natural infections. The same holds true for **equine rhinovirus,** which is incriminated as a minor cause of acute upper respiratory disease in horses.

Bibliography

Ditchfield, J., and MacPherson, L. W. The properties and classification of two new rhinoviruses recovered from horses in Toronto, Canada. *Cornell Vet* **55:** 181–189, 1965.

d. Calicivirus Infections Caliciviruses are closely related to picornaviruses and, originally, feline caliciviruses, which are the important members of the genus causing respiratory disease, were discussed as feline picornaviruses. **Feline calicivirus infection** is commonly manifest as an upper respiratory tract disease (see Rhinitis, Section II,D,1 of this chapter). Feline caliciviruses can replicate in a variety of tissues, but their pathogenic effects are usually limited to the oral and respiratory mucosa and to a lesser extent the conjunctiva. Clinical signs are principally fever, oral ulceration, rhinitis, conjunctivitis, and possibly pneumonia. The range and severity of lesions depend on the virulence and tropism of the particular strain of calicivirus and on the mode of infection. Ulceration of oral epithelium is a common finding in both natural and experimental infections and reflects the close relationship of feline caliciviruses to vesicular exanthema virus of swine. The ulcers, which occasionally are detected in the earlier transient vesicular stage, are most often present on the dorsal surface or lateral margins of the tongue and on the hard palate and external nares. Serous or mucoid rhinitis and conjunctivitis are less consistent findings but are more common in natural infections, and in experimental infections if the virus is administered intranasally rather than by aerosol exposure. Clinical signs of pneumonia may be present in natural infections, but affected cats usually recover within 7–10 days unless bacterial complications ensue.

Most information on the pneumonia caused by feline caliciviruses is derived from experiments using heavy exposure to aerosolized pneumotropic strains. This produces an exaggerated picture of lung lesions compared to natural infections. Nevertheless, certain strains of the virus have a strong tropism for alveolar type I epithelial cells. The resulting lesion is an acute to subacute interstitial pneumonia with little of the bronchiolitis produced by the viral infections described previously. Grossly, the pneumonia involves cranioventral margins of the lungs and possibly irregular foci elsewhere. Early lesions are bright red and become gray-red at the peak of consolidation (7 to 10 days) and thereafter become gray-tan as resolution occurs.

Histologically the lesion is an interstitial pneumonia initiated by virus-induced necrosis of alveolar type I epithelial cells. The epithelial necrosis is extensive from 12 to 96 hr after infection and is accompanied by exudation of serofibrinous fluid and large numbers of neutrophils. Hyaline membranes may be present. As the viral replication, necrosis, and acute inflammation subside, type II epithelial cells proliferate to line denuded alveolar walls, and the inflammatory cells become increasingly mononuclear. Between 7 and 10 days after infection, alveoli are epithelialized by type II cells, lumina contain mostly macrophages, and alveolar septa are thickened by accumulation of lymphocytes, plasma cells, and sometimes fibroblasts. Few residual lesions are present after 30 days other than scarring as the result of necrosis of alveolar walls and hemorrhage. The upper respiratory tract involvement in feline herpesvirus infections compared to the oral and pulmonary distribution of lesions in calicivirus infections is a useful differential feature. Specific diagnosis, however, requires demonstration of virus in tissues by immunofluorescence.

Bibliography

Langloss, J. M., Hoover, E. A., and Kahn, D. E. Diffuse alveolar damage in cats induced by nitrogen dioxide or calicivirus. *Am J Pathol* **89:** 637–648, 1977.

Langloss, J. M., Hoover, E. A., and Kahn, D. E. Ultrastructural morphogenesis of acute viral pneumonia produced by feline calicivirus. *Am J Vet Res* **39:** 1577–1583, 1978.

Ormerod, E., McCandlish, I. A. P., and Jarrett, O. Disease produced by feline calicivirus when administered to cats by aerosol or intranasal instillation. *Vet Rec* **104:** 65–69, 1979.

Wardley, R. C., and Povey, R. C. The pathology and sites of persistence associated with three different strains of feline calicivirus. *Res Vet Sci* **23:** 15–19, 1977.

e. Adenovirus Infections Adenoviruses have been isolated from most species of animals. They have differing virulence and tissue tropisms, but more often cause respiratory and enteric disease than other manifestations. The most pronounced feature of the pneumotropic strains is a necrotizing and proliferative bronchiolitis. Severe naturally occurring disease usually requires an immunodeficiency state.

Canine adenovirus type 1 is the cause of **infectious canine hepatitis** and is described with diseases of the liver (Chapter 2, Section X,B,1 of this volume). **Canine adenovirus 2** is more strictly associated with respiratory disease, but strain differences within both serotypes make their distinction not so clear-cut as once thought. The contributory role of the virus in causing infectious tracheobronchitis (kennel cough) has already been mentioned. Naturally occurring pulmonary disease caused by adenovirus in dogs is mostly found in conjunction with canine distemper or other conditions causing immunologic impairment. The salient features are necrotizing bronchiolitis and the presence of large, amphophilic, intranuclear inclusions in swollen nuclei of degenerating bronchiolar epithelial cells. Intranuclear inclusions are usually less common in alveolar and bronchial epithelial cells and alveolar macrophages. The inclusions either fill the nuclei or are separated by a narrow clear zone from the thickened nuclear membrane (Cowdry type A inclusion). Affected bronchioles are filled with debris of sloughed epithelium and neutrophils. When viral infection of alveolar cells is extensive, there is an accompanying exudate of serofibrinous material, neutrophils, erythrocytes, and macrophages. Alveolar epithelialization can be prominent after viral replication has peaked (~10 days). Interstitial thickening by mononuclear cells and neutrophils occurs but is not an impressive feature.

Equine adenovirus infection is widespread in horses but mainly causes disease in young Arabian foals with congenital, combined, or selective immunodeficiency disease. Pulmonary lesions are a combination of coalesced atelectatic and consolidated lobules in cranioventral regions; large amounts of lung may be affected. Mucopurulent exudate is frequently present in the airways. Histologically, the main lesion is a severe bronchiolitis, which varies from necrotizing to proliferative, depending on the age of the lesions and the proportion of epithelial cells infected with virus. In the early stage of severe infection, there is extensive necrosis and sloughing of bronchiolar epithelium (Fig. 6.60A). Later, bronchiolar epithelium is hyperplastic, and swollen superficial epithelial cells contain amphophilic intranuclear inclusion bodies. Large, indistinct, blue inclusions are present in nuclei of dead cells which have been sloughed into the lumen (Fig. 6.60B). The combination of sloughed or hyperplastic epithelium and luminal filling by cell debris and neutrophils causes bronchiolar obstruction that is responsible for the widespread alveolar atelectasis. The uncomplicated adenoviral lesion is sometimes limited to airways, without direct alveolar involvement. In other instances, there are intranuclear inclusions in alveolar epithelial cells and an alveolitis characterized mainly by accumulations of mac-

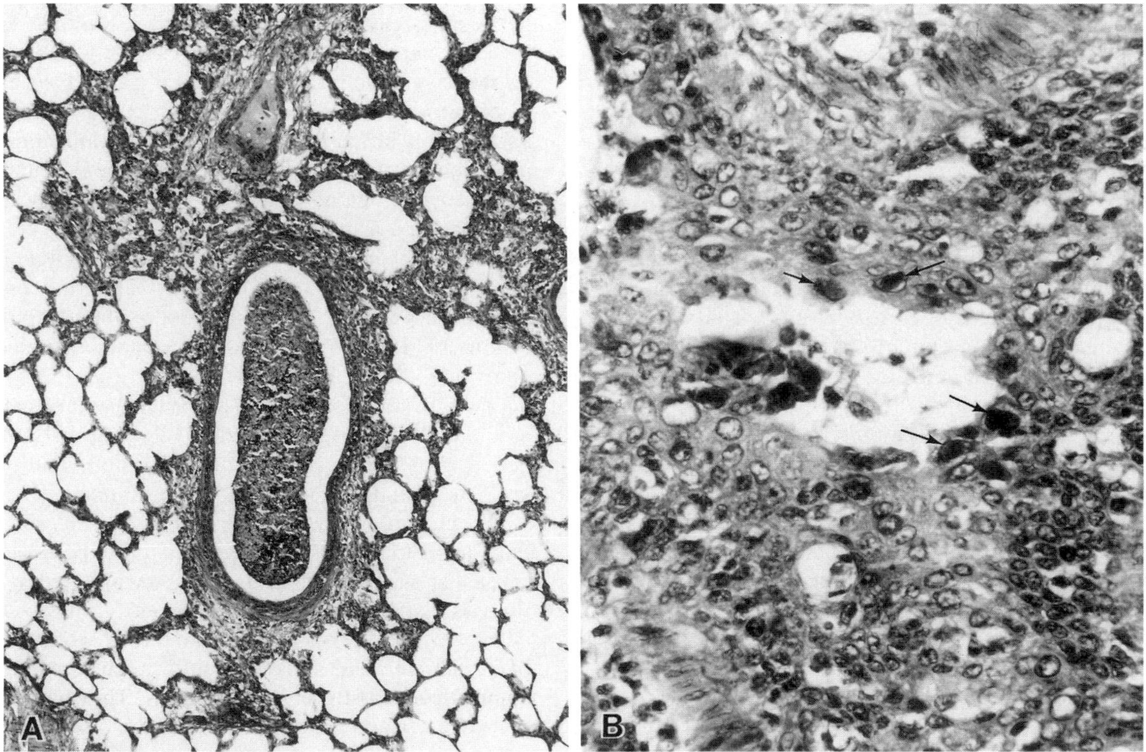

Fig. 6.60 Adenovirus infection in Arabian foal with combined immunodeficiency. (A) Acute necrotizing bronchiolitis. (B) Intranuclear inclusions (arrows) in superficial hyperplastic bronchiolar epithelium.

rophages and a variety of leukocytes. Epithelial lesions and inclusions may also be present in conjunctival and upper respiratory epithelium during the height of the disease. They can also occur in epithelium of the renal pelvis, ureters, urinary bladder, urethra, lacrimal and salivary glands, and pancreas. The viral bronchiolitis or bronchopneumonia and the associated immunodeficiency state may combine to lead to secondary bacterial pneumonia or *Pneumocystis* pneumonia.

A variety of epitheliotropic and endotheliotropic **bovine** and **ovine adenoviruses** have been isolated from ruminants. Circumstantial evidence indicates that certain serotypes of the bovine virus (particularly type 3) can cause mild respiratory or enteric disease or a combination of both. Bovine adenoviruses are not generally considered important pathogens; however, experimental infection of calves with epitheliotropic strains can cause necrotizing and proliferative bronchiolitis with intranuclear inclusions similar to the lesions occurring in foals. Only rarely are the characteristic lesions found in naturally occurring disease, usually in very young calves that lack colostral antibody or in which environmental stress or intercurrent diseases have impaired immune responses. A similar situation seems to exist in sheep. A noteworthy feature of the lesions caused by at least one strain of adenovirus from sheep is the exaggerated enlargement of both nucleus and cytoplasm of inclusion-bearing bronchiolar and alveolar epithelial cells. The pronounced cytomegaly can cause confusion with the cellular enlargement associated with cytomegalovirus infections.

Porcine adenoviruses studied so far appear to have less affinity for pulmonary epithelium than those from the species already mentioned. Limited experimental information indicates that pulmonary lesions are probably more a true interstitial pneumonia with alveolar septa thickened by proliferation of alveolar epithelial cells and accumulation of macrophages, lymphocytes, and plasma cells. Cells within alveolar septa, some possibly capillary endothelial cells, contain bluish intranuclear inclusions. Bronchiolar epithelial necrosis or hyperplasia is not a significant feature. Porcine adenoviruses have been associated with field cases of encephalitis or diarrhea but have not been established as an important cause of respiratory disease.

Bibliography

Belak, S. *et al*. Isolation of a pathogenic strain of ovine adenovirus type 5 and a comparison of its pathogenicity with that of another strain of the same serotype. *J Comp Pathol* **90:** 169–176, 1980.

Darbyshire, J. H. Bovine adenoviruses. *J Am Vet Med Assoc* **152:** 786–792, 1968.

Darbyshire, J. H. *et al*. Association of adenoviruses with bovine respiratory disease. *Nature* **208:** 307–308, 1965.

Darbyshire, J. H. *et al*. The pathogenesis and pathology of infection in calves with a strain of bovine adenovirus type 3. *Res Vet Sci* **7:** 81–93, 1966.

Davies, D. H., Dungworth, D. L., and Mariassy, A. T. Experimental adenovirus infection of lambs. *Vet Microbiol* **6:** 113–128, 1981.

Ducatelle, R. *et al*. Pathology of natural canine adenovirus pneumonia. *Res Vet Sci* **31:** 207–212, 1981.

Klein, M. The relationship of two bovine adenoviruses to human adenoviruses. *Ann N Y Acad Sci* **101:** 493–497, 1962.

McChesney, A. E. *et al*. Adenoviral infection in suckling Arabian foals. *Pathol Vet* **7:** 547–565, 1970.

McChesney, A. E., England, J. J., and Rich, L. J. Adenoviral infection in foals. *J Am Vet Med Assoc* **162:** 545–549, 1973.

Shadduck, J. A., Koestner, A., and Kasza, L. The lesions of porcine adenoviral infection in germ-free and pathogen-free pigs. *Pathol Vet* **4:** 537–552, 1967.

f. HERPESVIRUS INFECTIONS Members of this family are important causes of respiratory disease. Three of them are discussed with rhinitis: **inclusion-body rhinitis of swine, infectious bovine rhinotracheitis,** and **feline viral rhinotracheitis.** Another that is described elsewhere is **malignant catarrhal fever** (see The Alimentary System, Chapter 1 of this volume). **Pseudorabies (Aujeszky's disease)** mainly causes disease of the nervous system (see The Nervous System, Volume 1, Chapter 3) but certain strains of the virus can also cause rhinitis and pneumonia in swine. The severe acute lesion is hemorrhagic consolidation of cranioventral regions of the lung, which histologically has necrotizing lesions in bronchioles and adjacent alveoli as the principal features. Acidophilic or amphophilic intranuclear inclusions may be found in bronchiolar and alveolar epithelial cells early in the infection.

Canine herpesvirus is most important as a cause of fatal, generalized infection in neonatal puppies (see The Female Genital System, Volume 3, Chapter 4). It can occasionally be associated with usually nonfatal respiratory infection in older animals, either alone or with other infectious agents. The respiratory lesions are those to be expected from herpesviruses, namely a necrotizing rhinotracheitis and possibly bronchopneumonia. Acidophilic intranuclear inclusions can sometimes be found in epithelial cells in early lesions, more commonly in nasal and turbinate mucosa.

Equine herpesvirus 4 (rhinopneumonitis virus) is an important respiratory tract pathogen and, in contrast to equine herpesvirus 1, causes predominantly pulmonary lesions. The respiratory disease occurs independent of abortions caused by equine herpesvirus 1, and it now appears that different equine herpesviruses are specifically associated with each syndrome. For the role of equine herpesviruses 1 in causing genital lesions and abortion, see The Female Genital System (Volume 3, Chapter 4).

The clinical respiratory disease is seen mostly in weanling foals during the fall. It is characterized by slight fever, serous or catarrhal rhinitis, and conjunctivitis. Rarely, there is diarrhea and edema of the extremities. Recovery occurs in ~1 week but may be delayed when secondary bacterial infections supervene and cause mucopurulent or suppurative rhinitis and pharyngitis, or possibly pneumonia. The uncomplicated viral infection is not fatal even when severe, as it can be in young horses crowded in stockyards or stables. When fatalities occur, they are usually due to secondary suppurative bacterial bronchopneumonia. Intranuclear inclusions are extremely rare in postnatal respiratory infections.

Equine herpesvirus 2 (equine cytomegalovirus) has been isolated from normal and diseased respiratory tracts (including lymphofollicular pharyngitis and pneumonia), but its pathogenic importance is questionable.

Bibliography

Baskerville, A. The histopathology of pneumonia produced by aerosol infection of pigs with a strain of Aujeszky's disease virus. *Res Vet Sci* **12:** 590–592, 1971.

Baskerville, A. Ultrastructural changes in the pulmonary airways of pigs infected with a strain of Aujeszky's disease virus. *Res Vet Sci* **13:** 127–132, 1972.

Baskerville, A., McFerran, J. B., and Dow, C. Aujeszky's disease in pigs. *Vet Bull* **43:** 465–480, 1973.

Crandell, R. A. Pseudorabies (Aujeszky's disease). *Vet Clin North Am* (*Large Anim Pract*) **4:** 321–331, 1982.

Thompson, H., Wright, N. G., and Cornwell, H. J. C. Canine herpesvirus respiratory infection. *Res Vet Sci* **13:** 123–126, 1972.

g. PARVOVIRUS INFECTION **Canine parvovirus** is mainly a cause of enteritis and myocardial necrosis [see The Alimentary (Chapter 1 of this volume) and the Cardiovascular (Volume 3, Chapter 1) Systems]. Pulmonary lesions are usually those of severe acute to subacute pulmonary congestion and edema secondary to the myocardial damage. A true viral interstitial pneumonia is generally limited to very young pups (<2 weeks of age) in which there is generalized parvovirus infection. In such cases, basophilic intranuclear inclusions can be found in the vascular endothelium of many organs, including the lung. In the lung, viral infection of capillary endothelium, and perhaps alveolar epithelium, causes necrosis and accumulation of mixed inflammatory cells, mostly lymphocytes and monocytes. Alveolar edema is partly the result of local alveolar septal inflammation and partly cardiac failure.

Bibliography

Carpenter, J. L. *et al.* Intestinal and cardiopulmonary forms of parvovirus infection in a litter of pups. *J Am Vet Med Assoc* **176:** 1269–1273, 1980.

Lenghaus, C., and Studdert, M. J. Generalized parvovirus disease in neonatal pups. *J Am Vet Med Assoc* **181:** 41–45, 1982.

Robinson, W. R., Huxtable, C. R., and Pass, D. A. Canine parvoviral myocarditis: A morphological description of the natural disease. *Vet Pathol* **17:** 282–293,1980.

h. ORTHOREOVIRUS INFECTION Of the three serotypes of reovirus, one or more have been isolated from cattle, horses, sheep, pigs, dogs, and cats. They are associated with inapparent infection or a mild upper respiratory disease. Their roles as significant causes of, or predisposers to, pneumonia are not firmly established.

Bibliography

Baskerville, A., McFerran, J. B., and Connor, T. The pathology of experimental infection of pigs with type 1 reovirus of porcine origin. *Res Vet Sci* **12:** 172–174, 1971.

Lamont, P. H. *et al.* Pathogenesis and pathology of infection in calves with strains of reovirus types 1 and 2. *J Comp Pathol* **78:** 23–33, 1968.

Phillip, J. I. H. *et al.* Pathogenesis and pathology in calves of infection by *Bedsonia* alone and *Bedsonia* and reovirus together. *J Comp Pathol* **78:** 89–99, 1968.

i. RETROVIRUS INFECTIONS: OVINE PROGRESSIVE PNEUMONIA (MAEDI) Chronic progressive pneumonia (lymphoid interstitial pneumonia) of sheep is a slow virus infection of the ovine lung characterized by a gradually progressive interstitial pneumonia. It is caused by identical or very closely related strains of maedi–visna virus which belongs to the lentivirus subfamily of retroviruses. The name of the maedi–visna virus is derived from the fact that investigators in Iceland were the first to isolate the virus and demonstrate that the progressive pneumonia, referred to clinically as maedi (shortness of breath), and the meningoencephalitis, which they designated clinically as visna (wasting), were different manifestations of the same slow virus infection. For descriptions of visna, see The Nervous System (Volume 1, Chapter 3).

The pulmonary disease caused by the maedi–visna virus occurs widely throughout Europe, North America, Africa, and Asia and, until the development and use of serologic tests for detecting infected animals, was being spread further by importation of affected sheep. In addition to the terms ovine progressive pneumonia and maedi, the condition is known as **Graaff–Reinet** disease in the Republic of South Africa, ***zwoegerziekte*** in the Netherlands, and ***la bouhite*** in France.

The virus is spread by close contact among sheep and in milk from ewe to lamb. *In utero* infection can also occur. Infection of sheep is common in regions where the disease is endemic, but many go to slaughter without developing clinical signs. Because of the slow rate of progression of pulmonary lesions, clinical signs are uncommon until sheep reach 2 years of age. Evidence of disease is most frequent among sheep 5–10 years of age. The early signs are loss of weight and increased respiratory rate on exertion. Once signs begin, death usually occurs within ~6–8

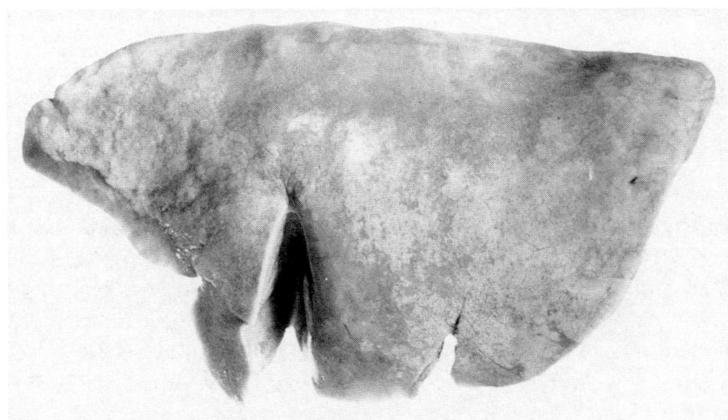

Fig. 6.61 Chronic progressive pneumonia (maedi). Sheep. Lungs fail to collapse and have widespread grayish mottling.

months because of continuing deterioration in condition and increasing respiratory difficulty.

The specific lesions of ovine progressive pneumonia occur in the lungs and their associated lymph nodes. Grossly, the lungs of severely affected sheep do not collapse fully when the thorax is opened, and sometimes the impressions of the ribs are retained. In cases uncomplicated by bronchopneumonia or abscessation, the lungs are mottled gray to grayish tan, and the pleura is smooth and glistening (Fig. 6.61). Lungs are much heavier than usual, often two or more times the normal weight. Close examination of the lung reveals that, although the lesions are widespread, there is relative sparing of the cranioventral regions in the absence of secondary bronchopneumonia. Least involved regions have an irregular grayish speckling against a light tan background. Greater involvement results in a reticular pattern, and in most severely affected regions there is homogeneous grayish consolidation. The lungs have a soft rubbery consistency or are moderately firm depending on the degree of confluence of the lesions. The cut surface is moist, but without oozing of free fluid. When complicated by bronchopneumonia, there are the typical cranioventral consolidations with pus-filled airways. There can also be coexistent lungworm lesions. A consistent gross finding in ovine progressive pneumonia is enlargement of bronchial and mediastinal lymph nodes, with soft grayish-white, homogeneous thickening of cortical regions on cut section.

Histologically, the most characteristic feature of ovine progressive pneumonia is the extensive lymphofollicular proliferations which occur predominantly in the perivascular, peribronchial, and peribronchiolar sheaths in association with the pulmonary lymphatics. The most consistent association is with pulmonary veins. Many of the lymphoid follicles contain germinal centers (Fig. 6.62A). These prominent lymphofollicular features have led to the designation, lymphoid interstitial pneumonia. The next most striking feature is hyperplasia of smooth muscle, which is most evident in the walls of terminal bronchioles and alveolar ducts, but also extends into the walls of neighboring alveoli (Fig. 6.62B). Alveolar septa are thickened by infiltrations of lymphocytes and macrophages, especially at the periphery of the lymphoid nodules. The amount of interstitial fibrosis is usually slight but tends to be exaggerated by collapse of small clusters of alveoli and apposition of their walls (microatelectasis). Hyperplasia of alveolar type II epithelial cells is not usually a prominent feature of ovine progressive pneumonia, in striking contrast to ovine pulmonary adenomatosis (see Neoplasms of the Lung, Section VI,J of this chapter). Partial or complete lining of alveoli by cuboidal type II cells does occur, but usually only in alveoli adjacent to the large interstitial lymphoid follicles or occasionally lining large cystlike spaces. Bronchiolar epithelial hyperplasia is also not a prominent feature of uncomplicated ovine progressive pneumonia, although collapsed airways have pleated epi-

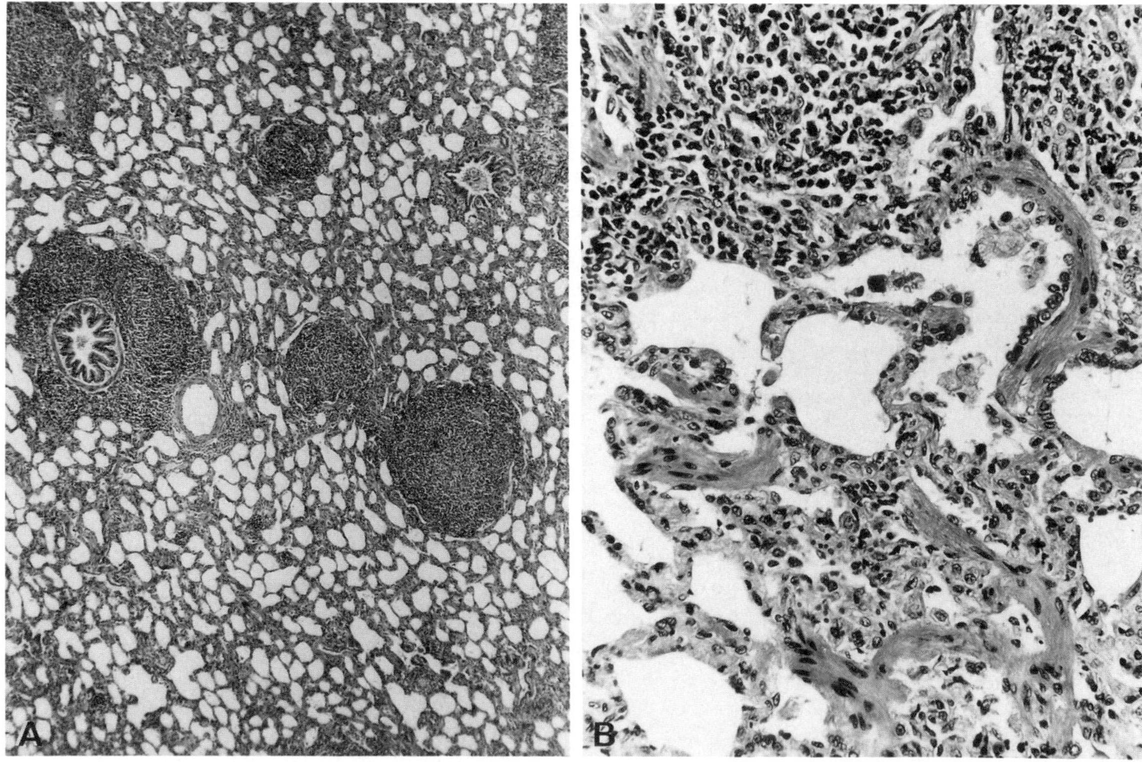

Fig. 6.62 (A) Chronic progressive pneumonia (maedi). Sheep. Diffuse thickening of alveolar walls and lymphofollicular accumulations around vessels and airways. (B) Hyperplasia of smooth muscle of terminal bronchioles and alveolar ducts.

thelium which can be mistaken for hyperplasia. The alveolar exudate in the uncomplicated disease is usually sparse and consists mainly of alveolar macrophages and small amounts of debris. Multinucleated macrophages are a variable feature. Suppurative lesions oriented on bronchioles indicate a secondary bacterial bronchopneumonia. Bronchial and mediastinal lymph nodes have a chronic hyperplastic lymphadenitis in which the main feature is pronounced follicular hyperplasia.

Pathogenesis of the disease involves infection of cells of the monocyte–macrophage lineage, possibly also a few T lymphocytes, with subsequent positive feedback established by macrophage-derived cytokines and the responding lymphoid cells releasing their cytokines in turn. There presumably is also low-grade involvement of an assortment of additional inflammatory mediators. In infected flocks, there is usually serologic evidence of infection of many animals and the maedi–visna virus can be isolated from both normal and diseased lungs. The diagnosis of ovine progressive pneumonia depends mainly on the presence of the characteristic lymphofollicular interstitial pneumonia.

Progressive pneumonia is a fairly common manifestation of disease in sheep long infected by the maedi–visna virus. Mastitis appears to be a more common manifestation if deliberately sought by postmortem examination. Chronic proliferative arthritis is less common than pneumonia and meningoencephalitis (visna) is the least frequent manifestation.

Caprine arthritis–encephalitis (CAE) is a disease complex in goats caused by a lentivirus antigenically closely related to the maedi–visna virus but separable on the basis of the large differences in nucleic acid sequences. The caprine virus has been studied mainly in reference to its ability to cause encephalitis and arthritis, as the name indicates [see The Nervous System (Volume 1, Chapter 3), and Bones and Joints (Volume 1, Chapter 1)]. An alternative term for the disease is viral leukoencephalomyelitis–arthritis. There are brief descriptions of a chronic interstitial pneumonia produced by the virus, but there has not been a detailed study of the pulmonary lesions. The virus also causes mastitis, so the range of organ involvement of the maedi–visna virus and CAE virus are the same. Naturally occurring chronic pneumonia in older goats often has two prominent features lacking in ovine progressive pneumonia. One is extensive alveolar filling mainly by dense, acidophilic, proteinaceous (lipoproteinaceous) material. The other is widespread lining of alveolar septa by alveolar type II epithelial cells. The pathogenesis of these components and their relationship to infection with the caprine arthritis–encephalitis virus remain to be determined.

Bibliography

Cutlip, R. C., Jackson, T. A., and Laird, G. A. Prevalence of ovine progressive pneumonia in a sampling of cull sheep from western and midwestern United States. *Am J Vet Res* **38:** 2091–2093, 1977.

Cutlip, R. C., Jackson, T. A., and Lehmkuhl, H. D. Lesions of ovine progressive pneumonia: Interstitial pneumonitis and encephalitis. *Am J Vet Res* **40:** 1370–1374, 1979.

Cutlip, R. C. *et al.* Effects on ovine fetuses of exposure to ovine progressive pneumonia virus. *Am J Vet Res* **43:** 82–85, 1982.

Georgsson, G., and Palsson, P. A. The histopathology of maedi: A slow viral pneumonia of sheep. *Vet Pathol* **8:** 63–80, 1971.

Gudnadottir, M., and Palsson, P. A. Host–virus interaction in visna infected sheep. *J Immunol* **95:** 1116–1120, 1965.

Gudnadottir, M., and Palsson, P. A. Transmission of maedi by inoculation of a virus grown in tissue culture from maedi-affected lungs. *J Infect Dis* **117:** 1–6, 1967.

Haase, A. T. The slow infection caused by visna virus. *Curr Top Microbiol Immunol* **72:** 101–156, 1975.

Lairmore, M. D., Rosadio, R. H., and DeMartini, J. C. Ovine lentivirus lymphoid interstitial pneumonia. Rapid induction in neonatal lambs. *Am J Pathol* **125:** 173–181, 1986.

Lucam, F. La "bouhite" ou "lymphomatose pulmonaire maligne du Mouton." *Rec Med Vet* **118:** 273–284, 1942.

Oliver, R. E. *et al.* Ovine progressive pneumonia: Pathologic and virologic studies on the naturally occurring disease. *Am J Vet Res* **42:** 1544–1559, 1981.

Perk, K. Slow virus infection of ovine lung. *Adv Vet Sci Comp Med* **26:** 267–288, 1982.

Rajya, B. S., and Singh, C. M. The pathology of pneumonia and associated respiratory disease of sheep and goats. I. Occurrence of jaagziekte and maedi in sheep and goats in India. *Am J Vet Res* **25:** 61–67, 1964.

Sigurdsson, B. Observations on three slow infections of sheep. *Br Vet J* **110:** 255–270, 1954.

Sigurdsson, B., Grimsson, H., and Palsson, P. A. Maedi, a chronic, progressive infection of sheep's lungs. *J Infect Dis* **90:** 233–241, 1952.

Sigurdsson, B., Palsson, P. A., and Tryggvadottir, A. Transmission experiments with maedi. *J Infect Dis* **93:** 166–175, 1953.

j. OTHER RESPIRATORY VIRUSES OF PIGS A **porcine respiratory coronavirus** emerged in Europe and Britain in 1986. The rapidity of spread suggested respiratory transmission, and this route is successful for experimental transmission. The natural infection has not been responsible for clinical disease; it is detected by seroconversion against the classical transmissible gastroenteritis coronavirus of pigs of which it is probably a derivative. The respiratory agent replicates in the epithelial lining of airways and in alveolar macrophages but is without significant tropism for intestinal mucosa. Experimental infection can cause severe illness and death from bronchopneumonia.

Porcine epidemic abortion and respiratory syndrome is a syndrome awaiting etiologic and pathologic clarification. The syndrome emerged in 1987 and has increased in importance as a cause of respiratory disease and pregnancy wastage in Canada, United States of America, Europe, and Britain. A virus designated as Lelystad agent and of undetermined taxonomic position is responsible for much of the European syndrome, whereas in North America the picture is somewhat clouded by other and mixed infections by such agents as *Haemophilus parasuis, Streptococcus suis, Pneumocystis,* swine influenza virus, encephalomyocarditis virus, and inclusion-body rhinitis virus.

The disease is expressed as pneumonia or as pregnancy wastage. The route of infection is respiratory, but pulmonary signs may be minimal in older pigs. The peak age for the respiratory disease is 4–10 weeks, in the range of 2–16 weeks. The lesions fit the description of bronchointerstitial pneumonia, which progresses in anteroventral lobes to suppurative bronchopneumonia and in the dorsal lobes to interstitial pneumonia with prominent epithelialization. Grossly, there is confluent consolidation of anterior lobes and ventral parts of the diaphragmatic lobes, together with lobular consolidation in dorsal areas. Often there is confluent consolidation of all lobes of both lungs.

In sows, infection is characterized by inappetence and fever, usually with brief but varying periods of blue discoloration of the ears, abdomen, and vulva. Infection in the pregnant sow during the first half of pregnancy (21–60 days of gestation) is followed by a return to estrus associated with embryonic death, absorption, or abortion, and in the last half of gestation by mummification, abortion, stillbirth, and the birth of live piglets, 50% of which may be nonviable. Piglets born alive are frequently weak, inappetent, and a high proportion die of respiratory disease. In contrast, feeder pigs are only transiently affected.

Bibliography

Cox, E., Hooybergh s, J., and Pensaert, M. B. Sites of replication of a porcine respiratory coronavirus related to transmissible gastroenteritis virus. *Res Vet Sci* **48:** 165–169, 1990.

McCullough, S. J. *et al.* Experimental transmission of mystery swine disease. *In* "EEC Seminar Report of the New Pig Diseases: Porcine Reproductive and Respiratory Syndrome (PRRS)," pp. 46–52, Brussels, 1991.

Morin, M. *et al.* Severe proliferative and necrotizing pneumonia in pigs: A newly recognized disease. *Can Vet J* **31:** 837–839, 1990.

Pol, J. M. A. *et al.* Pathological, ultrastructural, and immunohistochemical changes caused by Lelystad virus in experimentally induced infections of mystery swine disease [synonym: porcine epidemic abortion and respiratory syndrome (PEARS)]. *Vet Q* **13:** 137–143, 1991.

Terpstra, C., Wensvoort, G., and Pol, J. M. A. Experimental reproduction of porcine epidemic abortion and respiratory syndrome (mystery swine disease) by infection with Lelystad virus: Koch's postulates fulfilled. *Vet Q* **13:** 131–136, 1991.

Van Nieuwstadt, A. P., and Pol, J. M. A. Isolation of a TGE virus-related respiratory coronavirus causing fatal pneumonia in pigs. *Vet Rec* **124:** 43–44, 1989.

Wensvoort, G. *et al.* Mystery swine disease in the Netherlands: The isolation of Lelystad virus. *Vet Q* **13:** 121–130, 1991.

2. Bacterial Diseases

a. PASTEURELLOSIS The pasteurellae are strict parasites of animals, their usual habitat being the mucous membranes of the nasopharyngeal and oral regions. The type species is *Pasteurella multocida*. The other species of major importance for respiratory disease in domestic animals is *P. haemolytica*. A third, *P. pneumotropica*, can frequently be isolated from the pharynx of cats and may contaminate bite wounds made by cats.

The collective term pasteurellosis will be used in this section for infections by either *P. multocida* or *P. haemolytica*. Pasteurellosis may be manifested as a peracute or acute septicemia, or be slightly less acute and cause signs according to the organ in which the infection is localized. Thus, in the various species, pasteurellosis can take a variety of forms. It may be a primary infection, a contaminant of cutaneous or mucosal injuries, or a secondary infection, especially following viral disease of the respiratory tract.

Pasteurella multocida can be isolated from pathologic conditions in cattle, sheep, buffaloes, deer, pigs, rabbits, and other animals, and from a variety of birds, in which it causes fowl cholera. In the past, the different strains have been named for the species of host in which they are found, but it is current practice to regard these as types of the one species, *P. multocida*. Mammalian isolates of *P. multocida* are typed by biological characteristics (biotype) and serologically (serotype). The important strains are assigned on the basis of capsular antigens to one of five serotypes: A, B, D, E, and F. Further characterization can be made on the basis of the 11 somatic antigens. Types B and E are the cause of epidemic pasteurellosis, the classic hemorrhagic septicemia of cattle, sheep, goats, deer, and buffaloes. Type B is widespread in tropical Asia and Africa and in southern Europe. Type E occurs mainly in central Africa. Type A is ubiquitous and responsible for sporadic infections in many species; strains of this serotype are the ones usually isolated from pneumonia of cattle and fowl cholera and are sometimes found in pneumonia of swine. Type D is ubiquitous but has been found particularly in association with atrophic rhinitis and pneumonia in swine. It is also occasionally isolated from pneumonia in sheep.

Strains of *P. haemolytica* are also classified by biotype and serotype. The organism is weakly hemolytic, and as a rule is nonpathogenic for rodents. The two main biotypes are A (arabinose fermenters) and T (trehalose fermenters). There are 16 currently recognized serotypes based on analysis of capsular antigens, 12 in type A and 4 in type T. Type A1 is the usual cause of severe pneumonic pasteurellosis (shipping fever) of cattle. Type A strains are associated with pneumonia in sheep and septicemia in lambs before weaning. Type T strains cause septicemia in lambs past weaning age.

Pasteurella multocida and *P. haemolytica* are both members of the bacterial flora of normal nasopharyngeal and oral mucous membranes, with the former usually predominating. Outbreaks of disease caused by the organisms occur when local and systemic defense mechanisms are impaired and virulent strains of pasteurellae undergo massive proliferation prior to invading the nasopharyngeal mucosa or being inhaled in large numbers into the lung. Predisposing factors, such as the stress induced by transportation, crowding, climatic changes and poor management, or the damaging effects of respiratory viral infections, were mentioned previously (see Bronchopneumonia, Section VI,F,1 of this chapter). Effects of stress are mediated partly by adrenocorticosteroid release.

i. *Cattle* The major pasteurelloses of cattle are **hemorrhagic septicemia** and **pneumonic pasteurellosis.** Two other forms of pasteurellosis, meningitis in calves and mastitis in cows, occasionally are important in local situations. Meningeal pasteurellosis of calves is caused by *P. multocida,* and it is usually a disease of housed calves of 2–4 months of age. The reaction is fibrinopurulent and is sometimes accompanied by polyarthritis of the same type. Bovine mastitis is caused by either *P. multocida* or *P. haemolytica.* Sporadic, peracute, fatal mammary infections occur, caused by *P. haemolytica;* these infections are characterized by severe hemorrhagic inflammation of the parenchyma and a fibrinous and necrotizing inflammation of the ducts, quite similar to the peracute inflammation produced by coliform organisms. The pathway of infection is via the duct system. *Pasteurella multocida* can be responsible for outbreaks of mastitis in a herd. If the mastitis is acute, it may be progressive and result in fibrosis and atrophy. The route of infection is assumed to be through the ducts, and the source of infection, in some cases at least, is assumed to be the suckling calf. *Pasteurella haemolytica* is sometimes responsible for outbreaks of abortion in cattle in which there are no premonitory signs.

The classic form of bovine pasteurellosis is **hemorrhagic septicemia** caused by *P. multocida* types B or E. This disease was originally recognized in western Europe in the nineteenth century as a severe epidemic in deer; it later spread to cattle, wild and domestic pigs, and horses. It has been observed as an epidemic disease of cattle, sheep, and horses in the Argentine, in bison in the western United States, and it is the disease known as El Guedda of Syrian camels and barbone of Italian buffaloes. Hemorrhagic septicemia is now limited largely to tropical lands from Egypt to the Philippine Islands and in these regions is primarily a disease of buffaloes.

The most detailed descriptions are of the disease as it occurs in Asia, where outbreaks occur particularly during the rainy season. In intervening periods, the organism is apparently maintained in the nasopharyngeal regions of carrier cattle or buffaloes. The start of an outbreak depends on some stress disturbing the balance in a carrier animal. This results in extensive proliferation and dissemination of the organisms to susceptible contact animals.

Approximately 10% of animals survive subclinical infections and become immune, but once the infection is established clinically, the mortality is almost 100%, even though the bacteria may be killed by chemotherapy. This, together with the immense proliferation of organisms in the clinical disease, indicates that toxins, particularly endotoxins, are important in causing death.

Hemorrhagic septicemia is almost by definition a peracute disease with death often so early that few signs are observed. When observed clinically, there is high fever and rapid prostration, with profuse salivation. The saliva and feces contain large numbers of pasteurellae. The postmortem picture is characterized by petechial hemorrhages on the serous membranes and in the various organs, especially the lungs and muscles. Severe endotoxemia may cause an acute, fibrinohemorrhagic interstitial pneumonia. The lymph nodes are swollen and hemorrhagic, and there may be bloodstained fluid in the serous cavities. Acute gastroenteritis, which can be hemorrhagic, is often present. The spleen is not greatly enlarged, which is a point of differentiation from anthrax.

An edematous form of hemorrhagic septicemia may also be peracute. Edema of the throat is a regular part of hemorrhagic septicemia, and in some cases it can be unusually pronounced. It is characterized by extensive swelling of the subcutaneous tissues, especially of the throat, but it may affect the whole head, the tongue, or some other part of the body, such as the brisket or a limb. The swellings are produced by a copious, clotted, straw-colored exudate. The additional lesions in this form of pasteurellosis are those of hemorrhagic septicemia, although death may be caused by asphyxiation.

Pneumonic pasteurellosis refers to forms of pneumonia in which the predominant pulmonary damage is caused by pasteurellae. The most important form is the severe acute fibrinous or fibrinonecrotic pneumonia caused usually by *P. haemolytica* type A1. The pneumonia has a bronchopneumonic pattern or, in its most fulminating form, a lobar pattern. The frequent occurrence of this form of the disease in the period soon after transportation (shipping) and crowding of beef cattle led to the widespread use of the term shipping fever. This term emphasizes the major circumstances under which pneumonic pasteurellosis occurs, but cannot be used with precision as a synonym. Acute fibrinous broncho- or lobar pneumonia can also occur in very young calves, in older calves as an infection superimposed on enzootic pneumonia, and sporadically in cattle of any age. The fibrinous pneumonia is principally the result of rapid and massive proliferation of organisms. Although this is mostly associated with pathogenic strains of *P. haemolytica* in animals whose pulmonary defense has been compromised by various environmental stresses, and often a predisposing viral infection, it can also be caused by *P. multocida.* Occasionally *Haemophilus somnus* causes an indistinguishable lesion. Of the various viruses that have been incriminated as predisposing to the severe pasteurella pneumonia, parainfluenza 3 virus, BHV-1, and bovine respiratory syncytial virus are implicated most often.

The general features of fibrinous lobar pneumonia and bronchopneumonia have been described under those headings. In addition to the extensive reddish-black to grayish-brown cranioventral regions of consolidation with prominent gelatinous thickening of interlobular septa and fibrinous pleuritis, areas of coagulation necrosis are a characteristic feature. At their most prominent, they appear as irregular but sharply demarcated regions with thick white boundaries and sunken, deep red, central zones. Histologically, the necrotic regions are frequently seen to supervene as coagulation necrosis in previously pneumonic tissue. They usually contain very large numbers of bacteria, particularly at the periphery adjacent to the compacted debris of inflammatory cells that form the white boundary zones seen grossly. The cause of the necrosis is not fully determined. Although it has been attributed to thrombosis (infarction), the occurrence of thrombosed vessels is not consistent enough to be a satisfactory explanation, nor would it account for the necrosis sometimes cutting across interlobular septa into neighboring lobules (Fig. 6.63). In view of the massive numbers of bacteria present, it is much more likely that the necrosis is caused by the necrotizing effect of the large amounts of bacterial endotoxins and leukotoxins released locally and by the associated capillary thrombosis. Another characteristic histologic feature is the presence of clustered inflammatory cells with elongated or streaming nuclei (Fig. 6.41C). These are commonly referred to as oat cells. They seem to be an effect of bacterial toxins on leukocytes accumulating within inflamed alveoli. The extent to which they are derived from blood monocytes or neutrophils is not firmly established.

The less fulminating, fibrinous, or fibrinopurulent bronchopneumonias (Fig. 6.64) tend to be more often caused by *P. multocida* than by *P. haemolytica*. The nature of the pneumonia caused by pasteurellae depends on the rate and extent of bacterial proliferation and the amount of toxins released, which in turn depend on the virulence of the strain of organism and the degree to which the defenses of the host are impaired. Although in general *P. haemolytica* more often causes acute fibrinous lobar or bronchopneumonias, and *P. multocida* causes less acute fibrinopurulent bronchopneumonias, this generalization does not hold true in all circumstances, and intermediate lesions (Fig. 6.65) may be found among cases in the same outbreak.

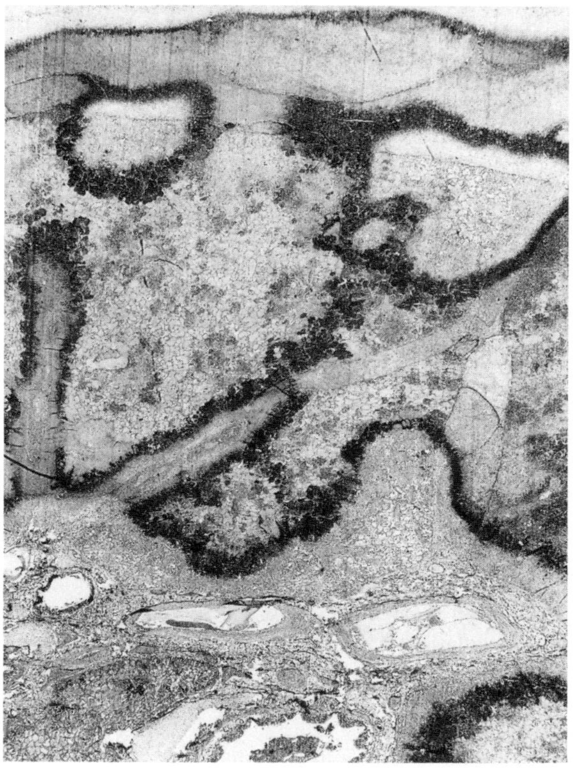

Fig. 6.63 Fibrinonecrotic pneumonia of pneumonic pasteurellosis. Ox. Large areas of pneumonic lung are necrotic and marginated by densely packed leukocytes.

Studies of the pathogenesis of the pneumonia caused by *P. haemolytica* have examined the relative roles of the endotoxins and leukotoxins produced by the bacteria and the various cells and corresponding cytokines and mediator cascades which amplify and are eventually responsible for most of the tissue damage. As far as toxic products of *P. haemolytica* are concerned, the relative importance of endotoxin and leukotoxin is not firmly established, but evidence to date supports the conclusion that, though both are involved, the endotoxin is more important. With regard to the cellular and humoral components involved, alveolar and intravascular macrophages appear to be initially involved, followed by neutrophil and platelet aggregation in alveolar capillaries. From there on, the mediators of inflammation and tissue damage would be those common to other forms of acute lung injury, particularly eicosanoids, TNFα, lysosomal proteases and reactive oxygen species. Macrophage-derived TNFα is probably an important initial component of the cytokine cascade because endotoxin is a potent stimulus for its production and release. Tumor necrosis factor-α enhances neutrophil adherence to capillary endothelium, stimulates neutrophil activity, and has a procoagulant effect, although it is not alone in these respects. The bovine pulmonary response to *P. haemolytica* is noteworthy for the predominance of fibrinous exudate. Alveolar macrophages from affected lungs have greatly increased procoagulant activity and greatly decreased profibrinolytic activity, and this, together with presence of antiplasmin and inhibitor of plasminogen activator in the acute alveolar exudate, could account for the large quantities of fibrin deposited within alveoli.

ii. *Sheep* There are several syndromes in sheep associated with *P. haemolytica* or *P. multocida*. Mastitis in ewes caused by *Pasteurella* spp. is discussed with The Female Genital System (Volume 3, Chapter 4). The principal forms of pasteurellosis in sheep are septicemia caused by *P. haemolytica* and sporadic or enzootic pneumonia, associated more often with *P. haemolytica* than with *P. multocida*.

Septicemia caused by *P. haemolytica*, biotype T, occurs mainly in weaned lambs during the fall months, but it can occur in other age groups and at other times of the year. Deaths, which seldom exceed 5% of the sheep at risk, usually follow within a few days of changes in pasture, feed, or other management practices.

The clinical syndrome is not specific. Signs of illness are vague and the usual course is short, with sudden death reminiscent of clostridial enterotoxemia. At necropsy, petechial and ecchymotic hemorrhages are usually present but sometimes are difficult to detect. They occur in subcutaneous tissues, particularly of the neck and thorax, in

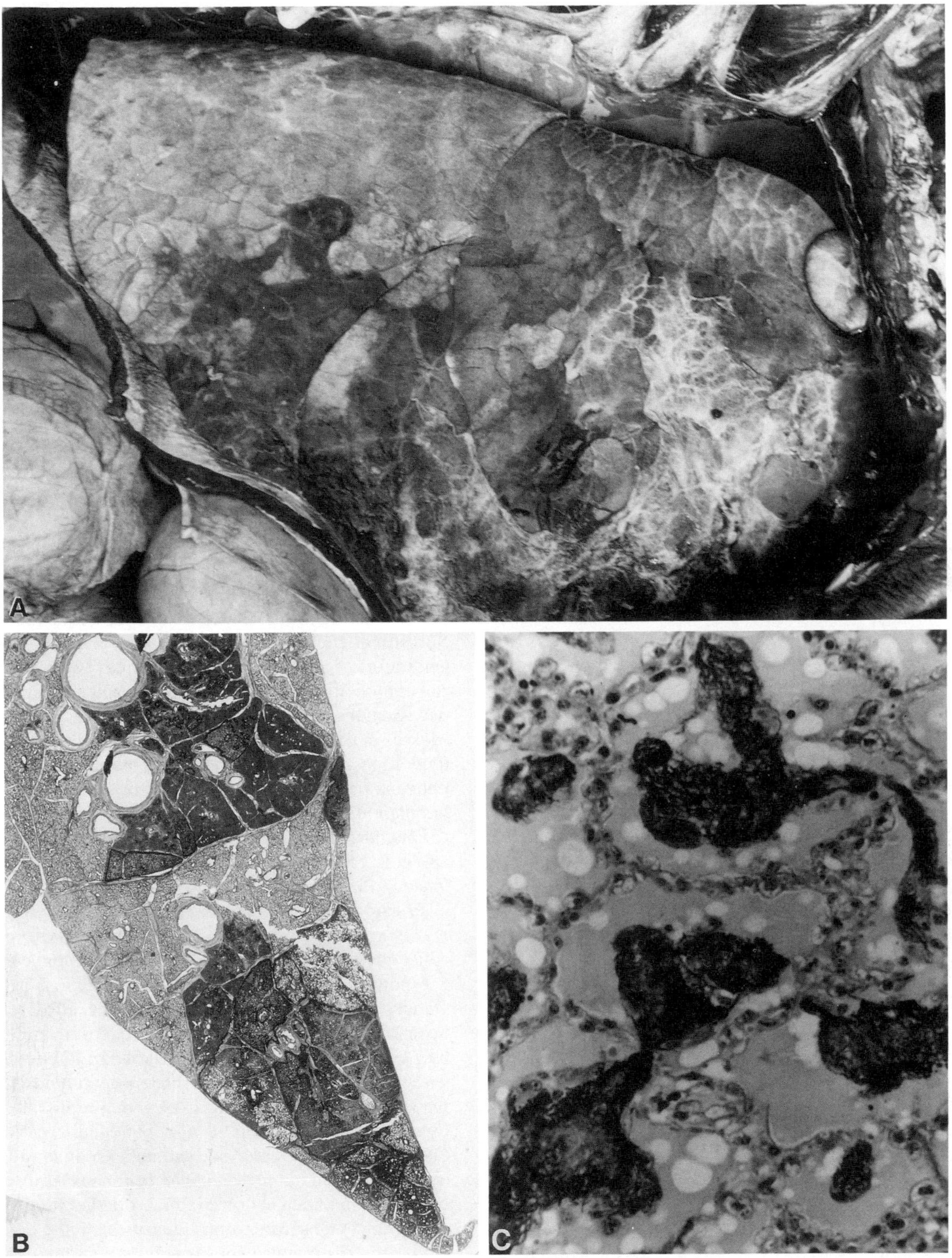

Fig. 6.64 (A) Fibrinous bronchopneumonia and pleuritis of pneumonic pasteurellosis. Ox. (B) Section of middle lobe in pasteurellosis. Ox. Irregular lobular involvement. (C) Intra-alveolar fibrin clumps connecting through pores of Kohn in alveolar septa. Fibrinous pneumonia. Ox.

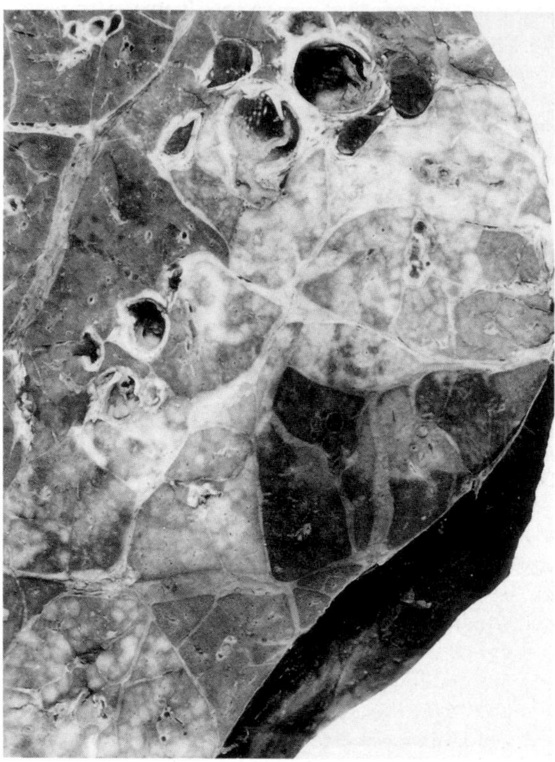

Fig. 6.65 Fibrinonecrotic pneumonia of pneumonic pasteurellosis. Ox. Marbled pattern produced by differing degrees and stages of consolidation.

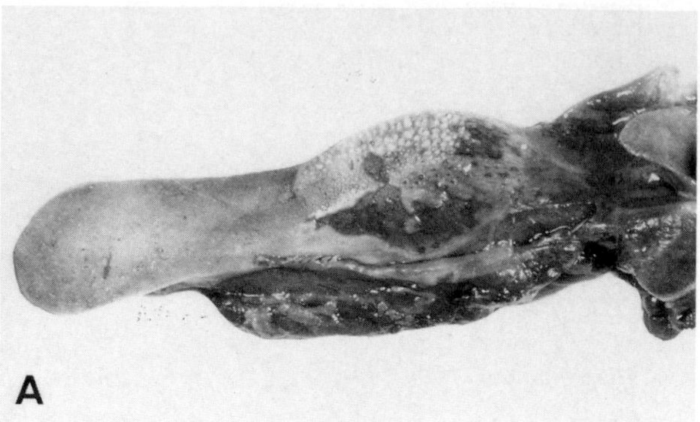

Fig. 6.66A *Pasteurella haemolytica* septicemia. Lamb. Ulceration of tongue.

intermuscular fascia, and in the pleura, epicardium, and mesentery. The lymph nodes are mainly affected in the throat and mesenteric regions, where they are hemorrhagic and edematous. Yellow plaques of necrotizing glossitis occur (Fig. 6.66A); pharyngitis is common, especially around tonsillar crypts; and ulcers may involve the esophageal mucosa (Fig. 6.66B). The abomasal, intestinal, and colonic mucosae sometimes have shallow ulcers (Fig. 6.66C). The lungs have diffuse, severe congestion and edema with abundant white or bloodstained foam in the airways. Discrete hemorrhagic foci (infarcts) can sometimes be seen scattered throughout the lungs. The liver is usually congested, and in some cases, there are many yellowish necrotic foci disseminated through the parenchyma. These are usually of miliary size but can be as large as 1 cm in diameter and surrounded by a narrow red border. Occasionally there is inflammation of joints, pericardium, meninges, and choroid plexus, but the development of these lesions requires that the course be a little longer than usual. These additional lesions are observed more frequently in the experimental disease, which is less fulminating than the natural one.

Microscopic examination of tissues reveals widespread bacterial embolism. The pale hepatic foci consist of colonies of bacteria with a surrounding ischemic zone. There may be thrombosis of the adjacent tributaries of the portal vein and small amounts of parenchymal necrosis, but generally there is little or no leukocytic response. This is probably related to the short course of the disease and partly the effects of bacterial toxin on the leukocytes. The pulmonary lesions are a combination of the effect of multiple bacterial emboli and the severe, diffuse pulmonary congestion and edema found in sheep dying suddenly of almost any cause. In the focal hemorrhagic lesions, masses of bacteria occluding capillaries are accompanied by hemorrhagic and fibrinous exudate into the alveoli. Sometimes there is a peripheral zone of necrosis and degenerating, spindle-shaped leukocytes. Occlusive bacterial emboli are regularly found in the spleen and adrenals, occasionally in the kidney, but are rare in other organs. Masses of bacteria adhere to the surface of the pharyngeal ulcerations and occlude underlying blood vessels and lymphatics. Peripheral and intermediate sinuses of the local lymph nodes also contain large numbers of bacteria within the hemorrhagic and edematous exudate. The principal site of bacterial proliferation and subsequent systemic invasion is believed to be the pharyngeal lesion.

Pneumonic pasteurellosis in sheep is usually caused by *P. haemolytica,* biotype A. The same biotype can also cause septicemia in the absence of pneumonia in lambs <2 months of age. The generalizations regarding circumstances giving rise to pneumonic pasteurellosis in cattle hold true for sheep. Most outbreaks occur in lambs during late spring and early summer. Sudden climatic changes, gathering, and handling are the most commonly recognized predisposing situations. Viral infection, particularly by parainfluenza-3 virus, is also believed to play a role. Other viruses implicated occasionally are respiratory syncytial virus and adenovirus. The lesions tend to be those of acute hemorrhagic or fibrinonecrotic lobar or bronchopneumonia and serofibrinous pleuritis in acute cases (Fig. 6.40), and fibrinopurulent bronchopneumonia leading to abscessation and fibrous pleural adhesions in subacute to chronic cases.

iii. *Swine* Pasteurellosis in swine is caused by *P. multocida*. The most common and important infections by *P. multocida* are usually those complicating mycoplasmal (enzootic) pneumonia and produce a chronic suppurative

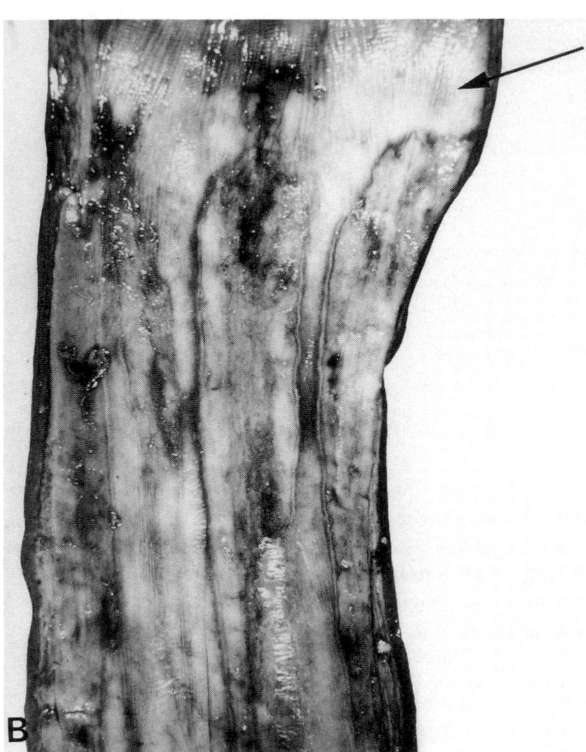

Fig. 6.66B *Pasteurella haemolytica* septicemia. Lamb. Ulceration of esophagus. Only small areas of intact esophageal epithelium remain (arrow).

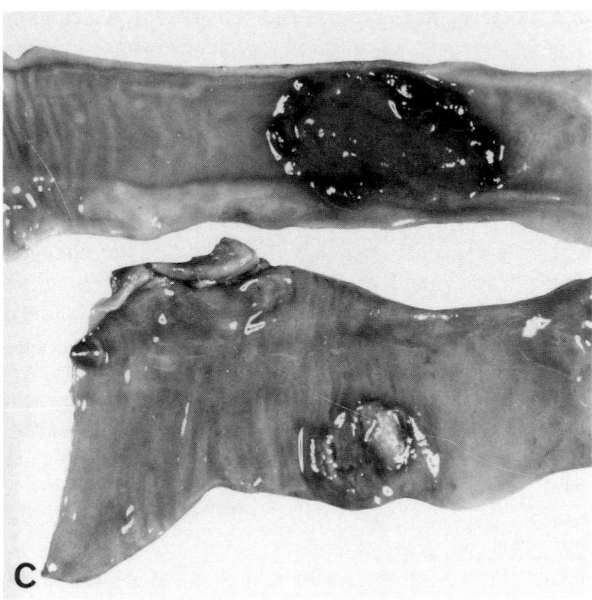

Fig. 6.66C *Pasteurella haemolytica* septicemia. Lamb. Ulceration of intestine.

bronchopneumonia with abscessation. Pleuritis frequently accompanies the pneumonia, and sometimes pericarditis also occurs. Septicemic pasteurellosis due to *P. multocida* is occasionally observed in neonatal pigs, and meningitis can also be present in the same age group. *Pasteurella haemolytica* rarely affects swine but has been recovered from aborted fetuses.

Septicemic disease without localization or distinctive lesions is seen in adult pigs, especially those that are specific pathogen free. The disease in these animals is peracute, and *P. multocida* can be recovered from all organs in large numbers. There is a report from India of a hemorrhagic septicemia type of pasteurellosis in pigs from which was isolated *P. multocida* type B.

Severe, acute, fibrinous pneumonias analogous to the more fulminating *Pasteurella* pneumonias in cattle and sheep are sometimes caused by *P. multocida* in pigs. As in cattle and sheep, stressing factors are usually involved. These are usually poor management and perhaps intercurrent infection by viruses such as swine influenza or hog cholera (swine fever).

The acute fibrinous or fibrinonecrotic pneumonia is similar in many respects to the lesion in cattle. The extensive gelatinous thickening of interlobular and subpleural tissues and the severe serofibrinous pleuritis lead to the term pleuropneumonia being used on occasion. In this connection, although epidemiologic patterns indicate that most severe pneumonias of the pleuropneumonia variety are caused by *Actinobacillus* (*Haemophilus*) *pleuropneumoniae,* there is no absolute separation between the severe pneumonia caused by the two organisms. Massive proliferation of a Gram-negative organism releasing abundant endotoxins and leukotoxins is common to both infections, hence a common pulmonary response.

In addition to the severe thoracic lesions in pneumonic pasteurellosis, there is often acute pharyngitis and inflammatory edema of the throat and yellow jaundicelike discoloration of the carcass of unknown cause. Severe pharyngitis can be necrotizing and ulcerative. A fibrinohemorrhagic polyarthritis may be present, and there is intense congestion of the gastric and intestinal mucosa. Complete recovery from pneumonic pasteurellosis seldom occurs in pigs. Animals which survive the acute disease tend to develop chronic lesions which are usually fatal in due course. In these, most obvious findings are polyarthritis, adhesive pericarditis, and pleuritis, and extensive areas of fibrotic lung, which contain numerous abscesses or fibrous capsules enclosing sequestrae or caseous detritus. As is usual in the fibrinous pneumonias caused by *Pasteurella* spp., the bacterium can often be cultured from the blood and other organs as well as the lung. The septicemic or bacteremic nature of the infection is revealed also by the recovery of the bacterium from aborted fetuses from pregnant sows which survive the acute disease.

The etiologic role of *P. multocida* in atrophic rhinitis of swine is discussed with that disease.

iv. *Other Species* *P. multocida* has been reported in fatal infections in horses, and the latter were included

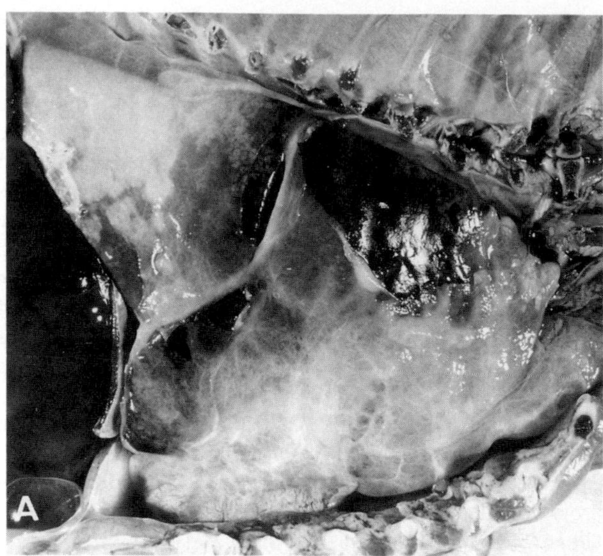

Fig. 6.67A Lung. Goat. Severe, acute pneumonia and pleuritis. *Pasteurella haemolytica.*

in the earliest reports of hemorrhagic septicemia from Europe. Pasteurellae may be found along with other bacteria in the fibrinous pneumonias which complicate infections of the upper respiratory tract in horses.

Pasteurella haemolytica causes sporadic cases and small outbreaks of acute pneumonia and pleuritis in goat kids (Fig. 6.67A). The disease usually occurs in late autumn and winter, and is characterized in an individual animal by a brief period of respiratory distress before death.

At postmortem, a sheet of yellow fibrin is loosely adherent to the pleural surfaces and between the cranial lobes of the lungs. These lobes are voluminous, firm, and dark red, with a transition to less firm tissue with mottled gray-pink discoloration in the caudal lobes. Acute diffuse bronchopneumonia is evident microscopically and is characterized by distended alveolar capillaries, and neutrophils and protein-rich exudate filling bronchioles and alveoli. There is usually little evidence of necrosis. In the caudal lobes, neutrophils fill the bronchioles and extend into the alveoli. Numerous bacteria are present in cranial lobes. It is not known whether a specific serotype of *P. haemolytica* is involved in this disease.

Pasteurella spp. are common inhabitants of the oral cavity of cats and dogs and are important as infections in bite wounds. Pulmonary infections with pasteurellae are uncommon in dogs and when present are usually found with other bacteria as complications of canine distemper and aspiration pneumonia. *Pasteurella multocida* causes meningitis and otitis media in cats. It is also commonly associated with pyothorax, often together with other bacteria, and probably results in many instances from penetration of the pleural cavity by a foreign body.

Bibliography

Bain, R. V. S. "Hemorrhagic Septicemia." Rome, Food and Agriculture Organization of the United Nations, 1963.

Biberstein, E. L., and Gills, M. G. The relation of antigenic types to the A and T types of *Pasteurella haemolytica. J Comp Pathol* **72:** 316–320, 1962.

Biberstein, E. L., and Kennedy, P. C. Septicemic pasteurellosis in lambs. *Am J Vet Res* **20:** 94–101, 1959.

Biberstein, E. L., and Thompson, D. A. Epidemiological studies on *Pasteurella haemolytica* in sheep. *J Comp Pathol* **76:** 83–94, 1966.

Breider, M. A. *et al.* Pulmonary lesions induced by *Pasteurella haemolytica* in neutrophil-sufficient and neutrophil-deficient calves. *Can J Vet Res* **52:** 205–209, 1988.

Carr, B. D. *et al.* The role of leukocytes in the pathogenesis of fibrin deposition in bovine acute lung injury. *Am J Pathol* **138:** 1191–1198, 1991.

Carter, G. R. A new serological type of *Pasteurella multocida* from central Africa. *Vet Rec* **73:** 1052, 1961.

Davies, D. H. *et al.* The pathogenesis of sequential infection with parainfluenza virus type 3 and and *Pasteurella haemolytica* in sheep. *Vet Microbiol* **6:** 173–182, 1981.

Davies, D. H., Herceg, M., and Thurley, D. C. Experimental infection of lambs with an adenovirus followed by *Pasteurella haemolytica. Vet Microbiol* **7:** 369–381, 1982.

Edwards, B. L. A note on haemorrhagic septicaemia in neonatal pigs. *Vet Rec* **71:** 208, 1959.

Friend, S. C., Thomson, R. G., and Wilkie, B. N. Pulmonary lesions induced by *Pasteurella hemolytica* in cattle. *Can J Comp Med* **41:** 219–223, 1977.

Gilmour, N. J. L. *Pasteurella haemolytica* infections in sheep. *Vet Q* **2:** 191–198, 1980.

Gourlay, R. N., Thomas, L. J., and Wyld, S. G. Experimental *Pasteurella multocida* pneumonia in calves. *Res Vet Sci* **47:** 185–189, 1989.

Haritani, M. *et al.* Immunoperoxidase evaluation of the relationship between necrotic lesions and causative bacteria in lungs of calves with naturally acquired pneumonia. *Am J Vet Res* **51:** 1975–1979, 1990.

Henning, M. W., and Brown, M. H. V. Pasteurellosis. An outbreak amongst sheep. *Onderstepoort J Vet Sci* **7:** 113–131, 1936.

Herceg, M., Thurley, D. C., and Davies, D. H. Oat cells in the pathology of ovine pneumonia-pleurisy. *N Z Vet J* **30:** 170–173, 1982.

Jericho, K. W. F. Histological changes in the respiratory tract of calves exposed to aerosols of bovine herpesvirus 1 and *Pasteurella haemolytica. J Comp Pathol* **93:** 73–82, 1983.

Jericho, K. W. F., Darcel, C. le Q., and Langford, E. V. Respiratory disease in calves produced with aerosols of parainfluenza-3 virus and *Pasteurella haemolytica. Can J Comp Med* **46:** 293–301, 1982.

Kielstein, P., Martin, J., and Janetschke, P. Experimentelle *Pasteurella multocida* Infektionen beim Schwein als ein Beitrag zur Atiologie der enzootischen Pneumonie des Schweines. *Arch Exp Vet Med* **31:** 609–619, 1977.

Lopez, A., Thomson, R. G., and Savan, M. The pulmonary clearance of *Pasteurella hemolytica* in calves infected with bovine parainfluenza-3 virus. *Can J Comp Med* **40:** 385–391, 1976.

Murty, D. K., and Kaushik, R. K. Studies on outbreak of acute swine pasteurellosis due to *Pasteurella multocida* type B (Carter, 1955). *Vet Rec* **77:** 411–416, 1965.

Namioka, S., Murata, M., and Bain, R. V. S. Serological studies on *Pasteurella multocida.* V. Some epizootiological findings resulting from O antigenic analysis. *Cornell Vet* **54:** 520–534, 1964.

Pijoan, C., and Ochoa, G. Interaction between a hog cholera vaccine strain and *Pasteurella multocida* in the production of porcine pneumonia. *J Comp Pathol* **88:** 167–170, 1978.

Rehmtulla, A. J., and Thomson, R. G. A review of the lesions of shipping fever of cattle. *Can Vet J* **22:** 1–8, 1981.

Rushton, B. *et al.* Pathology of an experimental infection of specific pathogen-free lambs with parainfluenza virus type 3 and *Pasteurella haemolytica*. *J Comp Pathol* **89:** 321–329, 1979.

Sharma, R., and Woldehiwet, Z. Increased susceptibility to *Pasteurella haemolytica* in lambs infected with bovine respiratory syncytial virus. *J Comp Pathol* **103:** 411–420, 1990.

Slocombe, R. F., Derksen, F. J., and Robinson, N. E. Comparison of pathophysiologic changes in the lungs of calves challenge exposed with *Escherichia coli*-derived endotoxin and *Pasteurella haemolytica,* alone or in combination. *Am J Vet Res* **50:** 701–707, 1989.

Slocombe, R. F. *et al.* Effect of *Pasteurella haemolytica*-derived endotoxin on pulmonary structure and function in calves. *Am J Vet Res* **51:** 433–438, 1990.

Smith, G. R. The pathogenicity of *Pasteurella haemolytica* for young lambs. *J Comp Pathol* **70:** 326–338, 1960.

Smith, G. R. The characteristics of two types of *Pasteurella haemolytica* associated with different pathological conditions in sheep. *J Pathol Bacteriol* **81:** 431–440, 1961.

Smith, G. R. Production of pneumonia in adult sheep with cultures of *Pasteurella haemolytica* type A. *J Comp Pathol* **74:** 241–249, 1964.

Smith, G. R. The pathogenicity of *Pasteurella multocida* in the production of porcine pneumonia. *J Comp Pathol* **88:** 167–170, 1978.

Thomas, L. H. *et al.* Evidence that blood-borne infection is involved in the pathogenesis of bovine pneumonic pasteurellosis. *Vet Pathol* **26:** 253–259, 1989.

Van den Ingh, T. S. G. A. M. *et al.* Pulmonary lesions induced by a *Pasteurella haemolytica* cytotoxin preparation in calves. *J Vet Med B* **37:** 297–308, 1990.

Whiteley, L. O. *et al.* Morphological and morphometrical analysis of the acute response of the bovine alveolar wall to *Pasteurella haemolytica* A1-derived endotoxin and leucotoxin. *J Comp Pathol* **104:** 23–32, 1991.

Wilkie, I. W. *et al.* The effect of *Pasteurella haemolytica* and the leukotoxin of *Pasteurella haemolytica* on bovine lung explants. *Can J Vet Res* **54:** 151–156, 1990.

Yates, W. D. G. A review of infectious bovine rhinotracheitis, shipping fever pneumonia, and viral–bacterial synergism in respiratory disease of cattle. *Can J Comp Med* **46:** 225–263, 1982.

b. *Haemophilus* AND *Haemophilus*-LIKE INFECTIONS The most important is porcine contagious pleuropneumonia, which is caused by *Actinobacillus* (*Haemophilus*) *pleuropneumoniae*. This disease has increased dramatically in major swine-raising areas of the world during recent years. The characteristic lesion is a severe fibrinonecrotic and hemorrhagic pneumonia with accompanying fibrinous pleuritis, hence the designation pleuropneumonia. *Actinobacillus pleuropneumoniae* is highly pathogenic and often appears capable of invading and rapidly proliferating within the lung in the absence of obvious predisposing factors. All aspects of pathogenesis of field outbreaks of the disease, however, are not understood.

There are twelve known antigenic varieties of *A. pleuropneumonia* based on capsular antigens, and protective immunization is serotype specific. There appear to be geographic differences in the distribution of serotypes and also differences in virulence between and within serotypes. The dynamics of the disease in infected herds are influenced by passive immunity in the young, which will persist for 8–12 weeks after peaking at ~4 weeks. Active infections in chronically infected herds, and seroconversion, begin in the period in which passive immunity is declining. Peak mortality occurs in the period from 10 to 16 weeks of age.

Factors in the bacterial virulence are not clear. The organism adheres poorly to tracheobronchial mucosa but adheres well to pulmonary tissue, which it must reach in droplet nuclei in inhaled air. The ability to adhere appears not to be related to serotype. The organism produces a hemolysin and a potent heat-labile cytotoxin with activity against endothelial cells and pulmonary alveolar macrophages. The local pathogenesis of the lesion will depend on complex interactions involving an activated coagulation system, direct cytotoxicity, early chemotaxis of neutrophils, and release by them of injurious hydrolases and free radicals, and impairment of macrophage clearing.

Contagious pleuropneumonia can affect pigs of any age but is more common from ~6 weeks to 6 months of age. The severe form of the disease occurs mostly in later stages of fattening and can cause a mortality in the 20–80% range. Peracute, acute, and subacute to chronic forms are recognized, the latter representing residual lesions of the acute disease. Deaths in the peracute and acute forms occur suddenly or after a short period of depression, fever, and possibly hemorrhage from nose and mouth. The main gross lesions are bloody nasal discharge, bloodstained foam in trachea and bronchi, and large regions of hemorrhagic or fibrinonecrotic pneumonia accompanied by fibrinous pleuritis. Since the tissue damage is caused by massive bacterial proliferation and release of toxins, the essential features are similar to those already described for fulminating pneumonic pasteurellosis in cattle, but vasculitis is an additional important feature. There is less tendency for the pneumonic foci caused by *A. pleuropneumoniae* to be limited to the cranioventral lung regions, however, presumably because of the greater virulence of the organism and the influence of vasculitis. Irregular, well-circumscribed regions of hemorrhagic consolidation or necrosis are commonly found in more dorsocaudal regions, especially surrounding major bronchi near the hilus of the lung (Fig. 6.67B). The foci of consolidation are also particularly prone to undergo sequestration, with the result that in subacute cases, there may be large foci of caseous or cavitating yellow-gray or tan necrotic debris surrounded by fibroblastic zones. Many of these can subsequently become abscesses through secondary contamination by *Actinomyces pyogenes, P. multocida, B. bronchiseptica,* Gram-negative enteric organisms, strep-

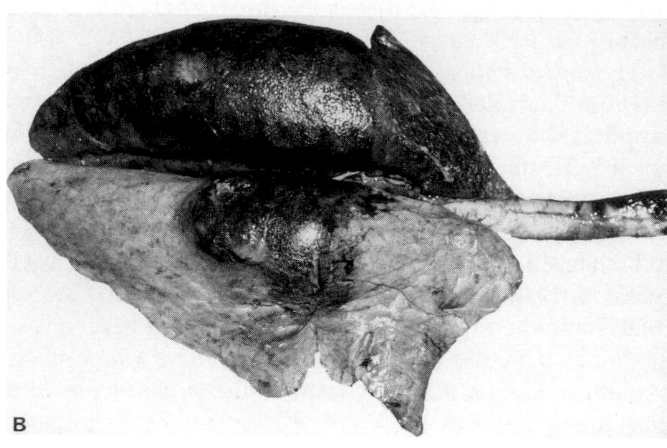

Fig. 6.67B Porcine contagious pleuropneumonia (*H. pleuropneumoniae*). Hemorrhagic consolidation and necrosis in dorsal and hilar regions with fibrinous pleuritis (Courtesy of B. W. Fenwick.)

tococci, or others. The end result can be a severely scarred, abscessed lung which is tightly bound to the thoracic wall by fibrous adhesions.

Extrapulmonary vascular lesions sometimes occur in acutely affected pigs, particularly in the kidneys. Hyaline thrombosis and fibrinoid necrosis of glomerular capillaries, afferent arterioles, and interlobular arteries indicate the probable effect of severe endotoxemia.

Other *Haemophilus* spp. can cause lung lesions. *Haemophilus parasuis* has been referred to as a synergistic infection with swine influenza. It causes a nonspecific suppurative bronchopneumonia. For its involvement in polyserositis and arthritis of swine, see Bones and Joints (Volume 1, Chapter 1). *Haemophilus somnus* is discussed with Diseases of the Nervous System (Volume 1, Chapter 3). It occasionally produces a lesion indistinguishable from the fibrinous lobar pneumonia of pneumonic pasteurellosis. More common descriptions of pneumonia associated with *H. somnus* in calves are of a subacute to chronic, fibrinopurulent, or purulent bronchopneumonia in which bronchiolar epithelial necrosis and bronchiolitis fibrosa obliterans are frequent features. Although *H. somnus* has been shown to be capable of causing some degree of bronchiolitis fibrosa obliterans experimentally, the obvious presence of this lesion in naturally occurring pneumonias should arouse the strong suspicion of a previous viral infection, such as by bovine respiratory syncytial virus. Vasculitis can also be found in pneumonia caused by *H. somnus,* but it is mostly a feature accompanying acute septicemic episodes or in acute experimental lesions resulting from endobronchial inoculation of the organism.

Bibliography

Andrews, J. J. *et al.* Microscopic lesions associated with the isolation of *Haemophilus somnus* from pneumonic bovine lungs. *Vet Pathol* **22:** 131–136, 1985.

Gogolewski, R. P. *et al.* Experimental *Haemophilus somnus* pneumonia in calves and immunoperoxidase localization of bacteria. *Vet Pathol* **24:** 250–256, 1987.

Gogolewski, R. P. *et al.* Pulmonary persistence of *Haemophilus somnus* in the presence of specific antibody. *J Clin Microbiol* **27:** 1767–1774, 1989.

Hani, H. *et al.* Zur *Haemophilus*-Pleuropneumonie beim Schwein. VI. Pathogenese. *Schweiz Arch Tierheilkd* **115:** 205–212, 1973.

Jackson, J. A., Andrews, J. J., and Hargis, J. W. Experimental *Haemophilus somnus* pneumonia in calves. *Vet Pathol* **24:** 129–134, 1987.

Liggett, A. D., and Harrison, L. R. Sequential study of lesion development in experimental *Haemophilus* pleuropneumonia. *Res Vet Sci* **423:** 204–221, 1987.

Martin, J. *et al.* Beitrag zur experimentellen *Haemophilus* Infektion (*Haemophilus parahaemolyticus, Haemophilus parasuis*) bei SPF-Ferkeln. 2. Mitteilung: vergleichende Pathologie und Histologie. *Arch Exp Vet Med* **31:** 347–357, 1977.

Nordstoga, K., and Fjolstad, M. The generalized Shwartzman reaction and *Haemophilus* infections in pigs. *Pathol Vet* **4:** 245–253, 1967.

Pattison, I. H., Howell, D. G., and Elliott, J. A *Haemophilus*-like organism isolated from pig lung and the associated pneumonic lesions. *J Comp Pathol* **67:** 320–330, 1957.

Potgieter, L. N. D. *et al.* Experimental bovine respiratory tract disease with *Haemophilus somnus*. *Vet Pathol* **25:** 124–130, 1988.

Shope, R. E. Porcine contagious pleuropneumonia. *J Exp Med* **119:** 357–375, 1964.

Watt, J. A. A. The isolation and cultural characteristics of an organism of the *Haemophilus* group in calf pneumonia. *J Comp Pathol* **62:** 102–107, 1952.

White, D. C. *et al.* Porcine contagious pleuropneumonia. *J Exp Med* **120:** 1–12, 1964.

c. BORDETELLOSIS *Bordetella bronchiseptica* is an obligate parasite of the upper respiratory tract of rodents, dogs, and pigs, and can occasionally be found in various other species. In dogs, it is involved in the causation of kennel cough and chronic bronchitis, as discussed previously. It is also frequently associated with the development of suppurative bronchopneumonia in dogs with interstitial pneumonia caused by the distemper virus. *Bordetella bronchiseptica* can also cause secondary bronchopneumonia in association with other diseases leading to reduced pulmonary defenses.

In swine, the role of *B. bronchiseptica* in the production of atrophic rhinitis has been dealt with under that heading. As a pulmonary pathogen, *B. bronchiseptica* is most important as the occasional cause of septicemia or severe bronchopneumonia in suckling pigs usually <3 weeks of age. Mortality can be high in these outbreaks. The bronchopneumonia is predominantly suppurative, affecting individual lobules or small groups of lobules in a scattered rather than confluent pattern, although mainly present in apical and cardiac lobes. Typically, it is associated with acute bronchitis and rapid onset of fibrosis, which is most evident in peribronchiolar sites. Fibrosis may extend to other interstitial regions when the amount of inflammation and exudation is severe. *Bordetella bronchiseptica* may also be a cause of suppurative bronchopneumonia in older pigs, mostly as a complication of mycoplasmal pneumonia in fattening animals.

Bordetella bronchiseptica has also been recorded as an occasional cause of suppurative bronchopneumonia in cats and foals.

Bordetella parapertussis has been implicated as one of the bacterial agents involved in the production of enzootic pneumonia in sheep, but its importance relative to other agents is not established.

Bibliography

Bemis, D. A., Greisen, H. A., and Appel, M. J. G. Pathogenesis of canine bordetellosis. *J Infect Dis* **135:** 753–762, 1977.

Duncan, J. R., Ramsey, F. K., and Switzer, W. P. Pathology of experimental *Bordetella bronchiseptica* infection in swine: Pneumonia. *Am J Vet Res* **27:** 467–472, 1966.

Dunne, H. W., Kradel, D. C., and Dotz, R. B. *Bordetella bronchiseptica* (*Brucella bronchiseptica*) in pneumonia in young pigs. *J Am Vet Med Assoc* **139:** 897–899, 1961.

Goodnow, R. D. Biology of *Bordetella bronchiseptica. Microbiol Rev* **44:** 722–738, 1980.

Koehne, G. W. *et al.* An outbreak of *Bordetella bronchiseptica* respiratory disease in foals. *Vet Med Small Anim Clin* **76:** 507–511, 1981.

L'Ecuyer, C., Roberts, E. D., and Switzer, W. P. An outbreak of *Bordetella bronchiseptica* pneumonia in swine. *Vet Med* **56:** 420–424, 1961.

Snyder, S. B. *et al.* Respiratory tract disease associated with *Bordetella bronchiseptica* infection in cats. *J Am Vet Med Assoc* **163:** 293–294, 1973.

d. TUBERCULOSIS Tuberculosis is typically a chronic infectious disease caused by bacteria of the genus *Mycobacterium*. Various forms of the disease have many features in common, but the exact pattern differs according to the species of *Mycobacterium* involved and the species of animal affected.

Tuberculosis is an ancient disease and is still widespread in some parts of the world. In many areas, however, the incidence of classic tuberculosis in humans and animals has been reduced to the point where mycobacterial disease is more often caused by atypical (nonmammalian) acid-fast bacilli. Infection and disease caused by these atypical mycobacteria are probably more widely recognized because they are no longer overshadowed by the classic disease and have been revealed for more detailed investigation. Changing environments and a susceptible population no longer provided with the cross-protection afforded by infection with the classic mycobacteria probably also play some role. The emergence of a wide range of mycobacteria as agents capable of causing disease has resulted in both diagnostic and taxonomic confusion. This is compounded by the large number of saprophytic mycobacteria now recognized and the lack of clear-cut separation between saprophytic and potentially pathogenic species. Assessment of the etiologic role of a mycobacterium isolated or identified in a particular case therefore needs to be made on the basis of specific evidence available for that case rather than on the basis of generalizations.

Mycobacteria are widely distributed in nature. Many are saprophytes, and some of these are opportunistic pathogens. Others, as far as is known, are strictly parasitic. Some of the pathogenic types cannot be cultivated *in vitro*, and those that can be cultivated generally grow slowly. For these reasons, taxonomic classification has been difficult. Currently, a variety of cultural and biological characteristics including serotyping, lipoprotein analyses, and phage typing are used in numerical classification schemes. More than 100 properties of new isolates can be subjected to computer analysis. A high degree of matching (>80% of characteristics) is used to group organisms together as the same species. Mycobacterial classification is still incomplete, however, so in the meantime, the following categorization puts the organisms into useful perspective. The listing is incomplete, and not all are of known veterinary significance.

The classical tubercle bacilli are *Mycobacterium tuberculosis* (human), *M. bovis* (bovine), and *M. avium* (avian). *Mycobacterium tuberculosis* and *M. bovis* are the principal, closely related mammalian pathogens. Two other closely related species are *M. microti* from voles and *M. africanum*. Differing strains of *M. avium* are now commonly included with strains of the very closely related *M. intracellulare* as the *M. avium–intracellulare* complex. To avoid confusion surrounding the term **tuberculosis,** convention limits it to diseases caused by *M. tuberculosis* or *M. bovis*. Other conditions are referred to as **mycobacteriosis,** qualified with the specific agent where known (e.g., avian mycobacteriosis when caused by *M. avium*). Atypical mycobacteriosis is sometimes used as a general term to cover all the diseases other than those caused by *M. tuberculosis* and *M. bovis*. In most veterinary literature, however, disease caused by *M. avium* is still included as one of the classic forms of tuberculosis, and this usage will be continued in this chapter.

Mycobacteria which can have an independent saprophytic existence in nature are widespread in soil and water, on vegetation, and in mucous membranes of the oropharynx. There are a large number of species whose taxonomic status is not fully established. When these organisms cause disease, it is usually in immunologically compromised hosts, and the manifestations are either cervical lymphadenitis, pulmonary lesions similar to tuberculosis, or cutaneous lesions associated with local penetration of organisms through wounds or abrasions of the skin. An example is *M. marinum,* which is abundant in pools in regions with temperate climates and causes tuberculous disease in fish and cutaneous ulcers in humans. This organism is grouped with the photochromogens (Runyon's group I) together with *M. kansasii*. The latter produces cervical lymphadenitis and pulmonary disease in humans, and has been isolated from cow's milk and from cattle in the United States and the Republic of South Africa. Scotochromogens produce pigment without photoactivation (Runyon's group II) and include *M. scrofulaceum,* which is closely related to the *M. avium–intracellulare* complex. These organisms have been isolated from disease in cattle and tuberculous-type lesions in dogs. Another member of the group, *M. aquae*, has been isolated from nodular lesions on the teats of cows. Nonphotochromogens (Runyon's group III) have organisms in the *M. avium–intracellulare* complex as the most important members. Organisms belonging to this complex have been isolated from tuberculin-sensitive cattle and pigs, and their pathogenicity has been assessed experimentally in calves and pigs. Some strains are virtually nonpathogenic, and others produce generalized disease.

Mycobacteria of group IV are rapid growers at room temperature, usually nonpigmented, and include many saprophytes. Within this group, *M. smegmatis* is one of the organisms isolated from tuberclelike lesions in lymph nodes of swine, and it has also been associated with development of bovine mastitis following its injection into the udder in oily infusions of penicillin. Another member, *M. fortuitum*, was initially isolated from lesions in bovine lymph nodes and is an occasional cause of mastitis in cattle. Members of this group, particularly *M. fortuitum*, *M. chelonei*, and *M. phlei* are the usual causes of cutaneous mycobacteriosis in cats and dogs. Further discussion of cutaneous lesions caused by mycobacteria, including those associated with *M. lepraemurium*, will be found in bacterial diseases of the skin (Volume 1, Chapter 5).

Other important distinct species of mycobacteria are *M. leprae* of human leprosy, *M. lepraemurium* (rat leprosy), and *M. paratuberculosis* (*johnei*). The last named causes Johne's disease in ruminants (see The Alimentary System, Chapter 1 of this volume).

It will be evident that the pathogenic mycobacteria present a wide range of specializations, from saprophytes to the extremes of parasitism represented by *M. leprae* and from a wide host range to infectivity for only specific hosts. As parasites, they are principally intracellular. They are mostly within macrophages in an association which does not necessarily cause their death or the death of the host cell. The lesions produced tend to be similar and of granulomatous type characterized by collections of macrophages, epithelioid cells, and giant cells. Additional components of inflammation and necrosis depend on the degree of cell-mediated response of the host against living bacilli with the corresponding production of cytokines and other inflammatory mediators. The phenomena of chronicity and latency are common to the mycobacterial infections. Both are related to the resistance of the organisms to phagocytic killing, to the slow growth of the organisms, and to the complex interactions between the organisms and the cellular immune system of the host.

The three main species of tubercle bacilli, *M. tuberculosis*, *M. bovis*, and *M. avium*, occur most frequently in their respective hosts, but cross-infections do occur, and various other species of animals are affected. Under natural conditions, *M. bovis* causes disease chiefly in cattle, humans, swine, and occasionally in horses, dogs, cats, and sheep; *M. avium* causes disease chiefly in birds and occasionally is found in cattle, swine, horses, sheep, and captive monkeys; *M. tuberculosis* is chiefly responsible for tuberculosis in humans, and occasionally infects pigs, captive monkeys, dogs, cats, cattle, and psittacine birds. The expression of tuberculosis in the various hosts usually differs somewhat according to the type of bacillus involved, as well as to other factors. Although the human and bovine bacilli can produce disease in a wide range of species under conditions of special exposure, they are each naturally maintained in only one species, the human bacillus in humans and the bovine in cattle. Thus, in the absence of infection from cattle, the bovine type disappears from the human and porcine populations. The situation with the *M. avium–intracellulare* complex is not so clear because of saprophyte members.

In addition to the hosts just mentioned, others of almost unlimited variety can be infected experimentally with one or more species of the tubercle bacilli. The differential pathogenicity of the organisms for guinea pigs, rabbits, and fowls was the original basis of the biological classification of organisms as to type in diagnostic laboratories. Fowls are highly susceptible to the avian types, but highly resistant to the mammalian types. The avian type will, with the usual test doses, produce progressive infection in rabbits, but only localized lesions in guinea pigs. For the differentiation of mammalian strains, the rabbit is usually used. In rabbits, the bovine bacillus, in the standard dose for the test, produces progressive infection which is fatal in 3 months; the human type does not kill rabbits although isolated tubercles can be found in various organs. The guinea pig is highly susceptible to both mammalian types and therefore useful for isolating the organisms.

The mycobacteria are nonmotile, non-spore–forming pleomorphic coccobacilli. They are Gram-positive but almost unstainable by the simpler bacterial stains because of their high content of lipids. They are routinely stained with hot carbol dyes, usually carbolfuchsin, and then resist decoloration by inorganic acids. This property of acid-fastness, or acid–alcohol fastness, of the stained bacilli depends on the amount and spatial arrangement of mycolic acids and their esters in the bacterial wall. Sometimes, in cultures or in old lesions, the organisms have a beaded or granulated appearance. This beading is partly caused by the presence of lipid droplets within the bacteria and is an indication of an unfavorable environment for organisms in the postexponential growth phase. Staining of the bacilli can be facilitated by incorporating a surface-active wetting agent, such as Tween 80, in the dyes. They are also demonstrable by fluorescence microscopy when stained by a fluorescent dye such as auramine.

Much attention has been given to the chemical composition of the mycobacteria, particularly the cell walls, in the interests of clarifying the pathogenesis of the lesions, perfecting diagnostic techniques, and developing vaccines. The chemical composition of the cell wall is dominated by complex lipids, which include glycolipids, peptidoglycolipids, lipopolysaccharides, lipoproteins, and waxes. The mycolic acids, on which acid-fastness depends, are among them. The precise role of the various lipids in contributing to the virulence and immunogenicity of the organisms is still unclear. The waxes, which are themselves composed of various proportions of lipids, glycolipids, and peptidoglycolipids depending on the species of mycobacterium, are important in the initial foreign-body type of macrophage response. Waxes, together with peptidoglycan (muramyl dipeptide) and various glycolipids, are responsible for most of the adjuvant activity of mycobacteria. Attraction of antigen-processing cells (macrophages) and presentation of antigen in appropriate surface configuration are major attributes of adjuvant activity. Increased glycolipid content of mycobacterial cell walls is associated with increased virulence. A close parallel is with the amount of cord factor (trehalose dimycolate). This correlates with the fact that in general the more acid-fast strains are more virulent. Other glycolipids (mycosides) appear to form a barrier against lysosomal digestion and partly explain the ability of the organisms to survive after phagocytosis by macrophages. Intracellular survival is also facilitated by the bacteria preventing fusion of phagosomes and lysosomes, possibly by secretion of cyclic adenosine monophosphate (AMP). The differing effectiveness of such mechanisms determines the relative ability of various mycobacteria to resist intracellular degradation.

Tuberculoproteins are the other major category of immunoreactive substances in mycobacteria. They provide most of the antigenic determinants, but in order for an animal to produce an immunologic response to these determinants, the adjuvant activity of the lipids and polysaccharides in the mycobacterial cell wall is needed. Purified protein derivatives from mycobacteria are capable of eliciting the delayed-type hypersensitivity once the animal is sensitized, however, and this is the basis of tuberculin testing. Both tuberculoproteins and the adjuvant lipids are present in infection, and the result is the development of both humoral and cell-mediated immune responses. The humoral antibodies can be demonstrated by serologic techniques but do not participate in pathogenesis of the characteristic lesions or in the production of immunity. Cell-mediated responses are responsible for both aspects of the disease.

Cell-mediated immunity and delayed-type hypersensitivity are expressions of immune responses mediated by lymphocytes, mostly T cells. Both manifestations usually develop simultaneously. They do not have identical mechanisms, however, because sometimes one is present without the other, and there is no quantitative relationship between them when both are present. The dissociation between the two types of responses appears likely to be explained on the basis of involvement by different subpopulations of T cells and corresponding sets of cytokines.

Cell-mediated immunity is effected by the enhanced ability of activated macrophages to phagocytose and kill bacilli. Macrophages are activated by cytokines secreted by specifically sensitized T lymphocytes, which respond to processed antigens released by previously infected macrophages. Most activated macrophages are derived from blood monocytes. Immunity to tuberculosis therefore is principally determined by the ability of macrophages to inhibit the growth of intracellular bacilli. Both innate (genetic) and acquired resistance are involved. Macrophages, for unexplained reasons, can also respond differently in organs such as the liver and kidney in the same animal. Since the balance between the virulence of the myobacteria and the ability of macrophages to kill them is often a precarious one, any compromise of the host's immune system is prone to precipitate or exacerbate the disease. This is revealed by the frequent clinical association of tuberculosis with immunosuppression caused by diseases, drugs, hormones, or malnutrition.

Delayed-type hypersensitivity is also mediated by cytokines released mainly from sensitized T cells in response to antigenic materials from the tubercle bacilli. The cytokines cause further accumulation of macrophages and lymphocytes. Release of cytotoxic factors and hydrolytic enzymes from macrophages is principally responsible for the caseation necrosis characteristic of many tuberculous lesions.

Functionally heterogeneous populations of lymphocytes and macrophages are present in tuberculous lesions. Relative numbers of the various subpopulations of these cells partly determine whether activation of macrophages and inhibition of bacterial growth (cell-mediated immunity) or a severe delayed-type hypersensitivity response is the dominant feature.

The importance of hypersensitivity in the pathogenesis of lesions of tuberculosis was first demonstrated by Koch in what is now known as the Koch phenomenon. If a normal guinea pig is inoculated subcutaneously with a culture of tubercle bacilli, generalization of the infection causes death in 2–3 months. At the site of inoculation, a hard nodule or tubercle develops in 10–14 days. This nodule soon breaks down to form an ulcer, which persists until the animal dies. If, however, the inoculation is made into a tuberculous guinea pig, the events are quite different. An acute response characterized by exudation and necrosis develops at the site of inoculation. The necrotic tissue soon sloughs, the lesion heals permanently and quickly, and the infection is not disseminated from it, even to the regional lymph node. The injected organisms which provoke the hypersensitivity reaction in the skin are fairly rapidly destroyed, but those in the primary lesions of the disease are not destroyed, and their persistence and proliferation may eventually kill the animal. Whether the hypersensitivity reaction is beneficial or harmful to the host depends on the circumstances. In common with most complex inflammatory conditions, there is a balance between inhibitory and amplifying factors. On the one hand, hypersensitivity to relatively small numbers of bacilli causes accelerated tubercle formation which enhances the killing of the organisms, and helps prevent reinfection or dissemination from the initial site of infection. On the other hand, the hypersensitivity response to large amounts of mycobacterial antigen causes extensive cell necrosis and tissue destruction, which is seriously detrimental. Liquefaction, which is brought about by hydrolytic enzymes of macrophages and possibly neutrophils, is the most harmful response. The bacilli multiply extracellularly in the liquefied material and are available in large numbers for dissemination through cavities, vessels, and airways. In summary, the final determinants of the nature and intensity of lesions are the mass of bacterial antigen presented to specifically reactive lymphocytes and the modifying influences of the structure of the tissue involved.

The lesions of tuberculosis are the prototype of granulomatous inflammation. The tuberculous granuloma (tubercle) is mainly cellular, and its development is frequently designated productive or proliferative in contrast to the more exudative type of lesion it occasionally causes.

When tubercle bacilli are initially implanted in tissue, they behave as relatively bland lipid-rich foreign particles would be expected to do and incite a foreign-body macrophage response. Bacilli are phagocytosed by macrophages, and if the resistance of the macrophages is adequate, the bacilli are eventually killed. If the balance tips the other way, however, the bacilli proliferate and are released from killed macrophages together with antigenic materials which sensitize attracted T lymphocytes. By the tenth day or so after exposure, by which time hypersensitivity is developing, many bacilli are present, and the tempo of events begins to quicken. Cytokines secreted by the sensitized T lymphocytes cause the attraction, proliferation, and activation of macrophages which are derived mostly from blood monocytes. In the infected foci, macrophages assume a distinctive appearance which causes them to be designated as epithelioid cells because of a vague histologic similarity to sheets of large epithelial cells. The epithelioid cells have large vesicular nuclei, and extensive pale cytoplasm with ill-defined borders. The epithelioid cells ultrastructurally are characterized by abundant organelles and extensive interdigitations of their plasma membranes. They contain ingested bacilli within their cytoplasm, and the structural changes indicate a heightened bactericidal activity. Mixed in with the epithelioid cells is a variable number of giant cells of the Langhans type (Fig. 6.68A). These are large cells with several eccentric nuclei and are formed by the fusion of macrophages. This admixture of epithelioid and giant cells forms the center of young tubercles. At the periphery is a narrow zone of lymphocyte, plasma cells, and unaltered monocytes. As the lesion progresses, the classic tubercle develops peripheral fibroplasia and central necrosis (Fig. 6.68B). These two features are not present in all tubercular infections; there are both species and individual variations. Encapsulating fibroplasia is more conspicuous in those individuals which have considerable powers of resistance, and it may, as tuberculous granulation tissue, overgrow and dominate the lesions. The development of central necrosis gives to the tubercle its high degree of histologic specificity. The necrosis is a product of cell-mediated hypersensitivity and is of caseous character. The necrotic material is most commonly inspissated into a yellowish cheesy mass, but may liquefy or calcify. Calcification is a characteristic development in some species of animals, but seldom observed in others.

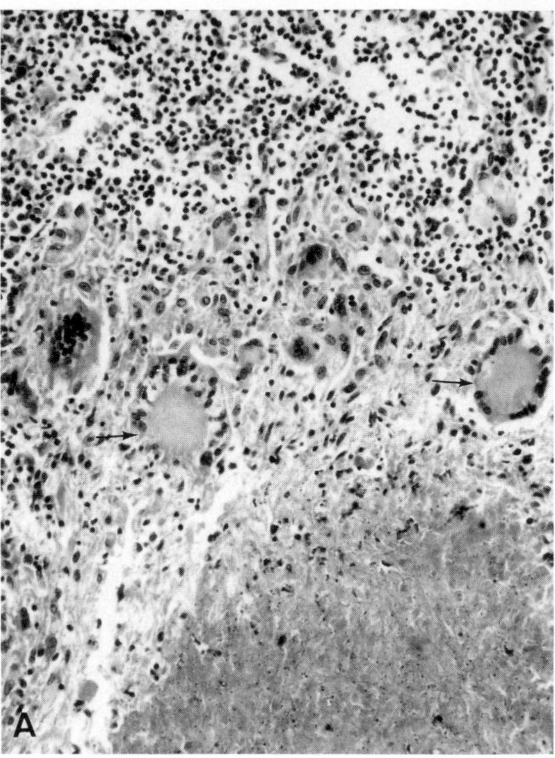

Fig. 6.68A Tuberculosis. Periphery of tubercle with Langhans' giant cells (arrows) and epithelioid cells bordering caseation necrosis.

The exudative type of lesion in tuberculosis usually develops acutely. The exudate is relatively voluminous and consists of fibrin and neutrophils as well as the usual mononuclear cells. Eventually, the exudate clots, and it too caseates. A combination of factors is usually regarded as responsible for the exudative lesions. Chief among them are rapid bacterial proliferation, presence of abundant reactive lymphocytes, and a site of localization in easily distensible or space-lining tissues.

There are various portals of entry available to the tubercle bacilli. Infection can occur congenitally by way of the umbilical veins, or postnatally through alimentary, respiratory, genital, or cutaneous routes. Growth of the original tubercle takes place by centrifugal expansion and by the development of satellite tubercles formed by spread of bacilli from the initial focus. The new tubercles may coalesce to produce large lesions. In a susceptible unsensitized animal, the bacilli spread rapidly, either free or in macrophages, along the lymphatics (Fig. 6.69) to the regional lymph nodes, where further tubercles develop. The combination of lesions in the initial focus and in the regional lymph node is known as the primary complex of Ranke. It is always present with first infection in animals, but both components may not be detectable because when infection occurs across a mucous membrane, such as of the pharynx or intestine, the initial lesion in the membrane may not be visible when the nodal lesions are present.

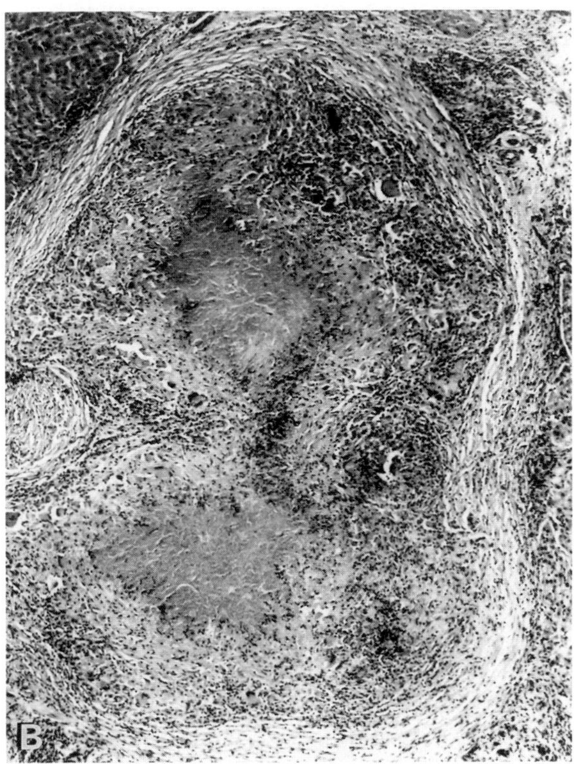

Fig. 6.68B Caseous tubercles with encapsulation. Liver. Sheep.

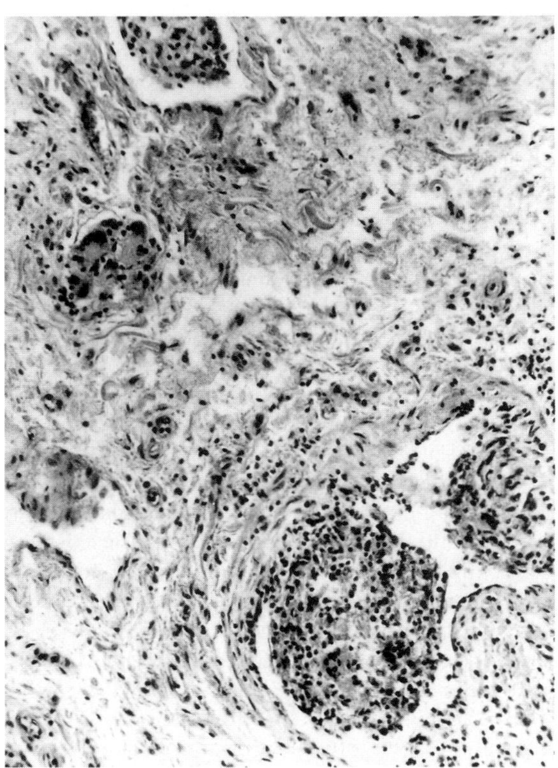

Fig. 6.69 Tuberculosis. Tuberculous lymphangitis. Liver. Pig.

The decision as to which lesions in a case of generalized tuberculosis constitute the primary complex is often impossible to make. The relative age of the lesions is an indication, as is their localization, because the site must be intimately related to one of the portals of entry.

As lesions develop in the regional lymph node, the infection passes successively from one node to another, and can eventually reach the blood, for potential widespread dissemination. Extensive hematogenous dissemination, however, is most frequently the result of breakdown of a blood vessel by an expanding caseating tubercle or cavitating lesion. The number of bacilli then released into the blood can be very large, and when these are removed by phagocytes in the various organs, a large number of small tubercles develop. The course of the disease after massive generalization is short, and the disease is then referred to as **miliary tuberculosis** because of the large number of tubercles the size of millet seeds. Hematogenous dissemination is, however, not always massive; the course then is much longer, and the metastatic foci are large and few or solitary. Some organs such as muscle, thyroid, and pancreas seldom develop lesions of hematogenous origin.

Spread can occur via natural passages. Common examples are spread from the kidney along the ureter to the bladder, from one bronchus to another by coughing and aspiration, or from the lungs to the intestine when infected sputum is swallowed. Rapid spread is possible in cavities such as the meningeal space and serous cavities of the trunk. Involvement of a serous membrane is usually by direct extension from an underlying lymph node or viscus. When the bacilli are freed on the serous surfaces, they are readily distributed by movements such as respiration and peristalsis.

i. *Cattle* Bovine tuberculosis has been, and in some areas remains, one of the most important diseases of cattle. In areas where the incidence is high, the disease is caused almost exclusively by *M. bovis*. When bovine tuberculosis is brought under control by eradication programs, however, the patterns of infection change, and the proportion of infections caused by the *M. avium–intracellulare* complex increases. Infections with *M. avium* usually have a benign self-limiting course. Often no lesions are detectable. If lesions develop, they are usually found in the mesenteric and retropharyngeal lymph nodes and are seldom >2 cm in diameter. They are usually caseous and encapsulated and may be either calcified or liquefied. There is commonly no spread from these sites, but sometimes initial lesions in intestinal mucosa are detected as focal thickenings. When extension of the avian-type infection occurs in cattle, the serous surfaces are most often involved. Occasionally, lesions may be found in the udder, lungs, liver, kidney, and spleen. The uterus is the most frequently involved organ in pregnant cows, and abortion or congenital disseminated tuberculosis in newborn calves can result. Large numbers of epithelioid cells are a regular feature of the histologic response, and pleomorphic acid-fast bacilli are abundant. The human bacilli, at most, cause small nonprogressive lesions in the lymph nodes of the pharynx, thorax, and mesentery.

The usual routes of infection by *M. bovis* are respiratory and alimentary. The unusual routes, which will be considered first, are cutaneous, congenital, and genital. **Infection via the skin** is rather rare. It requires that other primary cutaneous lesions be contaminated with the tubercle bacillus. The infection is limited to the initial site or may spread to the local lymph node. In **congenital** tuberculosis, the infection spreads via the umbilical vessels to the fetus. This route of infection is of some importance where the disease is common in cattle and where as many as 0.5% of newborn calves have been found to have tuberculosis. This route is of little significance in other species because only in cows is tuberculous endometritis common. When the primary complex is present in congenital infection of calves, it is in the liver and portal lymph nodes. But, as elsewhere, the complex may be apparently incomplete, and the lesions are found only in the nodes. In a fetus or calf of a few days of age, lesions in the portal node are assumed to be evidence of congenital infection; this is not necessarily the case in older calves because the portal node is also the regional node of the duodenum. Congenital tuberculosis in calves progresses quite rapidly, and the animals usually die in a few weeks or months. By that time, the disease has generalized, and lesions can be found especially in the lungs and regional lymph nodes, and in the spleen. Tuberculous lesions rarely occur in the spleen of adult cattle and when present, irrespective of the age of the animal, they are regarded as indicative of congenital infection. For congenital tuberculosis to occur, infection must be present in the uterus. Small tubercles can be found in the endometrium. Typical placental lesions are a slimy exudate separating the placenta from the endometrium and caseonecrotic foci in the cotyledons. Extensive areas of tuberculosis in the uterus result in repeated abortions. **Genital** infection occurs in cattle but is not common; its development requires that the sexual organs of either the female (usually uterus) or male (usually epididymis) are tuberculous. Mammary infusions used in the treatment of mastitis and contaminated with tubercle bacilli are responsible for occasional, but epidemiologically important, cases of tuberculosis of mammary gland.

Most bovine tuberculosis is acquired by inhalation or ingestion. Management factors and age at which the disease is contracted are major determinants of which route is the more probable. The location of the primary complex in the alimentary or respiratory tract can be helpful, but the evidence is sometimes not clear. The incidence of respiratory versus alimentary infection in postnatal calves is difficult to determine precisely, especially in very young calves, because it depends on whether involvement of the portal nodes, in the absence of intestinal or hepatic lesions, is taken to indicate alimentary or congenital infection. Primary complexes in the intestine are common in calves, particularly those which have been allowed to suck tuberculous udders or which have been given tuberculous milk to drink. Pulmonary complexes are also common in calves more than a few weeks of age. Pulmonary infections may well be more important than alimentary infections under crowded conditions. Tuberculosis of the anterior cervical nodes occurs with both aerogenous and alimentary routes of infection and is not, therefore, an indication of the route of infection.

Most cattle obtain their infections when they are older than 6 months. In these adult infections, the majority of lesions are in the retropharyngeal, mediastinal, and bronchial lymph nodes. When the lesions are limited to the retropharyngeal nodes, infection could be by either oral or nasal routes. Lesions are seldom found in the lungs with a frequency equal to their occurrence in the thoracic lymph nodes. This is probably because primary lesions in the pulmonary parenchyma can be very small and difficult to detect. In the very few series in which the examination has been thorough, the preponderance of primary complexes in the lung has been revealed. Intestinal infections do occur, and lesions in the mesenteric lymph nodes are common, but a significant proportion of these, perhaps most, are secondary infections which are established when sputum is swallowed.

In adult cattle, therefore, primary infection is usually in the lungs, and is caused by inhalation of infected droplet nuclei. The primary lesions may be single or multiple and may occur in any lobe, but they occur predominantly in a subpleural location in the dorsocaudal portions of the caudal lobes. There are almost always lesions in the regional lymph nodes, but they may be absent in some cases of chronic tuberculous pneumonia.

The **tuberculous pulmonary process** usually starts at the bronchiolar–alveolar junction and extends into the alveoli, so that it is initially sublobular or lobular. The histologic structure is typically tuberculous. There may be more than one focus within a lobule, giving a cloverleaf appearance, and more than one lobule can be involved (Fig. 6.70).

The initial lesions and their secondaries in the lymph

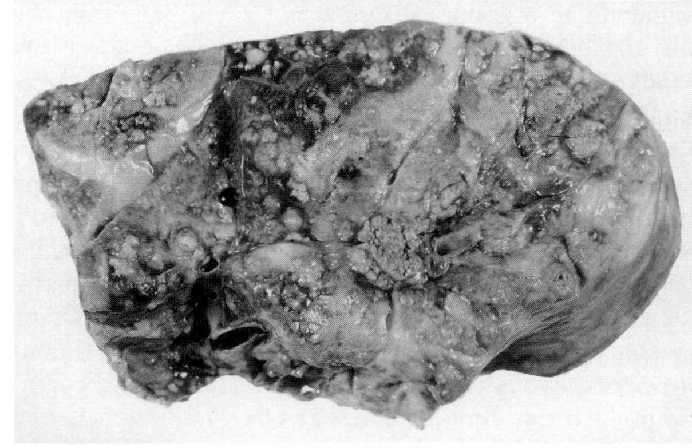

Fig. 6.70 Tuberculosis. Tuberculous bronchopneumonia. Ox. Larger granulomas (tubercles) have crumbly caseonecrotic centers.

nodes can heal completely, persist without progression, or progress. It is generally believed, on good but not certain grounds, that bovine tuberculosis most often progresses, with acquired cellular resistance slowing the progress considerably but not halting it.

The appearance of the pulmonary lesions varies with their age and rate of progress. The earliest lesions are not encapsulated, but are small and surrounded by condensed alveolar tissue. Even in these early lesions, the yellowish caseation and the calcification which are so characteristic of bovine tubercles can be seen. Caseated lesions can be encapsulated and heavily calcified. The capsules are not necessarily evidence of successful containment because many such nodules communicate with an airway and allow local dissemination. Multiple initial foci can coalesce to form large regions of caseating bronchopneumonia (Fig. 6.70), which in due course are usually encapsulated and calcified. Cavitations may form in any of these lesions, but they are never large because of the limitations imposed by the interlobular septa.

Dissemination of the infection within the lung can be by way of an intrapulmonary tuberculous lymphangitis but is mainly through the airways. The bronchogenic extension may be by direct contiguity, or it may be by aspiration of exudates, but in either case, what is initially a lobular type of lesion comes to involve much or all of a bronchopulmonary segment, or even most of a lobe. The reaction is the same as that in the primary lesion, although often more severely caseating. Depending on the rapidity and extent of spread, the lesions form a pattern of irregular caseous bronchopneumonia or more confluent caseous lobar pneumonia.

In association with chronic progressive pulmonary tuberculosis, it is common to find ulcers in the trachea and bronchi. These can arise by implantation of bacilli coughed up in the sputum or by progression of tuberculous lymphangitis. They begin as typical tubercles in the mucous membrane, especially near the bifurcation of the trachea, and are followed shortly by ulceration. Similar ulcers develop on the larynx by implantation of bacilli.

A feature of tuberculosis in cattle is the tendency to spread to the serous membranes (Fig. 6.71). This can take place by direct expansion of the original lesion, by lymphogenous extension from the lungs, by direct hematogenous dissemination, or by local expansion from a hematogenous focus in an adjacent organ. Once the tuberculous process breaches the serosa, the bacilli are distributed by respiratory movements and may be widely implanted. **Pleural tuberculosis** may be largely nodular, diffusely caseous, or of intermediate type. The affected areas of pleura, both visceral and parietal, are thickened by fibrous granulation tissue, and as a rule the tuberculous process does not invade the underlying tissue. The characteristic lesions are nodular and tend to occur in clusters. They may be sessile or pedunculated and frequently coalesce to form cauliflowerlike masses. In the early stages, they consist of reddish tags of granulation tissue containing typical tubercles and may be soft. Later, heavy calcification is

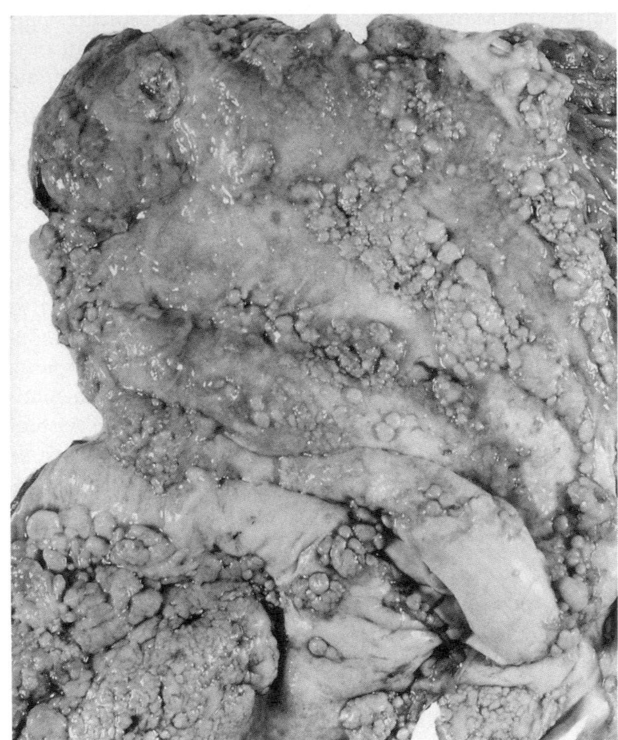

Fig. 6.71 Tuberculous peritonitis. Ox.

usual and is largely responsible for the term pearl disease. Caseous tuberculous pleuritis consists of large plaques of caseous exudate beneath which the pleura is uniformly thickened. Fibrin may be deposited on and between the plaques.

Generalization of the infection (dissemination to other organs) can occur early in the course of the disease (postprimary generalization) or late in the course of the disease (late generalization). In late generalization, it is assumed that the immunity the animal has acquired has broken down, thereby permitting wide spread. Generalization may be sudden and massive, when large numbers of the bacilli enter the blood stream (miliary tuberculosis), or it may be more protracted with fewer bacilli entering the circulation. The latter, whether early or late, is the more usual, and the lesions are larger and often of different ages.

In the respiratory pattern being described, the bacilli can enter the bloodstream in the lungs when the caseating process erodes a vessel, usually a small vein, or they may pass through the lymphatics and lymph nodes to the vena cava. In either event, the hematogenous metastases occur more frequently in the lung than elsewhere. Hematogenous metastases can also occur in most of the major organs and in lymph nodes, skeleton, and serous membranes, including the peritoneum, pericardium, and meninges. Organs such as salivary glands, pancreas, spleen, brain, myocardium, and muscles are rarely affected by hematogenous metastases in postnatal infections.

Miliary lesions in the lungs are associated with a fulminating course of the disease. The lesions are typical, small, grayish tubercles which are translucent at first but soon become caseous and centrally calcified. Hematogenous tubercles are diffusely scattered in both lungs although there is a tendency for them to be more numerous in the cranial portions. In slow or protracted generalization, which is the more usual type, the metastatic tubercles tend to be few in number, large, caseated, and calcified, and are often surrounded by a heavy capsule.

Tuberculosis of the **peritoneum** is less common than that of the pleura. It can arise in a number of ways. Peritonitis surrounding the liver is common in the congenital infection and is regarded as being of local and lymphatic spread. Peritonitis may also be hematogenous in the congenital disease as well as in postprimary and late generalization. Ulcerative intestinal tuberculosis which extends to the serosa is an important route of peritoneal infection in postnatal life. In adults, the intestinal lesions are usually secondary to respiratory lesions. Spread to the peritoneum from the uterus via the uterine tubes no doubt occurs, but the reverse is probably more common. The peritoneal lesions are similar to those of the pleura but are usually not so clearly nodular or pearly. They tend to be softer and more diffuse and to consist of extensive granulation tissue in which the tubercles are embedded (Fig. 6.71).

Hepatic lesions are hematogenous in origin. Infection arrives either through umbilical veins, as in congenital infections, through arteries as part of hematogenous dissemination, or through portal veins when lesions are present in the intestine. The hepatic foci may be miliary but, as elsewhere, it is more usual for the coarse nodular type of lesion to be present, sometimes only in one lobe. The portal lymph nodes are affected. The coarse nodular types of lesions occur in varying numbers and can be quite small or as large as 10 cm in diameter. They tend to be rounded and often project hemispherically above the surface. When sectioned, the nodules are seen to be enclosed by a heavy capsule, and the contents are bright yellow and caseous; the exudate may be inspissated and calcified or sometimes liquefied.

The **renal** lesions resemble in structure and type those of the liver. Miliary lesions are limited to the cortex, the initial development of the tubercles occurring in the interstitial tissue. The coarse nodular lesions may be multiple, but often they are limited to one or two adjacent lobules of the kidney. The caseating tubercles can be very large and may erode into the pelvis to cause a descending infection of the urinary tract. Frequently, the renal lymph nodes are concurrently involved.

Tuberculosis of the **skeleton** is usually hematogenous and occurs mainly in young animals. Its distribution is governed by the usual factors in hematogenous osteomyelitis. The lesions are most frequent in the vertebrae, ribs, and flat bones of the pelvis—all bones that are spongy and highly vascular. The epiphyseal–metaphyseal regions of long bones are also predilection sites. The osteomyelitis is in the form of miliary tubercles or large granulomas. Caseation is extensive in the granulomas, and there is a tendency to liquefaction resulting in the formation of tuberculous abscesses. The liquefied lesions especially tend to be progressive. They erode and fistulate through the cortex and erode the articular cartilages to produce tuberculous arthritis. Regenerative osteophyte formation is not prominent in tuberculosis as it is, for example, in actinomycosis. The predominantly erosive type of process is referred to as caries. Through the cortical fistulae, the infection spreads to the adjacent connective tissues and muscle. This is the usual pathogenesis of tuberculous myositis.

Tuberculosis in the **central nervous system** begins mainly as a meningitis and is more common in the cerebral than in the spinal meninges. Involvement of the spinal meninges may be direct from a vertebral osteomyelitis or hematogenous. Involvement of the cranial meninges is hematogenous, the initial lesions occurring usually in the basilar meninges and extending from there in the arachnoid spaces between the hemispheres and cerebellum, to the choroid plexuses and, to a limited extent, into the Virchow–Robin spaces and the brain itself. The meningeal lesions are similar to those of the serous membranes but are generally more exudative and necrotizing. Miliary or conglomerate tubercles are an uncommon development.

Tuberculous lesions, either small nodules or craterous ulcers, are occasionally found in the epithelium of the upper alimentary tract and abomasum. Whether primary or as endogenous secondaries, however, lesions in the alimentary lining membranes are uncommon. In contrast, the regional nodes, particularly of the retropharynx (Fig. 6.72) and mesentery, are often severely involved. In young calves, round or oval ulcers of small size may be found, especially in the ileum. These probably begin as small tubercles in the Peyer patches or solitary lymphoid nodules. Tubercles and ulcers can be found in the small intestine and cecum in adults, in which they frequently represent reinfection from the lungs. The ulcers vary in size and are either rounded or elongate in the axis of the intestine. The margins of the ulcers are distinct, firm, and raised. The bases are firm and usually covered with dry caseous exudate on granulation tissue speckled with tiny hemorrhages. Granulomas are sometimes visible in the draining lymphatics.

ii. *Horses* Horses apparently possess a high innate resistance to tubercle bacilli, because the disease is rare in them. Most infections involve *M. bovis*, but both *M. avium* and *M. tuberculosis* can produce localized or generalized disease. Many of the bovine strains recovered from horses are of lowered virulence when tested in laboratory animals.

The route of infection is almost exclusively alimentary. The primary complex is often incomplete, with large lesions in the retropharyngeal or mesenteric nodes but without an obvious primary focus in the related mucosa. In some cases, primary ulcers are present in the intestine. Bacilli of the *M. avium–intracellulare* complex sometimes produce a proliferative enteritis closely resembling Johne's disease of cattle. Lesions may be limited to the

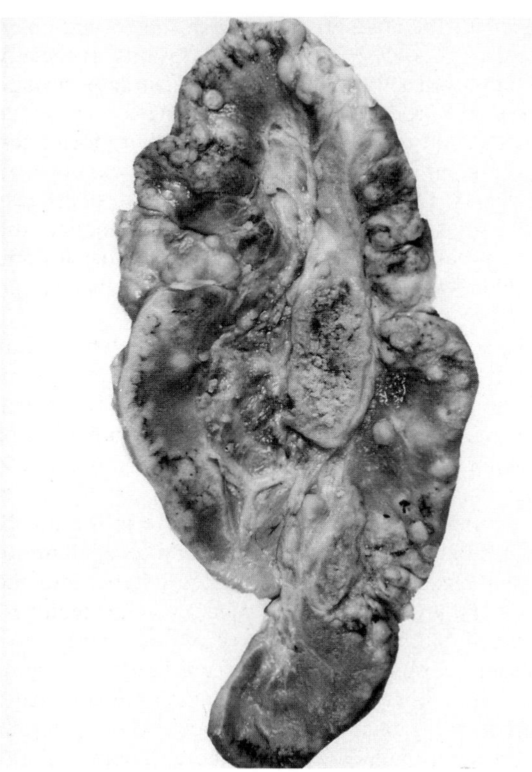

Fig. 6.72 Tuberculous lymphadenitis. Ox.

alimentary tract, but in fatal cases there is generalization with either miliary tubercles or scattered coarse nodular lesions. Secondary lesions have been described in the lungs, liver, spleen, serous membranes, mammary gland, and skin. They are unusual in the last two sites. Tuberculous changes in cervical vertebrae are repeatedly cited as being common in the disease in the horse, but this has not been thoroughly explored. If lesions occur in the central nervous system or genitalia, they are rare.

The lesions of tuberculosis in the horse often differ from those in cattle. Whereas extensive caseation and calcification are typical of bovine tubercles, the equine tubercles more commonly have a uniform, gray, smooth (lardaceous) appearance grossly resembling a sarcoma. Caseation does occur sometimes in the center of a lesion, but it is of minor degree, and calcification is rarely observable by the naked eye. Histologically, the early lesion is a tubercle which consists of macrophages, epithelioid cells, and few or many giant cells without a peripheral zone of lymphocytes. As the lesion progresses, it develops more and more proliferative fibrous tissue in which ill-defined tubercles are scattered. It is sometimes very difficult to find bacilli in these lesions, but the occasional tubercle which liquefies contains very large numbers. Pulmonary tuberculosis in horses is usually hematogenous and may be miliary or coarsely nodular. Usually there are miliary foci which appear like glassy dewdrops but are very firm. The coarse, nodular lesions, which grossly resemble sarcomas, are fewer and larger. Progression is by expansion of the lesion. Intrabronchial spread, which is so important in cattle, is of no significance in horses. The bronchial lymph nodes are invariably involved when the lung is; their appearance is that of a firm sarcoma, and corticomedullary distinction is lost.

When the primary lesions are found in the intestine, they take the form of tuberculous ulcers, which are more common in the large than in the small intestine. Tubercles in the liver and spleen are usually nodular rather than miliary. They can be extremely large and the organs correspondingly so; the spleen is more frequently affected than the liver. The lesions are of the usual lardaceous type. The serosal lesions, which are relatively common, are nodular and sometimes are accompanied by much effusion into the cavity.

iii. *Sheep and Goats* Sheep and goats do not appear to have any special resistance to tubercle bacilli, except possibly the human type, but tuberculosis in them is rare. It is usually caused by either *M. bovis* or *M. avium*. The main route of infection in goats, and possibly in sheep, is thought to be respiratory, because lesions are more common in the thorax than elsewhere. In general, tuberculosis in the small ruminants is similar in most respects to the disease in cattle.

iv. *Swine* Pigs are susceptible to all three major species of mycobacteria. The incidence of a particular species in any population of pigs depends largely on the species to which they are exposed and is, therefore, a reflection of the incidence of tuberculosis in associated cattle, poultry, or humans. *Mycobacterium bovis* is more capable of producing generalized disease than is the *M. avium–intracellulare* complex. *Mycobacterium tuberculosis* rarely spreads past the nodes local to the point of entry. Tuberculosis is seldom observed in pigs except at meat inspection and, because these animals are usually young, a local lymphadenitis is the extent of the disease usually observed.

Tuberculous infections of wounds, castration wounds especially, occur in swine, and occasionally the primary infection is respiratory. As a general rule, however, the route of infection is alimentary (Fig. 6.73). The primary complex in swine is seldom complete by gross inspection, but tubercles can usually be found microscopically in the mucosa of the pharynx or small intestine when gross lesions are present in the retropharyngeal, portal, or mesenteric nodes. Ulceration of a primary focus in a mucous membrane is rare.

There are certain differences between the lesions produced by the bovine and avian types of bacilli. The bovine bacilli produce caseocalcareous tubercles similar to those which occur in cattle, and the lesions are often surrounded by a fibrous capsule. In the liver, there is a tendency for the caseous centers to liquefy. The avian bacilli produce lesions which are proliferative in nature and consist of tuberculous granulation tissue resembling the lardaceous or sarcomatous lesions described in equine tuberculosis. Caseation is not a feature of these lesions, although it may

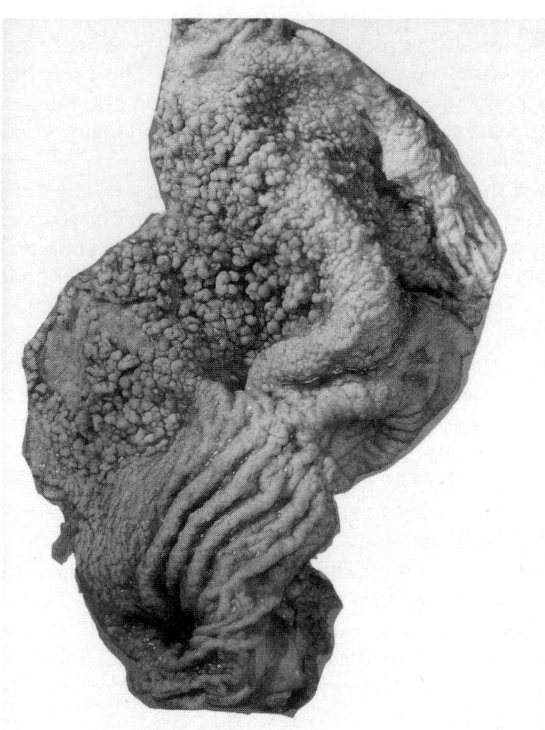

Fig. 6.73 Hypertrophic tuberculous gastritis caused by *M. bovis*. Pig.

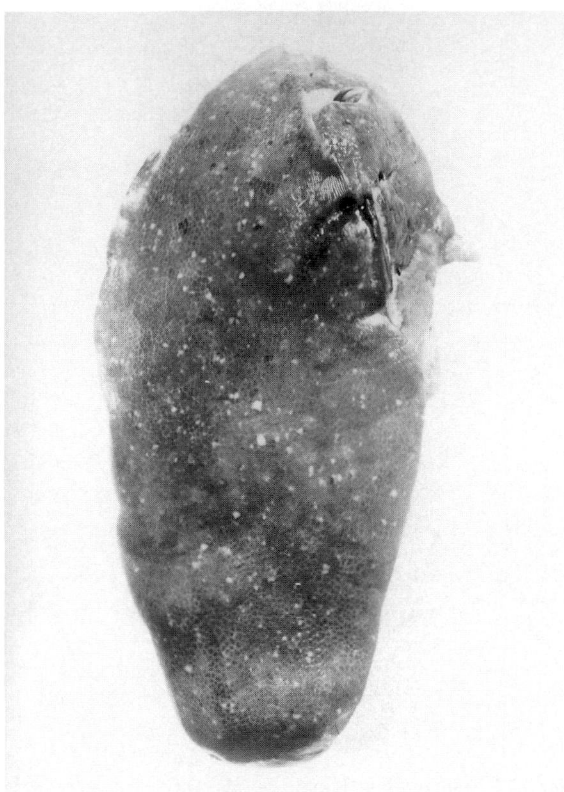

Fig. 6.74 Miliary tuberculosis of avian type in liver. Pig.

occur as minute foci, especially in the hepatic tubercles. There is little tendency for these caseous foci either to calcify or to liquefy, or for the lesions to be encapsulated. Affected lymph nodes are only slightly enlarged, and on cut surface they have a lardaceous appearance. The histologic appearance is of diffuse accumulations of macrophages, epithelioid cells, and Langhans' giant cells accompanied by extensive fibroplasia. The bacilli are numerous in these lesions, and they may also be recovered from nodes which appear grossly to be normal.

Pulmonary tuberculosis in swine is hematogenous and is usually of the miliary pattern. In some infections with the bovine bacillus, there is extensive consolidation of the cranial lobes resembling grossly the caseous bronchopneumonia of cattle, but histologically seen to be a confluence of numerous hematogenous tubercles. In this form of the pulmonary disease, there may be a tuberculous tracheitis. Miliary lesions in the lungs produced by the avian bacilli resemble dewdrops, and there appears to be a characteristic tendency for these to spread along the subpleural and septal lymphatics which are beaded by small tubercles.

The hepatic lesions produced by the bovine bacilli take the form of miliary or, more usually, coarse nodules. Those produced in the liver by the avian bacilli (Fig. 6.74) are quite different. The early lesions are scattered and miliary and are not discrete but blend peripherally with the portal stroma. The later lesions are merely an extension of this and, although softer, closely resemble the lesions of parasitic hepatitis produced by *Ascaris suum* and *Stephanurus dentatus*. Hepatic tuberculosis of avian type also cannot be distinguished grossly from the infiltrates of myeloid or lymphoid leukemia. Tuberculous granulation tissue spreads along the portal triads, surrounding and obliterating lobules, and at the periphery unites with the expansions of adjacent lesions. Typical tubercles do not occur.

Splenic lesions regularly occur in the generalized disease (Fig. 6.75). They project hemispherically above the surface, and their appearance, as previously indicated, depends on the type of bacilli present. Tuberculosis of the serous membranes is seldom observed in swine. Skeletal lesions, often confined to individual bones of the axial skeleton, are common. Tuberculous meningitis, primarily basilar in location, is relatively frequent in generalized infections by the bovine bacilli. The meningeal lesions in swine are more nodular than those in cattle, in which there tends to be diffuse exudation. Tubercles may also be found in the genital organs, skin, and eye.

v. *Cats and Dogs* Cats appear to be more susceptible to *M. bovis* than to *M. tuberculosis* or *M. avium*. The route of infection in cats is usually by ingestion of contaminated milk or possibly diseased wildlife. Dogs are susceptible to *M. bovis* and *M. tuberculosis*, and less so to *M. avium*. Dogs are more likely than cats to contract tuberculosis, usually by inhalation, in households with tubercu-

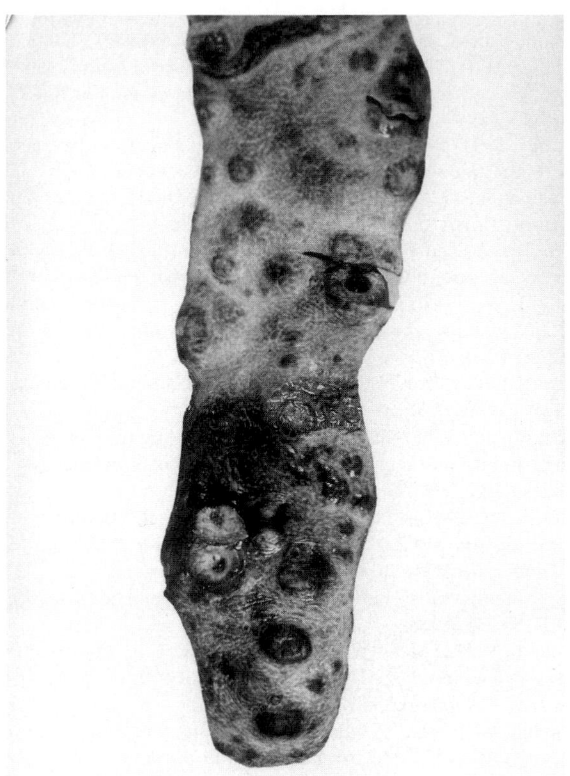

Fig. 6.75 Multiple tuberculous granulomas caused by *M. bovis* in spleen. Pig.

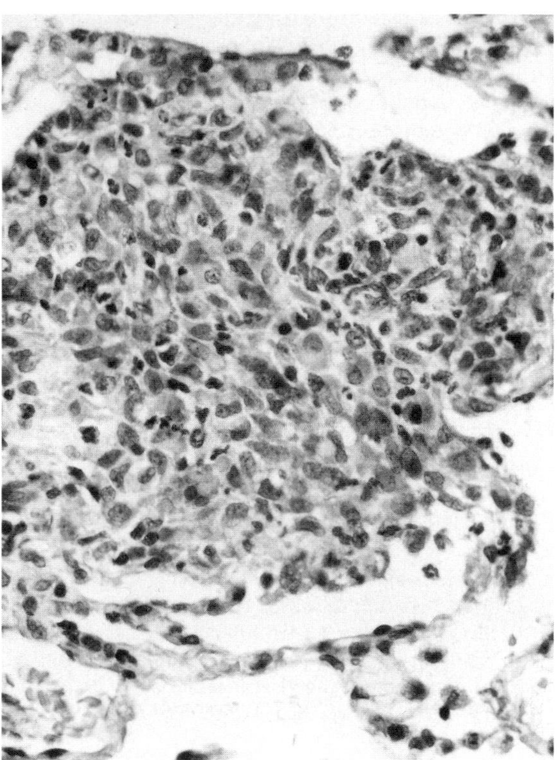

Fig. 6.76 Nonspecific appearance of pulmonary granuloma in disseminated (miliary) tuberculosis. Dog.

lous persons. Exposure of dogs to tuberculous cattle usually results in the alimentary form of the disease by ingestion of milk or other contaminated food.

The lesions of tuberculosis in carnivores differ from those in other species. Typical tubercles are not so common, and when they occur, caseation necrosis is not a prominent gross feature. More often there is a nonspecific granulation tissue in which macrophages are scattered at random and giant cells are rare (Fig. 6.76). The discrete tuberculous granulomas that do occur are composed principally of epithelioid cells surrounded by narrow zones of fibrous tissue in which there are scattered small collections of lymphocytes and plasma cells. Necrosis is often present in the centers of larger granulomas. Giant cells are rare or absent. The presence of central necrosis and fairly small numbers of acid-fast bacilli in lesions of cats helps to distinguish lesions of tuberculosis from those of feline leprosy.

The frequently sarcomatous gross appearance of the lesions can easily lead to misdiagnosis. This is particularly the case in cats. The pattern of pale homogeneous tissue causing enlargement and effacement of lymph nodes and present as diffuse or nodular lesions in the intestine and possibly other viscera can readily be mistaken grossly for lymphoma.

The primary foci in the lungs of dogs develop in most cases in the dorsal part of the caudal lobes. They appear as firm, pale, bulging nodules ~1–3 cm in size. The cut surface can be uniform, but frequently there is central liquefaction and a tendency to fistulate onto the pleura to produce serofibrinous or serohemorrhagic pleuritis. Metastatic nodules in the lung are usually few in number with an appearance similar to that of the primary foci. The bronchial lymph nodes are regularly involved. They are sometimes only moderately enlarged with softened necrotic areas on cut surfaces, but they may be very large and centrally liquefied. Dissemination within the lungs occurs quite rapidly and is predominantly intrabronchial with the production of a tuberculous bronchitis and bronchiolitis rather than a bronchopneumonia. The granulation tissue involves and destroys segments of the bronchial walls, and cavitation occurs by liquefaction and evacuation of exudate.

Pleuritis is particularly common in tuberculosis of dogs, and ascites is also likely to be present when the abdominal viscera are affected. The serosal lesions are not at all like those in cattle. Instead, there is diffuse or finely nodular pleural thickening by nonspecific granulation tissue. A large amount of serofibrinous exudate accumulates in the pleural cavity; this is often bloodstained. The pleural lesions may be unilateral or bilateral. Peritoneal tuberculosis accompanies lesions in the mesenteric nodes and liver and is accompanied by ascites. Large or small nodules of granulation tissue or a diffuse thickening occur on the visceral layers especially, and the omentum is often converted to a partially necrotic ropy mass in which there are very large numbers of bacilli. Tuberculous processes are seldom found in other organs, although involvement of the meninges, uveal tract of the eye, genitalia, bones, and skin have all been reported. Hypertrophic osteopathy is a possible sequel to pulmonary tuberculosis (see Bones and Joints, Volume 1, Chapter 1).

Bibliography

Amberson, J. B. A retrospect of tuberculosis: 1865–1965. *Am Rev Respir Dis* **93:** 343–351, 1966.

Armstrong, A. L., Dunbar, F. P., and Cocciatore, R. Comparative pathogenicity of *Mycobacterium avium* and Battey bacilli. *Am Rev Respir Dis* **95:** 20–32, 1967.

Bates, J. H., and Fitzhigh, J. K. Subdivision of the species *Mycobacterium tuberculosis* by mycobacteriophage typing. *Am Rev Respir Dis* **96:** 7–10, 1967.

Berthrong, M. The macrophage–tubercle bacillus relationship and resistance to tuberculosis. *Ann NY Acad Sci* **154:** 157–166, 1968.

Bull, L. B. Some comparative aspects of tuberculosis in lower animals. *Med J Aust* **2:** 827–830, 1937.

Collins, F. M., and Poulter, L. W. Effector and escape mechanisms in tuberculosis and leprosy. *In* "Immunological Aspects of Leprosy, Tuberculosis, and Leishmaniasis." D. P. Humber (ed.), pp. 97–113. Amsterdam, Oxford, Princeton; Excerpta Medica, 1981.

Cornell, R. L., and Griffith, A. S. Types of tubercle bacilli in swine tuberculosis. *J Comp Pathol* **43:** 56–62, 1930.

Daniel, T. M. The immune spectrum in patients with pulmonary tuberculosis. *Am Rev Respir Dis* **123:** 556–559, 1981.

Draper, P., and D'Arcy Hart, P. Phagosomes, lysosomes and mycobacteria: Cellular and microbial aspects. *In* "Mononuclear Phagocytes in Immunity, Infection, and Pathology." R. van Furth (ed.), pp. 575–594. Oxford, Blackwell Scientific Publishers, 1975.

Feldman, W. H. Generalized tuberculosis of swine due to avian tubercle bacilli. *J Am Vet Med Assoc* **92:** 681–685, 1938.

Fourie, P. J. J., De Wet, G. J., and VanDrimmelen, G. C. Tuberculosis in pigs caused by *M. tuberculosis* var. *hominis*. *J S Afr Vet Med Assoc* **21:** 70–73, 1950.

Francis, J. "Tuberculosis in Man and Animals." London, Cassell, 1958.

Glover, R. E. Infection of adult cattle with *M. tuberculosis avium*. *J Hyg Cambridge* **41:** 290–296, 1941.

Glover, R. E. Pulmonary versus alimentary infection in tuberculosis. *Vet Rec* **53:** 746–748, 1941.

Glover, R. E., Dobson, N., and Patterson, A. B. Tuberculosis in animals other than cattle. *Vet Rec* **61:** 875–881, 1949.

Griffith, A. S. Naturally acquired tuberculosis in various animals. Some unusual cases. *J Hyg Cambridge* **36:** 156–168, 1936.

Griffith, A. S. Types of tubercle bacillus in equine tuberculosis. *J Comp Pathol* **50:** 159–172, 1937.

Gunn, F. D. *et al.* Experimental pulmonary tuberculosis in the dog. *Am Rev Tuberculosis* **47:** 78–96, 1943.

Gwatkin, R., and Mitchell, C. A. Avian tuberculosis infection in swine. *Can J Comp Med* **16:** 345–347, 1952.

Innes, J. R. M. The pathology and pathogenesis of tuberculosis in domesticated animals compared with man. *Vet J* **96:** 42–50, 391–407, 1940.

Innes, J. R. M. Tuberculosis in the horse. *Br Vet J* **105:** 373–383, 1949.

Jarrett, W. F. H., and Lauder, I. A summary of the main points in tuberculosis in the dog and cat. *Vet Rec* **69:** 932–933, 1957.

Jennings, A. R. The distribution of tuberculosis lesions in the dog and cat, with reference to the pathogenesis. *Vet Rec* **61:** 380–384, 1949.

Lagrange, P. H. Tuberculosis: Immunologic and clinical aspects. *In* "Immunological Aspects of Leprosy, Tuberculosis, and Leishmaniasis." D. P. Humber (ed.), pp. 20–31. Amsterdam, Oxford, Princeton; Excerpta Medica, 1981.

Lesslie, I. W., and Birn, K. J. Tuberculosis in cattle caused by the avian type tubercle bacillus. *Vet Rec* **80:** 559–564, 1967.

Lesslie, I. W., Ford, E. J. H., and Linzell, H. L. Tuberculosis in goats caused by the avian-type tubercle bacillus. *Vet Rec* **72:** 25–27, 1960.

Liu, S. K., Weitzman, I., and Johnson, G. Canine tuberculosis. *J Am Vet Med Assoc* **177:** 164–167, 1980.

Lovell, R., and White, E. G. Naturally occurring tuberculosis in dogs and some other species. 1. Tuberculosis in dogs. *Br J Tuberculosis* **34:** 117–133, 1940.

Lovell, R., and White, E. G. Naturally occuring tuberculosis in dogs and some other species. 2. Animals other than dogs. *Br J Tuberculosis* **35:** 28–40, 1941.

Luke, D. Tuberculosis in the horse, pig, sheep, and goat. *Vet Rec* **70:** 529–536, 1958.

Mallmann, W. L., Mallmann, V. H., and Ray, J. A. Mycobacteriosis in swine caused by atypical mycobacteria. *Proc U S Livestock Sanit Assoc* **66:** 180–183, 1962.

Mallmann, W. L. *et al.* A study of pathogenicity of Runyon group III organisms isolated from bovine and porcine sources. *Am Rev Respir Dis* **92:** 82–84, 1965.

McKay, W. M. Congenital tuberculosis in bovines. *Vet J* **98:** 47–53, 1943.

M'Fadyean, J. Equine tuberculosis. *J Comp Pathol* **4:** 383–384, 1891.

Nieberle, K. Tuberkulose und Fleischhygiene. Jena, Germany, Fischer, 1938.

Nielsen, F. W., and Plum, N. Pulmonary tuberculosis in man as a source of infection for cattle. *Vet J* **96:** 6–18, 1940.

Orr, C. M., Kelly, D. F., and Lucke, V. M. Tuberculosis in cats: A report of two cases. *J Small Anim Pract* **21:** 247–253, 1980.

Ottosen, H. Histological studies on tuberculosis of bones in swine. *Skand Vet Tidskr* **32:** 65–77, 1942.

Plum, N. Tuberculosis abortion in cattle. *Acta Pathol Microbiol Scand (Suppl.)* **37:** 438–448, 1938.

Runyon, E. H. *Mycobacterium tuberculosis, M. bovis,* and *M. microti* species description. *Zentralblt Bakt Parasiten I* **204:** 415–413, 1967.

Scammon, L. A. *et al.* Nonchromogenic acid-fast bacilli isolated from tuberculous swine. Their relation to *M. avium* and the "Battey" type of unclassified mycobacteria. *Am Rev Respir Dis* **87:** 97–102, 1963.

Stamp, J. T. Tuberculosis of the bovine udder. *J Comp Pathol* **53:** 220–230, 1943.

Stamp, J. T. Bovine pulmonary tuberculosis. *J Comp Pathol* **58:** 9–23, 1948.

Wayne, L. G., Doubek, J. R., and Diaz, G. A. Classification and identification of mycobacteria. IV. Some important scotochromogens. *Am Rev Respir Dis* **96:** 88–95, 1967.

e. *Rhodococcus (Corynebacterium) equi* Infection

Rhodococcus equi is an important cause of pneumonia in foals. It can also cause intestinal and occasionally more widespread lesions. Bacteria of the *Corynebacterium, My-*

cobacterium, Nocardia, and closely related genera share the property of having cell walls containing complex lipids. The pathogenic features of *R. equi* infection therefore resemble those of mycobacteria. It is a facultative intracellular parasite of macrophages and causes a predominantly pyogranulomatous response characterized by abundant caseation necrosis. *Rhodococcus equi* is an inhabitant of both soil and the intestinal tract of mammals and birds. Whether it is a true soil saprophyte is still uncertain. Buildup of organisms in soil and dust occurs principally in association with the presence of carrier horses. This emphasizes the importance of its commensal status in the horse.

Pneumonia caused by *R. equi* generally causes clinical signs in foals 1–6 months of age, but the subacute to chronic nature of the lesion indicates that infection occurs well before clinical signs in most cases, and lesions can sometimes be found in foals dying for other reasons. Signs of the disease are fever, cough, nasal discharge, and increased respiratory rate. Because lesions are usually well advanced by the time the pneumonia is clinically apparent, mortality is commonly in the 40–80% range.

Characteristic gross lesions are multiple firm nodules of various sizes separated by congested and partly atelectatic lung. A typical feature is the very large size of many of the foci. There is sometimes evidence of their origin by coalescence of clustered small nodules. There is a tendency for more rapidly progressive lesions to be distributed widely throughout the lungs, and occasionally an acute clinical form in foals is associated with miliary pyogranulomatous foci. Lesions of slower, more insidious onset occupy cranioventral regions of the lungs, usually bilaterally, and therefore have the distribution pattern of a bronchopneumonia (Fig. 6.77A). The nodular lesions are often referred to as abscesses if circumscribed or as areas of suppurative bronchopneumonia if irregular and less well defined. They are, in fact, usually regions of caseation necrosis with either a slimy, homogeneous texture or a moist crumbly consistency with fluid-filled fissures. In most instances, there is no distinct fibrous tissue capsule surrounding the necrotic tissue (Fig. 6.77B).

Histologically, the lesions produced by *R. equi* are predominantly pyogranulomatous. Alveoli are filled with masses of macrophages containing many organisms (Fig. 6.77D). Giant cells containing organisms are common; neutrophils are less numerous. Lymphocytes and plasma cells are present in moderate numbers, mostly in alveolar septa and other interstitial zones. Necrosis of bacteria-laden macrophages and other cells involves local alveolar septa. Necrosis spreads gradually to affect large amounts of pulmonary parenchyma and produce the caseonecrotic foci seen macroscopically.

The bronchial lymph nodes are swollen and edematous. Sometimes they contain soft caseonecrotic foci. Histologically there is a pyogranulomatous lymphadenitis with similar components to the pneumonia. Pleuritis is uncommon, even when pulmonary involvement is extensive.

After the lungs, the next most frequent sites of lesions caused by *R. equi* in foals are the intestinal tract and mesenteric lymph nodes. Intestinal involvement may occur in upward of 50% percent of foals with pulmonary lesions, but intestinal lesions by themselves are uncommon. The intestinal lesion is an ulcerative enterocolitis (Fig. 6.77C), which mainly involves the cecum and colon. The mucosa has numerous, irregular but well-defined ulcers with fibrinonecrotic surfaces, red bases, and raised borders. Ulcers are based on lymphoid tissue, Peyer's patches in the ileum, and solitary nodules of the large intestine. Mesenteric lymph nodes are swollen and edematous. Those of the large intestine frequently contain caseonecrotic foci. Histologically, the main intestinal lesions are pyogranulomatous inflammation of lymphoid tissue and fibrinonecrotic ulceration of the overlying epithelium. Inflammatory cellular components are the same as those in the pulmonary lesions.

More widespread dissemination of infection in foals can occasionally give rise to suppurative arthritis, dermal abscesses, hepatic or splenic abscesses, vertebral abscesses, and hypopyon. *Rhodococcus equi* may also be a cause of ulcerative lymphangitis.

The pathogenesis of *R. equi* infection in foals is incompletely understood. The abundance of the organism in dusty environments where foals contract pneumonia, together with the predominant bronchopneumonic pattern of the disease, indicate that aerosol infection is the common route of pulmonary involvement. Aerosol exposure will produce the disease experimentally in foals to 2 weeks of age; later they become resistant, which suggests that susceptible animals may have delayed maturity of phagocytic cells. It also appears that the alimentary route of infection is the usual one for the intestinal form of the disease. Culture of the organism from parenchymal organs and occasional development of widespread lesions indicate that hematogenous dissemination also occurs. Infection of foals *in utero,* during birth, or through neonatal umbilical contamination are probably unimportant routes.

Rhodococcus equi has also been associated with metritis and abortion in mares, metritis in cows, pneumonia in calves, and tuberclelike lesions in lymph nodes of pigs and cattle. Its etiologic role in some of these instances is still questionable.

Bibliography

Ardans, A. A. *et al.* Studies of naturally occurring and experimental *Rhodococcus equi* (*Corynebacterium equi*) pneumonia in foals. *Proc Am Assoc Equine Pract* **32:** 129–144, 1987.

Holtman, D. R. *Corynebacterium equi* in chronic pneumonia of the calf. *J Bacteriol* **49:** 159–162, 1945.

Johnson, J. A., Prescott, J. F., and Markham, R. J. F. The pathology of experimental *Corynebacterium equi* infection in foals following intrabronchial challenge. *Vet Pathol* **20:** 440–449, 1983.

Johnson, J. A., Prescott, J. F., and Markham, R. J. F. The pathology of experimental *Corynebacterium equi* infection in foals following intragastric challenge. *Vet Pathol* **20:** 450–459, 1983.

Martens, R. J., Fiske, R. A., and Renshaw, H. W. Experimental

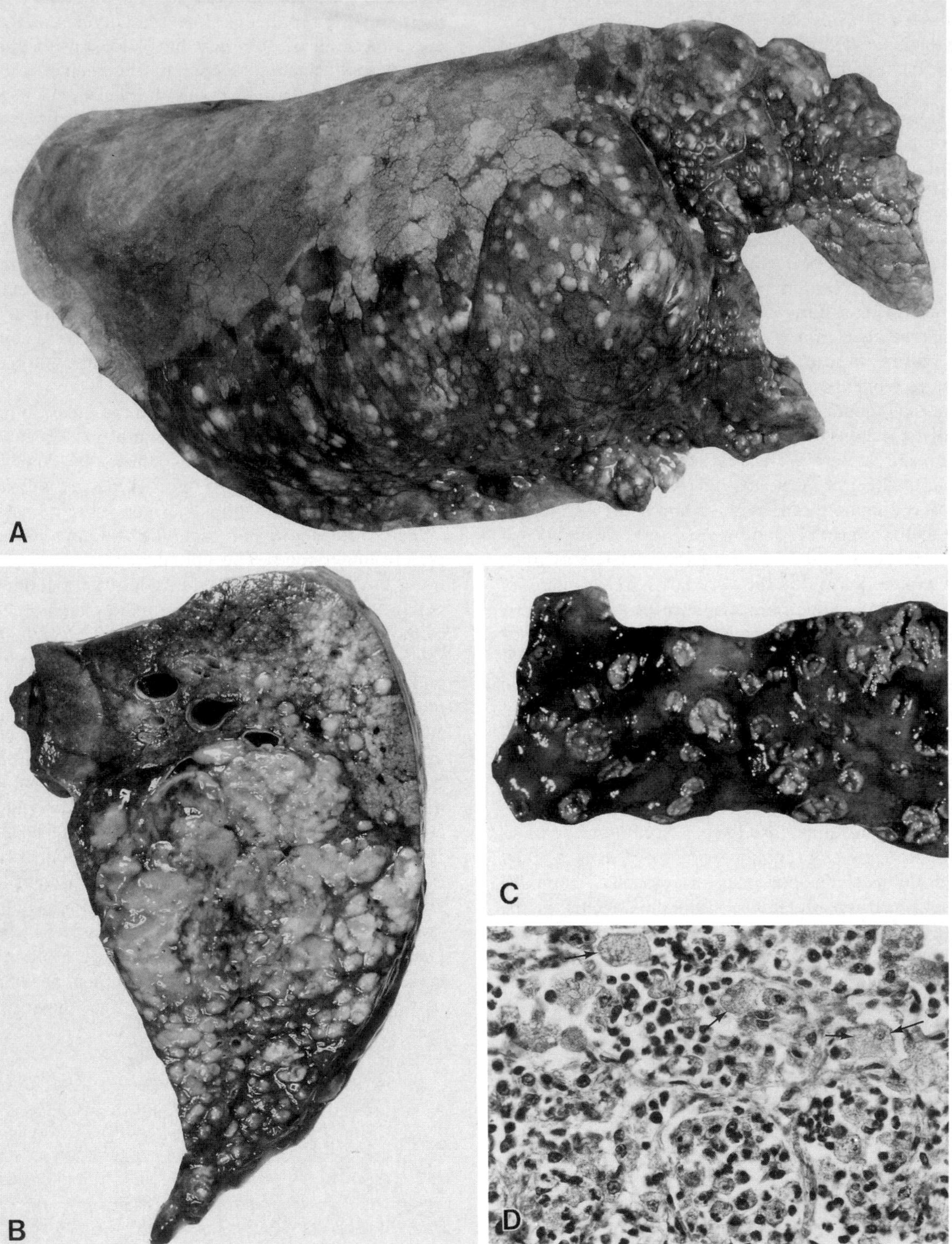

Fig. 6.77 (A) *Rhodococcus equi* infection. Foal. Extensive bronchopneumonia with multiple pyogranulomatous foci (abscesses). (B) Cross section of (A) showing variation in size and consistency of foci and absence of distinct capsules. (C) *Rhodococcus equi*. Multiple discrete ulcers in colon (Courtesy of J. A. Johnson and *Veterinary Pathology*.) (D) Alveoli filled by macrophages, which contain large numbers of *Rhodococcus equi* (arrows).

subacute foal pneumonia induced by aerosol administration of *Corynebacterium equi*. *Equine Vet J* **14:** 111–116, 1982.

Roberts, D. S. *Corynebacterium equi* infection in a sheep. *Aust Vet J* **33:** 21, 1957.

Smith, B. P., and Robinson, R. C. Studies of an outbreak of *Corynebacterium equi* pneumonia in foals. *Equine Vet J* **13:** 223–228, 1981.

Yager, J. A. The pathogenesis of *Rhodococcus equi* pneumonia in foals. *Vet Micro* **14:** 225-232, 1987.

Zink, M. C., Yager, J. A., and Smart, N. L. *Corynebacterium equi* infections in horses, 1958–1984: A review of 131 cases. *Can Vet J* **27:** 213–217, 1986.

f. OTHER BACTERIAL INFECTIONS A large variety of Gram-positive and Gram-negative bacteria can cause pneumonia, either singly or in mixed infections. They mostly cause a suppurative bronchopneumonia in lungs damaged by a preceding disease process such as a viral or mycoplasmal infection, or when pulmonary defenses are impaired for reasons outlined previously. There is considerable overlap among the bacteria found in the different species of animals, but the sets of organisms most commonly involved, and their relative importance, vary according to the species of animals affected. There is also some variation according to geographic location. Since the pneumonic lesions are relatively nonspecific, identification of causative agents must be by bacteriologic means, but, because bacteria can be opportunistic invaders of pneumonic tissue, isolation of an organism does not necessarily indicate a causal role. The presence of large numbers of a bacterial species in pure culture, or as the predominant agent, provides presumptive evidence of its importance in causing the pneumonic process. Difficulty in fulfilling Koch's postulates often leaves a measure of uncertainty even after considerable study. This was formerly the case for pneumonic pasteurellosis and still holds true for some of the mycoplasmal infections, as will be discussed later.

Pyogenic organisms, especially streptococci, staphylococci, *Actinomyces pyogenes, Pseudomonas aeruginosa,* and *Klebsiella pneumoniae,* are usually associated with suppurative bronchopneumonias, which may progress to abscessation. Either more virulent organisms or more severely compromised host defenses can lead to fibrinonecrotic or hemorrhagic pneumonias, such as the pneumonia caused by *Salmonella choleraesuis* in swine. This pneumonia can have the same appearance as pneumonic pasteurellosis in swine. In contrast, *Salmonella typhisuis* characteristically causes a chronic suppurative bronchopneumonia in which grossly there are large confluent regions of swollen, creamy-tan consolidation. On cut section, these appear smooth and homogeneous except where there are granular or friable foci of necrosis.

In addition to the bronchopneumonias, various bacteria cause interstitial pneumonia as part of a pyemia or septicemia. These are usually in very young animals and are most commonly caused by streptococci, *Escherichia coli* and, in foals and pigs, by *Actinobacillus* spp. *Actinobacillus* (*Shigella*) *equuli* in foals is typically associated with multifocal purulonecrotic foci, often recognizably involving small vessels. Fulminating systemic bacterial infections causing septicemias may be accompanied by little evidence of direct pulmonary involvement, or there may be a severe, diffuse, acute interstitial pneumonia with intravascular leukocyte sequestration, foci of alveolar wall necrosis, and widespread fibrinohemorrhagic exudation into alveoli. The acute interstitial pneumonia is particularly likely to be associated with the endotoxemias and septicemias caused by Gram-negative organisms such as *Salmonella* spp. (Fig. 6.78) and *E. coli.*

Finally, it is convenient to mention here that bacteria resembling *Pasteurella* spp. have been isolated from multifocal suppurative to pyogranulomatous interstitial pneumonia in several cats, a dog, and a tiger cub representing regions as far apart as California, Australia, and Northern Ireland. The bacteria are of uncertain taxonomic status and are currently referred to as eugonic fermenter-4 (EF-4). These organisms are present in the oral and nasopharyngeal flora of dogs and cats, and have been isolated from infected bite wounds in humans and animals. The pulmonary lesions are numerous, firm, cream-colored, or light tan nodules to 1 cm in diameter scattered throughout the pulmonary parenchyma. Histologically, they are foci of massive accumulations of neutrophils, monocytes, and macrophages which efface alveolar architecture and contain numerous bacterial colonies interspersed among them. Necrosis of inflammatory cells and alveolar walls occurs in foci of intense inflammation. The distribution of

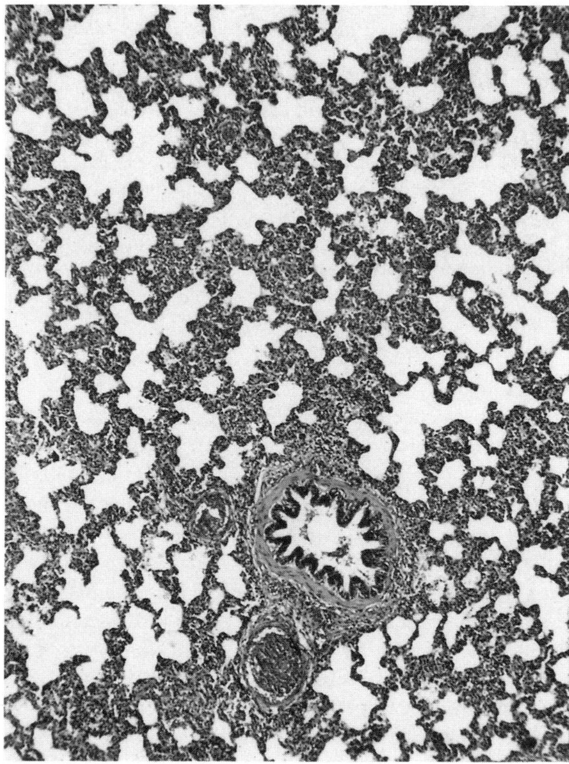

Fig. 6.78 Acute interstitial pneumonia in salmonellosis. Pig. Thickening of alveolar walls by leukocytes.

the lesions indicates a probable hematogenous origin, but the site of bacterial invasion of the bloodstream has not been identified to provide supporting evidence for this speculation.

Bibliography

Baskerville, A., and Dow, C. Pathology of experimental pneumonia in pigs produced by *Salmonella cholerae-suis*. *J Comp Pathol* **83:** 207–215, 1973.

Deem, D. A., and Harrington, D. D. *Nocardia brasiliensis* in a horse with pneumonia and pleuritis. *Cornell Vet* **70:** 321–328, 1980.

Dhanda, M. R., and Sekariah, P. C. Studies on pneumococcosis in domestic animals. 1. Isolation of *Streptococcus pneumoniae* from pneumonic lungs of sheep and goats. *Ind Vet J* **35:** 473–482, 1958.

Donald, L. G., and Mann, S. O. *Streptococcus pneumoniae* infection in calves. *Vet Rec* **62:** 257–258, 1950.

Garnett, N. L. *et al.* Hemorrhagic streptococcal pneumonia in newly procured research dogs. *J Am Vet Med Assoc* **181:** 1371–1374, 1982.

Gourlay, R. N., Flanagan, B. F., and Wyld, S. G. *Streptobacillus actinoides* (*Bacillus actinoides*): Isolation from pneumonic lungs of calves and pathogenicity studies in gnotobiotic calves. *Res Vet Sci* **32:** 27–34, 1982.

Hamdy, A. H., Pounden, W. D., and Ferguson, L. C. Microbial agents associated with pneumonia in slaughtered lambs. *Am J Vet Res* **20:** 87–90, 1959.

Jang, S. S. *et al.* Focal necrotizing pneumonia in cats associated with a Gram-negative eugonic fermenting bacterium. *Cornell Vet* **63:** 446–454, 1973.

McParland, P. J. *et al.* Pathological changes associated with group EF-4 bacteria in the lungs of a dog and a cat. *Vet Rec* **111:** 336–338, 1982.

Robertson, O. H., Coggeshall, L. T., and Terrell, E. E. Experimental *Pneumococcus* lobar pneumonia in the dog. *J Clin Invest* **12:** 433–493, 1933.

Sanford, S. E., and Tilker, A. M. E. *Streptococcus suis* type II-associated diseases in swine: Observations of a one-year study. *J Am Vet Med Assoc* **181:** 673–676, 1982.

Smith, T. The etiological relation of *Bacillus actinoides* to bronchopneumonia in calves. *J Exp Med* **33:** 441–469, 1921.

Stevenson, R. G. *Streptococcus zooepidemicus* infection in sheep. *Can J Comp Med* **38:** 243–250, 1974.

3. Mycoplasmal Diseases

Mycoplasmas are the smallest, free-living prokaryotes. They are placed in a separate class from other bacteria, mainly on the basis of their lacking the genetic capability to synthesize a cell wall (class Mollicutes, soft skinned). Lack of a cell wall results in extreme pleomorphism of the organisms. The type species of *Mycoplasma* is *Mycoplasma mycoides* subsp. *mycoides*. This organism was isolated from contagious bovine pleuropneumonia and therefore gave rise to the former designation of mycoplasmas as pleuropneumonialike organisms (PPLO).

It is difficult to prove a definite pathogenic role in the production of pneumonia for many infectious organisms. This is especially true for the mycoplasmas. They are ubiquitous inhabitants of moist mucosal surfaces, particularly of the respiratory tract, and are common opportunistic inhabitants of pneumonic lung. Proving the etiologic role of mycoplasmas isolated from pneumonic lung is complicated by several factors. Species of mycoplasmas vary in pathogenicity, and there is a tendency for the more virulent strains to be the most difficult to culture. This can divert attention to relatively nonpathogenic species. When a mycoplasma suspected of having a causal role is cultured, Koch's postulates are hard to fulfil because enhancing factors are usually involved in development of the naturally occurring disease. Simultaneous evaluation of the role of the mycoplasma and the nature and importance of enhancing factors, whether they are additional damaging agents or act by reducing pulmonary defenses in other ways, causes difficulty in designing experimental protocols that can convincingly demonstrate the mycoplasma's pathogenic importance. The degree of uncertainty regarding the significance of a species or strain of *Mycoplasma* is inversely proportional to its pathogenicity. Since establishment of a highly virulent species, *Mycoplasma mycoides* subsp. *mycoides,* as the causal agent of contagious bovine pleuropneumonia was difficult, it is easy to understand why considerable uncertainty still exists concerning the importance of many much less virulent species. A further source of uncertainty is the lack of understanding of the mechanisms by which mycoplasmas cause injury to tissues. The relative importance of a direct effect on cilia, effects on ciliated and other cells of proteolytic enzymes and membrane-associated toxins, macrophage–neutrophil interactions, and various immune-mediated responses are under investigation. The set of pathogenetic mechanisms appears to vary from one species of mycoplasma to another.

a. RESPIRATORY MYCOPLASMOSIS OF CATTLE There are two types of pneumonia associated with mycoplasmal infection in cattle. One is contagious bovine pleuropneumonia. The other is mycoplasmal bronchitis, bronchiolitis, and pneumonia of calves, an important component of enzootic pneumonia.

i. *Contagious Bovine Pleuropneumonia* Contagious bovine pleuropneumonia is caused by *Mycoplasma mycoides* subsp. *mycoides* (small-colony type). The small-colony designation is currently used to distinguish the organism causing bovine pleuropneumonia and *Mycoplasma mycoides* subsp. *mycoides* (large-colony type), which is a cause of disease in goats. Contagious bovine pleuropneumonia is characterized by a fibrinonecrotic pneumonia (Fig. 6.79A,B) with abundant serofibrinous pleuritis. Presence of necrotic material sequestered by fibrous capsules is a usual finding in subacute or chronic cases (Fig. 6.79C,D). The pattern of pneumonia is usually that of a lobar or bronchopneumonia (see Anatomic Patterns of Pneumonia, Section VI,F of this chapter). The lungs of cattle dying in the more acute stages of the disease typically have a marbled appearance in which relatively normal lobules are intermixed with lobules showing red or gray consolidation or necrosis. The marbled effect is heightened by the distension of interlobular septa and

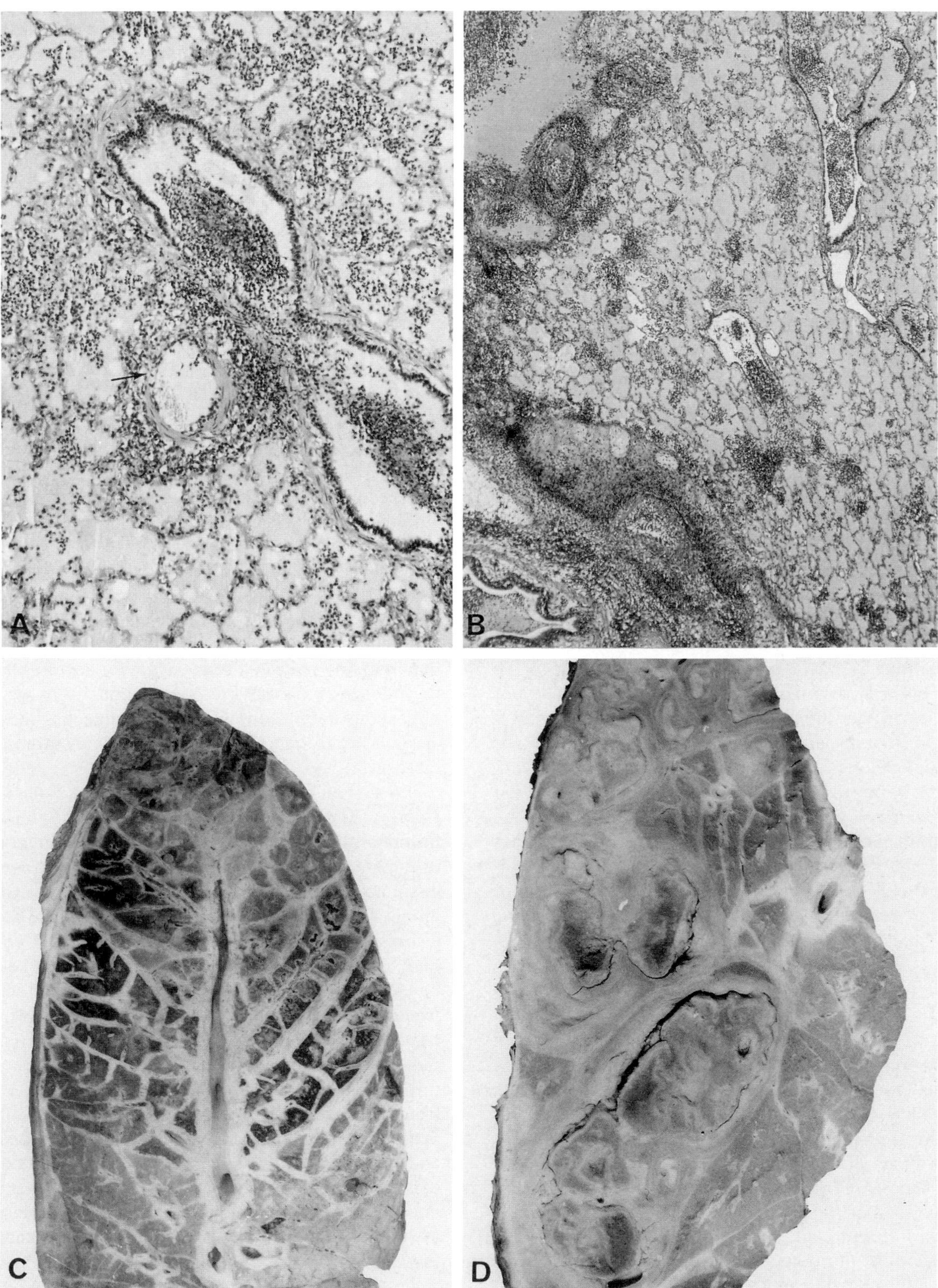

Fig. 6.79 Contagious bovine pleuropneumonia. (A) Acute arteritis (arrow) affecting portion of wall of peribronchial artery. (B) Acute fibrinonecrotic pneumonia with inflammation and necrosis within interlobular septa and peribronchial interstitium. (C) Scarring of distended interlobular septa in chronic disease. (D) Encapsulation of necrotic tissue (sequestra).

interstitium surrounding vessels and airways by broad bands of fibrinous exudate. It is also enhanced by the dense yellow-gray zones of packed inflammatory cells surrounding the necrotic areas. The fibrinonecrotic pneumonia and accompanying pleuritis of contagious bovine pleuropneumonia have features similar to those of the fibrinonecrotic pneumonia of acute pneumonic pasteurellosis. The marbled effect is more pronounced in contagious bovine pleuropneumonia, however, and the lesions are more prone to involve the caudal lobes. There is also a much greater frequency of development of sequestra in the mycoplasmal disease.

It appears that the disease originated in central Europe and remained endemic there until spread by the movement of cattle during the Napoleonic wars, and later by the growth in international commerce. Toward the end of the nineteenth century, it had become almost worldwide in distribution. It was eradicated from North America and much of Europe before the turn of the century and more recently appears to have been eradicated from Australia. It now occurs mostly in parts of Asia, central Africa, Spain, and Portugal. Enormous losses were reported from this disease in the nineteenth century, and in endemic areas the mortality rate among indigenous breeds of cattle is reported still to be more than 40%; in improved European breeds, the mortality in an unrestricted outbreak is not expected to exceed 10% of the animals. Species such as the buffalo, reindeer, and yak are susceptible to the disease, but are seldom affected. Sheep and goats do not appear to contract the natural disease caused by *M. mycoides* subsp. *mycoides* (small-colony type) and do not appear to develop the pulmonary disease after experimental infection, but they do develop a severe local reaction and septicemia if the organism is inoculated.

The transmission of infection requires close contact between infected and susceptible animals. It seems probable that the disease is transmitted by the inhalation of infected droplets exhaled by affected animals because the most reliable means of reproducing the disease experimentally is by endobronchial or aerosol exposure of susceptible cattle with suspensions of infected lung or organisms obtained from early subcultures. Factors other than the administration of the organism are evidently involved in determining whether cattle develop the disease, but exactly what these are is not known. Variations in innate susceptibility, interaction with other microorganisms or preexisting pneumonic lesions, and the state of pulmonary defenses have all been suggested as being important. It appears necessary for the organisms to reach the alveolar parenchyma, but the subsequent chain of pathogenetic events is still uncertain. It has been suggested that the acute vasculitis, fibrinous exudation, thrombosis, and necrosis are due in part to an Arthus-type or mixed hypersensitivity in animals with circulating antibodies capable of reacting with surface antigens on the mycoplasmas. Whatever the pathogenesis of the vasculitis, the thrombosis it can cause is to a large extent responsible for the infarction and sequestra formation.

The disease which can be produced in a percentage of animals following the aerosolization or endobronchial instillation of cultured organisms is similar to the natural disease, but the lesions are frequently small and multifocal and are not as likely to cause confluent consolidation of large regions of lung such as occurs in field outbreaks. Use of a suspension of infected lung is a more reliable method of reproducing the disease. Transmission experiments have confirmed that in an exposed population, 10–30% of the animals are refractory to infection. This resistance is native and not acquired by prior exposure to the organism. The natural incubation period is quite variable, but usually it is longer than 1 month. The clinical signs are those associated with fever and severe damage to lung and pleura, with a course of 2–8 weeks ending in death or slow recovery. Peracute cases which die in less than 1 week do occur. On the other hand, there are mild cases and some which are subclinical. Mortality can range from 10 to 70% in outbreaks. Slaughter of affected herds of cattle on occasion reveals frequency of pulmonary lesions approaching 90%, even though clinical signs may be obvious in only 30% of the animals at the time killing starts. There is no particular age distribution. Evidence of extrapulmonary localization may be observed in young calves as a polyarthritis, and in pregnant cows as abortion. As many as a third of cases that recover from the acute disease harbor residual infection in pulmonary sequestra. The organisms may remain viable in a sequestrum for several years. Cattle with sequestra that break down and discharge liquefied or caseous debris containing viable mycoplasmas into the airways are frequently the source of new outbreaks of the disease.

ii. *Mycoplasmal Bronchiolitis and Pneumonia of Calves* Mycoplasmal bronchitis and bronchiolitis or bronchointerstitial pneumonia is an important component of enzootic pneumonia of calves, which involves synergistic action of several infectious agents. Enzootic pneumonia will be discussed subsequently, but the pulmonary lesions attributable to mycoplasmas will be considered here. More than a dozen species of mycoplasmas can be isolated from bovine lungs, and mixed infections are frequent. The difficulties in proving pathogenetic significance for most of the mycoplasmas recovered from pneumonic lung were referred to earlier. Evidence supports the view that among the various mycoplasmas isolated from pneumonic calf lungs, *M. bovis* is at least moderately pathogenic. Others, such as *M. dispar, Ureaplasma* spp., and possibly *M. bovirhinis,* are generally accepted as being capable of producing slight subclinical bronchiolitis or pneumonia. A fifth species, *M. bovigenitalium,* is experimentally pathogenic for lung but is rarely isolated from the respiratory tract.

Experimentally, intratracheal inoculation of large doses of *M. bovis* culture causes suppurative bronchiolitis with peribronchiolar lymphoid hyperplasia. A majority of calves also have a bronchopneumonia characterized by small foci of coagulation necrosis surrounded by a zone of macrophages and plasma cells. The necrotic foci are associated with large numbers of *M. bovis* as revealed by immunoperoxidase labeling. *Mycoplasma bovis* is therefore more invasive and destructive than other mycoplasmas isolated from pneumonia in calves, and this is supported by the ability of the organism to cause mastitis and arthritis. Evidence that *M. bovis* is an important component in the complex etiology of enzootic pneumonia in calves will be referred to under that heading.

With the possible exception of *M. bovis,* mycoplasmas colonize the upper respiratory tract of calves soon after birth and extend to various depths of airways. They attach to the ciliated epithelial cells and, when present in large numbers, can be seen by electron microscopy to be packed two to three layers deep on and between the microvilli and base of the cilia. Their characteristic effect is to cause a chronic catarrhal bronchitis and bronchiolitis which, over the course of several months, leads to the development of prominent lymphofollicular sheaths around the airways. The term cuffing pneumonia is sometimes applied to lungs in which this is the predominant finding (Fig. 6.80).

The uncomplicated mycoplasmal lesion is usually inconspicuous. Grossly there are patchy, purple-red atelectatic foci in cranioventral regions of the lungs (Fig. 6.81A). More confluent, meaty consolidation is an indication of probable involvement by additional organisms. Microscopically, the lesion for the first several weeks after infection is a catarrhal bronchitis and bronchiolitis. Accumulations of neutrophils and mucus are present in the lumina of the airways, and there is increased prominence of bronchial submucosal glands and epithelial goblet cells. Moderate accumulations of lymphocytes and lesser numbers of plasma cells are found in the walls of the airways and around accompanying blood vessels. There is loss of cilia, and many ciliated cells have degenerative changes. Inflammation of alveoli adjacent to terminal bronchioles occurs in heavy experimental infections in colostrum-deprived, specific-pathogen-free calves and can probably occur in heavy natural infection. With the exception of necrotic foci caused by *M. bovis,* the alveolitis is nonspecific. There is a mixed intraluminal accumulation of neutrophils and alveolar macrophages with occasional plasma cells and giant cells. The alveolar septa appear thickened. This is partly because of accumulation of mononuclear cells within the septa but it often has a large artefactual component because of microatelectasis. Hyperplasia of alveolar type II cells can occur but is usually minimal in uncomplicated infections. More commonly, alveolar regions distal to occluded bronchioles are atelectatic rather than directly inflamed, and this correlates with the usual gross finding of atelectasis. The composite picture is of a bronchointerstitial pneumonia and partial atelectasis (Fig. 6.81B).

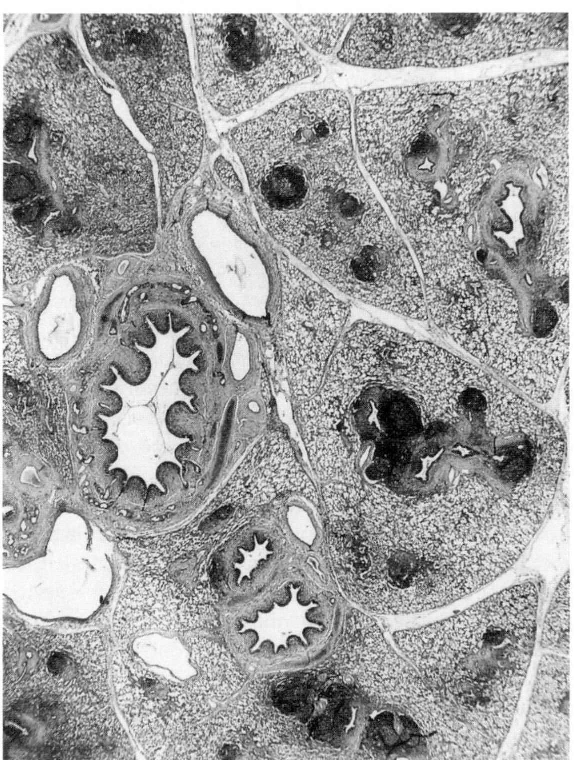

Fig. 6.80 Prominent lymphofollicular sheaths around bronchioles and vessels in chronic enzootic (cuffing) pneumonia. Calf.

Widespread lymphofollicular accumulations containing germinal centers develop slowly and are not usually present in calves <3 months of age. The follicular or ensheathing collars of lymphocytes extend into the lamina propria, often obliterate the bronchiolar smooth muscle, and cause narrowing of the bronchiolar lumina. This is the hallmark of cuffing pneumonia (Fig. 6.80). There is associated epithelial hyperplasia, including goblet cells, in bronchi and large bronchioles, and hypertrophy of bronchial submucosal glands. Alveolar regions are principally atelectatic because of bronchiolar occlusion by lymphofollicular accumulations and intraluminal exudate, but there may be an alveolitis as described for the earlier stages. The epithelium covering large lymphofollicular nodules in the submucosa of bronchi tends to assume the flattened appearance characteristic of lymphoepithelium.

Because the uncomplicated mycoplasmal lesion is rarely, if ever, lethal, it is usually detected as a cuffing type of pneumonia in slaughtered veal calves or in calves dying for other reasons. It can also be a component of other pneumonias of calves (see enzootic pneumonia of calves, in Section VI,H,7 of this Chapter). Other than the designation of cuffing pneumonia, various morphologic descriptors have been used. The most appropriate one for the airway lesion is chronic catarrhal bronchitis and bronchiolitis with lymphofollicular cuffing. When the inflammation extends to peribronchiolar alveoli, the general term bronchointerstitial pneumonia is applicable. Although the lesion is a chronic one, examination of the lungs of cattle older than 9–12 months indicates that it does gradually regress in most instances.

b. Respiratory Mycoplasmosis of Goats Mycoplasmas are an important cause of disease in goats. Various

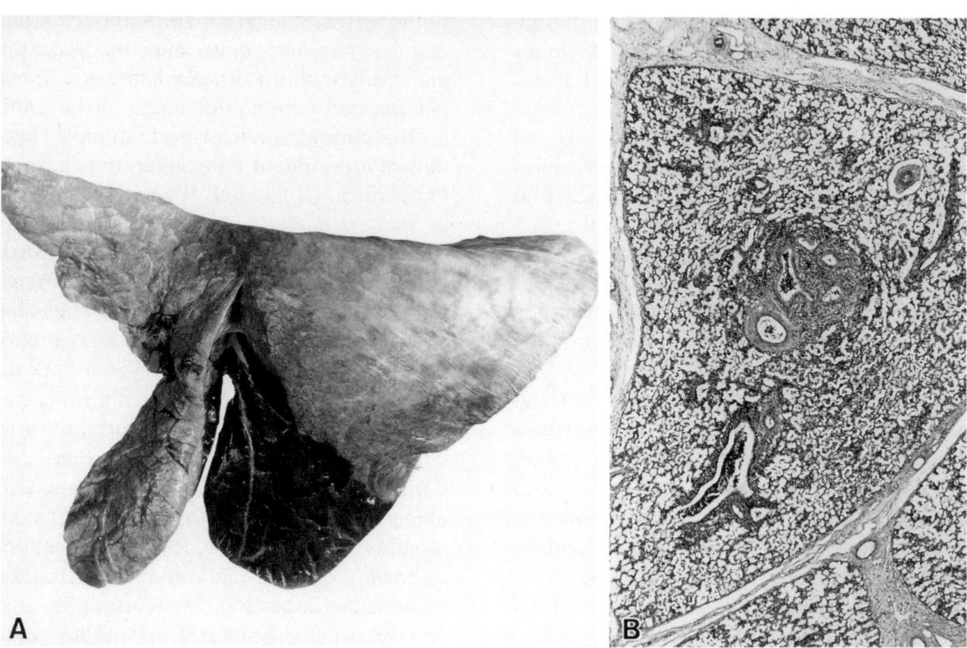

Fig. 6.81 (A) Atelectasis and consolidation of enzootic pneumonia. Calf. (B) Bronchointerstitial pneumonia and atelectasis associated with mycoplasma infection. Calf. (Courtesy of M. L. Anderson.)

species are responsible for pneumonia, mastitis, polyarthritis, keratoconjunctivitis, or a combination of these. Septicemic forms can also occur, mostly in young kids. Manifestations of mycoplasmosis vary according to prevalence of the various species and strains of mycoplasmas, the husbandry practices, and the presence of environmental influences or intercurrent diseases which act as predisposing factors.

Contagious caprine pleuropneumonia is the most important form of respiratory mycoplasmosis in goats. The disease occurs mainly in Africa, the Middle East, and western Asia. The prominent lesions are a severe fibrinous or fibrinonecrotic pneumonia and a profuse serofibrinous pleuritis. Fibrinous pericarditis is also common. Three species of *Mycoplasma* have been associated with severe outbreaks of caprine pleuropneumonia: *M. mycoides* subsp. *mycoides* (large-colony type), an unclassified organism referred to as *Mycoplasma* species F38, and *M. mycoides* subsp. *capri*. It is now generally accepted that *Mycoplasma* sp. F38, which was first isolated in Kenya, was the cause of the classic and highly contagious caprine pleuropneumonia reported from South Africa at the end of the nineteenth century. The main points of resemblance are a high degree of contagiousness for goats but not sheep or cattle, a fibrinous pleuropneumonia lacking conspicuous serofibrinous widening of interlobular septa, and absence of local inflammation when the organism is inoculated subcutaneously. *Mycoplasma mycoides* subsp. *mycoides* (large-colony type) and to a lesser extent *M. mycoides* subsp. *capri* appear to cause a form of caprine pleuropneumonia resembling the disease in cattle, in that there is often extensive widening of interlobular septa and peribronchial interstitium by serofibrinous exudate. They also seem to be less readily transmitted from goat to goat by contact. Sequestra are present in chronic stages of disease caused by all three mycoplasmas but are not so conspicuous a feature as in contagious bovine pleuropneumonia.

Mycoplasma mycoides subsp. *mycoides* (large-colony type) is found in widespread areas of the world where explosive outbreaks of caprine contagious pleuropneumonia do not occur. Syndromes caused by this organism vary and collectively they constitute the most important worldwide mycoplasmal diseases in goats. In North America and France, the organism causes severe disease with high mortality in kids. The predominant lesion is fibrinopurulent polyarthritis, but fibrinous pleuritis and pericarditis, acute interstitial pneumonia, and meningitis frequently accompany the severe mycoplasmemia. In older goats, less fulminating cases of mastitis, pneumonia, or arthritis are more usual. Peritonitis and abortion are occasional complications.

Various other mycoplasmas have been isolated from the lung. *Mycoplasma capricolum* is principally a cause of fibrinopurulent polyarthritis in kids. An acute diffuse interstitial pneumonia, such as occurs in other septicemias, occurs in the septicemia associated with acute polyarthritis in young kids. Mastitis can occur in milking females.

Other mycoplasmas, particularly *M. ovipneumoniae* and *M. bovis*, have been isolated from pneumonic lungs of goats. Their significance is uncertain. It is probable that they play a role similar to that of *M. dispar* in calves and *M. ovipneumoniae* in sheep by causing a mild, subacute to chronic catarrhal bronchiolitis or bronchointerstitial pneumonia and perhaps acting synergistically with other infectious agents to produce an enzootic type of pneumonia.

c. RESPIRATORY MYCOPLASMOSIS OF SHEEP The species most frequently isolated from lungs of sheep is *M. ovipneumoniae*. Most of the evidence indicates that it is one of the etiologic factors that combine to cause enzootic pneumonia of sheep, usually in association with *P. haemolytica*. Experimental studies using *M. ovipneumoniae* alone have been inconsistent and often difficult to interpret. There is sufficient evidence, however, to show that at least some strains of the organism can cause mild, subclinical lesions in a proportion of infected sheep. Lesions are principally chronic catarrhal bronchitis and bronchiolitis with development of lymphofollicular collars around the airways. The affected alveoli are mostly atelectatic because of bronchiolar obstruction, although a mild chronic alveolitis may be present. The role of *M. ovipneumoniae* therefore appears to be analogous to that of *M. dispar* in calves.

Mycoplasma mycoides subspecies of caprine origin experimentally cause fibrinous pneumonia and pleuritis in sheep. They are isolated only on rare occasions from naturally occurring outbreaks of pneumonia in sheep, and even in these instances, their etiologic importance is open to question because of the presence of *P. haemolytica*.

d. RESPIRATORY MYCOPLASMOSIS OF SWINE Mycoplasmas are by far the most important cause of enzootic pneumonia of pigs. In the absence of other proven etiologic agents, there is a tendency to regard mycoplasmas as the sole cause. It remains to be determined whether this is too sweeping a generalization. It is safe to say, however, that mycoplasmal pneumonia is the overwhelmingly preponderant form of enzootic pneumonia in pigs. Now that mycoplasmas are established as the main causative agents, the term **mycoplasmal pneumonia** replaces the earlier one, **virus pneumonia of pigs (enzootic virus pneumonia).**

Mycoplasma hyopneumoniae and *M. hyorhinis* are both established respiratory pathogens, with *M. hyopneumoniae* being the more important. A variety of other mycoplasmas such as *M. flocculare* and *Ureaplasma* spp. can also be isolated occasionally from enzootic pneumonia. Their relative importance in causing the disease is still under investigation.

Enzootic mycoplasmal pneumonia of swine is a chronic, usually nonfatal disease of young pigs. It is widespread throughout the world and in its most severe form can affect from 70 to 100% of pigs in a herd. Clinical expressions of the uncomplicated disease are coughing, unthriftiness, poor weight gain, and reduced food-conversion ratio. Because there is usually low mortality associated with mycoplasmal pneumonia, the lesions are generally seen in slaughtered animals or those dying from other diseases. When deaths do occur because of pneumonia, it is due mainly to superimposed bacterial infections. *Pasteurella multocida* is the most common secondary invader, but *Actinomyces pyogenes, Haemophilus* spp., streptococci, staphylococci, *Klebsiella* spp., and *Bordetella bronchiseptica* can be involved singly or in combination.

The characteristic gross feature of mycoplasmal pneumonia is confluent consolidation of cranioventral regions of the lungs (Fig. 6.82). When the amount of consolidation is small, it tends to affect portions of the right middle and right cranial lobes and the caudal portion of the left cranial lobe, but frequently there is bilateral involvement of more than 50% of cranial and middle lobes, together with the accessory lobe and cranioventral portions of caudal lobes. The consolidated lung ranges from dark red through grayish pink to more homogeneous gray according to the age of the lesion. This change occurs over the several-month course of disease. Even though there is often extensive confluent consolidation, careful examination reveals a regular pattern of small grayish nodules against a red background. This denotes the bronchiolar orientation of the inflammation. The cut surface of consolidated lung is moist and meaty, and mucopus is present in the airways. Minor mycoplasmal lesions are less characteristic and have a mosaic pattern of intermixed consolidated, atelectatic, hyperinflated, and more normal lobules. Occasional atelectatic lobules represent the minimal gross lesion. Sometimes, pale nodules indicating the presence of peribronchiolar lymphoid tissue can be detected in the centers of atelectatic lobules. Lesions of severe exudative bronchopneumonia or lobar pneumonia, especially with necrosis or abscessation, indicate secondary bacterial infection.

Mycoplasma hyopneumoniae can cause fibrinous or serofibrinous pleuritis and inflammation of other serous surfaces. When pleuritis is present, however, it is more probably associated with *M. hyorhinis* or infections complicated by *P. multocida* or *Haemophilus* spp. Pulmonary lymph nodes are enlarged by nonspecific hyperplastic lymphadenitis to a degree which corresponds to the extent and activity of pulmonary consolidation. On cut surface, they are moist, usually bulging, and sometimes hyperemic.

Histologically, mycoplasmal pneumonia in swine has the morphologic pattern of a catarrhal bronchointerstitial pneumonia (Fig. 6.83A), with development of prominent peribronchial, peribronchiolar, and perivascular accumulations of lymphoid tissue in the chronic stages. Thus there is a resemblance to the lesions caused by mycoplasmas associated with enzootic pneumonias in calves and lambs. The mycoplasmas of swine appear to be much more capable of eliciting chronic inflammation of the alveolar parenchyma without the assistance of other organisms, however, even though they mainly colonize the surface of ciliated cells in the airways as do the mycoplasmas of calves and lambs.

In the fully developed mycoplasmal pneumonia, there is extensive lymphoid hyperplasia around airways and their associated vessels. In severe cases, the lymphoid nodules or sheaths efface the muscularis mucosae and cause narrowing of the lumina of airways. Germinal centers may be present. The epithelium over prominent nod-

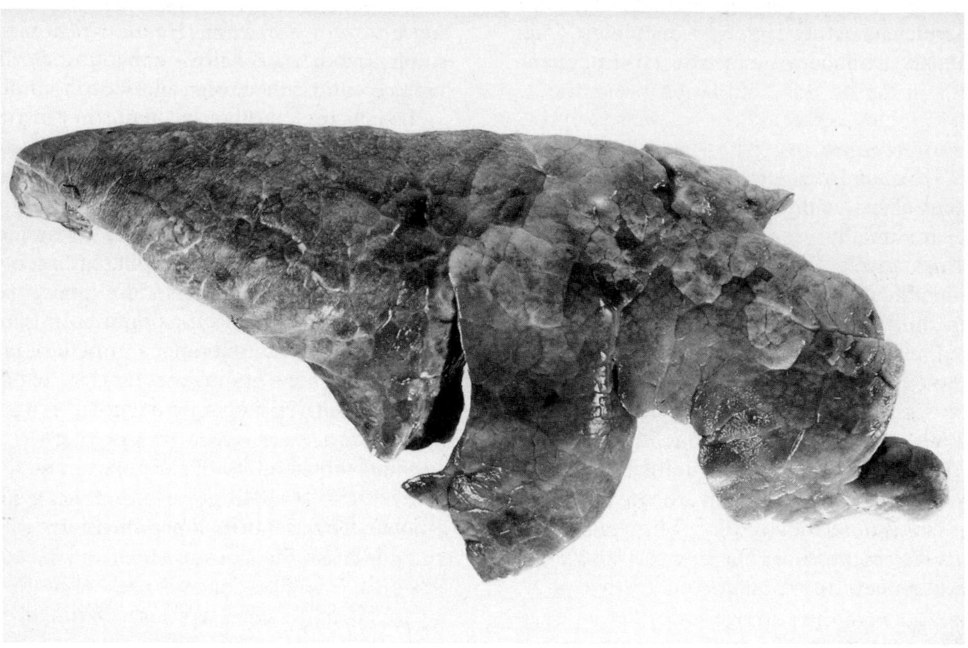

Fig. 6.82 Enzootic mycoplasmal pneumonia of swine. Confluent consolidation of cranioventral lobes. Multiple pale foci within affected lobules indicating bronchiolar orientation of the pneumonia.

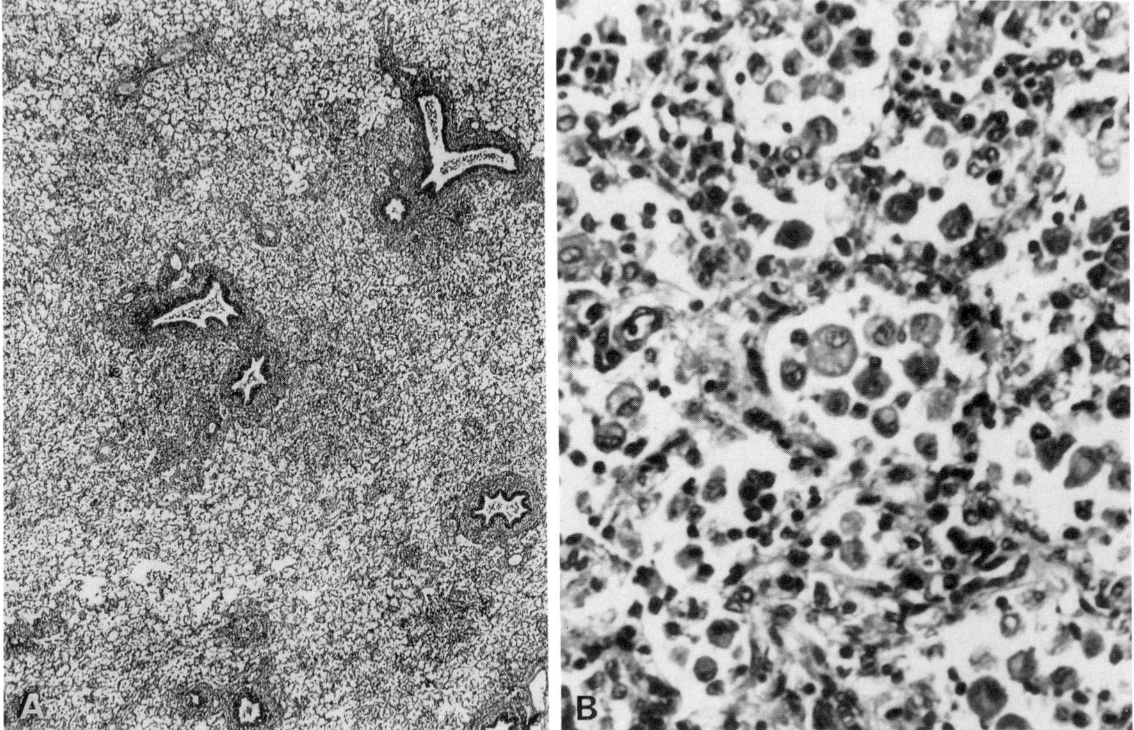

Fig. 6.83 (A) Enzootic mycoplasmal pneumonia of swine. Bronchointerstitial pattern of early lesion. (B) Peribronchiolar alveoli in (A) showing thickening of septa by lymphoid cells and macrophages within lumina.

ules is often degenerated or ulcerated. Elsewhere, there is epithelial hyperplasia, particularly in bronchioles. Cilia are absent from many surface regions. There is hyperplasia of goblet cells in the bronchi and larger bronchioles, and the bronchial submucosal glands are increased in size and number. The increased activity of mucus-secreting cells is responsible for the presence of large amounts of mucus or mucopus. The alveolitis component of the bronchointerstitial pneumonia consists of wide thickening of the septa of alveoli adjacent to bronchioles and accumulation of exudate in their lumina. The alveolar septa are thickened by accumulations of various-sized lymphocytes and small numbers of plasma cells. The intra-alveolar exudate consists predominantly of macrophages (Fig. 6.83B), but variable numbers of plasma cells, lymphocytes, and neutrophils are present. There is hyperplasia of type II alveolar epithelial cells of inflamed alveoli in established lesions. This can be difficult to detect histologically when alveolar architecture is obscured by absence of detectable demarcation between thickened alveolar septa and atelectatic or exudate-filled lumina.

Experimental studies of the pathogenesis of mycoplasmal pneumonia indicate that typical gross lesions do not occur until 2–4 weeks after infection. The rate of development of lesions is dependent on factors relating to the dose and strain of *Mycoplasma,* method of administration, and susceptibility of the pigs exposed. Inoculation of suspensions of lung containing mycoplasmas is a more reliable way of reproducing the disease, as is also the case with experimental production of respiratory mycoplasmosis in cattle, sheep, and goats. Young pigs naturally exposed to infectious aerosols soon after birth can develop lesions by the time they are 3–5 weeks of age. Initial lesions caused by the *Mycoplasma,* that is within a week after infection, are a neutrophilic bronchitis and bronchiolitis, and a mixed neutrophil and macrophage accumulation in adjacent alveoli. The numbers of neutrophils diminish, and the lymphoid cells increase over the subsequent several weeks to reach the fully developed stage of consolidation described earlier. There is conflicting evidence concerning persistence of the pneumonia after it has reached its peak some 5–6 weeks after infection. Estimations range from essentially complete resolution of uncomplicated mycoplasmal pneumonia within 2 months to no appreciable reduction in its extent even after 3 months. In view of the large number of variables in experimental and especially in field situations, the wide range in persistence is to be expected.

e. RESPIRATORY MYCOPLASMOSIS OF HORSES Although several mycoplasmas have been isolated from the respiratory tract of horses, particularly *Mycoplasma equirhinis* and *M. felis,* there have been no studies to determine whether any of them is capable of causing a subclinical bronchiolitis or bronchointerstitial pneumonia. *Mycoplasma felis* is believed to be a cause of pleuritis in the horse.

f. RESPIRATORY MYCOPLASMOSIS OF DOGS AND CATS Of the various mycoplasmas isolated from canine pneumonia, *M. cynos* experimentally is capable of causing a mild bronchointerstitial pneumonia similar to that produced by mycoplasmas in other species and is implicated in the pathogenesis of some cases of kennel cough. *Mycoplasma bovigenitalium* is also pathogenic, but to a lesser extent. The clinical significance of these mycoplasmas is doubtful, however, because they are usually isolated from severe exudative lesions in which pathogenic bacteria are also present, often in dogs with distemper.

Mycoplasma felis is an opportunistic pathogen of the conjunctiva in cats. Neither it nor the other mycoplasmas isolated from the respiratory tract of cats are recognized as significant respiratory tract pathogens.

Bibliography

Allan, E. M., and Pirie, H. M. Electron-microscopical observations on mycoplasmas in pneumonic calves. *J Med Microbiol* **10:** 469–472, 1977.

Alley, M. R., and Clarke, J. K. The experimental transmission of ovine chronic nonprogressive pneumonia. *N Z Vet J* **27:** 217–220, 1979.

Armstrong, C. H., and Friis, N. F. Isolation of *Mycoplasma flocculare* from swine in the U. S. *Am J Vet Res* **42:** 1030–1032, 1981.

Ball, H. J., and Bryson, D. G. Isolation of ureaplasmas from pneumonic dog lungs. *Vet Rec* **111:** 585, 1982.

Baskerville, A. Development of the early lesions in experimental enzootic pneumonia of pigs: An ultrastructural and histological study. *Res Vet Sci* **13:** 570–578, 1972.

Baskerville, A., and Wright, C. L. Ultrastructural changes in experimental enzootic pneumonia in pigs. *Res Vet Sci* **14:** 155–160, 1973.

Boidin, A. G., Cordy, D. R., and Adler, H. E. A pleuropneumonialike organism and a virus in ovine pneumonia in California. *Cornell Vet* **48:** 410–430, 1958.

Bolske, G., Nilsson, P. O., and Thunegard, E. Isolation of *Mycoplasma ovipneumoniae* from lambs with proliferative interstitial pneumonia. *Svensk Veterinartidning* **34:** 9–11, 1982.

Campbell, A. D. A preliminary note on the experimental reproduction of bovine pleuropneumonia. *J Coun Sci Industr Res Aust* **11:** 103–114, 1938.

DaMassa, A. J., Brooks, D. L., and Adler, H. E. Caprine mycoplasmosis: Widespread infection in goats with *Mycoplasma mycoides* subspecies *mycoides* (large-colony type). *Am J Vet Res* **44:** 322–325, 1983.

DaMassa, A. J. *et al.* Caprine mycoplasmosis: Acute pulmonary disease in newborn kids given *Mycoplasma capricolum* orally. *Aust Vet J* **60:** 125–126, 1983.

Daubney, R. Contagious bovine pleuropneumonia. Note on experimental production and infection by contact. *J Comp Pathol* **48:** 83–96, 1935.

Friis, N. F. *Mycoplasma dispar* as a causative agent in pneumonia of calves. *Acta Vet Scand* **21:** 34–42, 1980.

Goltz, J. P. *et al.* Experimental studies on the pathogenicity of *Mycoplasma ovipneumoniae* and *Mycoplasma arginini* for the respiratory tract of goats. *Can J Vet Res* **50:** 59–67, 1986.

Goodwin, R. F. W., and Whittlestone, P. A respiratory disease of pigs (type XI) differing from enzootic pneumonia. *J Comp Pathol* **72:** 389–410, 1962.

Goodwin, R. F. W., Pomeroy, A. P., and Whittlestone, P. Production of enzootic pneumonia in pigs with a mycoplasma. *Vet Rec* **77:** 1247–1249, 1965.

Goodwin, R. F. W., Pomeroy, A. P., and Whittlestone, P. Characterization of *Mycoplasma suipneumoniae:* A mycoplasma causing enzootic pneumonia of pigs. *J Hyg (Camb)* **65:** 85–96, 1967.

Gourlay, R. N., and Howard, C. J. Respiratory mycoplasmosis. *Adv Vet Sci Comp Med* **26:** 289–332, 1982.

Gourlay, R. N. *et al.* Pathogenicity of some *Mycoplasma* and *Acholeplasma* species in the lungs of gnotobiotic calves. *Res Vet Sci* **27:** 233–237, 1979.

Howard, C. J., Thomas, L. H., and Parsons, K. R. Comparative pathogenicity of *Mycoplasma bovis* and *Mycoplasma dispar* for the respiratory tract of calves. *Israel J Med Sci* **23:** 621–624, 1987.

Howard, C. J., Thomas, L. H., and Parsons, K. R. Immune response of cattle to respiratory mycoplasms. *Vet Immunol Immunopathol* **17:** 401–412, 1987.

Hutcheon, D. Contagious pleuropneumonia in Angora goats. *Vet J* **13:** 171–180, 1881.

Hutcheon, D. Contagious pleuropneumonia in goats at Cape Colony, South Africa. *Vet J* **29:** 299–404, 1889.

Jones, G. E., Gilmour, J. S., and Rae, A. G. II. The effects of different strains of *Mycoplasma ovipneumoniae* on specific-pathogen-free and conventionally reared lambs. *J Comp Pathol* **92:** 267–272, 1982.

Kaliner, G., and MacOwan, K. J. The pathology of experimental and natural contagious caprine pleuropneumonia in Kenya. *Zbl Vet Med B* **23:** 652–661, 1976.

Knudtson, W. U., Reed, D. E., and Daniels, G. Identification of Mycoplasmatales in pneumonic calf lungs. *Vet Micro* **11:** 79–91, 1986.

Longley, E. O. Contagious pleuropneumonia of goats. *Indian J Vet Sci* **10:** 127–197, 1940.

Mare, C. J., and Switzer, W. P. New species: *Mycoplasma hyopneumoniae,* a causative agent of virus pig pneumonia. *Vet Med Small Anim Clin* **60:** 841–846, 1965.

McMartin, D. A., MacOwan, K. J., and Swift, L. L. A century of classical contagious caprine pleuropneumonia from original description to aetiology. *Br Vet J* **136:** 507–515, 1980.

Mebus, C. A., and Underdahl, N. R. Scanning electron microscopy of trachea and bronchi from gnotobiotic pigs inoculated with *Mycoplasma hyopneumoniae*. *Am J Vet Res* **38:** 1249–1254, 1977.

Ojo, M. O. Caprine pneumonia. IV. Pathogenicity of *Mycoplasma mycoides* subspecies *capri* and caprine strains of *Mycoplasma mycoides* subspecies *mycoides* for goats. *J Comp Pathol* **86:** 519–529, 1976.

Ojo, M. O. Caprine pneumonia. *Vet Bull* **47:** 573–578, 1977.

Ojo, M. O., Kasali, O. B., and Ozoya, S. E. Pathogenicity of a caprine strain of *Mycoplasma mycoides* subspecies *mycoides* for cattle. *J Comp Pathol* **90:** 209–215, 1980.

Otte, E., and Peck, E. F. Observations on an outbreak of contagious pleuropneumonia of goats in Ethiopia. *Bull Epiz Dis Afr* **8:** 131–140, 1960.

Pattison, I. H. A histological study of a transmissible pneumonia of pigs characterised by extensive lymphoid hyperplasia. *Vet Rec* **68:** 490–494, 1956.

Roberts, E. D., Switzer, W. P., and Ramsey, F. K. Pathology of the visceral organs of swine inoculated with *Mycoplasma hyorhinis*. *Am J Vet Res* **24:** 9–18, 1963.

Rosendal, S. Canine mycoplasmas: Pathogenicity of mycoplasmas associated with distemper pneumonia. *J Infect Dis* **138:** 203–210, 1978.

Rosendal, S. Experimental infection of goats, sheep, and calves with the large-colony type of *Mycoplasma mycoides* subspecies *mycoides*. *Vet Pathol* **18:** 71–81, 1981.

Rosendal, S., and Vinther, O. Experimental mycoplasmal pneumonia in dogs: Electron microscopy of infected tissue. *Acta Pathol Microbiol Scand (B)* **85:** 462–465, 1977.

Shifrine, M., and Moulton, J. E. Infection of cattle with *Mycoplasma mycoides* by nasal instillation. *J Comp Pathol* **78:** 383–386, 1968.

Stevenson, R. G. Proliferative interstitial pneumonia in lambs. *Can Vet J* **18:** 313–317, 1977.

Sullivan, N. D., St. George, T. D., and Horsfall, N. A proliferative interstitial pneumonia of sheep associated with *Mycoplasma* infection. I. Natural history of the disease in a flock. 2. The experimental exposure of young lambs to infection. *Aust Vet J* **49:** 57–62, 63–68, 1973.

Underdahl, N. R., Kennedy, G. A., and Ramos, A. S. Duration of *Mycoplasma hyopneumoniae* infection in gnotobiotic pigs. *Can Vet J* **21:** 258–261, 1980.

Whittlestone, P. Enzootic pneumonia of pigs (EPP). *Adv Vet Sci Comp Med* **17:** 1–56, 1973.

Wilkinson, G. T. Mycoplasms of the cat. *Vet Ann* **20:** 145–150, 1980.

Woodhead, G. S. Some points in the morbid anatomy and histology of pleuro-pneumonia. *J Comp Pathol* **1:** 33–36, 123–133, 339–347, 1888.

4. Chlamydial Diseases

Indigenous strains of *Chlamydia psittaci* have been associated with respiratory disease in cats, cattle, sheep, goats, and horses. Feline *C. psittaci* was the first agent isolated from cats with conjunctivitis and respiratory disease, and therefore became known rather misleadingly as the feline pneumonitis agent. It is now recognized to be mainly a cause of chronic conjunctivitis, although it can cause transient rhinitis and subclinical bronchointerstitial pneumonia. Strains of *C. psittaci* can occasionally be isolated from pneumonia in cattle, sheep, and goats. The pneumonias are usually of the enzootic type and are sometimes accompanied by enteritis. Since the intestine is a major carrier site for chlamydiae, and they can readily be isolated from feces of ruminants, inhalation of dust contaminated with feces is assumed to be a source of respiratory infection.

In all the domestic animals studied, experimental pulmonary infection by indigenous strains of *C. psittaci* causes a mild, acute bronchointerstitial pneumonia, which resolves within 3–4 weeks unless secondary bacterial invasion occurs. The extent of the pneumonia varies according to the amount of inoculum and whether it is delivered by aerosol, intranasal, or intratracheal routes, but the course of the disease remains the same. There is an initial neutrophilic bronchiolitis and alveolitis, but by 5 days after infection there is predominance of macrophages in the alveolar exudate and extensive hyperplasia of alveolar type II epithelial cells. Moderate-sized cuffs of lymphoid cells are present around bronchioles and small blood vessels at the height of the lesion, and alveolar septa are thickened by a mixed infiltrate of mononuclear cells with a few neutrophils. A similar lesion, in which chlamyd-

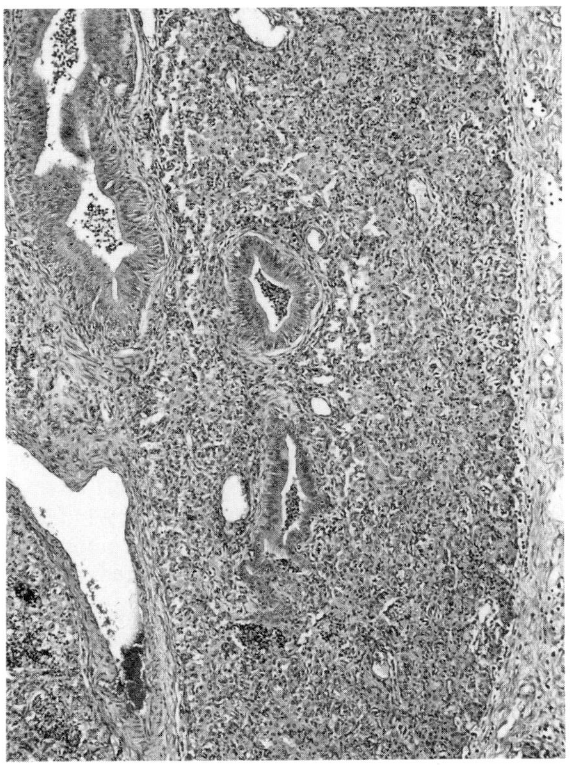

Fig. 6.84 Bronchointerstitial pneumonia caused by *Chlamydia psittaci* with epithelial hyperplasia of bronchioles and increased cellularity of atelectatic alveoli. Goat.

iae can be detected by immunofluorescence, is occasionally encountered in naturally occurring pneumonia in ruminants (Fig. 6.84). The chlamydiae are mostly destroyed during the acute phase of inflammation, which then subsides, and resolution can be complete within 3–4 weeks after experimental infection.

In assessing the importance of chlamydial infections in ruminants, it is important to note that they are usually capable of inducing only a transient inflammation. This is in contrast to mycoplasmas, which tend to persist on ciliated epithelium and cause chronic lesions. The part chlamydiae play in contributing to the cause of chronic enzootic pneumonia is therefore probably a relatively minor one.

Bibliography

Dungworth, D. L., and Cordy, D. R. The pathogenesis of ovine pneumonia. *J Comp Pathol* **72:** 49–79, 1962.

Hoover, E. A., Kahn, D. E., and Langloss, J. M. Experimentally induced feline chlamydial infection (feline pneumonitis). *Am J Vet Res* **39:** 541–548, 1978.

McChesney, S. L., England, J. J., and McChesney, A. E. *Chlamydia psittaci*-induced pneumonia in a horse. *Cornell Vet* **72:** 92–97, 1982.

Munro, R. *et al.* Pulmonary lesions in sheep following experimental infection by *Ehrlichia phagocytophilia* and *Chlamydia psittaci. J Comp Pathol* **92:** 117–129, 1982.

Omori, T., Ishii, S., and Matumoto, M. Miyagawanellosis of cattle in Japan. *Am J Vet Res* **21:** 564–573, 1960.

Ottosen, H. E. Pneumonitis in cattle. *Nord Vet Med* **9:** 569–589, 1957.

Smith, P. C., Cutlip, R. C., and Page, L. A. Pathogenicity of a strain of *Chlamydia psittaci* of bovine intestinal origin for neonatal calves. *Am J Vet Res* **34:** 615–618, 1973.

Storz, J., and Thornley, W. R. Serologische und aetiologische Studien uber die intestinale Psittakose-Lymphogranuloma-Infektion der Schafe. *Zentralblt Veterinaermed* **13:** 14–24, 1966.

York, C. J., and Baker, J. A. A new member of the psittacosis–lymphogranuloma group of viruses that causes infection in calves. *J Exp Med* **93:** 587–604, 1951.

5. *Rickettsial Diseases*

Several rickettsial and ehrlichial diseases can cause interstitial pneumonia as one of the manifestations of their systemic involvement. This is particularly true for organisms affecting vascular endothelium. The important organism of this type in animals is *Cowdria ruminantium* which causes heartwater in cattle, sheep, and goats (see The Cardiovascular System, Volume 3, Chapter 1). A mild interstitial pneumonia can be present in salmon poisoning of dogs caused by *Neorickettsia helminthoeca* (see The Alimentary System, Chapter 1, this volume).

6. *Pulmonary Mycoses*

a. Aspergillosis Fungi of the genus *Aspergillus* are ubiquitous, and exposure to the spores is an everyday matter. Nonetheless, established infections which produce disease are uncommon in mammals, although of great importance in birds. *Aspergillus fumigatus* is responsible for most infections in mammals, birds, and humans. Other species, including *A. flavus, A. niger,* and *A. nidulans,* occasionally act as pathogens.

Aspergillosis in animals is most often a respiratory infection initiated by inhaled spores. Moldy litter and feeds, especially hay and grain which have been damp and heated during storage, support an enormous growth of fungi, among which *A. fumigatus* can predominate. In view of the high rate of exposure that takes place among housed animals, it is perhaps surprising that more progressive infections are not detected. Very little is known concerning the pathogenesis of aspergillosis. It is generally assumed that a local or generalized immunodeficiency state or a breakdown of local barriers must exist for the organism to gain a foothold. Questions concerning the susceptibility of hosts, the number of spores necessary to initiate infection, toxigenicity of the organisms, and the role of immunity and hypersensitivity still have to be answered.

Aspergillosis can be a respiratory or placental disease in animals. Infections of either the upper or lower respiratory tract are sporadic in all species, but thus far infection of the pregnant uterus and fetus has been found mainly in cattle. The latter, which is described with diseases of the pregnant uterus (Volume 3, Chapter 4), is the more economically important of the two.

Aspergillosis of the respiratory tract appears often to

be a complication of some other debilitating disease, but there are cases in which no clear predisposition can be found. The infection may develop as an implantation on the mucous membrane of the nasal cavity, sinuses, guttural pouches, and tracheobronchial airways, or it may be in the form of a nodular bronchopneumonia. Secondary intestinal infections have been observed in cattle. When the fungi grow on a mucous membrane, they may be visible to the naked eye, first as a whitish growth and later as a powdery feltlike growth with a typical blue-green color produced by the conidia. These superficial colonies may develop after death, and the presence of colonies of the fungus on a mucosa is not significant unless there is tissue reaction. The usual reaction is caseating necrosis surrounded by a zone of hemorrhagic inflammation. Breakdown of these lesions in the walls of bronchi can result in bronchiectatic cavities.

The pulmonary lesions typically occur as one or many discrete gray-white nodules ~1–10 mm in diameter, with a narrow hyperemic rim. They may be obscured, especially in young animals, by severe pulmonary congestion. The nodules develop around fungal colonies which proliferate in the terminal bronchioles (Fig. 6.85B) and adjacent alveoli. The fungal colony consists of long branching, septate hyphae (Fig. 6.85A) and is surrounded by a zone of neutrophils, macrophages, and debris. The focus expands and compresses adjacent alveoli. The affected bronchioles contain plugs of purulent exudate. As is common in invasive fungal lesions of this type, occasional blood vessels are invaded, inflamed, and thrombosed. The nodules may become cavitated if they evacuate into airways. Chronic lesions are granulomatous. Macrophages and epithelioid cells predominate in the nodules and extensively infiltrate the septal tissues, and encapsulating fibroplasia is evident. Giant cells are not a significant part of the lesion, although they may be present later when the focus is being obliterated by fibrosis. Perhaps as an indication of host resistance, the form of the colonies changes in chronic infection. Instead of stretching out freely as long hyphae in all directions, as they do in early and progressive infections, the colonies become composed of shorter radiating hyphae which branch freely near their outer ends—the so-called actinomycotic forms of the fungus. Sometimes asteroid bodies can be found in the nodules and consist of small tangled remnants of the colony surrounded by radiating acidophilic clubs quite similar to those of the granules of actinomycosis (Fig. 6.85C). Dissemination of the infection from the pulmonary lesions can occur. Of the many organs, including the meninges, in which metastases develop, the kidney seems to be the most prone.

b. Mortierellosis Acute fatal mycotic pneumonia may be associated with placental infection by *Mortierella wolfii,* the most important cause of mycotic abortion of cattle

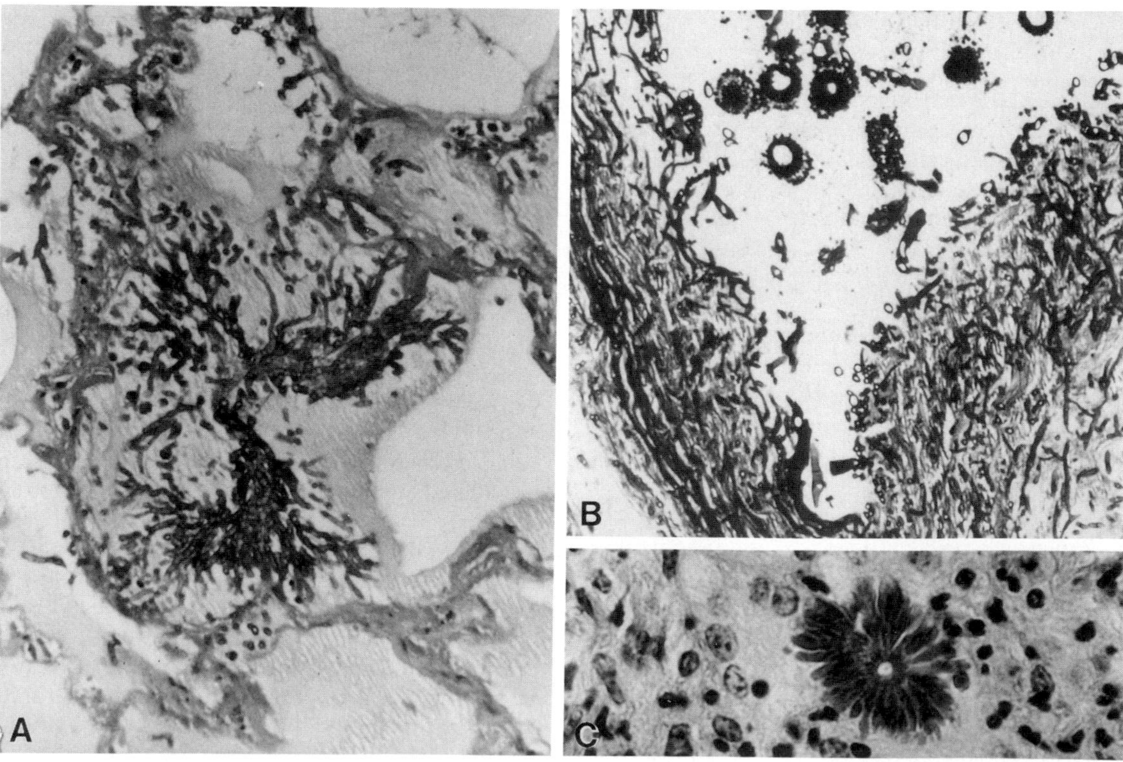

Fig. 6.85 (A) Branching septate hyphae of *Aspergillus fumigatus* in lung. Ox. (B) Mycelium invading bronchiolar wall and fruiting bodies in lumen. Pulmonary aspergillosis. Ox. (C) Chronic pulmonary aspergillosis. Ox. Clubs surrounding fungus in epithelioid cell granuloma.

in New Zealand. An acute fibrinonecrotic pneumonia can occur in infected cows at or within a few days of abortion or parturition. There is apparently extensive hematogenous dissemination of fungal elements when the placenta separates. This is followed by widespread vegetation of hyphae in pulmonary capillaries and larger vessels with resulting inflammation, thrombosis, and necrosis. Less severe pulmonary involvement leads to chronic, focal, granulomatous lesions.

Other fungi within the class Phycomycetes, such as *Mucor* and *Rhizopus* spp., are occasional opportunistic invaders of lung and are usually associated with nodular caseonecrotic or granulomatous lesions.

c. Blastomycosis Blastomycosis is a disseminated or localized mycotic infection caused by *Blastomyces dermatitidis*. It is a disease chiefly of humans and dogs in North America, Africa, Europe, and Asia. It occasionally occurs in cats, horses, and other species. The disease is sometimes referred to as North American blastomycosis to distinguish it from South American blastomycosis (*Blastomyces brasiliensis*) and European blastomycosis (*Cryptococcus neoformans*). The lesions are typically granulomatous or pyogranulomatous.

Blastomyces dermatitidis is a dimorphic fungus; in cultures at room temperature it produces a mycelial growth, whereas in tissues or culture at 37°C, it is yeastlike, 8–20 μm in diameter with a thick double-contoured wall, and reproduces by budding. The epidemiology of blastomycosis is obscure. The infection appears not to be contagious from animal to animal or animal to humans. The available evidence suggests that the source of infection is from growth on vegetation. In North America, most cases of the disease occur in the Mississippi–Ohio river basins and the central Atlantic states of the United States, and near the northern border of Ontario and Manitoba in Canada.

The disease in dogs is found predominantly in young males of large breeds. The lung is the most frequent site of primary involvement, but primary cutaneous infections are also found. Systemic dissemination often occurs and is particularly likely to cause clinical signs associated with lesions in lymph nodes, eyes, skin, subcutaneous tissue, bones and joints, and the urogenital tract. The pulmonary form of the disease is insidious in onset and has a chronic course which may last many months. The usual syndrome is one of a chronic debilitating disease with coughing, exercise intolerance, and terminal respiratory distress. The other clinical signs depend on the pattern of dissemination. The pulmonary lesions of fatal blastomycosis are multiple gray-white nodules of various sizes distributed throughout all lobes (Fig. 6.86). Superficial nodules produce elevations of the pleura, but it is exceptional for there to be pleuritis. When this does occur, it is because of fistulation from a mycotic abscess. Most pulmonary nodules are of firm granulomatous tissue, but some undergo central abscessation or caseation and then may fistulate into a bronchus or onto the pleura. Calcification is minimal or absent. Microscopically, the high frequency with which small lesions affect bronchioles and adjacent alveoli can be taken as evidence of aerogenous infection, although intrabronchial spread of organisms confuses the picture. The regional lymph nodes are consistently involved and contain granulomas, abscesses, or caseous foci. It is usual for the pulmonary nodules to be more or less of equivalent age, but it is sometimes possible to locate a larger, older caseous lesion in the lung and one in the corresponding lymph node, which together are probably comparable to the primary complex of tuberculosis.

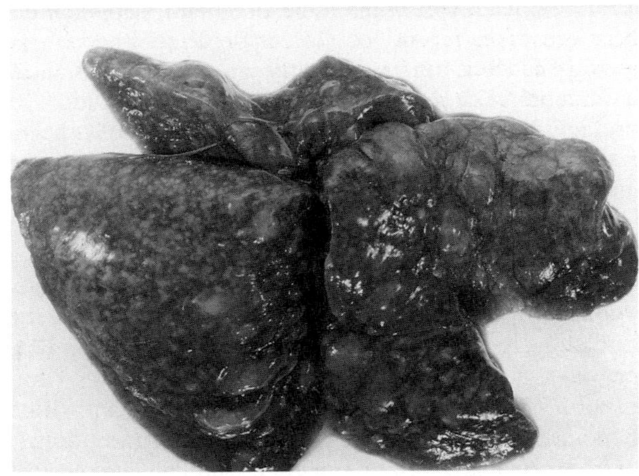

Fig. 6.86 Disseminated granulomatous foci of severe pulmonary blastomycosis. Dog.

Disseminated lesions take the same form as those in the lungs and have been observed in peripheral lymph nodes, eyes, skin, subcutaneous tissues, bones, and joints. Testes, prostate, brain, heart, liver, spleen, kidneys, intestines, and other organs are less commonly affected. The lesions are either typical granulomas with abundant epithelioid and giant cells or pyogranulomatous foci with central accumulation and necrosis of neutrophils and macrophages. The yeastlike fungi are plentiful and readily detected in the lesions, either free or in the cytoplasm of macrophages and giant cells. Identification of the organism and its characteristically broad-based, single-budding forms is aided by use of PAS or methenamine–silver stains.

The cutaneous lesions begin as papules, which soon develop into small abscesses with a surrounding inflammatory reaction. The lesions expand, with new small abscesses forming in the expanding margin of the papules while the central areas undergo some cicatrization. Microscopically, the abscesses and granulomas found within the skin and subcutis are of structure similar to that of the pulmonary lesions.

Pulmonary, cutaneous, or systemic blastomycosis occasionally occurs in cats, particularly in the Siamese breed. It has also been found rarely in horses and other species.

d. Cryptococcosis Cryptococcosis (European blastomycosis) is a subacute or chronic mycosis caused by

Cryptococcus neoformans. The organism is monomorphic, yeastlike, reproduces by single buds, and is ~4–8 μm in diameter, not including the large amount of capsular material. The disease has worldwide distribution. It may be a localized or disseminated disease, but it has a predilection for the respiratory system, particularly the nasal region, and for the central nervous system. All species of animals appear to be affected occasionally. Cats are affected more than other species.

There are several species in the genus, but only *C. neoformans* is a pathogen. It is distinguished from the nonpathogens by producing disease in experimental mice. The yeast is surrounded by a wide capsule, which is composed of mucopolysaccharides and, although cultivation of the organism is necessary for proper identification, a confident diagnosis can be made on pathologic material by identification of the capsule. The capsular material is sometimes copious enough to give the lesions a grossly mucinous texture, and it stains well with mucicarmine, the PAS reaction, or alcian blue. The capsule is wider in hydrated than in dehydrated sections. The organisms in wet mounts are not easily distinguished from erythrocytes or lymphocytes, but they are clearly evident by negative staining of the wide capsular zones with India ink or nigrosin.

The source of infection is generally believed to be soil, especially when enriched with pigeon or other bird droppings. Disease is sporadic and, as is usually true for the deep mycoses, the infection is not contagious. Cryptococci are natural saprophytes and only accidentally act as pathogens in animals with impaired local or systemic immunity. Debility, malnutrition, prolonged use of corticosteroids, and feline immunodeficiency virus infection are some of the conditions suspected of predisposing cats to cryptococcosis. Infection is acquired in most instances by inhalation of contaminated dust. The respiratory tract is the usual site of primary infection, with the nasal cavity more often affected than the lungs. The lungs are often stated to be the usual site for systemic dissemination of cryptococcal organisms, but the nasal region is probably the more important because its involvement leads much more frequently to hematogenous dissemination to central nervous system, eyes, lymph nodes, skin, and other organs than does pulmonary involvement (Fig. 6.87). There is also the possibility of local spread to the meninges and brain from nasal lesions. Local inoculation of the organism does not appear to be of general significance, although it has resulted in outbreaks of cryptococcal mastitis in cows (see The Female Genital System, Volume 3, Chapter 4). The cutaneous lesions, which are observed occasionally, may be primary or metastases following hematogenous dissemination from respiratory infection. The infection has a predilection for the central nervous system (Fig. 6.87A). Lesions can occur there without being grossly apparent in any other organ, but it is usual in the disseminated infection to find gross or microscopic lesions in some combination of the respiratory tract and other organs. Intraocular metastases may occur (Fig. 6.87B).

The cutaneous lesions of cryptococcosis take the form of firm, small nodules (Fig. 6.87C), which tend to ulcerate, discharge a small amount of serous exudate, and may then heal. In cats, the skin of the head is most commonly affected, but sometimes the lesions are distributed widely over the body. Nasal involvement was described earlier with granulomatous rhinitis. In the parenchymatous organs, the lesions are discrete, whitish, gelatinous foci, and may not be more than a few millimeters in diameter. Lesions in the meninges, brain, and cord also have a gelatinous character when they are visible, but often there are no significant gross changes. There may be some gelatinous areas in arachnoid spaces, especially around the larger vessels and in the cisterns, but the opacity of bacterial meningitis is seldom observed. The parenchymal lesions are chiefly in the peripheral gray matter and probably develop by extension of the lesions along the Virchow–Robin spaces (Fig. 6.87A).

The usual cryptococcal lesions are characterized histologically as having a soap-bubble appearance because of the unstained capsules of massed organisms. A profound cellular reaction is not typical, in contrast to other mycotic infections, and usually consists of a few macrophages, lymphocytes, and plasma cells (Fig. 6.87D). Vacuolated and degenerating macrophages may occasionally dominate the picture. Sometimes, particularly in lungs, the lesions become more typically granulomatous with numerous epithelioid and some giant cells. The lack of inflammation in regions such as the nasal cavity is probably because the capsular polysaccharide inhibits macrophages and antigen–antibody interactions. Caseation may occur in lesions in lymph nodes, but otherwise necrosis is not part of the reaction to these organisms.

When examined in sections stained by hematoxylin and eosin, the fungi appear as typical yeasts surrounded by a clear halo produced by unstained capsular substance. The capsular substance immediately around the organism is often condensed into an acidophilic rim. The free-lying organisms may calcify and stain intensely with hematoxylin.

e. Coccidioidomycosis This disease, which is caused by *Coccidioides immitis,* is important in humans but also occurs in animals in areas in which the infection is endemic. Most cases of coccidioidomycosis occur in the endemic area of the United States, which includes the arid parts of California, Arizona, and Texas. The disease is also endemic in portions of South and Central America. In arid regions, there is an association between the feces of desert rodents and high concentrations of the fungus. It is not clear to what extent numbers of organisms are increased by spherules excreted in the feces of the rodents as compared to the fecal matter enhancing vegetative growth of the organism in the soil. Vegetation of the fungus occurs in soil after rains, and subsequently, large numbers of infective arthroconidia (spores) are disseminated widely in wind-blown dust after the soil dries. It is estimated that most animals which live in endemic areas eventually become infected, but relatively few become clinically diseased.

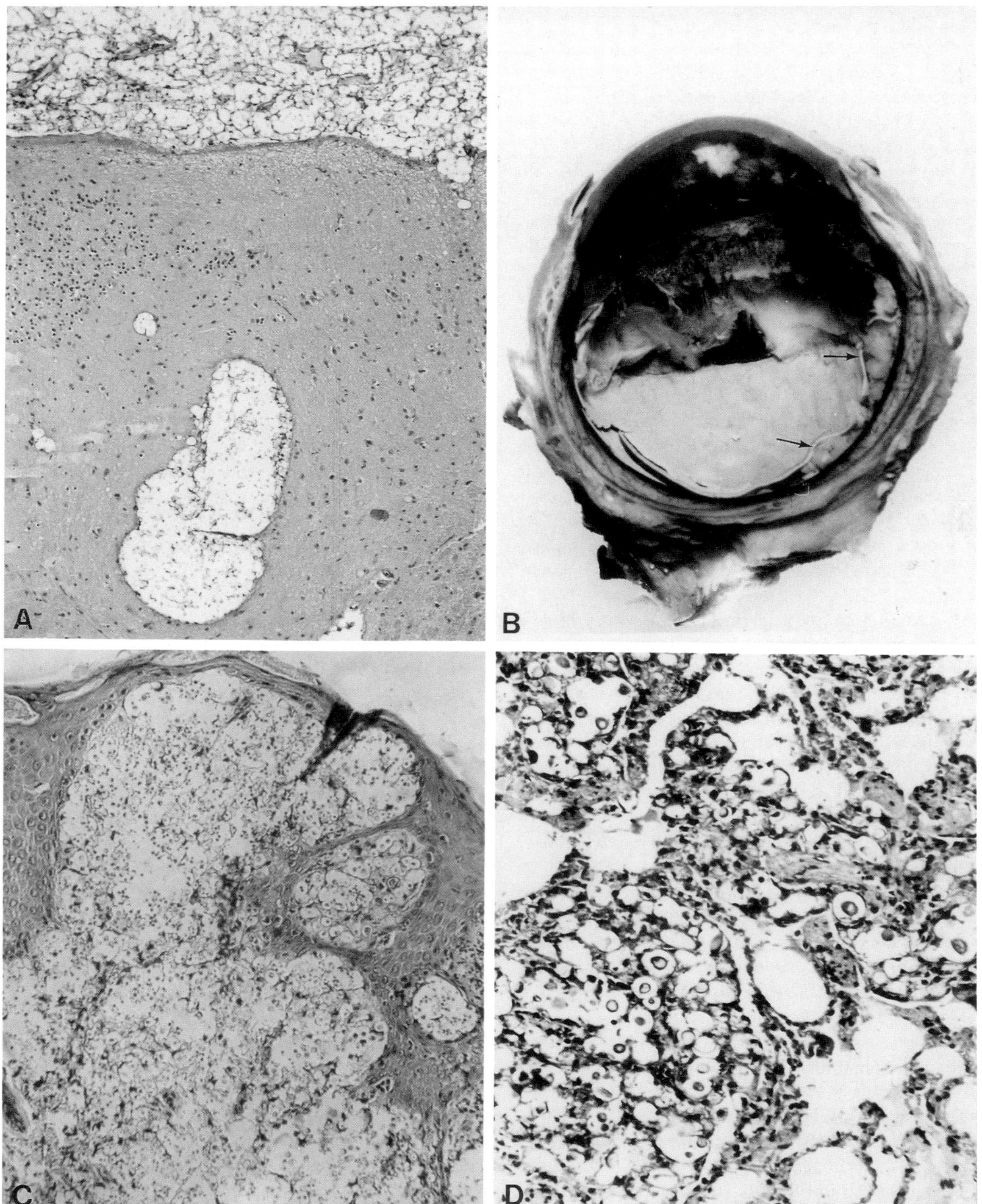

Fig. 6.87 (A) Cryptococcosis. Granulomatous meningitis with extension along Virchow–Robin space of penetrating vessel. Cat. Note characteristic soap-bubble appearance. (B) Cryptococcal choroiditis with exudative detachment of retina (arrows). Dog. (C) Cryptococcosis. Cutaneous lesion. Dog. (D) Yeastlike *C. neoformans* in pulmonary alveoli. Dog.

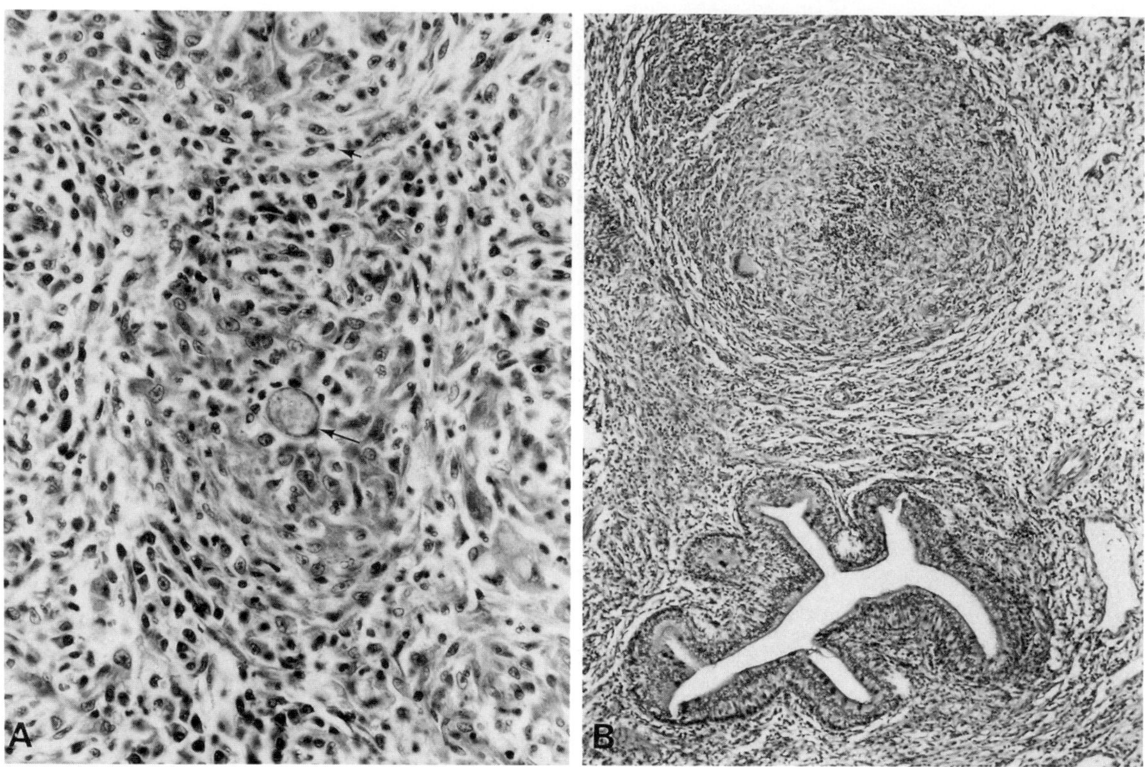

Fig. 6.88 Coccidioidomycosis. (A) Granulomatous pneumonia. Dog. Spherule (arrow) in center of small granuloma. (B) Pyogranuloma adjacent to bronchiole. Lung. Horse.

The fungus is dimorphic. In tissues, the distinctive form is a spherule (sporangium) which measures ~10–70 μm in diameter and has a thick, double-contoured wall (Fig. 6.88A). It is called a sporangium because reproduction in tissues is by endosporulation; the endospores are globose, 2–5 μm in diameter, and are released into the tissues in large numbers when a spherule ruptures. Mycelia are rare in animal tissues. On most artificial media, however, growth is mycelial. Reproduction in mycelial growth is by arthroconidia, which are produced in very large numbers along the hyphae. These arthroconidia are highly infective and easily detached from the mycelial growth.

Coccidioidomycosis is a primary respiratory infection (Fig. 6.88B). Local traumatic inoculation can occur and result in a fluctuating abscess, but dissemination from such a focus is unusual. The high susceptibility of the lungs to the establishment of infection can be demonstrated experimentally by intranasal insufflation of spores. The great majority of respiratory infections are benign and nonprogressive. This form in humans is known as San Joaquin Valley fever. A small percentage of the infections disseminate from the lung and the generalized disease is known as coccidioidal granuloma, with secondary lesions anywhere in the body. Among domestic animals, the disseminated disease has been observed mostly in dogs, and occasionally in horses, sheep, and cats. In these species, the lesions may be limited to the lungs and associated lymph nodes. In cattle and swine, lesions have so far been observed only in the lungs and their lymph nodes. The disease is common in cattle in endemic areas. As many as 20% of slaughtered cattle from feedlots in Arizona have lesions of the disease, but lesions are observed only in slaughtered animals. There is either a complete pulmonary complex or an incomplete complex with lesions only in the bronchial and mediastinal lymph nodes.

Dissemination is common only in dogs, and in this species, there is reported to be a predisposition for boxers and Doberman pinschers. The clinical signs frequently lack specificity and depend on the sites of active lesions. Persistent fever with one or more of respiratory abnormalities, shifting lameness, and the development of cutaneous nodules suggests the diagnosis in chronically ill dogs in endemic areas. The lameness is ephemeral when first seen, and radiographic evidence of the underlying osteomyelitis (Fig. 6.89A,B) is obvious only late in the course of disease. Usually the progressive debility leads to cachexia and eventual death, although recoveries do occur.

The lesions of coccidioidomycosis are granulomas or pyogranulomas (Fig. 6.88A,B). The granulomas are grayish white and usually nodular. There may be central caseation necrosis or liquefaction, but calcification is unusual. A common finding, particularly in the dog, is that large granulomatous nodules are composed of collections of discretely unitized small granulomas separated by fibrous tissue (Fig. 6.88A). The cellular reaction on the part of the host depends on the phase of the organism against which

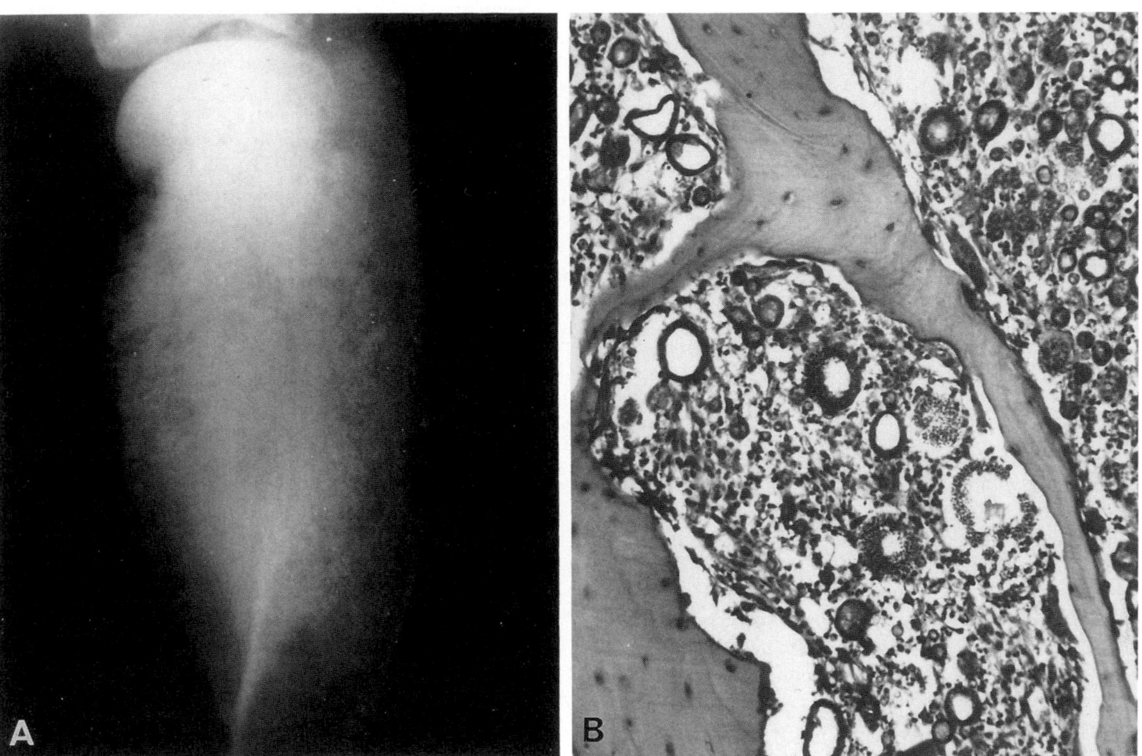

Fig. 6.89 (A) Coccidioidomycosis. Radiograph of coccidioidal osteomyelitis. Dog. (B) Granulomatous osteomyelitis from (A). There are spherules in various stages of their developmental cycle.

it is directed. Spores, whether endospores or the initial arthroconidia, provoke an acute exudative reaction in which neutrophils predominate. The larger spherules are usually surrounded by a wide zone of epithelioid cells mixed with a few giant cells, lymphocytes, and neutrophils. Because the organisms in any large focus are often in different phases of growth, there can be variations in the proportions of suppurative and granulomatous responses. In contained infections, however, the granulomatous response predominates, and it may then be difficult to find organisms. In such cases, they are most likely to be found in the cytoplasm of giant cells as large spherules which are either evacuated and crenated or contain endospores. Often in cattle, and occasionally in other species, the spherules become surrounded by a corona of acidophilic clubs similar to those which form around colonies of *Actinomyces bovis* and some other microorganisms. This is an indication of high host resistance.

A variety of other fungal diseases can affect the lung, the most important being histoplasmosis (see The Hematopoietic System, Volume 3, Chapter 2). Among the occasional opportunistic infections are sporotrichosis (*Sporothrix schenckii*), adiaspiromycosis (*Emmonsia* spp.) and geotrichosis (*Geotrichium candidum*).

Bibliography

Ajello, L. Comparative ecology of respiratory mycotic disease agents. *Bacteriol Rev* **31:** 6–24, 1967.

Austwick, P. K. C., Gitter, M., and Watkins, C. V. Pulmonary aspergillosis in lambs. *Vet Rec* **72:** 19–21, 1960.

Balwant, S., Chawla, R. S., and Sanota, P. Phycomycotic pneumonia in a pig. *Ind Vet J* **53:** 818, 1976.

Barron, C. N. Cryptococcosis in animals. *J Am Vet Med Assoc* **127:** 125–132, 1955.

Benbrook, E. A., Bryant, J. B., and Saunders, L. Z. A case of blastomycosis in the horse. *J Am Vet Med Assoc* **112:** 475–478, 1948.

Buchanan, C. A. Feline cryptococcosis: A case report and review. *Southwest Vet* **35:** 41–44, 1982.

Chauhan, H. V. S., and Dwivedi, P. Pneumomycosis in sheep and goats. *Vet Rec* **95:** 58–59, 1974.

Cordes, D. O., Dodd, D. C., and O'Hara, P. J. Acute mycotic pneumonia of cattle. *N Z Vet J* **12:** 101–104, 1964.

Cordes, D. O., Carter, M. E., and di Menna, M. E. Mycotic pneumonia and placentitis caused by *Mortierella wolfii*. II. Pathology of experimental infection in cattle. *Vet Pathol* **9:** 190–201, 1972.

Forbus, W. D., and Bestebreurtje, A. M. Coccidioidomycosis. A study of 95 cases of the disseminated type with special reference to the pathogenesis of the disease. *Milit Surg* **99:** 653–719, 1946.

Harrell, E. R., and Curtis, A. C. North American blastomycosis. *Am J Med* **27:** 750–766, 1959.

Hatkin, J. M., Phillips, W. E., and Utroska, W. R. Two cases of feline blastomycosis. *J Am Anim Hosp Assoc* **15:** 217–220, 1979.

Hilbert, B. J., Huxtable, C. R., and Pawley, S. E. Cryptococcal pneumonia in a horse. *Aust Vet J* **56:** 391–392, 1980.

Holzworth, J., and Coffin, D. L. Cryptococcosis in a cat. *Cornell Vet* **43:** 546–550, 1953.
Hugenholtz, P. G. *et al.* Experimental coccidioidomycosis in dogs. *Am J Vet Res* **19:** 433–439, 1958.
Ivanov, X. Ustilagineous pneumonia in cattle. The spores of *Ustilago maydis* as a pathogenic factor. *C R Acad Bulg Sci* **2:** 49–52, 1949.
Koller, L. D., and Helfer, D. H. Adiaspiromycosis in the lungs of a goat (associated with *Pieris japonica* poisoning). *J Am Vet Med Assoc* **173:** 80–81, 1978.
Koller, L. D., Patton, N. M., and Whitsett, D. K. Adiaspiromycosis in the lungs of a dog. *J Am Vet Med Assoc* **169:** 1316–1317, 1976.
Maddy, K. T. Coccidioidomycosis in animals. *Vet Med* **54:** 233–242, 1959.
Newberne, J. W., Neal, J. E., and Heath, M. K. Some clinical and microbiological observations in four cases of canine blastomycosis. *J Am Vet Med Assoc* **127:** 220–223, 1955.
Nyaga, P. N. *et al.* Canine pulmonary geotrichosis: Case report. *Kenya Vet* **4:** 6–9, 1980.
Pappagianis, D., and Kobayashi, G. S. Approaches to the physiology of *Coccidioides immitis*. *Ann N Y Acad Sci* **89:** 109–120, 1960.
Ramsey, F. K., and Carter, G. R. Canine blastomycosis in the United States. *J Am Vet Med Assoc* **120:** 93–98, 1952.
Robbins, E. S. North American blastomycosis in the dog. *J Am Vet Med Assoc* **125:** 391–397, 1954.
Ryan, M. J., and Wyand, D. S. *Cryptococcus* as a cause of neonatal pneumonia and abortion in two horses. *Vet Pathol* **18:** 270–272, 1981.
Saunders, L. Z. Systemic fungous infections in animals: A review. *Cornell Vet* **38:** 213–238, 1948.
Seibold, H. R. Systemic blastomycosis in dogs. *North Am Vet* **27:** 162–164, 1946.
Sharma, D. N., and Dwivedi, J. N. Pulmonary mycosis of sheep and goats in India. *Indian J Anim Sci* **47:** 808–813, 1977.
Smith, D. L. T., Fischer, J. B., and Barnum, D. A. Generalized *Cryptococcus neoformans* infection in a dog. *Can Med Assoc J* **72:** 18–20, 1955.
Smith, H. A. Coccidioidomycosis in animals. *Am J Pathol* **24:** 223–233, 1948.
Wilkinson, G. T. Feline cryptococcosis: A review and seven case reports. *J Small Anim Pract* **20:** 749–768, 1979.
Zontine, W. J. Coccidioidomycosis in the horse—a case report. *J Am Vet Med Assoc* **131:** 490–492, 1958.

f. *Pneumocystis carinii* *Pneumocystis carinii* is an organism of uncertain taxonomic status, which is widespread as a latent infection in the lungs of animals. It has been considered in the past to be either a fungus in the class Ascomycetes or a protozoan. Currently the evidence perhaps favors a fungal nature, but the issue is not resolved.

Pneumocystis carinii is an important cause of pneumonia in various forms of congenital or acquired immunodeficiency states in humans, particularly in association with human immunodeficiency virus infection. Latent infection in rats can be regularly converted to the active disease by

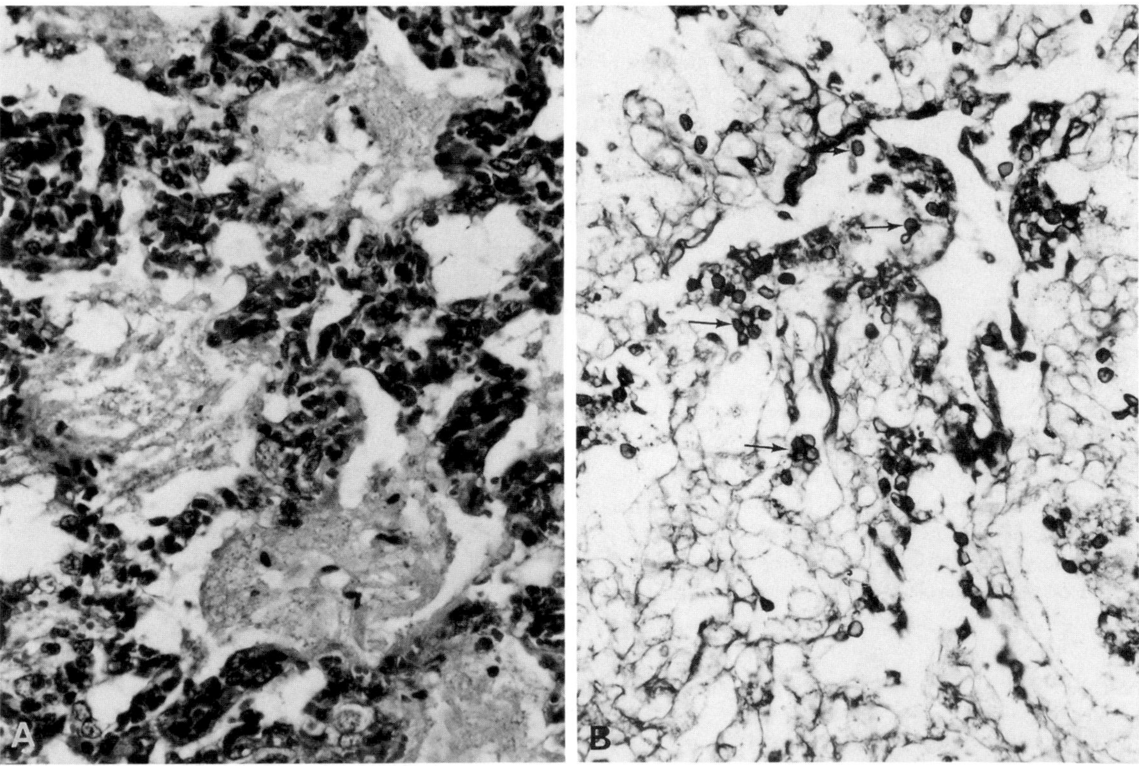

Fig. 6.90 Adenovirus infection in Arabian foal with combined immunodeficiency. *Pneumocystis* pneumonia complicating adenovirus infection. (A) Alveoli contain abundant foamy and granular acidophilic material. (B) *Pneumocystis carinii* organisms revealed by methenamine–silver stain (arrows).

administration of corticosteroids. *Pneumocystis* pneumonia has been recorded occasionally in the young dog, foal, goat, and pig as well as in laboratory animals. In horses, it appears mainly in Arabian foals with known or suspect congenital immunodeficiency, sometimes as a complication of adenovirus or other infectious pneumonia. Most of the reported canine cases have been in miniature dachshunds ranging from about 8 to 24 months in age, raising the possibility of a heritable immunodeficiency in this breed. Clinical signs are gradually increasing exercise intolerance, respiratory difficulties, and progressive loss of weight.

Gross lesions associated with *Pneumocystis* pneumonia are diffuse or patchy, red to yellow-brown regions of rubbery firmness or consolidation. The appearance may be modified by coexisting viral or bacterial pneumonia. Histologically, *P. carinii* causes a diffuse interstitial pneumonia in which the characteristic feature is prominent filling of alveoli by a foamy, pale acidophilic material (Fig. 6.90A). The amount of interstitial inflammation varies from minimal to moderate accumulation of lymphocytes, plasma cells, and macrophages. There are various degrees of hyperplasia of alveolar type II epithelial cells (epithelialization) and accumulation of macrophages within alveolar lumina. Fibrosis accompanies intense cellular inflammation within alveolar septa.

Pneumocystis carinii stains poorly with hematoxylin and eosin and is therefore easily overlooked. Its presence should be suspected when alveoli contain abundant, foamy, pale eosinophilic material, especially in the absence of significant inflammatory hallmarks. This is particularly important in young animals, in which there may be congenital, drug-induced, or disease-induced immunodeficiency. The foamy acidophilic material consists mainly of trophozoite and cyst forms of the organism. These may be seen as indistinct outlines of erythrocyte-sized structures, possibly with the presence of pale basophilic dots. The organism is best demonstrated histologically by methenamine–silver staining. This reveals the argyrophilic capsules of the cysts and trophozoites as round, distorted, or crescentic structures from 3 to 8 μm in width (Fig. 6.90B). The PAS stain is not so satisfactory for demonstration of the organism.

Current evidence indicates that *P. carinii* is mainly kept in check by alveolar macrophages in normal animals, but that this process fails in immunodeficient states. Progressive colonization of alveolar type I epithelial cells by *P. carinii* causes their necrosis and replacement by type II cells, with eventual filling of alveoli by the organisms and acellular material rich in alveolar surfactant lipid.

Bibliography

Bille-Hansen, V. *et al. Pneumocystis carinii* pneumonia in Danish piglets. *Vet Rec* **127:** 407–408, 1990.

Botha, W. S., and van Rensburg, I. B. J. Pneumocystosis: A chronic respiratory distress syndrome in the dog. *J S Afr Vet Assoc* **50:** 173–179, 1979.

Copland, J. W. Canine pneumonia caused by *Pneumocystis carinii*. *Aust Vet J* **50:** 515–518, 1974.

Farrow, B. R. H. *et al. Pneumocystis* pneumonia in the dog. *J Comp Pathol* **82:** 447–453, 1972.

Lanken, P. N. *et al.* Alveolar response to experimental *Pneumocystis carinii* pneumonia in the rat. *Am J Pathol* **99:** 561–578, 1980.

McConnell, E. E., Basson, P. A., and Pienaar, J. G. Pneumocystosis in a domestic goat. *Onderstepoort J Vet Res* **38:** 117–126, 1971.

Seibold, H. R., and Munnell, J. F. *Pneumocystis carinii* in a pig. *Vet Pathol* **14:** 89–91, 1977.

Shively, J. N. *et al. Pneumocystis carinii* pneumonia in two foals. *J Am Vet Med Assoc* **162:** 648–652, 1973.

Shively, J. N., Moe, K. K., and Dellers, R. W. Fine structure of spontaneous *Pneumocystis carinii* pulmonary infection in foals. *Cornell Vet* **64:** 72–88, 1974.

Walzer, P. D. *et al.* Growth characteristics and pathogenesis of experimental *Pneumocystis carinii* pneumonia. *Infect Immun* **27:** 928–937, 1980.

7. Enzootic Pneumonia

Enzootic pneumonia refers to pneumonia that is prevalent in groups of young animals maintained in close contact. It is mainly of importance in calves, lambs, and young pigs. Since it is an epidemiologic term, it allows considerable latitude in the morphologic and etiologic types of pneumonia it embraces. Both acute exudative bronchopneumonias and more chronic bronchointerstitial pneumonias have been included under the general designation of enzootic pneumonia, but the emphasis has differed according to the species of animal concerned, as will be evident from the following discussion.

Enzootic pneumonia of calves is a disease complex in intensively managed calves which is caused by the synergistic action of two or more of a wide variety of viruses, mycoplasmas and bacteria. The morphologic appearance of the pneumonia varies according to the mix of agents and the age of lesions encountered. The disease mainly affects calves <6 months of age and is of most importance as a cause of unthriftiness. Mortality is low unless there is a coincidence of highly pathogenic agents and predisposing factors associated with poor husbandry and possibly intercurrent disease.

Evidence to date indicates that the acute pneumonia is usually initiated by viral infection. More than one species of virus may be involved in an outbreak or even in a single calf. The relative importance of the 10 or so candidate viruses varies geographically to some extent. In general, respiratory syncytial and parainfluenza 3 viruses are considered to be most important. Infectious bovine rhinotracheitis virus, adenovirus, and the bovine virus diarrhea virus are the next most commonly mentioned. The lesions caused by those and the other viral respiratory pathogens were described earlier in this chapter. Although calves can die because of acute, uncomplicated viral lesions, most fatal cases have a superimposed acute bacterial bronchopneumonia or lobar pneumonia. These have the acute fibrinonecrotic to suppurative exudation characteristic of severe bacterial infection, particularly by *Pasteurella haemolytica* and *Pasteurella multocida*. More than 20 different species of bacteria have been isolated at various times, however, often in mixed infection. Next to *Pasteurella* spp., the most common are *Streptobacillus actinoides, Actinomyces pyogenes,* and *Escherichia coli.* Chlamydiae may also be involved occasionally. Since most fatal pneumonias are predominantly the result of bacterial activity, clearly establishing the initial role of viral infection can be difficult and requires attempts to isolate viruses by culture, to demonstrate their presence by immunofluorescence and electron microscopy, and to obtain serologic evidence of an active infection in the affected groups. Histologic search for inclusion bodies is usually unrewarding in fatal field cases, but pays dividends often enough to make the attempt necessary.

Mycoplasmas, especially *M. bovis, M. dispar,* and *Ureaplasma* spp., are implicated in contributing to the acute form of enzootic pneumonia, together with viruses and bacteria. *Mycoplasma bovis* has been established as an important pathogen in its own right. It is more invasive than other mycoplasmas isolated from enzootic pneumonia in calves and experimentally has been shown to cause an acute suppurative bronchopneumonia in which foci of coagulation necrosis are often present. These can to some extent be differentiated from the necrotic foci caused by *Pasteurella* spp., in that necrosis is a less dramatic feature of the *M. bovis*-induced lesion, fibrin deposition is not a significant feature, the necrotic zones do not cross interlobular septa, neutrophils are not a prominent component, and there is not the secondary alteration of leukocytes to form the fusiform oat cells. Immunoperoxidase labeling methods for detection of antigen in necrotic foci are an important diagnostic aid. Isolation of *M. bovis* has also been correlated with outbreaks of more severe enzootic pneumonia in some calf populations, although still as part of mixed infections. Foci of necrosis similar to those produced by experimental *M. bovis* infection are present in some of the naturally occurring cases.

Mycoplasmas are also important in causing the chronic form of enzootic pneumonia. This is the grayish-pink, meaty consolidation of cranioventral regions of the lung found in slaughtered veal calves or calves dying from other diseases. Histologically it is a chronic bronchointerstitial pneumonia with both exudative and proliferative components (see Mycoplasmal Bronchiolitis and Pneumonia of Calves, Section VI,H,3,a,ii of this chapter). This type of lesion appears to represent persistent infection by both the mycoplasmas and bacteria of species similar to those found in more acute lesions. The usual course of chronic enzootic pneumonia is that of a low-grade inflammatory lesion which resolves in several months to a year. The term cuffing pneumonia has been used for chronic enzootic pneumonia in which a dramatic feature is sheathing of small airways by lymphofollicular proliferations. Acute exudative bacterial pneumonia can supervene at any time and cause severe clinical disease or death if the calf's pulmonary defenses are impaired or there is additional infection by virulent pathogens. An alternative sequel is chronic suppurative bronchopneumonia with bronchiectasis, abscessation, and scarring.

Enzootic pneumonia of lambs has many similarities to enzootic pneumonia of calves. The acute form is manifest as pneumonic pasteurellosis, and has been described under that heading. The chronic, enzootic, bronchointerstitial pneumonia (Fig. 6.91) has features similar to those of enzootic mycoplasmal pneumonia of swine mentioned previously. Because the term enzootic pneumonia was used initially only for acute pneumonic pasteurellosis in sheep, various descriptive terms have been used for the chronic form. The most frequent ones are proliferative interstitial, proliferative exudative, atypical, and chronic nonprogressive. To avoid confusion, however, the chronic bronchointerstitial pneumonia of lambs should also be referred to as an enzootic pneumonia, just as it is in calves and pigs.

The causes of chronic enzootic pneumonia in lambs are not completely established. The disease can be regularly produced by intratracheal inoculation of a suspension of pneumonic lung. Attempts to produce the disease using various combinations of cultured microorganisms isolated from pneumonic lung have indicated that intratracheal or endobronchial inoculation of mixed strains of *Mycoplasma ovipneumoniae* and *Pasteurella haemolytica* is the most successful. *Bordetella parapertussis* is capable of producing a mild, acute bronchopneumonia, and the organism can be isolated frequently from cases of chronic enzootic pneumonia. It therefore seems that most cases of chronic enzootic pneumonia in lambs probably involve the synergistic action of *M. ovipneumoniae, P. haemolytica,* and *B. parapertussis.* One of these agents alone or in combination with other infectious agents may occasionally be responsible. The active pneumonic consolidation persists for ~3–12 weeks after infection and largely resolves within a few months unless acute bacterial exacerbations occur. Since the disease is not usually fatal, the characteristic cranioventral consolidations (Fig. 6.91A) are mostly seen in slaughtered lambs or those dying of other diseases.

Enzootic pneumonia of swine is generally held to be synonymous with enzootic mycoplasmal pneumonia (see Respiratory Mycoplasmosis of Swine, Section VI,H,3,d of this chapter).

Bibliography

Barr, J. *et al.* Enzootic pneumonia in calves. 1. The natural disease. *Vet Rec* **63:** 652–654, 1951.

Bryson, D. G. *et al.* Observations on outbreaks of respiratory disease in housed calves—(2) pathological and microbiological findings. *Vet Rec* **103:** 503–509, 1978.

Chen, W. *et al.* Pneumonia in lambs inoculated with *Bordetella parapertussis:* Bronchoalveolar lavage and ultrastructural studies. *Vet Pathol* **25:** 297–303, 1988.

Chen, W., Alley, M. R., and Manktelow, B. W. Pneumonia in lambs inoculated with *Bordetella parapertussis:* Clinical and pathological studies. *N Z Vet J* **36:** 138–142, 1988.

Davies, D. H., Jones, B. A. H., and Thurley, D. C. Infection of specific-pathogen-free lambs with parainfluenza virus type 3,

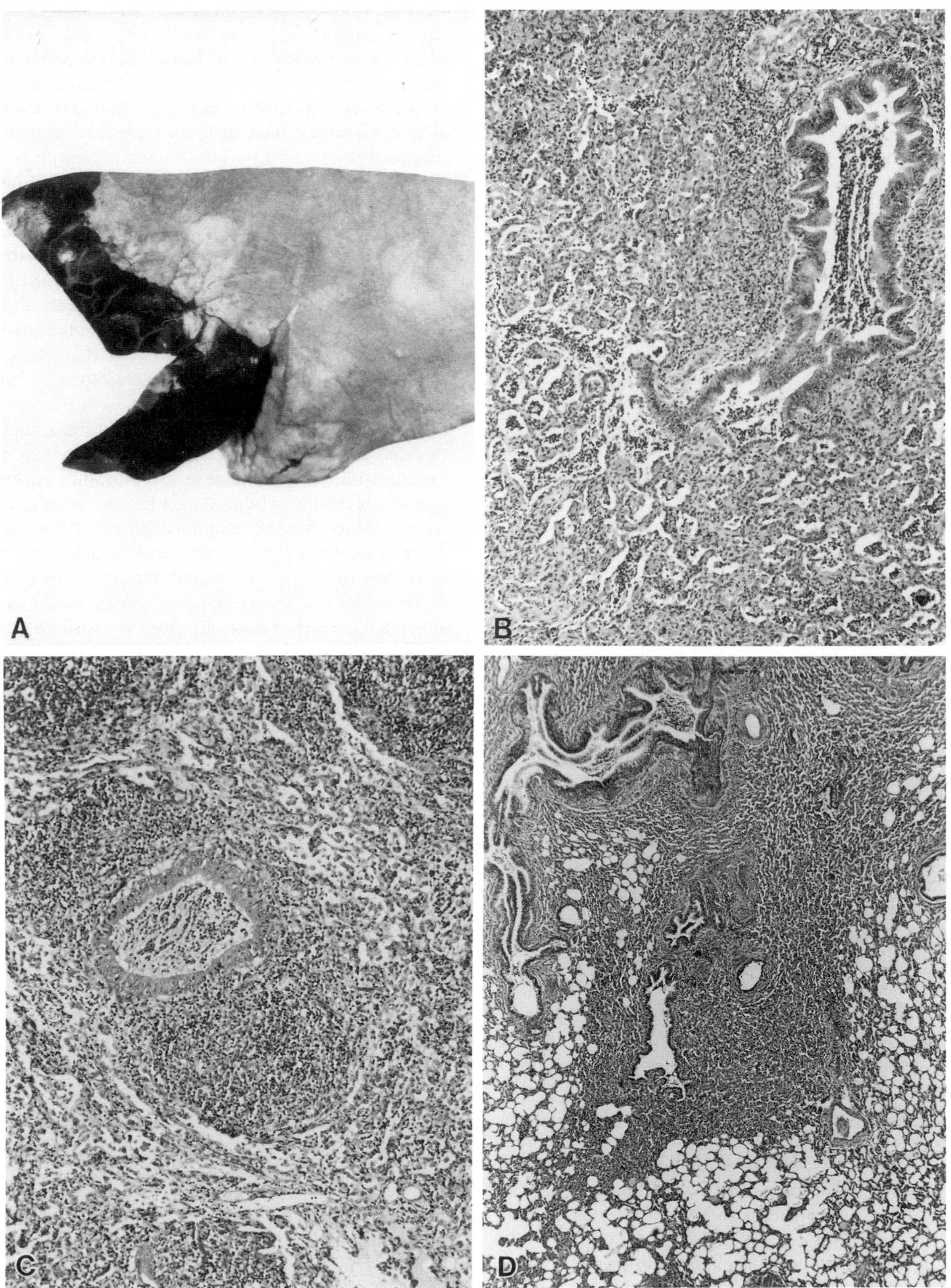

Fig. 6.91 Chronic enzootic pneumonia. Lamb. (A) Confluent cranioventral consolidation. (B) Histology of (A) showing bronchointerstitial pneumonia with mixed exudative and proliferative components. (C) Prominent peribronchiolar lymphofollicular nodules in chronic lesion. (D) Residual atelectasis in resolving pneumonia.

Pasteurella haemolytica, and *Mycoplasma ovipneumoniae. Vet Microbiol* **6:** 295–308, 1981.

Gilmour, J. S., Jones, G. E., and Rae, A. G. Experimental studies of chronic pneumonia of sheep. *Comp Immunol. Microbiol Infect Dis* **1:** 285–293, 1979.

Gilmour, J. S. *et al.* Long-term pathological and microbiological progress in sheep of experimental disease resembling atypical pneumonia. *J Comp Pathol* **92:** 229–238, 1982.

Gourlay, R. N., and Houghton, S. B. Experimental pneumonia in conventionally reared and gnotobiotic calves by dual infection with *Mycoplasma bovis* and *Pasteurella haemolytica. Res Vet Sci* **38:** 377–382, 1985.

Jarrett, W. F. H. The pathology of some types of pneumonia and associated pulmonary diseases of the calf. *Br Vet J* **112:** 431–452, 1956.

Jones, G. E., Gilmour, J. S., and Rae, A. G. I. The effect of *Mycoplasma ovipneumoniae* and *Pasteurella haemolytica* on specific-pathogen-free lambs. *J Comp Pathol* **92:** 261–266, 1982.

Omar, A. R. The aetiology and pathology of pneumonia in calves. *Vet Bull* **36:** 259–273, 1966.

Salisbury, R. M. Enzootic pneumonia of sheep in New Zealand. *N Z Vet J* **5:** 124–127, 1957.

Stamp, J. T., and Nisbet, D. I. Pneumonia of sheep. *J Comp Pathol* **73:** 319–328, 1963.

Thomas, L. H. *et al.* A search for new microorganisms in calf pneumonia by the inoculation of gnotobiotic calves. *Res Vet Sci* **33:** 170–182, 1982.

Thomas, L. H. *et al. Mycoplasma bovis* infection in gnotobiotic calves and combined infection with respiratory syncytial virus. *Vet Pathol* **23:** 571–578, 1986.

8. *Interstitial Pneumonia of Cattle*

The general features and wide range of causes of interstitial pneumonia were discussed in the section on Interstitial Pneumonia (Section VI,F,3 of this chapter). The condition in cattle is deserving of further mention, however, because of its frequency and the confusion concerning its causes.

Acute interstitial pneumonia is the result of acute diffuse damage to alveolar septa. Characteristic features in cattle are pulmonary hyperemia, alveolar edema, and hyaline membrane formation, hyperplasia of alveolar type II epithelial cells, and interstitial emphysema and edema. Other components may be present, such as larvae and eosinophils when migrating helminth larvae are the cause, but in general the lesion is nonspecific. Extensive interstitial emphysema and edema are usually found only in cows dying after a bout of severe, labored respiration. When this is prolonged, the interstitial emphysema can dissect through the mediastinum and reach subcutaneous regions of the back. Since the structure of the bovine lung predisposes it to the development of interstitial emphysema when there is severe pulmonary insufficiency and labored respiration for any cause, the diagnosis of acute interstitial pneumonia cannot be made solely on the basis of air in the pulmonary interstitium.

Various terms have been used for acute interstitial pneumonia in cattle, the most common one being atypical interstitial pneumonia, in recognition of the acute exudative nature of the process. Other terms have been used in certain geographic regions and have emphasized epidemiologic or morphologic features, the latter usually misleadingly. Examples are fog fever and acute bovine pulmonary emphysema and edema for pasture-associated acute interstitial pneumonia in Britain and the United States, respectively.

The pasture-associated condition usually occurs in adult, beef-type cattle soon after a change from sparse summer range or pasture to relatively lush pastures containing regrowth following removal of a crop for hay or silage. Cows dying of the disease have gross lesions dominated by interstitial emphysema and edema. Major airways contain abundant white foam. The pulmonary parenchyma is purplish to brownish red, depending on the acuteness of the disease, and affected lobules have a homogeneous, moist cut section and a soft rubbery texture (Fig. 6.42A,B). Irregular lobular or sublobular distribution of the lesions occurs to some extent. There is a tendency for most diffuse involvement to be found in dorsocaudal regions of the lungs. Histologically, the main features are as outlined previously, but hyperplasia of alveolar type II epithelial cells is not a pronounced feature until 4–6 days after the onset of the alveolar damage (Fig. 6.42C,D), and at this stage the term subacute can be used. Cows that survive the acute episode usually have residual interstitial fibrosis and some persistence of alveolar type II epithelial cells (Fig. 6.44).

The pasture-associated form of acute interstitial pneumonia is probably related to increased amounts of L-tryptophan in the ingested feed; the quantity of L-tryptophan can be sufficient to provide toxic levels of 3-methylindole under the special conditions of rumen fermentation occurring at the time of change in pasture. Acute interstitial pneumonia can also be caused by the pneumotoxic activity of (1) 4-ipomeanol and related furanoterpenoids from sweet potatoes spoiled by the mold *Fusarium solani;* (2) perilla ketone from purple mint (*Perilla frutescens*); and (3) an unidentified toxin from stinkwood (*Zieria arborescens*). The condition has also been reported following ingestion of garden beans contaminated with the mold *Fusarium semitectum*. Apart from chemical toxins, a similar lesion can be caused by massive invasion of the lungs by larvae of *Dictyocaulus viviparus* or, less commonly, *Ascaris suum* (see Parasitic Diseases of the Lungs, Section VI,I of this chapter).

Acute interstitial pneumonia also occurs occasionally in housed or feed-lot cattle. There is frequently an associated, more chronic, cranioventral bronchopneumonia. The factor or factors involved in the pathogenesis of the acute interstitial pneumonia occurring under these circumstances are not understood, however. The association of severe infection with bovine respiratory syncytial virus and acute interstitial emphysema, particularly in newly weaned calves in the fall, has given rise to the suggestion that the respiratory syncytial virus alone can cause an acute interstitial pneumonia under certain circumstances. This is not proven, and it is probable that a degree of acute alveolar damage and development of extensive interstitial emphysema can be final common events in cattle with various forms of severe primary pulmonary damage.

Chronic interstitial pneumonia in cattle occurs chiefly as a manifestation of **hypersensitivity pneumonitis.** This condition is also referred to as bovine farmer's lung or extrinsic allergic alveolitis and is caused by inhalation of dust from moldy hay which contains spores of *Micropolyspora faeni* and other thermophilic actinomycetes. The disease develops primarily in the winter in housed dairy animals. Death does not usually result from lesions occurring early in the disease. If lungs are available for examination, careful search reveals multiple, small, gray, subpleural foci and many pulmonary lobules with slightly pale, hyperinflated peripheral zones. Characteristic histologic lesions are a lymphocytic and plasmacytic bronchitis and bronchiolitis, often with severe obliterative bronchiolitis, the presence of scattered granulomas composed of epithelioid and giant cells, and thickening of alveolar septa by infiltration of lymphocytes, plasma cells, and macrophages. Eosinophils, globule leukocytes, and increased mast cells are usually present. Cattle are more likely to die as the result of severe, chronic disease. Additional features of severe interstitial fibrosis, accumulation of alveolar macrophages, and hyperplasia of alveolar type II epithelial cells are present in such cases. There can also be metaplasia of type II cells to ciliated or mucus-secreting cells. Vascular compromise can lead to pulmonary hypertension and cor pulmonale in a small proportion of cases. In these advanced cases, epithelioid granulomas are inconspicuous or absent. The lungs grossly are pale and heavy. Most severely affected lobules are yellow-white and fibrous or may show evidence of distortion and enlargement of airspaces by the scarring (honeycombing). Asteroids caused by *Aspergillus* spp. may also be present in these lungs because the conditions leading to heavy exposure to dusts containing *M. faeni* are also those in which large numbers of spores of *Aspergillus* spp. are present.

A chronic interstitial pneumonia (diffuse fibrosing alveolitis) similar to that occurring in dairy cattle with advanced hypersensitivity pneumonitis is sometimes seen in pastured beef cattle. Its cause remains undetermined.

Bibliography

Breeze, R. G. *et al.* The pathology of respiratory diseases of adult cattle in Britain. *Folia Veterinaria Latina* **5:** 95–128, 1975.

Dawson, C. O. *et al.* Studies on the incidence and titres of precipitatin antibody to *Micropolyspora faeni* in sera from adult cattle. *J Comp Pathol* **87:** 287–299, 1977.

Dickinson, E. O., Spencer, G. R., and Gorham, J. R. Experimental induction of an acute respiratory syndrome in cattle resembling bovine pulmonary emphysema. *Vet Rec* **80:** 487–487, 1967.

Doster, A. R. *et al.* Effects of 4-ipomeanol, a product from mold-damaged sweet potatoes, on the bovine lung. *Vet Pathol* **15:** 367–375, 1978.

Hammond, A. C. *et al.* 3-Methylindole and naturally occurring acute bovine pulmonary edema and emphysema. *Am J Vet Res* **40:** 1398–1401, 1979.

Logan, A. *et al.* Experimental production of diffuse pulmonary fibrosis and alveolitis in cattle: The effects of repeated dosage with 3-methylindole. *Res Vet Sci* **34:** 97–108, 1983.

Nicolet, J., de Haller, R., and Scholar, H. J. La pneumonie d'Uri: Une pneumonie allergique au foin moisi chez le bovin. *Pathol Microbiol* **34:** 252–253, 1969.

Nicolet, J., de Haller, R., and Herzog, J. Serological investigations of a bovine respiratory disease ("Urner Pneumonie") resembling farmer's lung. *Infect Immun* **6:** 38–42, 1972.

Piris, H. M., and Selman, I. E. A bovine disease resembling diffuse fibrosing alveolitis. *Proc R Soc Med* **65:** 987–990, 1972.

Wilkie, B. N. Bovine allergic pneumonitis: An acute outbreak associated with mouldy hay. *Can J Comp Med* **42:** 10–15, 1978.

Wilkie, B. N. Allergic respiratory disease. *Adv Vet Sci Comp Med* **26:** 233–266, 1982.

Wilson, B. J. *et al.* Perilla ketone: A potent lung toxin from the mint plant, *Perilla frutescens* Britton. *Science* **197:** 573–574, 1977.

Wiseman, A. *et al.* Bovine farmer's lung: A clinical syndrome in a herd of cattle. *Vet Rec* **93:** 410–417, 1973.

I. Parasitic Diseases of the Lungs

The lungs are at the crossroads of parasitic migrations, and the many parasites which pass through them cause various degrees of damage according to the nature and intensity of the host–parasite interaction. Usually, the lesions produced by transient parasites are of slight significance and are resolvable. There are exceptions, however. Severe and possibly fatal pulmonary lesions may develop if the migrating parasites are large in number or large in size, or especially when the host has a hypersensitivity reaction to them. Hypersensitivity occurs because of previous exposure of a natural host or because of infection of an unnatural host. *Ascaris suum,* because of its tremendous biotic potential, may migrate in huge numbers and sometimes kill pigs, which are its natural hosts. It can also cause death of cattle, which are its frequent unnatural host. The lesion is an acute, diffuse, eosinophilic, interstitial pneumonia associated with the presence of large numbers of larvae. The trematodes *Fasciola gigantica* and *F. hepatica* invade the lungs accidentally from the liver. Since they are large parasites which wander extensively, a small number of them in the lungs can produce extensive cavitations. In other instances, lesions caused by parasites may be of some importance for differential diagnosis even though not of much clinical significance. In this category are the worm nodules, such as those caused by migrating *Parascaris equorum* larvae in horses. Although distinctive when young by virtue of the mass of eosinophils present, when scarified and calcified they need to be differentiated from residual lesions of small abscesses or infectious granulomas such as occur in glanders.

The transient parasites with principal habitats in other organs are discussed elsewhere. Here we are mainly concerned with lungworms whose final habitat is the airways or, less commonly, the parenchyma of the lungs.

1. Dictyocaulus

The *Dictyocaulus* genus contains the most important lungworms. There are three species: *Dictyocaulus filaria* is parasitic in sheep, goats, and other small ruminants, *D. viviparus* is parasitic in cattle, and *D. arnfieldi* is parasitic in the horse and its relatives. The three species are similar morphologically and in the details of their life cycles; *D. filaria* will serve as the type for discussion.

Dictyocaulus filaria, the large lungworm of sheep and goats, is a slender, whitish worm 3–10 cm long. The adults live mainly in the small bronchi. The life cycle is direct. The eggs are embryonated when laid, and some of them hatch in the lungs. The eggs and larvae are expelled from the lung by coughing; most are subsequently swallowed. The eggs which have not hatched in the air passages hatch in the alimentary canal, and first-stage larvae are passed in the feces. Further development occurs on the ground and requires moisture and moderate to low temperatures. This explains why verminous pneumonia is predominantly a disease of cool, moist climates. The larvae can develop at temperatures as low as 5°C, and their viability is prolonged at these temperatures. The combination of long survival at low temperatures and long patent periods in the host endows these worms with the ability to persist in northern, cold latitudes.

The larvae undergo two molts on pasture in ~1 week. The third stage is infective, and infestation can occur only if the third-stage larvae are ingested by the final host. The infective larvae penetrate the wall of the intestine and migrate via the lymphatics to the local lymph nodes. In the abdominal lymph nodes, they undergo the third molt and then go by way of lymph and blood to the lungs. Some larvae accidentally take the portal route and are destroyed in the liver. Some, on reaching the lungs, continue into the systemic circulation and are lost except for those rare ones which pass the placenta and produce intrauterine infections in the fetus. The worms take ~1 month after larval ingestion to reach maturity in the lungs, and it is then that clinical signs are most common because of the development of parasitic bronchitis. Adult worms persist for ~3 months.

The life cycle of *D. viviparus* in cattle is a little shorter than that of *D. filaria* but is otherwise comparable. Adult worms can continue to lay eggs for 6 months, but most are expelled within 3 months. *Dictyocaulus arnfieldi* is mostly a patent infection in donkeys, but the worms can develop to maturity if horses or ponies are infected as young foals.

The lesions produced by *Dictyocaulus* spp. depend on the susceptibility of the host and on the number of invading larvae. Cattle and sheep are most susceptible to infection when they are first exposed to contaminated pastures, and therefore severe lesions and the clinical disease they cause are most commonly seen in animals <1 year of age where infection is endemic. Minor reaction occurs along the pathway of larval migration, but the important lesions are found in the lungs. The lesions in the pulmonary tissues can be considered in two main phases, between the time when the larvae reach the lung and the worms reach maturity (prepatent phase), and when the mature parasites are located in the bronchi (patent phase). In natural infections, these two phases overlap and are associated with hyperplastic lymphadenitis in the related nodes. The larvae arrive in the lungs from ~5 to 7 days after ingestion. Where they emerge from pulmonary capillaries, they cause microscopic foci of necrosis or rupture of alveolar walls with an infiltrate of eosinophils, neutrophils, macrophages, and a few giant cells. With more severe larval invasion, these foci become more numerous and larger. Mononuclear cells thicken the alveolar walls, and there is focal exudation of fibrin into alveoli together with the inflammatory cells. Eosinophils are a prominent feature of the reaction. Various degrees of hyperplasia of alveolar type II epithelial cells also occur. The larvae, some of them dead, can be found in the alveoli. When the number of larvae is large, the foci of acute interstitial pneumonia may be visible grossly as small lobular or sublobular areas which are slightly depressed, purplish, and distributed widely throughout the lungs.

By about the tenth day, many of the larvae have gained the terminal bronchioles. Frothy fluid is present in the bronchi and, in very heavy infestations, there is often edema and emphysema of the interlobular septa. Eosinophils invade the septal tissues in large numbers and follow the larvae into the bronchioles. Most of the bronchioles contain plugs of exudate composed largely of eosinophils. Neutrophils, lymphocytes, and macrophages are present in smaller numbers in both the lumina and walls of the bronchioles. Death can occur at this time in very heavy infections. The early bronchiolar epithelial response is of degeneration and sloughing, but subsequently hyperplasia and metaplasia also occur. As the worms reach maturity, beginning ~4 weeks after infection, emphasis shifts to the bronchial lesion, and some resolution of the initial alveolar lesion occurs. The mature, threadlike worms in the bronchi and perhaps caudal trachea are easy to see in moderate to severe infections. Although the early development of lungworms can take place in all lobes, dorsocaudal and ventrocaudal regions are most affected. Mature worms are most numerous in the dorsocaudal bronchi of the caudal lobes, and in light infections may be found only in these regions. The worms are usually bathed in mucinous, foamy bronchial exudate. In some cases, there may be no superficial indications of the worms except for failure of the lungs to collapse. It is usual for gross lesions to be present in patent infections, however. Typically, there are large wedge-shaped areas of dark red or grayish consolidated lung at the posterior border of the caudal lobes (Fig. 6.92). These consolidated areas have firm consistency and are slightly depressed below the surface of surrounding inflated or sometimes hyperinflated lung. Patchy consolidation may also occur in other dorsocaudal regions and, with severe involvement, can be found on cut section in much of the pulmonary tissue surrounding larger bronchi. There is no pleuritis.

The adult worms cause chronic catarrhal and eosinophilic bronchitis and bronchiolitis. The epithelium of bronchi is thickened and hyperplastic. Increase in the proportion of mucus-producing cells is a prominent feature.

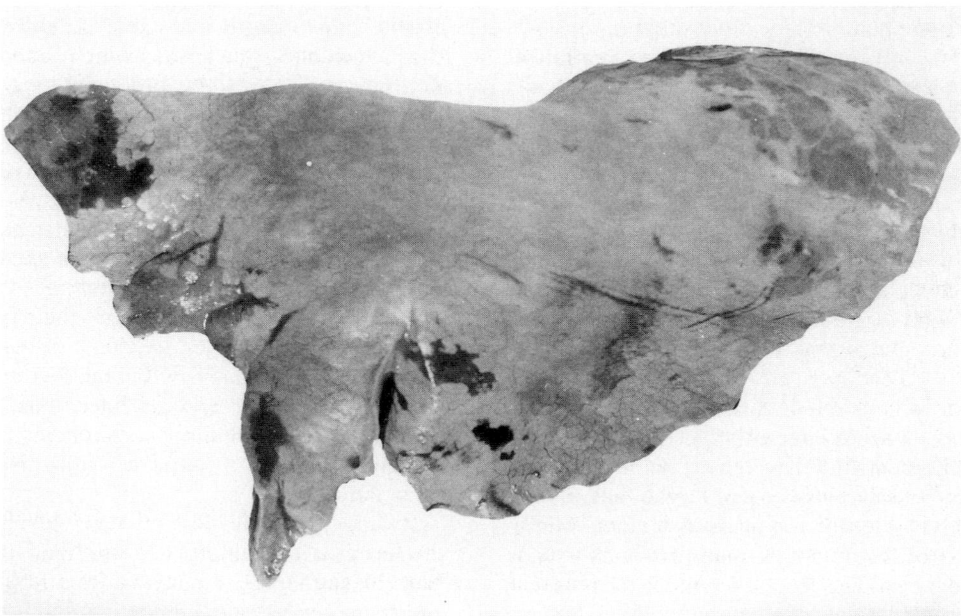

Fig. 6.92 Verminous pneumonia. Bronchopneumonia caused by *Dictyocaulus filaria* in dorsocaudal region of caudal lobe (unrelated areas of atelectasis and enzootic pneumonia in cranioventral regions). Sheep.

Elsewhere there may be ulceration or occasionally squamous metaplasia. The epithelium and lamina propria are infiltrated by mixed leukocytes, with a preponderance of eosinophils, and there is hyperplastic bronchus-associated lymphoid tissue. The lumina contain adult worms, plugs of mucus, numerous leukocytes, eggs, and larvae. Components of the verminous bronchiolitis are similar, but there is also a tendency for obliterative bronchiolitis to occur. The hyperplasia of bronchiolar smooth muscle, increase in peribronchiolar fibrous tissue, and proliferation of lymphoid cells in bronchiolar walls also assume relatively greater prominence (Fig. 6.93).

The parenchymal lesions which accompany the bronchitis caused by the adult worms are compounded mostly of atelectasis secondary to the bronchiolitis and of pneumonia which is provoked by aspirated eggs and newly hatched larvae. It is complicated in some cases by bacteria. Granulomas are frequently present around fragments of discarded cuticle, eggs, or dead larvae. The alveoli, which are partially collapsed, contain many giant cells and vacuolated macrophages. Their walls are thickened by cellular infiltration and slight fibroplasia and may be more or less completely covered by low cuboidal epithelium. Toward the end of the patent period, the alveolar reaction subsides and resolution begins, especially in the periphery of the lobules. Around the bronchioles, however, many of the alveoli are permanently obliterated by the organizing peribronchiolar reaction. The lymphoid nodules which develop in the walls of bronchi and bronchioles are not generally so conspicuous as those occurring in chronic mycoplasmal infection. In resolving lesions, however, when worms are no longer present, there is no clear mor-

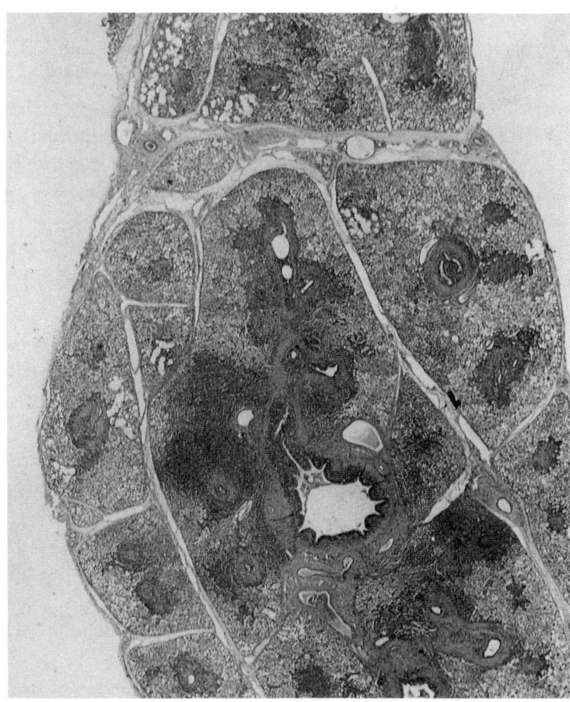

Fig. 6.93 Verminous pneumonia. Residual lesions caused by *Dictyocaulus filaria*. Sheep. Note the obliterative bronchiolitis and prominent hyperplasia of bronchiolar smooth muscle with lymphofollicular cuffing.

phologic distinction. A useful clue to separate these two major causes of lymphoid proliferation is that the airways mainly affected by mycoplasma are in cranioventral regions, whereas those affected by lungworms in ruminants are dorsocaudal.

Two features of the lesions caused by *D. viviparus* in cattle deserve special mention. The first is that extremely severe damage is associated with pulmonary edema and interstitial emphysema. The interstitial emphysema is secondary to severe pulmonary dysfunction and forced expiratory efforts in lungs with nonuniform lobular emptying of air during expiration together with bronchiolar obstruction and probably bronchospasm. In fatal cases, interstitial emphysema may be the most obvious gross finding and therefore lead to confusion with the interstitial emphysema accompanying acute interstitial pneumonia of toxic origin. This is particularly likely when the pulmonary damage is caused by massive invasion of larvae, and mature worms are not yet present for gross detection. Microscopic detection of larvae and immature worms usually provides the diagnosis. The second feature is the presence in the lungs of older animals of scattered nodules 2–4 mm in diameter. The nodules are homogeneously gray, or gray with a greenish center. The gray tissue represents dense accumulations of lymphocytes and possibly plasma cells, and the greenish center is the degenerating larval or adult worm surrounded by eosinophils, macrophages, and giant cells. The nodules are an indication of reinfection of an immune animal, vaccination with x-irradiated larvae or anthelmintic treatment.

Dictyocaulus arnfieldi is a lungworm mainly of donkeys and survives for long periods without causing undue clinical signs. The gross lesions are scattered discrete foci of hyperinflated pulmonary parenchyma, mostly in caudal lobes. In the center of the lesions are small bronchi packed with coiled adult worms. Histologically, the worms are associated with a chronic catarrhal bronchitis. Goblet cell hyperplasia and extensive lymphoid cell infiltration of the walls are the main features. Adult worms cause relatively little luminal response, whereas first-stage larvae stimulate an intense mucopurulent reaction. There is also a chronic catarrhal and eosinophilic bronchiolitis of bronchioles distal to affected bronchi. Alveoli are reported to be hyperinflated, but it is uncertain to what extent this reflects true *in vivo* hyperinflation as opposed to air trapping and failure to collapse when the lungs are examined after death. Infection of adult horses with *D. arnfieldi* usually results in failure of the worm to develop to sexual maturity. The lesions are similar to those described for the donkey and are occasionally associated with chronic coughing and abnormal sounds on auscultation.

2. Protostrongylus

The most common and important member of the genus is *P. rufescens*. Whereas *Dictyocaulus* species have direct life cycles, *Protostrongylus rufescens* and the other worms to be discussed have indirect life cycles.

Protostrongylus rufescens is parasitic in sheep, goats, and deer. The adults are smaller than *D. filaria*, being from 16 to 35 mm in length. They are reddish and mainly inhabit the bronchioles. The lesions which accompany the infection are similar to those produced by *D. filaria* but are less numerous, lobular in size, and located chiefly in the periphery of the caudal lobes. The lesions are not readily distinguished grossly from those produced by *Muellerius capillaris*. The first-stage larvae are passed in the feces and enter the intermediate hosts, which are various genera of land snails, by boring through the foot. Two molts occur in the snail and the infective third-stage larvae develop in 2 weeks. Sheep and goats obtain the parasites by eating the snails.

Neostrongylus linearis is a species comparable to *P. rufescens*. It is common in western Europe and probably elsewhere, but is confused with other small lungworms of sheep.

3. *Muellerius* and *Cystocaulus*

Cystocaulus ocreatus (*C. nigrescens*) is little studied, but it is stated to resemble *Muellerius* spp. in the details of life cycle and pathogenicity.

Muellerius capillaris, which is parasitic in sheep and goats, is the most common and ubiquitous of the lungworms. The species is sometimes referred to as the nodular lungworm because the adults live in the alveolar parenchyma and almost always provoke an enveloping granulomatous response. The adult worms are found on rare occasions in the bronchioles. There is usually no clinical evidence of respiratory disease in sheep even when the number of nodules is large. Sometimes they become confluent. Diminished weight gains have been recorded in heavily infested lambs, and it has been postulated that the worms predispose to pulmonary bacterial and viral infections.

The eggs are laid and hatch in the nodules. This requires that the sexes be paired in the nodules. Often this does not occur, and therefore the examination of feces for larvae may give no indication of the degree of pulmonary parasitism. The first-stage larvae break out of tissues into the airways and are eventually passed with feces or mucus. The intermediate hosts are various slugs and snails. The infective stage is reached after two molts in the intermediate host, and the life cycle is completed when sheep and goats swallow the intermediate hosts. The larvae migrate to the lungs, presumably via the lymphatic pathway, and break out into the alveoli. As a consequence of this type of life cycle, infections are acquired gradually, and large worm burdens are seldom observed in animals <6 months of age. On the other hand, heavy infections are not common in old sheep and goats.

The nodules produced by these parasites represent lesions of multifocal interstitial pneumonia. They may occur anywhere in the lung, but most of them are located beneath the pleura of dorsal regions of the caudal lobes (Figs. 6.94, 6.95) so that the severity of infestation can be assessed quite accurately by superficial inspection. Why there should be this predilection for the subpleural tissues is not

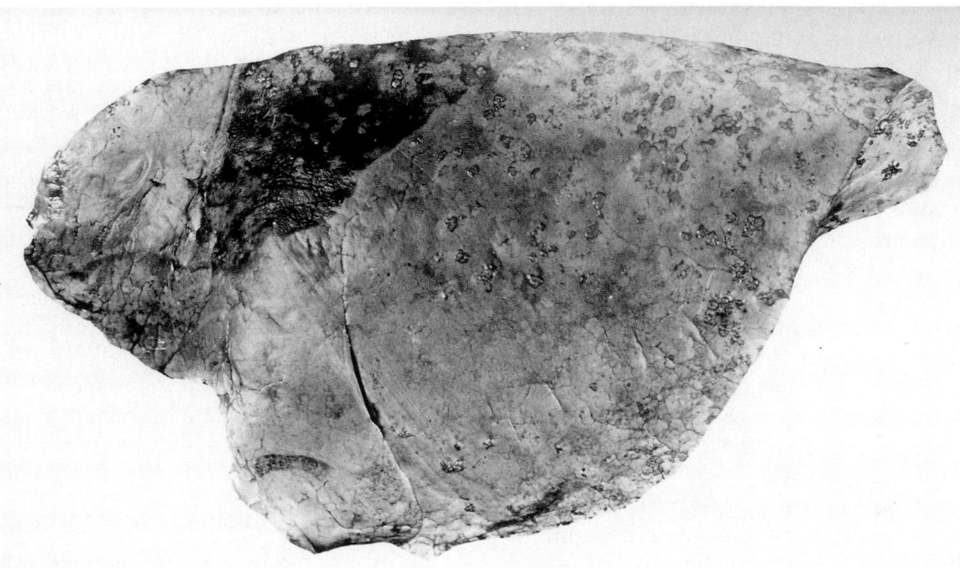

Fig. 6.94 Verminous pneumonia. Multifocal subpleural nodules of interstitial pneumonia produced by *Muellerius capillaris*. Sheep.

known. The nodules range in size from 1 mm to several centimeters. They are soft and hemorrhagic early in an infection. Later they are greenish gray and project above the pleural surface of adjacent lung at necropsy. Some of them become calcified. Similar nodules are present in various numbers in the bronchial and mesenteric lymph nodes. Sheep are rather tolerant of initial exposure and readily develop patent infections. With repeated exposure, sheep become resistant and inhibit fourth-stage larval migration or development. Immature adults may have their development checked, or mature worms may cease

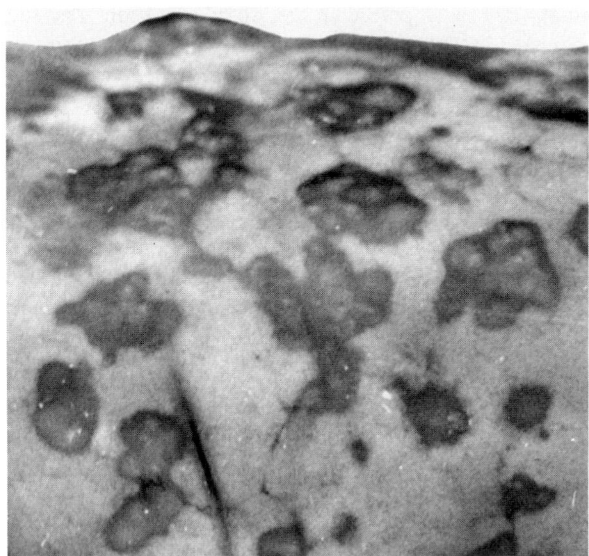

Fig. 6.95 Subpleural nodules produced by *Muellerius capillaris*. Sheep.

reproduction in a resistant animal. The cellular reaction reflects the stage of the parasite present and resistance of the host. The earliest form of nodule is produced by the fourth-stage larvae when they enter the lungs, and usually consists of little more than groups of alveoli which are mechanically disrupted. There may be little cellular reaction to these larvae of the first infestation, but an eosinophilic infiltration may accompany later ones. The adult worms also disrupt the alveolar septa. The eggs and first-stage larvae lie in the alveolar spaces and provoke little inflammatory response, although there is a mild fibrous thickening of the alveolar septa with infiltrated lymphocytes in the septa and around the blood vessels and bronchioles. In older animals, presumably as a result of developing resistance, the cellular reaction is more marked, especially to the first-stage larvae and the adults (Fig. 6.96). There are intense foci of infiltrated eosinophils around the larvae; the alveolar spaces become crowded with macrophages and some giant cells, and the distorted alveolar walls are thickened by fibrous tissue. The larvae which escape into small bronchioles are enclosed in plugs of mucus and cellular debris. The epithelium of the bronchioles is hyperplastic, and the muscularis, much thickened. When the larvae leave the nodules, the cellular reaction subsides, but the thickening of the alveolar septa persists because of patchy or diffuse fibromuscular hyperplasia. An intense reaction also occurs to the adult worms. There are large numbers of eosinophils, a narrow zone of epithelioid and giant cells, and peripheral fibroblastic tissue. The cellular debris becomes calcified, particularly when the worms die, and these calcified nodules persist indefinitely as spherical masses of calcium salts surrounded by a fibrous capsule. Not all the calcification, however, occurs about adult worms. Some is precipitated

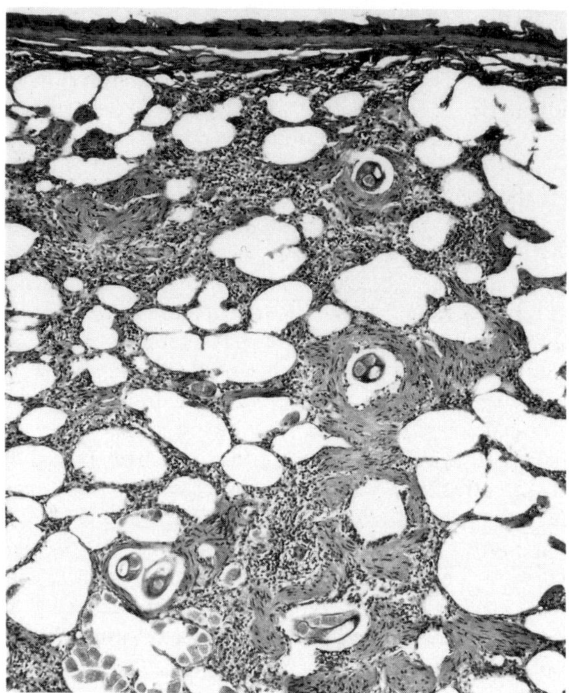

Fig. 6.96 Verminous pneumonia. Moderate reaction of *Muellerius capillaris*. Sheep. Adults lie in bronchioles and alveolar ducts and are associated with muscular hyperplasia. Eggs and first-stage larvae have provoked a chronic interstitial pneumonia.

in the inspissated mucus which collects in obstructed bronchial glands, and some in mucus and debris which accumulate in the bronchioles.

An extensive diffuse interstitial pneumonia has been associated with *Muellerius* infection in goats, but in such cases it is often impossible to assess the possible role of concurrent infection with *Mycoplasma* spp. or the caprine arthritis–encephalomyelitis virus.

4. Metastrongylus

There are three important species of the genus, *M. elongatus* (*apri*), *M. pudendotectus,* and *M. salmi,* and they are all parasitic in the bronchi and bronchioles of pigs. They are believed to be responsible for the occasional transmission of the virus of swine influenza. The adult worms are white, threadlike, and from 14 to 60 mm in length, depending on species and sex. In heavy infections, which are mostly in young pigs, they may be found in all lobes of the lung. When there are fewer worms, particularly as occurs in older animals, the worms may be restricted to airways along the ventrocaudal borders of the caudal lobes. These apparently are areas of predilection or residual infestation. The eggs are laid in the bronchi, and a few of them hatch there, but most hatch after passing to the exterior in the feces. The first-stage larvae are inactive and are capable of prolonged survival in moist conditions. Their further development depends on ingestion by earthworms, which are the intermediate hosts. The larvae develop to the third, infective stage in ~10 days and then remain quiescent unless the earthworm is eaten by a pig. The larvae may survive for as long as 18 months in the earthworms and, by that time, some thousands of them may be accumulated by a single worm without doing it any harm. Migration within the pig is through the lymphatics from the intestine to the lungs. Some larvae pass through the liver and produce a focal hepatitis for which the larvae of *Ascaris suum* are, however, more usually responsible.

Even with heavy adult infestations, gross lesions are inconspicuous and are seldom as extensive as those produced in ruminants by *Dictyocaulus* spp. In light infections, the worms live in the smallest airways, and on superficial examination of the lungs, the presence of the parasites frequently is indicated only by grayish nodules 1–3 mm in diameter and by hyperinflated lobules along the ventrocaudal margins of the caudal lobes (Fig. 6.97).

Histologically, the lesions are basically the same as those produced by *Dictyocaulus* spp. The initial lesions are multiple foci of intense accumulations of eosinophils surrounding larvae in alveoli. Subsequently, when reproduction is active, a granulomatous alveolar response occurs to the eggs and larvae. The prepatent period for *Metastrongylus* spp. is ~25 days, after which the rate of egg production rapidly reaches a peak and then subsides to a low level. At this later stage, the adults persist mainly in the bronchioles and small bronchi and provoke a chronic

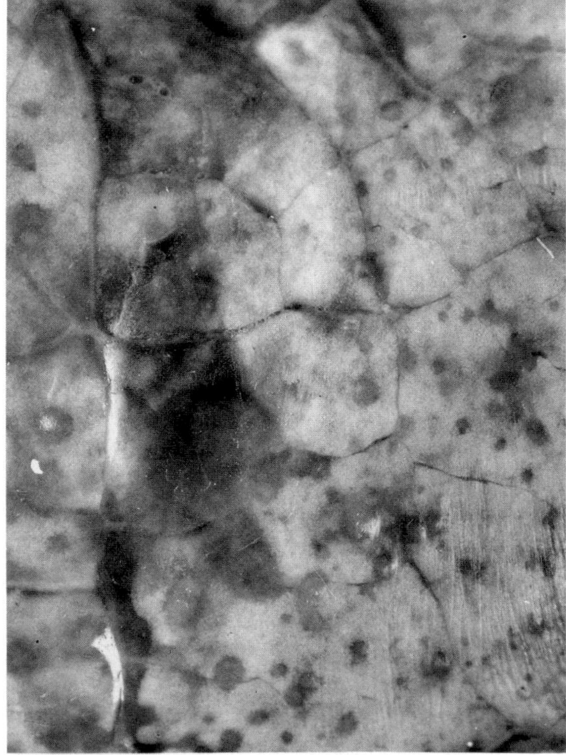

Fig. 6.97 Verminous pneumonia. Multiple subpleural nodules produced by *Metastrongylus* spp. Pig.

catarrhal and eosinophilic bronchiolitis and bronchitis with the features as described for *Dictyocaulus* infection in ruminants. Large lymphofollicular nodules are mainly responsible for the grayish nodules visible grossly.

5. Crenosoma

Crenosoma vulpis is a common lungworm of foxes, but it also occurs in other Canidae. It is occasionally found in dogs that have access to the snails and slugs which are intermediate hosts. The adult worms live in bronchioles and small bronchi. The gross lesions usually observed in dogs are grayish consolidations in dorsal regions of the caudal lobes. Histologically, the lesions caused by adult worms are catarrhal, eosinophilic bronchitis and bronchiolitis closely resembling those caused by *Dictyocaulus* spp. in ruminants.

6. Filaroides

a. *Filaroides* (*Anafilaroides*) *rostratus* This parasite of cats appears to have very limited distribution since it has been recorded mainly from Sri Lanka. In that its final habitat is the walls of large airways, it resembles *Filaroides osleri* of dogs (see Parasitic Diseases of the Larynx and Trachea, Section IV,E of this chapter). It does not form nodules, however, but causes sinuous thickenings of the bronchial walls. When the infective larvae invade the bronchial walls, they provoke only slight cellular response. The adults develop in cystic spaces which are probably dilated lymphatics and which cause displacement of the surrounding tissues. The worms are viviparous, and the larvae escape to the bronchiolar lumen where they provoke a catarrhal bronchitis. The adults remain alive for ~1 year, and possibly for much longer. When they die, they provoke an intense infiltration of neutrophils and may calcify. There is residual fibrosis in the bronchial wall. The larvae are passed in the feces and develop to the infective stage in a variety of molluscs. They can probably survive for a long time in the intermediate hosts, and the capacity for survival and dissemination is increased by the fortuitous use of transport hosts, such as mice and chickens.

There are other species of lungworms in cats which are probably similar to *F. rostratus,* but virtually the only details concerning them are taxonomic. *Vogeloides massinoi* (*Osleroides massino*) lives in the bronchial wall. *Vogeloides ramanujacharii* occurs in cats in India. *Troglostrongylus brevior* occurs in cats in the Middle East and is known to use snails as intermediate hosts.

b. *Filaroides hirthi* Two similar filarid worms have been recorded as inhabiting the pulmonary parenchyma of dogs, *Filaroides hirthi* and *F. milksi*. Original reports were of *F. milksi,* but more recent descriptions have been of a worm that, although it closely resembles *F. milksi,* has been assigned to a separate species, *F. hirthi*. This description summarizes the current knowledge concerning *F. hirthi,* leaving the taxonomic and pathogenic uncertainties surrounding *F. milksi* for future clarification.

Adult *F. hirthi,* which are 6–10 mm in length, live in alveoli and respiratory bronchioles. Clinical signs of infection are rare, and evidence of the worms' presence is usually limited to the incidental finding at necropsy of tan, green, or gray subpleural nodules 1–5 mm in diameter. The nodules are widely scattered over subpleural regions, the numbers varying with the severity of infection. Histologically, there is little response to living adult worms (Fig. 6.98A), but a severe granulomatous response featuring many eosinophils occurs around dead or degenerating worms (Fig. 6.98B). Larvae provoke a more acute neutrophilic reaction. Foci of granulomatous interstitial pneumonia can often be found in which worm remnants may no longer be identified. Killing the worms with anthelmintic is particularly prone to cause the severe response.

Filaroides hirthi has a direct life cycle, like that of *F. osleri*. Infective first-stage larvae are passed in the feces and usually the infection is passed from dam to pups. Infection is mostly reported to occur in colonies of beagles reared for experimental studies in which lungs are routinely given thorough examinations. The incidence of *F. hirthi* in the canine population at large is not known. There are a few single-case reports of dogs with lethal infection, however, so it is probably more widespread than realized. The fatalities have been caused by severe, miliary granulomatous pneumonia with a superimposed acute exudative component associated with huge numbers of worms and

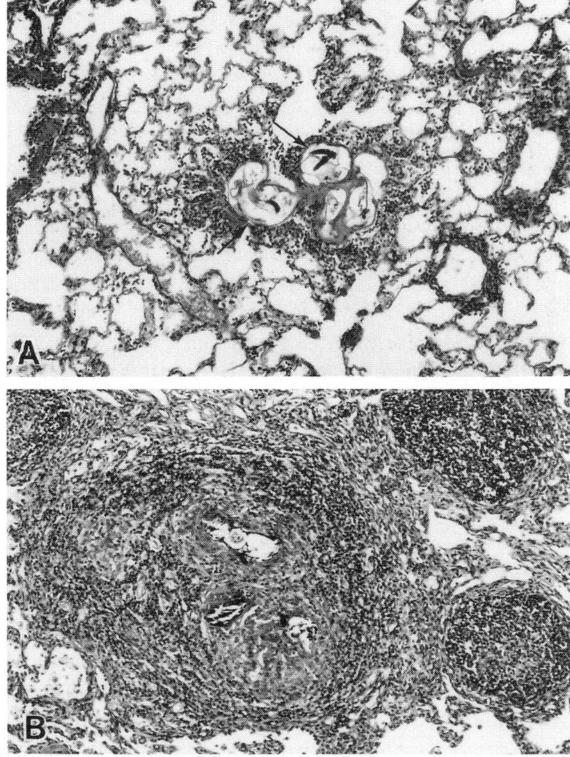

Fig. 6.98 Verminous pneumonia. Dog. (A) Eosinophilic and lymphocytic interstitial reaction to adult *Filaroides hirthi* (arrow). (B) Severe granulomatous response surrounding dead *F. hirthi*.

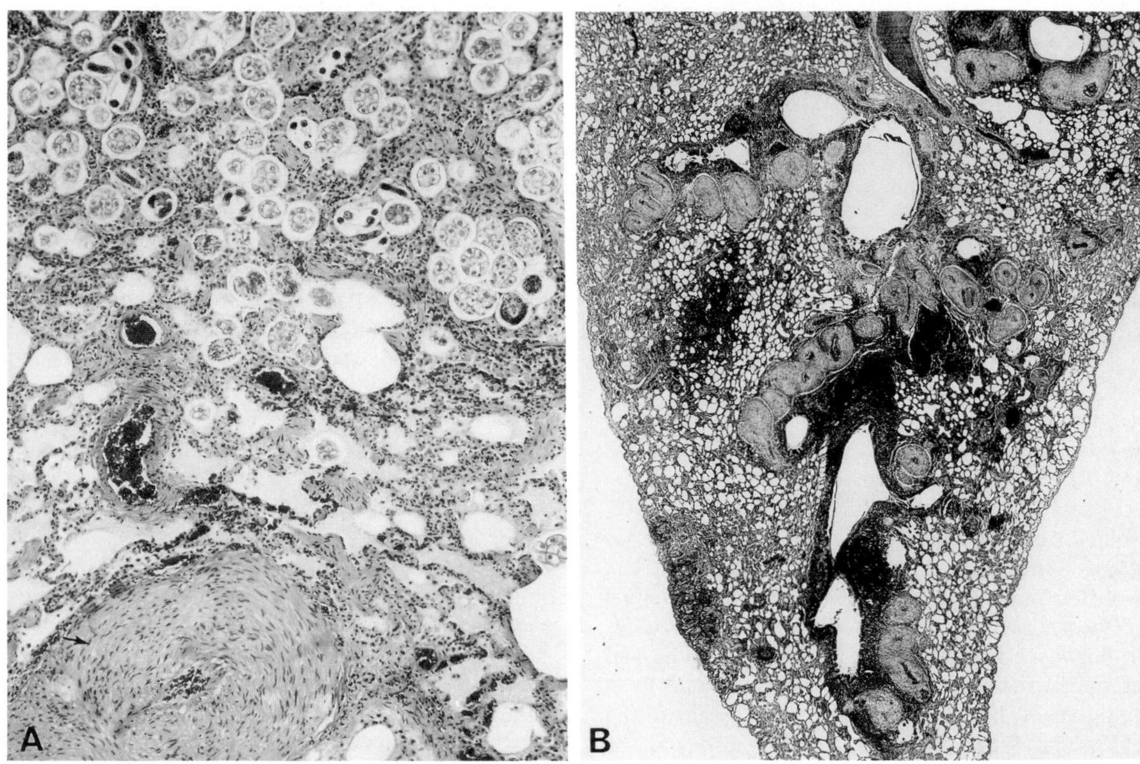

Fig. 6.99 Verminous pneumonia. Cat. (A) Granulomatous interstitial pneumonia provoked by eggs and larvae of *Aelurostrongylus abstrusus*. Note hyperplasia of smooth muscle of pulmonary artery (arrow). (B) Residual lesions of *A. abstrusus*. Tortuous, hypertrophied arteries have infiltration of walls by eosinophils.

larvae. This type of hyperinfection and probable autoinfection seems to occur in dogs with drug- or disease-induced immunosuppression.

7. Aelurostrongylus abstrusus

Aelurostrongylus abstrusus is a widespread lungworm of the cat. The adults live in the respiratory bronchioles and alveolar ducts. The eggs form nodular deposits in alveoli and hatch to give first-stage larvae which reach the airways and are eventually passed in the feces. The indirect life cycle involves various snails and slugs as intermediate hosts and birds, rodents, frogs, and lizards as transport hosts. The life cycle can be completed if a cat eats either an intermediate host or a transport host.

The extent to which infective larvae reach the lungs in the blood or by migration through peritoneal and pleural cavities is not certain. Worms reach maturity ~5–6 weeks after ingestion of the third-stage larvae. The pulmonary lesions are quite characteristic, usually being in the form of nodules 1–10 mm in diameter, which represent nests of eggs and larvae (Fig. 6.99A). These nodules, which are yellowish and firm, are scattered throughout the parenchyma but are more common in the peripheral parts of the lungs and usually project from the surface of the deflated lung. A small amount of creamy exudate containing numerous eggs and larvae can be expressed from the cut surface of incised nodules. Severe, confluent consolidation caused by heavy infections of *A. abstrusus* can produce clinical signs of chronic coughing and perhaps progressive loss of weight. Occasionally death occurs when there is secondary infection.

Microscopically, the eggs and larvae are visible in the alveolar spaces with some disruption of alveolar septa. They are surrounded by dense collections of mixed mononuclear cells with some giant cells. The latter are more numerous around dead or disintegrating larvae. Eosinophils and neutrophils are mostly a feature of early infection. Lymphocytic nodules form around vessels and airways (Fig. 6.99B). Necrosis and calcification seldom occur. In older lesions from which eggs and larvae have disappeared, the alveoli remain epithelialized for a time, and the septa are persistently thickened by fibrous tissue and smooth muscle. This fibromuscular hyperplasia is often focal and barely appreciable, but in some cases is diffuse and rigid enough to produce a rubbery consistency.

Hypertrophy and hyperplasia of the smooth muscle in the walls of the bronchioles and alveolar ducts occurs early in the course of the infestation and is progressive, but is not so well developed as is the increase in smooth muscle in the media of small pulmonary arteries and arterioles. The presence of one or more of adult worms, eggs, or larvae in the bronchioles is associated with a chronic catarrhal and eosinophilic bronchiolitis similar to that caused by *Dictyocaulus* spp. in ruminants. A prominent

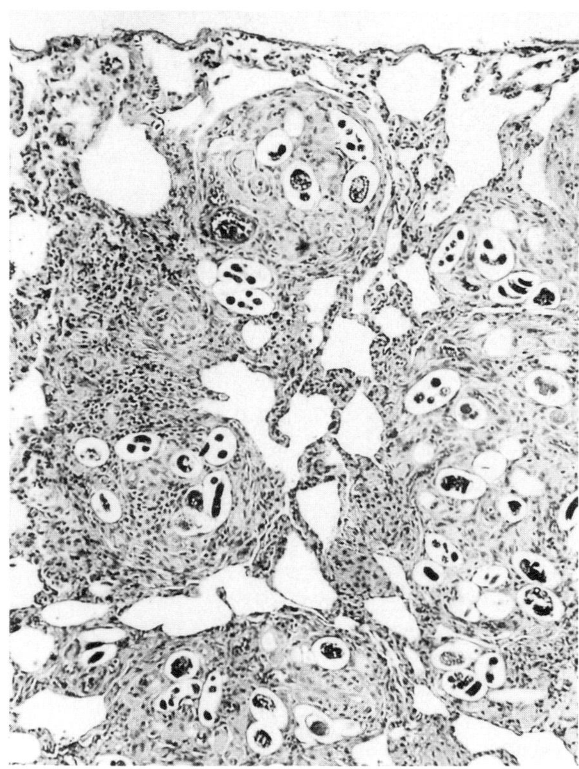

Fig. 6.100 Verminous pneumonia. Chronic interstitial pneumonia with prominent fibrosis surrounding eggs and larvae of *Angiostrongylus vasorum*. Dog.

component is the hyperplasia of submucosal glands, which are a usual but generally inconspicuous feature of small airways of cats.

The most active phase of the parasite is 6–12 weeks after infection, and this is associated with the peak pulmonary response. Adult worms can persist as long as 9 months. Although the granulomatous alveolitis and catarrhal bronchiolitis gradually regress, the hypertrophy and hyperplasia of smooth muscle in arteries, bronchioles, and alveolar ducts persist. The association between *Aleurostrongylus* infection and the dramatic muscular thickening of the walls of pulmonary arteries has been the subject of controversy. The evidence indicates that hyperplasia and hypertrophy of smooth muscle in pulmonary arteries is a common finding in cats of all ages for reasons which are obscure.

8. Angiostrongylus

Angiostrongylus vasorum is a parasite of the pulmonary arteries and the right ventricle of dogs and foxes. The adult worms are 15–25 mm in length. They cause a proliferative endoarteritis, but the more severe damage is caused by eggs which lodge in arterioles and capillaries. They and the larvae which hatch from them provoke chronic inflammation in which fibroplasia predominates (Fig. 6.100). The larvae break into the alveoli, migrate in the respiratory passages, and are eliminated in the feces. Various snails and slugs serve as intermediate hosts.

In the acute form of the disease, with heavy infestations of larvae in alveoli, the fatal outcome is in large part attributable to pulmonary edema and pneumonia. The chronic expression of the disease is largely one of congestive cardiac failure, secondary to obliterative and thrombotic vasculitis, organizing infarcts, and progressive granulomatous response to eggs and larvae. Inflammation and scarring of alveolar walls leads to distortion and enlargement of remaining airspaces, which can result in a foam-rubber appearance. This is sometimes referred to as emphysema but is more a form of honeycombing than emphysema in the conventional sense.

Because of their similar location, there is overlap in the types of abnormalities caused by *A. vasorum* and *Dirofilaria immitis* (see The Cardiovascular System, Volume 3, Chapter 1).

9. Paragonimus

Of the trematodes, the only genus which has its final habitat in the lungs is *Paragonimus*. Several species have been described for the genus. The important ones are *P. westermanii* (the oriental lung fluke) in the Far East and *P. kellicotti* in America. For the latter species, mink and other fish-eating carnivores are regarded as being the usual hosts. The fluke is not selective in its final hosts, however, and has also been found in humans, swine, and ruminants. Among domestic animals, it is most commonly found in cats. Its natural habitat is the lung, but aberrant localizations have included the nervous system.

The life cycle of the parasite is typical of the cycles of the trematodes (see *Fasciola hepatica* in The Liver and Biliary System, Chapter 2, Section X,D,3 of this volume). The first intermediate hosts are small aquatic snails. The second intermediate host is a freshwater crab or crayfish. When the crayfish is eaten by the final host, the metacercariae are liberated in the intestine and migrate across the peritoneal and pleural cavities to the lungs. Their passage through the pleura is marked by multiple small hemorrhages and foci of eosinophilic and fibrinous pleuritis, which heal as small umbilicate scars (Fig. 6.101A). The adult flukes are ovoid, reddish brown, and as long as 7 mm. They are found, usually in pairs, in inflammatory cysts in the pulmonary parenchyma (Fig. 6.101B) and occasionally in the bronchi. The cysts are more common in the caudal lobes, particularly the right side. They are spherical, ~10–15 mm in diameter, and dark red-brown. Their size and the fact that surrounding lung is frequently atelectatic give them a distinctive appearance. The cysts frequently communicate with bronchioles. Rupture of cysts on the pleural surface and resulting pneumothorax is a rare complication. The cysts become progressively surrounded by fibrous tissue and partially lined by bronchiolar epithelium. Eosinophilic, granulomatous pneumonia develops around degenerating eggs adjacent to the cysts containing flukes (Fig. 6.101C). There is also a chronic catarrhal, eosinophilic bronchiolitis with smooth

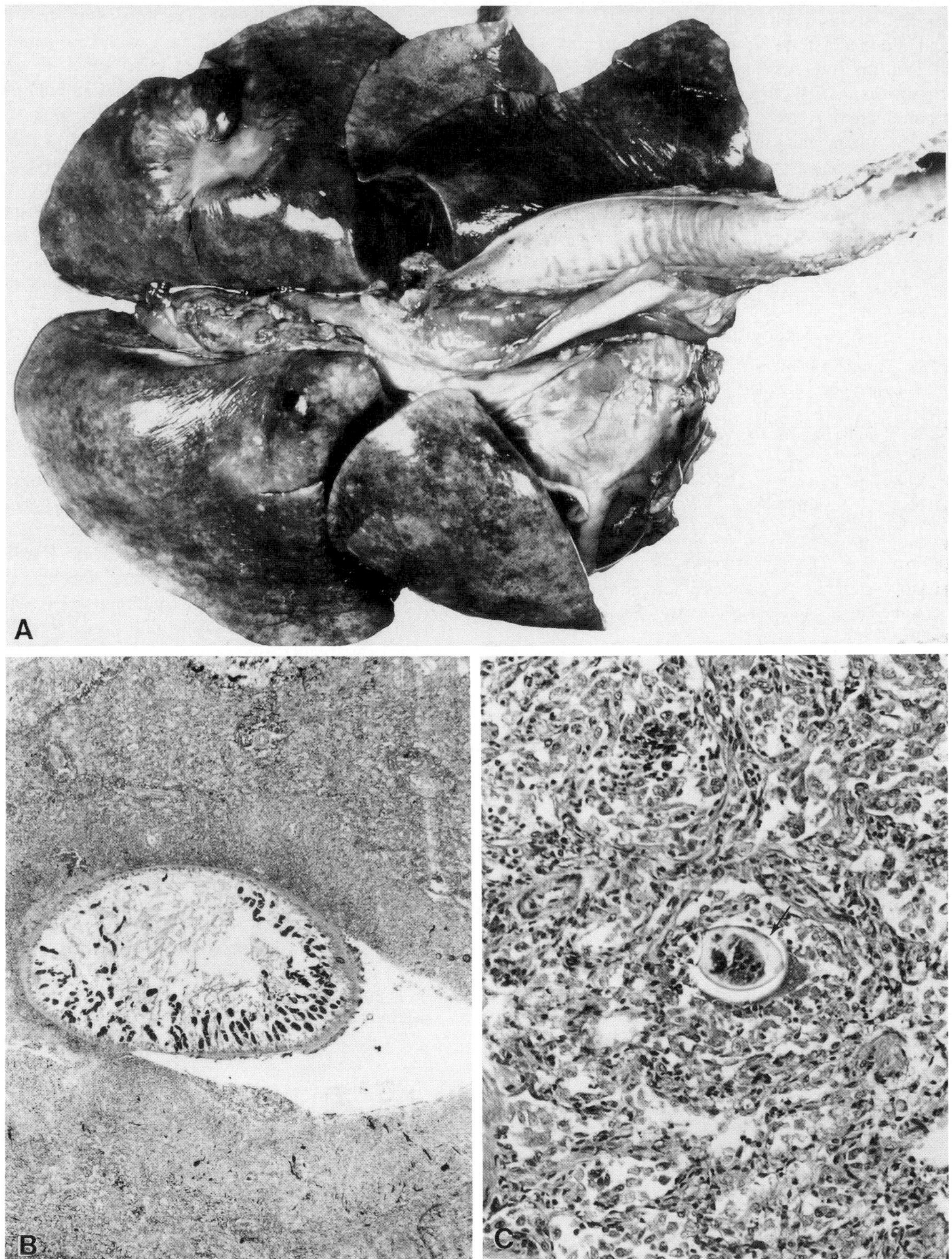

Fig. 6.101A Paragonimiasis. Dog. (A) Residual scar on surface of left caudal lobe. (B) *Paragonimus kellicotti* in inflammatory cyst in pulmonary parenchyma. (C) Granulomatous pneumonia surrounding distinctive operculate egg (arrow).

muscle hyperplasia. Clusters of eggs, which occasionally are visible grossly as yellowish-brown streaks, occur in subpleural and mediastinal lymphatics and cause a granulomatous pleuritis and lymphangitis. The large operculate eggs are quite distinctive (Fig. 6.101C); in old lesions only fractured shells may remain.

Various protozoa are capable of causing interstitial pneumonia, most notably *Toxoplasma gondii* (see The Alimentary System, Chapter 1 of this volume). *Sarcocystis* spp. also produce a multifocal interstitial pneumonia as part of the widespread multiplication of tachyzoites in vascular endothelium during acute sarcocystosis in herbivores (see Muscle and Tendons, Volume 1, Chapter 2).

Bibliography

Alden, C. L., Gay, S., and Adkins, A. Pulmonary trematodiasis in a cat: A case report. *Vet Med Small Anim Clin* **75:** 612–617, 1980.

Alwar, V. S., Lalitha, C. M., and Seneviratna, P. *Vogeloides ramanujacharii* n. sp., a new lungworm from the domestic cat (*Felis catus* Linne), in India. *Ind Vet J* **35:** 1–5, 1958.

Ameel, D. J. *Paragonimus*, its life history and distribution in North America and its taxonomy. *Am J Hyg* **19:** 279–317, 1934.

Atwell, R. B., and Carlisle, C. H. The distribution of filariae, superficial lung lesions, and pulmonary arterial lesions following chemotherapy in canine dirofilariasis. *J Small Anim Pract* **23:** 667–673, 1982.

Bailey, W. S., and Williams. A. G. Verminous pneumonia in the cat. *Vet Med* **44:** 267–269, 1949.

Beaver, P. C. Larva migrans. *Exp Parasitol* **5:** 587–621, 1956.

Benakhla, A. Pneumonie vermineuse ovine a *Muellerius capillaris* ou mulleriose ovine. *Ann Med Vet* **125:** 177–189, 1981.

Beresford-Jones, W. P. Observations on *Muellerius capillaris* (Muller, 1889) Cameron, 1927. III. Experimental infection of sheep. *Res Vet Sci* **8:** 272–279, 1967.

Breeze, R. Parasitic bronchitis and pneumonia. *Vet Clin North Am Food Anim Pract* **1:** 277–287, 1985.

Castleman, W. L., and Wong, M. M. Light and electron microscopic pulmonary lesions associated with retained microfilariae in canine occult dirofilariasis. *Vet Pathol* **19:** 355–364, 1982.

Chu, C. C. Pathological changes of paragonimiasis: Preliminary observations on 30 dogs. *Chin J Pathol* **3:** 163–165, 1957.

Clayton, H. M., and Duncan, J. L. Natural infection with *Dictyocaulus arnfieldi* in pony and donkey foals. *Res Vet Sci* **31:** 278–280, 1981.

Cohrs, P. *Paragonimus westermanii* und primares Plattenepithelkarzinom in der Lunge. *Beitr Pathol Anat* **81:** 101–120, 1928.

Craig, T. M. *et al*. Fatal *Filaroides hirthi* infection in a dog. *J Am Vet Med Assoc* **172:** 1096–1098, 1978.

Cuille, J., and Darraspen, E. De la strongylose cardio-pulmonaire du chien. *Rev Gen Med Vet* **39:** 625–639, 694–710, 753–765, 1930.

Daubney, R. The life histories of *Dictyocaulus filaria* and *Dictyocaulus viviparus*. *J Comp Pathol* **33:** 225–266, 1920.

Davtjan, E. A. Ein neuer Nematode aus den Lungen der Hauskatze. *Osleroides massino*, nov. sp. *Dtsch Tierearztl Wochenschr* **41:** 372–374, 1933.

Djafar, M. I., Swanson, L. E., and Becker, R. B. Lungworm infections in calves. *J Am Vet Med Assoc* **136:** 200–204, 1960.

Dubey, J. P. *et al*. Sarcocystosis in goats: Clinical signs and pathologic and hematologic findings. *J Am Vet Med Assoc* **178:** 683–699, 1981.

Dunn, D. R. The pig lungworm (*Metastrongylus* spp.). 2. Experimental infection of pigs with *M. apri*. *Br Vet J* **112:** 327–337, 1956.

Dunn. D. R., Gentles, M. A., and White, E. G. Studies on the pig lungworm (*Metastrongylus* spp.). 1. Observations on natural infection in the pig in Great Britain. *Br Vet J* **111:** 271–281, 1955.

Garlick, N. L. Canine pulmonary acariasis. *Can Pract* **4:** 42–47, 1977.

Hare, T. Chronic tracheobronchitis of the dog due to *Oslerus osleri*. *Vet Rec* **11:** 1074–1075, 1931.

Hieronymi, E. Zur Entwicklung von *Aelurostrongylus abstrusus* in der Katzenlunge. *Tierarztl Umsch* **8:** 8230–233, 1953.

Hirth, R. S., and Hottendorf, G. H. Lesions produced by a new lungworm in beagle dogs. *Vet Pathol* **10:** 385–407, 1973.

Hobmaier, A., and Hobmaier, M. Die Entwicklung des Lungenwurmes des Schafes, *Dictyocaulus filaria*, Ausserhalb und Innerhalb des Tierkorpers. *Munch Tieraztl Wschr* **80:** 621–625, 1929.

Hoover, E. A., and Dubey, J. P. Pathogenesis of experimental pulmonary paragonimiasis in cats. *Am J Vet Res* **39:** 1872–1882, 1978.

Jarrett, W. F. H., McIntyre, W. I. M., and Urquhart, G. M. Recent work on husk. A preliminary report on an atypical pneumonia. *Vet Rec* **65:** 153–156, 1953.

Jarrett, W. R. H., McIntyre, W. I. M., and Urquhart, G. M. The pathology of experimental bovine parasitic bronchitis. *J Pathol Bacteriol* **73:** 183–193, 1957.

Jarrett, W. F. H. *et al*. Symposium on husk. 1. The disease process. *Vet Rec* **72:** 1066–1068, 1960.

Kassai, T. Die synonymie des *Cystocaulus ocreatus*. *Acta Vet Hung* **7:** 157–163, 1957.

Kassai, T. Vizsgalatok a juhok gocos tudofergessegerol. 4. Resz vizsgalat a *Cystocaulus ocreatus* pathogenitasarol. (Nodular verminous pneumonia in sheep. 4. *Cystocaulus ocreatus* infestation.) *Mag Allator Lapja* **12:** 333–337, 1957.

Li, P. L. A histopathologic study of small lungworm infection in sheep and goats with special reference to muscular hypertrophy of the lungs. *J Pathol Bacteriol* **58:** 373–379, 1946.

Mackenzie, A. Studies on lungworm infection of pigs. II. Lesions in experimental infections. *Vet Rec* **70:** 903–906, 1958.

Mackenzie, A. Pathological changes in lungworm infestation in two cats with special reference to changes in pulmonary arterial branches. *Res Vet Sci* **1:** 255–258, 1960.

Mackerras, M. J. Observations on the life history of the cat lungworm *Aelurostrongylus abstrusus* (Railliet, 1898) (Nematoda: Metastrongylidae). *Aust J Zool* **5:** 188–195, 1957.

Mackerras, M. J., and Sandars, D. F. The life history of the rat-lungworm, *Angiostrongylus cantonensis* (Chen) (Nematoda: Metastrongylidae). *Aust J Zool* **3:** 1–21, 1955.

McLennan, M. W., Humphris, R. B., and Rac, R. *Ascaris suum* pneumonia in cattle. *Aust Vet J* **50:** 266–268, 1974.

Michel, J. F., and Coates, G. H. D. An experimental outbreak of husk among previously parasitised cattle. *Vet Rec* **70:** 554–556, 1958.

Nicholls, J. M. *et al*. A pathological study of the lungs of foals infected experimentally with *Parascaris equorum*. *J Comp Pathol* **88:** 261–274, 1978.

Nicholls, J. M., Duncan, J. L., and Grieg, W. A. Lungworm (*Dictyocaulus arnfieldi*) infection in the horse. *Vet Rec* **102:** 216–217, 1978.

Nicholls, J. M. *et al.* Lungworm (*Dictyocaulus arnfieldi*) infection in donkeys. *Vet Rec* **104:** 567–570, 1979.

Nielsen, S. W. Canine paragonimiasis. *North Am Vet* **36:** 659–662, 1955.

Nimmo, J. S. Six cases of verminous pneumonia (*Muellerius* sp.) in goats. *Can Vet J* **20:** 49–52, 1979.

Parker, G.A. *et al.* Pathogenesis of acute toxoplasmosis in specific-pathogen-free cats. *Vet Pathol* **18:** 786–803, 1981.

Pirie, H. M. The pulmonary lesions characteristic of parasitic bronchitis and the commoner pneumonias of adult cattle in Britain. *In* "Respiratory Diseases in Cattle." W. B. Martin (ed.), The Hague, Boston, London; Martinus Nijhoff, 1978.

Prestwood, A. K. *et al.* Experimental canine angiostrongylosis. I. Pathological manifestations. *J Am Anim Hosp Assoc* **17:** 491–497, 1981.

Rose, J. H. Site of development of the lungworm *Muellerius capillaris* in experimentally infected lambs. *J Comp Pathol* **68:** 359–362, 1958.

Rose, J. H. Experimental infection of lambs with *Muellerius capillaris*. *J Comp Pathol* **69:** 414–422, 1959.

Saito, M., and Oishi, J. Natural infection of *Paragonimus ohirai* in pigs. *Med Biol (Tokyo)* **16:** 142–145, 1950.

Schnieder, T., Kaup, F.-J., and Drommer, W. Morphological investigations on the pathology of *Dictyocaulus viviparus* infections in cattle. *Parasitol Res* **77:** 260–265, 1991.

Schwartz, B., and Alicata, J. E. *Ascaris* larvae as a cause of liver and lung lesions in swine. *J Parasitol* **19:** 17–24, 1932.

Schwartz, B., and Alicata, J. E. Life history of lungworms parasitic in swine. *U S Dept Agric Tech Bull* **456:** 1934.

Seneviratna, P. Parasitic bronchitis in cats due to the nematode *Anafilaroides rostratus,* Gerichter, 1949. *J Comp Pathol* **68:** 352–357, 1958.

Sharma, D. N., and Dwivedi, J. N. Pulmonary schistosomiasis in sheep and goats due to *Schistosoma indicum* in India. *J Comp Pathol* **86:** 449–454, 1976.

Soliman, K. N. Observations on the orientation of certain lungworms in the respiratory tract and on their feeding habits. *Br Vet J* **107:** 274–278, 1951.

Soliman, K. N. Migration route of *Dictyocaulus viviparus* and *D. filaria* infective larvae to the lungs. *J Comp Pathol* **63:** 75–84, 1953.

Soulsby, E. J. L. "Helminths, Arthropods, and Protozoa of Domesticated Animals." Philadelphia, Pennsylvania, Lea & Febiger, 1982.

Srihakim, S., and Swerczek, T. W. Pathologic changes and pathogenesis of *Parascaris equorum* in parasite-free pony foals. *Am J Vet Res* **39:** 1155–1160, 1978.

Stockdale, P. H. G. Pulmonary pathology associated with metastrongyloid infections. *Br Vet J* **132:** 595–608, 1976.

Supperer, R. *Capillaria bohmi* sp. nov., eine neue Harrwurmart aus den Stirnhohlen des Fuchses. *Z Parasitenk* **16:** 51–55, 1953.

Wetzel, R. Zur Biologie des Fuchslungenwurmes *Crenosoma vulpis*. *Arch Wiss Prakt Tierheilk* **75:** 445–460, 1940.

Whitlock, J. H. A description of a new dog lungworm. *Wien Tieraerztl Mschr* **43:** 731–739, 1956.

Wirth, D. Lungenwurmkrankheit des Hundes. *Wien Tieraerztl Mschr* **34:** 768–771, 1947.

J. Neoplastic Diseases of the Lungs

Primary pulmonary tumors are rare in domestic animals. Metastatic lesions are relatively common, however, because of the vulnerability of the lungs to tumor emboli. In view of the much greater frequency of metastatic tumors, and because their gross and microscopic patterns can sometimes be difficult or impossible to distinguish from those of a primary tumor, an important part of the diagnosis of a primary lung tumor is thorough examination to exclude possible primary sites elsewhere in the body.

1. Primary Tumors

The rarity of primary pulmonary tumors in domestic animals is in contrast to their frequency in humans. This can probably be accounted for by the lack of carcinogenic stimuli from cigarette smoke or occupationally related chemicals in animals, and by the absence of large numbers of aged individuals. Primary tumors are encountered more often in dogs and cats than in other species. Reported incidence for the dog is ~4–5 per 100,000 animals in the population per year. The frequency based on postmortem examination varies with the population sampled, but as many as 1% of dogs necropsied have been recorded as having primary tumors of the lung. Comparable statistics for the cat indicate a frequency of approximately half that of the dog.

Neoplasms can arise from any of the tissues present in the lung, but with few exceptions, the significant ones arise from pulmonary epithelium. Classification of epithelial tumors of the lung is complicated by the recognition that what were once looked on as specific cell types can undergo metaplasia (transdifferentiation) in both inflammatory and neoplastic lesions. The histologic appearance of cells in a tumor is therefore not certain evidence of histogenetic origin. Thus there can be no absolutely rigid histogenetic classification. With this in mind, the following classification provides a useful working basis for categorization:

Primary Epithelial Tumors of the Lung

- Bronchial papilloma
- Bronchial gland adenoma
- Bronchogenic carcinoma
  - Squamous cell (epidermoid) carcinoma
  - Adenocarcinoma
  - Adenosquamous carcinoma
  - Undifferentiated (anaplastic) carcinoma
    - Small-cell type
    - Large-cell type
- Bronchioloalveolar tumor
  - Adenoma
  - Carcinoma
- Carcinoid

This classification serves as a framework for categorizing primary epithelial lung tumors across a range of species. Modifications are sometimes necessary, especially in domestic animals in which tumors are often well advanced when examined. In dogs and cats, for instance, clinically significant adenocarcinomas have frequently undergone sufficient phenotypic alterations that it is no longer possible to classify them as either bronchogenic (arising from major airways) or bronchioloalveolar (arising from small airways or alveolar parenchyma). The tumors usually develop in more peripheral lung regions, which is a feature of bronchioloalveolar tumors. Their distorted, invasive, papillary, and acinar pattern, however, is distinct from the orderly alveolar pattern seen in the typical bronchioloalveolar tumors which are usually found incidentally at necropsy.

Most pulmonary tumors in domestic animals are adenocarcinomas of bronchogenic or bronchioloalveolar origin. Adenosquamous carcinomas are the next most common, at least in the dog. Squamous cell carcinomas are occasionally found. Other varieties are extremely rare. Affected animals are usually middle-aged to old, with the mean age in dogs and cats being ~10–12 years.

Bronchogenic carcinomas are conventionally subdivided into squamous cell (epidermoid), adenocarcinoma, adenosquamous carcinoma, and undifferentiated forms. There is a strong tendency for both glandular and squamous components to occur in the same tumor (Fig. 6.102A). Sometimes these are mixed with more anaplastic regions. When both glandular and squamous components have cytologic and behavioral features of malignancy, the tumors should be designated adenosquamous. This has practical value because these adenosquamous carcinomas are among the most invasive of all the pulmonary carcinomas. Squamous cell and undifferentiated carcinomas are especially prone to arise from major airways and therefore have a more central (hilar) location in the lung. The bronchogenic carcinoma is typically a large, irregular, pale, fleshy mass with ill-defined border and possibly satellite nodules. More distant intrapulmonary metastasis can occur in the same or opposite lung. Consistency ranges from firm to soft and friable. Mucinous, cystic, or hemorrhagic and necrotic regions are sometimes present in the center of large, bulky masses. Occasionally, highly malignant infiltrative tumors cause more diffuse, discolored, rubbery, or solid regions that cannot be distinguished grossly from pneumonia. Squamous cell carcinomas have a preponderance of large cells with vesicular nuclei and abundant faintly granular acidophilic cytoplasm. Intercellular bridges can often be detected, but keratinization is usually limited to individual cells with intracytoplasmic clumps of keratin. Bronchogenic adenocarcinomas are invasive and destructive. They have disordered acinar, papillary, solid, or mixed patterns (Fig. 6.102B). Adenosquamous carcinomas have intermixed squamous components and glandular components (Fig. 6.102A). Differentiation from metastatic adenocarcinomas is often difficult.

Undifferentiated (anaplastic) carcinomas are the most rare variety in animals. Those recorded have mainly been of the small-cell type. This type can be further subdivided into round (oat cell), fusiform, and polygonal forms according to the appearance of the component cells. The so-

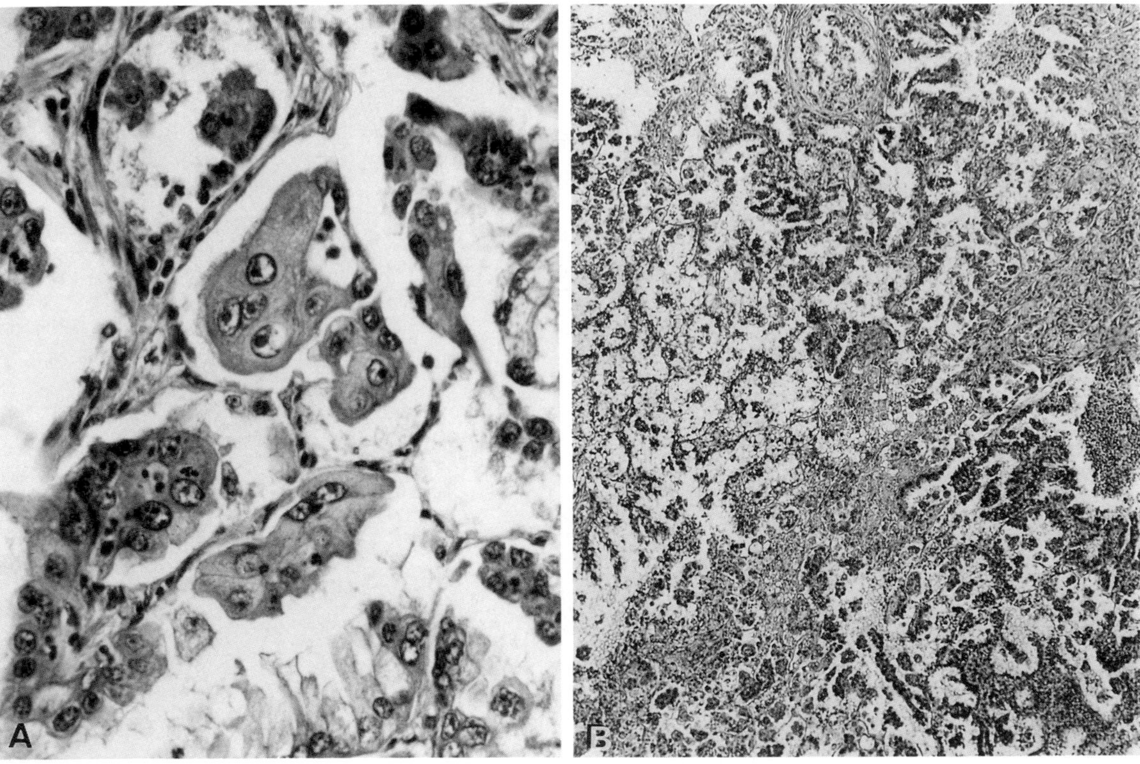

Fig. 6.102 (A) Adenosquamous carcinoma. Dog. (B) Invasive and destructive pattern of bronchogenic adenocarcinoma. Cat.

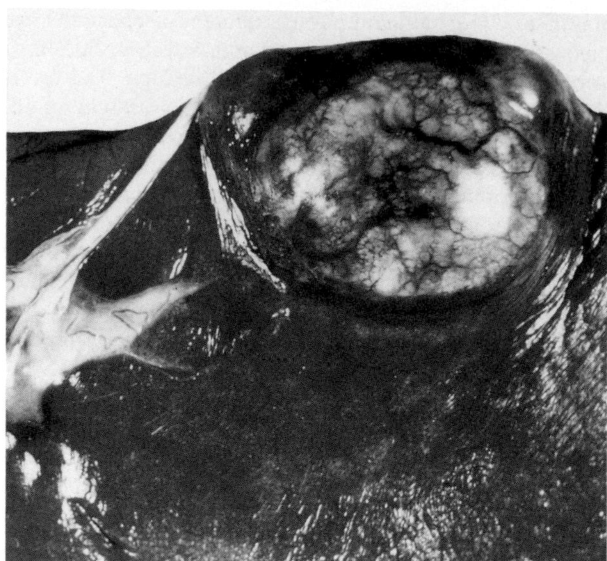

Fig. 6.103 Solitary, peripheral bronchioloalveolar tumor. Dog. (Courtesy of S. W. Nielsen.)

called oat cell carcinoma has ill-defined clusters of small round or oval cells resembling lymphocytes because of their hyperchromatic nuclei and small amounts of cytoplasm. In humans, the small-cell anaplastic tumors appear to arise from solitary neuroendocrine cells or formed neuroepithelial bodies, as do carcinoids. They are therefore particularly likely to be associated with paraneoplastic syndromes caused by secretion of polypeptide hormones [e.g., adrenocorticotropic hormone (ACTH), antidiuretic hormone (ADH), calcitonin] or biogenic amines (e.g., serotonin). Paraneoplastic syndromes accompanying primary pulmonary tumors do not appear to have been identified in animals.

In general, squamous cell, adenosquamous, and undifferentiated carcinomas are more malignant than adenocarcinomas, but all have a strong predilection for spread through intrapulmonary lymphatics. Dissemination through airways to alveoli also occurs. Metastasis can also take place to thoracic lymph nodes, abdominal nodes, and kidneys, liver, brain, heart, and bones.

Bronchioloalveolar tumors originate from either secretory bronchiolar (Clara) cells or alveolar type II epithelial cells. Because of the close phenotypic relationship between these two cell types, it is not surprising that histologic and ultrastructural examination sometimes reveals both cell types in the same tumor. Bronchioloalveolar tumors are found most often in dogs, occasionally as an incidental finding at necropsy. They compose over half the tumors found in some surveys of primary pulmonary tumors of dogs. Typically, they occur as solitary nodules in the periphery of the lung (Fig. 6.103). Occasionally there are multiple nodules. The more benign tumors (adenomas) grow slowly by peripheral expansion and compression of surrounding parenchyma. Centers of large nodules frequently become necrotic. Other tumors, in which the neoplastic cells spread peripherally over alveolar walls, have the characteristics of low-grade adenocarcinomas. Less frequently, there is a rapidly spreading diffuse or disseminated multifocal type (Fig. 6.104). Histologically, the special feature of bronchioloalveolar tumors is the regular alveolar pattern and preservation of pulmonary architecture (Fig. 6.105). The preexisting alveolar stroma becomes lined by cuboidal or columnar epithelium, often with small papillary projections into the alveolar lumina.

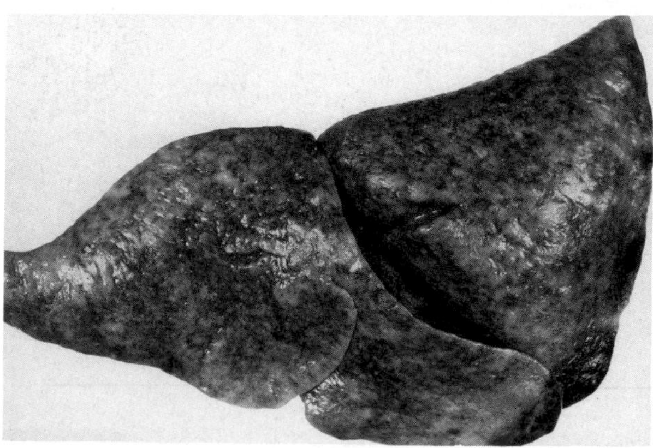

Fig. 6.104 Widespread multifocal involvement in bronchioloalveolar carcinoma. Dog.

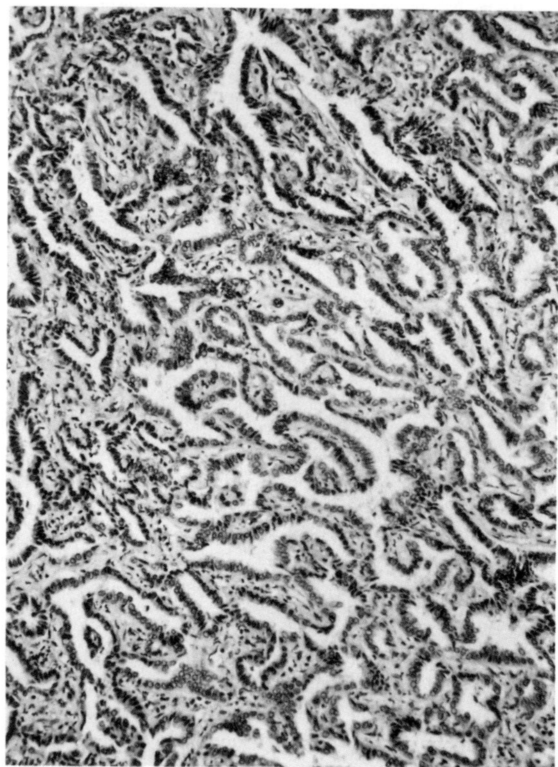

Fig. 6.105 Histology of bronchioloalveolar tumor showing regular pattern of spaces lined by cuboidal to low columnar epithelium. Dog.

As with many tumors, there is difficulty in clearly separating benign and malignant bronchioloalveolar tumors. Because there seems to be potential for eventual development of malignant behavior, there is often no attempt to categorize them as adenomas or carcinomas, but to regard them all as low-grade carcinomas unless there is clear evidence of highly aggressive behavior.

There are two major pitfalls in the diagnosis of bronchioloalveolar tumors. One is that the hyperplasia of bronchiolar and alveolar type II epithelial cells, which is frequently caused by chronic inflammation of the bronchioloalveolar junction, can be mistaken for neoplastic proliferation. The other is that rapidly invasive spread of neoplastic cells from either a bronchogenic adenocarcinoma or a metastasis from elsewhere in the body can sometimes mimic the regular pattern of a bronchioloalveolar carcinoma. Exclusion of alternative primary sites is therefore an integral part of the diagnosis of bronchioloalveolar tumors, especially the multinodular or diffuse varieties.

The difficulty of classifying advanced adenocarcinomas as bronchogenic or bronchioloalveolar was referred to earlier. In such cases, the tumors should be classified on the basis of morphologic pattern as adenocarcinomas without attempt to specify the site of origin. As an indication of how this works in practice, a review of 22 clinically detected pulmonary carcinomas in dogs revealed 13 adenocarcinomas (8 predominantly papillary, 5 mucin-secreting), 5 adenosquamous carcinomas, 2 bronchioloalveolar adenocarcinomas, 1 bronchioloalveolar adenoma and 1 large-cell undifferentiated carcinoma. A prominent feature of most adenocarcinomas was presence of tall columnar neoplastic cells. Five of the 13 adenocarcinomas each had a few small foci where squamous phenotypic expression occurred, even though this was not prominent enough to warrant a diagnosis of adenosquamous carcinoma.

Pulmonary adenomatosis of sheep is an infectious form of bronchioloalveolar tumor with the behavioral characteristics of a low-grade carcinoma. For this reason, it is now referred to as **pulmonary carcinomatosis.** The cause is reasonably established as a type B/D retrovirus, but reproduction by purified, cloned virus has not yet been reported. The term *jaagsiekte* appeared in original descriptions of the disease from South Africa, *jaagsiekte* being the Afrikaans word for driving sickness.

Pulmonary carcinomatosis occurs in many sheep-raising areas of the world. It is most important under conditions of intensive management, which favor aerosol transmission of the causative virus. The disease is less common where populations of sheep are dispersed, and it can escape detection for a time, as happened in the United States. The condition belongs in the category of slow virus diseases. Lesions develop slowly with the result that the disease has an insidious onset. Clinical signs are not apparent for several months to several years and therefore are seen only in adult sheep. Early signs of the disease are coughing and exercise intolerance. Later there are also crackles and wheezes associated with the production of abundant watery exudate. The exudate is discharged from the nose, especially when the head is lowered, and is an important diagnostic clinical feature.

Early gross lesions are scattered, small gray-white nodules, sometimes with surrounding hyperinflated zones (Fig. 6.106). Sheep with clinical signs have extensive nodular and confluent firm gray lesions affecting much of the pulmonary tissue. The lungs are heavy and fail to collapse. The cut surface is moist and reveals the basic nodularity of the lesion, even in regions where they coalesce. The centers of advanced lesions lose their friability and become fibrotic. There can be coexisting bronchopneumonia, verminous pneumonia, chronic progressive pneumonia (maedi) or combinations of these. This has been a source of considerable confusion in the past, particularly when the viruses causing chronic progressive pneumonia and pulmonary carcinomatosis were both present in the same flock. The lesions of chronic progressive pneumonia and pulmonary carcinomatosis are quite different histologically.

The characteristic histologic lesion of pulmonary carcinomatosis consists of multiple proliferative foci of cuboidal or columnar cells which line alveoli and form papillary projections into their lumina (Fig. 6.107A,B). Continued proliferation obscures this pattern, and fibroplasia often occurs in more disorganized and degenerative regions. Early and uncomplicated proliferative lesions are not associated with significant accumulations of inflammatory

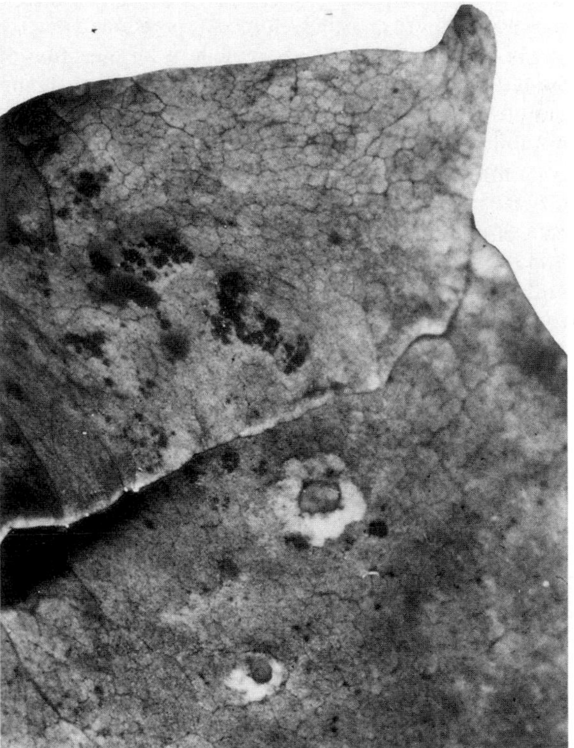

Fig. 6.106 Isolated subpleural nodules present in early case of pulmonary carcinomatosis (*jaagsiekte*). Sheep.

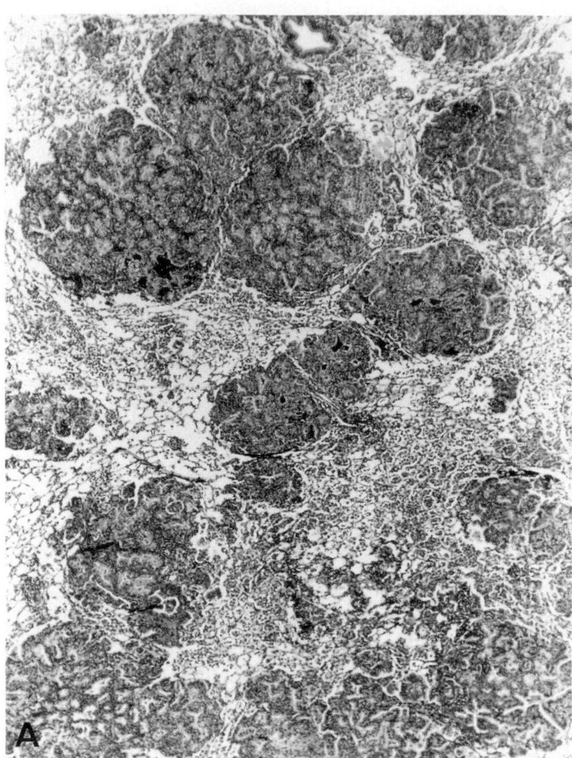

Fig. 6.107A Multiple discrete tumor nodules with acinar and papillary patterns in pulmonary carcinomatosis. Sheep.

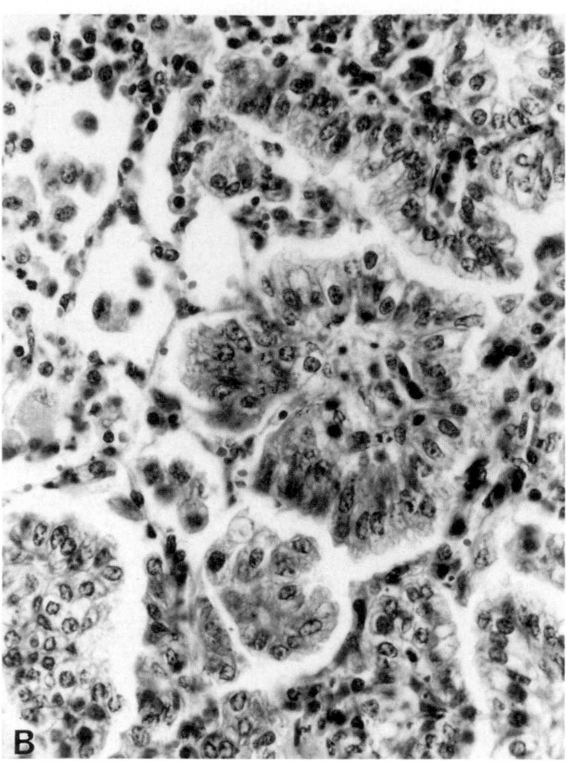

Fig. 6.107B Higher magnification of (A) showing columnar cells lining alveolar walls and forming papillae within lumina. [(A) and (B) courtesy of K. Perk and *Advances in Veterinary Science*.]

cells, although there is usually some aggregation of macrophages in alveolar lumina. The papillary proliferation of cuboidal or columnar epithelium in the absence of significant interstitial inflammation is in marked contrast to the lymphofollicular interstitial pneumonia of chronic progressive pneumonia (maedi) in which alveolar epithelial hyperplasia is an inconstant and relatively minor feature.

The papillary proliferations involve both alveoli and bronchioles in many nodules. Ultrastructurally the cuboidal cells usually have lamellar bodies characteristic of alveolar type II cells, whereas the columnar cells have secretory granules and glycogen compatible with origin from secretory bronchiolar epithelial (Clara) cells. The potentially carcinomatous nature of this infectious bronchioloalveolar tumor is confirmed by the occasional finding of metastatic foci in the bronchial or mediastinal lymph nodes.

Carcinoids have been reported to occur in lungs of animals but have not yet been adequately documented. Carcinoids in humans originate from neuroendocrine components of major airways. They have an endocrine pattern of nests or ribbons of uniform cells separated by well-vascularized stroma. The cells are round to polygonal. They have relatively small nuclei and abundant, pale, acidophilic cytoplasm. Ultrastructurally their neuroendocrine derivation is revealed by large numbers of small, dense, secretory granules. Immunocytochemical labeling reveals the presence of functional markers such as gastrin-releasing peptide, neuron-specific enolase, chromogranin, and serotonin. It is probable that carcinoids occur in animals, albeit extremely rarely.

Granular cell tumors (myoblastomas) are the only neoplasm of mesenchymal origin deserving special mention. These are tumors which were originally thought to be derived from myoblasts but are now believed to originate from a fibroblastlike cell which is related to the progenitor of Schwann cells. Although granular cell tumors can occur in various tissues, there is a difference in predilection sites among species. All granular cell tumors found to date in the lungs of animals have been in horses, and in fact this is the most frequently reported primary pulmonary tumor of the horse in recent years. The tumors have occurred in older horses and either were associated with coughing and pulmonary insufficiency or were found as incidental lesions at slaughter. Gross lesions are usually multiple discrete or semiconfluent nodules which have a tendency to be associated with major bronchi and to cause obstruction by bulging into their lumina. The lesions are limited to one lung in most instances, more often the right one. The main histologic feature of the tumor is lobular aggregation of large, round to polyhedral cells with abundant acidophilic granular cytoplasm (Fig. 6.108A,B). The lobules are surrounded and dissected by fibrovascular stroma. The cytoplasmic granules in the tumor cells are

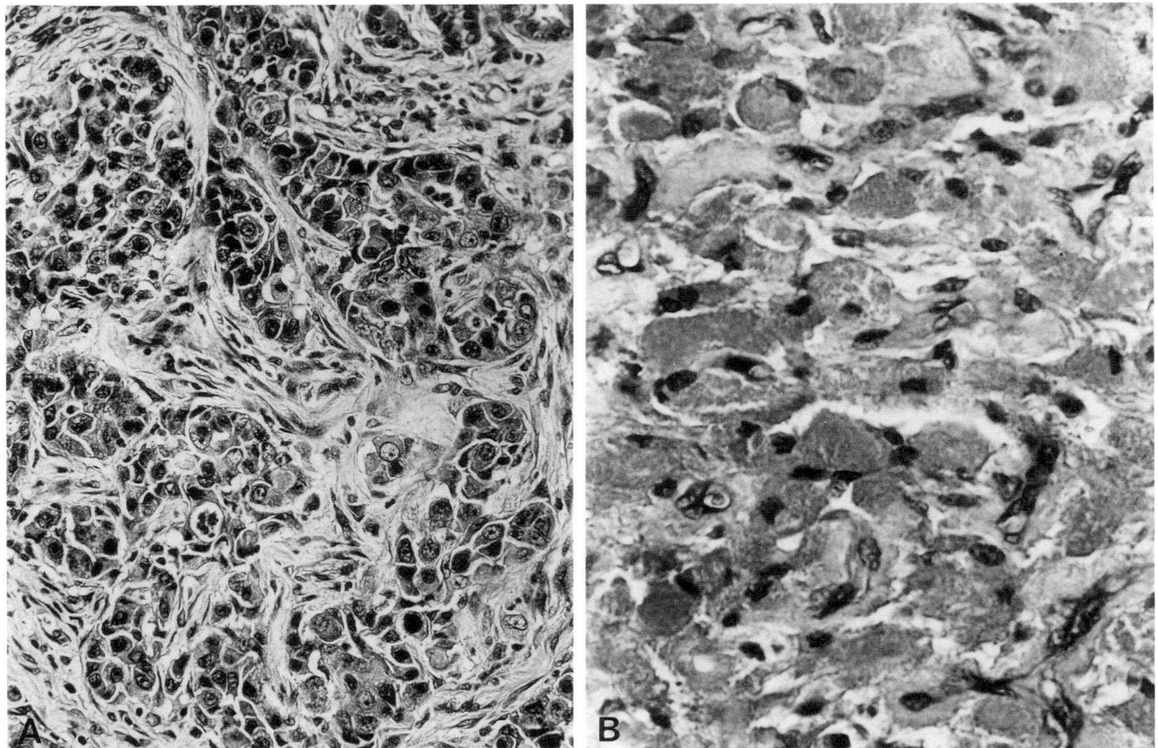

Fig. 6.108 (A) Granular cell tumor of the lung. Horse. (B) Higher magnification of (A) showing cells with abundant acidophilic granular cytoplam.

PAS positive and have characteristic ultrastructural features.

Lymphomatoid granulomatosis refers to a rare condition of dogs in which there is extensive infiltration of one or more lobes of the lung by accumulations of mixed atypical lymphoreticular cells. The cells have a pronounced tendency to invade the walls of vessels (Fig. 6.109A) and airways. The few reported cases have been in young dogs. Cells composing the neoplasm are of various types. Large histiocytic and plasmacytoid forms predominate (Fig. 6.109B), but binucleate cells, eosinophils, lymphocytes, and plasma cells are often also present. A network of fibrous stroma runs throughout the tumor. Mitotic figures are plentiful. The exact nature of the condition is not known, but evidence is emerging that lymphomatoid granulomatosis in dogs is a pleocellular form of T-cell lymphoma. It is important, however, not to use this diagnosis for generally unclassifiable tumors of the lung or for more usual forms of lymphoma in which there is extensive invasion of perivascular and peribronchial regions of the lung by the neoplastic lymphoid cells.

2. *Metastatic Tumors*

Many types of malignant tumors can metastasize to the lungs. Mammary carcinomas are among the most frequent in dogs and cats (Fig. 6.110A), uterine adenocarcinomas, in cattle (Fig. 6.110B), and malignant melanoma, in the horse. Carcinomas originating in endocrine gland or skin are also a common source. Osteosarcomas, hemangiosarcomas, and fibrosarcomas are frequent varieties of sarcoma. The most easily recognizable pattern of metastatic tumors is of multiple nodules scattered throughout the pulmonary parenchyma, without great variation in size range (Fig. 6.110A). The presence of a few gross lesions, especially if there is great discrepancy in size, requires careful analysis of all gross and microscopic findings to provide the best chance of making an unequivocal distinction between metastatic foci and primary pulmonary tumor. The probability of neoplastic foci in the lungs being metastases is increased if the animal is a young one. Sometimes, microscopic examination is needed to differentiate neoplastic nodules and multifocal granulomas.

Microscopically, metastatic tumors usually resemble the primary lesions, although they may be either better or less differentiated. Presence of tumor cells within arteries is an important indicator of metastatic origin, although this can be difficult to identify in some instances. This is particularly so where scirrhous response around invaded lymphatics gives them a superficial resemblance to thick-walled blood vessels.

In some cases where there is fulminating metastasis, there is no gross evidence of solid neoplastic infiltrations, merely tan discoloration of the lung and slightly increased firmness. Microscopically, however, widespread vascular embolization by anaplastic cells is seen (Fig. 6.110C) with early invasion of alveoli and lymphatics. Regardless of

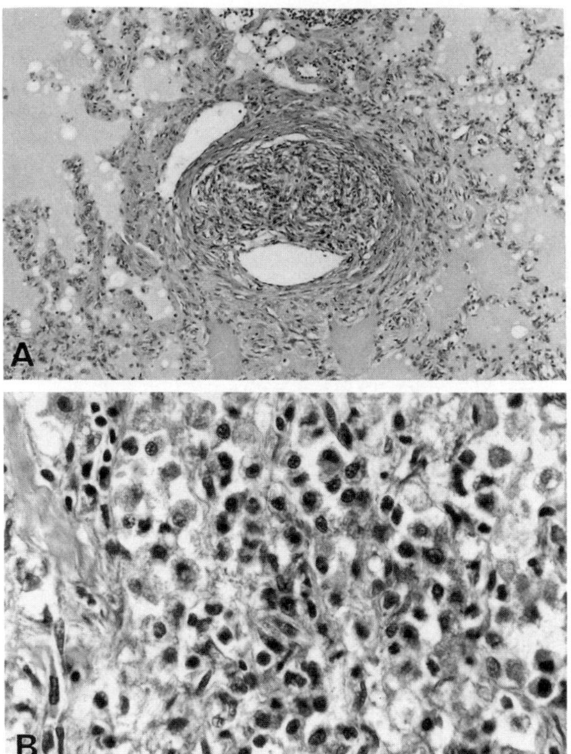

Fig. 6.109 (A) Eccentric invasion of intima of small artery in lymphomatoid granulomatosis. Dog. (B) Predominance of histiocytic and plasmacytoid cells in lymphomatoid granulomatosis. Dog.

source or initial pattern of pulmonary involvement, highly malignant tumors have a predilection for widespread dissemination through intrapulmonary lymphatics.

Bibliography

Blakemore, F., and Bosworth, T. J. The occurrence of jaagziekte in England. *Vet Rec* **53:** 35–37, 1941.

Carpenter, R. H., and Hansen, J. F. Diffuse pulmonary bronchiolo-alveolar carcinoma in a cat. *Calif Vet* **36**(4): 11–14, 1982.

Cuba-Caparo, A. La poliadenomatosis pulmonar del carnero. (Pulmonary adenomatosis in sheep.) *Bol Esc Nacl Ciencias Vet* **1:** 27–57, 1945.

Cutlip, R. C., and Young, S. Sheep pulmonary adenomatosis (jaagsiekte) in the United States. *Am J Vet Res* **43:** 2108–2113, 1982.

Dungal, N. Experiments with jaagsiekte. *Am J Pathol* **22:** 737–759, 1946.

Ferri, A. G., and Tausk, E. Primary pulmonary carcinomas of the dog. *J Comp Pathol* **65:** 159–167, 1955.

Geisel, O. Primare Lungensarkome beim Hund. *Berl Muench Tieraerztl Wochenschr* **93:** 174–177, 1980.

Gould, V. E. *et al.* Neuroendocrine components of the bronchopulmonary tract: Hyperplasias, dysplasias, and neoplasms. *Lab Invest* **49:** 519–537, 1983.

Hod, I. *et al.* Lung carcinoma of sheep (jaagsiekte). III. Lymph node, blood, and immunoglobulin. *J Natl Cancer Inst* **48:** 487–507, 1972.

Hod, I., Herz, A., and Zimber, A. Pulmonary carcinoma (jaagsiekte) of sheep: Ultrastructural study of early and advanced tumor lesions. *Am J Pathol* **86:** 545–558, 1977.

Lucke, V. M. *et al.* A lymphomatoid granulomatosis of the lungs in young dogs. *Vet Pathol* **16:** 405–412, 1979.

Markson, L. M., and Terlecki, S. The experimental transmission of ovine pulmonary adenomatosis. *Pathol Vet* **1:** 269–288, 1964.

Martin, W. B. *et al.* Experimental production of sheep pulmonary adenomatosis (jaagsiekte). *Nature* **264:** 183–184, 1976.

Monlux, A. W. *et al.* Adenocarcinoma of the uterus of the cow—differentiation of its pulmonary metastases from primary lung tumors. *Am J Vet Res* **17:** 45–73, 1956.

Monlux, W. S. Primary pulmonary neoplasms in domestic animals. *Southwest Vet* (*Suppl.*) 1–39, 1952.

Moulton, J. E., von Tscharner, C., and Schneider, R. Classification of lung carcinomas in the dog and cat. *Vet Pathol* **18:** 513–528, 1981.

Murphy, J. R., Breeze, R. G., and McPherson, E. A. Myxoma of the equine respiratory tract. *Mod Vet Pract* **59:** 529–532, 1978.

Nickels, F. A., Brown, C. M., and Breeze, R. G. Myoblastoma: Equine granular cell tumor. *Mod Vet Pract* **61:** 593–596, 1980.

Nielsen, S. W., and Horava, A. Primary pulmonary tumors of the dog, a report of sixteen cases. *Am J Vet Res* **21:** 813–830, 1969.

Nisbet, D. I. *et al.* Ultrastructure of sheep pulmonary adenomatosis (jaagsiekte). *J Pathol* **103:** 157–162, 1971.

Parker, G. A. *et al.* Granular cell tumour (myoblastoma) in the lung of a horse. *J Comp Pathol* **89:** 421–430, 1979.

Parodi, A. L., Tassin, P., and Rigoulet, J. Myoblastome a cellules granuleuses. Trois nouvelles observations a localisation pulmonaire chez le cheval. *Recueil Med Vet* **150:** 489–494, 1974.

Perk, K. Slow virus infection of ovine lung. *Adv Vet Sci Comp Med* **26:** 267–288, 1982.

Perk, K. *et al.* Lung carcinoma of sheep (jaagsiekte). II. Histogenesis of the tumor. *J Natl Cancer Inst* **47:** 197–205, 1971.

Sanford, S. E., and Bundza, A. Multicentric bronchiolo-alveolar neoplasm in a steer. *Vet Pathol* **19:** 95–97, 1982.

Sjolte, I. P. Primare miligne Tumoren der Lungen bei Tieren. *Virchows Arch* **312:** 35–63, 1944.

Stunzi, H. Das epidermoide Lungenkarzinom des Hundes als Vergleichsobjekt fur das Raucherkarzinom des Menschen. *Schweiz Arch Tierheilkd* **113:** 311–319, 1971.

Stunzi, H. Das anaplastische Lungenkarzinom des Hundes. *Vet Pathol* **10:** 102–113, 1973.

Stunzi, H., Head, K. W., and Nielsen, S. W. Tumors of the lung. *Bull WHO* **50:** 9–20, 1974.

Theilen, G. H., and Madewell, B. R. Tumors of the respiratory tract and thorax. *In* "Veterinary Cancer Medicine," G. H. Theilen and B. R. Madewell (eds.). Philadelphia, Pennsylvania, Lea & Febiger, 1979.

Troy, M. A. Bronchogenic carcinoma in the cat. *J Am Vet Med Assoc* **126:** 410–411, 1955.

Turk, M. A. M., and Breeze, R. G. Histochemical and ultrastructural features of an equine pulmonary granular cell tumour (myoblastoma). *J Comp Pathol* **91:** 471–481, 1981.

Verwoerd, O. W., and Williamson, A. L. Preliminary characterization of newly isolated ovine retrovirus causing jaagsiekte, a pulmonary adenomatosis. *In* "Advances in Comparative Leukemia Research 1981," D. S. Yohn and J. R. Blakeslee (eds.). New York, Elsevier Biomedical, 1982.

Verwoerd, O. W., Williamson, A. L., and De Villiers, E. M.

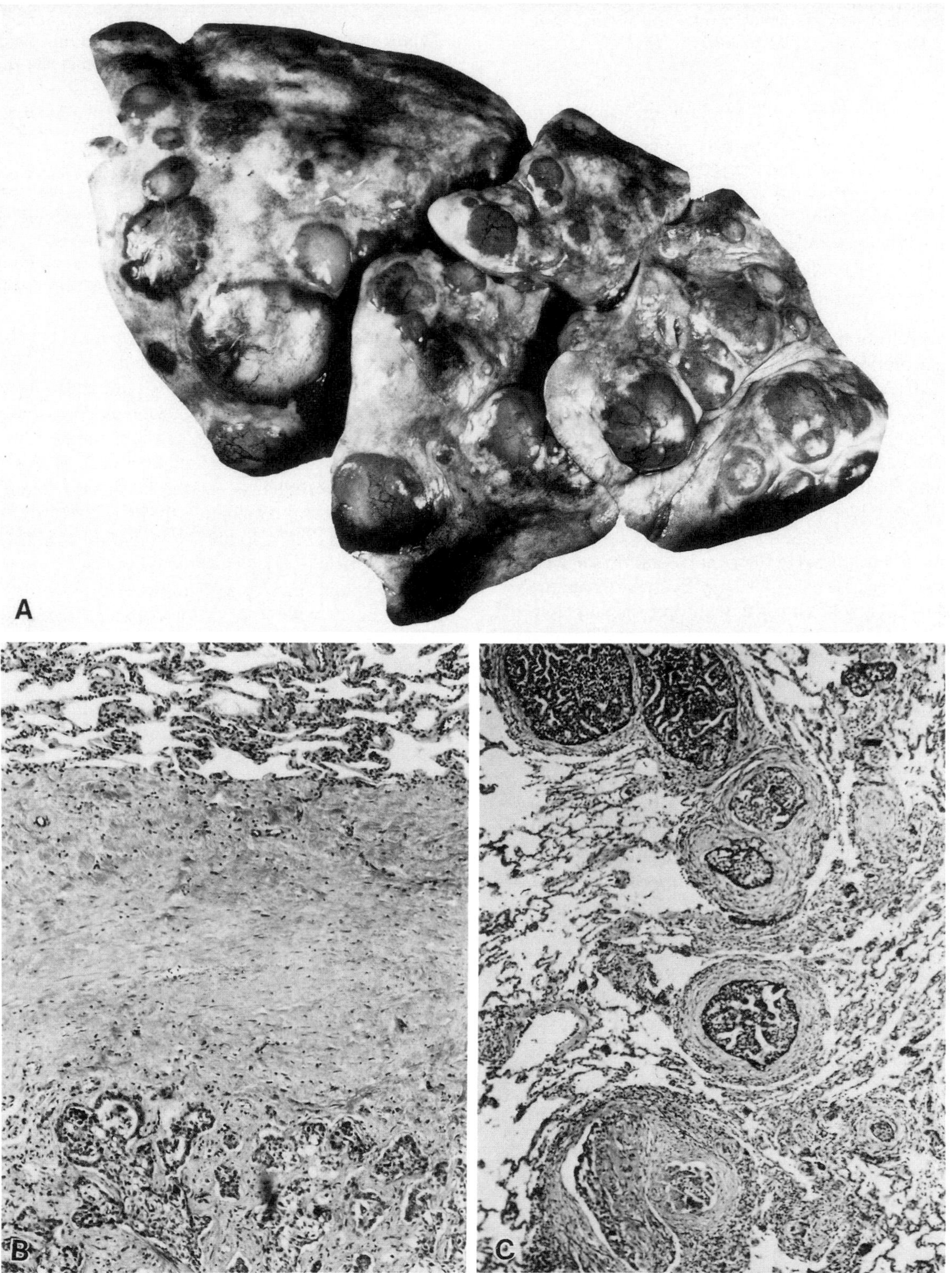

Fig. 6.110 (A) Metastatic nodules of mammary adenocarcinoma. Dog. (B) Metastatic uterine adenocarcinoma with extensive scirrhous response. Cow. (C) Multiple foci of malignant mammary adenocarcinoma resulting from neoplastic embolization of pulmonary vessels. Dog.

Aetiology of jaagsiekte: Transmission by means of subcellular fractions and evidence for involvment of a retrovirus. *Onderstepoort J Vet Res* **47:** 275–280, 1980.

VII. Pleura and Mediastinum

Pleural abnormalities are usually secondary to lesions in tissues or organs forming the pleural cavity, especially the lung, or are part of more generalized disorders.

Congenital anomalies of the pleura and mediastinum are of little significance unless associated with a condition such as congenital diaphragmatic hernia. Congenital cysts may occasionally be found in the anterior mediastinum, mostly of brachycephalic dogs, and are presumed to be vestiges of the branchial pouches. Usually they are detected microscopically as cystic spaces lined by a single layer of cuboidal epithelium, often in close association with thymic tissues. Cysts of ~1 cm or more in diameter can be seen grossly as thin-walled structures containing clear, light yellow fluid. Air- or fluid-filled cysts in the caudal mediastinum are more likely to be of bronchogenic origin and can be large enough to cause pulmonary insufficiency.

Degenerative changes in the pleura occur in some cases of uremia in dogs (see The Urinary System, Chapter 5 of this volume). They are most evident in parietal pleura of the intercostal spaces, particularly the second, third, and fourth. Mineralization centered on degenerate subpleural elastin and collagen fibers is visible as white horizontal striations.

Pneumothorax refers to the presence of air or gas in the pleural cavities. Air in the cavities allows the lungs to collapse to a degree proportional to the amount of air present. A normal subatmospheric pressure can be assumed to have been present at necropsy if the diaphragm moves caudally when the thorax is pierced and air is allowed to enter. In small animals, pneumothorax can be detected by opening the chest under water and observing the escape of air bubbles.

Pneumothorax can be spontaneous or traumatic. Spontaneous pneumothorax is rare. It may complicate any pulmonary disease which leads to rupture of pulmonary parenchyma at the pleural surface. It is most often associated with rupture of emphysematous bullae. Less commonly it follows rupture of a cavitated abscess or pyogranuloma that communicates with an airway, or rupture of a parasitic cyst such as can occur in paragonimiasis. Traumatic pneumothorax is usually the result of accidental perforation of the thoracic wall or rupture of lung and visceral pleura. Air which tracks through the pulmonary interstitium to the mediastinum (pneumomediastinum) does not usually escape into the pleural cavities unless there is traumatic rupture of the mediastinum.

Traumatic pneumothorax can also be a complication of cardiac resuscitation or biopsy of the lung. Whatever the cause of pneumothorax, if entry of air stops before there is critical reduction of pulmonary function, the air is slowly resorbed.

A. *Noninflammatory Pleural Effusions*

Hydrothorax is the accumulation of edema fluid in the thoracic cavities. It is usually bilateral and has the same wide range of causes as edema of the lung or elsewhere. The fluid is clear, watery, and ranges from almost colorless to light yellow. Large amounts of it are present when there is widespread neoplastic involvement of pleural surfaces or when lymphatic drainage is impeded by neoplastic enlargement of the thymus or cranial mediastinal lymph nodes.

Hydrothorax may be present in cases of congestive heart failure, particularly in dogs, cats, and cattle. It is also present in severe anemias or in hypoproteinemias associated with the nephrotic syndrome, hepatopathy, protein-losing enteropathy, or malnutrition. Hydrothorax is also a feature of specific diseases or syndromes such as mulberry heart disease in swine, black disease in sheep, African horsesickness, and ANTU poisoning. Chronic hydrothorax causes pleural opacity because of reactive hyperplasia of mesothelial cells and fibrous thickening of the underlying pleural connective tissue.

Chylothorax refers to the accumulation of milky fluid in the thorax (Fig. 6.111). The fluid is lipid-rich lymph, which can be distinguished from other turbid effusions by extraction of the fat with ether or by staining the droplets with a sudanophilic dye. Occasionally the source of the chylothorax is traced to rupture of the thoracic or right lym-

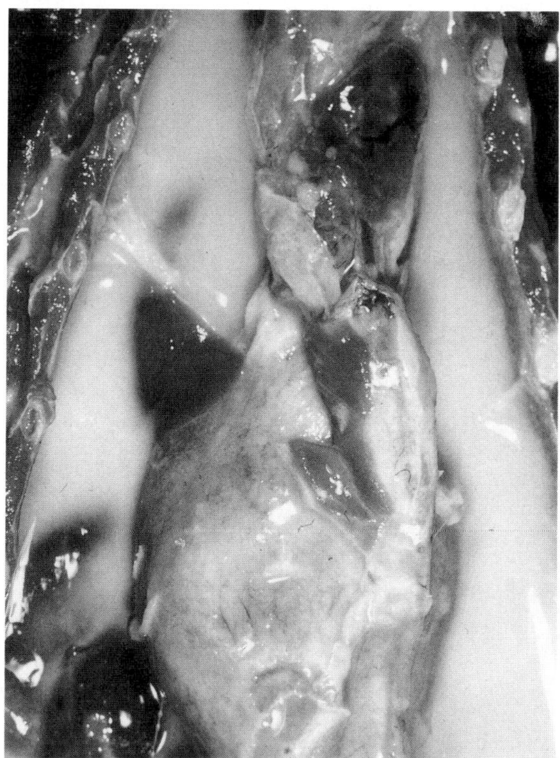

Fig. 6.111 Chylothorax. Cat.

phatic ducts. This is presumed to be the case in the many instances in which the origin is not found. The most common association of chylothorax is with a traumatic event, bouts of severe coughing, or tumors in the cranial mediastinum.

Hemothorax is the presence of blood in the pleural cavities. It is most often the result of traumatic rupture of blood vessels, but it can also be caused by erosion of the wall of a vessel by an inflammatory or neoplastic process. Less common causes are diseases in which there is a clotting disorder. Hemorrhage may also arise from highly vascularized tumors (e.g., hemangiosarcoma) or inflammatory processes such as pleural tuberculosis in dogs. Chronic hydrothorax may lead to the development of well-vascularized papillae on the pleura, and rupture of these may cause the effusion to resemble blood.

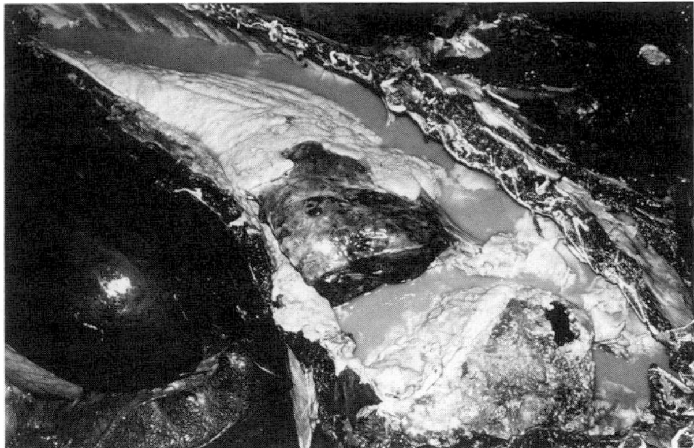

Fig. 6.112 Severe fibrinopurulent pleuritis and pyothorax. Horse.

B. Pleuritis

Inflammation of the pleura (pleuritis) is the most commonly encountered abnormality. It is usually secondary to pneumonia (see Anatomic Patterns of Pneumonia, Section VI,F of this chapter). Other pathways by which inflammatory agents reach the pleura are the bloodstream, lymphatic permeation from the peritoneal cavity, traumatic penetration from outside the chest or from the esophagus or abdominal viscus such as the bovine reticulum, or direct extension from a mediastinal abscess or esophagitis. The agents causing pleuritis as part of blood-borne infections vary with species of animal affected. *Haemophilus* spp. are commonly the cause in swine, as are mycoplasmas in swine and goats. *Chlamydia psittaci* is occasionally involved in ruminants. The virus of feline infectious peritonitis is the most common cause in cats. Pleural defenses against microorganisms are much less effective than those of the lung. Even a few organisms reaching the pleural surfaces are therefore apt to have serious consequences in contrast to the result of a similar exposure in the lungs. The reactions of the pleura to inflammation are the same as those of the pericardium (see The Cardiovascular System, Volume 3, Chapter 1).

Abundant purulent effusion into the pleural sacs is designated as **pyothorax** or **thoracic empyema.** The condition can occur in any animal, but is of most clinical significance in horses, dogs, and cats. It can be caused by pyogenic organisms reaching the pleural cavities by any of the pathways mentioned previously, but the relative importance of the pathways and the mix of organisms involved vary with the species of animal. Most cases of serofibrinous effusion or pyothorax in the horse are secondary to either pneumonia or pulmonary abscessation. The exudate is usually thin and dirty yellow (Fig. 6.112) and may be either unilateral or bilateral. Streptococci are the organisms most consistently isolated, sometimes in mixed infections with *E. coli, Klebsiella* spp., *Pasteurella* spp., *Pseudomonas* spp. or staphylococci. *Pasteurella* spp., staphylococci, and *Bacteroides* spp. are isolated in pure culture on occasion. *Mycoplasma felis* has been added to the list of possible agents. There is failure to culture organisms from the pleural effusion in as many as 50% of cases, however. In horses, exudative pleuritis occurs most often in racehorses, and in many cases the onset is associated with stress of traveling, training, or racing.

Pyothorax unassociated with significant pneumonia occurs in dogs, mostly in sporting breeds with access to rural environments. It particularly affects dogs which are used for hunting or are in training. The exudate is unilateral or bilateral, more commonly the latter. It is usually blood stained and viscous or flocculent but may be creamy or darkly serofibrinous. Yellowish sulfur granules may be present in the bloodstained pus. The pleural surfaces are thickened and velvety red or grayish yellow and fibrotic, depending on age and nature of the lesion. The cranial mediastinum is the main site of thickening. *Actinomyces, Nocardia,* and *Bacteroides* spp. are the most frequently recovered organisms, and these are commonly associated with the presence of sulfur granules and a characteristic pyogranulomatous pleuritis and mediastinitis (Fig. 6.113). Mixed infections are common, however, and a variety of other organisms can be present, including *Corynebacterium* spp., *Pasteurella* spp., *E. coli, Fusobacterium necrophorum, Pseudomonas* spp., and streptococci. The pathogenesis of the lesion is uncertain, but the circumstantial evidence supports the belief that infection reaches the pleural cavity in most instances by way of migrating grass awns or florets. It is next to impossible to find plant material in the copious pleural exudate, but there is sometimes an association with subcutaneous abscesses or fistulous tracts compatible with migration of grass awns, and affected dogs are those with greatest exposure to the species of grasses responsible for invasion of body orifices and subcutis. The damage caused by the migrating grass awns also seems particularly favorable for growth of the actinomycetes.

Pyothorax is fairly common in cats (Fig. 6.114). The pus is usually creamy yellow or grayish brown. As in dogs, it is more often bilateral than unilateral. Various bacteria are responsible, often in mixed infection. *Pasteurella mul-*

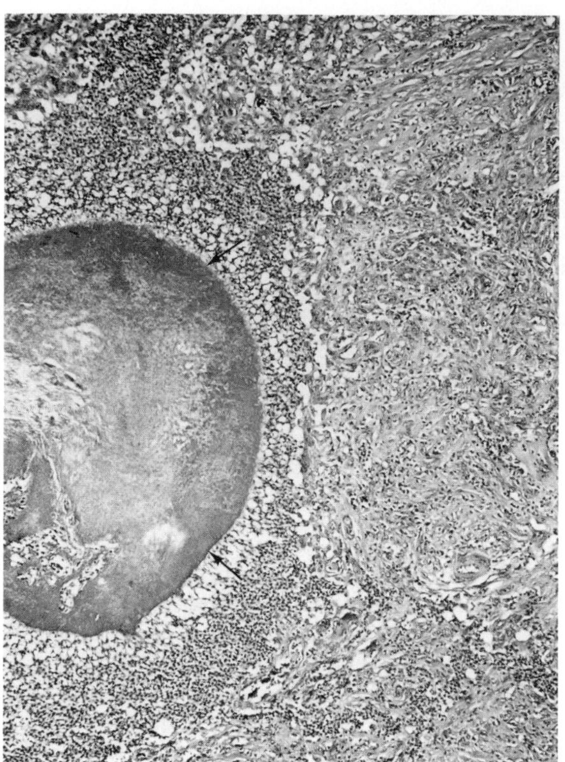

Fig. 6.113 Pyogranulomatous pleuritis caused by *Actinomyces* sp. Dog. Note the large bacterial colony (arrows).

tocida, various Gram-negative enteric bacteria, streptococci, and staphylococci have been isolated. *Actinomyces, Nocardia,* and *Bacteroides* spp. are recovered on occasion, but much less consistently than in dogs. There are few pointers regarding the pathogenesis of the condition in cats. Although it is speculated that infection could gain access by penetration of a foreign body from the external surface or esophagus, or by a penetrating bite wound, there are few data available.

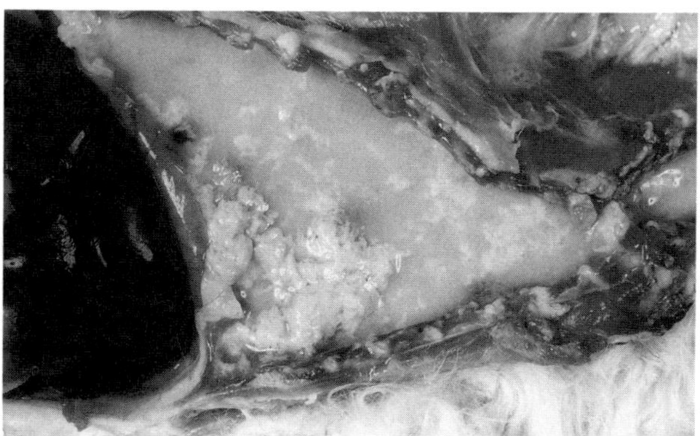

Fig. 6.114 Pyothorax. Cat.

C. Neoplastic Diseases of the Pleura

Primary pleural tumors are rare. The specific type is the pleural mesothelioma, which has been found in the cow, dog, cat, horse, and goat. Mesotheliomas arise from the pericardial and peritoneal surfaces, as well as from the pleura (see The Peritoneum, Retroperitoneum, and Mesentery, Chapter 4 of this volume). There is one report of ferruginous bodies being present in significantly greater numbers in the lungs of a small series of dogs with mesotheliomas. Ferruginous bodies are fine fibers irregularly coated by ferritin and amorphous protein. The cores are most commonly asbestos fibers, and therefore the numbers of ferruginous bodies are usually accepted as an index of exposure to asbestos. The finding of increased numbers in the lungs of dogs with mesotheliomas suggests that inhalation of asbestos fibers could be related to the development of mesotheliomas in this species, as it is in humans.

Primary tumors can also arise from the chest wall and mediastinal tissues. Tumors of bone and cartilage, nerve sheaths, thymus, lymph nodes, and ectopic glandular tissue are discussed elsewhere.

Secondary tumors of the pleura are also uncommon, but transpleural dissemination of carcinomas and sarcomas occasionally occurs by extension from the lungs, chest wall, or mediastinum. Carcinomas from the abdominal cavity can reach the pleura by penetrating diaphragmatic lymphatics.

Bibliography

Creighton, S. R., and Wilkins, R. J. Thoracic effusion in the cat. Etiology and diagnostic features. *J Am Anim Hosp Assoc* **11:** 66–76, 1975.

Gruffydd-Jones, T. J., and Flecknell, P. A. The prognosis and treatment related to the gross appearance and laboratory characteristics of pathological thoracic fluids in the cat. *J Small Anim Pract* **19:** 315–328, 1978.

Harbison, M. L., and Godleski, J. J. Malignant mesothelioma in urban dogs. *Vet Pathol* **20:** 531–540, 1983.

Kramer, J. W., Nickels, F. A., and Bell, T. Cytology of diffuse mesothelioma in the thorax of a horse. *Equine Vet J* **8:** 81–83, 1976.

McCullagh, K. G., Mews, A. R., and Pinsent, P. J. N. Diffuse pleural mesothelioma in a goat. *Vet Pathol* **16:** 119–121, 1979.

Nicholson, F. R., and Horne, R. D. Grass awn penetration in the dog. *Auburn Vet* **29:** 59–65, 1973.

Prasse, K. W., and Duncan, J. R. Laboratory diagnosis of pleural and peritoneal effusions. *Vet Clin North Am (Small Anim Pract)* **6**(4): 625–636, 1976.

Quick, C. B. Chylothorax: A review. *J Am Anim Hosp Assoc* **16:** 23–29, 1980.

Raphel, C. F., and Beech, J. Pleuritis and pleural effusion of the horse. *Proc Am Assoc Equine Pract* **27:** 17–25, 1982.

Raphel, C. F., and Beech, J. Pleuritis secondary to pneumonia or lung abscessation in 90 horses. *J Am Vet Med Assoc* **181:** 808–810, 1982.

Robertson, S. A. *et al.* Thoracic empyema in the dog; a report of twenty-two cases. *J Small Anim Pract* **24:** 103–119, 1983.

Smith, B. P. Pleuritis and pleural effusion in the horse: A study of 37 cases. *J Am Vet Med Assoc* **170:** 208–211, 1977.

Straub, R. *et al.* Mesothelioma of the pleura in a horse. *Schweiz Arch Tierheilkd* **116:** 207–211, 1974.

Thrall, D. E., and Goldschmidt, M. H. Mesothelioma in the dog: Six case reports. *J Am Vet Radiol Soc* **19:** 197–115, 1978.

von Recum, A. F. The mediastinum and hemothorax, pyothorax, and pneumothorax in the dog. *J Am Vet Med Assoc* **171:** 531–533, 1977.

Wheeldon, E. B., Mariassy, A. T., and McSporran, K. D. The pleura: A combined light-microscopic and scanning and transmission electron microscopic study in the sheep. II. Response to injury. *Exp Lung Res* **5:** 125–140, 1983.

ACKNOWLEDGMENTS

I am grateful to W.L. Castleman for his review of portions of the manuscript and provision of relevant illustrations. I am deeply indebted to Anja Sterner-Kock and Colleen Prather for assistance with bibliographic searches and to Lucy Day for keeping straight the revisions to the manuscript. Much of the credit for the quality of the photographic plates belongs to Andrej T. Mariassy.

Index

Boldface, major discussion; f, figure; t, table

A

D

E

F

H

I

J

K

L

M

N

O

P

Q

R

S

T

U

Z

ISBN 0-12-391606-2